Essentials of
Oral Pathology

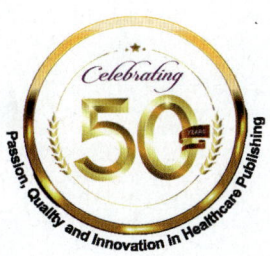

*Take up one idea.
Make that one idea your life—think of it, dream of it,
live on that idea.
Let the brain, muscles, nerves, every part of your
body, be full of that idea, and just leave every other idea alone.
This is the way to success.*

—**Swami Vivekananda**

Essentials of
Oral Pathology

FOURTH EDITION

Swapan Kumar Purkait MDS
Professor and Postgraduate Teacher
Department of Oral and Maxillofacial Pathology
Buddha Institute of Dental Sciences and Hospital
Patna, Bihar, India.

Forewords
RR Paul
Jay Gopal Ray
Tamal Kanti Pal

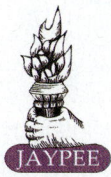

JAYPEE BROTHERS MEDICAL PUBLISHERS
The Health Sciences Publisher
New Delhi | London | Panama

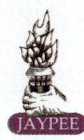
Jaypee Brothers Medical Publishers (P) Ltd

Headquarters
Jaypee Brothers Medical Publishers (P) Ltd
4838/24, Ansari Road, Daryaganj
New Delhi 110 002, India
Phone: +91-11-43574357
Fax: +91-11-43574314
Email: jaypee@jaypeebrothers.com

Overseas Offices

J.P. Medical Ltd
83 Victoria Street, London
SW1H 0HW (UK)
Phone: +44 20 3170 8910
Fax: +44 (0)20 3008 6180
Email: info@jpmedpub.com

Jaypee-Highlights Medical Publishers Inc
City of Knowledge, Bld. 235, 2nd Floor, Clayton
Panama City, Panama
Phone: +1 507-301-0496
Fax: +1 507-301-0499
Email: cservice@jphmedical.com

Jaypee Brothers Medical Publishers (P) Ltd
Bhotahity, Kathmandu
Nepal
Phone: +977-9741283608
Email: kathmandu@jaypeebrothers.com

Website: www.jaypeebrothers.com
Website: www.jaypeedigital.com

© 2019, Jaypee Brothers Medical Publishers

The views and opinions expressed in this book are solely those of the original contributor(s)/author(s) and do not necessarily represent those of editor(s) of the book.

All rights reserved. No part of this publication may be reproduced, stored or transmitted in any form or by any means, electronic, mechanical, photocopying, recording or otherwise, without the prior permission in writing of the publishers.

All brand names and product names used in this book are trade names, service marks, trademarks or registered trademarks of their respective owners. The publisher is not associated with any product or vendor mentioned in this book.

Medical knowledge and practice change constantly. This book is designed to provide accurate, authoritative information about the subject matter in question. However, readers are advised to check the most current information available on procedures included and check information from the manufacturer of each product to be administered, to verify the recommended dose, formula, method and duration of administration, adverse effects and contraindications. It is the responsibility of the practitioner to take all appropriate safety precautions. Neither the publisher nor the author(s)/editor(s) assume any liability for any injury and/or damage to persons or property arising from or related to use of material in this book.

This book is sold on the understanding that the publisher is not engaged in providing professional medical services. If such advice or services are required, the services of a competent medical professional should be sought.

Every effort has been made where necessary to contact holders of copyright to obtain permission to reproduce copyright material. If any have been inadvertently overlooked, the publisher will be pleased to make the necessary arrangements at the first opportunity. The **CD/DVD-ROM** (if any) provided in the sealed envelope with this book is complimentary and free of cost. **Not meant for sale.**

Inquiries for bulk sales may be solicited at: jaypee@jaypeebrothers.com

Essentials of Oral Pathology

First Edition: 1999

Second Edition: 2003

Third Edition: 2011

Fourth Edition: **2019**

ISBN: 978-93-5270-570-2

Printed at: Samrat Offset Pvt. Ltd.

Dedicated to

*My children Prithu and Pubali
and my wife Maitreyee*

FOREWORD

Today, our society needs not just a dental surgeon, but a medically competent dental surgeon. Oral pathology is undoubtedly the most integral subject of teaching in dental curriculum which bridges the gap between the medical and dental sciences. But, the available textbooks in this field of oral pathology are so voluminous that it becomes virtually impossible for dental students to gather comprehensive knowledge out of those textbooks during their BDS course of studies. In view of this, the book *Essentials of Oral Pathology* by Dr Swapan Kumar Purkait seems to fill this lacuna admirably. I am sure this book will also be immense importance to the general dental practitioners too.

RR Paul MDS Oral Pathology (Mum) PhD (Kol)
Deputy Director and Incharge (R&D)
Ex-Professor, Ex-Principal, Postgraduate Teacher and Head
Department of Oral and Maxillofacial Pathology
Guru Nanak Institute of Dental Sciences and Research
Kolkata, West Bengal, India
Ex-Member: Dental Council of India, New Delhi

FOREWORD

It gives me immense pleasure to introduce the fourth edition of *Essentials of Oral Pathology* by Dr Swapan Kumar Purkait to the budding graduates of dentistry. Oral and maxillofacial pathology is a specialty of dentistry and a very fundamental subject for all the students contemplating to practice clinical dentistry at large.

The purpose of this edition remains the same, i.e. to provide the reader with a comprehensive discussion of a wide variety of diseases that affects the maxillofacial region. The previous editions have been well accepted and thousands of students were benefitted so far by reading the same.

The immense effort put in by the author in bringing out this edition is highly commendable. We all trust in the basic philosophy that education brings knowledge with consistent effort and knowledge when properly nurtured brings wisdom. Similarly, this book has also grown qualitatively and refined with every new edition.

This book has twenty-three chapters, illustrations and photographs arranged systematically to fit in with the course and curriculum for undergraduate teaching; though much emphasis is not given on in-depth detail of molecular and biochemical aspects of modern diagnostic pathology, since this book has been written keeping in mind the need of undergraduate students only.

Finally, I wish Dr Purkait all success in life and my deepest regards to him for sharing his knowledge with the students. I conclude by saying "Man is not immortal but remains immortal through his work". I am sure all of us will be benefitted by this book.

Jay Gopal Ray MDS (Oral Pathology) PhD
Head
Department of Oral Pathology
Burdwan Dental College and Hospital
Bardhaman, West Bengal, India
Formerly, Postgraduate Teacher and Head
Department of Oral Pathology
Dr R Ahmed Dental College and Hospital
Kolkata, West Bengal, India

FOREWORD

There is an ongoing search for an improved approach to deliver oral healthcare to all human across the globe. The gap between the reality and expectations in oral healthcare system has become wider and this disparity, however, lies with the failure of transforming fundamental biological science into own clinical practice.

Oral pathology is one of the basic sciences in dentistry, the thorough understanding of which can certainly bring about qualitative changes in our clinical approaches towards amelioration of disease entity, providing both early intervention with better therapeutics and preventions. With this mission in mind, Dr Swapan Kumar Purkait, an eminent oral pathologist, has strived for fourth edition of his book *Essentials of Oral Pathology*.

It is with great pleasure and profound satisfaction, I have gone through the entire edition and found it to be very informative and useful for pursuing undergraduate studies. This is a wonderful piece of work with simple language and lucid presentation also, easy for students to assimilate and reproduce. Several new pages have been added to this new edition to incorporate current contents and references and other chapters are thoroughly updated throughout. New chapters like Diseases of Temporomandibular Joint, Syndromes Related to Oral Diseases, and Important Classifications of Oral Diseases will certainly enrich the readers.

The breakneck increase in information and indecent speed of expanding knowledge have paved the way for the fourth edition to come out. I am sure that this book will find its own place in dental profession and the readers shall have ready access to a comprehensive reference that enables rapid retrieval of integrated and relevant information on the subject.

Tamal Kanti Pal
MDS PhD Cert Implant, New York University, USA
Professor for PhD Studies
JIS University

Formerly, Principal
Guru Nanak Institute of Dental Sciences and Research
Kolkata, West Bengal, India

PREFACE TO THE FOURTH EDITION

The first edition of *Essentials of Oral Pathology* was published in the year 1999, the second edition in 2003 followed by the third edition in 2011 and now we have the fourth edition of the book; it's been a wonderful journey over these years and I am really grateful to my publisher, my teachers, colleagues, friends and specially the students for the success of the book. Every new edition of a book is made for making improvements and innovations in the various aspects of its presentation, and this edition will be unique due to the incorporation of numerous clinical and radiographic images and a large number of photomicrographs, which I hope will help the students in understanding this highly dynamic subject better. Oral pathology is a vast science and it is also rapidly expanding, especially with the incorporation of immunohistochemistry, forensic odontology and genetics, to name a few, which make learning the subject all the more challenging. Moreover, basic knowledge in oral pathology is essential for professionals in all the specialties in dentistry as it provides the clue to the very basic understanding about oral diseases and their correct diagnoses. Hence, I hope this book will be helpful not only to the students of this particular specialty, but also to the people of dentistry in general. In this fourth edition, the chapters have been revised and relevant changes are made but the organization of the text and the simplicity of presentation, which have been the hallmark of this book throughout, have been preserved. I once again sincerely request the teachers, friends and students of oral pathology to express their views about this book and also kindly provide me with constructive suggestions as to how this book can further be improved. I hope students will like this new edition as much as they liked the three previous editions.

Swapan Kumar Purkait

PREFACE TO THE FIRST EDITION

Oral pathology is an important branch of dentistry and although there are few good textbooks available in the subject, *Essentials of Oral Pathology* has been written with a view to present the subject to the students in a more simplified but comprehensive manner.

I hope the book will fulfill the need of the students by giving them relevant guidance in their day-to-day learning process as well as during their preparation for examination and above all, with the book in hand, students will find the subject easy to handle.

As no one is perfect in absolute sense, I also humbly accept my limitations regarding shortcomings in the book and therefore, I sincerely welcome the valuable suggestions from my senior colleagues and students regarding what further should be done to improve this book.

Swapan Kumar Purkait

ACKNOWLEDGMENTS

This book has been accomplished with the help of many people from all over the country and I am indebted to all of them for their kind gesture. First of all I wish to thank and express my sincere regards to my teachers Dr RR Paul, Dr (Mrs) Kabita Chatterjee and Dr Tamal Kanti Pal for their constant encouragement and inspirations.

Special thanks to Dr Jay Gopal Ray for his continuous encouragement and whole-hearted support; he has been a true mentor for me all the time from the beginning of this work.

I am indebted to the management of Buddha Institute of Dental Sciences and Hospital, where I am presently working, specially to Mr RK Singh (Secretary) and Dr (Prof) Binoy Kumar Singh our Vice-Principal and Dr (Prof) Surendra Prasad our Principal who always extended their kind support and encouragement.

I am thankful to my student Dr Sumanta Kumar Kolay (Oral Pathologist) for his continuous support, suggestions and encouragement extended as always from the inception of this book. Deepest thanks to my wife Maitreyee, my daughter Pubali and my son Prithu for their never-ending support and love which gave me the energy to continue with the work since the publication of the first edition up to this level. Mr Suman Kumar Guha and Mr Sutripta Sur who have done a great job in making the computer-generated graphic illustrations, making the index for the book and designing of the tables used in the book.

My seniors and friends have always stood behind me and gave their kind support to enhance my confidence and my special thanks to Dr Alok Banerjee, Dr Tushar Deb, Dr Debasis Banerjee, Dr Chaitanya Babu, Dr Anjana Majumder, Dr Jayanta Bhattacharya, Dr Mrs Mousumi Pal, Dr Asit Paul, Dr Chitrita Gupta Mukherjee, Dr Uday Mukherjee, Dr Anindita Banerjee, Dr KP Das, Dr Bijoy Das, Dr SR Karmakar, Dr Sanjib Mitra, Dr Arup Ghosh, Dr Samindra Sengupta, Dr Neeta Mohanty, Dr Ruchi Bhuyan, Dr Bindu Nair, Dr Partha Chakraborty (Pediatric Surgeon), Dr Shila Datta, Dr Jayanta Chatterjee, Dr Sumit Majumder, Dr A Mamud, Dr Dipto Dey, Dr Sourav Bhattacharjee, Dr Sandip Ghose, Dr Dipankar Samaddar, Dr (Col) Inrdanil Mukhopadhyaya, Dr Hiralal Ash, Dr Manas De, Dr Nitubrata Biswas, Dr Rajarshi Banerjee, Dr Ajay Shahi (Oral Surgeon), Dr Narendra Nath Singh, Dr Virendra Prajapati (Oral Surgeon), Dr Tarun Santra, Dr Shikar Kumar, Dr Chikoy Wang, Dr Rajat Kumar Singh, Dr JN Shukla, Dr Veeranna Ramesh, Dr Abhishek Laha, Dr Sudheer KH, Dr Archana Sudheer, Dr Suma, Dr Ranjan Ghosh, Dr Basudeb Mahato, Dr Badal Sarkar, Dr Sanchita Samanta, Dr Somnath Paul, Dr Saikat Paul, Dr Sarita Singh, Dr Manisha Singh, Dr Ananjan Chatterjee, Dr Shashi Ranjan, Dr Amesh Golwara, Dr Rajat Sahgal, Dr Prabhat Kumar Singh, Dr Sujay Kumar Sinha, Dr Tushar, Dr Garima Mangal, Dr Sadanand Dungryanaik, Dr Shovendu Jha, Dr Anand Kumar (Oral Medicine), Dr Kumar Arunesh, Dr Madhumita Bhattacharjee, Dr Harsha Vardhan Choudhary, and Mrs Gopa Roy.

Special thanks to Dr (Prof) Keya Basu (Head, Department of Pathology, National Medical College, Kolkata), Dr Subhankar Mukherjee, (Faculty, National Medical College, Kolkata), and Dr Sudhakar Rao (Eminent Dermatologist) for their kind help and inspiration.

Heartiest thanks to my students and colleagues Dr Sunil Thapar, Dr Pradip Kr Jha, Dr Madhuresh Kumar, Dr Suwasini, Dr Somes Ranjan Das, Dr Manish Kumar, Dr Jyoti Prakash, Dr Abhijit Pratap Singh, Dr Priyasree, Dr Debeswar Das, Dr Suchita Sinha, Dr Kumar Viswajit for their whole hearted support and encouragement.

We are thankful to Shri Jitendar P Vij (Group Chairman), Mr Ankit Vij (Managing Director), Mr MS Mani (Group President), Ms Pooja Bhandari (Production Head), Ms Sunita Katla (Executive Assistant to Group Chairman and Publishing Manager), Mr Rajesh Sharma (Production Coordinator), Dr Sneha Kashyap (Development Editor), Ms Seema Dogra (Cover Visualizer), Mr Dinesh Bhardwaj (DTP Operator), Mr Binay Kumar (Proofreader), Mr Ratan Lal (Graphic Designer), and team members of Jaypee Brothers Medical Publishers (P) Ltd, New Delhi, India, for all their support and work in this project. Moreover, Mr Gupta and Mr Sabyasachi Hazra of Kolkata Branch are real friends in need for me at all times, many thanks to them.

Last but not least, I sincerely thank the students and teachers of Oral and Maxillofacial Pathology, who have made the 1st, 2nd and 3rd editions of the book successful and this 4th edition would not have been possible without their acceptance and appreciation.

If someone's name has inadvertently not been included in this column of acknowledgments, I sincerely apologize for that.

CONTENTS

1. Developmental Anomalies of Oral and Paraoral Structures 1
Anomalies of Lips and Palate 2
- Lip Pits and Fistulas 2   ❑ Double Lip 2   ❑ Frenal Tag 3
- Hereditary Intestinal Polyposis Syndrome 3   ❑ Oral Melanotic Macule 4
- Uvula Elongata 5   ❑ Cheilitis Glandularis 5   ❑ Cheilitis Granulomatosa 7

Anomalies of the Oral Mucosa 8
- Fordyce's Granules 8   ❑ Focal Epithelial Hyperplasia 9   ❑ White Sponge Nevus 10

Developmental Defects of the Gingivae 11
- Fibromatosis Gingivae 11   ❑ Retrocuspid Papilla 12

Developmental Anomalies Involving the Jawbone 12
- Agnathia 12   ❑ Micrognathia 12   ❑ Macrognathia 13   ❑ Facial Hemihypertrophy 14
- Facial Hemiatrophy 15   ❑ Torus in the Jaws 16   ❑ Orofacial Clefts 16
- Cleft Lip and Cleft Palate 16   ❑ Cleft in Lower Lip and Mandible 21

Developmental Anomalies of the Tongue 21
- Aglossia 21   ❑ Microglossia 22   ❑ Macroglossia 22   ❑ Ankyloglossia 24
- Cleft Tongue 24   ❑ Fissured Tongue 25
- Median Rhomboid Glossitis or Glossal Central Papillary Atrophy 25   ❑ Lingual Varices 27
- Geographic Tongue or Benign Migratory Glossitis 27   ❑ Hairy Tongue 29
- Lingual Thyroid Nodule 29   ❑ Thyroglossal Tract Cyst 30

Anomalies of Oral Lymphoid Tissue 31
- Reactive Lymphoid Aggregates 31   ❑ Lymphoepithelial Cyst 31
- Angiolymphoid Hyperplasia with Eosinophilia 32

Developmental Anomalies Involving Oral Hard Tissues 32
- Abnormalities of Teeth 32

Disturbance in Size of Teeth 32
- Microdontia 32   ❑ Macrodontia 34

Disturbance in Number of Teeth 35
- Anodontia 35   ❑ Supernumerary Teeth 36

Disturbances in Eruption of Teeth 38
- Types of Eruption Abnormalities 39   ❑ Premature Eruption 39
- Delayed Eruption 39   ❑ Impacted Teeth 40

Disturbances in the Shape of Teeth 41
- Gemination 41   ❑ Fusion 41   ❑ Concrescence 43   ❑ Dilaceration 44
- Taurodontism 45   ❑ Dens in Dente 46   ❑ Dens Evaginatus 48   ❑ Talon Cusp 48
- Enamel Pearl 49

Disturbance in the Structure of Teeth 50
- Disturbance in the Structure of Enamel 50

Acquired Disturbances of Enamel 50
- Focal Enamel Hypoplasia 50   ❑ Idiopathic Enamel Opacities 50
- Generalized Enamel Hypoplasia 51

Effect of Individual Systemic Conditions on Enamel Hypoplasia 51
- Nutritional Deficiency 51   ❑ Congenital Syphilis 51   ❑ Hypocalcemia 52
- Exanthematous Disease 52   ❑ Birth Injuries and Low Birthweight 52
- Fluorides and Mottling 52

Hereditary Disturbance of Enamel Formation 53
- Amelogenesis Imperfecta 53
- Syndrome Associated Enamel Defects 55

Disturbances in Structure of Dentin 56
- Dentinogenesis Imperfecta 56
- Dentinal Abnormality due to Systemic or Environmental Disturbances 60
- Dentin Dysplasia 60
- Regional Odontodysplasia 62

Disturbance in Structure of Cementum 63
- Hypercementosis 63
- Hypocementosis 64

2. Benign and Malignant Neoplasms of the Oral Cavity 67

Neoplasm 67
- Definition 67
- Local Invasion 67
- Metastasis 68
- Classification of Oral Neoplasms 68
- Benign Neoplasms of the Epithelial Tissue Origin 71
- Malignant Neoplasms of the Epithelial Tissue Origin 77
- Clinical Staging of Carcinomas of Head and Neck 101
- Second Primary Tumors in Squamous Cell Carcinoma 102
- Screening Tests for Squamous Cell Carcinoma 103
- Special Investigations in Oral Cancer 103
- Prevention of Oral Cancer 104

Basal Cell Carcinoma 104
- Definition 104
- Origin 104
- Etiology 104
- Clinical Features 104
- Presentation 105
- Histopathology 105
- Differential Diagnosis 106
- Treatment 106

Verrucous Carcinoma 106
- Definition 106
- Etiology 106
- Clinical Features 106
- Presentation 106
- Histopathology 107
- Differential Diagnosis 109
- Treatment 109

Malignant Melanoma 109
- Definition 109
- Clinical Features 109
- Clinical Types of Melanoma 109
- Presentation 110
- Histopathology 111
- Differential Diagnosis 112
- Treatment 112

Primary Intra-alveolar Carcinoma 112
- Definition 112
- Origin 112

Neoplasms of Mesenchymal Tissue Origin: Benign Neoplasms of Fibrous Connective Tissue 112
- Fibroma 112
- Desmoplastic Fibroma 114
- Giant Cell Fibroma 115
- Myofibroma 115
- Peripheral Ossifying Fibroma 116
- Central Ossifying Fibroma 117

Giant Cells 120
- Peripheral Giant Cell Granuloma 120
- Central Giant Cell Granuloma 123
- Benign Fibrous Histiocytoma 126
- Myxoma 127
- Nodular Fasciitis 128

Benign Neoplasm of Adipose Tissue Origin 129
- Lipoma 129

Benign Neoplasm of Vascular Tissue Origin 131
- Hemangioma 131

Benign Neoplasm of Lymphatic Vessels 136
- Lymphangioma 136
- Cystic Hygroma 137

Benign Neoplasm of Bone 138
- Osteoma 138
- Osteoid Osteoma/Osteoblastoma 140

Benign Neoplasm of Cartilage Tissue 141
- Chondroma 141
- Benign Chondroblastoma 142

Benign Neoplasm of Smooth Muscles 143
- Leiomyoma 143

Benign Neoplasm of Striated Muscle 114
- Rhabdomyoma 144   □ Granular Cell Tumor/Granular Cell Myoblastoma 145

Benign Neoplasms of Neural Tissue 146
- Neurilemmoma 146   □ Neurofibroma 149
- Melanotic Neuroectodermal Tumor of Infancy 151   □ Traumatic Neuroma 152

Neoplasm of the Mixed Tissue 153
- Teratoma 153

Malignant Neoplasms of Mesenchymal Tissue 154
- Fibrosarcoma 154   □ Malignant Fibrous Histiocytoma 156   □ Liposarcoma 157
- Hemangioendothelioma 158   □ Hemangiopericytoma 159   □ Kaposi's Sarcoma 160
- Ewing's Sarcoma/Ewing's Tumor 162   □ Staging System for Bone Cancer Including Ewing Tumor: By American Joint Committee on Cancer 164
- Stages 164   □ Chondrosarcoma 165   □ Osteosarcoma 169
- Lymphomas 173   □ Multiple Myeloma 183   □ Solitary Plasmacytoma 187
- Leiomyosarcoma 187   □ Rhabdomyosarcoma 188   □ Neurogenic Sarcoma 189
- Metastatic Tumors of the Jaws 190

3. Oral Precancerous Lesions and Conditions   197
- Precancerous Lesion 197   □ Precancerous Condition 197   □ Leukoplakia 197
- Tobacco Pouch Keratosis 208   □ Oral Hairy Leukoplakia 208   □ Leukoedema 209
- Carcinoma in Situ 210   □ Erythroplakia 211   □ Stomatitis Nicotina 213
- Oral Submucous Fibrosis 214   □ Sideropenic Dysphagia 220   □ Lichen Planus 220
- Lichenoid Reactions 227

4. Diseases of the Salivary Glands   229
- Classification of Salivary Gland Diseases 230
- Developmental Anomalies of the Salivary Gland 230
- Reactive Lesions of the Salivary Gland 232   □ Infective Lesions 237
- Immune-mediated Disease 238   □ Miscellaneous Disorders of Salivary Gland 242
- Neoplasm of the Salivary Glands 244   □ Malignant Salivary Gland Neoplasms 254
- Histopathology 256   □ TNM Classification of Carcinomas of the Salivary Glands 264

5. Odontogenic Neoplasms   268
- Definition 268   □ Formation of Dental Papilla 268
- Dental Follicle 269   □ Formation of Root 269   □ Neoplasms of Debatable Origin 269

Ameloblastoma 269
- Definition 269   □ Etiology 270   □ Histogenesis of Ameloblastoma 270
- Clinical Features   □ Clinical Presentation 270   □ Radiological Features 272
- Differential Diagnosis 272   □ Macroscopic Features 273
- Histopathological Features 273   □ Plexiform Ameloblastoma 273
- Follicular Ameloblastoma 273   □ Other Histological Patterns of Ameloblastoma 274

Unicystic Ameloblastoma 277
- Origin 277   □ Clinical Presentation 277   □ Radiographic Finding 277
- Histopathology 277   □ Differential Diagnosis 279

Adenomatoid Odontogenic Tumor 279
- Definition 279   □ Origin 279   □ Clinical Features 279   □ Clinical Presentation 280
- Radiological Features 280   □ Macroscopic Features 281   □ Differential Diagnosis 281
- Histopathological Features 281

Calcifying Epithelial Odontogenic Tumor/Pindborg's Tumor 282
- Origin 283
- Clinical Features 283
- Clinical Presentation 283
- Radiological Features 284
- Differential Diagnosis 284
- Histopathological Features 284

Dentinogenic Ghost-cell Tumor 285

Squamous Odontogenic Tumor/Benign Epithelial Odontogenic Tumor 286
- Definition 286
- Origin 286
- Clinical Features 286
- Presentation 286
- Radiographic Features 286
- Histopathology 287
- Differential Diagnosis 288

Ameloblastic Fibroma 288
- Clinical Features 288
- Clinical Presentation 288
- Radiological Features 288
- Histopathological Features 288

Ameloblastic Fibro-odontome 289
- Clinical Features 289
- Clinical Presentation 289
- Radiological Appearance 290
- Histopathology 290
- Treatment 290

Odontomes 290
- Definition 290
- Types 290
- Clinical Features 290
- Clinical Presentation 290
- Radiological Features 291
- Differential Diagnosis 291
- Histopathology 293
- Treatment 293

Odontogenic Fibroma 293
- Definition 293

Peripheral Odontogenic Fibroma 293
- Definition 293
- Origin 293
- Clinical Features 293
- Histopathology 293
- Differential Diagnosis 293
- Treatment 293

Central Odontogenic Fibroma 294
- Definition 294
- Clinical Features 294
- Radiographic Features 294
- Histological Presentation 294
- Differential Diagnosis 295
- Treatment 295

Odontogenic Myxoma 295
- Definition 295
- Origin 295
- Clinical Features 295
- Presentation 295
- Radiographic Features 295
- Macroscopic Appearance 296
- Histological Presentation 296
- Differential Diagnosis 296
- Treatment 296

Periapical Cemental Dysplasia 296
- Clinical Features 296
- Clinical Presentations 296
- Radiological Features 296
- Histopathology 297
- Differential Diagnosis 297
- Treatment 297

Central Cementifying Fibroma 297

Familial Gigantiform Cementoma 297
- Definition 297
- Origin 298
- Clinical Features 298
- Radiographic Features 298
- Histological Presentation 298
- Differential Diagnosis 298
- Treatment 299

Cementoblastoma 299
- Clinical Features 299
- Origin 299
- Clinical Presentation 299
- Radiological Features 299
- Macroscopy 300
- Histopathology 300
- Differential Diagnosis 300
- Treatment 300

Malignant Odontogenic Neoplasms 300
- Malignant Ameloblastoma 300
- Ameloblastic Carcinoma 300
- Odontogenic Carcinoma 301
- Clinical Features 301
- Radiographic Features 301
- Histopathology 302
- Treatment 302
- Odontogenic Sarcomas 302
- Clear Cell Odontogenic Carcinoma 302
- Clinical Features 302
- Clinical Presentation 302
- Radiological Finding 302
- Histological Presentation 302
- Treatment 302
- Primary Intra-alveolar Carcinoma 302

6. Cysts of the Oral Region — 306
- Definition 306 □ Classification of Cysts 306

Odontogenic Cysts 308
- Odontogenic Keratocyst/Primordial Cyst 308 □ Dentigerous Cyst 318
- Radicular Cyst 324 □ Eruption Cyst 331 □ Lateral Periodontal Cyst 332
- Dental Lamina Cyst (Gingival Cyst) of the Newborn 333 □ Gingival Cysts of the Adult 334
- Sialo-Odontogenic Cysts/Glandular Odontogenic Cyst 335
- Botryoid Odontogenic Cysts 336
- Calcifying Epithelial Odontogenic Cyst/Gorlin Cyst 337 □ Paradental Cyst 340

Nonodontogenic Cysts 340
- Globulomaxillary Cyst 340 □ Nasolabial Cyst/Nasoalveolar Cyst 341
- Nasopalatine Duct Cyst 342 □ Solitary Bone Cyst 344 □ Stafne's Bone Cyst 345
- Treatment 346 □ Aneurysmal Bone Cyst 346 □ Cyst of the Salivary Gland 347
- Ranula 350 □ Dermoid Cyst 351 □ Surgical Ciliated Cyst of Maxilla 352

7. Regressive Alterations of Teeth — 355
Attrition of Teeth 355
- Definition 355 □ Types of Attrition 355 □ Causes of Pathological Attrition 356
- Clinical Features of Attrition 356 □ Treatment 357

Abrasion of Teeth 357
- Definition 357 □ Etiology and Pathogenesis 357 □ Causes of Abrasion 357
- Treatment 359

Tooth Abfraction 359
- Definition □ Forces Causing Abfraction 359 □ Clinical Features 359

Erosion of Teeth 359
- Definition 359 □ Etiologic Factors for Erosion 360 □ Clinical Features of Erosion 360
- Treatment 361

Resorption of Teeth 361
- Definition 361 □ Types of Root Resorption of Teeth 361

Pulp Calcification 365
- Definition 365 □ Pathogenesis of Pulp Calcification 365 □ Types 366
- Types of Pulp Stones 366 □ Clinical Symptoms 366 □ Diagnosis 366
- Clinical Significance of Pulp Calcifications 367

Hypercementosis 367
- Definition 367 □ Etiology of Hypercementosis 367 □ Clinical Features 367
- Radiographic Features 367 □ Microscopy 367 □ Clinical Significance 367

Age Changes in Teeth 368
- Changes in Enamel 368 □ Changes in Dentin 368 □ Changes in Cementum 368
- Changes in Pulp 368

Cementicles 368
- Pathogenesis 368

8. Bacterial, Viral and Fungal Infections — 370
Specific Bacterial Infections 370
- Tuberculosis 370 □ Syphilis 373 □ Gonorrhea 378 □ Actinomycosis 379
- Streptococcal Infections 381 □ Diphtheria 382 □ Sarcoidosis 383
- Leprosy/Hansen Disease 384 □ Tetanus 385 □ Midline Lethal Granuloma 387
- Wegener's Granulomatosis 387 □ Noma 387 □ Pyogenic Granuloma 388

Viral Infections 390
- Acquired Immunodeficiency Syndrome 390 □ Herpes Virus Infections 398
- Herpes Simplex Virus Type–I Infections 398 □ Herpes Simplex Virus Type-II Infections 401

- Herpes Zoster 401 - Cytomegalovirus Infection 404
- Epstein–Barr Virus Infections 405 - Human Papillomavirus Infection 405
- Paramyxovirus Infection 406 - Coxsackie Virus Infections 407

Fungal Infection 413
- Candidiasis 413 - Deep Fungal Infections 417 - Oral Myasis 420

9. Dental Caries 426
- Definition of Dental Caries 426 - Epidemiology of Dental Caries 426
- Pathophysiology of Dental Caries 427 - Contributing Factors in Dental Caries 434
- Clinical Aspects of Dental Caries 437 - Histopathological Aspect of Dental Caries 441
- Protective Responses of Dentin and Pulp Against Caries 444 - Caries Activity Tests 444
- Methods of Caries Prevention 446 - Caries Vaccine 446

10. Disease of Dentin-pulp Complex and Periapical Tissues 450
Pulpal Diseases 450
- Introduction 450 - Dentin-pulp Complex 450 - Etiology of Pulpal Diseases 451
- Classification of the Pulpal Diseases 451 - Diagnosis of Pulpal Diseases 457

Diseases of the Periapical Tissues 458
- Primary Acute Apical Periodontitis 458 - Periapical Granuloma 458
- Acute Exacerbation of Chronic Periapical Granuloma/Abscess 460
- Periapical Abscess 460 - Osteomyelitis 463 - Endodontic-Periodontic Lesions 474

11. Spread of the Oral Infection 477
- Important Factors for Odontogenic Infections 477

Space Infections 477
- Space Infections Related to Maxilla 478 - Space Infections Related to Mandible 479

Cellulitis 483
- Definition 483 - Pathogenesis 483 - Clinical Features 483
- Histopathologic Features 485 - Treatment 485

Ludwig's Angina 485
- Definition 485 - Causative Microorganisms 485 - Pathogenesis of Ludwig's Angina 485 - Clinical Features 485 - Diagnosis 486

Cavernous Sinus Thrombosis 486
- Definition 486 - Routes of Spread of Infections 486 - Clinical Features 487
- Treatment 487

Maxillary Sinusitis 487
- Definition 487 - Etiology 487 - Clinical Features 487 - Radiological Features 487
- Histological Features 488 - Treatment 488

Focal Infection 488
- Definition 488 - Mechanism of Focal Infection 488
- Common Consequences of "Focal Infections" from the Orofacial Region 488

12. Physical and Chemical Injuries of the Oral Cavity 491
Physical Injuries 491
- Fractures of Teeth 491 - Root Fracture 491 - Cemental Tear 491
- Bruxism 491 - Ankylosis of Teeth 493 - Submerged Teeth 493
- Toothbrush Injury 494 - Toothpick Injury 494 - Linea Alba 494
- Traumatic Atrophic Glossitis 494 - Traumatic Ulcer 495 - Factitious Injuries 495
- Denture Related Injuries or Lesions 496 - Electrical Burns in the Mouth 497
- Thermal Burns in Mouth 497 - Radiation Injuries 498 - Osteoradionecrosis 502
- Laser Radiation 503

Chemical Injuries 503
- Congenital Porphyria 503   - Biliary Atresia 503   - Erythroblastosis Fetalis 504
- Fluorosis 504   - Oral Manifestations of Various Metal Poisoning 504
- Oral Manifestations of Cytotoxic Drug Therapy 504
- Oral Manifestations of Tetracycline Staining 505   - Angioneurotic Edema 506
- Chemical Burns 506   - Chemical Burns due to Other Medicaments 506

13. Biopsy and Healing of Oral Wounds 509
Biopsy 509
- Definition 509   - Indications of Biopsy 509   - Contraindications of Biopsy 510
- Types of Biopsy 510   - Procedure of Tissue Biopsy 514   - Labelling of Specimen 515
- Biopsy Report 515

Healing of Oral Wounds 516
- Healing of Biopsy Wound 518   - Healing of Gingivectomy Wound 518
- Healing of the Extraction Wound 519   - Healing of the Fractured Jawbone 521
- Healing around Osteointegrated Implants 523

14. Oral Aspects of Metabolic Disorders 526
Disturbances in Mineral Metabolism 526
- Calcium 526   - Phosphorus 528   - Iron 528   - Zinc 529

Disturbance in Vitamin Metabolism 529
- Vitamin D 529   - Vitamin A 531   - Vitamin E 531   - Vitamin B Complex 531
- Vitamin C 532   - Vitamin K 533

Disturbances in Protein Metabolism 533
- Amyloidosis 533   - Porphyria 534

Disturbances in Carbohydrate Metabolism 535
- Hurler's Syndrome 535

Disturbances in Lipid Metabolism 535
- Hand-Schuller-Christian Disease 535   - Eosinophilic Granuloma 536
- Letterer-Siwe Disease 536   - Gaucher's Disease 537   - Niemann-Pick Disease 537

Disturbances in Hormone Metabolism 537
- Hypopituitarism 537   - Pituitary Insufficiency in Adults 537
- Diabetes Insipidus 538   - Hyperpituitarism 538   - Pituitary Gigantism 538
- Acromegaly 539   - Hypothyroidism 539   - Cretinism 540   - Myxedema 540
- Hyperthyroidism 541   - Hyperparathyroidism 541   - Hypoparathyroidism 543
- Adrenal Hormones 544   - Waterhouse–Friderichsen Syndrome 545
- Chronic Adrenocortical Insufficiency 545   - Pancreatic Hormone 547
- Hypoglycemia 549   - Progeria 549   - Imbalance of Sex Hormones 549

15. Diseases of Bone 552
- Basic Structure and Function of Bone 552
- Paget's Disease of Bone 553   - Fibrous Dysplasia of Bone 558
- Cherubism/Familial Fibrous Dysplasia or Disseminated Juvenile Fibrous Dysplasia 563
- Osteogenesis Imperfecta 566   - Cleidocranial Dysplasia 568
- Osteopetrosis/Marble Bone Disease/Albers–Schönberg Disease 570
- Marfan Syndrome 571   - Down Syndrome 572   - Infantile Cortical Hyperostosis 573
- Mandibulofacial Dysostosis 574   - Achondroplasia 574   - Massive Osteolysis 575

16. Diseases of Temporomandibular Joint 578
- Developmental Disorders 578   - Traumatic Disorders 578
- Inflammatory Disorders 581

17. Oral Aspects of Hematological Disorders — 586
- Pernicious Anemia 586
- Iron Deficiency Anemia 588
- Aplastic Anemia 589
- Hemolytic Anemia 589
- Thalassemias 590
- Sickle Cell Anemia 592
- Erythroblastosis Fetalis 596
- Polycythemia Vera 593
- Leukemias 594
- Agranulocytosis 596
- Cyclic Neutropenia 597
- Purpura 598
- Hemophilia or Royal Disease 600

18. Periodontal Diseases — 606
- Epidemiology 606
- Pathogenesis of Periodontal Disease 610
- Clinical Features of Periodontitis 612
- Gingival Hyperplasia 614
- Desquamative Gingivitis 617
- Acute Necrotizing Ulcerative Gingivitis/Vincent's Disease/Trench Mouth 617
- Lateral Periodontal Abscess 619
- Pericoronitis 620
- Staining of Teeth 620

19. Oral Aspects of Dermatological Disorders — 623
- Hereditary Ectodermal Dysplasia 623
- Psoriasis 625
- Pityriasis Rosea 626
- Histopathology 626
- Incontinentia Pigmenti 626
- Erythema Multiforme 627
- Dermatitis Herpetiformis 630
- Keratosis Follicularis 630
- Acanthosis Nigricans 631
- Dyskeratosis Congenita 631
- White Sponge Nevus 632
- Polymyositis 633
- Autoimmunity 633
- Pemphigus 635
- Pemphigoid 641
- Epidermolysis Bullosa 644
- Lupus Erythematosus 646
- Scleroderma 651
- Ehlers–Danlos Syndrome 654

20. Diseases of the Nerves and Muscles — 658
Diseases of the Nerves 658
- Trigeminal Neuralgia 658
- Sphenopalatine Neuralgia 660
- Glossodynia and Glossopyrosis 661
- Auriculotemporal Syndrome 661
- Glossopharyngeal Neuralgia 662
- Bell's Palsy 662
- Causalgia 663
- Eagle's Syndrome 664

Disease of the Muscles 664
- Generalized Familial Muscular Dystrophy 664
- Myasthenia Gravis 665
- Myositis Ossificans 665

21. Oral Manifestations of Generalized Diseases — 668
- Vitamin Deficiencies 668
- Important Causes of Lymphadenopathy 668
- Blood Dyscrasias 669
- Metabolic Disorders 670
- Heavy Metal Poisoning 670
- Endocrine Disturbances 671
- Granulomatous Diseases 672
- Dermatological Diseases 672
- Bone Diseases 673
- Acute Lethal Type Infectious Diseases 673
- Helminthic Diseases 673
- Renal Diseases 674
- Neural Diseases 674
- Sexually Transmitted Diseases 674
- Cardiovascular Diseases 675
- Genetic Disorders 675
- Allergic Conditions 675
- General Manifestations of Oral Diseases 675

22. Syndromes Related to Oral Diseases — 677
- Definition of Syndrome 677

23. Important Classifications of Oral Diseases — 688
- White Lesions of the Oral Cavity 688
- Red-Blue Lesions of the Oral Cavity 688
- Pigmented Lesions of the Oral Cavity 689
- Classification of Vesiculobullous Diseases 689
- Classification of Ulcerative Conditions 690
- Classification of Discoloration of Tooth 690
- Classification of Giant Cell Lesions 690

- Classification of Verrucal-Papillary Lesions of Oral Cavity 691
- Classification of Fibro-osseous Lesions 691
- Classification of Vascular Tissue Diseases 691
- Classification of Diseases of the Hemopoietic Tissues and Lymphoreticular System 691
- Classification of Stomatitis 691
- Classification of Severe Infections of the Orofacial Tissues 692
- Classification of Chronic Orofacial Pain 692
- Classification of Diseases of Tongue 692
- Classification of Gingival Enlargements 693
- Classification of Taste Disorders 693
- Classification of Neck Swellings 693
- Classification of Yellow Conditions of Oral Mucosa 694
- Anatomic Radiolucencies of Jaw Bones 694
- Radiolucent Lesions of the Periapical Region 694
- Classification of Pericoronal Radiolucent Lesions 694
- Classification of Interradicular Radiolucent Lesions 694
- Classification of Multilocular Radiolucent Lesions of the Jaws 695
- Mixed Radiolucent-Radiopaque Lesions Associated with Teeth 695
- Mixed Radiolucent-Radiopaque Lesions not Necessarily Associated with Teeth 695
- Multiple Separate Radiopaque Lesions of the Jaws 695
- Generalized Radiopacities of the Jaws 695
- Classification of Causes of Trismus 696
- Classification of Hamartomatous Lesions of Oral and Maxillofacial Region 696
- Classification of Oral Granular Cell Lesions Including Odontogenic and Nonodontogenic Tumors 696
- Classification of Granulomatous Diseases 697

Index 699

CHAPTER 1

Developmental Anomalies of Oral and Paraoral Structures

INTRODUCTION

Development of face, jawbones, and teeth are highly complex processes, which begin during the early part of embryonic life with simultaneous growth and merger of multiple tissue processes. Any malformation or defect resulting from the disturbance of growth and development of an organ in the body is known as a developmental anomaly (*an "anomaly" literally means deviation from normal*), and a large number of such developmental defects or anomalies may affect the body in general and oral structures in particular. The oral and paraoral developmental anomalies mostly occur due to disturbance in the growth of tissue processes or failure of their fusion at the right time during the embryonic life. Manifestations of such defects are evident either at birth or sometimes after birth, which often have some serious implications in the further growth and function of the involved organ during the later stages of life (Table 1.1).

Moreover, in the orofacial region, developmental anomalies affecting the teeth are seen more often than probably any other defects in the oral cavity. Disorders of development of teeth may be due to abnormalities in the differentiation of the dental lamina and tooth germs (abnormal morphodifferentiation); which results in various anomalous defects in the number, size and form of teeth. Besides this, abnormalities in histodifferentiation may also cause defective formation of dental hard tissues, resulting in the structural disturbance in the constitutional elements of teeth.

Disturbance in histodifferentiation often occurs at a later stage of tooth development as compared to the disturbance of morphodifferentiation.

Table 1.1: Types of developmental anomalies.

Types	Description
Congenital anomalies	The defects, which are present at birth or before birth during the intrauterine life, are known as congenital anomalies
Hereditary developmental anomalies	When certain defects are inherited by the offspring from either of the parents, it is called hereditary anomaly. Such types of anomalies are always transmitted through genes
Acquired anomalies	Acquired anomalies develop during intrauterine life due to some pathological environmental conditions. They are not transmitted through genes
Hamartomatous anomalies	• A hamartoma can be defined as an excessive, focal overgrowth of mature, normal cells and tissues, which are native to that particular anatomic location • Developmental abnormalities occurring due to such hamartomatous change in the tissue are known as hamartomatous developmental anomalies
Idiopathic anomalies	Developmental abnormalities of unknown cause are called idiopathic anomalies

ANOMALIES OF LIPS AND PALATE

■ LIP PITS AND FISTULAS

Definition
Lip and commissural pits are congenital mucosal invaginations, which involve either the lower or upper lips or the labial commissural area.

Origin
Development of upper lip begins during the 6th week and 7th week of intrauterine life; a "pit" in the lip develops due to formation of a notch, which causes fixation of tissue at the base of the notch at the early stage of labial development. The condition may also arise due to failure of a complete union of the embryonic lateral sulci of the lip, which persist in the later life.

Clinical Features

Lip Pits

- The lip pit is a small mucosal depression over the lip, which can be either unilateral or bilateral and are more commonly seen on the lower lip.
- These pits can be up to 3–4 mm in diameter and may have a depth of up to 2 cm.
- Lip pit occurs more commonly among females and their frequency ranges from 1:75,000 to 1:100,000 among Caucasians.
- Congenital lip pits may occur either as an isolated condition or they may be associated with cleft lip and/or cleft palate (van der Woude's syndrome or lip pit syndrome).
- The opening of a lip pit often appears as a circular or transverse slit; moreover, a lip pit opening may be located at the apex of a nipple-like elevation.
- Mucous secretion is often seen at the opening of those pits, which communicate with an underlying minor salivary gland (because the salivary gland orifices open into these pits and saliva exudes through them).

Commissural Pits

- The commissural pits, measure from 1 mm to 4 mm in diameter, are found either bilaterally or unilaterally and often they have a familial tendency. These are seen more often in males than in females.
- Commissural pits can occur in association with multiple preauricular pits.
- Unlike lip pits, the commissural pits are more frequent among males and black people are affected more often than whites.
- In both lip and commissural pits, there are no signs of inflammation or ulceration and both conditions are harmless.
- Sometimes, minor salivary glands may secrete at the bottom of these pits and salivary fluids often come out as the pit is squeezed.

Treatment
While commissural pits require no treatment, the lip pits are sometimes surgically excised for cosmetic reason.

■ DOUBLE LIP

Double lip is a rare developmental anomaly characterized by a horizontal fold of excess or redundant tissue, on the inner aspect (mucosal side) of the lip. It probably forms due to persistence of a sulcus between pars glabrosa and pars villosa of the lip during development (Fig. 1.1).

Acquired cases of double lip may develop due to trauma.

Clinical Features

- Double lip is an oral anomaly, which can be either a congenital or an acquired one, the acquired type occurs mostly due to trauma.
- The condition clinically appears as a "cupid's bow" when the lip is tense, but it is not visible when the lip is at rest.
- Double lip in association with blepharochalasis (dropping of the upper eyelid) and nontoxic thyroid enlargement are known as Ascher's syndrome.

Developmental Anomalies of Oral and Paraoral Structures

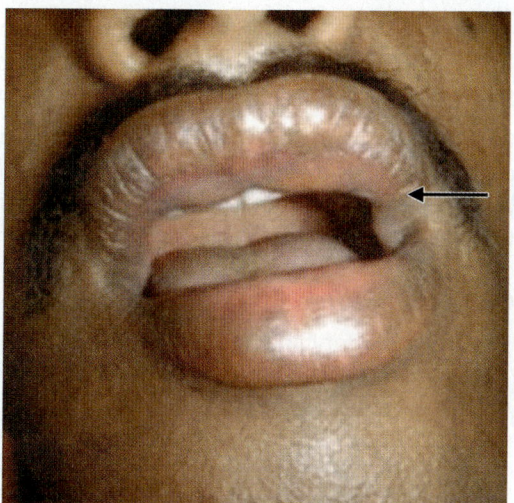

Fig. 1.1: Double lip (involving upper lip).

- Clinically, a double vermilion border is apparent with a transverse furrow between the two borders, when the patient smiles.

Treatment
Although, it is excised sometimes for cosmetic reasons, double lip mostly requires no treatment.

FRENAL TAG
Definition
Frenal attachments are thin folds of mucous membrane with enclosed muscle fibers that attach the lips to the alveolar mucosa and the periosteum. The most important among them are the maxillary labial frenum, mandibular labial frenum and the lingual frenum; the purpose of them is to provide stability to both lips and the tongue while performing different oral functions.

Frenal tag is a redundant piece of mucosal tissue, which projects from the maxillary labial frenum.

Clinical Features
- It is a familial condition and seems to be inherited as autosomal dominant trait.
- The shape and size of frenal tag varies from patient to patient and is clinically asymptomatic.
- Sometimes, the condition is mistaken for a fibrous hyperplasia caused by local injury or irritation.

Treatment
No treatment is required.

HEREDITARY INTESTINAL POLYPOSIS (PEUTZ–JEGHERS) SYNDROME
Definition
Peutz–Jeghers syndrome is a hereditary condition characterized by gastrointestinal hamartomatous polyposis in association with mucocutaneous pigmentations.

The disease is transmitted either through an autosomal dominant gene, or it can occur spontaneously. Although pigmentation is an important feature of this disease, the primary disorder is actually not of the melanocyte system.

Clinical Features
- Peutz–Jeghers syndrome begins in infancy (2nd and 3rd decades of life) and there is no sex predilection.
- Patients almost always have a positive history of the disease in the family.
- There are multifocal melanin pigmentations in the perioral locations, which often manifest as discrete, brown to bluish-black or purple-black macules on the skin.
- The size of the macule varies from 1 mm to 5 mm in diameter and these macules often group around the oral, nasal and orbital orifices.
- The pigmentation is most intense at the vermilion border of the lower lip and it often extends both to the facial skin as well as into the oral mucosa (crosses vermilion border in about 94% cases).
- Buccal mucosa is the most frequently involved intraoral site, followed by palate, gingiva, tongue and floor of the mouth, etc.

- Sometimes, these macules can be seen over the hands and feet as well.
- The skin pigmentations tend to fade away in adult life, while the mucosal pigmentations continue to persist.
- Intestinal polyposis is the other very important feature of Peutz–Jeghers syndrome besides the melanotic pigmentations. Although the polyps occur throughout the small intestine, colon and stomach are more commonly affected.
- Presence of these polyps can cause recurrent abdominal pain (in patients younger than 25 years of age), unexplained rectal bleeding and prolapse of tissue from rectum with diarrhea.
- Occasionally, intussusceptions (invagination or infolding of one part of intestine into another) and intestinal obstruction may cause even death.
- The syndrome can also cause precocious puberty, menstrual disturbances in females, gynecomastia in males and development of testicular mass, etc.

Key Points of Peutz–Jeghers Syndrome

- Melanin pigmentations of the vermillion border.
- Multiple intestinal polyps.
- Recurrent abdominal pain and obstruction.
- Precocious puberty in some cases.

Histopathology

Histologic examination of the oral macular lesions exhibits excessive accumulation of melanin granules in the basal cell layer.

Differential Diagnosis

- Albright syndrome
- Addison's disease
- Oral melanotic macule.

Treatment

No treatment is required for the oral and perioral melanotic macules. However, surgical intervention may be required for the intestinal polyps causing intussusceptions.

ORAL MELANOTIC MACULE (EPHELIS)

Definition

Oral melanotic macule is an idiopathic benign pigmented lesion of oral cavity; characterized by increased focal melanin pigmentations in the oral mucosa (Fig. 1.2).

Clinical Features

- Oral melanotic macules present small, flat, well-circumscribed, asymptomatic areas in the oral mucosa.
- These are seen commonly on the vermilion border of the lip (mostly lower lip) near the midline. Intraorally, the gingiva, buccal mucosa and the palate are the most frequently involved sites.
- Most of the lesions are less than 1 cm in diameter or sometimes little more and their color ranges from brown, black, or bluish green, etc.
- There is no specific age group for this condition; however, middle-aged females are most often affected.
- The conditions are asymptomatic and have no malignant potential.

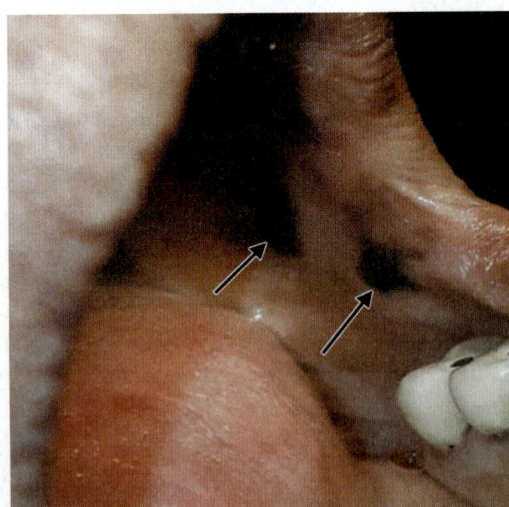

Fig. 1.2: Oral melanotic macule.

Histopathology
- Microscopically, oral melanotic macule presents diffuse accumulations of melanin granules in the basal keratinocytes and the lamina propria.
- The lesions do not evolve from proliferation of melanocytes, and there is no risk of malignant transformation in them.
- Occasionally, melanin incontinence is observed with pigmented granules being seen in subepithelial melanophages.
- Melanophagocytosis can also be seen.

Differential Diagnosis
- Superficial melanoma
- Blue nevi
- Amalgam tattoo
- Addison's disease
- Peutz–Jeghers syndrome.

Treatment
The persistent, innocuous-looking lesions do not require any treatment; however, biopsy is mandatory for a definitive diagnosis of the condition as well as to rule out any possibility of malignant melanoma.

■ UVULA ELONGATA
Definition
Uvula enlongata is a developmental anomaly characterized by abnormally long uvula, which touches or hangs lower than the base of the tongue (Fig. 1.3).

Clinical Features
- The condition is usually seen at birth and sometimes it has a familial tendency for occurrence.
- It is seen more frequently among females than males.
- Although it is mostly asymptomatic, some sensitive patients may cough or gag when the elongated uvula touches the epiglottis or the base of the tongue.

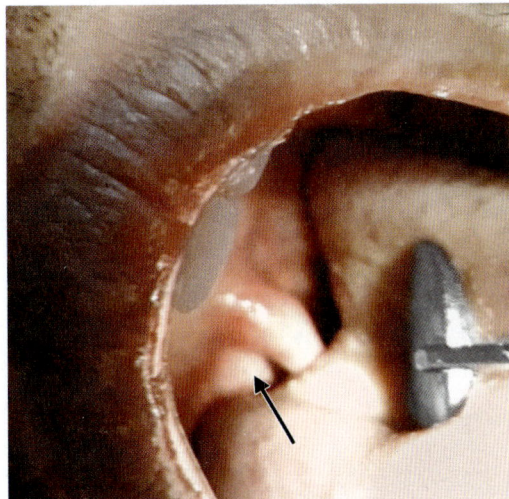

Fig. 1.3: Uvula elongata.

Differential Diagnosis
Neoplasms of the uvula.

Treatment
In most of the cases, no treatment is required.

■ CHEILITIS GLANDULARIS
Definition
Cheilitis glandularis is an uncommon, fundamentally benign, developmental anomaly of the lips characterized by chronic, progressive enlargement of the labial salivary glands (Fig. 1.4).

Etiology
- Chronic exposure to sun (actinic damage), wind and dust
- Factitial injury
- Infection, e.g. HIV
- Neoplasm, especially squamous cell carcinoma
- Use of tobacco
- Emotional stress
- Heredity

Recent investigations indicate that overexposure to sun with superimposed bacterial infection is the more likely cause of this condition.

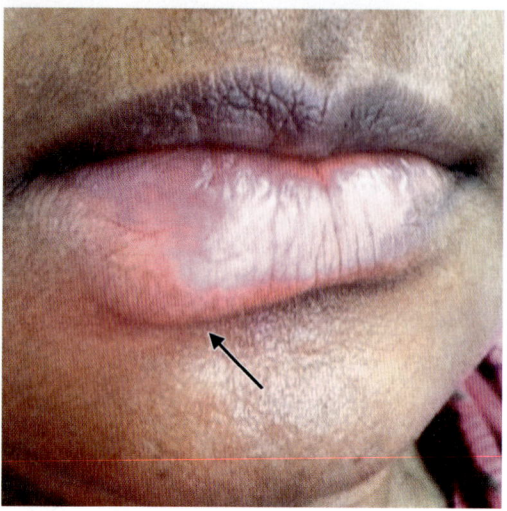

Fig. 1.4: Cheilitis glandularis.

- Few cases of cheilitis glandularis may undergo malignant transformation and produce carcinoma of the lip.

> **Key Points of Cheilitis Glandularis**
> ❖ Swelling of the lip due to enlargement of the minor salivary glands.
> ❖ Lower lip involved more frequently.
> ❖ Lip is everted with multiple fistulas found on the surface.
> ❖ Exudation on the lip surface with occasional erosion, ulceration and crusting.
> ❖ It is predominantly caused by sun, dust exposure, stress and tobacco use.
> ❖ Increased risk of malignant transformation.

Clinical Features

- Cheilitis glandularis commonly occurs among middle-aged or elderly adults and often there is a male predilection.
- Inflammatory enlargement of the superficial or deep minor salivary glands of the lip often causes progressive, multinodular swelling.
- There may be secretion of clear, viscous exudates from the minor salivary duct openings on the labial mucosa.
- Enlargement of the labial salivary glands often causes eversion and induration of the lower lip.
- Lower lip is involved more often than the upper lip and the vermilion borders as well as the labial mucosa are of normal color.
- However, in many cases, the lip shows diffuse keratosis with scaling of the surface.
- Patient sometimes complains of burning discomfort or a feeling of rawness in the lip.
- When the lip is everted due to swelling of the glands, its surface often reveals multiple pits or fistulas representing dilated and inflamed minor salivary duct openings.
- Externalization and chronic exposure of the delicate labial mucosa often result in erosion, ulceration, crusting and infection, etc.

Types

Clinically, cheilitis glandularis can be of three basic types:
1. The simple type
2. The superficial suppurative type
3. The deep suppurative type.

The simple type is the most common variant of the disease and it presents multiple, painless, pinhead size swellings on the lip with central depression.

The superficial suppurative type of cheilitis glandularis presents painless swelling of the lip with induration, areas of shallow ulcerations and crusting.

The deep suppurative type is characterized by deep-seated inflammation, abscess formation in the lip with development of fistulas tracts. The disease often heals by scarring.

Differential Diagnosis

- Cheilitis granulomatosa
- Crohn's disease
- Bacterial infection (Elephantiasis nostras verrucosa)
- Actinic cheilitis
- Squamous cell carcinoma
- Eczematous cheilitis
- Chronic factitial injury.

Histopathology

- The surface epithelium can be either normal or hyperkeratotic.

- The underlying salivary gland tissue shows hypertrophy and inflammation with distention of acini.
- Squamous metaplasia of the ductal epithelium may be seen.
- Dysplastic changes can be noted in some cases especially in type II and type III cases with increased risk of malignant transformation.

Treatment

Biopsy is mandatory especially in suspected cases, where the lip shows excessive or ulcerations.

Lesions with premalignant changes should be treated by surgical stripping.

CHEILITIS GRANULOMATOSA

Cheilitis granulomatosa is an atypical granulomatous disease of the lip, the origin of which is not clearly understood (Fig. 1.5).

Pathogenesis

As mentioned above, the exact cause of cheilitis granulomatosa is not known. Some investigators believe it as a regional form of sarcoidosis or Crohn's disease, while others suggest it as a granulomatous lesion of allergic origin.

Clinical Features

- Children and young adults commonly develop this disease (median age 25 years) and usually there is a female predominance.
- Either lower or upper or both lips show a sudden diffuse, nontender, nodular enlargement, which involves the entire lip.
- Generally, the lower lip is enlarged on a more regular basis.
- The swelling is usually painless, firm and exhibits no pitting upon pressure.
- There is no sign of inflammation or ulceration on the surface of involved lips in the initial stage.
- During the early stage, the disease is sometimes accompanied by fever, malaise and visual disturbance, etc. Regional lymph nodes are enlarged in about 50% cases.
- The initial swelling subsides within few hours or days; however, with more and more attacks of the disease, the swelling tends to become larger in size and persists longer and eventually become permanent.
- Enlarged lips often create some cosmetic problems due to the presence of several cracks and fissures on the surface along with a reddish-brown discoloration.
- Patient may also have difficulties during eating, drinking or talking.
- Few lesions may exhibit scaling, fissuring and vesicle or pustule formation at the vermilion border. The fissured lip is often painful and is firm and rubbery in consistency.
- Patients sometimes complain of decreased salivary secretion and loss of taste sensation.
- Cheilitis granulomatosa in association with facial paralysis and fissured tongue constitutes the "Melkersson–Rosenthal syndrome".

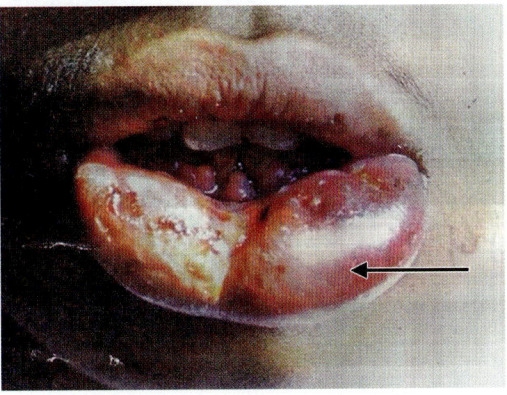

Fig. 1.5: Chelitis granulomatosa.

Key Points of Cheilitis Granulomatosa

- ❖ Diffuse, firm, painless swelling of the lip with difficulty in eating, drinking and talking.
- ❖ Granulomatous inflammation or allergy is the suspected underlying cause.
- ❖ Cheilitis granulomatosa, facial paralysis and scrotal tongue constitute Melkersson–Rosenthal syndrome.

Histopathological Features

- Microscopically, cheilitis granulomatosa shows granulomatous inflammation of the lip with infiltration by chronic inflammatory cells, chiefly lymphocytes, plasma cells and histiocytes.
- The multinodular, noncaseating granulomas are often located close to the blood vessels and these are composed of epitheloid cells and swirled collagen fascicles with interspersed Langhans type of multinucleated giant cells.
- Generalized edema and dilated blood vessels are present throughout the connective tissue.

Differential Diagnosis

- Sarcoidosis
- Cheilitis glandularis
- Angioneurotic edema
- Leprosy
- Crohn's disease
- Traumatic injury

Treatment

- Intralesional injection of steroid (Triamcinolone) may result in reduction in the size of the lesion.
- Surgical excision of the granulomas may be effective but often there is recurrence.

ANOMALIES OF THE ORAL MUCOSA

FORDYCE'S GRANULES

Definition

Sebaceous glands are normal structures of skin but sometimes they may be ectopically present in the oral and genital mucosa. Fordyce's granules are ectopic collections of sebaceous glands in the oral mucosa, generally unassociated with hair follicles (Figs. 1.6 and 1.7).

Clinical Features

- Fordyce's granules are mostly seen in adult life and there is often a male predilection.

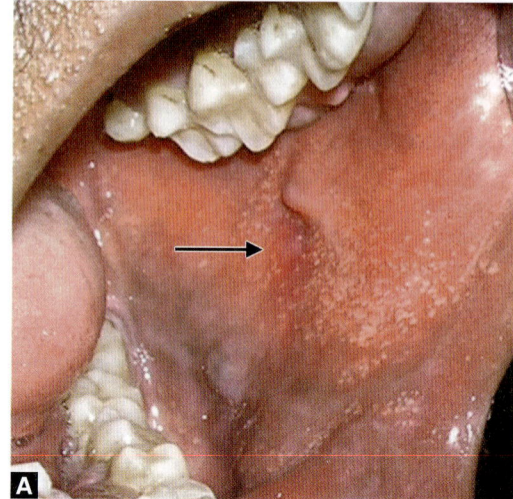
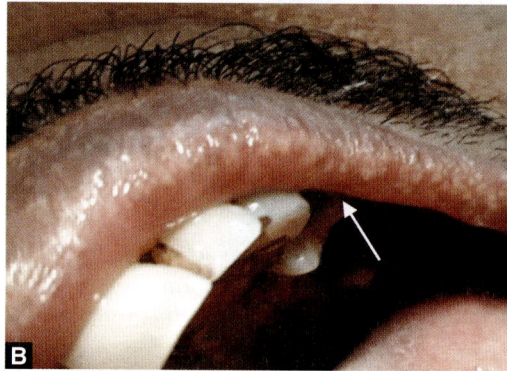

Figs. 1.6A and B: Fordyce's granules: (A) Cheek; (B) Lip.

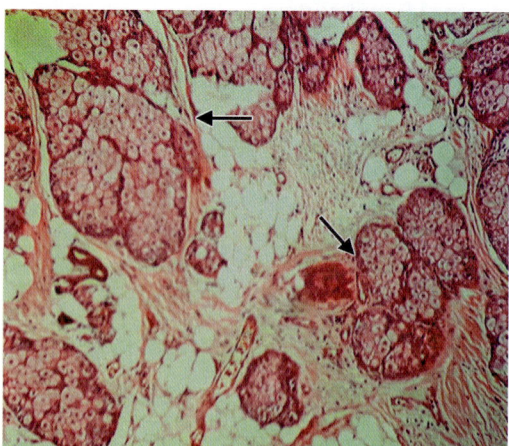

Fig. 1.7: Photomicrograph of Fordyce's granules showing lobules of sebaceous glands.

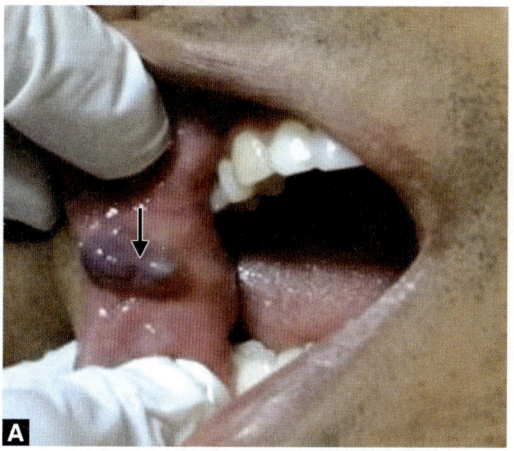
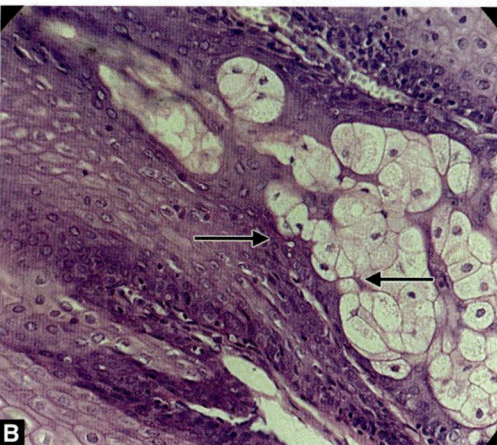

Figs. 1.8A and B: (A) Sebaceous adenoma on the cheek; (B) Histopathology of the same tumor.

- They commonly occur in a bilaterally symmetrical pattern over the buccal mucosa, labial mucosa and vermilion border of upper lip. Fordyce's granules are seen rarely in lower lip.
- Fordyce's granules can also be present in many extraoral locations such as the esophagus, genitalia, nipples, palms and the parotid glands, etc.
- The number and size of tend to increase with age.
- Fordyce's granules clinically appear as soft, creamy-white or yellowish spots or clusters on the oral muocsa, often measuring about 1–2 mm in diameter.
- These spots often have a typical "rice-like" or "milia-like" appearance and sometimes, cluster of these granules may form slightly raised confluent plaques with a creamy appearance.
- Fordyce's granules are completely asymptomatic conditions and in most of the cases, patients are not aware of their presence in the mouth.

Histopathology

- Histologically, Fordyce's granules exhibit typical sebaceous glands (with no associated hair follicles); these glands are located superficially, quite close to the surface epithelium and they open directly onto the surface epithelium by short, keratinized ducts.
- Each gland is composed of 1–5 lobules, which have flat and darkly stained peripheral cells and lipid-rich pale type cells at the center (Figs. 1.8A and B).
- Secretions from these sebaceous glands flow through small ducts, which open directly on to the oral mucosa. The duct may show keratin plugging.

Key Points of Fordyce's Granules
- These are ectopic collections of sebaceous glands in the oral cavity (normal location is skin).
- Appear as multiple, yellowish, milia-like discrete granules on the buccal mucosa (bilaterally).
- Sebaceous cyst may develop from them.

Treatment
No treatment is required for this condition. However, on rare occasions, sebaceous cysts or adenomas may develop from the preexisting Fordyce's granules.

FOCAL EPITHELIAL HYPERPLASIA

Definition
Focal epithelial hyperplasia (commonly known as Heck's disease) is a condition characterized by multiple papillary or sessile hyperplastic areas in the oral mucosa.

Clinical Features
- The disease commonly occurs among children between the ages of 3 years and 18 years and there is no sex predilection.
- Clinically, focal epithelial hyperplasia presents multiple, small, pedunculated, polypoid or nodular soft tissue growths in the oral cavity.
- They also can appear as well demarcated, slightly raised plaques.
- Sometimes several hyperplastic lesions may cluster together to produce a typical "cobblestone" appearance.
- Labial and buccal mucosa are the most common sites and lower lip is more frequently affected than the upper. However, the disease can also involve the tongue, gingiva and anterior faucial pillars, etc.
- Individual lesions measure about 1–5 mm in diameter and are either white or pink in color.
- Most of the lesions regress spontaneously after about 4–6 months and occasionally few lesions can recur.

Differential Diagnosis
- Leukoplakia
- Psoriasis
- Keratoacanthoma
- Veruciform xanthoma.

Histopathology
- Focal epithelial hyperplasia histologically shows hyperparakeratosis of the covering epithelium with extensive acanthosis (increased thickening of the spinus cell layer).
- The epithelial cells of the upper spinus layer show enlarged nuclei and vacuolated clear cytoplasms (koilocytes).
- Deeper layer of epithelium reveals thickening, elongation and even fusion of the rete pegs.
- Basal cell layer of the epithelium exhibit increased mitotic activity.

Since focal epithelial hyperplasia is a harmless, self-regressing condition, it usually requires no treatment.

WHITE SPONGE NEVUS

Definition
White sponge nevus or Cannon's disease is a congenital mucosal abnormality, which appears to follow an autosomal dominant hereditary pattern and manifests as a white lesion of the oral mucosa.

Pathogenesis
- This condition is transmitted as an autosomal dominant trait with incomplete penetrance and variable expressivity.
- Mutations in the genes coding for keratins 4 and 13 have been identified, suggesting the disorder as a hereditary keratin defect.
- The heaping up of cells on the surface of the epithelium also suggests the possibility of an impaired normal desquamation process of the superficial strata of cells.

Clinical Features
- White sponge nevus has its onset mostly during childhood. Some lesions are congenital and are present at birth and few lesions may even initiate during the adolescent period.
- There is no sex predilection, several members of the same family are often affected.
- The intraoral lesions are almost always bilateral and are mostly found over the buccal mucosa and tongue. Occasionally, the vestibular mucosa, palate, gingiva and floor of the mouth, etc. are also affected.
- Clinically, white sponge nevus presents a thick, bilateral, asymptomatic, deeply folded or corrugated white or gray lesion on the oral mucosa.
- The surface of the lesion is soft, uneven and has a shaggy appearance with a spongy consistency.
- The lesions can be either diffuse or patchy and have a translucent opalescence similar to that of leukodema.

Histopathology

- White sponge nevus histologically shows marked thickening of the epithelium with mild to moderate hyperparakeratinization, acanthosis and spongiosis.
- Marked intracellular edema of the spinus and parakeratinized cell layer of the epithelium is an important characteristic feature of the disease.
- The cells with intracellular edema show vacuolated cytoplasms and shrunken (pyknotic) nuclei.
- Interestingly, under microscope only, the cell walls and the pyknotic nuclei at the centers of the cells are visible, which often give rise to a so-called "basket weave" appearance.
- Parakeratin plugging is another important finding in white sponge nevus, which runs the surface and extends deep into the spinus layer.

Electron Microscopic Study

Ultrastructural studies of white sponge nevus reveal that some cells of the spinus layer differentiate early and become enriched with tonofilaments.

Differential Diagnosis

- Leukoplakia
- Hereditary intraepithelial dyskeratosis
- Lichen planus
- Candidiasis
- Leukodema.

Treatment

No treatment is required for this disease.

DEVELOPMENTAL DEFECTS OF THE GINGIVAE

■ FIBROMATOSIS GINGIVAE

Definition

Fibromatosis gingivae are rare, benign, diffuse, noninflammatory hyperplasia of the gingival tissue, which sometimes cover the entire teeth.

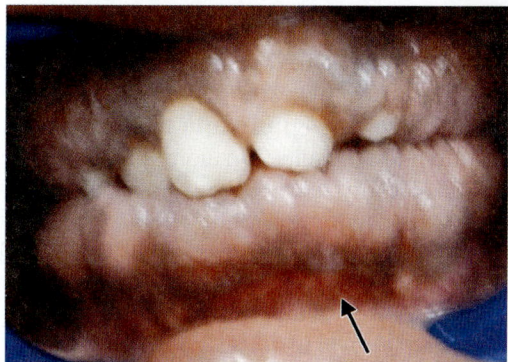

Fig. 1.9: Fibromatosis gingivae.

It is a hereditary condition, which is transmitted as an autosomal dominant trait (Fig. 1.9).

Clinical Features

- Clinically, the disease is characterized by dense, diffuse, smooth or nodular overgrowth of the gingival tissue.
- The gingival enlargement mostly appears in young children or it may be present even at birth; however, in some cases the swelling may not be noticed until the adult life.
- Both sexes are equally affected in gingival fibromatosis.
- The gingiva shows multinodular enlargements, especially in the interdental papilla regions.
- The gingival tissue changes become obvious soon after the eruption of the deciduous teeth.
- The hyperplastic tissue is firm, painless and retains the normal coral pink color of gingiva.
- Sometimes, the markedly enlarged gingiva may cover the entire crown of the erupted teeth. The eruption process of teeth is, however, normal.
- Occasionally, the condition is associated with hypertrichosis, epilepsy and mental retardation, etc.
- Gingival fibromatosis can also be associated with other syndromes, e.g. Cowden's syndrome and Rutherford's syndrome (features of individual syndrome are given in the relevant chapter dealing with syndromes).

Histopathology

Histopathologically, gingival fibromatosis presents the following features:
- The covering epithelium is hyperplastic and often exhibits thin elongated rete pegs.
- The fibrous connective tissue consists mainly of course bundles of collagen fibers with scattered mature spindle-shaped fibroblasts few of which are multinucleated.

Differential Diagnosis

- Phenytoin (Dilantin) sodium induced gingival hyperplasia
- Generalized hyperplastic gingivitis
- Leukemic infiltration of the gingiva.

History of familial involvement is extremely important in making the diagnosis of the disease.

Treatment

Periodic gingivectomy with placement of gingival acrylic splints for cosmetic and functional reasons.

■ RETROCUSPID PAPILLA

Retrocuspid papilla is a slightly raised area of mandibular alveolar mucosa, which as the name implies, is commonly located lingual to the cuspids. This structure measures about 2–4 mm and is often present bilaterally between the marginal gingiva and the mucogingival junctions.

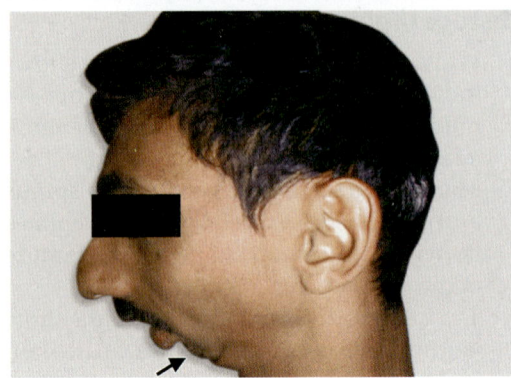

Fig. 1.10: Micrognathia of mandible.

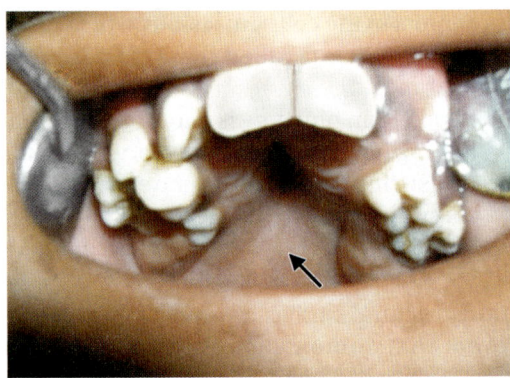

Fig. 1.11: Micrognathia of maxilla with high-arched palate.

DEVELOPMENTAL ANOMALIES INVOLVING THE JAWBONE

■ AGNATHIA

Agnathia refers to the complete failure of development of jawbone, involving either maxilla or mandible or even both the jaws. It is an extremely rare condition, however, often a portion of the jawbone, e.g. premaxilla, condyle, or ramus, etc. can be developmentally missing.

■ MICROGNATHIA

Micrognathia is an orofacial anomaly characterized by development of jaws, which are unusually smaller than normal (Figs. 1.10 and 1.11).

Causes

- Pierre Robin syndrome
- Hallermann–Streiff syndrome
- Trisomy 13
- Trisomy 18
- Turner syndrome
- Marfan syndrome
- Progeria.

Types

Micrognathia can be of two types:
1. Pseudomicrognathia
2. True micrognathia.

Pseudomicrognathia: It is a condition where normal-sized jawbone appears to look smaller when compared with the opposing jaw. A jawbone of standard size may appear smaller, if the opposite jaw is larger than normal or if it is positioned more posteriorly in relation to the skull.

True micrognathia: It is the condition, where the jawbone is actually smaller than normal and it can be either a congenital or an acquired problem.

The congenital micrognathia may follow a hereditary pattern and it often occurs in association with other congenital diseases, such as Pierre Robin syndrome or congenital heart disease, etc.

Congenitally, missing premaxilla often leads to maxillary micrognathia and patients with this anomaly show retracted middle third of the face.

Congenital mandibular micrognathia may occur due to posterior positioning of the condyle in relation to the skull.

Acquired micrognathia mostly occurs due to trauma or severe infections in the orofacial region especially in younger age. Ankylosis of the temporomandibular joint in young individuals often leads to mandibular micrognathia with retruded chin.

Clinical Features

- Micrognathia often results in defective alignment of teeth, crowding and malocclusion, etc.
- Retruded chin with small face
- Difficulty in feeding the children
- Difficulty in proper articulation and speech.

■ MACROGNATHIA

Macrognathia is a developmental anomaly characterized by abnormally large jaws. The condition can affect both the jaws at a time but more often it involves either maxilla or mandible (Fig. 1.12).

Types

True macrognathia: When the jawbone is abnormally large in size in true sense, it is called true macrognathia.

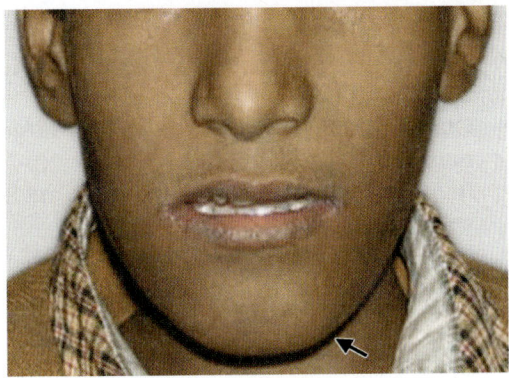

Fig. 1.12: Mandibular macrognathia.

Pseudomacrognathia: A normal-sized jaw may look larger when the opposing jaw is smaller than normal in size. This condition is known as pseudomacrognathia.

Common Causes of True Macrognathia

- *Pituitary gigantism*: It is often associated with abnormally large jawbones. Both are affected in gigantism.
- *Paget's disease of bone*: Paget's disease often causes increase in the size of maxilla.
- *Acromegaly*: Progressive increase in the size of mandible occurs in cases of acromegally.
- *Hereditary causes*: Mandibular prognathism often occurs hereditarily.

Mandibular prognathism may occur due to anterior positioning of the lower jaw in relation to the cranium, even though the exact size of the jaw is normal.

However, there are certain factors, which cause mandibular prognathism and thereby create an appearance of mandibular macrognathia.

These factors are as follows:
- Increased length of the body of mandible
- Decreased maxillary length
- Posterior positioning of the maxilla in relation to the cranium
- Prominent chin button
- Varying soft-tissue contours.

Clinical Features

- Mandibular protrusion (when mandible is affected)
- Gummy smile (mostly due to very large maxillary)
- Ramus of mandible forms a less steep angle with body of the mandible
- Excessive condylar growth
- Prominent chin.

Treatment

Surgical correction (osteotomy) for both functional and esthetic reasons.

FACIAL HEMIHYPERTROPHY

Definition

Facial hemihypertrophy is a developmental condition characterized by disproportionate unilateral enlargement of the face.

Although most humans exhibit some degrees of facial asymmetry only few individuals actually develop clinically significant facial hemihypertrophy (Figs. 1.13 to 1.15).

Etiology

Although, a number of factors have been proposed to explain this condition, the most important ones appear to be vascular and neurogenic disturbances that cause an increased neurovascular supply to the affected side of the face resulting in its overgrowth.

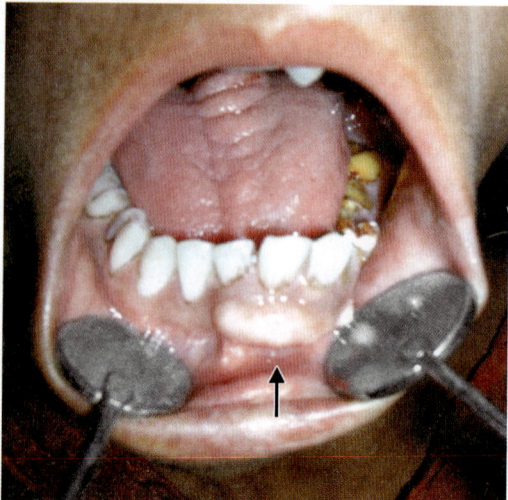

Fig. 1.14: Facial hemihypertrophy with overgrowth of mandible on left side.

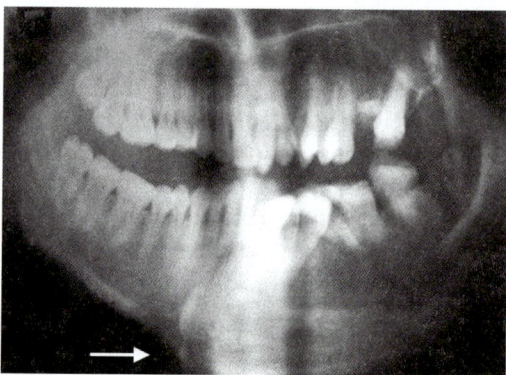

Fig. 1.15: Radiograph of facial hemihypertrophy (left side).

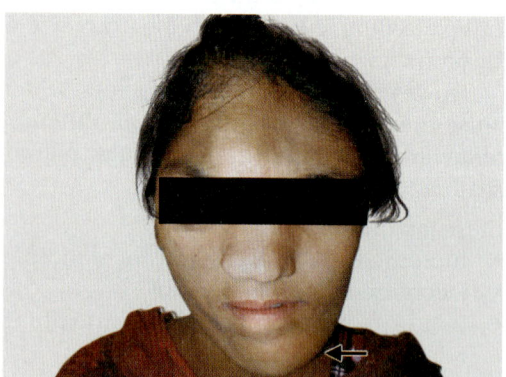

Fig. 1.13: Facial hemihypertrophy of left side.

Clinical Features

Facial hemihypertrophy clinically exhibits the following features:
- Unilateral enlargement of the facial soft tissues, bones and teeth.
- Either side of the face can be affected and there is a slight female predilection for this condition.
- The asymmetry is more specifically noticed in the frontal bone, maxilla, palate, mandible, alveolar process, condyles and the associated soft tissues.

- The skin is thick and coarse on the affected side and also there is presence of thick and abundant hair (hypertrichosis).
- The sebaceous and sweat glands on the affected side show excessive secretions.
- The ear and eye on the affected side may also be enlarged.
- Unilateral enlargement of the cerebral hemisphere may cause mental retardation and seizure in about 15–20% cases.
- There can be an increased incidence of certain systemic conditions in facial hemihypertrophy such as Wilms' tumor, tumor of kidney, adrenocortical tumor and hepatoblastoma, etc.

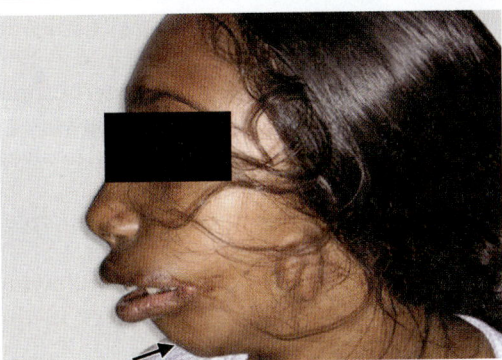

Fig. 1.16: Facial hemiatrophy showing defect in the cranial bone also.

Oral Manifestations

- Unilateral macroglossia with an increase in the size of the fungiform papilla is often seen.
- Crowns and roots of teeth, especially of the permanent teeth are often enlarged on the affected side.
- The teeth on the affected side may also erupt prematurely.
- There is often early shedding of deciduous teeth on the affected side.
- The jawbone proper is larger and thicker on the affected side.
- Because of the osseous and dental asymmetries malocclusion often develops.

Treatment

No treatment is usually required for facial hemihypertrophy. However, selective surgical treatments may be performed.

FACIAL HEMIATROPHY

Definition

Facial hemiatrophy, also known as Parry-Romberg syndrome, is a developmental anomaly characterized by progressive decrease in the size of one side of the face due to atrophy of the facial structures (Figs. 1.16 and 1.17).

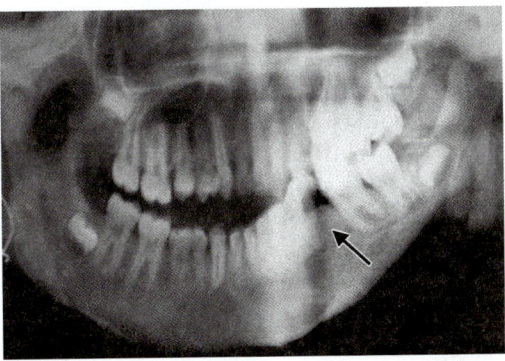

Fig. 1.17: Radiograph of facial hemiatrophy with smaller size of jaw and teeth on the affected side.

Etiology

The exact etiology of the disease is not known, however, certain possible factors have been identified which include:
- Peripheral nerve dysfunction
- Trauma
- Heredity
- Peripheral trigeminal neuritis
- Infection
- Regional systematic sclerosis.

Clinical Features

- The condition usually begins in the first or second decade of life. Many cases may be present since birth.
- Initially, a slightly depressed vertical furrow or line is noticed at the midline of the forehead and eyebrow.

- As the condition progresses, facial tissues on the affected side including the skin, subcutaneous tissue, muscle and bone, etc. become atrophic, resulting in facial deformity.
- Usually, the left side of the face is involved more often than the right side.
- Affected side of the face shows hyperpigmentation of skin with loss of hair.
- Severe cases may often result in following of the cheek and depressed eye in the orbit.
- Other features associated with facial hemiatrophy include trigeminal neuralgia, contralateral Jacksonian epilepsy and ocular and hair changes.

Oral Manifestations
- Intraoral tissues on the affected side exhibit an overall atrophy.
- Delayed development of the jawbone.
- Tooth eruption on the affected side may also be retarded.
- Teeth on the affected side often have shorter crowns and roots.
- Development of the roots of teeth on the affected side is also delayed.

Treatment
There is no effective treatment for facial hemiatrophy. Progression of the condition ceases after certain age and it remains static thereafter for the remaining part of life.

■ TORUS IN THE JAWS
Torus (plural is tori) is a developmental anomaly of the jaws; characterized by localized bony overgrowths or protuberances on the inner aspect of maxilla or mandible. These lesions often believed to be hereditary in origin and they occur more often in men than in women. Mandiblular tori are seen more often bilaterally on the lingual aspect and, in maxilla, these are seen in the midportion of the hard palate (Fig. 1.18).

In most cases, tori are asymptomatic; however, larger growths may cause some discomfort while taking foods and often they cause difficulty in denture wearing. Treatment is done by surgical removal of the lesion or reshaping of the bone.

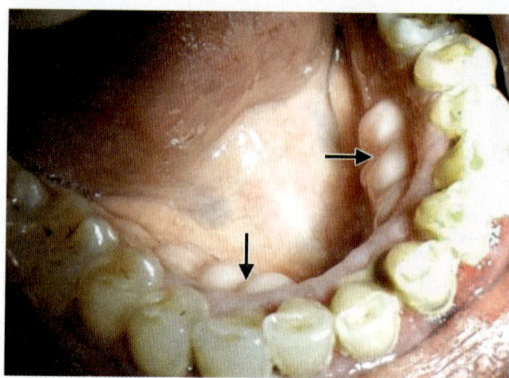

Fig. 1.18: Torus mandibularis.

■ OROFACIAL CLEFTS
Orofacial clefts are gaps or openings created due to incomplete fusion of various embryonic processes during the intrauterine life; these are quiet common entities especially in the lips and palate regions. Clefts may also involve mandible, tongue and nose, etc. (Tables 1.2 and 1.3).

■ CLEFT LIP AND CLEFT PALATE
Development of upper lip occurs during the 6th week and 7th week of intrauterine life with the fusion of both median nasal processes and the maxillary processes. Cleft lip and palate are the most common developmental defects in the head and neck region.

Definition
The primary palate is formed by the fusion of *median nasal processes of either side*, which later on gives rise to premaxilla (the anterior most part of maxilla holding central and lateral incisor teeth of both sides). The secondary palate is formed by the *fusion of both palatal shelves, which are formed from the maxillary processes*.

Table 1.2: Different processes involved in the formation of oral structures.

Processes	Oral structures
Median nasal processes	Midportion of upper lip and primary palate (premaxilla).
Lateral nasal process	Alae of the nose
Maxillary processes	Lateral portion of the upper lip and secondary palate
Mandibular processes	Lower jaw and lower lip
Maxillary and mandibular processes together	Lateral part of face

Table 1.3: Classification of cleft lip and cleft palate.

Davis and Ritchie classification	• *Group I*: Clefts anterior to the alveolus (unilateral, median, or bilateral cleft lip). • *Group II*: Post-alveolar clefts (Cleft palate alone, soft palate alone, soft palate and hard palate, or submucous cleft).
Veau classification	• *Group I (A)*: Defects of the soft palate only. • *Group II (B)*: Defects involving the hard palate and soft palate. • *Group III(C)*: Defects involving the soft palate to the alveolus, usually involving the lip. • *Group IV (D)*: Complete bilateral clefts.
Kernahan and Stark symbolic classification	• *Areas 1 and 4*: Lip. • *Areas 2 and 5*: Alveolus. • *Areas 3 and 6*: Palate between alveolus and the incisive foramen. • *Areas 7 and 8*: Hard palate. • *Area 9*: Soft palate.
International confederation of plastic and reconstructive surgery classification	• *Group I*: Defects of the lip or alveolus. • *Group II*: Clefts of the secondary palate (hard palate, soft palate, or both). • *Group III*: Any combination of clefts involving the primary and secondary palates.

Cleft lip: It is a developmental anomaly characterized by a wedge-shaped gap or opening in the lip, which results from failure of two parts of the lip to fuse together at the time of development. Cleft lip actually occurs in case the median nasal process does not fuse properly with the maxillary process during the embryonic development.

This defect is more commonly seen in upper lip as compared to the lower.

Cleft palate: It is a developmental defect, which occurs due lack of fusion between two palatal shelves with the premaxilla (*it involves the nonunion of median nasal processes and the maxillary processes*). Cleft in the palate leads to communication between oral and the nasal cavity.

These developmental defects often have very serious impacts on the growth, development and functions of the involved facial organ. Moreover, such defects can jeopardize the appearance of the face and badly affect the personality of the patient as well.

Etiology

The etiology of cleft lip and cleft palate covers both hereditary and environmental factors (Box 1.1).

Hereditary Factors

Different studies indicate that nearly 40% of cleft lip cases with or without cleft palate are hereditary in origin. Heredity also plays role in the development of about 20% cases of isolated cleft palate.

> **Box 1.1** Congenital malformations causing clefts in the orofacial region.
>
> - Cleft lip
> - Clefts of the primary palate
> - Cleft of the secondary palate
> - Mandibular cleft
> - Oblique facial cleft
> - Submucosal cleft palate
> - Bifid uvula
> - Pits of the lip

Moreover, research also indicates that cleft lip or cleft palate of hereditary origin can occur either due to polygenic influence or monogenic influence.

- *Polygenic inheritance*: If the origin of the disease is influenced by several different genes acting together. It is presumed that every individual carries some genetic liability for clefting and only if the combined liabilities of both the parents exceed a minimum threshold level, then clefting occurs in their offspring.
- *Monogenic inheritance of cleft lip and cleft palate*: When clefting is influenced by only a single gene, it is called monogenic defect.

Environmental Factors

- Nutritional factors, such as deficiency of or excess of vitamin A and deficiency of riboflavin.
- Maternal smoking (during pregnancy) is a very high risk factor.
- Psychogenic, emotional or traumatic stress in pregnant mothers
- Relative ischemia to the area due to defective vascular supply
- Mechanical obstruction by enlarged tongue
- High dose of steroid therapy during pregnancy
- Localized mucopolysaccharide metabolism defect in the area
- Infections
- Substances, such as alcohol, drugs or toxins in the circulation
- Pathological conditions like Streeter's fetal dysplasia
- Lack of inherent developmental force.

Pathogenesis

Cleft lip and cleft palate usually develop due to incomplete obliteration and maturation of different embryonic processes, which are associated with the formation of normal lip and palate.

- Mandibular cleft (lower lip and/or mandibular bone) usually occurs either due to failure of the copula to form the mandibular arch or due to persistence of the central groove of the mandibular process. Mandibular clefts are mostly midline defects.
- Cleft of the upper lip and premaxilla occur due to failure of mesodermal penetration and subsequent obliteration of the ectodermal grooves between the median nasal process, lateral nasal process and the maxillary process, which occurs during the 7th week of intrauterine life.
- The tongue occupies the space between two palatal halves during the initial phase of development. However, 9th and 10th weeks of intrauterine life are associated with mandibular enlargement and gradual downward movement of the tongue.
- If the tongue does not move downwards sufficiently, the palatal shelves remain separated and do not rotate to their horizontal position; this causes lack of fusion between the palatal shelves resulting in clefts.
- Palatal fusion occurs anteroposteriorly and is completed in between 11th week and 12th week of the intrauterine life.
- Isolated cleft of the palate develops due to the failure of fusion between two palatal shelves in the midline.

Incidence

Incidence varies with racial and geographic background. Incidence of cleft lip and/or cleft palate is about 1 in 800 childbirths (range in 1:500–1:2,500). It is interesting to note that when a couple have their first baby born with the defect of either cleft lip or cleft palate or both, their second baby will carry a 1% risk of having the same defect (Table 1.4 and Figs. 1.19A to C).

Developmental Anomalies of Oral and Paraoral Structures

Table 1.4: Average frequency of development of cleft lip and palate.

Isolated cleft lip	25% cases
Isolated cleft palate	30% cases
Cleft lip and cleft palate together	45% cases

Common Syndromes Associated with Cleft Palate

- Pierre Robin syndrome
- Goldenhar syndrome
- Median cleft face syndrome
- Oral facial digital syndrome
- Apert's syndrome
- Cleidocranial dysplasia
- Scheuthauer–Marie–Sainton syndrome
- Nager syndrome
- Elsahy–Waters syndrome
- Crouzon syndrome
- Larsen syndrome
- Treacher–Collins syndrome
- Marfan syndrome
- Otopalatodigital syndrome
- Down syndrome
- Edwards syndrome.

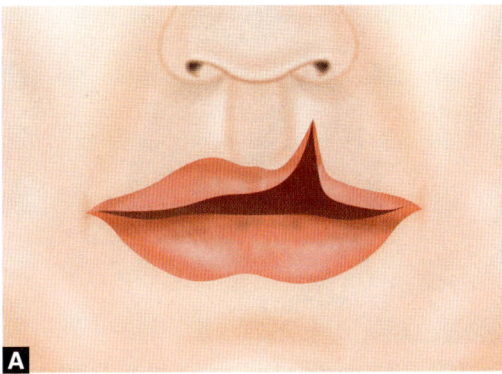
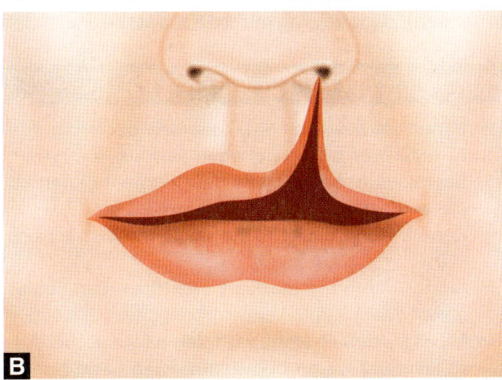
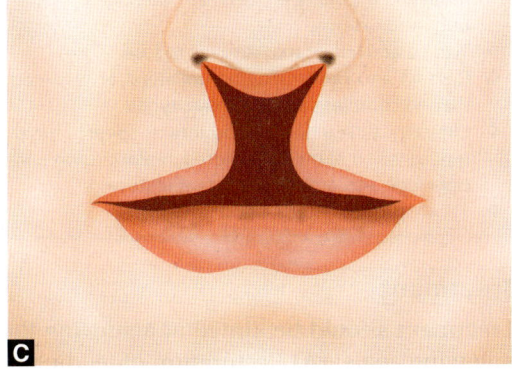

Figs. 1.19A to C: Spectrum of defect in cleft lip and cleft palate: (A) Isolated cleft lip; (B) Unilateral cleft lip and palate; (C) Bilateral cleft lip and palate.

Clinical Features

- These defects occur more commonly among male people; most common type of cleft in both sexes combined is cleft lip and palate.
- Most common type of isolated cleft lip only is unilateral complete type and the mildest form of cleft palate is the cleft uvula (Fig. 1.20).
- Clefting involves left side of the face more often than the right side.
- A complete cleft lip may extend upward and involve the nostril (incomplete cleft lip does not involve the nostril). Such cases may cause

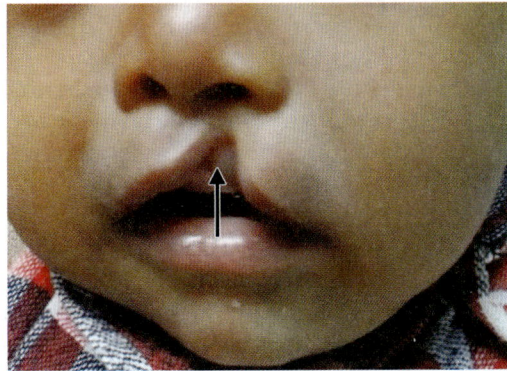

Fig. 1.20: Isolated cleft in upper lip.

- deflection of nasal tip towards the noncleft side and larger nares on the clefted side.
- Cleft palate may involve both hard and soft palates or the soft palate alone. In some cleft palate cases, the defect may be entirely submucosal where the overlying mucosa is intact.
- As cleft palate creates a communication between the oral and the nasal cavities, patients often feel difficulty in taking foods and drinks due to nasal reflux or regurgitation.
- Breastfeeding is impossible to babies having cleft lip or cleft palate, as they cannot generate sufficient suction as well as the problem of nasal regurgitation of the milk.
- Cleft palate may extend into the alveolar bone in anterior maxilla and cause displacement of the lateral incisor and canine teeth, some teeth can be missing (especially lateral incisors); upper anterior teeth are often misplaced, deformed or impacted; and in some cases, supernumerary teeth can be formed.
- Bony deficiency of upper jaw may cause retrusion of maxilla with narrow arched palate.
- Bilateral complete cleft is the worst situation where complete separation of the anterior palate occurs, which projects towards the midportion of the lip and is attached only by the nasal septum. There may be deflection of nasal tip towards the noncleft side and larger naris on the cleft side (Fig. 1.21).
- Increased susceptibility to middle ear infections via the auditory tube.
- Difficulty is correct phonation and articulation of speech.
- There may be associated major congenital defects in the body including heart defects, spina bifida, and mental deficiency, etc.
- Mental trauma to the child due to the unusual appearance as well as due to the speech problems, which often prevents them from mixing with other children freely.
- Improper or untimely surgical correction of these defects may also cause persistence of some ugly appearance and defective speech (Figs. 1.22A and B).

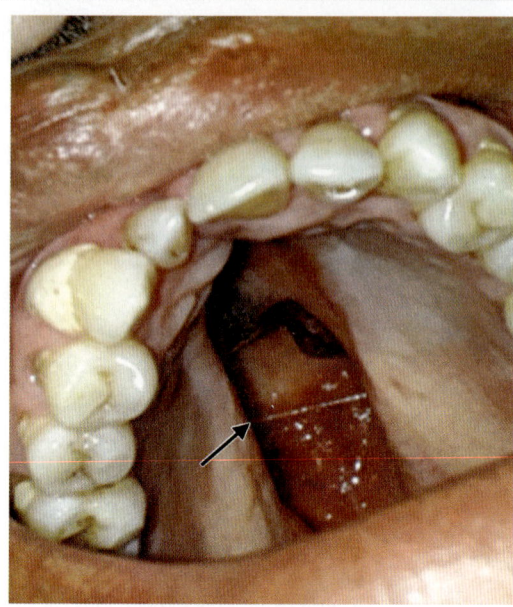

Fig. 1.21: Unilateral cleft lip (repaired) and cleft palate (untreated); also showing microdontia at the site of cleft.

Key Points of Cleft Lip and Cleft Palate

- Important developmental anomaly occurring due to failure of fusion between various embryonic processes associated with development of normal lips and palate.
- Genetic abnormality is the single most important cause.
- More common in maxillary arch than mandibular arch.
- Maxillary cleft lip along with cleft palate occurs due to failure of fusion between median nasal, lateral nasal and maxillary processes in varying combinations and extents.
- Two palatal halves may also fail to fuse.
- Cleft lip and palate may be unilateral or bilateral; may be complete or incomplete types.
- Clinically, difficulties in food intake, speech, nasal regurgitation of milk in children, malocclusion and poor look, etc. are the important features.
- Timely surgical intervention is required.

Treatment

Treatment should be aimed at achieving the following goals: (A) Restoration of feeding to the child; (B) Proper development of speech; (C) Prevention of maxillary arch collapse; and (D) Cosmetic repair of the face and lips.

Developmental Anomalies of Oral and Paraoral Structures

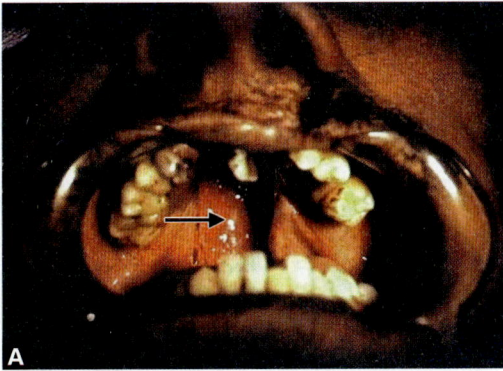
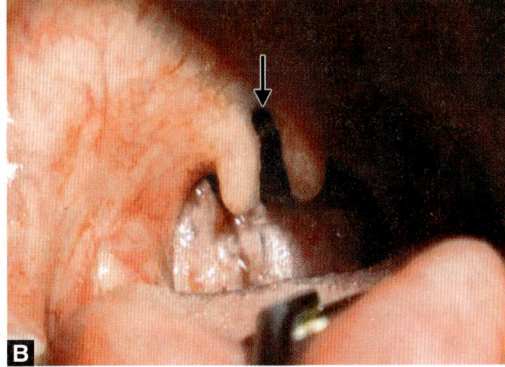

Figs. 1.22A and B: (A) Bilateral complete cleft lip and cleft palate; (B) Cleft (bifid) uvula.

- Cleft lip should be treated surgically within 4–6 months of age of the child.
- Generally, cleft palates are corrected surgically at the age of around 12 months. Delay in treatment can interfere with development of speech and also puts the child into more psychological stress.
- Obturators may be given in untreated adult patients with palatal clefts; this appliance helps in keeping the palatal clefts closed and thereby helps in speech and taking food.

■ CLEFT IN LOWER LIP AND MANDIBLE

Mandibular clefts are very rare anomalies, which occur due to failure of fusion of the two mandibular processes on either side. There may be a cleft in the lower lip only or it can involve both lower lip as well as the mandible; and in most cases, the clefts occur in the midline. Tongue is often involved with presence of cleft tongue and fixation of the tip to the alveolar ridge in the midline (Figs. 1.23A and B).

DEVELOPMENTAL ANOMALIES OF THE TONGUE

■ AGLOSSIA

Aglossia is an extremely rare congenital defect characterized by complete failure of development of tongue. Sometimes, it occurs in association with aglossia-adactylia syndrome characterized by congenital absence or severe hypoplasia of tongue with absence of the digits.

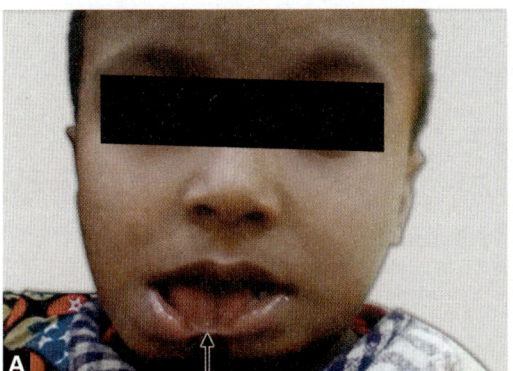
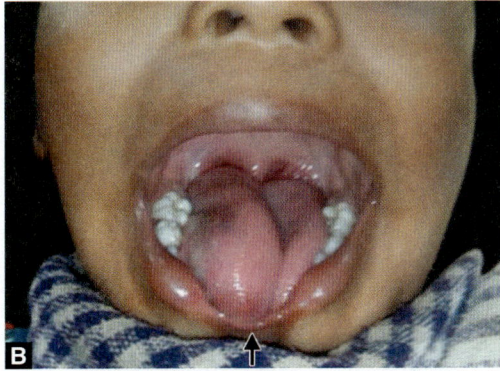

Figs. 1.23A and B: Cleft in: (A) Mandible; (B) Lower lip.

MICROGLOSSIA

- Microglossia is a rare congenital anomaly in which only a tiny or rudimentary tongue develops in the oral cavity (Fig. 1.24). Although microglossia may develop as an isolated case but in most cases, it occurs in association with other congenital anomalies, e.g. oromandibular limb hypogenesis syndrome or hypoglossia-hypodactylia syndrome, etc.
- However, patients with microglossia do not have severe speech difficulties or difficulty in taking food.
- Small children often have problem in sucking milk.
- Since the size of the tongue often determines the growth and size of the mandibular arch, in case of microglossia, the length of the mandibular arch is often smaller.

MACROGLOSSIA

Macroglossia is a relatively common condition characterized by an abnormally large tongue in the oral cavity.

Types

Macroglossia can be either congenital or acquired (secondary) in nature.

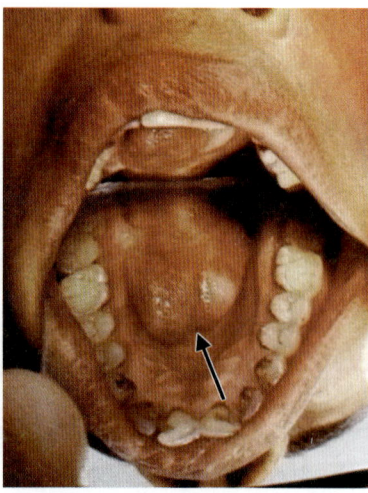

Fig. 1.24: Microglossia with bifid tongue.

Causes

Causes of macroglossia are listed in Box 1.2.

Box 1.2	Causes of macroglossia.

A. Causes of Congenital Macroglossia
- Idiopathic muscle hypertrophy causing overdevelopment of the tongue musculature.
- Lysosomal storage diseases:
  - Hurler syndrome
  - Hunter syndrome
  - Maroteaux–Lamy syndrome
- Down syndrome
- Beckwith's hypoglycemic syndrome
- Multiple endocrine neoplasia syndrome
- Lingual thyroid nodule
- Gargolysm
- Trisomy
- Neonatal diabetes mellitus

B. Causes of Acquired (Secondary) Macroglossia
Tumors in the tongue
- Lymphangioma
- Hemangioma
- Neurofibromatosis
- Carcinoma
- Plasmacytoma
- Metastatic tumors

Infiltrative diseases:
- Amyloidosis
- Sarcoidosis

Systemic conditions:
- Uremia
- Iatrogenic macroglossia

Traumatic conditions:
- Surgery
- Hemorrhage
- Tongue biting
- Intubation injury
- Radiation injury

Endocrine disorders:
- Acromegaly
- Cretinism
- Hypothyroidism
- Diabetes
- Myxedema

Obstructive lesions in the tongue: Lymphatic obstruction of the tongue by any malignant tumor.
Inflammatory conditions of tongue:
- Syphilis
- Ludwig's angina
- Pemphigus
- Tuberculosis
- Smallpox

Contd...

Contd...
- Scurvy
- Actinomycosis
- Typhoid
- Pellagra

Cystic lesions in the tongue:
- Dermoid cyst
- Epidermoid cyst

Relative Macroglossia

Relative macroglossia is a condition in which a normal-sized tongue appears abnormally large if it is particularly enclosed within a small oral cavity. It happens mostly in cases of maxillary retrusion or in cases of restricted growth of nasopharynx.

Lymphangioma restricted to the tongue or in continuity with a cystic hygroma of the neck is the most common cause of macroglossia.

Apparent Macroglossia

Apparent macroglossia is a condition, where the tongue appears abnormally large due to poor muscular control of the tongue, although there is no real increase in the bulk of the tongue tissue. Apparent macroglossia is often seen in cretinism and in "Happy puppet" syndrome.

Clinical Features

- Macroglossia causes displacement of teeth and malocclusion as the enlarged tongue creates continuous pressure or thrust on the teeth.
- It may disturb the process of speech and food intake to some extent.
- The lateral margin of the tongue exhibits scalloping or indentations as the tongue is always pressed against the teeth.

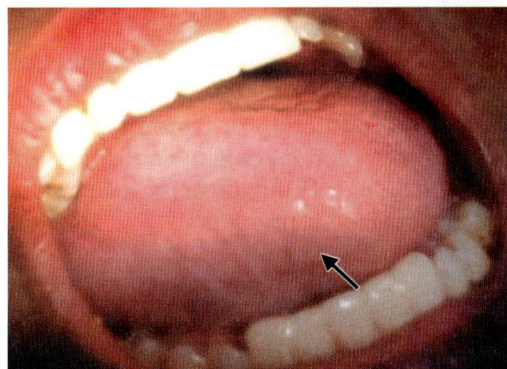

Fig. 1.25: Macroglossia.

- Children with macroglossia often develop tongue-thrusting habits, which may lead to malocclusion, open bite and diastema formation, etc.
- Macroglossia developing in adult people (as in acromegaly or in tumors, etc.) may produce spacing of teeth and distortion of the mandibular arch (Table 1.5 and Fig. 1.25).
- Blockage of the pharyngeal airway due to macroglossia may result in a condition called "obstruction sleep apnea", which is characterized by intermittent cessation of respiration during sleep.
- Macroglossia can also be an important component of "Beckwith's hypoglycemic syndrome, which features—neonatal hypoglycemia, mild microcephaly, umbilical hernia, high birth weight and postnatal somatic gigantism.
- Edentulous patients with macroglossia often have difficulty in wearing dentures.

Table 1.5: Macroglossia: The tongue characteristics in different underlying diseases.

Various diseases	Tongue characteristics
Lymphangioma	Pebbly surface with multiple vesicle-like blebs
Hypothyroidism	Diffuse enlargement with smooth surface
Neurofibromatosis and amyloidosis	Swelling with multinodular surface
Down syndrome	Enlarged tongue with papillary fissured surface
Hemifacial hyperplasia	Unilateral enlargement of tongue

Treatment
- Removal of the primary cause, whenever possible.
- Surgical reduction or trimming may be required when macroglossia disturbs the oropharyngeal function or is causing some major cosmetic problems.

ANKYLOGLOSSIA (TONGUE-TIE)

Definition
Ankyloglossia can be defined as a congenital developmental condition characterized by fixation of the tongue to the floor of the mouth; causing restricted tongue mobility. *During functional movements, the tip of the normal tongue should touch the anterior palate but in case of ankyloglossia, it fails to reach up to that limit.*

Possible Causes of Development
- *Developmental cause*: Due to a short, thick lingual frenum and frenum that attaches too near to the tip of tongue.
- *Other causes*: Trauma and cocaine abuse by pregnant mother.

Types
- *Complete ankyloglossia*: Frenum is totally absent and tongue fully fixed to the floor of mouth.
- *Partial ankyloglossia*: Frenum is present but is much shorter.

Complete ankyloglossia is an extremely rare condition; however, partial ankyloglossia, which is otherwise known as "tongue-tie" is a relatively common developmental anomaly of the tongue. The tongue-tie occurs either due to a short and thick lingual frenulum (a membrane connecting the undersurface of the tongue to the floor of the mouth) or due to a frenulum, which attaches too near to the tip of the tongue (Fig. 1.26).

Clinical Features
- Ankyloglossia affects the males more frequently than females (2.6:1).

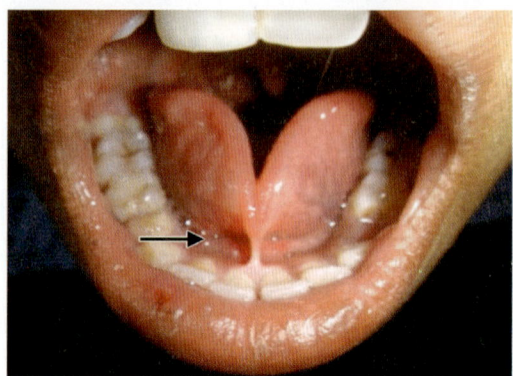

Fig. 1.26: Tongue-tie.

- Most affected individuals can perform tongue functions almost normally. However, restricted tongue mobility in ankyloglossia may cause the following problems—
  - Speech defect—patient cannot properly pronunciate certain consonants and diphthongs, such as *L, R, T, D, N, TH, SH, Z,* etc.
  - Patient often pronunciates the word "lemonade" as wemonade.
  - Difficulty in sucking breast milk for infants.
  - Gingival recession and diastema in lower incisors due to tension in the anterior lingual gingiva.
  - Difficulty in swallowing food and maintaining oral hygiene.
  - Difficulty in kissing, licking one's lips, eating ice-cream cones and performing tongue tricks.

Treatment
Partial ankyloglossia in most of the cases does not require any treatment; however, in severe cases of ankyloglossia, surgical correction (frenectomy) of the lingual frenulum is done to free the tongue.

CLEFT TONGUE (BIFID TONGUE)
Developmental disturbance may sometimes cause partial or complete cleft in the tongue.

Although a complete cleft or bifid tongue is a rare congenital anomaly; however, a partially cleft tongue is more frequently encountered.

Cleft tongue usually develops due to partial or complete failure of union between the two lateral lingual swellings during embryogenesis. Incomplete cleft in the tongue develops due to failure of mesenchymal tissue proliferation that obliterates the groove.

Partial cleft tongue clinically exhibits a deep groove in the midline, while the bifid tongue shows a complete cleft along its long axis. Cleft tongue, in most of the cases, is an asymptomatic condition, although sometimes irritation can be felt due to accumulation of food debris or microorganisms at the bottom of the cleft.

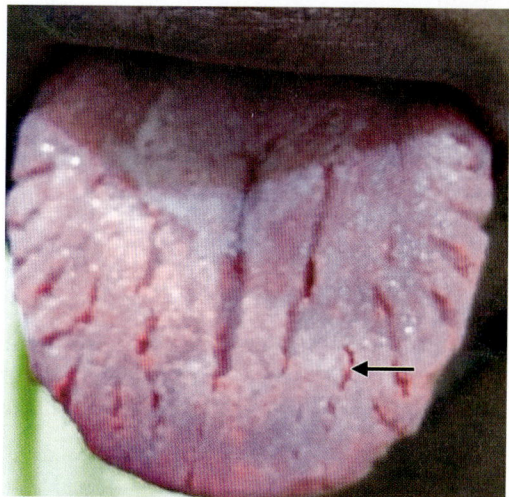

Fig. 1.27: Fissured (scrotal) tongue.

■ FISSURED TONGUE (SCROTAL TONGUE/PLICATED TONGUE/ FURROWED TONGUE)

Fissured tongue is a congenital developmental malformation, characterized by presence of numerous shallow or deep groves (fissures) on the dorsal and lateral surface of the tongue.

Etiology

The exact etiology for this condition is not known; however, the following factors are often suspected:
- Genetic defect (polygenic or autosomal mode of inheritance)
- Vitamin deficiency
- Trauma
- It may be a normal variation of tongue architecture.

Clinical Features

- Slightly more common among males.
- Usually, there is no clinical symptom in fissured tongue but collection of food debris and microorganisms in the fissures or groves may sometimes cause discomfort.
- Similar discomfort may also be felt when fissured tongue occurs in association with geographic tongue.
- The fissures or groves often radiate from a central groove on the dorsal surface in an oblique direction.
- The large and deep fissures may be interconnected and they separate the dorsum of the tongue into multiple lobules.
- The average depth of individual fissure is about 6 millimeters.
- The disease often occurs in association with Melkersson–Rosenthal syndrome and some investigators believe that fissured tongue can be a feature of benign migratory glossitis (Fig. 1.27).

Treatment

No treatment is required for fissured tongue except brushing of the tongue to eliminate the debris that irritates.

■ MEDIAN RHOMBOID GLOSSITIS OR GLOSSAL CENTRAL PAPILLARY ATROPHY

Definition

Median rhomboid glossitis forms an "erythematous patch" of papillary atrophy in the mid-dorsal surface of tongue, near the junction of the anterior two-thirds and posterior one-third area.

Etiopathogenesis

In the past, median rhomboid glossitis was thought to represent a developmental defect of the tongue, presumably arising as a result of persistence of the "tuberculum impar" on the surface of dorsum of the tongue.

During normal embryogenesis, however, the tuberculum impar should retrude and is overgrown by the lateral lingual swellings.

In recent times, median rhomboid glossitis is no longer believed to be a developmental defect of tongue, and it is thought to occur as a result of chronic infection by *Candida albicans*.

Clinical Features

Age: The condition is mostly seen among adults (30–50 years) and is rarely found among children.

Sex: Median rhomboid glossitis is seen more frequently among males (M:F=3:1).

Site: The lesion is located immediately anterior to the foramen cecum and the circumvallate papillae, in the midline on the dorsurm of tongue (at the junction of the anterior two-third and posterior one-third areas).

Presentation (Fig. 1.28)

- The median rhomboid glossitis starts as a narrow, mildly erythematous area located along the median fissure on the dorsum of the tongue just anterior to the circumvallate papilla.
- The lesion finally appears as a diamond or lozenge-shaped area devoid papilla and it is clinically asymptomatic and often remains unnoticed by the patient for many years.
- It enlarges slowly and the fully developed lesion of median rhomboid glossitis reaches to a size of little less than 2 cm in diameter. Its color varies from pale pink to bright red and occasionally, there is presence of a white halo.
- The surface is usually smooth, flat or slightly raised and is sometimes fissured

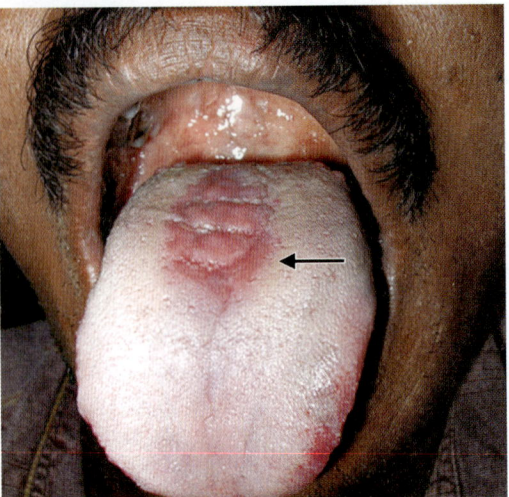

Fig. 1.28: Median rhomboid glossitis.

or lobulated; often it resembles chronic hyperplastic candidiasis.
- Median rhomboid glossitis is usually asymptomatic but occasionally it may cause slight soreness or burning sensation.
- The lesion is clinically suspicious and it is often mistaken for carcinoma of the tongue.

Key Points of Median Rhomboid Glossitis

- Diamond or lozenge-shaped depapillated area on the mid dorsum of the tongue, anterior to the circumvalate papilla.
- Color is erythematous and surface is generally smooth.
- Condition is asymptomatic with occasional irritations.
- Superficial candidiasis may be present.
- Often mistaken for carcinoma, but it is an innocent developmental anomaly.

Differential Diagnosis

- Squamous cell carcinoma
- 'Gumma' of tertiary syphilis
- Granular cell tumor
- Lingual thyroid nodule
- Tuberculous granuloma

Histopathology

Microscopically, median rhomboid glossitis presents the following features:

- Mild to severe parakeratosis of the surface epithelium, which lacks both filiform and fungiform papillae.
- There may be presence of psoriasiform hyperplasia or occasionally pseudoepitheliomatous hyperplasia.
- Superficial layer of the epithelium often shows presence of numerous candidal hyphae and neutrophilic infiltration.

Treatment

No treatment is basically required for this lesion. Antifungal agents and antiseptic gurgles are used to relieve the erythema and irritation in the area.

■ LINGUAL VARICES

Definition

A varix is a dilated, tortuous vein which is often subjected to increased hydrostatic pressure but is poorly supported by the surrounding tissue.

Clinical Features

- Varicosities can be observed in many oral locations like ventral surface of tongue, floor of the mouth, lips, buccal mucosa and the commissure, etc.
- Among all these intraoral locations, ventral surface of tongue and floor of the mouth are the most common sites for oral varices.
- Clinically lingual varices appear as small, round, purplish nodules, lateral to the sublingual vein, which is usually also deflected (Fig. 1.29).
- Thrombosis can occur occasionally in these varicose veins; however, only rarely, there are any clinical symptoms.
- In case of lingual varices, there is absence of any similar lesion in the skin and other mucosal locations.
- The lesion interestingly has no bleeding tendency either.
- Presence of lingual varices before the age of 50 years indicates premature aging.

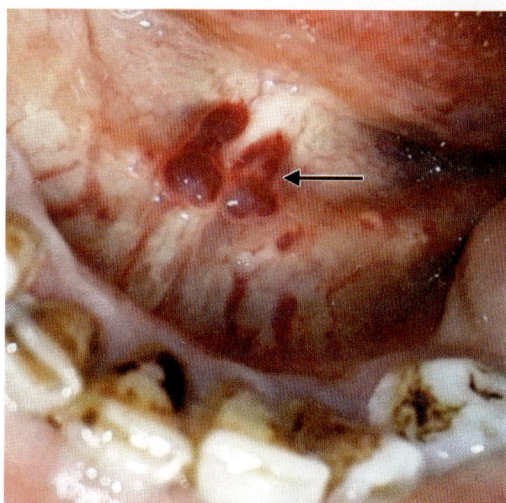

Fig. 1.29: Lingual varices.

- Sometimes, lingual varices can be indistinguishable from hereditary hemorrhagic telangiectasia.

Treatment

No treatment is required for lingual varices.

■ GEOGRAPHIC TONGUE OR BENIGN MIGRATORY GLOSSITIS

Definition

Geographic tongue is the multifocal, patchy irregular areas of depapillation of tongue characterized by frequent remissions and recurrences.

Etiology

The exact etiology of geographic tongue is not known; however, patients often have a positive family history of the similar problem for generations. However, many investigators believe that emotional stress, asthma, eczema and allergy may also precipitate this condition.

Clinical Features (Fig. 1.30)

- The condition occurs in about 1–2% of the population.
- It can be seen among children as well as adults and there is a slight female predilection.

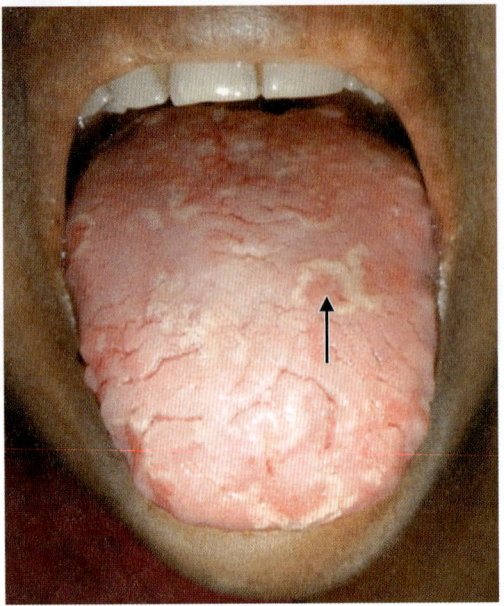

Fig. 1.30: Geographic tongue.

of the term "geographic tongue" for the condition.
- The condition is mostly painless and asymptomatic, however on few occasions, it may produce soreness or burning sensation (glossodynia) particularly during taking spicy or citrus foods.
- Occasionally, these lesions may occur in association with scrotal tongue or psoriasis.

> **Key Points of Geographic Tongue**
> ❖ Developmental anomaly characterized by multiple, irregular, patchy, depapillated areas on the dorsum of the tongue.
> ❖ The patch heals up at one location only to reappear at a newer location; apparently exhibiting a sense of "migration".
> ❖ The lesions have irregular border and are often surrounded by a white line at the periphery.
> ❖ Patches exhibit loss of filiform papilla but fungiform papillae are retained which appear as elevated, red rods.
> ❖ Mostly asymptomatic but occasional burning sensations; no treatment required.

- Geographic tongue clinically presents multiple, irregular, well-demarcated, smooth patchy erythematous areas on the dorsum of the tongue with desquamation of the filiform papilla.
- At the periphery, these lesions are often surrounded by a well-defined, slightly raised, yellowish-white, serpiginous line on the dorsum of the tongue.
- Although the filiform papillae are absent in the desquamated zone, the fungiform papillae remain present, which appear as few red dots, projecting from the surface.
- The lesions heal centrally and spread centrifugally, and they may even sometimes involve the ventral surface of the tongue.
- Remission of the initial lesion is always followed by fresh recurrent lesion at a new location over the tongue. Because of this tendency for migration of the lesion from one area to the other, it is often called "migratory glossitis".
- Moreover, the benign migratory glossitis lesion mimics the continental outlines on the globe and this also makes frequent use

Histopathology

- Geographic tongue microscopically shows hyperparakeratinization of the covering epithelium of tongue with loss of filiform papilla.
- Intercellular edema and accumulation of neutrophil polymorphs (so called spongiotic abscess) is often seen in the superficial layers of the epithelium.
- Mild inflammatory cell infiltration is present in the underlying connective tissue.

Differential Diagnosis

- Psoriasis
- Lichenoid reactions
- Reiter's syndrome
- Chronic hyperplastic candidosis
- Familiar dysautonomia.

Treatment

There is no specific treatment for geographic tongue. Heavy doses of vitamins may produce some results in few cases.

HAIRY TONGUE

Definition

Hairy tongue is an unusual condition, which occurs due to hypertrophy of the filiform papilla of tongue along with loss of normal desquamation process. The abnormal hair-like growth of the papilla eventually leads to formation of a pigmented, thick, matted layer on the tongue surface often heavily coated with bacteria and fungi (Fig. 1.31).

Etiology

- Poor oral hygiene
- Fungal infections
- Prolonged use of antibiotics
- Heavy smoking
- Excessive use of antiseptic mouthwashes
- Chronic illness
- Lack of toothbrushing and consumption of soft foods with little or no roughage.

Clinical Features

- Hairy tongue commonly affects the mid dorsum of the tongue.
- Hypertrophy of the filiform papilla produces a thick matted layer on the dorsal surface.
- Hairy tongue in extreme cases may produce a thick, leathery coating on the tongue surface and this condition is often known as "earthy or encrusted tongue".
- Hypertrophied filiform papilla may grow up to half a centimeter long, which often brushes the soft palate and produces gagging sensations.
- Hairy tongue in many cases produces halitosis.
- There can be irritation to the tongue due to accumulation of food debris and microorganisms.

Differential Diagnosis

- Candidiasis
- Leukoplakia
- Lichen planus
- Oral hairy leukoplakia.

Treatment

- Cleaning and scraping of the tongue
- Application of topical keratolytic agents
- Consumption of yoghurt
- The affected tongue papilla often rapidly returns to normal when long-term antibiotics or other drugs are discontinued.

LINGUAL THYROID NODULE

Definition

Accessory accumulation of functional thyroid gland tissue within the body of the tongue is called lingual thyroid nodule.

Pathogenesis

Embryologically, thyroid gland develops as an endodermal downgrowth at the site of the foramen cecum. It then migrates inferiorly along the thyroglossal tract to its ultimate destination in the anterolateral surface of the trachea of the anterior neck. If all or part of the thyroid analog fails to migrate, then lingual thyroid nodule develops, which is characterized by a mass of thyroid tissue on the midposterior dorsum of the tongue.

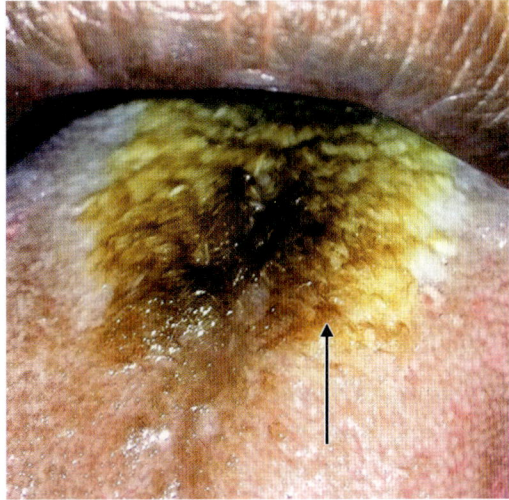

Fig. 1.31: Hairy tongue.

Clinical Features
- Lingual thyroid nodule is predominantly seen in females and it becomes clinically apparent usually during puberty or adolescence.
- In the tongue, thyroid tissue appears as a deep-seated, nodular, exophytic mass, measuring about 2–3 cm in diameter and is located posterior to the foramen cecum mostly in the midline.
- Symptoms may vary, which include change of voice (dysphonia), bleeding, pain, difficulty in swallowing (dysphagia), respiratory obstruction (dyspnea) and a feeling of tightness in the throat.

Histopathology
Histologically, most cases of lingual thyroid nodules are composed of normal mature thyroid tissue, although embryonic or fetal thyroid gland tissues may also be seen.

Differential Diagnosis
- Thyroglossal tract cyst
- Neoplasms.

Diagnosis
Diagnostic procedures include:
- Iodine-131 and technetium scans.
- Preoperative biopsy from the thyroid nodule.

Treatment
Surgical Excision

Lingual thyroid nodules can be excised only if a normal thyroid gland is present in the neck. If the secretion from the thyroid gland in the neck is subnormal, then thyroid replacement therapy may be required.

■ THYROGLOSSAL TRACT CYST

Definition
The thyroglossal tract cyst is an uncommon developmental cystic lesion arising from the embryonic remnants of the thyroglossal tract. It develops on the midline of the neck, anywhere between the base of the tongue above and the thyroid gland.

Origin
- The thyroglossal tract cyst arises from the remnants of the embryonic thyroglossal tract, which had not become obliterated.
- Initiation of the process of cyst development is triggered by infection of the lymphoid tissue in the area of the remnants, through drainage from upper respiratory tract infection.

Clinical Features
- The cyst occurs primarily in children and young adults.
- It presents as a slow enlarging, asymptomatic mobile swelling involving the midline of the anterior neck above the thyroid gland.
- The firm cystic mass may vary in size from a few millimeters to several centimeters.
- When seen in the region of the tongue, it appears as a dome-shaped compressible lesion.
- The cyst moves during swallowing.
- A small percentage of these cysts can occur within the tongue and these lesions may produce dysphagia.

Histopathology
- The cyst is usually lined by stratified squamous epithelium or ciliated columnar epithelium or transitional epithelium or a mixture of any of these epithelial types.
- The lining epithelium of the cyst often occurs in association with follicles of the glandular thyroid epithelium.

Differential Diagnosis
- Lingual thyroid nodule
- Mesenchymal neoplasms
- Dermoid cysts
- Epidermoid cyst.

Treatment

Thyroglossal tract cyst should be surgically excised along with the tract.

ANOMALIES OF ORAL LYMPHOID TISSUE

■ REACTIVE LYMPHOID AGGREGATES

The oropharyngeal lymphoid tissue is primarily distributed in a circular arrangement called the "Waldeyer ring" in the posterior region of the mouth. It consists of three main masses of lymphoid tissue namely, the paired palatine tonsils, the pharyngeal tonsils (adenoids) and the lingual tonsils.

Besides this, lymphoid tissues may also be found in a variety of intraoral locations like the buccal mucosa, soft palate, floor of the mouth and gingiva, etc.

Reactive hyperplasias may occur in lymphoid tissue in any of these locations. Lingual tonsil is one of the largest oral lymphoid aggregates, and its common location is the posterior part of the tongue. It may extend anteriorly up to the region of the foliate papilla and reactive lymphoid hyperplasia of the lingual tonsil in this location is sometimes termed as "foliate papillitis".

When inflamed, the lingual tonsils produce swelling, erythema of the overlying mucosa and pain or discomfort, etc. especially during swallowing. There can be diagnostic confusion if the involvement is unilateral rather than bilateral.

■ LYMPHOEPITHELIAL CYST (BRANCHIAL CYST)

Definition

Lymphoepithelial cyst is the term used to describe cystic lesion previously classified as branchial cyst. It is a developmental cyst with an uncertain pathogenesis.

Clinical Features

Age: Lymphoepithelial cysts occur during late childhood or early adulthood.

Sex: It occurs more frequently among males than females.

Site: The most common location is the lateral aspect of the neck, anterior to the sternomastoid muscle.

Intraoral lymphoepithelial cysts are uncommon lesions but whenever they occur, these lesions involve floor of the mouth in 50% cases and ventral and posterolateral surface of tongue in 40% cases.

Clinical Presentation

- Lymphoepithelial cyst generally presents as an asymptomatic, circumscribed, movable swelling on the lateral aspect of the neck anterior to the sternomastoid muscle.
- Intraorally, it commonly appears as a small, slow enlarging, elevated, yellowish-pink nodule.
- The cysts may be unilateral or bilateral and may be tendered on palpation.

Histopathology

- Histologically, the lesion consists of a cystic cavity lined by thin stratified squamous epithelium.
- The cyst is generally embedded in a circumscribed mass of lymphoid tissue, which typically exhibits discrete follicles of the lymph node pattern.

Pathogenesis

Lymphoepithelial cyst is probably derived from epithelium entrapped within lymphoid tissues of the neck during embryologic development of the cervical sinuses or second branchial clefts or pouches.

Differential Diagnosis

- Inflammatory lesions
- Teratoma
- Warthin's tumor
- Dermoid cyst
- Neoplasms of the minor salivary gland

Treatment

The intraoral counterpart of lymphoepithelial cyst is treated by conservative surgery. Recurrence is usually rare.

■ ANGIOLYMPHOID HYPERPLASIA WITH EOSINOPHILIA

Definition

This is a benign condition characterized by subcutaneous nodular aggregates of lymphocytes and eosinophils, regional lymphadenopathy and peripheral blood eosinophilia.

Clinical Features

Age: Mean age of occurrence is about 35 years.
Sex: More common among males.
Site: Although 85% of the lesions usually occur in the head and neck area, oral lesions are rare.
   Lower lip is the most common site.

Presentation

- The lesion clinically presents a slow enlarging, painless submucosal nodule.
- It measures about 1.5 cm in diameter and is movable.
- In about 40% cases, eosinophilia is detected in peripheral blood examination.
- Some of the patients may exhibit multiple lesions in the oral cavity.

Histopathology

- Microscopically, angiolymphoid hyperplasia with eosinophilia reveals a circumscribed lesion, which is grossly separable from the surrounding tissue.
- A nodular mass of hyperplastic lymphoid tissue is seen with well-defined lymphoid follicles.

Treatment

- Surgical excision
- Intralesional steroid therapy may produce some response.

DEVELOPMENTAL ANOMALIES INVOLVING ORAL HARD TISSUES

■ ABNORMALITIES OF TEETH

Teeth develop from the cooperative interaction of two germ layers: (1) ectoderm and (2) ectomesenchyme. The tooth development begins at about the 6th week of the intrauterine life when few cells of the oral ectoderm undergo proliferation and eventually result in the formation of the dental lamina. The odontogenic cells (tooth forming cells) emerge from dental lamina and the later event constitutes the beginning of tooth development. The enamel develops from the ectoderm while the dentin, pulp, cementum, periodontal ligament and alveolar bone develop from the ectomesenchyme. The development of tooth occurs in several stages, namely:

- The stage of initiation (bud stage)
- The stage of proliferation (cap stage)
- The stage of histodifferentiation (bell stage)
- The stage of morphodifferentiation
- The stage of apposition
- The stage of calcification, and
- The stage of eruption.

Developmental anomalies may occur during any of these developmental stages of tooth formation, which are, manifested clinically in the later life once the tooth is fully formed. These anomalies of tooth can occur either due to genetic factors or due to some environmental factors.

DISTURBANCE IN SIZE OF TEETH

■ MICRODONTIA

Definitions

Microdontia is the condition in which one or more teeth are smaller than normal in size. When all teeth are involved, it is called generalized microdontia and when only a few teeth are involved it is called localized or focal microdontia (Figs. 1.32 and 1.33).

Developmental Anomalies of Oral and Paraoral Structures

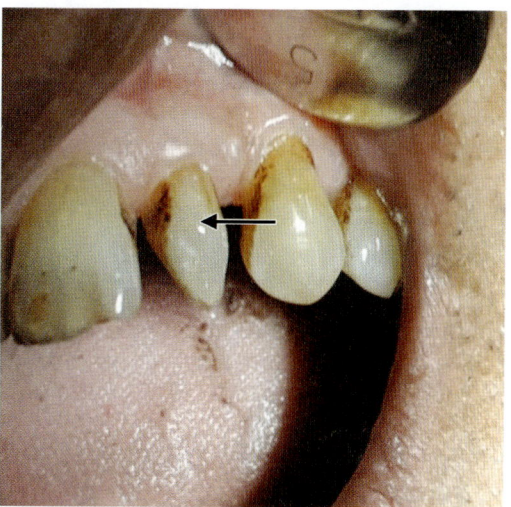

Fig. 1.32: Microdontia of lateral incisor (peg-lateral).

- Congenital syphilis
- Hypopituitarism
- Peg-shaped laterals
- Supernumerary teeth
- Idiopathic.

Types

True Generalized Microdontia

- When all the teeth in both arches are uniformly and measurably smaller than normal the condition is known as true generalized microdontia.
- This is an extremely uncommon condition and can be seen in pituitary dwarfism.
- True generalized microdontia can also be associated with other congenital defects like Down syndrome and congenital heart disease, etc.

Relative Generalized Microdontia

- Relative generalized microdontia is the condition in which teeth of normal size may look smaller, if they are placed in an abnormally large maxilla or mandible.
- In such cases larger size of the jaws give an illusion of microdontia although the teeth are not really small.

Causes

- Genetic factor—microdontia is predominantly a genetic disorder, which is caused by a faulty gene and occurs more often in the children of relative parents
- Dens invaginatus
- Cleft lip and cleft palate
- Hereditary ectodermal dysplasia
- Radiotherapy during pregnancy

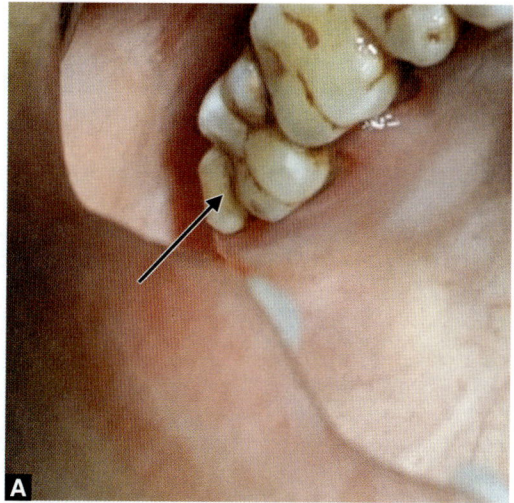
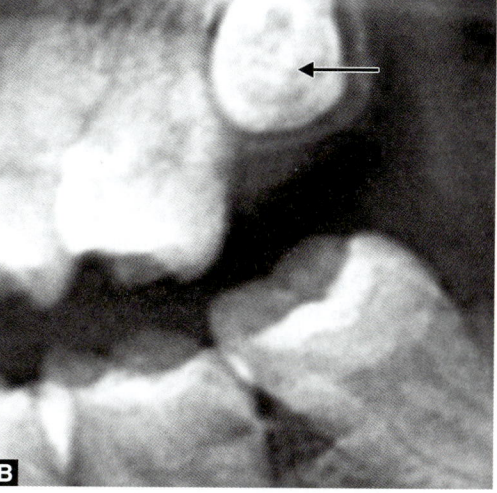

Figs. 1.33A and B: Microdontia: (A) Microdontia of upper third molar; (B) X-ray showing microdontia of upper third molar.

Focal Microdontia
- When one or two teeth in the jaw are measurably smaller in size while rest of the teeth are normal, the condition is called focal microdontia.
- Microdontia involving one or two teeth in the dental arch is far more common than the generalized types.
- The affected teeth are often present symmetrically in the jaw and in addition to being miniature in size, these teeth often exhibit alteration in their shape as well.
- Maxillary lateral incisors and maxillary third molars are the most frequently involved teeth in focal microdontia.
- When maxillary lateral incisors are involved, the teeth often appear "cone" or "peg"-shaped and are often designated as peg laterals. These teeth often give a peculiar facial expression of the patient.
- Maxillary and mandibular second premolars may sometimes exhibit microdontia.
- Supernumerary teeth are almost always smaller than the normal teeth and are often conical in shape.

Examples
- Smaller teeth can be seen in the affected side of the jaw in facial hemiatrophy.
- In case of gemination or twinning one single tooth germ splits into two, during development and gives rise to two separate teeth, which are always smaller than normal.
- Small, conical teeth are often seen in hereditary ectodermal dysplasia.
- Multiple miniature teeth can be found in compound odontomes and in teratoma.
- A retained deciduous tooth within the permanent dentition may give an illusion of focal microdontia.

Clinical Significance
- In microdontia, teeth are often spaced which may be disturbing cosmetically.
- There may be difficulty in speech and taking food.
- When shapes of these teeth are also altered along with microdontia (e.g. peg laterals), it will require immediate correction.

■ MACRODONTIA

Definition
Macrodontia is a condition in which teeth in the jaws are measurably larger than normal in size. This is a far less common anomaly of tooth than microdontia (Figs. 1.34 and 1.35).

Causes
- Pituitary gigantism
- Fusion of teeth
- Facial hemihypertrophy
- Idiopathic.

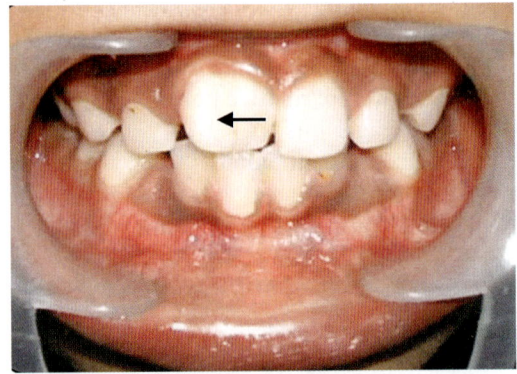

Fig. 1.34: Macrodontia of upper central incisor.

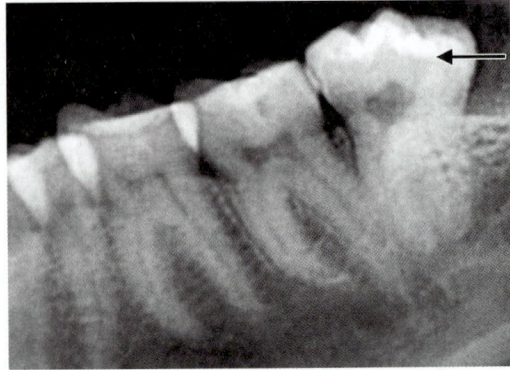

Fig. 1.35: Macrodontia of the mandibular third molars.

Types

Macrodontia can be of three types, which are as follows:
1. *True generalized macrodontia*: When all the teeth in both arches are measurably larger than normal, can be seen infrequently in case of pituitary gigantism.
2. *Relative generalized macrodontia*: Relative generalized macrodontia is used to designate a condition in which the normal sized teeth appear somewhat larger because of the smaller jaw size.
3. *Focal or localized macrodontia*: Localized macrodontia is occasionally seen on the affected side of the mouth with hemifacial hypertrophy. Macrodontia of individual tooth is a rare entity and it mostly affects the incisors. However focal macrodontia should not be confused with "fusion" of teeth, (in which two adjacent teeth unite together to form a single large tooth).

DISTURBANCE IN NUMBER OF TEETH

ANODONTIA

Definition

Anodontia can be defined as a condition in which there is congenital absence of teeth in the oral cavity (Figs. 1.36 and 1.37).

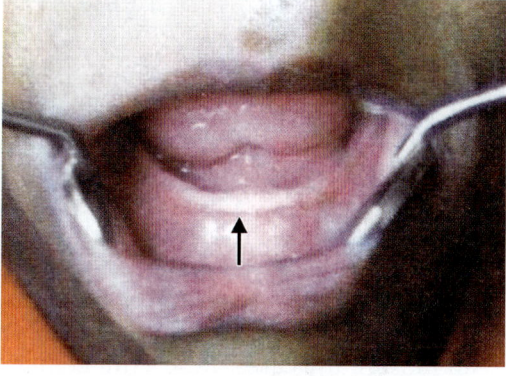

Fig. 1.36: Complete (total) anodontia.

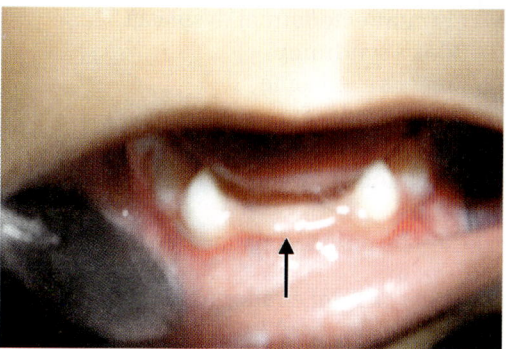

Fig. 1.37: Partial anodontia with missing lower incisors.

Types

Anodontia can be of two types:
1. *Complete or total anodontia*: Congenital absence of all teeth (Fig. 1.37).
2. *Partial anodontia or oligodontia or hypodontia*: Congenital absence of one or few teeth (Fig. 1.37).

Anodontia can further be divided into the following types:
- *True anodontia*: True anodontia occurs due to failure of development or formation of tooth in the jawbone.
- *Pseudoanodontia*: Refers to the condition in which the teeth are actually present within the jawbone but are not clinically visible in the mouth, as they have not erupted. Examples of pseudoanodontia can be impacted teeth or submerged teeth, etc.
- *False anodontia*: False anodontia is the condition in which the teeth are missing in the oral cavity because of their previous extraction or exfoliation.

Etiology

- Idiopathic anodontia
- Hereditary anodontia
- Environmental factor
- Ectodermal dysplasia
- Incontinentia pigmenti
- Hyalinosis cutis mucosae
- Mandibulo-oculofacial dyscephaly

- Chondroectodermal dysplasia
- Book's syndrome
- Rieger's syndrome
- Down syndrome
- Syndrome associated anodontia
- Radiation injury to the developing tooth germs
- Cleft lip and cleft palate.

Complete or Total Anodontia

Total anodontia is a rare condition in which there is neither any deciduous tooth nor any permanent tooth present in the oral cavity.
- It is usually seen in association with hereditary ectodermal dysplasia.
- Complete anodontia sometimes occur among children those who have received high doses of radiation to the jaws as infants for therapeutic reasons.

High doses of radiation cause destruction of tooth germs resulting in complete failure of tooth formation in future, moreover even a very lower dose may cause cessation of odontogenesis.

Partial Anodontia

Partial anodontia is a much more common phenomenon and is characterized by congenital absence of one or few teeth. This condition is also known as hypodontia or oligodontia. The condition is more commonly seen in permanent dentition.

In partial anodontia, when a deciduous tooth is congenitally absent it is very much likely that its permanent successor will also be missing thereby suggesting some genetic influence.

A familial tendency for congenitally absent teeth is a well-recognized phenomenon.

Commonly missing teeth in partial anodontia:
- In partial anodontia, any tooth can be congenitally missing; however, it is often noticed that certain teeth tend to be absent more often than others.
- The third molars (any one or all four of them) are the most frequently observed congenitally missing teeth.
- Maxillary lateral incisors and mandibular premolars are the next most common group of teeth, which are often congenitally absent.
- When deciduous teeth are involved it partial anodontia, the maxillary lateral incisors are most likely to be affected.
- It should be noted that mandibular first molars and mandibular lateral incisors are the teeth, which are least likely to be missing during anodontia.

SUPERNUMERARY TEETH

Definition

Presence of any extratooth or teeth in the dental arch, in addition to the normal series of teeth is known as supernumerary teeth. The condition is also known as hyperdontia or polydontia. Supernumerary teeth occur less frequently than the anodontia. These teeth may erupt spontaneously in the oral cavity or they may be impacted and are detected incidentally during routine radiographic examinations.

Etiology

- Heredity, these are more commonly seen among the family members of the affected individual as compared to the general population.
- Dichotomy (division into two) of the tooth bud.
- Localized conditioned hyperactivity of the dental lamina.
- Fragmentation of the dental lamina during development of cleft lip and cleft palate.
- The supernumerary tooth can occur in both males as well as in females.
- Morphologically sometimes these teeth may look like molars, premolar or like incisors, etc. depending upon their location or sometimes they may have an altogether different morphologic appearance. However in most of the cases these extrateeth are much more smaller in size (miniature form) than their normal counterparts.

Developmental Anomalies of Oral and Paraoral Structures

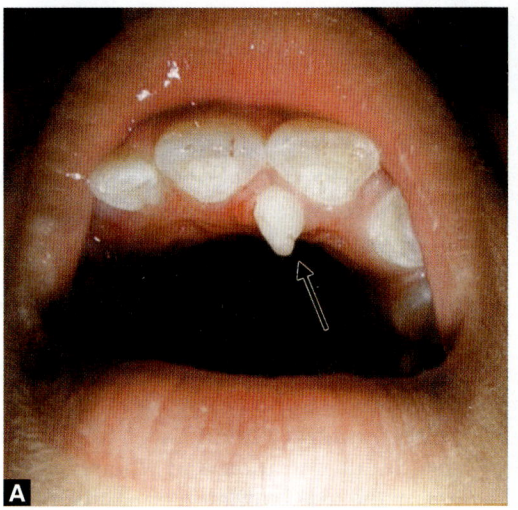
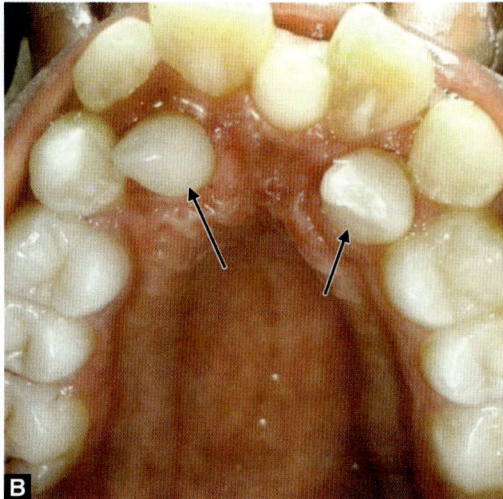

Figs. 1.38A and B: Supernumerary teeth (mesiodens): (A) Mesiodens on the palatal aspect of upper central incisors; (B) Multiple supernumerary teeth.

Common Locations

- These are far more common in maxilla (90%) as compared to mandible.
- Supernumerary teeth are more often seen in maxillary permanent dentition and are rarely seen in deciduous dentition.

Types

According to the Site

Mesiodens: Mesiodens are the most common of all supernumerary teeth and these are located in the midline, on the palatal aspect, between the roots of two upper central incisors (Figs. 1.38A and B).

Peridens (extra premolars): Supernumerary teeth present on the buccal or lingual aspect of premolar teeth (Fig. 1.39).

Paramolars: These are also extra molar teeth, which are usually located either in the buccal or in the lingual aspect of the normal molars (Fig. 1.40).

Distomolars: Distomolars are supernumerary molars, which are usually located on the distal aspect of the regular molar teeth in the dental arch.

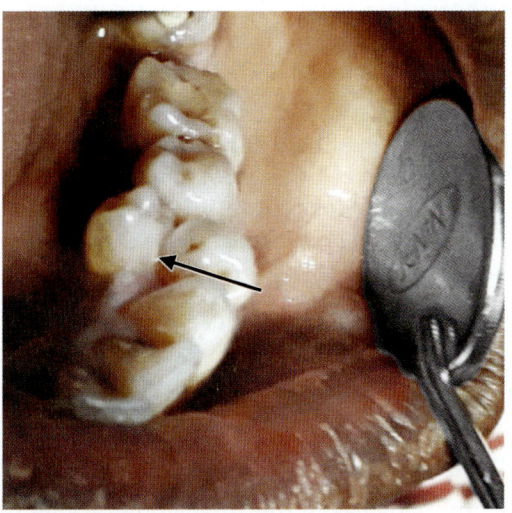

Fig. 1.39: Supernumerary teeth (peridens). Supernumerary teeth lingual to lower premolars

Extralateral incisors: Although rare, extralateral incisor teeth can be present and they are more common in the maxillary arch.

According to Morphology

Conical type: These supernumerary teeth are small, often peg-shaped and mostly seen in the permanent dentition, i.e. mesiodens.

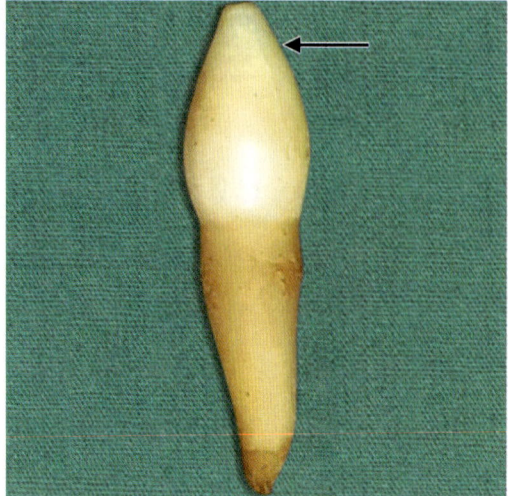

Fig. 1.40: Small conical-shaped tooth (extracted mesiodens).

Tuberculate type: These supernumerary teeth posses more than one cusp or tubercle, are often barrel-shaped and may be invaginated.

Supplemental type: This type of supernumerary tooth shows duplication (similarity in appearance) of any normal tooth in the dental arch. Most common example is the one which resembles permanent maxillary lateral incisor.

Odontome associated: These supernumerary teeth occur in association with compound odontome as multiple miniature teeth inside the tumor.

Clinical Features

- In many cases, the supernumerary teeth remain clinically asymptomatic.
- The supernumerary tooth may develop as a single one or they may be multiple in numbers, moreover these teeth can be either unilateral or bilateral.
- The extra tooth may be either erupted or impacted in the oral cavity and both upper and lower jaw can be affected.
- Supernumerary teeth may sometimes produce crowding or malocclusion and they often cause cosmetic problems.
- They may cause rotation, protrusion or displacement of the normal teeth.
- In many instances, these teeth are responsible for either failure of eruption or delayed eruption of other normal teeth.
- In many cases these extrateeth may be either directly or indirectly responsible for increased caries incidence and periodontal problems.
- Multiple supernumerary teeth (most of them are impacted), may occur in association with conditions like cleidocranial dysplasia or Gardner's syndrome, etc.
- Supernumerary teeth can occur in the deciduous dentition and whenever they occur, the most common one is the maxillary lateral incisor.
- Supernumerary teeth may initiate the development of some pathological conditions in the jaw, e.g. dentigerous cyst may develop in relation to an impacted supernumerary tooth.
- Supernumerary teeth may sometimes occur in association with cleft palate; moreover, presence of these extra teeth often creates problem in the surgical correction of cleft palate itself.
- These extrateeth often cause root resorption of the neighboring normal teeth in the jaw.

Treatment

Supernumerary teeth are mostly nonfunctional and they should be extracted especially if they are causing displacement or delayed eruption of the normal teeth.

DISTURBANCES IN ERUPTION OF TEETH

Eruption is the process in which the developing teeth move from their area of formation inside the jaw into the oral cavity to become a part of the dental arch.

When the eruption of tooth occurs in the mouth either much before or long after the expected normal time, then we can consider that an eruption abnormally exists.

TYPES OF ERUPTION ABNORMALITIES
- Premature eruption
- Delayed eruption
- Impacted teeth
- Embedded teeth
- Eruption sequestrum.

PREMATURE ERUPTION

Definition
Premature eruption can be defined as a situation when a tooth erupts into the oral cavity much before its normal time of eruption (Figs. 1.41A and B).

Types
- *Natal teeth*: These are erupted deciduous teeth present at birth.
- *Neonatal teeth*: These are deciduous teeth, which erupt within the first 30 days of life.

Commonly Involved Teeth
- Premature eruption usually involves only one or two teeth, most commonly the deciduous mandibular central incisors.
- Natal or neonatal teeth are not supernumerary teeth, in fact they are part of the normal component of deciduous dentition and therefore, these teeth should be preserved in the mouth if possible.

DELAYED ERUPTION

Definition
Delayed eruption refers to the first appearance of the teeth in the oral cavity at a much later time than what is normally expected.
This is can involve both deciduous as well as the permanent dentition.

Factors Causing Delayed Eruption of Tooth

Systemic factors:
- Decreased secretion of growth hormone in early life, resulting in a small jaw with insufficient space for eruption of all teeth.
- Rickets
- Failure of timely resorption of deciduous teeth with delayed eruption of the permanent successors.
- Cleidocranial dysplasia
- Cretinism
- Ionizing radiation in the jaw in early life.
- Fetal alcohol syndrome—occurs due to maternal alcoholism and it causes delayed eruption of teeth and mottled opacity of enamel at the incisal margin.

Local factors:
- Obstruction from an impacted tooth or a supernumerary tooth.

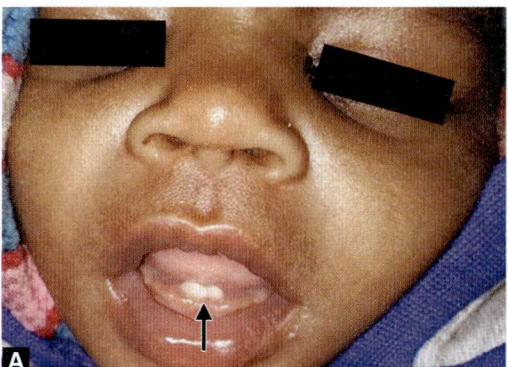
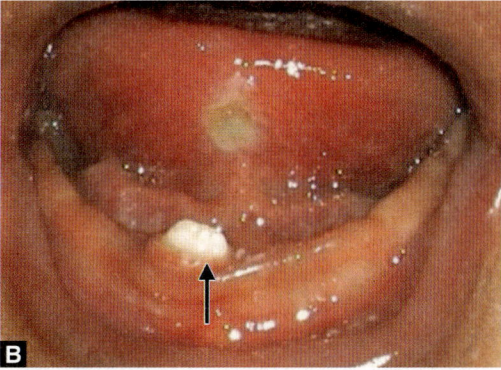

Figs. 1.41A and B: (A) Neonatal teeth in a 2-month-old baby; (B) Single neonatal tooth in another baby.

- Obstruction from a tumor or cyst in the jaw
- Abnormal position of the crypt.
- Retained deciduous teeth
- Gingival fibromatosis
- Cleft lip and cleft palate
- Premature loss of primary teeth.
- Fracture of jaw during the time of eruption of teeth.
- Crowding of teeth showing delayed eruption.

IMPACTED TEETH

Definition

Impaction is defined as the cessation of eruption of tooth caused by a clinically and radiographically detectable physical barrier in the eruption path or by an ectopic position of the tooth (Figs. 1.42 and 1.43).

Factors Causing Impaction of Tooth

- *Micrognathia*: A smaller jaw cannot afford to accommodate all the teeth, hence few of them may become impacted.
- Malocclusion
- *Rotation of teeth*: Rotation results in eruption of a tooth at a different angulation in the jaw, which results in impaction of such tooth.
- *Premature exfoliation of deciduous teeth*: It causes partial closure of space in the alveolar ridge.
- *Retained deciduous tooth*: An abnormally retained deciduous tooth may resist the eruption of its permanent counterpart.
- *Supernumerary tooth*: A supernumerary tooth may sometimes obstruct the pathway for eruption of other teeth resulting in their impaction.
- *Odontogenic cyst (e.g. keratocyst)*: It may act as a physical barrier and result in the impaction of tooth.
- *Odontogenic tumor (e.g. odontome)*: It also may results in impaction of a tooth by acting as physical barrier in the path of eruption.
- *Cleft palate*: In many cases, teeth may be impacted in the area of cleft palate.
- Nonodontogenic tumors or cysts
- *Cleidocranial dysplasia*: This disease entity is often associated with multiple impactions.
- *Gardner's syndrome*: It is also associated with multiple impacted teeth.
- *Amelogenesis imperfecta*: Impacted teeth are also seen in various forms of amelogenesis imperfecta.

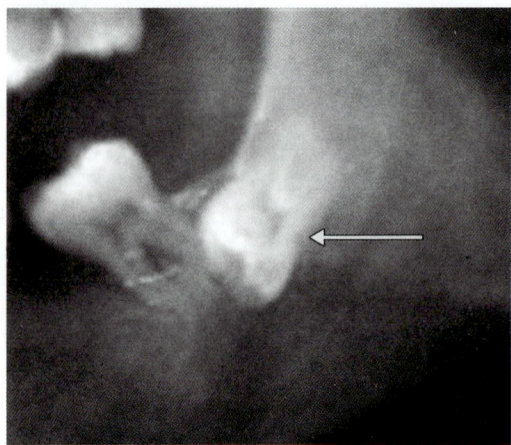

Fig. 1.43: Impacted third molars.

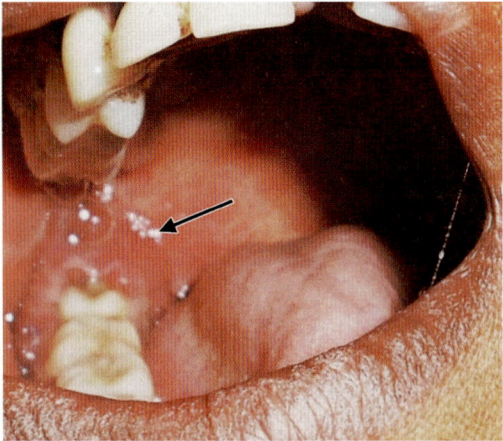

Fig. 1.42: Pericoronoitis due to impacted lower third molar.

Teeth which may be Commonly Impacted

- Although, virtually any tooth can be impacted, the most common impacted

teeth are the mandibular and maxillary third molars.
- The next common teeth are the mandibular second premolars and maxillary canines.
- The supernumerary teeth can be impacted in many cases.

Submerged tooth: When there is cessation of eruption of a deciduous tooth after gingival emergence, it is called a submerged tooth. The occlusal surface of the tooth lies above the gingiva but below the occlusal plane of the remaining teeth.

Embedded tooth: When an individual tooth fails to erupt for no apparent cause, it is called an embedded tooth. The tooth lies below the gum line and there is no physical barrier present as may be seen in case of impaction.

DISTURBANCES IN THE SHAPE OF TEETH

■ GEMINATION (TWINNING)

Definition

Gemination is a developmental anomaly characterized by a partial cleavage in a single tooth germ resulting in the formation of an anomalous tooth with two partially separated crowns and one root. It is therefore an abortive attempt at division of one tooth into two.

The term twinning refers to the complete and equal division of a single tooth germ that result in the formation of one normal and one supernumerary tooth.
- Gemination affects both deciduous as well as the permanent dentition.
- There is no sex predilection.
- Geminated tooth often shows doubling of both the crown as well as the root.
- Gemination mostly affects the deciduous mandibular incisors and permanent maxillary incisors.
- Clinically the geminated tooth reveals either an extremely widened crown or their can actually be an indentation or groove delineating the two crown forms.

Problems in gemination: The following problems can occur due to gemination of tooth:
- Tooth malposition
- Spacing of teeth
- Dental arch asymmetry
- Cosmetic problems
- Periodontal problems
- Increased caries susceptibility
- Disturbance in the eruption of adjacent teeth.

Treatment

Since gemination produces some cosmetic disturbance, construction of esthetic crown or bridge may be necessary for cosmetic rehabilitation.

■ FUSION

Definition

Fusion can be defined as the union of two adjacent normally separated tooth germs at the level of dentin during development.

Fusion results in one anomalous large tooth formation in place of two normal regular sized teeth and the tooth have either a single enlarged root or two roots. One of the most important criteria for fusion is that the fused tooth must exhibit confluent dentin (Figs. 1.44 and 1.45).

Causes
- Hereditary cause
- Trauma during development of teeth
- Physical force or pressure causing contact between two adjacent tooth germs.

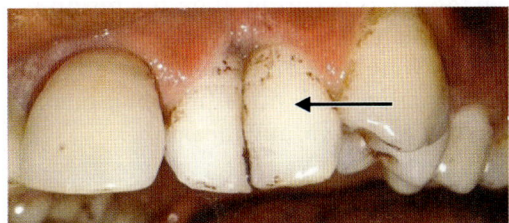

Fig. 1.44: Fusion of teeth.

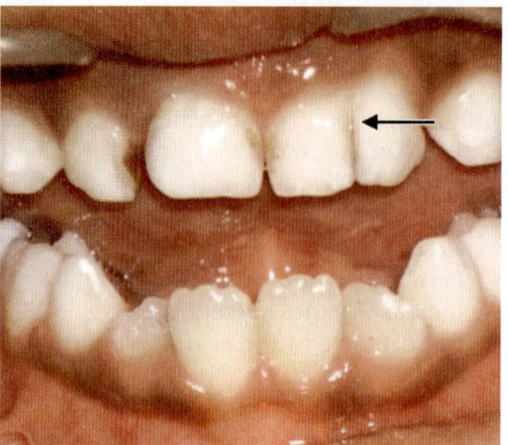

Fig. 1.45: Fusion of incisors teeth.

separate crowns and the fusion process may be limited to the roots only, with pulp canals either fused or separate. This condition is called incomplete fusion.

Radiographic Features

Radiographs can be immensely helpful in determining the complete or incomplete fusion. Complete fusion gives rise to the development of a single large tooth with single root canal (Figs. 1.46 and 1.47).

Clinical Features

- Both deciduous as well as permanent teeth can be affected in case of fusion, although it is more common in deciduous teeth.
- Fusion can occur between two normal teeth or between one normal and one supernumerary tooth.
- In both dentitions, the incisor teeth are more frequently affected.
- Fusion can be complete or incomplete and its extent will depend on the stage of odontogenesis at which the fusion took place.
- In case of fusion between two adjacent deciduous teeth, the resultant fused tooth may not exfoliate normally and thus may interfere with the eruption of the permanent successor.

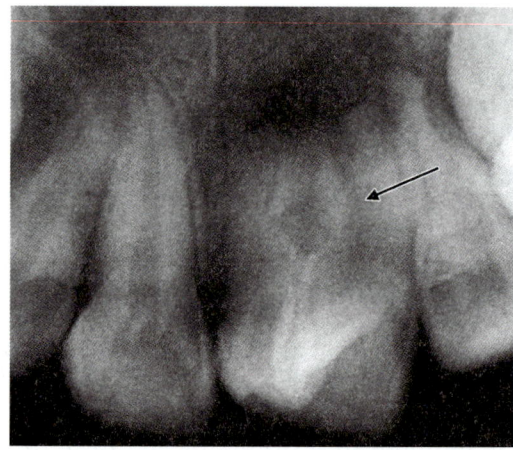

Fig. 1.46: Radiograph of fusion of teeth

Complete Fusion

If fusion begins before the calcification of the tooth has occurred, then the fusion will be complete and the fused tooth crown will incorporate all components of both the participating teeth including their enamel, dentin, cementum, and the pulp.

Incomplete Fusion

If fusion begins in the later stages of tooth development, then the fused tooth may exhibit

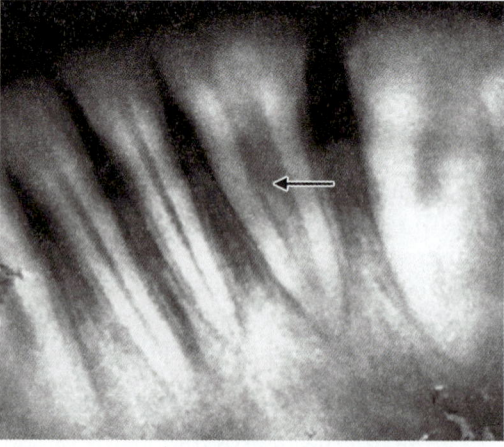

Fig. 1.47: X-ray showing confluence or merger of dentin of two separate teeth.

Clinical Complications

Fusion often creates the following problems:
- There can be spacing or diastema formation between the teeth.
- There can be crowding of teeth in the arch.
- Esthetic problems.
- Periodontal complication.
- Fusion can be differentiated from gemination by counting the number of teeth in the arch, since in case of fusion there will be one tooth less in the dental arch. However, in case of twining there will be one extra-tooth in the dental arch.

Treatment

Depending upon the extent of clinical problem, fabrication of cosmetic crowns or bridges may be necessary for esthetic recovery in case of fusion.

■ CONCRESCENCE

Definition

Union of the roots of two or more adjoining completely formed teeth along the line of cementum is known as concrescence.

This is a type of fusion, which is limited only to the roots of the teeth and it occurs due to deposition of cementum after the root formation of the involved teeth have been completed (Figs. 1.48 and 1.49).

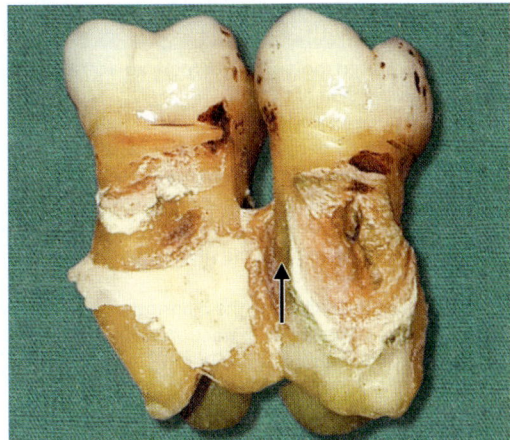

Fig. 1.49: Concrescence of molar teeth.

Etiology

- Traumatic injury
- Crowding of teeth
- Hypercementosis associated with chronic inflammation.

Pathogenesis

The condition is thought to occur as a result of traumatic injury to the jaw, which causes loss of interdental bone and brings the roots of the neighboring teeth in close proximity to one another. Finally such fusion occurs between the roots of two or more such separate teeth due to deposition of cementum between them.

Clinical Features

- Concrescence represents an acquired defect and it can occur in both erupted and unerupted teeth.
- There is no sex predilection.
- In case of concrescence, union never takes place between the enamel, dentin or the pulp of the involved teeth except cementum.
- In concrescence, the union mostly occurs between two teeth; however, there may be cases where union occurs between multiple teeth.
- Permanent maxillary molars are more often affected than any other teeth.

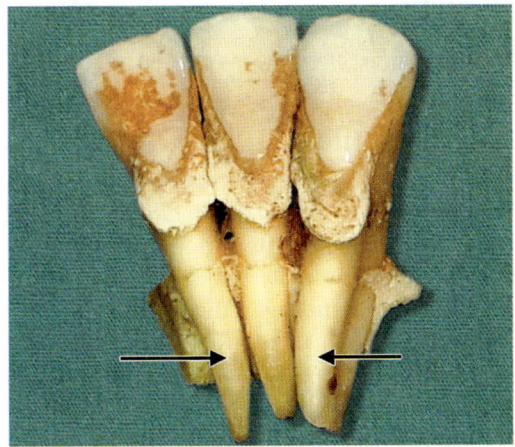

Fig. 1.48: Concrescence in lower incisors.

> **Key Points of Concrescence**
> - Union between roots of two or more adjacent teeth (radicular version of fusion).
> - It occurs due to deposition of cementum causing obliteration of periodontal ligament space with subsequent union between adjacent teeth.
> - It develops only after the root completion of teeth has occurred.
> - Trauma is believed to be the single most important underlying cause.
> - X-ray helps in confirming the diagnosis.
> - May cause difficulty in extraction of the affected teeth in undiagnosed cases.

- Concrescence rarely involves the deciduous dentition.
- Concrescence frequently occurs in those areas of the dental arch where the roots of the neighboring teeth are anatomically placed close to one another (e.g. between maxillary second and third molars).

Radiographic Features

Radiographs reveal obliteration of periodontal ligament space in the interradicular areas of teeth.

Clinical Significance

The clinical significance of concrescence relates primarily to its radiographic diagnosis before planning a tooth extraction. Because in undiagnosed cases attempted extraction of the affected tooth may cause trauma to the jaw or may result in removal of many teeth instead of one.

DILACERATION

Definition

Dilaceration is a developmental disturbance in the shape of tooth, it refers to a severe angulation or a sharp bend or curve in the root or crown of a formed tooth.

The bend is mostly located at the junction between the crown and the root of the tooth; in other cases it may be located at the mid portion of the root or sometimes even near the root apex.

In dilacerations the bend in the tooth sometimes can be as stiff as 90°. When the bend is restricted only to the root portion of the tooth the condition is known as "flexion" (Figs. 1.50A to C).

Pathogenesis

- It is generally believed that trauma to a partially calcified tooth may cause displacement of the hard calcified portion of the tooth away from its normal axis and later on, the unclassified portion develops with an unusual angulation.
- Injury to a deciduous tooth may push a partly formed permanent tooth further down apically into the jaw and as a result a bend in the permanent tooth develops.
- Some investigators believe that trauma is not always an essential factor for the development of dilacerations and according to them the anomaly occurs as a result of continued root formation during a curved or tortuous path of eruption.

> **Key Points of Dilacerations**
> - Developmental anomaly of tooth characterized by a sharp bend or curve along the length of the tooth.
> - Injury to the deciduous tooth with subsequent pressure on the developing permanent tooth is the most likely cause.
> - The affected often looks "hook-shaped" due to curving of the root.
> - X-ray is very useful for diagnosis.
> - They may get broken during removal.

Clinical Features

- Dilaceration may involve any tooth belonging to either the deciduous as well as the permanent dentition.
- The tooth typically looks "hook-shaped" due to the bending in the root.

Dilaceration in a tooth can easily be detected by radiographs and care should be taken during extraction of such teeth. Since these teeth are more prone to fracture during removal.

TAURODONTISM

Definition

Taurodontism or "bull-like" tooth is a peculiar morphoanatomical defect, in which the crown portion of the tooth is enlarged at the expanse of its roots. The condition generally affects the multirooted teeth and the involved teeth have larger crown and extremely large pulp chamber; moreover, the pulpal floor or the furcation area is apically displaced (Figs. 1.51 and 1.52).

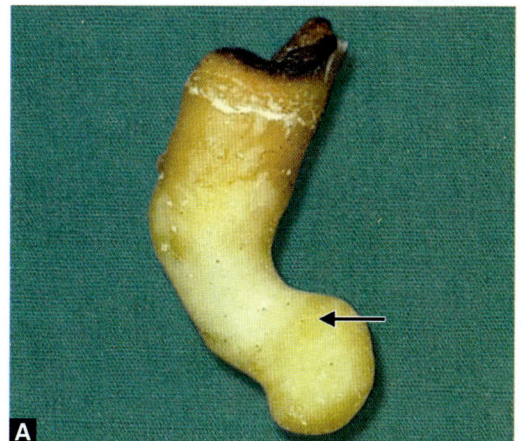
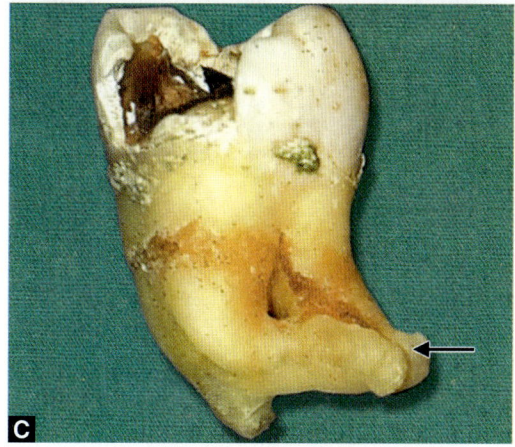

Figs. 1.50A to C: Dilaceration of teeth.

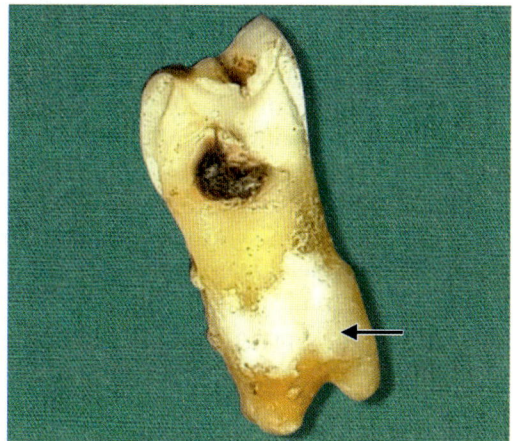

Fig. 1.51: Taurodontism I.

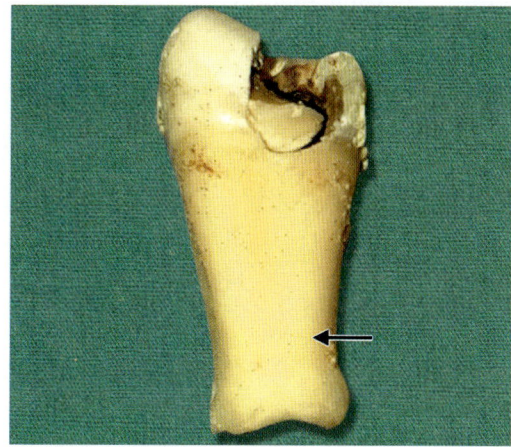

Fig. 1.52: Taurodontism II.

Pathogenesis

This is a hereditary condition, which probably occurs due to failure of the epithelial root sheath of Hertwig to invaginate at the proper horizontal level during tooth development.

Clinical Features

- The affected tooth in taurodontism exhibits large crown with elongated pulp chamber and short rudimentary root.
- The affected tooth is usually rectangular in shape with minimum constriction at the cervical area (bull-like tooth).
- Moreover, the furcation area of the tooth is so much apically placed that the root lengths could be only few millimeters only.
- This dental anomaly may sometimes be associated with some craniofacial deformities, e.g. Down syndrome, Klinefelter syndrome, amelogenesis imperfecta, and poly-X syndrome, etc.
- Patients with hypodontia may have taurodontism in about 30% cases.

Treatment

No treatment is required for taurodontism; however, this anomaly can pose some difficulty during root canal treatments.

■ DENS IN DENTE (DENS INVAGINATUS)

Definition

Dens in dente refers to a folding or invagination on the surface of the tooth toward the pulp; which begins before the calcification of the tooth and eventually after calcification the defect produces a typical appearance of a "tooth within a tooth".

The defect in generally localized to a single tooth and interestingly maxillary lateral incisors are more often affected than any other tooth in the dental arch (Figs. 1.53 to 1.55).

Types

Dens in dente is often broadly divided into two types—(1) coronal type, and (2) radicular type.

Coronal type: Coronal type of dens in dente occurs when the invagination or folding occurs on the crown portion of the tooth. The coronal type is further divided into three subtypes, which are as follows:

1. *Type I*: The invagination within the crown of the tooth.
2. *Type II*: The invagination extends below the cementoenamel junction (CEJ) of

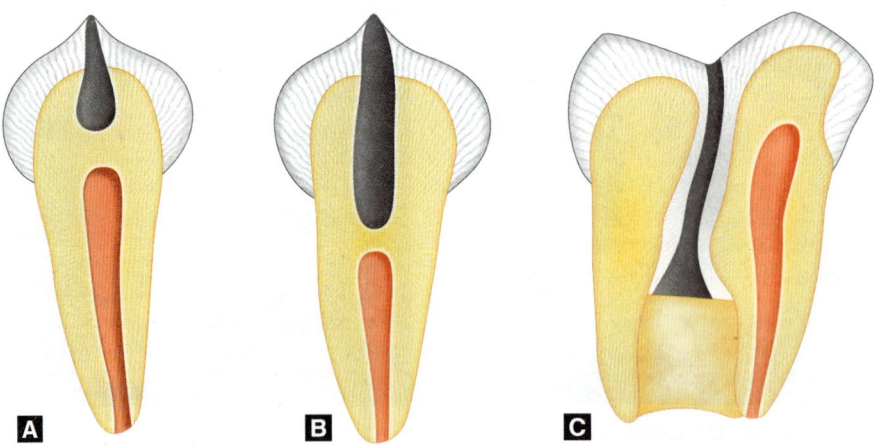

Figs. 1.53A to C: Dens in dente Types I, II and III (left to right).

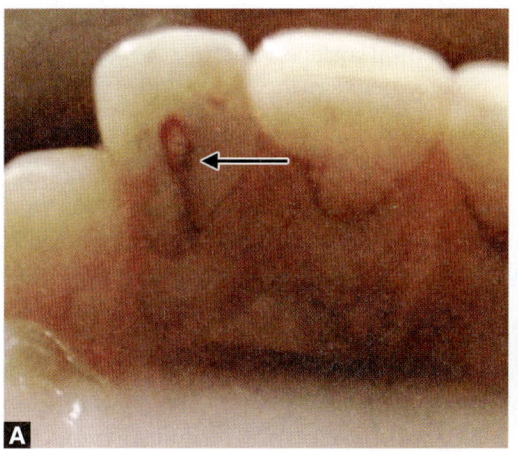
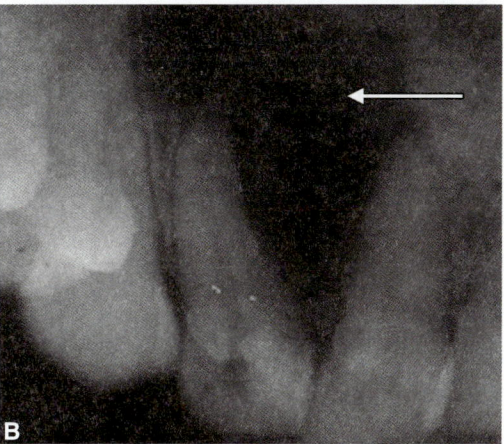

Figs. 1.54A and B: Dens in dente.

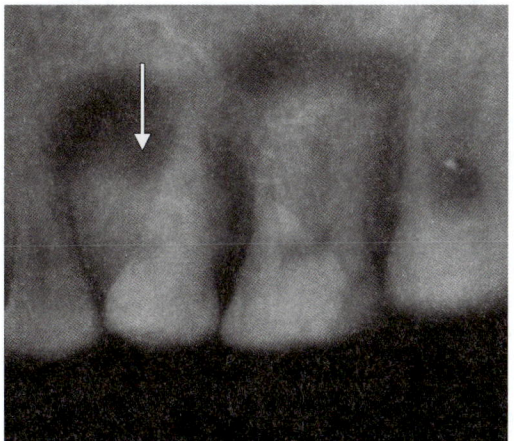

Fig. 1.55: Radicular dens in dente.

tooth but, it may or may not communicate with the pulp.
3. *Type III*: The invagination extends through the root and perforates in the apical or lateral radicular area.

Radicular type: In case of dens in dente if the invagination occurs in the root portion of the tooth it is called the radicular type and the condition presumably occurs due to folding of the Hertwig's sheath during the development of root.

Clinical Forms

Depending upon the extent or depth of the invagination toward the pulp, the dens in dente presents several clinical forms and these are mostly determined by radiographs.

Mild form: This form of dens in dente is characterized by the presence of a deeply invaginated or accentuated lingual pit area.

Intermediate form: Intermediate form of dens in dente radiographically reveals a small, pear-shaped invagination of the enamel and dentin into the pulp chamber, this produces a typical appearance of "tooth with in a tooth".

Extreme form: In this form of dens in dente the invagination extends beyond the pulp chamber in the root of the affected tooth. This condition is sometimes known as "dilated odontomes".

Clinical Significance

Since the base of the pit or the deep invagination in dens in dente is composed of a thin and often defective layer of enamel and dentin, this makes the tooth extremely vulnerable to caries soon after the tooth erupts into the oral cavity.

As a result most of the teeth with dens in dente frequently develop pulpitis, pulp necrosis, periapical cysts or periapical abscesses, etc.

Treatment

Early detection of the condition and restoration of the defect is the best treatment. In case of pulp involvement, endodontic treatment should be attempted. However in more severe form of the defect, extraction of the affected tooth should be done.

■ DENS EVAGINATUS

Definition

Dens evaginatus is a rare developmental anomaly of tooth, in which a focal area of the crown projects outward and gives rise to a "globe-shaped" or "nipple-shaped" protuberance on the occlusal surface. The projected portion often appears as an extra cusp or tubercle (Fig. 1.56).

Pathogenesis

Dens evaginatus probably develops as a result of excessive localized elongation and proliferation of the inner enamel epithelium as well as the odontogenic mesenchyme into the dental organ. The condition usually occurs during the early stage of tooth development.

Clinical Features

- Dens evaginatus primarily affects the premolars and the affected tooth exhibits a globe-shaped extra cusp or bump on the occlusal surface, which is often centrally located between the buccal and lingual cusps.
- The condition can also affect the molars, canines or even the incisors. In such cases, the defect may occur either unilaterally or bilaterally.
- Dens evaginatus is commonly seen among Chinese, Japanese, Filipino, American-Indians, and occasionally Caucasians.
- Clinically, this defect may sometimes interfere with tooth eruption and in such cases there may be incomplete eruption of tooth or displacement of tooth with occlusal disharmony.
- Since the extracusp contains a vital pulp horn, its attrition, fracture or deliberate cutting may result in pulp exposure with pain, pulpitis, and the other associated symptoms.

Treatment

The condition usually does not require any treatment as long as it is asymptomatic. In case of occusal disharmony, minor reduction should be attempted. However, in case of exposure or fracture of the extra cusp, endodontic treatment of the tooth should be done.

■ TALON CUSP

Definition

Talon cusp is an anomalous projection from the lingual aspect of the maxillary and mandibular permanent incisors. A "talon" is the claw of a bird of prey and the name talon cusp has evolved since this anomalous structure often resembles an "eagle's talon" (Figs. 1.57 and 1.58).

Clinical Features

- This abnormal cusp arises from the cingulum area of incisor teeth, which extends up to the incisal edge as a prominent T-shaped projection.
- It is usually an asymptomatic condition however; in some cases, it may cause

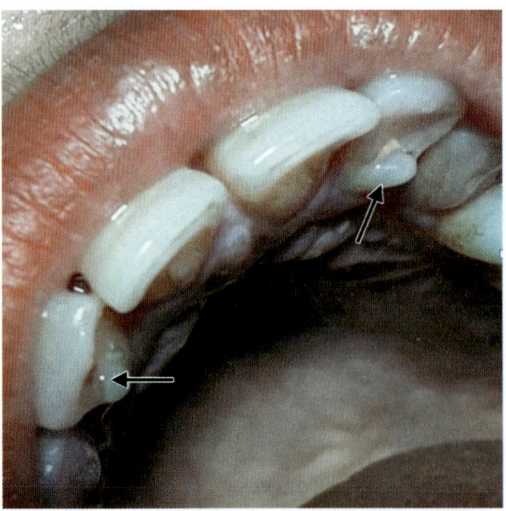

Fig. 1.56: Dens evaginatus of maxillary lateral incisors.

Developmental Anomalies of Oral and Paraoral Structures

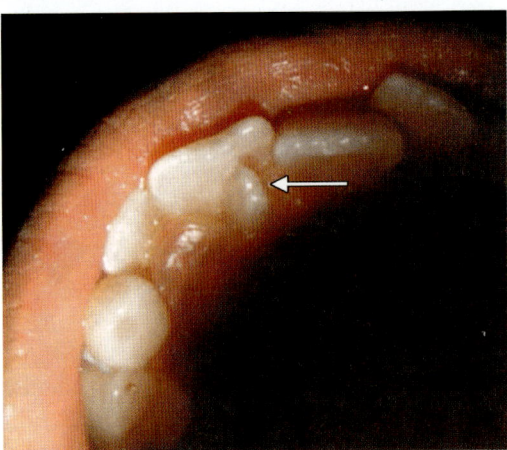

Fig. 1.57: Talon cusp-I.

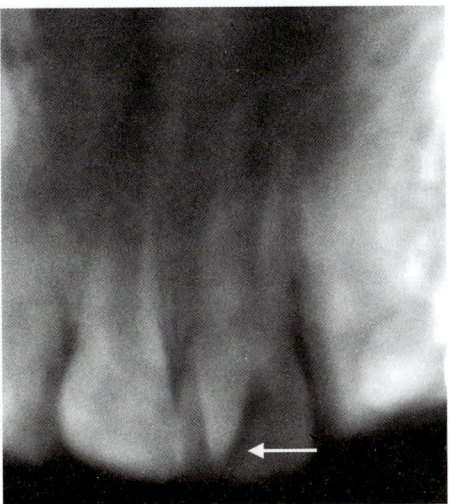

Fig. 1.58: Talon cusp X-ray.

problems like poor esthetics, increased susceptibility to trauma, caries and occlusal disharmony, etc.
- The projected structure in talon cusp usually consists of normal appearing enamel and dentin; moreover, in few cases there can be presence of vital pulp tissue as well.
- Wearing or deliberate grinding of talon cusp may lead to pulp exposure and pain.
- Occasionally, lingual pits develop on either side of the talon cusp.
- This anomaly is often seen in patients suffering from Rubinstein–Taybi syndrome.

Treatment

Whenever the lingual pits are present restorative treatments should be done to prevent caries.

ENAMEL PEARL

Enamel pearls are white, dome-shaped calcified projections of enamel, usually located at the furcation areas of the molar teeth.

Maxillary molars are more frequently affected than any other teeth.

Enamel pearls are radiographically seen as 1–3 mm round radiopaque areas at the furcation region of tooth.

General Causes of Malformed Crown of Tooth

- Supernumerary tooth
- Peg-shaped laterals
- Environmental enamel hypoplasia
- Dens invaginatus
- Dens evaginatus
- Turner's tooth
- Fusion of tooth
- Gemination of tooth
- Talon cusp
- Ghost tooth
- Congenital syphilis
- Vitamin-D resistant rickets
- Amelogenesis imperfecta
- Dentinogenesis imperfecta
- Renal osteodystrophy
- Hypoparathyroidism
- Epidermolysis bullosa
- Radiotherapy during infancy.

Histologically, these are composed of normal appearing enamel, sometimes with a central core of dentin.

It is believed that the epithelial component of root sheath of Hertwig may sometimes retain its ameloblastic potential and therefore may synthesize enamel in some focal areas in place of cementum. This gives rise to the formation of enamel pearl.

DISTURBANCE IN THE STRUCTURE OF TEETH

DISTURBANCE IN THE STRUCTURE OF ENAMEL

During the process of enamel formation, the ameloblast cells are susceptible to various external factors, which can damage the ameloblast cells and thus disturb the process of amelogenesis. The effect of disturbed amelogenesis is reflected on the surface enamel after the tooth erupts in the oral cavity.

Defect in the enamel due to disturbance during its formative process can be either qualitative or it can be quantitative.

- Quantitatively defective enamel having normal thickness is known as enamel hypoplasia.
- Qualitatively defective enamel having normal thickness is called enamel hypocalcification.

The type of developmental defect in enamel depends upon which factor was responsible for the defective amelogenesis and moreover the disturbance occurred during which stage of enamel synthesis (Table 1.6).

ACQUIRED DISTURBANCES OF ENAMEL

FOCAL ENAMEL HYPOPLASIA

When local infection or trauma causes damage to the ameloblast cells during odontogenesis, it may result in defects in enamel formation in isolated permanent tooth and this phenomenon is often known as focal enamel hypoplasia.

- This is probably the most common form of enamel hypoplasia among all the varieties, which occurs in permanent tooth due to

Table 1.6: Defective amelogenesis.

Responsible factors	Developmental defects
Matrix formation	Enamel hypoplasia
Initial mineralization	Enamel hypocalcification
Enamel maturation	Enamel hypomineralization

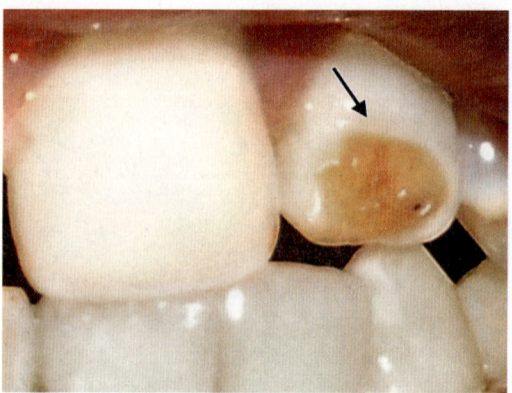

Fig. 1.59: Turner's tooth.

periapical inflammation or trauma from the infected deciduous teeth.
- It is believed that trauma or infection from the overlying deciduous tooth cause damage to the ameloblast cells and result in the enamel defect in the underlying permanent successors.
- The enamel defect is called "Turner's hypoplasia" and the tooth affected in this process is commonly known as the "Turner's tooth" (Fig. 1.59).
- "Turner's hypoplasia" is most commonly seen in mandibular first premolars, as the deciduous first molars are the most susceptible teeth to have apical inflammation (mostly due to caries). Anterior teeth are less frequently affected because of their early crown completion as compared to premolars and molars.
- Depending on the severity of the injury, the crown of the Turner's tooth may only have a small area of enamel hypoplasia that is relatively smooth with some pitting on the surface.
- However, in very severe cases, the crown is grossly deformed and exhibits severe pitting with a yellowish or brownish discoloration of the surface.

IDIOPATHIC ENAMEL OPACITIES

This condition is characterized by white opaque spots on the smooth surface enamel,

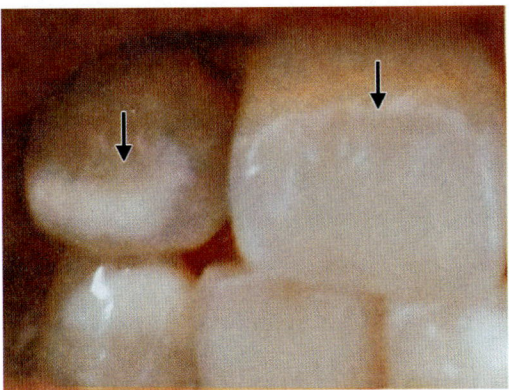

Fig. 1.60: Idiopathic enamel opacity.

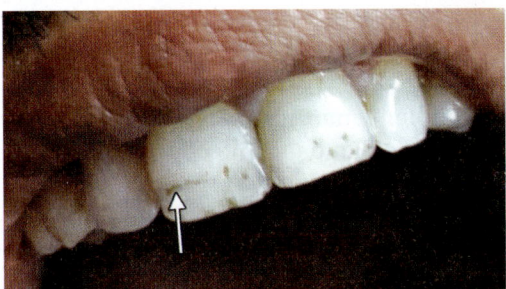

Fig. 1.61: Enamel hypoplasia (pitting type).

which occur due to some unknown cause (Fig. 1.60).

- Some of these spots may eventually turn brown after the tooth is erupted in the mouth.
- Enamel opacities may affect deciduous as well as permanent dentition and maxillary central incisor is the most frequently involved tooth.
- Histologically these opaque spots represent the area of hypomineralization.

GENERALIZED ENAMEL HYPOPLASIA

A short-term systemic or environmental disturbance in the functioning of ameloblasts at a specific period of time during odontogenesis often manifests clinically as a horizontal line of small pits or grooves on the enamel surface.

This line on the tooth surface indicates the zone of enamel hypoplasia and it corresponds to the time of development and the duration of the insult.

If the duration of the systemic or environmental insult is brief, the line of hypoplasia on the enamel surface will be narrow, whereas a prolonged insult may produce a wider zone of hypoplasia and also affect more number of teeth as well.

It has been observed from different clinical studies that generalized enamel hypoplasia due to systemic or environmental disturbances usually involves those teeth, which develop in children during their first year of life. That is why the teeth like permanent incisors, cuspids, and the first molars are often affected by generalized enamel hypoplasia (Fig. 1.61).

Whereas the teeth like premolars, second molars and third molars are seldom affected by this defect since formation of the teeth begins usually 3 years after birth or even later.

EFFECT OF INDIVIDUAL SYSTEMIC CONDITIONS ON ENAMEL HYPOPLASIA

NUTRITIONAL DEFICIENCY

Since ameloblasts are amongst the most sensitive cells in the body in terms of metabolic requirements and any serious nutritional deficiency occurring during odontogenesis may result in generalized enamel hypoplasia of teeth.

- Deficiency of vitamin A, C, and D often causes injury to the ameloblast cells and results in enamel hypoplasia.
- Hypoplasia of enamel due to nutritional deficiency commonly affects the central and lateral incisors, the cuspids, and the first molars.
- The teeth exhibit variable degrees of pitting on the enamel surface.

CONGENITAL SYPHILIS

Enamel hypoplasia resulting from congenital syphilis is a well-known phenomenon.

- The disease is contracted by the child in utero from a mother, who had active infection with *Treponema pallidum*.

- In syphilis, the infection is diffuse in nature and it can involve virtually any organ of the body. However, certain body tissues like the bone, nerves and the teeth are more susceptible to this infection as compared to other tissues of the body.
- The disease produces characteristic hypoplastic change in the enamel of permanent incisors and first molars due to infection to the developing tooth germ by treponemal spirochetes.
- The organism causes inflammation of the tooth germ during the morphodifferentiation stage resulting in hyperplasia in the epithelium of the enamel organ.
- Because of the inflammation of the tooth germ and subsequent hyperplastic change in the enamel organ, enamel hypoplasia results often in association with some specific morphologic changes in the affected tooth.
- In congenital syphilis, the affected permanent incisors exhibit tapering of the mesial and distal surfaces toward the incisal edge rather than toward the cervical margin and this gives a typical "screwdriver" appearance of these teeth.
- Moreover, these teeth also have a central notch at their incisal edge and hence are called "Hutchinson's incisors". These changes are more pronounced in maxillary central incisors.
- The lateral incisors in congenital syphilis are usually "peg-shaped" and are called "peg-laterals".
- Congenital syphilis also produces some classic changes is molar teeth (usually the first molars), which are characterized by a crumpled and discolored occlusal surface and occlusal two-thirds area of the crown.
- The affected teeth are often covered by a globular mass of enamel and such teeth are popularly known as "Moon molars" or "Mulberry molars".

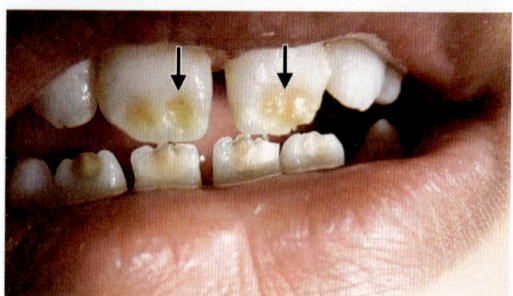

Fig. 1.62: Generalized enamel hypoplasia.

■ HYPOCALCEMIA

Enamel hypoplasia may result from hypocalcemia secondary to vitamin D deficiency and the defect is usually pitting type (Fig. 1.62).

■ EXANTHEMATOUS DISEASE

Exanthematous diseases are a group of diseases caused by a number of viruses but these have a prominent common feature of skin eruption and rash, e.g. smallpox, chickenpox, cowpox, measles, and rubella.

- Severe form of these diseases in childhood often cause generalized enamel hypoplasia and it probably happens due to prolonged high fever associated with the infection, which may result in injury to the ameloblast cells.
- Similar type of enamel hypoplasia can also occur in rickets and in congenital hypoparathyroidism.

■ BIRTH INJURIES AND LOW BIRTHWEIGHT

Enamel hypoplasia is a common developmental anomaly in case of birth injuries and it might result from a transient cessation of ameloblastic activity at the time of injury during labor.

■ FLUORIDES AND MOTTLING

If fluoride levels in the drinking water exceeds 1 ppm (parts per million), it can cause mottling of enamel. Mottling is a type of enamel hypoplasia,

Developmental Anomalies of Oral and Paraoral Structures

Table 1.7: Effects of raised fluoride levels on enamel and bone.

Fluoride level	Effects	Clinical appearance
0.5–1.5 ppm	On the higher side, few people have very mild defects	Non-detectable
2.5 ppm	Mild defects in most and moderate defect in few people	Noticeable white spots
4.4 ppm	Moderate to severe defects in nearly all patients	Opaque and pitted
6 ppm	All patients affected	Severe disfigurement of tooth
8 ppm	Osteosclerosis of bone	Skeletal deformity with increased bone density seen in the X-rays

which occurs as a result of damage to the ameloblast cells due to fluoride toxicity when the ion is absorbed in the body at a very high concentration. Besides causing damage to the enamel forming cells the excess fluorides also cause disturbance in the calcification process of enamel and mottling actually results from this dual effect of fluoride toxicity (Table 1.7).

Clinical Features of Mottling of Enamel

- Excessive amount of fluoride in drinking water causes sclerosis of the skeleton, which is characterized by calcification of the muscles and ligaments (especially intervertebral muscles and ligaments) with stiffening of the body and pain. The bone changes include increased thickening and mineralization similar to that of Paget's disease of bone.
- Mottling (a condition of spotting with patches of color) is a generalized disturbance affecting all those teeth exposed to excess fluoride during odontogenesis or development of tooth (Fig. 1.63).
- The condition does not affect adults.
- Mostly the permanent dentition is affected and the involvement of deciduous teeth is rare.
- The mottled teeth often have chalky or typical "paper white" opaque enamel with areas of flecking or pitting.
- The damage can be extensive in some teeth, which exhibit fracturing of enamel with an associated brown or black pigmentation.
- Mottled teeth are less susceptible to caries.

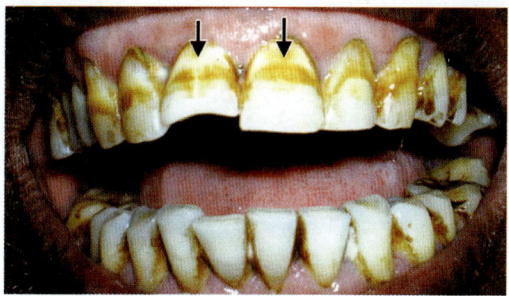

Fig. 1.63: Mottling of teeth.

HEREDITARY DISTURBANCE OF ENAMEL FORMATION

■ AMELOGENESIS IMPERFECTA

Definition

Amelogenesis imperfecta is a heterogeneous group of hereditary disorders of enamel formation, affecting both deciduous and the permanent dentition.

The disease involves only the ectodermal component of the tooth (i.e. enamel) while the mesodermal structures of tooth, (e.g. dentin, cementum, and pulp), etc. always remain normal.

Types

Normally, the process of enamel formation progresses through three stages:
1. Stage of enamel matrix formation
2. Stage of early mineralization
3. Stage of enamel maturation.

Amelogenesis imperfecta may set in during any stage of enamel formation. Four basic types of the disease have been identified,

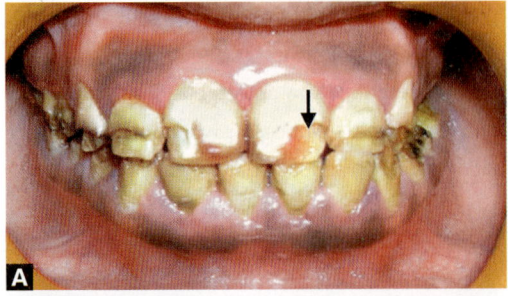

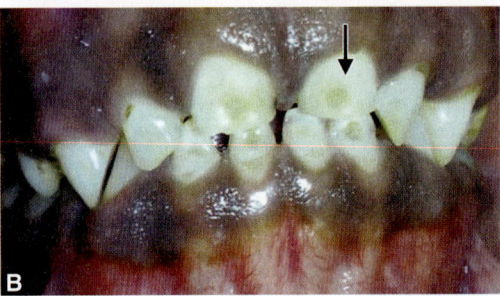

Figs. 1.64A and B: (A) Amelogenesis imperfecta–hypomaturation type; (B) Hypoplastic type.

which corresponds with four developmental stages of enamel (Figs. 1.64A and B).
Type I: Hypoplastic type of amelogenesis imperfecta.
Type II: Hypomaturation type of amelogenesis imperfecta.
Type III: Hypocalcification type of amelogenesis imperfecta.
Type IV: Hypomaturation–hypoplastic type with taurodontism.

Hypoplastic Type

The enamel thickness is usually far below normal in hypoplastic type of amelogenesis imperfecta since the disease affects the stage of matrix formation. The teeth exhibit either complete absence of enamel from the crown surface or there may be a very thin layer of enamel on some focal areas of crown.

Hypomaturation Type

This type occurs due to interruption in the process of maturation of enamel. Here, the enamel is of normal thickness but it does not have the normal hardness and translucency (snow-capped tooth). The enamel color is often yellow-white or yellow-brown and it can be pierced with an explorer tip with firm pressure.

Hypocalcification Type

Hypocalcification type of amelogenesis imperfecta represents the disturbance in the process of early mineralization of the enamel.

In this type of amelogenesis imperfecta, the enamel is of normal thickness but is soft and can be easily removed with a blunt instrument.

Hypomaturation–hypoplastic Type with Taurodontism

This is a rare condition where taurodontism is reported in association with amelogenesis imperfecta.

Clinical Features

- Amelogenesis imperfecta affects both deciduous as well as the permanent dentition.
- Sex predilection varies according to the mode of inheritance.
- The color of the teeth is mostly chalky white (opaque white) but sometimes it can be yellow or even dark brown.
- Besides the discoloration, these teeth are sensitive and are prone to disintegration.
- The contact points in the proximal surfaces are mostly open either due to lack of formation or early loss of enamel.
- The occlusal surfaces and the incisal edges of the teeth are often severely abraded.
- Sometimes, the tooth may be completely devoid of enamel, which results in severe abrasion of the dentin.
- In some patients, the enamel may have a cheesy consistency which is easily removable from the tooth surface with dental explorers.
- Amelogenesis imperfecta can be associated with retained deciduous tooth and delayed eruption of permanent tooth.

- Alteration in the eruption pattern of teeth in amelogenesis imperfecta may further result in the development of anterior-open bite.
- On rare occasions, the enamel may look almost normal except the presence of few grooves and wrinkles on its surface.
- Amelogenesis imperfecta does not increase the susceptibility of the teeth to dental caries.
- In the mildest form of hypomaturation type, the enamel is of near normal hardness and the teeth exhibit some white opaque flecks at the incisal margins. These types of teeth are known as "snow-capped teeth".

Radiographic Features

In amelogenesis imperfecta, the thickness and radiodensity of enamel varies greatly. The tooth may be completely devoid of enamel and wherever the enamel is present, it is very thin and found mostly on the tip of the cusps and on the interproximal areas.
- In hypoplastic type, the radiodensity of the enamel is usually greater than the adjacent dentin.
- The radiodensity of enamel in hypomaturation type is almost equal to that of the normal dentin.

Key Points of Amelogenesis Imperfecta
- This is the hereditary enamel hypoplasia characterized by little or no formation of enamel.
- The disease has four types—(1) hypoplastic type, (2) hypomaturation type, (3) hypocalcification type, and (4) hypomaturation–hypoplastic type with taurodontism.
- Thin layer of soft or cheesy enamel often present on the tooth surface; (predominantly on the cuspal and incisal areas), even the hard enamel whichever is present can be easily removed by dental explorers.
- The tooth often has a chalky discoloration.
- Lack of enamel results in severe abrasions of tooth.
- Besides enamel other structures of tooth, e.g. dentin, cementum and pulp are absolutely normal.

Histopathology

Histologically, the enamel in hypoplastic type of amelogenesis imperfecta exhibits lack of differentiation of the ameloblast cells with little or no matrix formation.

The enamel in hypocalcification type shows defective matrix structure and abnormal or subnormal mineral deposition.

The hypomaturation type reveals alteration in the enamel rod and rod-sheath structures.

The dentin and pulp chamber appear normal.

Treatment

There is no definitive treatment for amelogenesis imperfecta, composite veneering can be done to improve overall esthetics of teeth.

SYNDROME ASSOCIATED ENAMEL DEFECTS

A large number of syndromes and pathological conditions have been identified, which are often associated with hereditary enamel defects. In the following section few such syndromes or conditions have been discussed.

Epidermolysis bullosa: It is a bullous disease of the skin and mucous membrane. Dental defects associated with this condition include—enamel hypoplasia with random pitting.

Morquio's syndrome (mucopolysaccharidoses type IV): Dental defects which occur in association with this syndrome include:
- Enamel hypoplasia with pointed peak-like cusp tips.
- Gray colored teeth with vertically oriented pits on the surface.

Sanfilippo's syndrome (mucopolysaccharidoses type III): This syndrome presents features like-loss of enamel from the dentinal surfaces, defective formation of dentin and obliteration of pulp chambers.

Oculodento-osseous dysplasia: Dental defects in this syndrome include the following:
- Thick mandibular bone.
- Multifocal enamel hypoplasia of the tooth surface with pitting.
- Moth-eaten radiographic appearance of the teeth.

Table 1.8: Classification of developmental defects in dentin.

Local causes	General causes
Trauma in the deciduous tooth causing *"Turner's tooth"*	A. *Dentinogenesis imperfecta*:
	Type I: Dentinogenesis imperfecta associated with osteogenesis imperfecta
	Type II: Dentinogenesis imperfecta not associated with osteogenesis imperfecta (only teeth are affected)
	Type III: Dentinogenesis imperfecta of Brandywine type
	B. *Dentin dysplasia*:
	Type I: Radicular dentin dysplasia (rootless teeth)
	Type II: Coronal dentin dysplasia
	C. *Environmental/systemic*:
	Vitamin D—dependent rickets
	Vitamin D—resistant rickets (hypophosphatemia)
	Hypophosphatasia
	Juvenile hypoparathyroidism
	Other mineral deficiencies
	Drugs, e.g. chemotherapeutic agents

Classification of Developmental Defects in Dentin

Classification of developmental defects in dentin has been described in Table 1.8.

DISTURBANCES IN STRUCTURE OF DENTIN

Dentin is the first formed dental hard tissue and it is produced by the specialized odontogenic mesenchymal cells called the odontoblasts. These dentin forming cells or odontoblasts are derived from the mesenchymal cells of the dental papilla under the influence of the internal enamel epithelium. In the initial stage of dentin formation a collagenous matrix is formed, which is embedded in a ground substance rich in glycosaminoglycans (GAG). When sufficient thickness the dentin matrix is laid down the odontoblast cells migrate through it centripetally and their processes remain in the matrix, which begin to mineralize later. Mineralization of dentin is initiated by the formation of small crystallines, which subsequently grow and fuse together to form discrete calcific globules called calcospherites.

Most of the factors causing interference in the process of dentinogenesis are genetic in nature. However, there are some environmental factors as well, which can also cause disturbance in the normal dentin formation.

■ DENTINOGENESIS IMPERFECTA (HEREDITARY OPALESCENT DENTIN)

Definition

Dentinogenesis imperfecta is an inherited disorder of dentin formation, characterized by excessive formation of defective dentin, which results in obliteration of pulp chambers and root canals of tooth. The condition affects both deciduous as well as the permanent dentition and it usually exhibits an autosomal dominant mode of transmission.

Classification

Shields Classification

The disorder has been classified into three types:

1. *Type I*: Dentinogenesis imperfecta associated with osteogenesis imperfecta.
2. *Type II*: Dentinogenesis imperfecta not associated with osteogenesis imperfecta.

3. *Type III*: Dentinogenesis imperfecta of "Brandywine type".

Witkop Classification

- Dentinogenesis imperfecta
- Hereditary opalescent dentin
- Brandywine type.

Type I: Dentinogenesis imperfecta associated with osteogenesis imperfecta:
- This type is usually inherited as an autosomal dominant trait and it characteristically shows "defects both in dentin and bone".
- It involves the deciduous teeth more often (and more severely) than the permanent teeth.
- Teeth will usually have an opalescent color (as seen in type II as well).
- Patients will exhibit features of osteogenesis imperfecta (since both conditions occur together), which include bluish selera of the eyes, Wormian skull bones with several bony defects and increased tendency for fractures.
- It is important to note that not all cases of osteogenesis imperfecta will be associated with dentinogenesis imperfecta.
- Moreover, there is no correlation between dentinogenesis imperfecta and the severity of the osseous defects present in osteogenesis imperfecta.

Type II: Dentinogenesis imperfecta not associated with osteogenesis imperfecta
- This type of dentinogenesis imperfecta is often known as "hereditary opalescent dentin" and it shows defect only in dentin but not in bone (Figs. 1.65 and 1.66).
- It is the most common type among all the three forms of the disease, having incidence rate about 1 in 8,000 people.
- The condition is inherited as an autosomal dominant trait and unlike type I, there is no bony abnormality.
- Involves deciduous and permanent teeth with equal frequency.

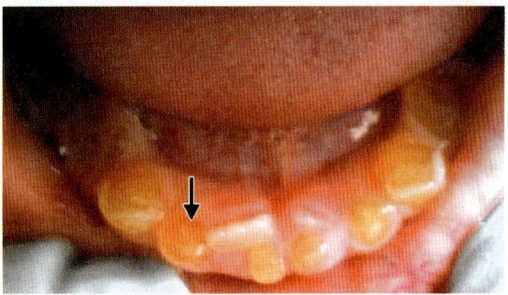

Fig. 1.65: Dentinogenesis imperfecta involving deciduous teeth and showing typical "opalescent" dentin.

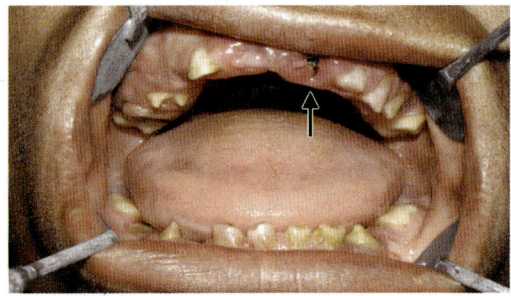

Fig. 1.66: Dentinogenesis imperfecta in permanent teeth.

Type III: Dentinogenesis imperfecta of "Brandywine type"
- Type III dentinogenesis imperfecta is a rare condition and is inherited as an autosomal dominant trait; this type also exhibits defect only in dentin and not in bone.
- It is commonly seen in a racial isolate area in the state of Maryland and deciduous teeth mostly affected.
- It characteristically shows lack of dentin formation resulting in an empty, enlarged pulp chamber and root canal (shell tooth) *(unlike type I and type II, which show overproduction of dentin causing obliteration of pulp chamber and root canals)*
- Clinically, the disease is same as type I and type II variants, however, it often exhibits multiple pulp exposures and periapical lesions in deciduous teeth.
- Presence of little or no dentin in the tooth with large pulp chamber; results in a classic

"shell tooth" appearance of the affected tooth.
- Both "shell tooth" and "pink tooth" have enlarged pulp chambers; but the shell tooth develops due to lack of dentin formation, while the pink tooth forms due to dentin resorption.

Clinical Features
- In all three types of dentinogenesis imperfecta both deciduous and permanent dentitions are affected.
- The condition affects males and females with almost equal frequency.
- On eruption, the teeth exhibit a normal contour but they have an opalescent "amber-like" appearance.
- Few days after eruption, the teeth may achieve an almost normal color, following which they become translucent.
- Finally, the teeth become either gray or yellowish-brown in color with a bluish reflection from the enamel.
- The teeth in dentinogenesis imperfecta often have "tulip" shape, which is characterized by a broad or bulbous crown and a narrow constricted cervical area.
- The overlying enamel is structurally normal in most cases, however, this enamel fractures rapidly from the dentin surface, soon after the teeth erupt in the oral cavity (early enamel loss is due to poor bonding between the enamel and dentin at the dentinoenamel junction, where the scalloping is absent).
- Early loss of enamel often results in severe attrition of the teeth, moreover, the deciduous teeth exfoliate early.
- Teeth are not particularly sensitive even when most of the surface enamel is lost, it happens since the dentinal tubules are haphazardly arranged and most of them are devoid of the odontoblastic processes.
- Although the dentin is soft and easily penetrable in dentinogenesis imperfecta, these teeth are not caries prone. The possible reason could be the structural change in the dentin itself, which provides little scope for the entry of the cariogenic microorganisms into the tooth since most of the dentinal tubules are obliterated in this disease.
- Type III cases of dentinogenesis imperfecta are often associated with multiple pulp exposures (mostly due to attrition) and periapical pathology.

Radiographic Features
Radiographically dentinogenesis imperfecta reveals the following features:

Type I and Type II Dentinogenesis Imperfecta
- Both forms are radiographically similar and they often exhibit "bulbous" or "bell-shaped" crowns of the teeth with abnormally constricted cervical areas.
- The roots of the teeth are thin, short, and spiked.
- Depending on the age of the patient, the teeth exhibit varying degrees of obliteration (opacification) of the coronal as well as the radicular pulp chamber, due to continued deposition of secondary dentin.
- The cementum, periodontal ligament and the alveolar bone radiographically appear normal.

Type III Dentinogenesis Imperfecta
- It exhibits extremely large pulp chambers and root canals, surrounded by a thin shell of dentin; hence, these affected teeth are called "shell" teeth (Fig. 1.67).
- These teeth frequently exhibit multiple pulp exposure and associated periapical pathology.

Histopathology
- Histologically, the enamel appears normal in dentinogenesis imperfecta.

Developmental Anomalies of Oral and Paraoral Structures

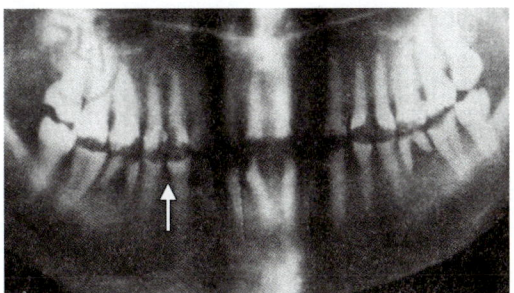

Fig. 1.67: Radiograph of dentinogenesis imperfecta showing severe attrition and obliteration of pulp chambers of teeth.

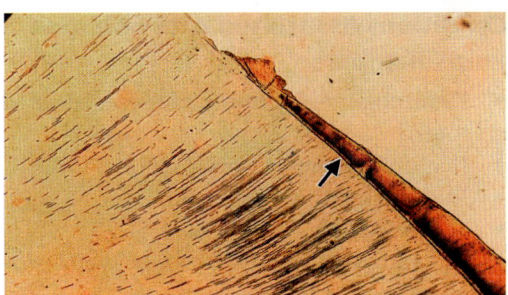

Fig. 1.68: Photomicrograph of dentinogenesis imperfecta showing loss of scalloping at the dentinoenamel (DE) junction.

- The mantle dentin (a narrow zone of dentin immediately beneath the enamel) is also nearly normal.
- The major parts of the remaining dentin are severely dysplastic and exhibit vast areas of amorphous matrix with globular or interglobular foci of mineralization.
- The dentinal tubules are far less in number per square unit area of dentin as compared to the normal dentin.
- These tubules are often distorted, irregular in shape, widely spaced and are often larger in size.
- In many cases the odontoblastic processes are absent in the dentinal tubules, instead there can be presence of some degenerating cellular debris inside these tubules.
- There may be large areas of atubular dentin present along with areas of noncalcified matrix.
- Degenerating odontoblasts are often trapped inside the dentin matrix.
- The pulp chamber and root canals are often obliterated by abnormal secondary dentin deposition.
- The dentinoenamel junction appears smooth or flattened instead of being scalloped (Fig. 1.68). This abnormal configuration is mostly responsible for the early loss of enamel from the tooth surface in dentinogenesis imperfecta.

Key Points of Dentinogenesis Imperfecta

- This is a hereditary defect of dentin characterized by increased, abnormal synthesis of dentin in the tooth with presence of normal enamel.
- The disease occurs in three forms—type I, type II, and type III.
- The affected teeth have an opalescent hue with amberlike color after eruption; with time they become brown or gray with a bluish reflection from enamel.
- Dentinoenamel junction is flat instead of scalloped and it causes poor locking between enamel and dentin; because of this tooth enamel is quickly lost from the dentin surfaces.
- Teeth in dentinogenesis imperfecta often exhibit severe abrasions.
- Tooth has narrow constricted cervical area.
- Type I and type II show obliteration of pulp chamber due to abnormal dentin formations. Type III shows abnormally large pulp chamber (shell tooth).

Biochemical Property of Dentin

- Biochemical analysis of the dentin in dentinogenesis imperfecta reveals increased water content and decreased mineral content.
- The microhardness of the dentin is low as compared to the normal dentin.

Treatment

The treatment in dentinogenesis imperfecta is mostly aimed at preventing excessive tooth attrition and improving esthetics of the patients. Metal and ceramic crowns are given.

Conditions Associated with Enlarged Pulp Chambers

- Dentinogenesis imperfecta type III (shell tooth)
- Regional odontodysplasia (ghost tooth)
- Internal resorption of tooth
- Taurodontism
- Vitamin D-resistant rickets (high pulp horns)
- Hypophosphatasia
- Dentin dysplasia type II.

DENTINAL ABNORMALITY DUE TO SYSTEMIC OR ENVIRONMENTAL DISTURBANCES

The environmental or systemic conditions, which can affect dentinogenesis are as follows:
- Vitamin D-dependent rickets
- Vitamin D-resistant rickets
- Cytotoxic drugs
- Juvenile hypoparathyroidism
- Hypophosphatasia
- Dentin dysplasia type II (thistle-tube pulp).

Vitamin D-dependent Rickets

Dentinal Changes

Dentinal changes in this disease include the following:
- The width or thickness of the predentin is increased
- Improper and incomplete calcification of the regular dentin
- Thick band-like areas of interglobular dentin can be seen histologically, which correspond to the periods of active phase of the disease.

Vitamin D-resistant Rickets (Hypophosphatemia)

Dentinal Changes

- Increased amount of interglobular dentin formation.
- These teeth exhibit large pulp chambers and long pulp horns. The later may even extend to the dentinoenamel junction as narrow clefts.
- The overlying enamel is defective and shows numerous cracks, which can serve as the direct pathways for entry of microorganisms into the pulp.
- Many such teeth with this defect often exhibit pulpitis and periapical lesions even in the absence of caries.

Hypophosphatasia

Dentinal Changes

- Increased formation of interglobular dentin
- Widening of the predentine.

Cytotoxic Agents

Presence of many prominent incremental lines in the dentin, which often correspond to the periods of the drug (cytotoxic) administration.

Juvenile Hypoparathyroidism

Dentinal changes include:
- Presence of small sized teeth in the arch
- Hypoplastic enamel
- Multiple prominent incremental lines can be seen in the dentine
- Roots of the teeth are small
- Histologically radicular dentine reveals many structural abnormally and there can be areas of vascular inclusions in the dentine.

DENTIN DYSPLASIA

Definition

Dentin dysplasia is an autosomal dominant inherited disorder characterized by defective dentine formation and abnormal pulpal morphology; however, the enamel in such teeth is absolutely normal. The condition is also known as "rootless teeth".

Types

The condition is classified into two types:
1. Type I or radicular dentin dysplasia
2. Type II or coronal dentin dysplasia.

Dentin Dysplasia Type I (Radicular)

Dentin dysplasia type I represents a peculiar disturbance in the development of radicular dentin.

Clinical features

- There is no sex predilection.
- Although, both types of dentin dysplasias are rare entities; however, type I dentin dysplasia is far more common than type II.
- The anomaly affects both deciduous as well as permanent dentitions.
- Although the roots of the teeth are defective, the crown portions are normal both structurally and morphologically.
- The color of the teeth is usually normal but in some cases the crowns of the teeth reveal a slight bluish or brownish translucency at the cervical region.
- Unlike dentinogenesis imperfecta, the enamel does not chip off from the crown surface.
- The teeth usually erupt at the normal time, although in some cases there can be delayed eruption.
- Because of the presence of functionally unstable short roots, the affected teeth often exhibit severe mobility and they may even exfoliate prematurely due to minor trauma.
- Dentin dysplasia type I can occur in association with diffuse generalized osteosclerosis (Figs. 1.69 and 1.70).

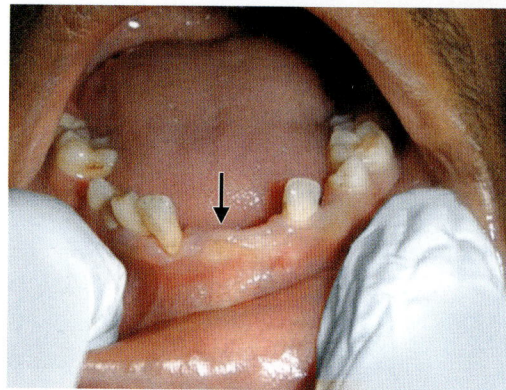

Fig. 1.69: Dentin dysplasia type I—premature loss of teeth.

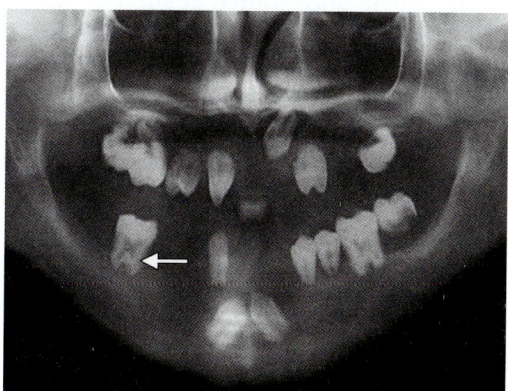

Fig. 1.70: Dentin dysplasia type I- teeth with extremely short roots or "rootless teeth".

Radiographic features

- The roots of the teeth are characteristically malformed, short, blunt or conical.
- Although presence of rudimentary roots is common, in many cases the teeth may be completely devoid of roots.
- The deciduous teeth often exhibit total obliteration of the pulp chambers and root canals.
- The permanent teeth also present pulp obliterations but there may be presence of very thin crescent-shaped remnants of the pulp.
- Obliteration of the pulp chamber in the affected teeth may occur even before the teeth erupt in the oral cavity.
- The mandibular molars often exhibit characteristic "W"-shaped roots.
- Periapical radiolucencies of unknown etiology (e.g. periapical cyst, abscess or granuloma, etc.) may be found in many normal appearing teeth.

Histopathology

- The enamel and mantle dentins are normal.
- The remaining coronal and radicular dentin appear as a fused nodular mass comprising of tubular dentin, osteodentin and amorphous dentin mass.

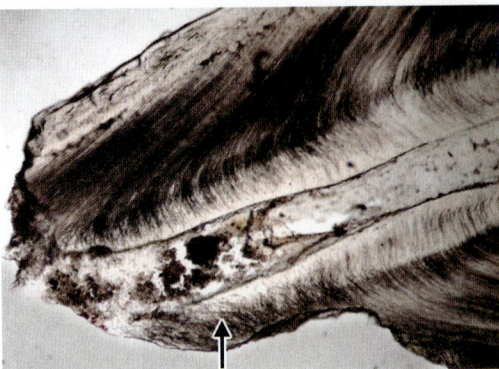

Fig. 1.71: Defective dentin in dentin dysplasia type I—appearing as "lava flowing around boulders".

- Histologic appearance of such defective mass of dentinal tissue often resembles, what is called "a series of sand dunes" or "lava flowing around boulders" (Fig. 1.71).
- Remnants of pulp tissue may occasionally be seen between the normal and the abnormal dentinal tissue.

Pathogenesis

Dentin dysplasia type I develops probably due to a defect in the epithelial root sheath of Hertwig, which fragments and becomes incorporated into the dental papilla, where it induces formation of dysplastic dentin.

Treatment

No specific treatment is available. These teeth also do not serve as good abutments since their roots are very short.

Dentin Dysplasia Type II (Coronal)

Definition

It is an inherited autosomal dominant disorder of dentine, which mostly affects the coronal dentine.

Clinical features
- Both deciduous and permanent teeth are affected in this disorder.
- The permanent teeth are of normal color, whereas the deciduous teeth exhibit an "amber-gray" color with some translucent or opalescent appearance.
- There is no sex predilection.

Radiographic features
- The deciduous teeth in dentin dysplasia type II reveals obliterated pulp chambers and root canals, thereby resembling dentinogenesis imperfecta.
- Permanent teeth exhibit large pulp chambers with a typical "thistle-tube" appearance.
- Pulpal obliteration occurs only after tooth eruption.
- The roots of the deciduous and the permanent teeth are usually of normal shape and length.
- Unlike dentinogenesis imperfecta there is no cervical constriction of the teeth in dentin dysplasia type II.
- The pulp chambers in permanent teeth are abnormally large instead of being obliterated and have a typical flame shape.
- The pulp chamber contains many pulp stones or denticles.
- Root canals may be partially obliterated in the apical third region.

Histopathology
- The deciduous teeth exhibit a dense amorphous mass of dentin, which contains only few haphazardly arranged dentinal tubules.
- The permanent teeth show normal dentinal structures but may have the presence of abnormal globular or interglobular dentin near the pulpal third area and in the roots.
- The pulp chambers exhibit the presence of numerous pulp stones.

Treatment and prognosis

No special treatment is required in case of dentin dysplasia type II. Prognosis is good for the permanent teeth since their root length is essentially normal.

REGIONAL ODONTODYSPLASIA (GHOST TEETH)

Definition

Regional odontodysplasia is an unique nonhereditary developmental disturbance of teeth, characterized by defective formation of both ectodermal and mesodermal structures of tooth, e.g. enamel and dentin, along with the pulp.

Clinical Features

- Both permanent and deciduous dentitions are affected in this disease although it is more common in permanent anteriors (central incisors, lateral incisors, and canines).
- There is no sex predilection.
- The maxillary teeth are affected more often than the mandibular teeth; the affected teeth are more caries prone.
- The disease is called regional, since it affects several contiguous teeth in a single quadrant of the jaw.
- It frequently occurs unilaterally, often affecting certain parts of maxilla.
- The affected teeth show either delayed eruption or a complete failure of eruption.
- These teeth are often small and mottled; these deformed teeth often have a soft leathery surface and are yellowish-brown in color.
- Gingival swelling adjacent to the affected teeth is common finding.

Radiographic Features

- The hard tissues of the teeth like enamel, dentin, and cementum are all hypoplastic and hypocalcified in this disease; which make these teeth look unusually subdued and less radio-dens (ghost teeth).
- The enamel and dentin are very thin and radiographic distinction between these two structures is impossible, this accounts for the "ghostly" appearance of the involved teeth.

Histopathology

- The enamel layer is attenuated and disrupted.
- Dentin is very thin and globular, and exhibits irregular tubules and a wide predentine layer.
- Large pulp chamber exhibits numerous pulpal calcifications.

Treatment

Extraction of the affected teeth and fabrication of a suitable prosthesis is usually recommended.

Conditions Associated with Malformation of the Roots of Teeth

- Dilaceration
- Hypercementosis
- Concrescence
- Supernumerary roots
- Taurodontism
- Enamel pearl
- Benign cementoblastoma
- Dentinogenesis imperfecta
- Dentin dysplasia type I
- Radiotherapy during childhood
- External resorption of tooth.

DISTURBANCE IN STRUCTURE OF CEMENTUM

Cementum is the odontogenic mesenchymal tissue, which covers the root surface of teeth. There are two types of cemental tissues found:

1. *The acellular or primary cementum*—which covers the coronal one-third of the roots.
2. *The cellular or secondary cementum*: It covers the apical two-thirds and furcation areas of the teeth. The cellular cementum often has a thicker layer and it continues to form throughout the life of the tooth.

There are two main types of defects seen in the cementum:
 i. Hypercementosis
 ii. Hypocementosis.

HYPERCEMENTOSIS

Definition

It represents an increased and abnormal thickness of the cementum, which results from abnormal cementogenesis (Fig. 1.72).

Etiology

- *Periapical inflammation*: Periapical inflammation causes cemental opposition on the root. This may result in either a generalized

64 Essentials of Oral Pathology

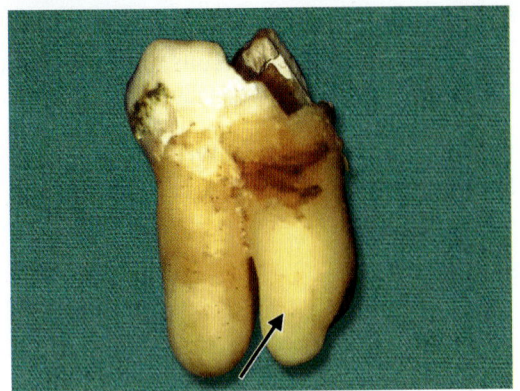

Fig. 1.72: Hypercementosis.

increase in the thickness of cementum or a localized "knob-like" enlargement.
- *Mechanical stimulation*: Although excessive mechanical forces applied to a tooth produce cemental resorption but forces below a certain threshold level may stimulate cemental apposition and subsequent hypercementosis.
- *Nonfunctional and unerupted teeth*: These teeth sometimes show cemental resorption but excessive apposition of cementum is also possible.
- *Paget's disease of bone*: Hypercementosis is a common feature of Paget's disease of bone. The cementum in this disease is very thick and it often has a mosaic pattern.
- *Root ankylosis and concrescence*: Teeth in these conditions may be associated with hypercementosis.

Typical radiographic changes in various tooth abnormalities have been described in Table 1.9.

HYPOCEMENTOSIS

Hypocementosis or acementosis is a rare developmental anomaly of tooth characterized by lack of cementum formation in the tooth (Fig. 1.73).

Causes
- Cleidocranial dysplasia
- Hypophosphatasia.

Hypocementosis prevents the normal development of the periodontal attachment or

Table 1.9: Typical radiographic changes in various tooth abnormalities.

Diseases	Characteristics
Gemination (incomplete)	Two crowns with one root
Dilacerations	Sharp bend in the tooth (mostly root)
Dens in dente	Tooth within a tooth
Taurodontism	Large crown with small root, too much apically placed bifurcation
Concrescence	Joining of roots of many teeth with obliteration of periodontal ligament space
Amelogenesis imperfecta	Little or no enamel on tooth
Dentinogenesis imperfecta	Obliteration of pulp chamber
Dentinogenesis imperfecta type III	Abnormally large pulp with thin shell of enamel and dentin surrounding the pulp
Ghost tooth	Decreased radiodensity of tooth; abnormally large pulp chamber
Dentin dysplasia	Abnormally short, blunt root, molar roots appear "w" shaped
Hypercementosis	Bulbous root
Supernumerary tooth	Mostly small and conical shaped
Pit and fissure caries	Triangular-shaped radiolucency with its base toward dentinoenamel (DE) junction
Smooth surface caries	Triangular-shaped radiolucency with its base toward surface of the tooth
External resorption of tooth	Moth-eaten irregular destruction of root surface.
Internal resorption	Well-defined spherical radioluceny of dentine in continuation with the pulp
Compound odontome	Multiple miniature teeth projecting from a single focus

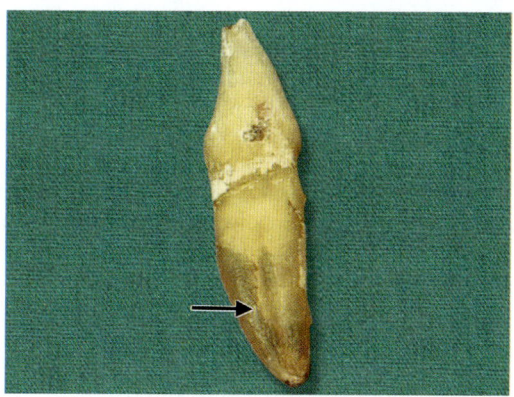

Fig. 1.73: Hypocementosis

even the normal dentin formation. Premature loss of few or all deciduous and permanent teeth may occur in this disease.

BIBLIOGRAPHY

1. Albery EH, Hathorn IS, Pigott RW. Cleft lip and palate: A team approach. Bristol: John Wright and Sons; 1986.
2. Aldred M, Crawford P. Register of developmental dental anomalies. Br Dent J. 1989;167:370.
3. Amaratunga AN, Chandrasekera A. Incidence of cleft lip and palate in Sri Lanka. J Oral Maxillofac Surg. 1989;47:559-61.
4. Berg KL. Tongue-tie (ankyloglossia) and breastfeeding: a review. J Hum Lact. 1990;6:109-12.
5. Berman FR, Fay JT. The retrocuspid papillae. A clinical survey. Oral Surg Oral Med Oral Pathol. 1976;42:80-5.
6. Bowden DE, Goose DH. Inheritance of tooth size in Liverpool families. J Med Genet. 1969;6:55-8.
7. Brauer JC, Blackstone CH. Dental aspects of congenital syphilis. J Am Dent Assoc. 1941;28:1633-9.
8. Buchner A, Hansen LS. Melanotic macule of the oral mucosa: A clinicopathologic study of 105 cases. Oral Surg Oral Med Oral Pathol. 1979;48:244-9.
9. Burton DJ, Saffos RO, Scheffer RB. Multiple bilateral dens indente as a factor in the aetiology of multiple periapical lesions. Oral Surg Oral med Oral Pathol. 1980;49:496-9.
10. Chandra S, Chawla HS. Prevalence of anodontia among Lucknow city school children. J Indian Dent Assoc. 1975;47:489-96.
11. Chapman CJ. Ethnic differences in the incidence of cleft lip and/or cleft palate in Aukland, 1960-1976. N Z Med J. 1983;96:327-9.
12. Chawla HS, Tiwari A, Gopalakrishnan NS. Talon cusps—a prevalence study. J Indian Soc Pedod Prev Dent. 1983;1:28-34.
13. Clayton JM. Congenital dental anomalies occurring in 3,557 children. J Dent Child. 1956;23:206-18.
14. Dolan EA, Riski JE, Mason RM. Macroglossia: clinical considerations. Int J Orofacial Myology. 1989;15:4-7.
15. Ettinger RL, Manderson RD. A clinical study of sublingual varices. Oral Surg Oral Med Oral Pathol. 1974;38:540-5.
16. Everett FG, Wescott WB. Commissural lip pits. Oral Surg Oral Med Oral Pathol. 1961;38:540-5.
17. Ferraz JA, Pecora JD. Three rooted mandibular molars in patients of Mongolian, Caucasian and Negro origin. Braz Dent J. 1993;3:113-7.
18. Gardner DG, Girgis SS. Taurodontism, shovel-shaped incisors and the Klinefelter syndrome. Dental J. 1978;44:372-3.
19. Gardner DG. The dentinal changes in regional odontodysplasia. Oral Surg. 1974;38:887-97.
20. Goh EH. Lingual thyroids. Singapore Med J. 1971;12:46-9.
21. Grahnen H. Hypodontia in the permanent dentition. A clinical and genetically investigation. Odontol Revy. 1956;7:1-100.
22. Harris EF, Friend GW, Tolley EA. Enhanced prevalence of ankyloglossia with maternal cocaine use. Cleft Palate Craniofac. 1992;29:72-6.
23. Heys FM, Blattner RJ, Robinson HB. Osteogenesis imperfecta and odontogenesis imperfecta: clinical and genetic aspects in eighteen families. J Paediatr. 1960;56:230-5.
24. Horowitz HS. Fluoride and enamel defects. Adv Dent Res. 1989;3:143-6.
25. Jones AW. Dental morphology in people of Mongoloid origin. Odontostomatol Trop. 1981;4:165-9.
26. Kalter H, Warkany J. Congenital malformations. Etiologic factors and their role in prevention. N Engl J Med. 1983;308:424-31,491-7.
27. Kaul V, Prakash S. Morphologic features of Jat dentition. Am J Phys Anthropol. 1981;54:123-7.
28. King NM, Brook AH. A prevalence study of enamel defects among young adults in Hong Kong: use of the FDI Index. N Z Dent J. 1984;80:47-9.

29. Kulid JC, Weller RN. Treatment considerations in dens invaginatus. J Endod. 1989;15:323-5.
30. Levitas TC. Germination, fusion, twinning and concrescence. J Dent Child. 1965;32:93-100.
31. Li Y, Navia JM, Bian JY. Prevalence and distribution of developmental enamel defects in primary dentition of Chinese children 3–5 years old. Community Dent Oral Epidemiol. 1995;23:72-9.
32. Ligh RQ. Coronal dilaceration. Oral Surg Med Oral Pathol. 1981;51:567.
33. Lum YM, Lim ST. Four cases of congenitally missing permanent cuspids. Singapore Dent J. 1976;2:49-51.
34. Lustmann J, Klein H, Ulmansky M. Odontodysplasia. Report of two cases and review of the literature. Oral Surg Oral Med Oral Pathol. 1975;39:781-93.
35. MacDonald-Jankowski DS. Multiple dental developmental anomalies. Dentomaxillofac Radiol. 1991;20:166-8.
36. Macfarlane JD, Swart JG. Dental aspects of hypophosphatasia: A case report, family study, and literature review. Oral Surg Oral Med Oral Pathol. 1989;67:521-6.
37. Meares N, Bradue S, Burgess K. Massive macroglossia as a presenting feature of hypothyroid-associated pericardial effusion. Chest. 1993;104:1632-3.
38. Melhado RM, Mathews G, Conrado LA. Bilateral germination. Oral Surg. 1982;54:605.
39. Menezes DM. Opacities and hypoplasia in the enamel of Burmese children from a low fluoride area. J Dent. 1976;4:71-2.
40. Midtbø M, Halse A. Tooth crown size and morphology in Turner Syndrome. Acta Odontol Scand. 1994;52:7-19.
41. Miles AE. Sebaceous glands in the lip and cheek mucosa of man. Br Dent J. 1958;105:235-48.
42. Oehlers FA. Dens invaginatus. Oral Surg. 1957;10:130-216.
43. Oehlers FA. The radicular variety of dens invaginatus. Oral Surg. 1958;11:1251-60.
44. Padgham ND, Bingham BJ, Purdue BN. Episodic macroglossia in Down's syndrome. J Laryngol Otol. 1990;104:494-6.
45. Papanayotou PH, Hatziotis JC. Ascher's syndrome: report of a case. Oral Surg Oral Med Oral Pathol. 1973;35:467.
46. Patel JR. Transposition and microdontia. Oral Surg Oral Med Oral Pathol. 1993;76:129.
47. Prabhu SR, Daftary DK, Dholakia HM. Chondroectodermal dysplasis (Ellisvan Creveld syndrome): report of two cases. J Oral Surg. 1978;36:631-7.
48. Rhodus NL. An actively secreting Fordyce granule: A case report. Clin Prev Dent. 1986;8:24-6.
49. Ross RB, Johnson MC. Cleft lip and palate. Baltimore: Williams and Wilkins; 1972.
50. Rusmah M. Talon cusp in Malaysia. Aust Dent J. 1991;36:11-4.
51. Sidhu SS, Deshmukh RN. Submucous cleft palate anomaly in India—a hospital based study. J Pierre Fauchard Acad. 1978;1:61-4.
52. Steidler NF, Radden BG, Reade PC. Dentinal dysplasia: a clinicopathological study of eight cases and review of the literature. Br J Oral Maxillofac Surg. 1984;22:274-86.
53. Suckling GW. Developmental defects of enamel: Historical and present day perspective of their pathogenesis. Avd Dent Res. 1989;3:87-94.
54. Sundell S, Koch G. Hereditary amelogenesis imperfecta. Swed Dent J. 1983;9:157-69.
55. Varrela J, Alvesalo L. Taurodontism in females with extra X chromosomes. J Craniofac Genet Dev Biol. 1989;9:129-33.
56. Warden PJ. Ankylossia: a review of the literature. Gen Dent. 1991;39:252-3.
57. Weiss LS, White JA. Macroglossia: A review. J La State Med Soc. 1990;142;13-6.
58. Winter GB, Brook AH. Enamel hypoplasia and anomalies of the enamel. Dent Clin North Am. 1975;19:3-24.
59. Witkop CJ. Clinical aspects of dental anomalies. Int Dent J. 1976;26:378-90.
60. Witkop CJ. Hereditary defects of dentin. Dent Clin North Am. 1975;9:25-45.

CHAPTER 2

Benign and Malignant Neoplasms of the Oral Cavity

NEOPLASM (TUMOR)

DEFINITION

A neoplasm is an abnormal mass of tissue, the growth of which exceeds and is incoordinated with that of the surrounding normal tissues and persists in the same excessive manner after cessation of the stimuli that evoked the change (Rupert Willis 1950).

Important characteristics of a neoplasm:
- Abnormal growth—due to multiplication of cells that cannot be controlled
- Ceaseless—growth of a neoplasm never ends
- Purposeless—it is an unnecessary mass of cells
- Uncoordinated—growth pattern of tissue/cells is far in excess than that of the surrounding normal tissue
- Cessation of stimuli—a neoplasm continues to grow even after the stimulus or the initiating factor is removed.

Neoplasms can occur from virtually any tissue anywhere in the body and the oral cavity is an important location where a large variety of neoplasms often develop with diverse pathogenicity.

The modern classification of oral neoplasms is based primarily on the structural basis or in other words, several neoplastic conditions are put into different categories on the basis of their tissue of origin.

Depending on the pathologic state, the oral neoplasms can be divided into two broad categories or groups, namely:
1. Benign neoplasm
2. Malignant neoplasm

In the following section, we will see how a benign neoplasm may differ clinicopathologically from its malignant counterpart (Table 2.1).

Generally, the benign tumor is designated by attaching the suffix "oma" to the cell type from which it arises. For example, a benign tumor arising from the fibrous tissue is called a "fibroma" while a benign cartilaginous tumor is called a "chondroma". A benign epithelial tumor arising from the gland is known as "adenoma".

A malignant tumor arising from the epithelial tissue is called "carcinoma" and a malignant tumor arising from the connective tissue is known as "sarcoma". Recent literatures have documented about another malignancy, which is called "carcinosarcoma" and it is characterized by simultaneous malignant transformation of both the epithelial and mesenchymal components of the tissue.

LOCAL INVASION

When a tumor penetrates into the adjoining tissues due to its increased rate of growth, it is known as invasion. Most of the malignant tumors as well as few benign tumors show this behavior. Invasion is an important pathological

Table 2.1: Difference between benign and malignant neoplasms.

	Features	Benign	Malignant
On the basis of clinical features	Size of the tumor	Usually small	Usually large
	Rate of growth	Slow	Very fast
	Pain	Absent	Mostly painful
	Hemorrhage	Not usual	Very common
	Ulceration	Absent	Present
	Paresthesia	Does not occur	Commonly occurs
	Induration	Absent	It is often present
	Symptoms	Asymptomatic	Always symptomatic
	Superadded infection	Usually absent	Commonly present
	Necrotic areas	Usually absent	Commonly present
	Metastasis	Usually Absent	Very common
On the basis of histopathologic features	Cell multiplication rate	Slow	Very fast
	Cell maturation	Good	Cells are often immature
	Cell uniformity	Uniform	Irregular size and shape
	Cell morphology	Not changed	Normal cell morphology is lost
	Cell function	Restored	Mostly lost
	Stroma	Almost normal	Exhibits invasion
	Tissue architecture	Intact	Mostly lost or altered
	Capsule	(Resembles normal tissue) Usually present	Absent
Prognosis		Good	Mostly poor

change in any malignant neoplasm, which determines the future course of the neoplasm as well as the prognosis.

METASTASIS

Metastasis can be defined as the distant spread of tumor cells anywhere in the body away from its primary location. This is an important characteristic of the malignant tumor. The tumor which occurs initially is called the primary tumor; while the newly formed tumor developing as a result of metastasis at a distant site is called the metastatic or secondary tumor.

During metastasis, the tumor cells spread either via the lymphatic channels or the blood vessels, besides this, in some cases, the metastatic cells can spread via the nerve sheath or even through other natural tissue spaces. With some exceptions, the carcinomas generally metastasize via lymphatic channels while the sarcomas metastasize via blood vessels.

CLASSIFICATION OF ORAL NEOPLASMS (TUMORS)

In the oral cavity, several types of neoplasms often develop and these entire varieties of neoplastic lesions are broadly divided into two categories:
1. Odontogenic neoplasm and
2. Nonodontogenic neoplasms.

Odontogenic neoplasms: These are a group of neoplastic conditions either benign or malignant, which develop from the dental formative tissues or their remnants.

Nonodontogenic neoplasms: These are the neoplastic lesions, which arise from virtually any tissue in the oral cavity excepting from those arising from the dental formative organs.

The nonodontogenic neoplasms can develop from several tissues like skin or mucous membrane, fibrous connective

Table 2.2: Neoplasms of epithelial tissue origin.

Benign neoplasms	Malignant neoplasms
Papilloma	Basal cell carcinoma
Keratoacanthoma	Squamous cell carcinoma
Pigmented cellular nevus	Verrucous carcinoma
Papillary hyperplasia	• Adenoid squamous cell carcinoma • Adenosquamous cell carcinoma • Malignant melanoma • Spindle cell carcinoma • Primary intra-alveolar carcinoma • Multicentric oral carcinoma

tissue, blood vessels, muscles, bone, cartilage, neural tissue and lymphoid tissue, etc. It is important to remember that unlike the odontogenic neoplasms which can arise only in the oral cavity or its surrounding areas, the nonodontogenic neoplasms are not always confined to the oral region, rather they can develop in other parts of the body as well.

Classification of Oral Nonodontogenic Neoplasms

The neoplasms of epithelial tissue origin and neoplasms of mesenchymal tissue origin are given in Tables 2.2 and 2.3, respectively.

Table 2.3: Neoplasms of mesenchymal tissue origin.

Benign neoplasms	Malignant neoplasms
Neoplasms of fibrous connective tissue	Neoplasms of fibrous connective tissue
Fibroma	Fibrosarcoma
Fibromatosis	Malignant fibrous
Desmoplastic fibroma	Histiocytoma
Pyogenic granuloma	
Fibroepithelial polyp	
Giant cell fibroma	
Peripheral ossifying fibroma	
Central ossifying fibroma	
Peripheral giant cell granuloma	
Central giant cell granuloma	
Benign fibrous histiocytoma	
Nodular fasciitis	
Myxoma	
Neoplasms of adipose tissue	Neoplasms of adipose tissue
Lipoma	Liposarcoma
Angiolipoma	
Neoplasms of vascular tissue	Neoplasms of vascular tissue
Hemangioma	Hemangiopericytoma
Lymphangioma	Hemangioendothelioma
Juvenile angiofibroma	Angiosarcoma
Hereditary hemorrhagic telangiectasia	Kimura's disease
Glomus tumor	

Contd...

Contd...

Benign neoplasms	Malignant neoplasms
Neoplasms of osseous tissue	**Neoplasms of osseous tissue**
Osteoma	Osteosarcoma
Osteomatosis	Parosteal osteosarcoma
Osteoid osteoma	Ewing's sarcoma
Osteoblastoma	
Osteoclastoma	
Torus palatinus	
Torus mandibularis	
Neoplasms of cartilaginous tissue	**Neoplasms of cartilaginous tissue**
Chondroma	Chondrosarcoma
Chondroblastoma	Mesenchymal
Chondromyxoid fibroma	Chondrosarcoma
Neoplasms of neural tissue	**Neoplasms of neural tissue**
Neurolemmoma	Neurosarcoma
Neurofibroma	Olfactory neuroblastoma
Neurofibromatosis	
Multiple endocrine neoplasia syndrome	
Melanotic neuroectodermal tumor of infancy	
Neuroblastoma	
Ganglioneuroma	
Traumatic neuroma	
Plexiform neuroma	
Neoplasms of smooth muscle tissue	**Neoplasms of smooth muscle tissue**
Leiomyoma	Leiomyosarcoma
Angiomyoma	Angiomyosarcoma
Neoplasms of striated muscle tissue	**Neoplasms of striated muscle tissue**
Rhabdomyoma	Rhabdomyosarcoma
Granular cell myoblastoma	
Congenital epulis of newborn	
Neoplasms of lymphoid tissue	**Neoplasms of lymphoid tissue**
No benign neoplasm	Hodgkin's lymphoma
	Non-Hodgkin's lymphoma
	Burkitt's lymphoma
	Mycosis fungoides
	Leukemias
	Multiple myeloma
	Plasmacytoma
Neoplasms of mixed tissue	**Neoplasms of mixed tissue**
Teratoma	
Neoplasms of salivary gland tissue	**Neoplasms of salivary gland tissue**
See the chapter of *Salivary Gland Neoplasm* (Chapter 4)	

BENIGN NEOPLASMS OF THE EPITHELIAL TISSUE ORIGIN

Papilloma

Definition

Papilloma is a common benign neoplasm of the oral cavity, arising from the epithelial tissue. It is characterized by an exophytic papillary growth with a typical "cauliflower like" appearance.

This lesion constitutes about 2% of all oral neoplasms and it is believed by many investigators that they are caused by human papilloma virus (HPV).

HPV virus subtypes 6 and 11 frequently detected from neoplastic tissues of papilloma.

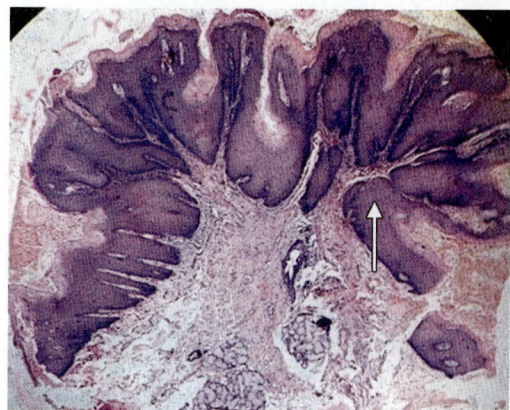

Fig. 2.2: Histopathology of papilloma (low power).

Clinical Features

- *Age*: Any age but mostly third, fourth and fifth decade
- *Sex*: Both sexes are equally affected
- *Site*: Tongue, lips, buccal mucosa, gingiva, hard and soft plate, etc.

Clinical Presentation (Figs. 2.1 and 2.2)

- Clinically, papilloma appears as a slow growing, exophytic, soft, usually pedunculated, painless, nodular growth often with a typical "cauliflower-like" appearance.
- Papillomas often characteristically have numerous finger-like projections on their surface, which can be either blunt or pointed.
- Because of these projections, the papilloma often appears as an ovoid swelling with a rough, corrugated surface.
- The size of the lesion is usually small and that varies from few millimeters to about one centimeter in diameter.
- The base of the lesion can be either pedunculated or sessile (broad based) but papilloma is mostly a well-circumscribed growth.
- The lesion is mostly white in color and is firm in consistency as the surface is highly keratinized.
- On rare occasions, papillomas may grow in an inwardly direction (inverted type) instead of growing in the usual exophytic manner. Such lesions are mostly

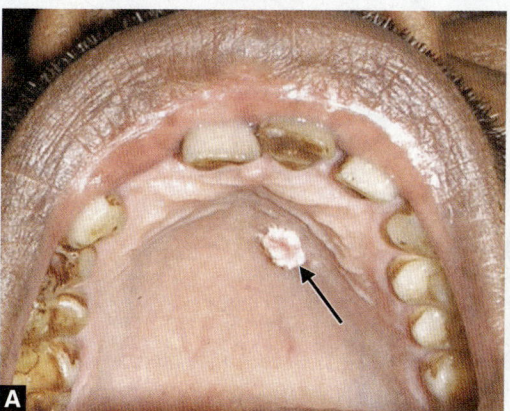
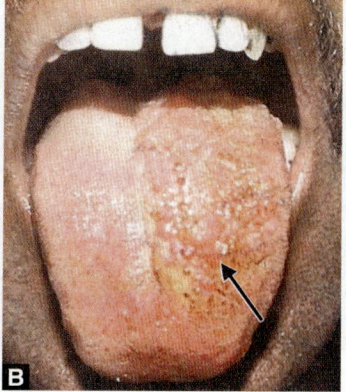

Figs. 2.1A and B: (A) Papilloma on the palate; (B) Papillomatosis of tongue.

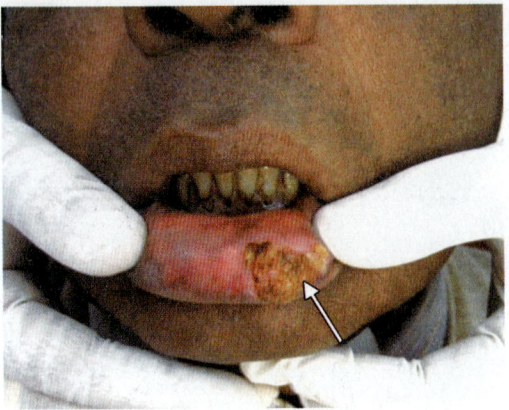

Fig. 2.3: Keratoacanthoma of lower lip.

seen in the lateral nasal wall, paranasal sinuses and in the maxillary antrum, etc. Moreover, they have great tendency for local destruction and malignant transformation.
- Multiple papillomas may sometimes coalesce together and form a large lesion in the oral cavity and the condition is commonly known as "papillomatosis" (Figs. 2.3 and 2.4).
- Papillomatosis of oral mucosa may sometimes occur in association with skin disorders, e.g. focal dermal hypoplasia syndrome, nevus unius lateris, Cowden syndrome and acanthosis nigricans, etc.

Histopathological Features

Microscopically, papillomas present the following features:
- Proliferating keratinized stratified squamous epithelium in the form of multiple fingers-like projections.
- Every single finger-like projection has a fibrovascular connective tissue core in the center, which contains few inflammatory cells.
- The covering squamous epithelium shows hyperkeratosis and acanthosis. Thickening of the keratin is seen in lesions which are clinically whiter.
- In the spinous cell layer "koilocytes" are sometimes seen, these are virus-altered epithelial clear cells with small dark (pyknotic) nuclei surrounded by clear halos.
- There can be little cellular atypia in some papillomas, however, the dysplastic changes in the epithelium is rarely found.
- Papilloma is not a premalignant lesion and malignant transformation in preexisting oral papillomas has not been documented.

Differential Diagnosis

- Verruca vulgaris
- Focal dermal hyperplasia
- Verruciform xanthoma
- Verrucous carcinoma
- Condyloma acuminatum.

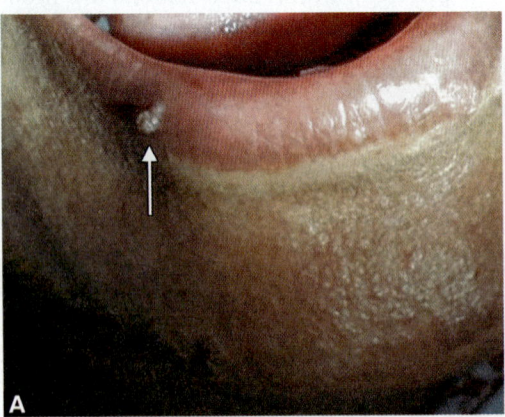
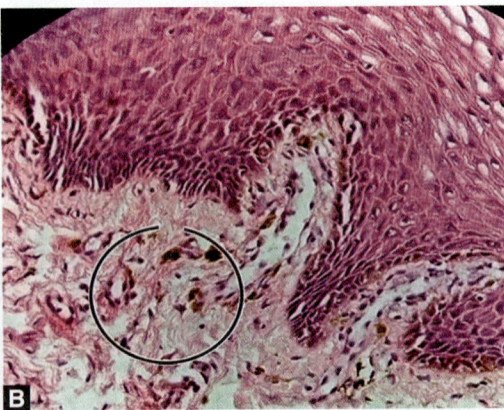

Figs. 2.4A and B: (A) Nevus on the lip; (B) Nevus cells.

Treatment
Conservative surgical excision of the lesion including the base is the common treatment. Recurrence is rare.

Keratoacanthoma (Self-healing Cancer)
Definition
Keratoacanthoma is a benign endophytic epithelial tissue neoplasm with profound clinical and histological resemblance to well-differentiated squamous cell carcinoma (SCC). It commonly occurs in the sun-exposed skin of the face and it usually appears as a circumscribed keratin filled crater.

Origin
Keratoacanthoma of the skin surfaces probably develops from the hair follicles above the sebaceous glands.

On the mucosal surfaces these lesions are extremely rare but if they occur at all, they probably develop from the superficial epithelium of the sebaceous ducts.

Causes
- Chronic sun exposure
- HPV infection (especially types—9, 11, 13, 16, 18, 25, 33, 37 and d5)
- Immunosuppression
- *Heredity*: Chromosomal aberrations such as gains on 8q, 1p, and 9q with deletions on 3p, 9p, 19p, and 19q.
- Trauma.

Clinical Features
- *Age*: Middle-aged adults are frequently affected between the age group of 50 years and 70 years
- *Sex*: Male to female ratio in this tumor is about 2:1
- *Site*: Keratoacanthoma chiefly develops over the sun-exposed skin surface of the lips (both upper and lower lips) near the outer edge of vermilion border. Besides this, the lesion can also occur on the cheeks, nose, eyelids and ear. Intraoral lesions of keratoacanthoma are rare, although few have been reported in the palate and gingiva.

Presentation (Fig. 2.3)
- Keratoacanthoma initially begins as a small, red macule that soon turns into a well-circumscribed, elevated and umbilicated, crater-like lesion with a central depression.
- The lesion is firm, painless and sessile in nature; and can be single or multiple in number.
- The fully developed lesion of keratoacanthoma clinically presents a well-circumscribed, elevated nodule, which has a sharply delineated, rolled margin and a central keratotic core.
- Clinically, the outer surface of the lesion shows normal skin color or slight erythema, while the central keratin plug appears yellow, brown or black with an irregular crusted appearance.
- The disease is often painful and sometimes it may have an associated lymphadenopathy.

Stages of Development of Keratoacanthoma
- *Growth phase*: The lesion initiates as a small lump or a bud like growth on the sun-exposed skin surface of the face, it grows rapidly and achieves the maximum size (1–2 cm in diameter) over a period of about 4–8 weeks.
- *Stationary phase*: After the initial growth, the disease remains static for an indefinite period of up to 4–8 weeks and then it starts to regress spontaneously.
- *Involution phase*: Within the next 6–12 months time, the lesion regresses completely leaving only a small depressed scar.

Muir–Torre syndrome: Gastrointestinal carcinoma, keratoacanthoma, and sebaceous neoplasm.

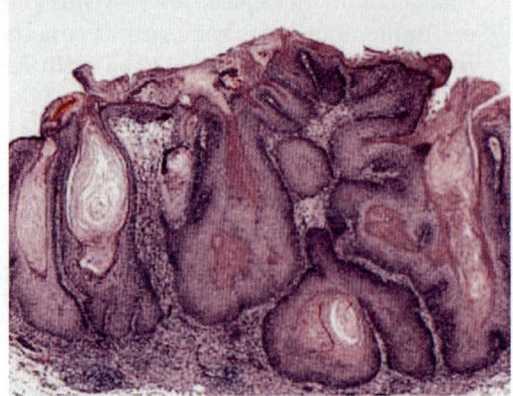

Fig. 2.5: Photomicrograph of keratoacanthoma.

Histopathology (Fig. 2.5)

- Keratoacanthoma clinically and histologically appears very similar to well-differentiated SCC and because of this, it is often known as "self-healing" cancer (Box 2.1).
- The cells appear mature and often there is individual cell keratinization and even keratin pearl formation in the tumor.
- The lesion consists of a thick hyperkeratinized covering epithelium with a central zone of keratin or parakeratin plugging.
- Pseudoepitheliomatous hyperplasia may be observed in some cases.
- Pathognomonic nonmalignant feature of this neoplasm can be identified at the margin, where the lesion shows a crater-like area, plugged with keratin and is surrounded by hyperplastic normal epithelium.
- This abrupt transition of the normal surrounding epithelium at the margin of the crater-like area is an important diagnostic clue for keratoacanthoma.
- Although, keratoacanthomas are benign and self-limiting conditions, serial sectioning is always required of the available tissue sample for confirmation of the diagnosis.
- Moreover, careful long-term follow-up evaluations are necessary since the neoplasm is often confused with SCC.

Differential Diagnosis

- Basal cell carcinoma
- Squamous cell carcinoma.

Treatment

Surgical excision is the treatment of choice for keratoacanthoma, usually before the lesion reaches its maximum size of 2–2.5 cm diameter. Waiting for spontaneous regression of the lesion is not advisable for the following reasons:

- Confusion with SCC
- The scar developing after spontaneous regression is depressed and cosmetically unacceptable
- Surgical treatment always provides good tissue specimen for confirmation of the diagnosis.

Pigmented Cellular Nevus

Definition of Nevus

The term "nevus" has got several meanings; in *Latin* nevus means birth marks, however, the common lay term used for nevus is "mole". A nevus can be defined as a congenital, developmental, tumor-like malformation of the skin or mucous membrane; which are often present at birth or they can be seen any time after birth (Box 2.2).

Oral nevi are much rarer than their cutaneous counterparts with a prevalence of 0.1% among the general population; Women are affected twice as common as men and most cases are seen in the third and fourth decades. In the mouth these are commonly seen in the hard palate, buccal and labial mucosa.

Box 2.1 The distinction between keratoacanthoma and squamous cell carcinoma.

- The epithelium in this neoplasm exhibits a pseudocarcinomatous rather than a true carcinomatous growth pattern
- Dyskeratosis is always absent in keratoacanthoma
- The epithelium is composed of well-differentiated spinous cells with abundant cytoplasm, minimal nuclear pleomorphism, infrequent mitotic figures and no abnormal mitosis

Benign and Malignant Neoplasms of the Oral Cavity

> **Box 2.2** Different types of nevi.
> - Intradermal (intramucosal) nevus
> - Junctional nevus
> - Compound nevus
> - Blue nevus
> - Halo nevus (halo mole)

Nevus is composed of "nevus cells" which are neuroectodermal in origin, these cells, except for their tendency to form cell nests and their less prominent dendritic processes, are nothing but melanocytes or their precursors. After their formation, nevus cells migrate through the peripheral nerves and finally reach to the basal layer of the skin or mucous membrane (*See* Figs. 2.4A and B).

The function of nevus cells is to produce melanin, this pigment, after being synthesized within the nevus cells is passed on to the adjacent keratinocytes of the oral mucous membrane.

Intradermal (Intramucosal) Nevus

The term intradermal nevus and intramucosal nevus are synonymous, the former occurs on the skin surfaces while the later occurs over the mucous membrane.

Clinical Features

- Intradermal nevus is a very common lesion of the skin (comprise more than 50% of all types of nevi) and it usually occurs in children
- This lesion is often referred to as common "mole"
- Intradermal nevus clinically appears as a raised or flat area on the skin surface, with a typical tan or dark brown color
- The mucosal lesions clinically appear as asymptomatic, slightly elevated papules or flat macules with a pigmented surface
- The color of these nevi varies from brown to black
- The intraoral lesions are often slow growing and their size is usually less than 1 cm in diameter.

Histopathology

- Microscopically intramucosal nevus reveals clusters or nests of nevus cells which are confined within the connective tissue.
- The cells may appear as epithelioid cells or lymphocyte like cells; however few cells may be even spindle-shaped.
- Multiple multinucleated giant cells may be found in some cases.
- Intramucosal nevus often characteristically presents a narrow zone of connective tissue devoid of nevus cells, which separates the zone of nevus cells from the overlying epithelium.
- The amount of melanin produced by these nevus cells varies; some cells are heavily pigmented whereas other cells are almost nonpigmented.

Treatment

Intramucosal nevi usually do not require any treatment. However, when these lesions are subjected to persistent trauma during mastication, surgical excision should be preferred. Once excised, they usually do not recur.

Junctional Nevus

Clinical Features

- Junctional nevus is usually a less common variety as compared to the intradermal nevus.
- It appears as an asymptomatic, brown or black macule, affecting both skin as well as the oral mucosal surfaces.
- Intraorally these lesions are commonly seen over the hard palate and gingiva.

Histopathology

- Histologically, junctional nevus reveals focal areas of proliferating nevus cells or in some cases clusters of cells at the basement membrane zone of the epithelium.
- The cluster of nevus cells is often specifically present at the apex of the epithelial rete-pegs.

Treatment

Junctional nevus should be excised surgically. Postsurgical recurrence is uncommon.

Compound Nevus

The compound nevus characteristically presents the combined features of intradermal nevus and the junctional nevus.

Clinical Features

- This lesion occurs far more commonly in skin as compared to the oral mucosa
- Intraorally they appear as pigmented papules or macules over the hard palate or the gingiva.

Histopathology

Microscopically, compound nevus reveals the presence of nevus cells, which are distributed both in the basal layer of the epithelium as well as in the adjacent superficial connective tissue.

Treatment

Surgical excision is the treatment of choice for compound nevus.

Blue Nevus

Blue nevus is a relatively common pigmented lesion of the oral cavity.
- Two major types are recognized—(1) the common blue nevus and (2) the cellular blue nevus.
- The common blue nevus is the second most frequent melanocytic nevus encountered in the mouth.

Clinical Features

- Clinically, it often appears either as a dome-shaped, dark blue papule or as a flat pigmented macule over the skin or the oral mucous membrane.
- Intraoral blue nevi are commonly seen on the mucosal surfaces of the hard palate.

Histopathology

- Instead of being round or epithelioid in shape, the cells of blue nevus are usually elongated, bipolar and spindle-shaped.
- Sometimes, fusiform dendritic cells can also be present in these lesions.
- The spindle-shaped cells are mostly oriented parallel to the overlying epithelium and are not arranged in clusters.
- Few pigmented macrophages may be present among these dendritic nevus cells and they are known as "melanophages".

Treatment

Blue nevus often clinically resembles a melanoma and therefore surgical excision of the lesion with subsequent histopathological evaluation blue nevi do not have much tendency to undergo malignant transformation.

Halo Mole (Halo Nevus)

It is a peculiar nevus on the skin, which characteristically has a white ring around it; (also known as Sutton nevus or leukoderma aquisitum centrifugum) (Fig. 2.6).

It develops like any other nevus of the skin with the typical nevus cell being present in it, but later on, an autoimmune reaction develops against the nevus to destroy it, and there is activation of cytotoxic T lymphocytes, which start destroying the nevus cells. The white ring is

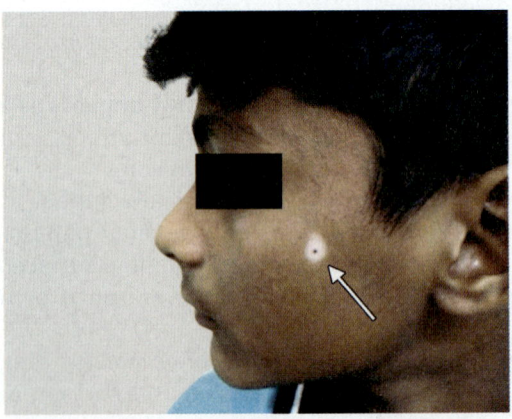

Fig. 2.6: Halo nevus on the facial skin.

> **Box 2.3** Symptoms of malignant transformation in a preexisting nevus.
>
> - Sudden faster rate of growth
> - Size becoming much more than 5 mm in diameter
> - Asymmetric growth pattern
> - Irregular border of the lesion
> - Sudden change of color (becoming darker in color).
> - Development of surface ulceration and pain (sometimes)
>
> *(Histopathological confirmation is always required)*

created due to the elimination of the pigmented cells at the periphery of the nevus (Box 2.3).

MALIGNANT NEOPLASMS OF THE EPITHELIAL TISSUE ORIGIN

Squamous Cell Carcinoma

Definition

Squamous cell carcinoma is the most common malignant epithelial tissue neoplasm of the oral cavity, which is derived from the stratified squamous epithelium. Since oral SCCs constitute bulk of the oral malignancies (above 90%) it is thus commonly referred to as oral cancer (although there are several other malignancies of the oral cavity besides SCC).

Epidemiology

- SCC is also termed as epidermoid carcinoma and it is by far the most common malignant neoplasm of the oral cavity.
- The incidence of oral SCC varies in different countries and also in different population groups. It represents the eleventh most common cancer in males and the sixteenth most common in females.
- On an average, oral SCCs represent about 3% of all cancers in males and about 2% of all cancers in females.
- This disease is responsible for 2% of all annual deaths in males and 1% of all annual deaths in females.
- The incidence of oral cancer varies in different countries depending upon the frequency of tobacco usage and other related habits throughout the world.
- The general trend indicates that the incidence of oral SCC increases alarmingly in the societies, where extensive tobacco use begins in the early life and is continued for a longer period.
- The incidence of oral SCC increases with age and most of the cases occur usually after the age of 40 years.
- Although, oral SCCs can arise from virtually any intraoral site, but they develop more frequently from the lower lip, lateral borders of the tongue, buccal mucosa and floor of the mouth, etc.
- According to this ICD classification, oral cancers are numerically categorized in the following manner:
  - Lip cancer–ICD No. 140
  - Tongue cancer–ICD No. 141
  - Cancer of the gingiva and alveolar mucosa–ICD No. 143
  - Cancer of the floor of the mouth–ICD No. 144
  - Cancer of other parts of the mouth–ICD No. 145.
- The annual age-adjusted incidence rates of oral cancer per 100,000 (one lakh) population varies from continents to continents, from countries to countries and also from places to places within the same country.
- In Europe, it varies from 2.0, in UK to 9.4, in France, in USA it varies from 4.4, in Columbia to 13.4 in Canada.
- In Asia, the annual incidence rates of oral cancer per 100,000 population vary from 1.6 in Japan to as high as 13.5 in India.
- In Sri Lanka, the oral cancers constitute about 40% of all malignancies.
- In the Manipuri districts in India, the annual incidence rate of oral cancer is about 21.4 per 100,000 population (Wahi 1968).
- Survey among textile mill workers in Ahmedabad (Gujarat), India, indicates that

- the average incidence rate of oral cancer among individuals above 35 years of age is 25 per 100,000 population (Malaowalla et al.).
- Recent trends besides few exceptions indicate that the incidence and mortality rates of oral cancer are declining and it can be due to the reduced exposure to various etiological agents.

Etiology of Oral Cancer

A large number of etiological factors have been implicated in the development of oral cancer, specifically the oral SCCs, these include the following:
- Tobacco smoking
  - Cigarettes
  - Beedies
  - Pipes
  - Cigars
  - Reverse smoking
- Use of smokeless tobacco
  - Snuff dipping
  - Tobacco sachets (*Gutkha*)
  - Tobacco chewing
  - Tobacco as a toothpaste
- Consumption of alcohol
  - Drinking spirits
  - Drinking wines
  - Drinking beers
  - Tobacco and alcohol synergism (smoking and chewing tobacco with drinking of alcohol)
- Diet and nutrition
  - Vitamin A, B-complex and C deficiency
  - Nutritional deficiency with alcoholism
- Dental factors
  - Chronic irritation from broken teeth
  - Ill-fitting or broken prosthesis
- Radiations
  - Actinic radiation, X-ray radiation
- Viral infections
  - Herpes simplex virus (HSV)
  - Human papilloma virus (HPV)
  - Human immunodeficiency virus (HIV)
  - Epstein-Barr virus (EBV)
- Immunosuppression
  - AIDS
  - Organ transplants
- Chronic infections
  - Candidiasis
  - Syphilis
- Occupational hazards
  - Woolen textile workers
- Genetic factors
  - Oncogenes
  - Tumor-suppressor genes
- Preexisting oral diseases
  - Lichen planus
  - Plummer–Vinson syndrome
  - Oral submucous fibrosis
  - Leukoplakia
  - Discoid lupus erythematosus.

Role of Tobacco in Oral Cancer

- One person dies in every 10 seconds in the world due to the use of tobacco.
- Epidemiological and experimental studies categorically indicate that tobacco plays an important role in the development oral cancer.
- Tobacco is used in various smoking forms such as cigarettes, cigars, pipes and *beedies*, etc.
- It can also be used in smokeless forms like paan-beetel quid, snuff, tobacco sachets (*khaini*), *zarda* and other popular forms.

Factors Influencing the Carcinogenic Effect of Tobacco

- Frequency of smoking—number of cigarette or Pipe used per day (smoking 40 or more cigarettes per day increases 10–20 times more cancer risk).
- Duration of smoking—habit continued for how many years.
- Age of beginning of the habit—smoking from a younger age has more risk.
- Composition of tobacco—variation in tar, nicotine and nitrosamine content, e.g. "beedi" (country made cigarette) is made up of crude form of tobacco containing more harmful chemicals and it has no filter.

- Manufacturing technique of tobacco—curing technique used by the manufacturer.
- Species of tobacco—different species content different amount of nicotine.
- Method of smoking technique used by the patient—conventional smoking or reverse smoking (if burning end of the cigarette is kept inside the mouth while smoking; the heat inside mouth from burning cigarette cause damage to mucosa and is an additional risk factor besides the effect of tobacco). Conventional smokers have more cancer risk than nonsmokers while reverse smokers have even more risk than conventional smokers.
- Additional habits—cancer risk increases significantly is smoking is coupled with other habits especially alcohol (tobacco-alcohol synergism).

Mechanism of Action of Tobacco in Carcinogenesis

There are about 300 carcinogens found in tobacco smoke, which include: aromatic hydrocarbon benzopyrene and tobacco specific nitrosamines (TsNs), N-nitrosonornicotine (NNN), N-nitrosopyrrolidine (NPYR), N-nitrosodimethylamine (NDMA), etc. In our body these carcinogenic agents produce DNA adduct (it is a piece of DNA covalently bonded to a cancer causing chemical) called O-6-methylguanine, which interferes with the DNA replication and thereby cause mutation. Mutations open the floodgate of molecular chain of events leading eventually to carcinogenic change in cells.

Research indicates that excessive use of tobacco, heavy consumption of alcohol and poor diet together cause increased incidence of oral cancer.

Smokeless Tobacco-betel Quid (Paan) and Other Chewing Habits

- Chewing of paan is a popular habit all over the world and it is practiced by over 200 million people in different countries.
- This habit is particularly more common in Southeast Asia and India.
- *Paan* is made up of several ingredients like betel nut, lime, tobacco, catechu and other spices, which are wrapped within a betel leaf.
- The carcinogenic effect of paan chewing could be due to the presence of tobacco as one of its main ingredients (Fig. 2.7).
- Moreover, the possible interactions between different ingredients of *paan* may results in the formation of some chemicals which might be harmful, for example, shaked lime used in pan may hydrolyze one of the alkaloids of the betel nut called arecoline to produce arecoidene, the later is experimentally proved to be carcinogenic.
- The habit of placing a mixture of tobacco and lime (commonly known as *khaini*) in oral vestibule is a popular practice in India and Pakistan, which contributes to the occurrence of large number of oral and oropharyngeal cancer cases.
- Tobacco users can develop oral cancers in their mouth either as direct lesions (de novo lesions) or such habits may result in the development of precancerous lesions in their mouth like oral submucous fibrosis or leukoplakia, etc. which may turn into malignancy in future, if the habits are continued for long.

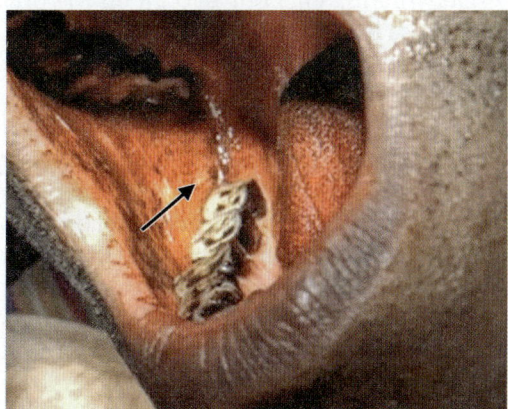

Fig. 2.7: Mucosal changes due to "*paan*" chewing.

Alcohol

- Several epidemiological studies have indicated about alcohol as a possible risk factor for oral cancer.
- Both the quantity and quality of alcohol consumed and duration of the habit are crucial factors in this regard. People consuming more amount of alcohol per day, for more number of years will have an increased risk for developing oral cancer than others.
- Inferior quality of the alcohol also increases the risk of oral cancer since these liquors may contain some carcinogenic byproducts.
- Many studies have shown a marked increase in the relative risk of oral cancer when smoking and drinking are practiced together, suggesting a synergistic effect.

Mechanism of Action of Alcohol in Carcinogenesis

- Alcohol acts as a solvent and breaks down the bigger particles of tobacco; thereby facilitates penetration of carcinogens (especially nitrosonornicotine) across the oral mucous membrane.
- Alcohol can cause atrophic change in the oral mucosa, thus make the tissue more vulnerable to the effect of other carcinogenic agents.
- Dehydrating effect of alcohol on the oral mucosa increases the risk of tissue injury, which may further enhance the risk of cancer.
    - Long-term alcoholic habit often produces cirrhosis of liver; this disease in turn increases the risk of oral cancers since the damaged liver cannot detoxify the carcinogenic chemicals in the blood.
- Chronic alcoholics from poor socioeconomic status often fail to get adequate nutritious food (as financial resources are limited and more of it being drained toward the addiction). This in the long run causes lack of immunity with more risk of cancer.

Diet and Nutrition

- Iron deficiency anemia often causes dysphagia, glossitis and atrophy of the oral mucosa; these changes may increase the risk of malignant transformation of oral mucosa in presence of other carcinogenic agents.
- Deficiencies of certain dietary factors like vitamin A, D, C and E, etc. may cause atrophy of the oral epithelium and thereby make the tissue more vulnerable to various carcinogenic agents.
- Fresh fruits and vegetables (rich in carotene) provide increased protection against cancer of the mouth, pharynx and larynx, etc.
- Deficiency of certain trace elements like zinc, manganese, magnesium and molybdenum, etc. disturbs the structural integrity of the oral epithelial tissue, as a result of which, the epithelium becomes more vulnerable to the free radical injury. The later may cause development of oral cancer.

Dental Factors

- Ill-fitting dentures, poor oral hygiene, faulty restorations, sharp or broken teeth, etc. cause persistent irritation and trauma to the oral mucosa and therefore may act as possible predisposing factors in this development of oral cancer.
- Moreover, carcinogenic potential of tobacco and/or alcohol may be increased significantly in the presence of these orodental factors.
- Chronic oral sepsis is another important contributing factor in the development of oral cancer.

Ultraviolet Radiation

- Ultraviolet radiation (UV rays) are part of the "sunrays" and are believed to be responsible for the development of carcinoma of the skin and lips. This type of cancer happens more in fair-skinned people, especially those who are engaged in outdoor activities (both recreational and professional) of longer

durations, e.g. farming, forestry, postal delivery, outdoor games and fishing, etc.
- UV ray induced carcinomas are less common among the black or the brown skinned people; it is mainly because of two reasons:
  - *Their skin is more protected by heavy melanin pigmentations.*
  - *Outdoor recreational activities are less due to extremely hot weather conditions.*
- Lip cancer is the most common lesion caused by ultraviolet radiation; the lesion often begins as "solar keratosis" (a type of premalignant lesion) on the lip, near the vermilion border. If left untreated these lesions may gradually turn into SCCs.

Ionizing Radiation

Squamous cell carcinoma may develop in those areas of the oral cavity, which were exposed to long-term radiation therapy in the past.

Viruses

It is often believed that the oncogenic viruses can initiate oncogenesis by altering the DNA and the chromosomal structure of the infected cells and also by inducing some proliferative changes in the host cells.

The common viruses which might be having some oncogenic potential are as follows:
- Human papilloma virus
- Herpes simplex virus
- Epstein-Barr virus
- Human immunodeficiency virus.

Immunosuppression

- Immunosuppression may be associated with an increased risk of oral cancer and it can be seen in patients with HIV infection, who often develop Kaposi sarcoma and oral SCC.
- HIV infected patients often develop oral cancers at an early age (as compared to the normal age of occurrence for these tumors) and moreover, these tumors develop without the presence of any tobacco or alcohol related habits.
- Increased risk of oral cancers has been reported in patients receiving immunosuppressive drugs following renal or other organ transplant treatments.

Chronic Oral Infections

Candidiasis:
- Chronic oral candidiasis may occur in association with leukoplakia, the later disease often undergoes malignant transformation.
- It is believed that candidal infections probably act as cofactors in the transformation of oral premalignant lesions into oral SCCs.

Syphilis: Tertiary syphilis has often been linked with oral SCCs, particularly the lip or tongue lesions. Studies indicate that long standing syphilitic infections may cause atrophy of the oral epithelium and thus increases the carcinogenic effects of tobacco, alcohol and other agents.

Atmospheric Pollution

Vehicular and industrial exhausts contain excessive amount of harmful chemicals, e.g. sulfur, nitrogen, carbon monoxide, carbon dioxide and several hydrocarbons; these agents increase the risk of oral cancer among people living in cities or in industrial areas.

Occupational Hazards

Exposure to hazardous chemicals such as nitrosamines and polycyclic aromatic hydrocarbons, etc. make people susceptible to oral cancers.

The people of the following profession or trade are often considered to be in high-risk category:
- Textile workers those who are regularly exposed to particles created by the initial carding of raw cotton wool are especially at risk for this disease.

- People working in rubber, asbestos, woods or chemical industries.
- People in printing trade and others who may be regularly exposed to gas and soot.
- Heavy metal factory workers.

Genetic Factor (Oncogenes and Tumor Suppressor Genes)

Oral cancers occur due to the uncontrolled neoplastic proliferation of cells as a result of some abnormal genetic activity.

It is a multi-step event involving multiple sequential mutations to the genes, which regulate the system of cell growth and cell multiplication.

Oncogenes

- The specific gene loci responsible for producing proteins that can upset the normal replication cycle of cells are known as "oncogenes". When oncogenes are stimulated to overproduce proteins that stimulate the process of mitosis, the result is neoplastic growth.
- Alteration in the oncogene activity may be associated with environmental factors such as tobacco habits, alcohol, radiation hazards, nutritional deficiency and chronic infections, etc.

Tumor Suppressor Genes

- These are suppressor gene loci responsible for producing proteins, which can stop or control unnecessary cell cycling.
- Neoplastic growths can occur if there is deactivation of these tumor suppressor genes.
- Most commonly mutated gene in cancer cell is *p53*.

Preexisting Oral Lesions

There can be few oral lesions, from which oral SCCs may sometimes develop and these lesions include the following:
- Erythroplakia
- Oral submucous fibrous
- Oral lichen planus
- Oral leukoplakia
- Plummer–Vinsons syndrome
- Epidermolysis bullosa
- Discoid lupus erythematosus
- Xenoderma pigmentosum.

Clinical Features of Oral Squamous Cell Carcinoma

- *Age*: Carcinomas mostly occur in the older age while sarcomas occur in the younger age. 4th, 5th, 6th and 7th decade of life is the common age range for oral SCC.
- *Sex*: The disease affects male people more after than the females and it happens because male people are more frequently exposed to the various deleterious oral habits.
- *Sites*: The incidence of oral SCCs in various anatomic locations is significantly different, some oral sites are relatively immune to the disease while other sites are particularly more prone to it. Among all oral anatomic areas, lower lip is the most common site, the second most common site is the lateral borders of the tongue. Among all intraoral sites, dorsum of the tongue and hard palate are the least common sites for oral SCC.

Relative incidence of squamous cell carcinoma in various oral sites: Taking into account of the incidence rates of cancer in different intraoral sites given in Table 2.4, a horse-shoe shaped imaginary zone can be drowned, which will indicate the more prone oral sites for this disease. The zone includes the following areas—anterior floor of the mouth, lateral borders of the tongue, tonsillar pillars and lateral part of soft palate.

Clinical Presentation of Oral Squamous Cell Carcinoma

Oral SCC has a number of different clinical features depending upon its location and its duration of presence.
- The most common early appearance of oral SCC could be extensive oral leukoplakia and erythroplakia.

Benign and Malignant Neoplasms of the Oral Cavity

Table 2.4: Relative incidence of squamous cell carcinoma in various oral sites.

Site		Relative incidence
Lower lip		35%
Lateral/ventral tongue		25%
Floor of the mouth		20%
Soft palate (near the tonsillar pillars)		15%
Gingiva/alveolar ridge		4%
Buccal mucosa (above occlusal line)		1%

- The initial lesion may also present an asymptomatic, white or red, variegated patch or a nodule or fissure over the oral mucosa.
- Initially the condition is usually painless and quite innocuous looking; however an early biopsy often reveals the real nature of this disease.
- More advanced lesions present either as a fast enlarging, exophytic or invasive ulcer or sometimes as a large tumor mass or a verrucous growth.

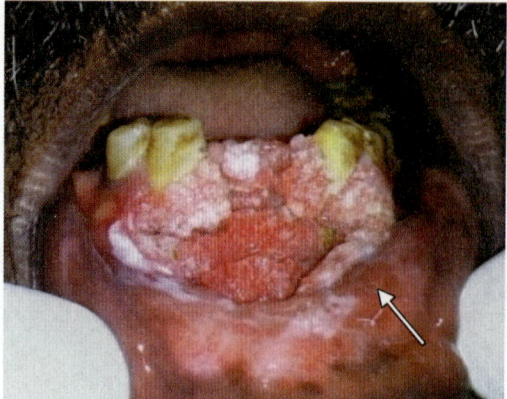

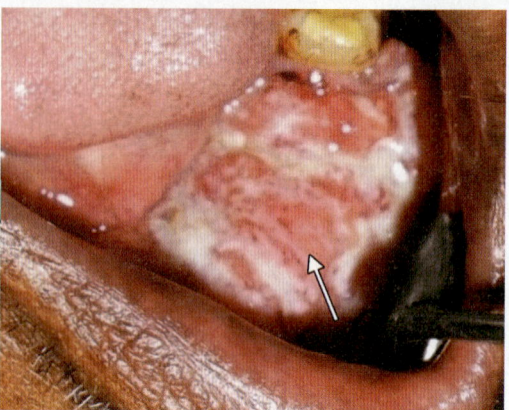

Fig. 2.8: Carcinoma showing indurated and everted ulcer.

Fig. 2.9: Carcinoma in floor of the mouth with superadded candidal infection.

- The ulcerated lesion often shows *persistent induration* around the periphery with an *elevated and everted margin (Fig. 2.8)*.
- The induration (hardness at the border of the lesion on palpation) is caused by infiltration of the tumor cells deep into the surrounding tissues.
- Moreover the elevated and everted margin of the lesion occurs due to an increased rate of growth of the malignant epithelial cells (because of the extensive mitosis) as compared to the surrounding normal epithelium.
- In many cases, there is presence of superadded candidal infections due to decreased immune response of the affected individual (Fig. 2.9).
- The lesion can be painful either due to secondary infection or due to involvement of the peripheral nerves by the tumor cells.
- The lesion can also bleed easily due to increased vascularity (tumor angiogenesis) and surface ulceration.
- Floor of the mouth lesions often cause fixation of the tongue to the underlying structures causing difficulty in speech and inability to open the mouth (trismus).
- When malignant tumor cells invade into the alveolar bone of either maxilla or mandible, they effectively cause resorption of the bone leading to mobility or exfoliation of regional teeth.
- In mandibular lesions, involvement of inferior alveolar nerve often causes paresthesia of the lower teeth and the lower lip.
- Tumor cells often spread to the regional lymph nodes and the affected nodes become enlarged, tender and fixed; some of these nodes can be stony hard in consistency as well.
- In squamous cell carcinoma, the first affected lymph node is called the "sentinel lymph node" (Fig. 2.10).

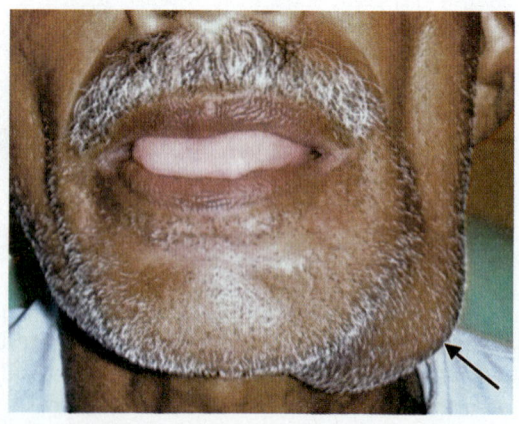

Fig. 2.10: Carcinoma spreading into the submandibular lymph node.

- In oral SCC, enlarged lymph nodes do not always indicate metastatic spread of the tumor cells, since this enlargement of lymph nodes may also represent only nonspecific reactive hyperplasias.
- Extensive maxillary lesions may often invade into the maxillary antrum, which often results in nasal bleeding (epistaxis) and pressure sensation in the eyeball.
- Untreated lesions of SCC may sometimes destroy the oral tissues and extend into the skin on the outer surface of the face to produce a nodular or lobulated growth on the facial skin, which appears as an extraoral discharging sinus (Fig. 2.11).
- Involvement of facial skin is significant in SCC, since it indicates a very poor prognosis of the tumor.
- Long standing oral SCCs also produce severe facial disfigurement, difficulty in taking food (dysphagia) and difficulty in phonation, etc.
- Pathological fracture (fracture occurring in a bone due any pathological condition weakening it) of the jaw bone may sometimes occur in untreated cases due to extensive destruction of the bone by the tumor.
- Untreated patients mostly die of cachexia, hemorrhage, secondary infections, aspiration bronchopneumonia and multiorgan failure, etc.

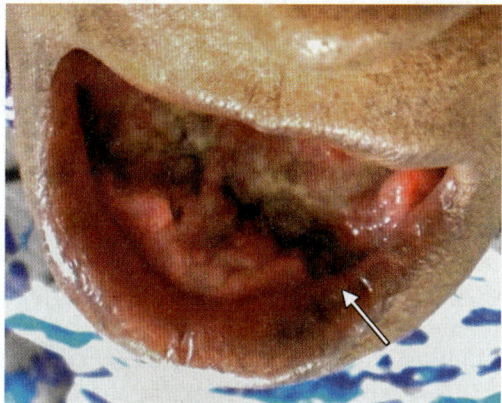

Fig. 2.11: Carcinoma causing destructive, infiltrative growth.

Special Aspects of Oral Cancer

Multiple cancer: Multiple cancer refers to the condition in which a patient develops cancer in multiple organs of the body at a time. For example, a patient with oral SCC may also have cancer of the small intestine, cancer in the lung and in the kidney, etc.

Multicentric cancer: Multicentric cancer means occurrence of two or more separate malignant lesions within a single organ or area of the body, which develop either concurrently (synchronous) or subsequently (metachronous). For example, a patient with tongue cancer may also separately have cancer of the lip or of the buccal mucosa or soft palate, etc. All these malignant lesions may occur either simultaneously or they can develop at certain time intervals.

Oral multicentric cancers probably occur as a result of the phenomenon called "field cancerization", in which a large wide area of the oral epithelium becomes vulnerable to cancer either by itself or by the influence of certain carcinogenic agents.

Key Points of Squamous Cell Carcinoma

- Fast enlarging, exophytic swelling or a large ulcer, which does not respond to conventional therapies.
- Few lesions may appear as extensive leukoplakic or erythroplakic patches.
- The ulcer is indurated or everted, painful and bleeds frequently.
- Difficulty in speech, difficulty in taking food and difficulty in opening the mouth.
- Regional lymph nodes are enlarged, tendered, and are often fixed.
- Regional teeth are often mobile and these can exfoliate spontaneously.
- Regional lymph nodes are often enlarged, tendered and fixed; sometimes they can be "stony hard".
- Most of the lesions exhibit superadded candidal infections.
- There may be anesthesia or paresthesia of the affected area.
- Severe weakening of the jawbone with occasional pathological fractures.
- Long standing lesions may spread extraorally by perforating the facial skin.
- Maxillary lesions can invade the antrum and cause pain, swelling and nasal bleeding, etc.

Oral Cancer in Different Intraoral Locations or Subsites

Separate descriptions of oral SCCs occurring at different intraoral sites may be necessary since this can help in gathering reliable informations regarding variations in the etiology, clinical features and prognosis of the disease.

Carcinoma of the Lip

- Squamous cell carcinoma of the lip accounts for about 30–40% of all oral cancers and in most of the cases, it is caused by actinic radiation.
- Carcinomas of the lip (Figs. 2.12A and B) account for about 12% of all head and neck cancers and about 21.5% of all intraoral cancers.
- The lesion occurs more commonly among males as compared to females (uncommon

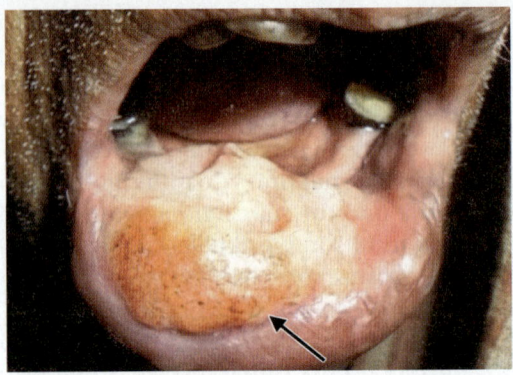

Fig. 2.13: Carcinoma of the lip.

in females) and most often the patients are in their fifth to eighth decade of life. However, several cases are also found in young patients below 40 years of age.
- Among the lip carcinomas (Fig. 2.13), the lower lip is affected in about 85–95% cases; the upper lip is affected in only about 2–7% cases, while the vermilion border is affected in about 1–4% cases.
- The lesions are mostly preceded by the presence of long standing keratotic leukoplakia or actinic cheilitis, etc. which are characterized by innocuous looking white plaques on the lip.
- The ulcer spreads diffusely and the lip becomes everted; and later on the ulcer develops a rolled border with induration of the surrounding tissue.
- Pain, bleeding and paresthesia are common features of lip carcinoma, moreover patient often have difficulty in speech, difficulty in taking food and inability to close the mouth.
- Most lesions in lip carcinoma are small and measure about below 2 cm in diameter; however some lesions can be extremely large, which extend either to the facial skin in the adjacent area or to the underlying connective tissue or bone.
- Lip carcinomas are slow to metastasize, however long standing, untreated cases may metastasize to submental lymph nodes and also to the submandibular nodes.

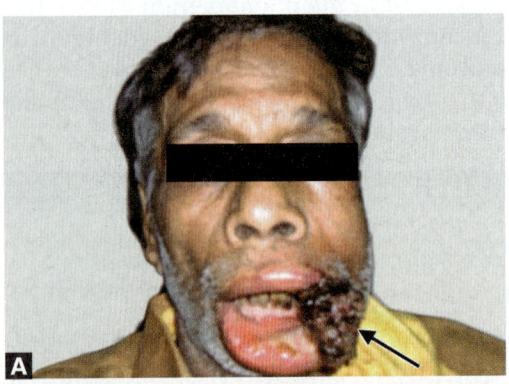
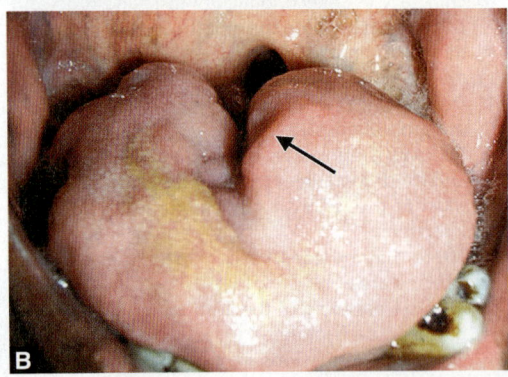

Figs. 2.12A and B: (A) Squamous cell carcinoma causing a massive extraoral growth; (B) Oropharyngeal carcinoma.

- Carcinoma of the lower lip and commissure are often associated with skin pigmentations.
- Histologically, lip carcinomas are mostly well-differentiated malignancies (85% cases) and if the treatment is done before the metastasis has taken place, prognosis could be as good as 100%.

Carcinoma of the Tongue

Tongue is anatomically divided into two parts—(1) anterior two-thirds area (movable tongue), and (2) posterior one-third area (base). Anterior two-thirds area is the portion lying anterior to the line of circumvallate papilla on the top and the junction of the ventral surface of tongue to the floor of the mouth below. The posterior one-third area of the tongue is the portion extending from the circumvallate papilla to the junction with the epiglottic vallecula and it includes the pharyngoepiglottic and glossoepiglottic folds.

Carcinoma of the tongue constitutes about 50% of all oral malignancies and out of this, about 25% cases affect the lateral borders of posterior one-third area of the tongue and 75% lesions occur on the anterior two-thirds area.

- The lateral borders of the tongue and the anterior, right and left floor of the mouth, the retromolar pad and the adjacent parts of the soft palate constitute a "U" shaped zone in the oral cavity, which is considered to be a high-risk area for the development of SCC (Fig. 2.14).
- The dorsum of the tongue is a relatively resistant site for the initiation of oral cancer, although extension from adjacent areas frequently occurs.
- The initial lesions often appear as painless, erythematous macules or nodules or fissured areas over the tongue. There may be some cases of nonhealing ulcers on the lateral border.
- In some cases, the lesion can appear only as an extensive leukoplakic patch, which

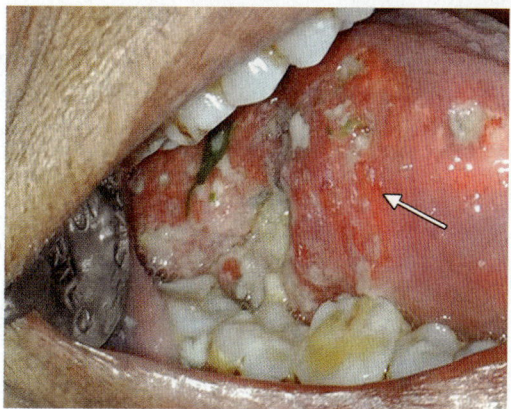

Fig. 2.14: Carcinoma of the posterolateral border of tongue.

later on ulcerates and gives rise to a raised, painful and indurated lesion.
- The advanced lesions often produce fast enlarging, painful, exophytic and large, extensively indurated ulcers with elevated and everted margin.
- SCC of tongue in advanced stages often spreads to involve the adjacent areas like gingiva, floor of the mouth, base of the tongue and mandible, etc.
- Tongue lesions usually have excessive bleeding tendency upon slight provocation and often there is presence of superadded candidal infection.
- Squamous cell carcinomas often cause fixation of the tongue to the floor of the mouth, which results in difficulty speech and swallowing, etc.
- Paresthesia of the tongue frequently occurs due to invasion of the lingual nerve by tumor cells.
- Tumor cells from the anterior two-thirds area of tongue often spread via lymphatics to submandibular, mid-anterior jugular and subdigastric lymph nodes.
- Long standing invasive lesions of posterior one-third area of tongue may spread to any of the following areas, e.g. towards the anterior part of tongue, pre-epiglottic space, pharyngeal or laryngeal wall and the mandible, etc.

Table 2.5: Lymph node metastasis with zonal variation in tongue carcinoma.

Spreading from the area of tongue	Targeted lymph nodes
• Anterior two-thirds area • Tip of the tongue • Posterior part of tongue	• Submandibular, mid-anterior jugular and subdigastric lymph nodes • Submental and to the jugulo-omohyoid lymph nodes • Submandibular and jugulodigastric lymph nodes (ipsilateral or contralateral side)

- Untreated tumors at the tip of tongue tend to spread to the submental and to the jugulo-omohyoid lymph nodes (Table 2.5).
- Tumors at the posterior part of the tongue usually spread to the submandibular and jugulodigastric lymph nodes of either the ipsilateral or the contralateral side.
- Tongue carcinomas have tremendous tendency for metastasis to the neck; the metastatic lymph nodes are enlarged, tendered and are often fixed to the surrounding tissue.
- Tongue lesion extending to the floor of mouth often increases the possibility of nodal metastasis; moreover lesions which cross the median longitudinal raphe can cause contralateral or bilateral nodal involvement.
- Sometimes distant metastasis may occur and in such cases, the malignant tumor cells often spread to the bone or lung or to the brain, etc.
- The prognosis of tongue carcinoma is often excellent if an early diagnosis is made and prompt treatment could be given.

Carcinoma of the Floor of the Mouth

Floor of the mouth is the mucosal area spreading over anterior and lateral floor of the oral cavity. Anteriorly and laterally it is bordered by the lingual surface of lower alveolar ridge, its posterior boundary is formed by the base of tongue and anterior tonsillar pillar. The lingual frenulum divides the floor of mouth into right and left halves, moreover from the front up to the posterior edge of lower second molar is called the anterior zone and the area behind that is called the posterior zone of floor of the mouth.

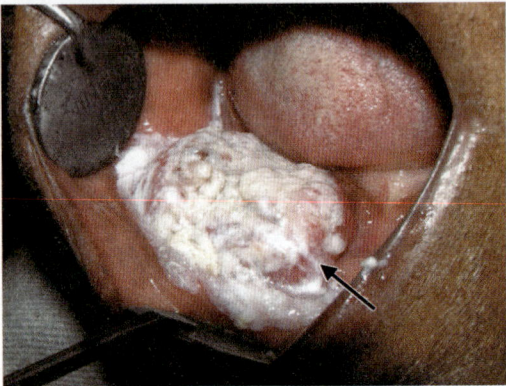

Fig. 2.15: Squamous cell carcinoma of floor of the mouth.

Floor of the mouth can be the site of about 20% of all oral carcinomas and moreover, it is the third most common location of all intraoral SCCs.

- Carcinomas of the floor of the mouth mostly occur in the anterior part (72% cases), near the opening of the Wharton's duct (Fig. 2.15).
- There is absolute male predominance.
- Almost all the patients are either heavy smokers or alcoholics or both.
- The initial lesions often appear either as erythroplakia or speckled leukoplakia; or a "sore spot" as described by most patients. These lesions gradually undergo central ulceration and exhibit induration at the periphery.
- Carcinomas of the floor of the mouth are among the most fatal and aggressive lesions of oral cavity as they can spread easily to the adjoining structures; moreover as it is the area of rich lymphatic drainage and up to 40% patients have nodal involvement during first reporting.

- The advanced lesions become nodular, ulcerated or indurated, and extension of the tumor cells to the deeper tissues of the tongue often results in fixation of the later.
- These lesions can also extend to the adjoining gingival tissues and cause pain, swelling and bleeding of the gingiva with mobility of the regional teeth.
- SCCs of the floor of the mouth usually spread to the submandibular lymph nodes. Distant metastasis is also a common.

Carcinoma of the Palate

Palate is divided into two parts, anteriorly hard palate and posteriorly soft palate. From the inner aspect of superior alveolar ridge up to the posterior edge of palatine bone is the hard palate and from there up to the end of uvula is the soft palate (Fig. 2.16).
- Squamous cell carcinomas affect the soft palate in about 75% cases and hard palate in nearly 25% cases.
- History often reveals that most of these patients with carcinoma of the soft palate are heavy smokers with high affinity toward alcohol.
- Clinically the lesions often appear either as mixed red-white patchy areas or extensive erythroplakic plaques with late ulceration.
- Invasion into deeper structures occurs usually before the surface ulceration begins.

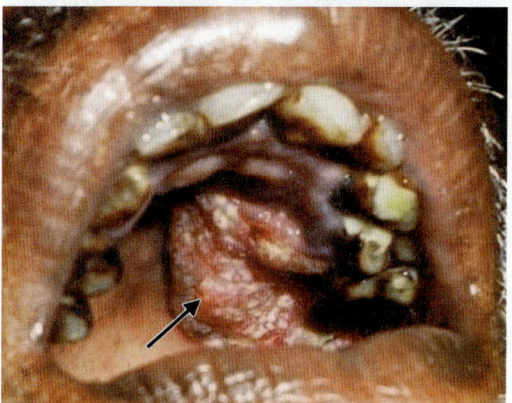

Fig. 2.16: Carcinoma of the palate.

- Carcinoma of the hard palate is fairly common in the Indian population, especially among reverse smokers.
- Carcinomas of the hard palate mostly occur as lateral ulcers in the glandular zone and these lesions often invade into the underlying bone, floor of the nasal cavity, maxillary antrum, gingiva and the soft palate, etc.
- These tumors generally spread to the internal jugular and submandibular lymph nodes.

Carcinoma of the Buccal Mucosa

Buccal mucosa is that part of oral epithelium which covers the inner aspect of cheeks and lips.

It is a common site for the occurrence of SCC especially among people of the Indian subcontinent.

Such higher incidences of SCC can be attributed to the widespread use of betel nut and tobacco in various forms among the people of this region.
- Carcinoma of the buccal mucosa frequently occurs in the posterior part of the buccal mucosa.
- Clinically, these lesions often present as white speckled patch or small nodule or well-defined ulcer with surrounding induration or may be as verrucous type of growth.
- Exophytic ulcers are commonly seen in the commissural areas while deep excavating lesions are mostly seen in the area along the occlusal line of buccal mucosa.
- In the advanced stage of the disease or in untreated cases, the lesion often presents large, painful, indurated ulcers, which may perforate the cheek and reach to the external surface of the face as a nodular protruding mass (Fig. 2.17).
- Lesions from this area can also spread to the underlying bone or to the pharyngomaxillary fossa or to the muscles, etc.
- Buccal mucosal carcinomas often metastasize to the submandibular lymph nodes. Recurrence after treatment is also very high.

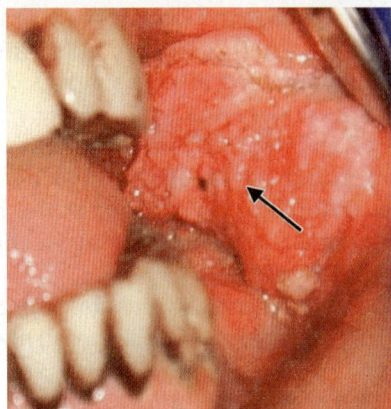

Fig. 2.17: Carcinoma of buccal mucosa with exophytic growth.

Carcinoma of the Gingiva/Alveolar Ridge

Carcinoma of the gingiva and alveolar ridge (both upper and lower) represents approximately about 4–6% of all oral carcinomas (Fig. 2.18). The most common predisposing factor is tobacco and betel nut chewing.

- Mandibular gingiva is affected more often (70%) than the maxillary gingiva (30%) and elderly people (predominantly males) are commonly affected usually after the age of 60 years.
- Attached gingiva is affected more than the free gingiva and edentulous people develop the disease more often than the dentulous people.
- The initial lesion appears either as a verrucous leukoplakia or as a small ulceration with indurated margin.
- Early invasion of the bone takes place, mostly via the periodontal ligament and this causes extensive mobility and premature loss of the regional teeth.
- Extraction of tooth often leads to early bone invasion, which causes nonhealing or delayed healing of the extraction socket.
- Mandibular lesions often extend to the adjoining structures, e.g. labial mucosa, tongue, bone, floor of the mouth and the retromolar areas.
- Carcinoma of the maxillary gingiva often extends to hard palate, maxillary antrum, buccal mucosa, lip and facial skin, etc.
- Metastasis occurs often to the submandibular and deep cervical lymph nodes.

Carcinoma of the Maxillary Antrum

Squamous cell carcinomas sometime involve the maxillary antrum (Fig. 2.19) and these lesions often present the following features:

- Pain and heaviness of the upper face on the involved side, with occasional epistaxis.
- Anesthesia or paresthesia of the affected area is very common.
- There can be pain in the upper molar teeth with pressure sensation on the eyeball.

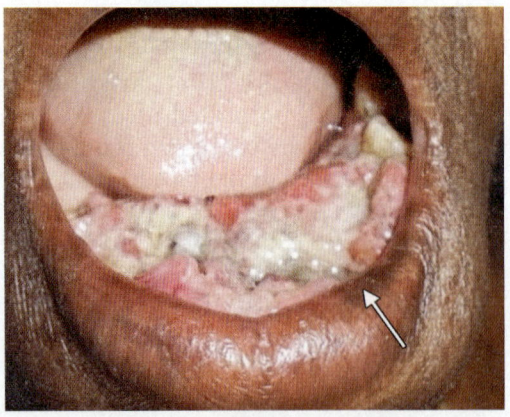

Fig. 2.18: Carcinoma of gingiva.

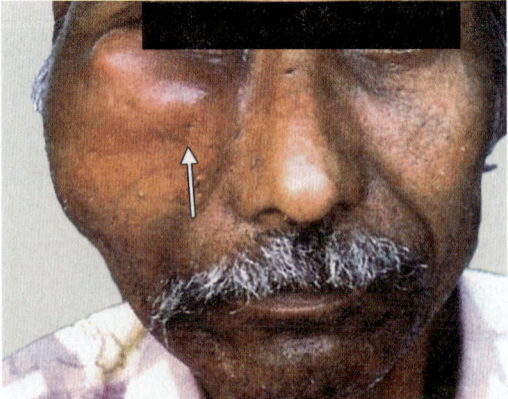

Fig. 2.19: Carcinoma of the maxillary antrum with large swelling in the infraorbital area.

- Edentulous patients often feel pain and discomfort under the artificial denture.
- In advanced stages of the disease, there can be mobility of the upper molar teeth as well as swelling of the face.
- Radiograph (Waters' view) often reveals clouding of the antral space and sometimes destruction of the bony walls of the antrum.

Differential Diagnosis of Squamous Cell Carcinoma

A large numbers of neoplastic or non-neoplastic lesions often resemble SCC (Box 2.4, Figs. 2.20 and 2.21):
- Malignant melanoma
- Keratoacanthoma

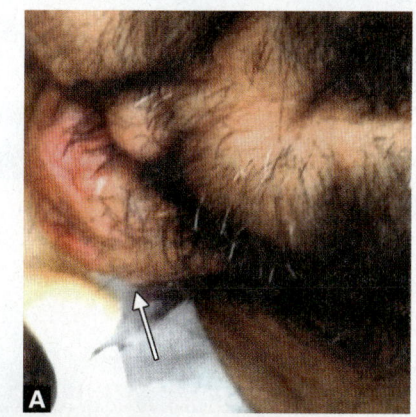

Box 2.4	Consequences of delay in diagnosis and treatment of oral cancers.

Oral cancers (SCC) are highly destructive lesions, therefore early detection and prompt are extremely important to contain the disease to whatever extent possible. Delay in diagnosis and treatment often lead to the following consequences:
- Growth of enormous size of tumor with massive local tissue destruction
- Involvement of vital structures like–nerves, muscles and major vessels
- Nerve involvement causes anesthesia or paresthesia in the region, muscle involvement causes lack of movement and loss of function of the affected organs and encroachment or perforation of major vessels often leads to fatal bleeding or hemorrhage
- Untreated tumor of mouth can perforate the mouth and can spread extraorally
- Large oral lesions often spread to the maxillary antrum, oropharynx and esophagus, etc.
- Long standing oral lesions may involve the jawbones, which produces osteomyelitis and pathological fractures
- Involvement of extraoral skin in squamous cell carcinoma often indicates a poor prognosis
- Untreated oral cancers obviously have more risk for local or distant metastasis
- Difficulty in food intake leads to malnutrition and cachexia
- Loss of immunity and secondary systemic infection in oral cancer can cause pneumonia and septicemia, etc.

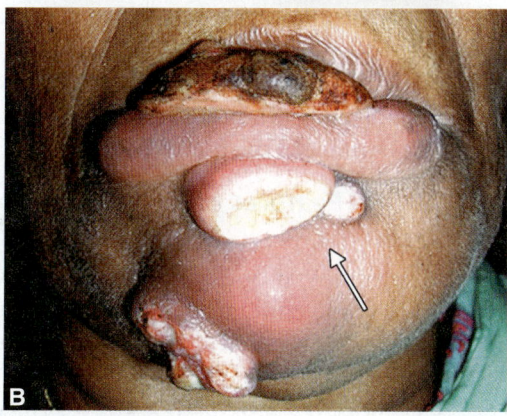

Figs. 2.20A and B: Extraoral spread of SCC with perforation of face and involvement of skin (both images).

- Lymphoma
- Verrucous carcinoma
- Adenocarcinoma
- Adenosquamous carcinoma
- Mucoepidermoid carcinoma
- Carcinoma ex pleomorphic adenoma
- Granular cell tumor with pseudoepitheliomatous hyperplasia
- Neuroendocrine carcinoma
- Epithelial overgrowths at the periphery of a nonmalignant chronic ulcer
- Metastatic tumor from a primary lesion located elsewhere in the body
- Tangential sectioning of hyperplastic oral epithelium, which often microscopically looks like an invading SCC

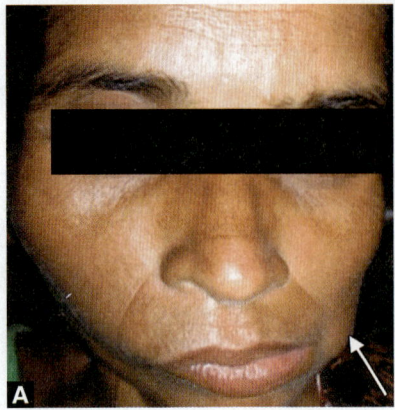 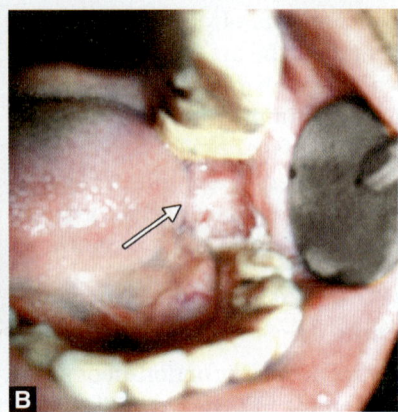

Figs. 2.21A and B: Squamous cell carcinoma causing pathological fracture of jawbone (both images).

- Organ of Chievitz often resembles SCC (it is seen in the bucco-temporalis fascia on the medial surface of the mandible).

Radiological Features of Squamous Cell Carcinoma

Variable degrees of bone destruction may occur when malignant cells of the squamous cell carcinoma invade into the jaw bones (Box 2.5). This type of bony involvement can be seen more frequently, if the primary tumor occurs in gingiva or alveolar ridge or in the floor of the mouth, which extends to the jaw bone. Moreover, metastatic carcinomas also frequently affect the jawbone and cause bony changes which could be detected by radiographs (Fig. 2.22).

Radiographic Features of Jaw Malignancy

- Radiographically the involved bone often exhibits large, irregular and ill-defined radiolucent areas with a typical "moth-eaten" appearance (Fig. 2.23; Boxes 2.6 and 2.7).
- Border of the lesion is often hazy and not clearly demarcated.

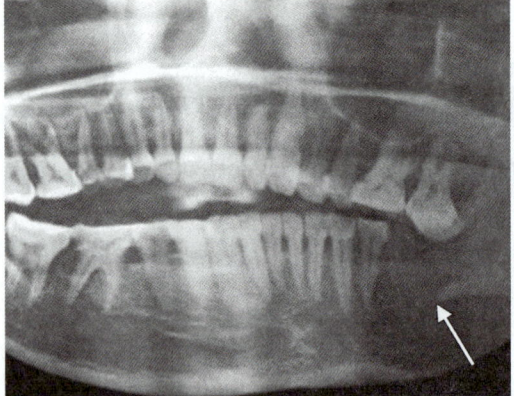

Fig. 2.22: Pathological fracture of mandible in SCC.

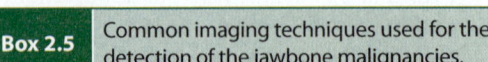

| Box 2.5 | Common imaging techniques used for the detection of the jawbone malignancies. |

- Anteroposterior (AP) and posteroanterior (PA) view radiograph of the jaw
- Orthopantomogram of the jaw (OPG)
- Standard occlusal radiograph of the jaw
- Water's view radiograph of the jaw
- Intraoral periapical (IOPA) radiograph of the jaw
- CT Scan of the jaw and skull
- CBCT
- Magnetic resonance imaging (MRI)

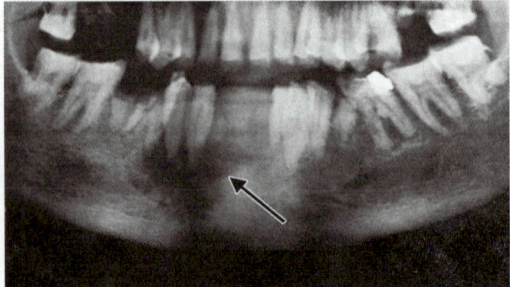

Fig. 2.23: Carcinoma of jaws showing "moth-eaten" radiolucency.

Benign and Malignant Neoplasms of the Oral Cavity

Box 2.6	Involvement of jawbones in oral carcinomas.

- Carcinoma of the surface epithelium infiltrating into the underlying tissue and eventually invading the bone
- Metastatic carcinoma from other organs reaching into the jawbone and making secondary tumor
- Primary intra-alveolar carcinoma developing from entrapped epithelium (in the sutural areas) within the jawbone
- Carcinomas developing from the preexisting lining epithelium of jaw cysts
- Malignant transformation of benign oral tumors e.g. ameloblastic carcinoma
- Intra-osseous mucoepidermoid carcinoma of the jawbone

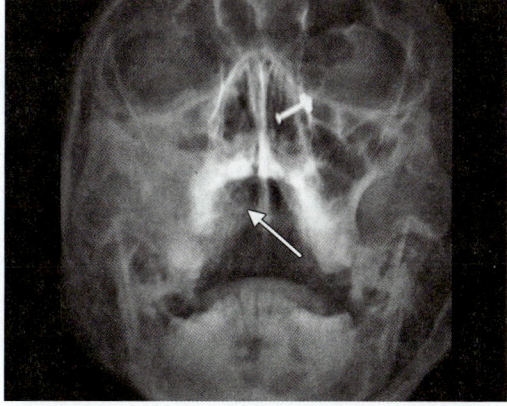

Fig. 2.24: Carcinoma of right maxillary antrum causing "antral clouding".

Box 2.7	Diseases showing "moth-eaten" radiographic appearance.

- Multiple myeloma
- Primary lymphoma of bone
- Ewing's sarcoma
- Osteomyelitis
- Squamous cell carcinoma (when invading bone)
- Eosinophilic granuloma
- Metastatic tumors
- Malignant fibrous histiocytoma
- Burkitt's lymphoma

- Irregular expansion and destruction of the cortical plates of the jawbone is common.
- Destruction of the interdental or inter-radicular bone may be seen frequently and this causes expansion of the periodontal ligament space in the localized area, displacement or exfoliation of the regional teeth.
- In advanced cases, the bone destruction could be so extensive that it may lead to pathological fractures of the affected jawbone.
- Clouding of the maxillary antrum and destruction of the lateral antral wall is commonly seen in case of antral carcinoma (Fig. 2.24).

Histopathology

Histopathology is the most important tool for making the diagnosis of SCCs. It is performed by obtaining a biopsy from the representative site of an existing lesion with subsequent histopathological evaluation.

Microscopically SCC is characterized by the following:

- *Excessive mitosis*: Increased proliferation of malignant squamous epithelial cells (keratinocytes) due to increased and often abnormal mitosis. The tumor cells exhibit varying grades of squamous differentiation.
- *Invasion*: Invasive growth of the tumor manifested by breakdown of the basement membrane and the growth of islands, cords or single (dyscohesive) tumor cells into the subepithelial connective tissue stroma. Large tumors often invade deeper structures, i.e. muscle, cartilage or bone. Perineural invasion and invasion of the lymphatic or blood vessels are often seen (Fig. 2.25).
- *Metastasis*: Malignant tumor cells of squamous cell carcinoma have a strong potential to spread into distant sites or organs in the body.

Malignant cells in SCC exhibit variable degrees of *cellular pleomorphism and nuclear hyperchromatism*. Besides this, there can be other neoplastic changes in these cells which include—increased nuclear-cytoplasmic ratio, individual cell keratinization, etc. The connective tissue stroma into which the tumor cells infiltrate

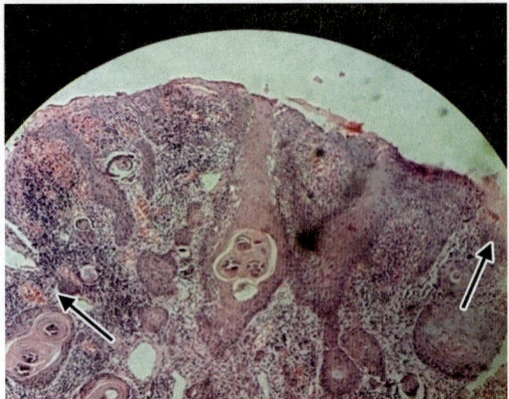

Fig. 2.25: Early invasive squamous cell carcinoma.

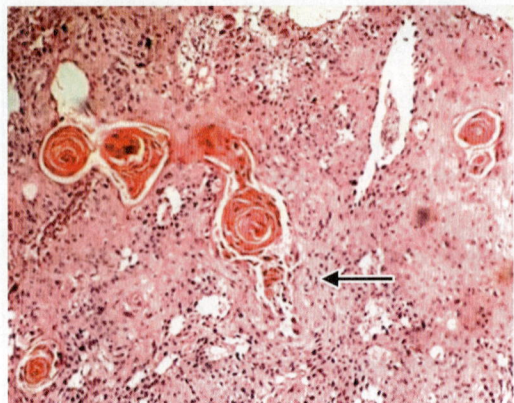

Fig. 2.26: Well-differentiated squamous cell carcinoma showing epithelial islands.

generally shows intense inflammatory cell infiltration mostly by the lymphocytes and the plasma cells.

Histologic Grading (Differentiation) of Squamous Cell Carcinomas

Differentiation: It refers to the extent to which the tumor cells resemble their mother cells (cell of origin) both structurally and functionally. According to the characteristics of the neoplastic cells, squamous cell carcinomas are traditionally graded into:
- Well-differentiated squamous cell carcinoma
- Moderately-differentiated squamous cell carcinoma, and
- Poorly-differentiated squamous cell carcinoma.

The criteria for grading are: (a) the degree of differentiation (b) nuclear pleomorphism and (c) mitotic activity.

Well-differentiated squamous cell carcinoma:
- Most of the SCCs histologically belong to the well-differentiated category (about 80%).
- Well-differentiated SCCs closely resemble normal squamous epithelium and they exhibit excessive proliferation of large, *keratinocyte-like squamous cells* and some *small basal-type cells*.
- There are prominent intercellular bridges and often full keratinizations; mitotic activities are scanty.
- The tumor cells form many large epithelial islands within the connective tissue stroma, which are bordered at the periphery by the basal cells and there is progressive differentiation as well as maturation of the tumor epithelial cells at the center of the islands (Fig. 2.26).
- Large amount of keratin (it a special fibrous protein normally produced by the keratinocytes) in the form of "keratin pearls" at the center of the island.
- SCC often exhibits desmoplastic stromal reactions characterized by proliferation of myofibroblasts, excessive deposition of extracellular matrix and neovascularization. The desmoplastic stromal reaction is a definite indicator of invasive carcinoma (it is not seen in epithelial dysplasia). This reaction is more pronounced in well differentiated SCC and less in moderately or poorly differentiated SCC. Intensity of desmoplasia is inversely proportional to the density of stromal lymphocytic infiltration (Table 2.6).
- Squamous cell carcinoma of well-differentiated type is usually associated with a better prognosis.

Benign and Malignant Neoplasms of the Oral Cavity

Table 2.6: Invasion patterns and their significance in squamous cell carcinoma (SCC).

When tumor cells invade into the underlying stroma the advancing area or the *"tumor-host interface"* is called the *invasive front* and its characteristics often vary.	
Expansive growth pattern of invasion	This type of invasion characteristically exhibits many large tumor islands spreading over a large area with well-defined pushing margins. This pattern is associated with better prognosis.
Infiltrative growth pattern of invasion	Characterized by small, scattered irregular cords or small group of invading tumor cell with poorly defined infiltrative margins. This type of invasion is more aggressive in nature and related to poor prognosis of the tumor.

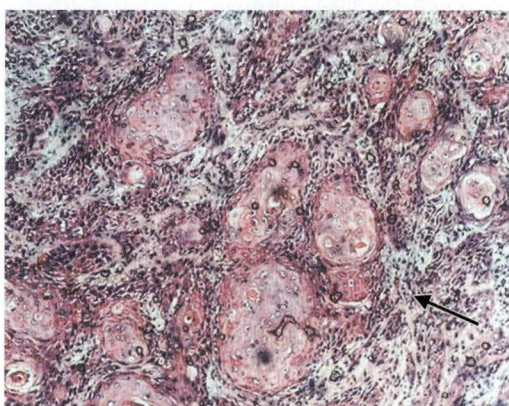

Fig. 2.27: Photomicrograph of moderately differentiated squamous cell carcinoma.

Key Points of Histopathological Aspect of Squamous Cell Carcinoma

- Excessive proliferation of malignant epithelial cells.
- There will be cellular pleomorphism, nuclear hyperchromatism and increased abnormal mitosis of the malignant epithelial cells.
- Formation of epithelial islands and keratin pearls.
- Malignant cells invade into the underlying connective tissue by breaking the basement membrane.
- The well-differentiated squamous cell carcinoma exhibits cells which resemble their mother cells (stratified squamous epithelial cells) both structurally and functionally.
- The well-differentiated cells produce large amounts of keratin in the form of "keratin pearls"; also produce large epithelial islands and prominent intercellular bridges.
- The moderately differentiated squamous cell carcinoma produces keratin pearls and their rate of mitosis is faster, the malignant cells resemble the mother cells but not as convincingly as the well-differentiated type.
- Poorly differentiated squamous cell carcinoma reveals extremely high rate of mitotic cell divisions, the cells look immature, there is no keratin pearl formations and nor any intercellular bridges.
- The poorly differentiated squamous cell carcinomas are difficult to diagnose as the cells have no structural or functional resemblance to their mother cells.

Moderately-differentiated Squamous Cell Carcinoma (Fig. 2.27)

In moderately-differentiated squamous cell carcinoma, the tumor exhibits the following characteristics:

- The tumor cells are less mature than those of the well-differentiated SCC.
- The cells exhibit more nuclear pleomorphism and more mitosis, including abnormal mitosis.
- There is usually far less keratinization.
- Formation of epithelial islands are diminished
- Fewer tendencies shown by the malignant cells to produce normal stratification.

However, despite their significant deviation from normal, the tumor cells of moderately differentiated SCC *still resemble their mother cells*. Moderately-differentiated SCC also carries a reasonably good prognosis.

Poorly-differentiated Squamous Cell Carcinoma (Fig. 2.28)

Poorly-differentiated SCC has the following important characteristics:

- The basal cells predominate in this tumor, with a very high mitotic rate including abnormal mitoses.
- Tumor cells produce very little keratin or no keratin at all.

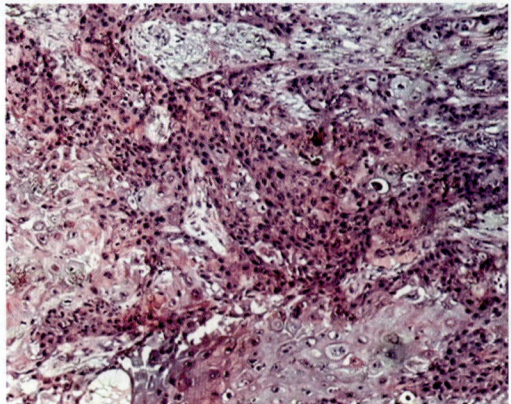

Fig. 2.28: Photomicrograph of poorly-differentiated squamous cell carcinoma.

Different Variants of Squamous Cell Carcinoma

Spindle Cell Carcinoma (Carcinosarcoma/Sarcomatoid Carcinoma)

Spindle cell carcinoma (SpCC) is a *biphasic tumor* composed of conventional SCC and a malignant spindle cell component; it probably originates from non-committed stem cells capable of forming both epithelial and mesenchymal components (Figs. 2.29 and 2.30).

Clinically the tumor shows a polypoid or pedunculated growth with frequent surface ulceration.

- Intercellular bridges between cells are also rarely seen.
- Cells are extremely immature and often exhibit infiltrative growth pattern.
- Connective tissue stroma appears to be bland with very less chronic inflammatory cell reaction.
- Tumor cells hardly bear any structural or functional resemblance whatsoever to their mother cells.

Diagnosis of poorly differentiated SCC often requires special investigative procedures like immunohistochemistry and flow cytometry, etc.

These tumors always have a very poor prognosis (Box 2.8).

Box 2.8	Factors determining the poor prognosis in squamous cell carcinoma (SCC).

- Poorly differentiated tumors
- Late diagnosis or delay in treatment
- Increased size and depth of tumor
- Infiltrative pattern of invasion of the tumor cells.
- Less number of immune cells (lymphocyte, plasma cell and macrophage) in the tumor.
- Extraoral spread of the tumor with involvement facial skin
- Extracapsular spread of tumor cells in nodal metastasis
- Distant metastasis especially in the vital organs, e.g. brain, liver and lung, etc.

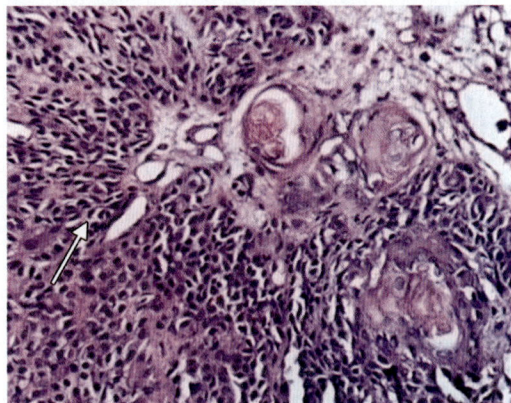

Fig. 2.29: Photomicrograph of spindle cell carcinoma.

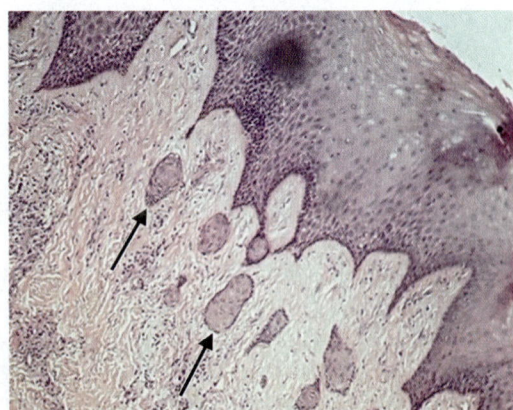

Fig. 2.30: Photomicrograph of tangential section of epithelium.

Histologically SpCC exhibits two cellular components—(1) Conventional *SCC component* showing features of invasive SCC, and (2) *Spindle cell component* (more predominant type) showing malignant spindle cells with hyperchromatic nuclei, prominent nucleoli and increased abnormal mitosis. These spindle cells are typically arranged in "fascicles or whorls" and as a result SpCC may resemble a fibrosarcoma or malignant fibrous histiocytoma.

Papillary Squamous Cell Carcinoma

Papillary squamous cell carcinoma (PSCC) is a rare variant of squamous cell carcinoma, which characteristically shows a *typical papillary growth pattern*. The tumor clinically presents a small, papillary, friable and soft growth. Histologically PSCC shows many papillary growths; each papilla has a central fibrovascular core covered by neoplastic squamous or basaloid or pleomorphic cells with little or no keratin formation.

Basaloid Squamous Cell Carcinoma

Basaloid squamous cell carcinoma (BSCC) is poorly differentiated variant of SCC, composed of both "basaloid cell" and "conventional malignant squamous cell".

Adenoid Squamous Cell Carcinoma

Adenoid SCC is a histologic variant of SCC, it resembles a conventional SCC, however due to acantholysis of the malignant squamous cells multiple pseudoluminae (duct/cavity) are formed which gives a glandular appearance to the tumor (Fig. 2.31).

Adenosquamous Cell Carcinoma

Adenosquamous cells carcinoma (ASC) is an interesting type of rare aggressive malignant neoplasm, which has the presence of *both SCC and adenocarcinoma (Fig. 2.32)*.

Microscopically there is presence of two components—(1) conventional SCC and (2) adenocarcinoma. The SCC component is mostly present in the superficial part of the tumor, while the adenocarcinoma component

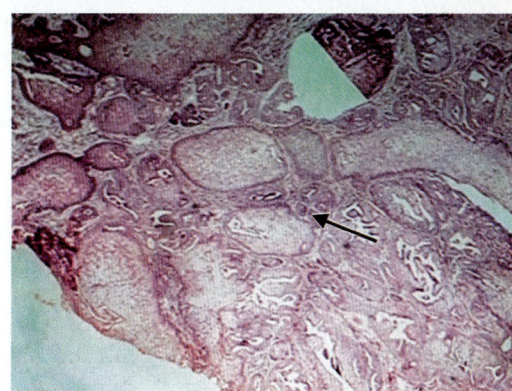

Fig. 2.31: Photomicrograph of adenomatoid squamous cell carcinoma.

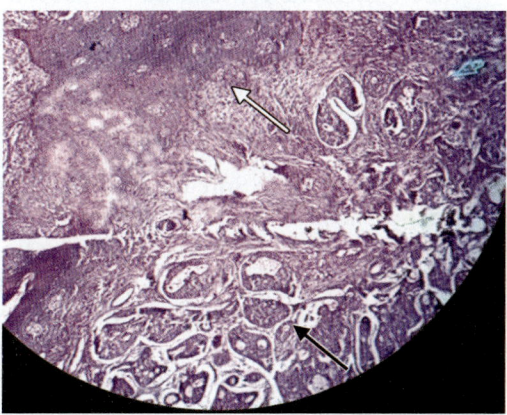

Fig. 2.32: Photomicrograph of adenosquamous cell carcinoma showing both SCC (White arrow) and adenocarcinoma (Black arrow).

present in the deeper part; the later often consists of tubular or ductal structures.

Lymphoepithelial Carcinoma

Lymphoepithelial carcinoma (LEC) is a poorly differentiated or undifferentiated variant of SCC which characteristically exhibits dense lymphocytic stromal infiltration. This tumor is also called "nasopharyngeal-type carcinoma" since it often closely resembles the conventional nasopharyngeal carcinoma.

Metastasis in Squamous Cell Carcinoma

Definition of metastasis: Spread of cancer cells from a primary tumor to distant organ or organs of the body with formation of a new tumor there is called *metastasis*. When there is more than one metastasis, they are called *metastases*.

Routes of Metastasis

Malignant tumor cells spread to the distant organs via the following routes:
- *Direct extension*: Tumor spreads by simply invading into other organs.
- *Lymphatic route*: Tumor cells move via the lymphatic channels (mostly carcinomas take this route).
- *Hematogenous route*: Cells spread via the blood vessels and capillaries (sarcomas as well as SCCs often spread via this route).

It is to be noted that cancer cells easily invade the thin-walled lymphatic vessels, capillaries and veins, etc. whereas the thicker walled arterioles and arteries are relatively resistant to such invasions.
- *Perineural sheath*: Spread of tumor cells through the perineural spaces and spread both proximally and distally along the nerve fiber. The distance traveled by the tumor cells in route is often less as compared to lymphatic or hematogenous spreads. Perineural invasion of tumor is often associated with pain and paresthesia (any tumor can take this route but most common is adenoid cystic carcinoma).
- *Tissue spaces*: Tumors cells easily spread through various tissue spaces as these are areas of least resistance.
- *Intraspinal seeding*: Spread of tumor cells through spinal canal via the Batson plexus of veins.

Factors primarily determining the distant metastasis in oral SCC:
- If the primary tumor is located in a highly vascular area (e.g. base of tongue).
- If the tumor cells are poorly differentiated.

Distant metastasis in cases of oral SCC should generally be considered when tumor *spreads below the clavicle*; and it can result due to both lymphatic and hematogenous spread.

> **Box 2.9** Lymph nodes where metastasis of oral squamous cell carcinoma (SCC) commonly occur.
>
> - Submandibular lymph nodes—about 32% cases
> - Submental nodes about—12% cases
> - Superior deep cervical nodes about—10% cases
> - Jugulodigastric and jugulo-omohyoid nodes about—30% cases
> - Midcervical lymph nodes about—4% cases.
> - Posterior supraclavicular nodes about—2% cases

- Lymphogenic spread results in spread of tumor to distant lymph nodes, e.g. mediastinal, axillary and inguinal nodes (Box 2.9).
- Hematogenous spread of oral SCC often results in metastasis to lung, liver, bones, skin and brain, etc.

Mechanism of metastasis (Flowchart 2.1, Table 2.7):
- Malignant cells gradually loose the intercellular bridges and are not bound to one another as seen in normal epithelium.
- These free malignant cells destroy the basement membrane and invade into the underlying connective tissue stroma.
- Inside the stroma, the malignant cells invade into vessels for further travel into distant organs; generally the carcinoma cells take the lymphatic route while the sarcomatous cells take route via blood vessels.
- Tumor angiogenesis or neovascularization is the phenomenon in which new blood vessels form within the tumor which additionally facilitates the spread of tumor cells.
- Once the tumor cells get inside the lymphatic vessel, they are easily carried into the regional lymph nodes; here some cells are implanted and start multiplying within the node; while other cells move further down the line till they reach to a suitable distal organ, e.g. lung, bone, liver, brain and skin, etc.
- As mitosis continues and tumor cell numbers hugely increased within the lymph node, the affected node becomes palpable, enlarged and firm/hard in consistency; some may be even "stony hard".

Flowchart 2.1: Step-by-step events in metastasis of squamous cell carcinoma (SCC).

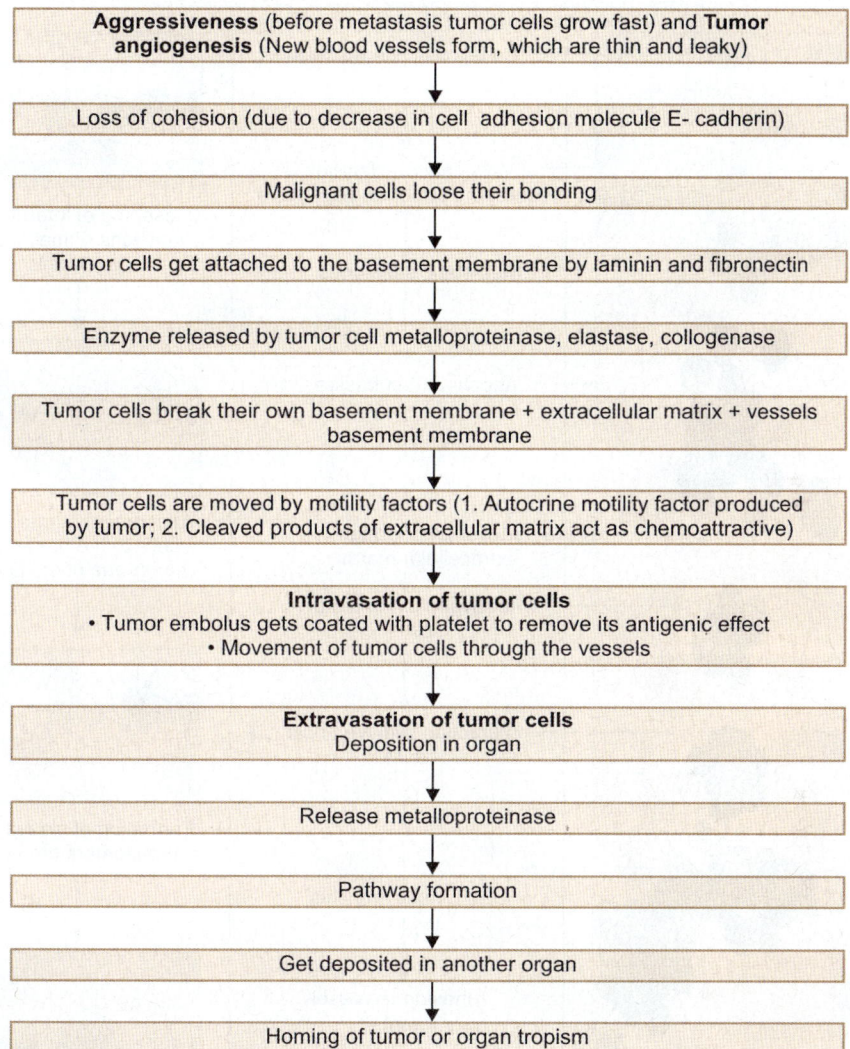

- Over the period, the tumor cells destroy the nodal structure and penetrate through the nodal capsule and spread into the surrounding tissue, this is known as extracapsular spread (ECS).
- ECS often leads to fixation of the involved node to the surrounding tissue.
- Bilateral involvement of the lymph nodes is uncommon unless the tumor is very large and it crosses the midline.
- Metastasis through blood vessels or perineural infiltration is rare in oral SCC.

Micrometastasis: It is defined as the microscopic deposit of malignant cells (smaller than 2–3 mm) within the tissue spaces; that are segregated from the primary tumor. Since there is no specific blood supply to these tumor cells, they depend only on passive diffusion of oxygen and nutrition for survival; thus majority of such cells are destroyed and

Table 2.7: Step-by-step mechanism of metastasis.

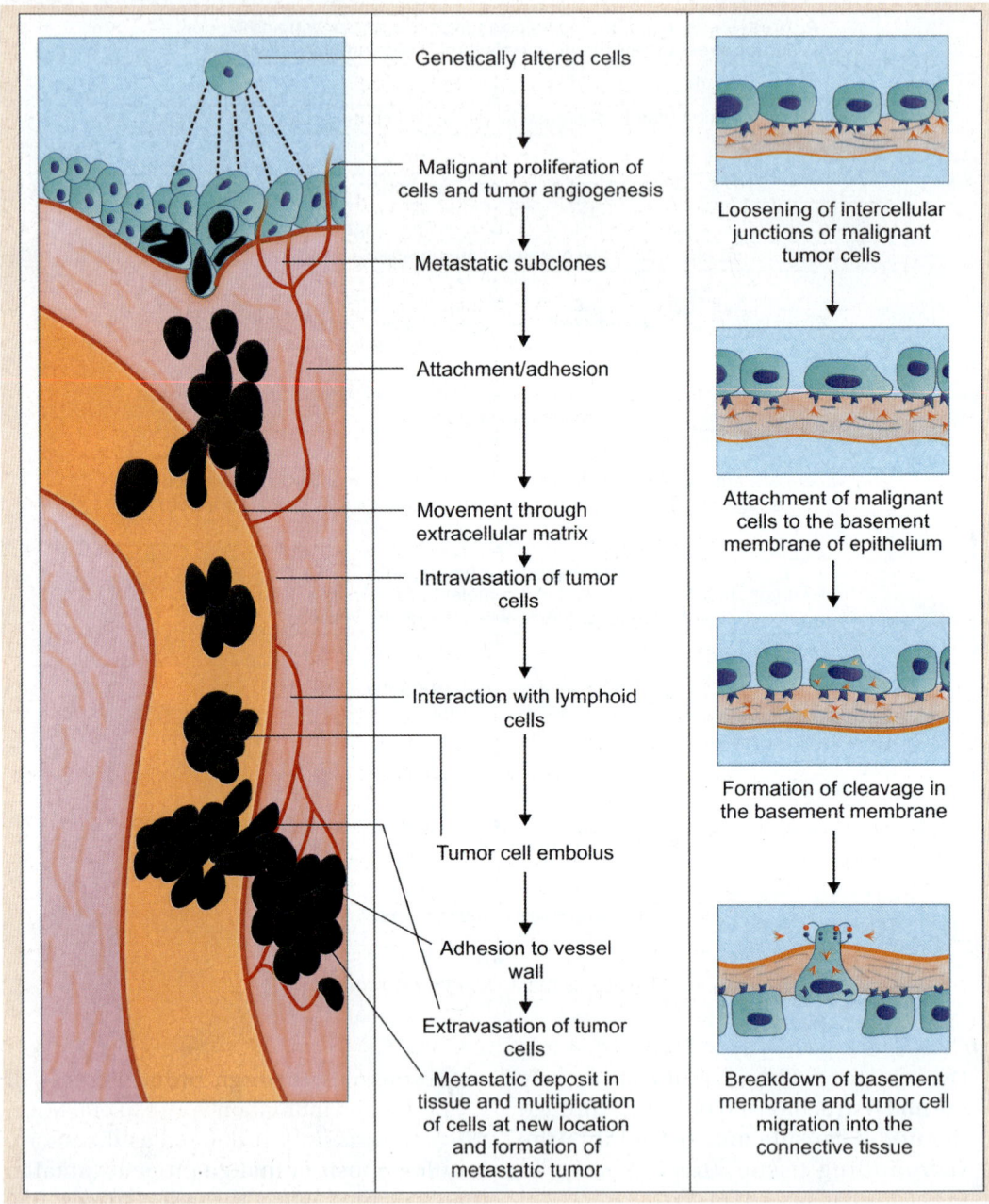

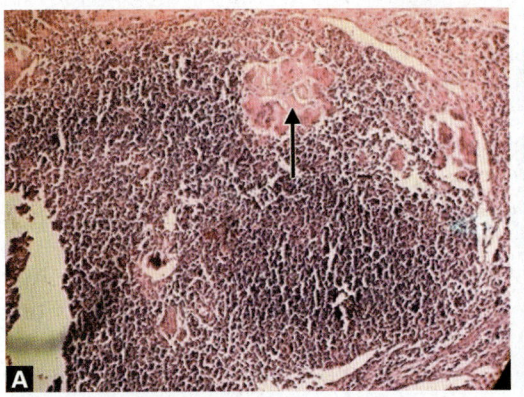 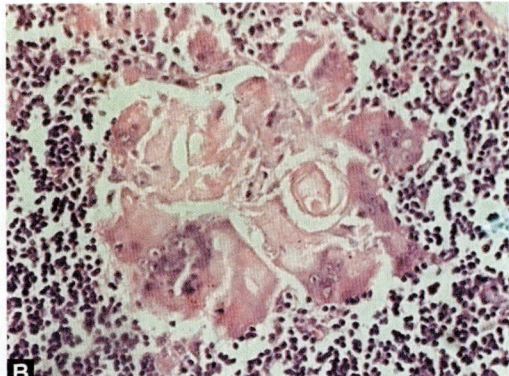

Figs. 2.33A and B: Photomicrograph of metastatic lymph node in SCC: (A) Low power; (B) High power.

while only few cells may survive to continue to multiply and produce a metastatic focus (Figs. 2.33A and B).

CLINICAL STAGING OF CARCINOMAS OF HEAD AND NECK (TNM SYSTEM)

In a patient with carcinoma, clinical staging is used to designate the extent of the disease and to determine the most appropriate treatment necessary for that patient during that particular stage of the disease. Finally the method helps in making an overall evaluation regarding the prognosis of the disease.

TNM system is the most popular system for describing the anatomical extent of disease is based on the assessment of three components (Table 2.8):
- T—the extent of the primary tumor
- N—the absence or presence and extent of regional lymph node metastasis
- M—the absence or presence of distant metastasis.

TNM SYSTEM: For the Cancer of Lip and Oral Cavity (ICD-O-3 C00, C02-006)*

T–Primary tumor
TX: Primary tumor cannot be assessed
To: No evidence of primary tumor
TIS: Carcinoma-in-situ.
T1: Tumor 2 cm or less in greatest dimension and 5 mm or less depth of invasion.

Table 2.8: Tumor-node-metastasis (TNM) classification of malignant tumors.

Stage	T	N	M
Stage 0	Tis	N0	M0
Stage I	T1	N0	M0
Stage II	T2	N0	M0
Stage III	T3	N0	M0
	T1,T2,T3	N1	M0
Stage IVA	T4a	N0 N1	M0
	T1, T2, T3, T4a	N2	M0
Sage IVB	Any T	N3	M0
	T4b	Any N	M0
Stage IVC	Any T	Any N	M1

T2: Tumor 2 cm or less in greatest dimension and more than 5 mm but no more than 10 mm depth of invasion or tumor more than 2 cm but not more than 4 cm in greatest dimension and depth of invasion no more than 10 mm.

T3: Tumor more than 4 cm in greatest dimension or more than 10mm depth of invasion.

T4a (Lip): Tumor invades through cortical bone, inferior alveolar nerve, floor of mouth, or skin (of the chin and nose).

T4a (Oral cavity): Tumor invades through the cortical bone of the mandible or maxillary sinus, or invades the skin of the face.

T4b (Lip and oral cavity): Tumor invades masticator space, pterygoid plates, or skull base, or encases internal carotid artery.

N–Regional lymph node

NX: Regional lymph nodes cannot be assessed
N0: No regional lymph node metastasis
N1: Metastasis in single ipsilateral lymph node, 3 cm or less in greatest dimension without extranodal extension
N2: Lymph node metastasis described as:
N2a: Metastasis in single ipsilateral lymph node, more than 3 cm but not more than 6 cm in greatest dimension without extranodal extension.
N2b: Metastasis in multiple ipsilateral lymph nodes, none more than 6 cm in greatest dimension without extranodal extension.
N2c: Metastasis in bilateral or contralateral lymph nodes, none more than 6 cm in greatest dimension without extranodal extension.
N3a: Metastasis in a lymph node, more than 6 cm in greatest dimension without extranodal extension.
N2b: Metastasis in a single or multiple lymph nodes with clinical extranodal extension.

M–Distant metastasis

Mo: No distant metastasis
M1: Distant metastasis

*(Source: Erierley JD, Gospodarowicz MK, Wittekind C. TNM Classification of malignant tumors, 8th edition. West Sussex: Wiley-Blackwell; 2017.)

SECOND PRIMARY TUMORS IN SQUAMOUS CELL CARCINOMA

A patient with oral SCC can have a *"second primary tumor (SPT)"* in the body at a separate site from the primary (or the first) tumor. These tumors occur especially in patients with long history of excessive tobacco and alcohol abuse if the primary SCC is present in mouth, pharynx and esophagus then the SPT is generally develops in and around the same site. If the primary tumor is present in the larynx then the SPT often develops in the lung.

SPTs are put into different categories according to their time of diagnosis:
- *Simultaneous SPT*: If the second tumor is diagnosed at the time when the primary tumor is detected.
- *Synchronous SPT*: Second tumor diagnosed within 6 months after the primary tumor.
- *Metachronous SPT*: Second tumor diagnosed more than 6 months after the primary tumor.

The prognosis SPT is often poorer than the primary SCC.

Immune Response in Cancer

Both cell mediated and humoral immunity play important roles in malignancy:
- Humoral immunity comes into effect with the production of specific immunoglobulins against the tumor cells.
- Cell mediated immunity can be demonstrated in malignancy by activation of lymphokines, increased formation of cytotoxic T cells and stimulation of DNA synthesis, etc.

Survival of Cancer Cells against the Immune Surveillance System of the Body

Despite having an effective immune system in place, the malignant tumor cells still manage to grow in the following mechanisms:
- *Higher rate of mitosis*: The rate of malignant cell proliferation is sometimes so high that few cells remain undetected and they manage to "sneak through" the immune surveillance system.
- *Hiding from the defense cells*: The circulating tumor antigens often create a "smoke-screen" coating on the lymphoid (immune) cells and thus prevent them from attacking the tumor cells.
- *Suppression of immunity*: Some tumors release cytokines, e.g. transforming growth factor (TGF-β), which suppresses the cell mediated immunity.

- *Low immunogenicity of few tumor cells*: Poor immunogenicity of tumor cells or lower levels of expression of class I MHC molecules by them, often make the tumor cells non-recognizable to the immune system.

SCREENING TESTS FOR SQUAMOUS CELL CARCINOMA

Exfoliative Cytology

Exfoliative cytology can often be helpful in making the diagnosis of oral SCC. This method is not an alternative but an adjunct to the system of standard histopathology.

Toluidine Blue Test

It is an *in vivo* test for detection of dysplastic lesions.

Methods
First of all, the surface of the suspected lesion is gently painted with 1% aqueous solution of toluidine blue and then after 10 seconds, decolorization of the surface is done with 1% acetic acid solution.

Results
If the color of toluidine blue is retained, malignancy or dysplasia is suspected in the lesion. If the color is washed away following application of acetic acid solution, the lesion should be considered nonmalignant.

Acridine-binding method
In this method the uptake of acriflavine by the desquamated buccal cells are measured.

Since the DNA content of the dysplastic cells are more, they will be stained more intensely than normal cells.

Brush Biopsy

Brush biopsy is a useful screening method in SCC, in this technique a round stiff bristle brush is rotated vigorously in one particular spot of a suspected lesion till bleeding starts. Because of this rotation, cells from the surface as well as the subsurface layer of the lesion will be collected by the brush, which are then transferred onto a slide and viewed microscopically after the smear is prepared.

SPECIAL INVESTIGATIONS IN ORAL CANCER

Special investigations like immunocytochemistry, flow cytometry and DNA probe analysis may be necessary for the detection of some poorly differentiated oral cancers which cannot be diagnosed by conventional histopathology or cytology, etc.

Tumor Markers

When a tumor develops in the body, certain tumor markers are produced in the blood in response to it. Carcinoembryonic antigen (CEA) and alpha-fetoprotein are two important such tumor markers.

The presence of these tumor markers in blood indicates that there is a tumor developing somewhere in the body or it might have already developed. These tumor markers disappear from blood once the tumor is surgically removed or treated by other means. However, they can reappear once again if the tumor recurs.

Treatment

Squamous cell carcinomas of the oral cavity are usually treated by surgical excision, radiotherapy and chemotherapy, etc.

Depending upon the size, the anatomical location and the histological gradation of the tumor, surgical treatment may consist of either only local excision or a combination of local excision and regional lymph node dissection.

Survival

Since most of the oral SCCs are well differentiated (about 80% lesions), prognosis is often expected to be good for them. Unfortunately however, excepting the lip carcinomas, most of the other intraoral cancers have a rather poor prognosis and it is mostly due to their late diagnosis and failure of initiating prompt treatment.

The survival rates for oral SCCs depend on the clinical staging of the disease, degree of differentiation of the tumor cells and the specific intraoral site of involvement.

According to one study (Hibbert et al., 1983), the overall 5-year survival rate of oral SCC is under 55%. According to Herkey (1979), the survival rate is equal among men and women in case of lip cancers. However, the survival rate is always better for women in case of other intraoral cancers as compared to men.

PREVENTION OF ORAL CANCER

Nowadays the evidence is overwhelming that tobacco chewing and smoking are the major causes of oral cancer.

Methods of Prevention

Primary Prevention

In primary prevention, the risk of cancer development is minimized by avoiding the exposure to tobacco and other deleterious habits.

Secondary Prevention

This form of prevention includes early detection and treatment of already developed cancer cases and prompts management of potentially risky precancerous lesions and conditions.

BASAL CELL CARCINOMA (RODENT ULCER/JACOB ULCER)

DEFINITION

Basal cell carcinoma is a common, locally aggressive, non-metastasizing malignant neoplasm of the skin, which is usually composed of medullary pattern of basaloid cells. It is the most common skin cancer, as well as the most common of all cancers (Box 2.10).

(A rodent is a small furry mammal whose teeth never stop growing. Rodent species includes mice, rats, squirrels and beavers, etc.)

Box 2.10	Types of basal cell carcinoma.
• Nodular basal cell carcinoma • Pigmented basal cell carcinoma • Basosquamous type basal cell carcinoma • Superficial basal cell carcinoma • Nodular basal cell carcinoma • Morpheaform of basal cell carcinoma • Infiltrating basal cell carcinoma	

ORIGIN

The disease arises from either the basal layer of epidermis or from the hair follicles and it affects the facial skin more often than any other part of the body.

ETIOLOGY

Chronic occupational or recreational exposure to direct sunlight (actinic radiation).

In the tropical black populations, this lesion is very uncommon and it could be attributed to the natural pigmentation of the skin of these people, which provide adequate protection from actinic radiation and thereby prevent the development of basal cell carcinoma among them.

CLINICAL FEATURES

- *Age*: Basal cell carcinoma develops mostly in middle-aged people, preferably in the 4th decade of life.
- *Sex*: Males are more commonly affected than females.
- *Geographical area*: The incidence of basal cell carcinoma is particularly high in geographic areas with high temperature and low humidity. For this reason large numbers of cases have been reported from Queensland in Australia and Arizona in United States.
- *Site*: The neoplasm commonly occurs (over 85% cases) over the hair-bearing areas of facial skin (especially the mucocutaneous areas) in blonde, white males (Fig. 2.34).

Benign and Malignant Neoplasms of the Oral Cavity

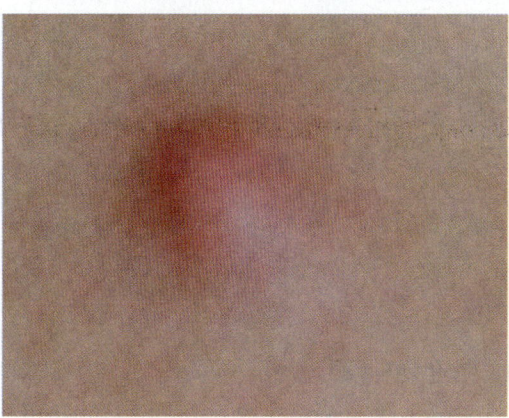

Fig. 2.34: Basal cell carcinoma of skin.

The orofacial areas particularly vulnerable to these lesions are the upper lip, nasolabial folds, periorbital region, cheek, forehead and ear, etc.

The lesion does not arise from the oral mucous membrane; however it can sometimes invade the mucous membrane by directly spreading from the adjacent skin.

PRESENTATION

- The neoplasm initiates as a slow growing, firm, slightly elevated, small nodules or papules (often called "pearly or waxy papules" containing prominent blood vessels.
- Few lesions are flat and exhibit red (flesh-like) or brown colored small growth.
- It gradually enlarges and develops a central crusted ulcer with an elevated, smooth, rolled border.
- The lesion may heal partially by scarring in the central area but it keeps on spreading centrifugally.
- One or more telangiectatic blood vessels may be seen coursing over the lesion and moreover, a characteristic pearly opalescence is noticed when the tumor is digitally pressed.
- Local invasion into the bone, facial sinuses and other structures.
- Distant metastasis is rare.
- The synonym "rodent ulcer" is given to this tumor since it makes a slow but relentless progress over months or years and increases in size by invading and destroying the adjoining tissues.
- There may be intermittent bleeding from the ulcer.

HISTOPATHOLOGY

- Histologically, basal cell carcinoma is characterized by neoplastic proliferation of basaloid epithelial cells in the form of multiple solid islands or strands (Fig. 2.35).
- These cells arise from the basal cell layer of the epidermis and they invade into the underlying dermis.
- The cells in the periphery of the tumor islands are columnar in shape and they often resemble basal layer of the oral epithelium with hyperchromatic nuclei.
- These tumor cells do not show any feature of abnormal mitosis.
- The cells are uniform in shape and size, and in their staining reaction. Moreover, these cells often have a palisaded arrangement.
- The central cells of the tumor islands may be polyhedral, oval, round or even spindle shaped.
- Intercellular bridges are often absent in routine tissue sections and apoptosis

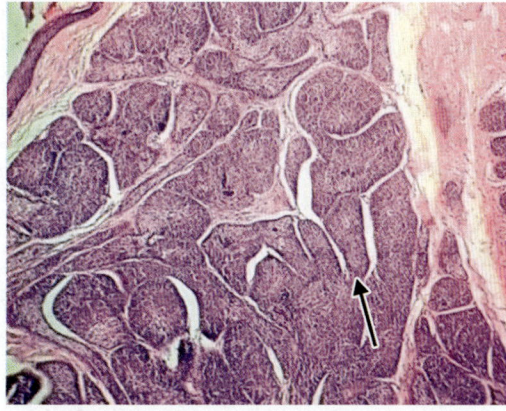

Fig. 2.35: Photomicrograph of basal cell carcinoma.

(individual cell death) of the tumor cells are commonly seen.

DIFFERENTIAL DIAGNOSIS

The following lesions are included in the differential diagnosis of basal cell carcinoma:
- Ameloblastoma
- Salivary gland neoplasms
- Squamous cell carcinoma.

TREATMENT

Surgical excision or electrocautery along with radiotherapy is the treatment of choice. Prognosis is extremely good and cure rate is about 95%.

VERRUCOUS CARCINOMA (SNUFF DIPPER'S CANCER; ACKERMAN'S TUMOR)

DEFINITION

Verrucous carcinoma is a diffuse, papillary, non-metastasizing, well-differentiated malignant neoplasm of the oral epithelium.

It is also known as "Ackerman's tumor" since it was first recognized as a distinct entity by Ackerman in 1948. According to the biological nature, verrucous carcinoma stands between benign hyperplasia of squamous epithelium and the conventional SCC.

ETIOLOGY

Verrucous carcinoma commonly occurs in people with "Paan" and tobacco chewing and snuffs dipping habits (that is why it also called the "snuff dipper's cancer"). Human papilloma virus (HPV type 16 and 18) is also implicated as a possible etiologic factor (Box 2.11).

CLINICAL FEATURES

- *Age*: The tumor usually affects individuals over 60 years of age and never before 35 years of age (between 50 years and 80 years).
- *Sex*: Predominantly affects males.
- *Site*: Intraorally buccal mucosa accounts for more than half of the cases, other common intraoral locations include gingiva and alveolar mucosa. Hard-palate and floor of the mouth.

Box 2.11	Lesions in which keratin horns may be present.

- Verrucous carcinoma
- Seborrheic keratosis
- Actinic keratosis
- Squamous cell carcinoma

PRESENTATION

- Clinically verrucous carcinoma presents slow enlarging, large, broad-based exophytic neoplasm with a white to tan, heavily keratotic and warty surface.
- The surface of the lesion is often raised and "pebbly" or sometimes it is "warty" and shows multiple rouge-like folds with deep clefts in between.
- The fully developed tumor appears as an exophytic, grayish-red, bulky lesion with a rough shaggy fungating surface.
- Excessive accumulation of compact keratin may sometimes result in the development of hard elevated projections from the surface of the lesion, which are called "keratin horns" (since they resemble the animal "horns").
- In verrucous carcinoma, majority of the lesions are exophytic and well circumscribed in nature; however, there can be few lesions which are of invasive type and they quickly invade into the underlying tissues including the bone.
- The lesions on the buccal mucosa are sometimes very extensive and they often cause pain, tenderness and difficulty in taking food.
- Verrucous carcinoma of the gingiva or the alveolar mucosa rapidly becomes fixed to the underlying periosteum (Figs. 2.36 and 2.37).
- The regional lymph nodes are often enlarged and tendered. However, these features are only due to the inflammatory reactions in the lymph nodes as a result of

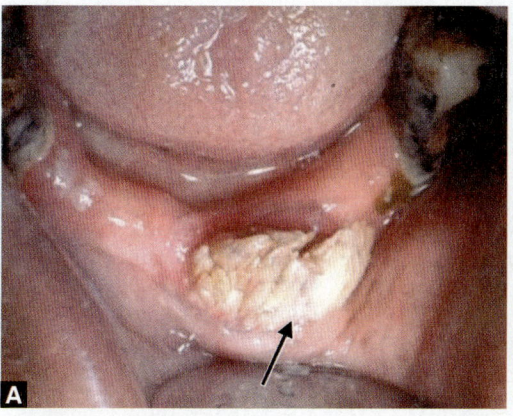
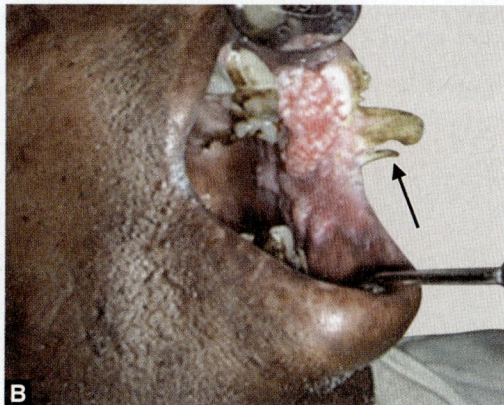

Figs. 2.36A and B: Verrucous carcinoma with (A) typical warty growth and (B) the "keratin horn".

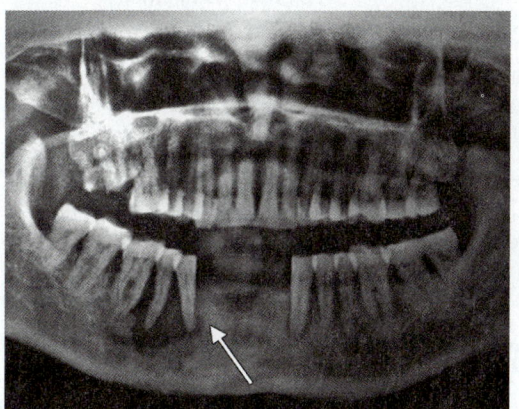

Fig. 2.37: Verrucous carcinoma of gingiva causing local invasion and irregular destruction bone.

secondary infection and are not due to the metastatic spread of the tumor cells.

The important differences between SCC and verrucous carcinoma are given in Table 2.9.

HISTOPATHOLOGY

Histologically verrucous carcinoma presents the following features:
- The tumor is composed of highly differentiated malignant epithelial cells, which proliferate as broadly papillary structures.
- Verrucous carcinoma is a low-grade malignancy and the neoplastic cells often lack the usual cytologic criteria of malignancy.
- The hyperplastic epithelium often exhibits a papillary surface, being covered by a thick layer of parakeratin.
- The continuity of the surface is maintained by filiform processes of well differentiated squamous cells and these processes often resemble "church spires".
- The lesion is slow growing and the neoplastic cells spread laterally more rather than vertically.
- Massively enlarged, bulb-like or "elephant foot-like" acanthotic rete-ridges are seen, which often invaginate into the underlying connective tissue stroma (Figs. 2.38 and 2.39).
- The bulbous rete-ridges of the epithelium tend to project into the underlying connective tissue at more or less the same level and this is known as "pushing margin".
- Many deep cleft-like spaces lined by thick layer of parakeratin, often extend from the surface of the epithelium and project deep into the center of the bulbous rete rides, this phenomenon is known as "parakeratin-plugging."
- The basement membrane is almost always intact and the underlying connective tissue shows an intense inflammatory reaction, with numerous chronic inflammatory cell infiltrations in the area.

Table 2.9: Major differences between squamous cell carcinoma (SCC) and verrucous carcinoma.

	Squamous cell carcinoma	Verrucous carcinoma
Clinical	• Exophytic growth or ulcer with indurated margin • Tobacco smoking, chewing, alcohol, and local irritation are causative factors • Very fast growing and more invasive • Average size of the lesion is larger • Color of the surface is mostly red • Surface whiteness is mostly due to superadded candidiasis. • Lymph node enlargement is due to metastasis. • SCC does not covert into verrucous CA • Prognosis is relatively poor	• Diffuse, white, papillary growth • Pan chewing and snuff dipping are main causative factors • Slow growing and only locally destructive • Average size smaller • Surface color is white • Due to excessive keratinization • Lymph node enlargement is inflammatory • Verrucous CA converts into SCC if not treated • Prognosis is good
Histopathological	• Epithelium shows severe dysplasia • It is a high grade malignancy • Basement membrane is broken causing invasion of tumor cells • Tumor cells spread vertically and laterally • Bulbous, elephant-foot like rete-pegs not seen • Abnormally high rate of mitotic activity in tumor cells • Keratin pearls present • Parakeratin plugging absent • Large islands of malignant epithelium seen in connective tissue	• Epithelium rarely shows dysplasia • Low grade malignancy • Basement membrane is intact and there is no invasion • Tumor cells spread only laterally • Elephant foot-like rete-pegs seen • Mitotic activity rare • Keratin pearls absent • Paraheratin plugging is present • Epithelial islands in connective tissue not seen

- Long-standing verrucous carcinoma lesions sometimes cause compression of the underlying superficial muscle bundles and saucerization of the cortical bone.

- If left untreated for years together, focal areas of neoplastic cells within verrucous carcinoma may turn into invasive SCC and cause metastasis.

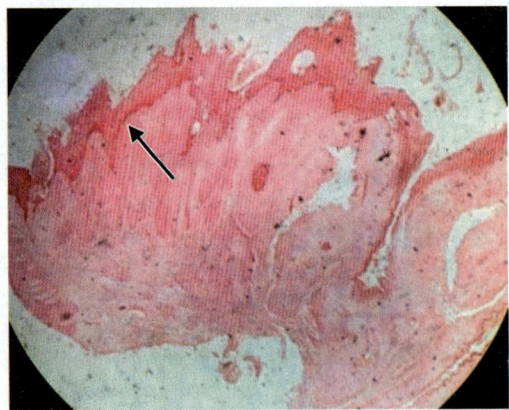

Fig. 2.38: Photomicrograph of verrucous carcinoma showing "church spires" like filiform processes.

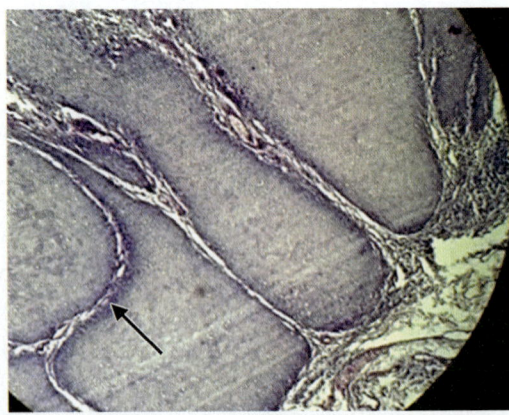

Fig. 2.39: Photomicrograph of verrucous carcinoma showing "elephant foot-like broad" rete-pegs with "pushing margins".

- A hybrid or mixed type of lesion is sometimes seen, which is a combination of both verrucous carcinoma and the conventional invasive SCC. Such types of tumor are to be treated aggressively as they can cause metastasis.

■ DIFFERENTIAL DIAGNOSIS
- Papillary hyperplasia
- Verrucous leukoplakia
- Pyostomatitis vegetans
- Squamous cell carcinoma
- Chronic hyperplastic candidiasis
- Pseudoepitheliomatous hyperplasia.

■ TREATMENT
Surgical excision or laser therapy. Prognosis is good. Anaplastic transformation may sometimes be seen following radiotherapy in verrucous carcinoma.

MALIGNANT MELANOMA

■ DEFINITION
These are malignant neoplasms arising from melanocytes of the skin or mucous membrane; their origin is strongly linked to acquired mutations caused by exposure to UV radiation in sunlight.

Malignant melanomas can develop either as "de novo" lesions or they form due to the malignant transformation of the preexisting "nevi". The neoplasms commonly have an initial radial growth phase, which is followed by a vertical growth phase.

Malignant melanomas are biologically the most unpredictable tumors and are recognized as the most aggressive as well as deadly among all malignant tumors occurring in humans (Box 2.12). It is the third most common cancer of skin.

■ CLINICAL FEATURES
- *Age*: Ranges between 20 years and 90 years of age, however maximum number of cases develops in the 5th to 7th decade of life.

Box 2.12 Predisposing factors in melanoma.
- Sun exposure
- Exposure to artificial ultraviolet rays
- Fair skin, red hair and freckles
- Genetic (familial) factor
- Higher socioeconomic status with regular holidaying habit

- *Sex*: Both sexes are affected but there is a slight male predilection.
- *Sites*: up to 70% lesions occur in the skin, particularly the sun exposed skin of the fair skinned races.

Oral cavity is the primary site for 0.2–8% of all melanomas. These lesions most frequently affect the hard palate and maxillary alveolar ridge or gingiva. However, the lips, lower jaw, floor of the mouth, tongue, buccal mucosa and parotid glands are also sometimes affected. For malignant melanomas the other susceptible mucosal areas include the eyes, vulva and vagina, anus and rectum, and upper respiratory tract, etc.

■ CLINICAL TYPES OF MELANOMA
- *Superficial spreading melanoma*: This type mostly shows radial growth phase, however in long standing lesions vertical growth phase may be seen.
- *Nodular melanoma*: Nodular lesions exhibit only vertical growth phase and are often deeply pigmented.
- *Lentigo maligna melanoma*: Also known as "melanotic freckle of Hutchinson", it characteristically develops as a macular lesion over the malar region, mostly among Caucasian females.
- *Acral lentiginous melanoma*: This lesion occurs as a macular, lentiginous pigmented area around a nodule and is commonly seen over the palms and soles, and fingers and toes.
- *Mucosal lentiginous melanoma*: These are aggressive lesions and are commonly seen on the mucosal surfaces of eye, respiratory tract, esophagus, oral cavity and genitourinary system, etc.

- *Amelanotic melanoma*: Instead of being dark brown or bluish black as the conventional melanomas look like, these lesions appear red or reddish or pinkish due to lack of melanin pigmentations. The malignant melanocytes in these lesions are so poorly differentiated that they cannot produce melanin pigments and hence are called "amelanotic melanomas".

■ PRESENTATION (FIGS. 2.40A AND B)

- Oral melanomas initiate as macular pigmented focal lesions.
- In melanoma, most of the lesions are pigmented excepting few nonpigmented lesions which are referred to as "amelanotic melanomas", and which appear as "slightly" inflamed-looking areas.
- The pigmented lesions may exhibit striking color variations; the lesions may be dark-brown, bluish-black, red, gray or simply black in appearance.
- The initial macular lesions grow very rapidly and often result in a large, painful, diffuse mass.
- Surface ulceration is very common and besides this, hemorrhage, paresthesia and superficial fungal infections are often present.
- The border of melanoma is irregular and often notched; it is an important

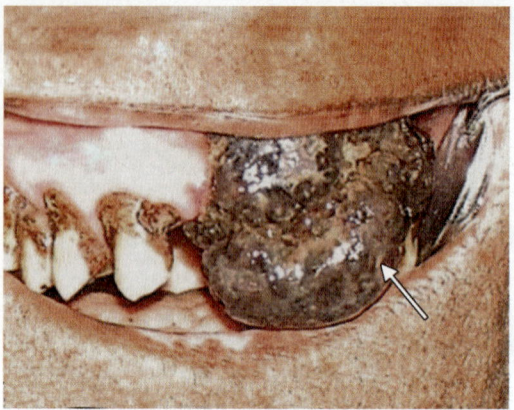

Fig. 2.41: Malignant melanoma of the buccal mucosa.

characteristic for the tumor since the benign nevi will have smooth, round and uniform border.
- As the tumor continues to grow, small satellite lesions can develop at the margin of the primary tumor.
- Unlike other epithelial malignant tumors, melanomas exhibit little or no induration at the periphery.
- Oral melanomas often cause rapid invasion and extensive destruction of bone (Fig. 2.41). This often results in loosening and exfoliation of the regional teeth in the jaw.
- Widespread dissemination of the tumor cells occurs frequently in the lymph nodes

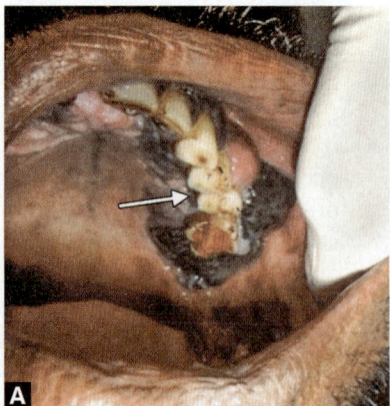 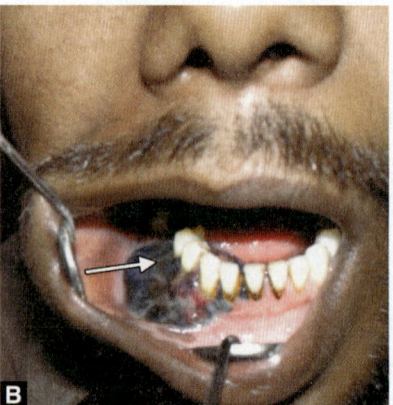

Figs. 2.40A and B: Malignant melanoma of upper and lower alveolar ridge.

Benign and Malignant Neoplasms of the Oral Cavity

> **Box 2.13** *ABCDE*—rule in the clinical diagnosis of melanoma.
>
> - *A*symmetry—due to irregular and uncontrolled growth pattern, one half of the lesion does not match the other half
> - *B*order irregularity—with blurred, notched, or ragged edges
> - *C*olor irregularity—due to variation in melanin formation, a single tumor often exhibit difference in color in its different parts (colors ranging from brown to black, even tan, red, white or blue, etc.)
> - *D*iameter—greater than 6 mm, high rate of growth in itself is also a sign
> - *E*levation—a raised surface can also be a sign

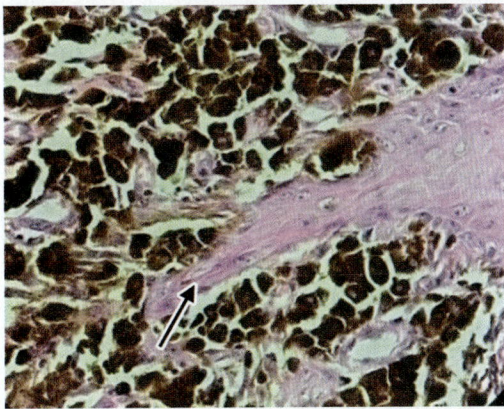

Fig. 2.43: Photomicrograph of malignant melanoma (high power).

as well as in the distant sites, e.g. the lung, liver, bone and brain, etc.
- Survival rates for oral melanomas are extremely low and only less than 5% patients remain alive for 5 years (Box 2.13).

■ HISTOPATHOLOGY (FIG. 2.42)
- Microscopically, malignant melanoma reveals excessive proliferation of neoplastic melanocytes in the form of large masses within the dermis or epidermis (Fig. 2.43).
- These malignant melanocytes often exhibit extensive cellular pleomorphism and nuclear hyperchromatism.

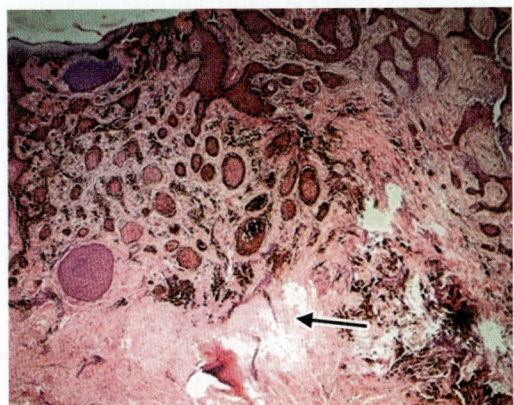

Fig. 2.42: Photomicrograph of malignant melanoma (low power).

- The individual melanoma cells are much larger than the normal melanocytes or those found in the nevi, they have large nuclei with irregular contours, clumped chromatin at the periphery of the nuclear membrane and prominent eosinophilic (red) nucleoli.
- The cells may be round, polyhedral or fusiform in nature and these are either mono-nucleated or multinucleated.
- Mitotic activity is usually numerous and these tumor cells often produce huge amounts of melanin pigments.
- However, in some lesions melanin production by the tumor cells can be very little and on few occasions there can be virtually no melanin production.

According to the arrangement of the tumor cells, malignant melanomas can be divided into three specific histologic patterns:
1. Hutchinson's freckle type
2. Superficial spreading type
3. Invasive type.

Hutchinson's Freckle Type
- Histologically, these lesions are characterized by proliferation of pleomorphic, palisaded, malignant melanocytes in a horizontal direction along the epidermal-dermal junction.

- These atypical tumor cells do not invade into the upper layers of the epithelium.

Superficial Spreading Type

This type of melanoma is histologically characterized by the presence of numerous, large, atypical melanocytes, which proliferate superficially and remain within the epithelial layer.

Invasive Type

- The invasive types of melanoma are usually nodular lesions and are characterized by vertical pattern of growth of the malignant, melanocytes, which frequently invade the underlying connective tissue.
- In invasive type of melanoma, the risk of metastasis increases with increase in the depth of invasion of the tumor cells into the connective tissue; (the depth of invasion is the vertical distance between granular cell layer of the surface epithelium above and the deepest level of tumor cells in the connective tissue below, this measurement is known as "Breslow thickness").

■ DIFFERENTIAL DIAGNOSIS

- Kaposi's sarcoma
- Pigmented basal cell carcinoma
- Hemangioma
- Seborrheic keratitis
- Amalgam tattoo
- Hereditary hemorrhagic telangiectasia
- Benign intraoral nevus
- Hematoma
- Venous lake
- Oral melanotic macule
- Dermatofibroma.

Grades of Malignant Melanoma

Depending upon the depth unto which the malignant cells have invaded or infiltrated into the connective tissue, malignant melanomas are categorized into 5 grades (Table 2.10).

Table 2.10: Grades of malignant melanoma.

Grade I	Malignant cells are confined within the epithelium
Grade II	Malignant cells have invaded into the papillary dermis
Grade III	Malignant cells have invaded up to the level of reticular dermis
Grade IV	Malignant cells have completely invaded the reticular dermis
Grade V	Malignant cells have extended into the subcutaneous fat

■ TREATMENT

The key to the successful treatment of malignant melanoma is early diagnosis as long as the lesion remains in the radial growth phase. Radical surgery with prophylactic neck dissection is often advised. Regardless of the treatment modalities, the tumors in the vertical growth phase often exhibit very poor prognosis.

PRIMARY INTRA-ALVEOLAR CARCINOMA

■ DEFINITION

These are rare malignant neoplasms of epithelial tissue origin, which develop as central jaw lesions with no indication that they have originated from the surface epithelium or they have metastasized from other distant sites.

■ ORIGIN

The tumor arises from the cell rests of the odontogenic epithelium or from the epithelial remnants at the site of fusion between two embryonic processes.

NEOPLASMS OF MESENCHYMAL TISSUE ORIGIN: BENIGN NEOPLASMS OF FIBROUS CONNECTIVE TISSUE

■ FIBROMA

Definition

Fibroma is a benign neoplasm of fibrous connective tissue origin. It is characterized by excessive proliferation of neoplastic fibroblast cells with synthesis of large amount of collagen true fibromas are extremely rare.

Clinical Features

- *Age*: Fibromas commonly develop in the 3rd, 4th and 5th decade of life.
- *Sex*: They are more common among females.
- *Site*: Intraoral fibromas are most commonly seen on the buccal mucosa along the plane of occlusion; besides that they may develop from the gingiva, buccal mucosa, tongue, lips and palate, etc.

Clinical Presentation (Figs. 2.44 and 2.45)

- Clinically, fibromas appear as small, asymptomatic, round or oval, well-circumscribed, slow enlarging, nodular growths in the oral cavity.
- The size varies between 1 cm and 2 cm in diameter.
- These lesions can be either pedunculated or sessile and their surface is usually smooth.
- On palpation, these lesions are either soft or firm in consistency and the overlying covering epithelium often appears normal in color. The color may be gray-brown in black patients.

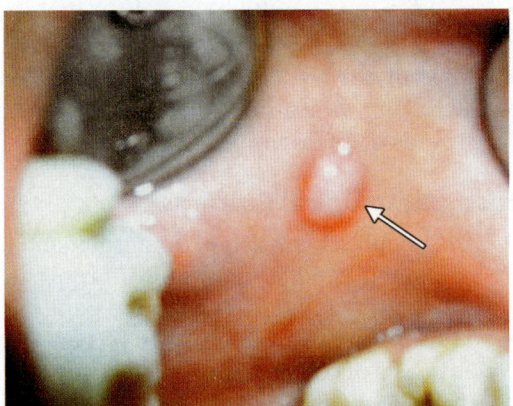

Fig. 2.44: Fibroma.

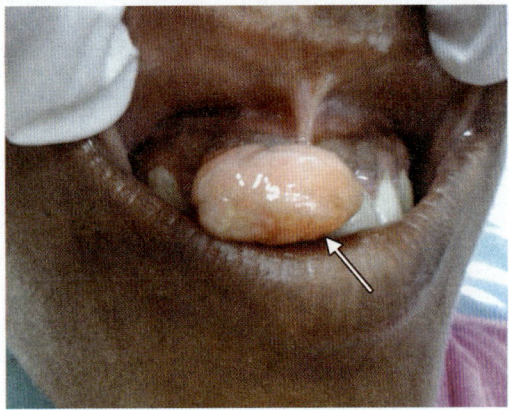

Fig. 2.45: Irritation fibroma.

- Persistent trauma or injury to these lesions often causes pain, inflammation or surface ulceration, etc.
- Sometimes, the surface may be hyperkeratotic.

Differential Diagnosis

- Giant cell fibroma
- Neurofibroma
- Peripheral giant cell granuloma
- Peripheral ossifying fibroma
- Mucoceles
- Salivary gland (minor) neoplasms
- Peripheral odontogenic neoplasm

Histopathology

- Histologically, the neoplasm reveals unencapsulated, solid, nodular mass of dense and sometimes hyalinized connective tissue, which is often arranged in haphazard fascicles (Fig. 2.46).
- The proliferating neoplastic fibroblast cells are large in numbers and they exhibit production of excessive amount of collagen.
- The neoplastic fibroblast cells often appear "spindle-shaped" and they have prominent hyperchromatic nuclei.
- Thick bundles of collagen fiber are characteristically present throughout the lesion. Sometimes, concentric layers of

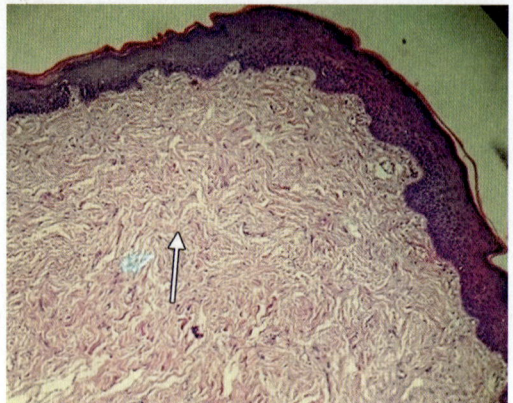

Fig. 2.46: Photomicrograph of irritation fibroma.

collagen fibers may produce a capsule or pseudocapsule around the periphery of the lesion.
- The overlying epithelium is thin and it often shows flattening of the rete pegs. Sometimes it may be hyperplastic or hyperkeratotic.
- Connective tissue stroma is relatively avascular and in some lesions there may be presence of small foci of calcified or ossified tissue within it.

Treatment
By surgical excision.

DESMOPLASTIC FIBROMA

Definition
These are rare benign primary fibroblastic neoplasms arising from the mesenchymal tissue of the jawbone. It is a locally aggressive, intraosseous lesion with high tendency of local recurrence.

Clinical Features
- *Age*: 1st, 2nd and 3rd decade of life. Older patients are rarely affected.
- *Sex*: Both sexes are equally affected.
- *Site*: Mandible is affected more often than maxilla and majority of the lesions occur posterior to the premolar region.

Clinical Presentation
- These intraosseous fibromas are generally asymptomatic neoplasms, however some lesions may produce painless swelling in the jaw.
- Long standing lesions may cause expansion or perforation of the cortical plates of jaw bone.
- Few lesions even corrode through the cortical bone of the jaw and protrude outside as a soft tissue lump.
- Few lesions are locally infiltrative and may cause painful swelling in the jawbone.

Radiographic Features
- Radiographically desmoplastic fibromas reveal unilocular or occasionally multilocular, well-defined, radiolucent areas in the bone.
- Occasionally these lesions can be poorly defined and in most of the cases there is resorption of the roots of the adjoining teeth.

Differential Diagnosis
- Ameloblastoma
- Central giant cell granuloma
- Myxoma
- Central ossifying fibroma.

Macroscopic Features
- Small, circumscribed growth of fibrous tissue, which is firm in consistency.
- The cut surface of the lesion appears as a grayish-white mass, with interlacing strands of fibers running across it.

Histopathological Features
- The neoplasm consists of numerous small, elongated, proliferating young fibroblasts, which are arranged in a whorled pattern.
- The neoplastic cells produce varying amounts of collagen fibers in the tumor.
- In some areas of the tumor, the collagen fibers produce thick bundles and in these

areas the fibroblast cells are only few in numbers.
- In other areas, the fibroblasts are numerous and there is only little amount of collagen present. Intratumor ossification is usually not seen.
- The collagen fibers are usually thin and delicate with fasciculation, often these collagen bundles produce a "herring-bone" or "chevron" or "stori-form" configuration.
- In some cases the tumor mass may extend into the adjacent normal tissues by perforating the cortical plates of bone.

Treatment

Radical surgery is not indicated for the treatment of desmoplastic fibromas. Local excision and curettage can be enough. However even in properly treated cases recurrence is expected in about 25% cases.

GIANT CELL FIBROMA

Definition

Giant cell fibromas are distinct neoplastic entities which arise from the fibrous connective tissue.

Clinical Features

- *Age*: Most of the giant cell fibromas develop in the 1st, 2nd or 3rd decade of life. (Mostly diagnosed in persons aged between 10 years and 30 years).
- *Sex*: Slightly more prevalent among females.
- *Site*: Maxillary or mandibular gingiva is most frequently affected.

Presentation

The unique clinical characteristic of the lesion is its asymptomatic, pedunculated type of nodular growth. Sometimes it can be sessile.
- The lesion usually has a papillary or warty (bosselated) surface and thus sometimes can be mistaken for a papilloma.
- The size is generally less than 1 cm in diameter.
- Some tumors may present a painless, nonulcerated growth and it generally measures about less than 1 cm in size.

Differential Diagnosis

- Squamous papilloma
- Fibroepithelial polyp
- Peripheral giant cell granuloma
- Irritation fibroma.

Histopathology

- Giant cell fibroma microscopically presents an unencapsulated mass of fibrous connective tissue.
- Often there are numerous, actively proliferating, large, plump spindle-shaped or stellate fibroblasts in the tumor with formation of several collagen bundles.
- Presence of multiple multinucleated fibroblastic giant cells is the hallmark in the histopathology of this lesion.

Treatment

By conservative surgical excision. Recurrence is rare.

MYOFIBROMA

Definition

Myofibroma is a rare benign solitary neoplasm characterized by proliferation of spindle shaped myofibroblasts (cells with both smooth muscle and fibroblastic features).

Clinical Features

- *Age*: Children and young adults.
- *Sex*: Both sexes equally affected.
- *Site*: Lips, cheek, tongue and mandible, etc.

Clinical Presentation

Myofibroma typically produces a slow enlarging, painless, well circumscribed mass. Some lesions can be fast enlarging and when multiple myofibromas occur the condition is known as "myofibromatosis". Intraosseous lesions cause bony hard swelling with expansion of cortical plates of the jaw.

Radiographic Features
Intraosseous myofibromas cause unilocular or multilocular radiolucent areas in the jaw with poorly defined borders.

Histopathological Features
Neoplastic proliferation of spindle shaped myofibroblast cells containing tapered or blunt nuclei. Some areas of the tumor is highly cellular, while the other areas are hyalinized with little cellularity. The central area often has a hemangiopericytoma like appearance.

Treatment
By local excision.

■ PERIPHERAL OSSIFYING FIBROMA

Definition
Peripheral ossifying fibroma is an exophytic nodular growth, which commonly occurs on the gingiva and is consisting mostly of hyperplastic connective tissue with focal areas of bone.

Origin
The neoplasm develops as a result of reactive proliferation of either the periodontal or the periosteal tissues. Since both the periodontal and the periosteal tissues contain cells which have some osteogenic potential.

Clinical Features
- *Age*: It predominantly occurs among children and young adults.
- *Sex*: More common among females.
- *Site*: Peripheral ossifying fibromas occur exclusively on the gingiva (mostly on the superficial part of the interdental papilla). More than half of the cases occur within the incisor-cuspid area and lesions have slight predilection for the maxillary arch.

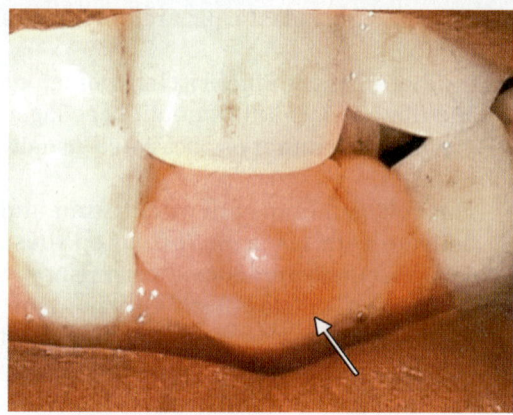

Fig. 2.47: Peripheral ossifying fibroma.

Presentation (Fig. 2.47)
- The neoplasm clinically presents a small, painless, lobulated or nodular swelling on the gingiva.
- It can be either pedunculated or sessile growth, which typically projects from the interdental papilla.
- The overlying mucosa often appears normal, although in some cases it appears reddish.
- The surface of the lesion is usually smooth, although in some cases there can be ulceration on the surface.
- The regional teeth are mostly unaffected. However, there can be migration or loosening of teeth in few cases due to pressure from of the lesion.
- These lesions are either hard or firm on palpation and often they are fixed to the underlying tissue.
- Most lesions are less than 2 cm in diameter, although larger lesions may occasionally develop.

Radiographic Features
Radiograph often reveals the presence of some radiopaque foci within tumor mass, having varying radiodensities (Fig. 2.48).

Histopathology
- Histologically peripheral-ossifying fibroma exhibits diffuse sheets of proliferating,

Benign and Malignant Neoplasms of the Oral Cavity

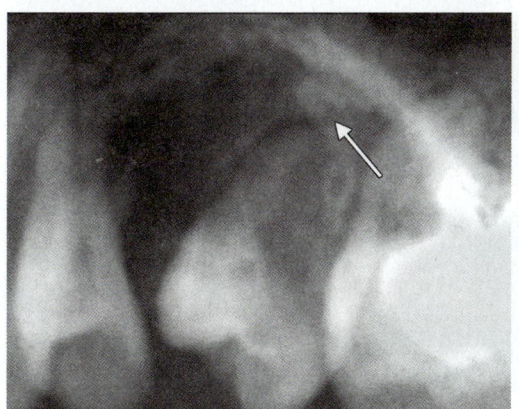

Fig. 2.48: Radiograph of peripheral ossifying fibroma.

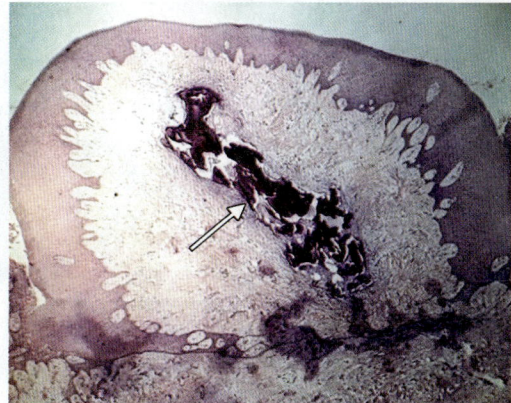

Fig. 2.49: Photomicrograph of peripheral ossifying fibroma.

immature fibroblasts with plump monomorphic nuclei.
- Varying amounts of calcified materials are often present in the lesion, which may be osteoid, cementoid or dystrophic in nature.
- The osteoids can be of varying shape and size; and are often randomly deposited within the fibrous tissue mass.
- The remaining area (other than the area of calcification) of the tumor resembles simple fibroma.
- The covering epithelium appears normal but sometimes it can be ulcerated.
- The bone within the neoplasm is generally of woven or trabecular type, however on rare occasions, thick mature foci of bony trabeculae may be present within the lesion (Fig. 2.49).
- On few occasions multinucleated giant cells can be present in the neoplasm in association with the calcified tissue.
- There is no capsule in this tumor and the hypercellular zone gradually merges with the normal healthy fibrous tissue at the periphery.

Differential Diagnosis
- Peripheral giant cell granuloma
- Fibroma
- Fibroepithelial polyp
- Peripheral ameloblastoma
- Peripheral odontogenic fibroma
- Pyogenic granuloma
- Inflammatory gingival hyperplasia.

Treatment
By surgical excision down to the periosteum along with thorough curettage. The associated teeth are preserved.

■ CENTRAL OSSIFYING FIBROMA

Definition
Central ossifying fibroma represents a well-demarcated, encapsulated, expansile, central jaw lesion that is composed of cellular fibrous tissue, with spherical calcifications and irregular randomly oriented bony structures.

Clinical Features
- *Age*: Greatest numbers of cases occur in children and young adults.
- *Sex*: More predilections for females.
- *Site*: Mandible is far more commonly affected than maxilla. The disease often involves posterior to the canine area (Figs. 2.50A and B).

Presentation (Fig. 2.51)
Central ossifying fibroma clinically presents the following features:
- There will be a localized, painless, non-tendered, bony hard swelling in the jaw (Fig. 2.52).

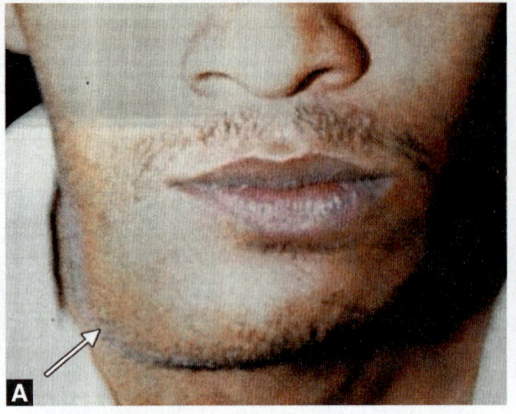 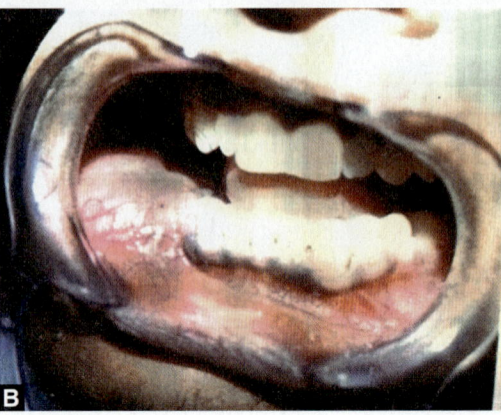

Figs. 2.50A and B: (A) Central ossifying fibroma of mandible; (B) Intraoral view of the same patient.

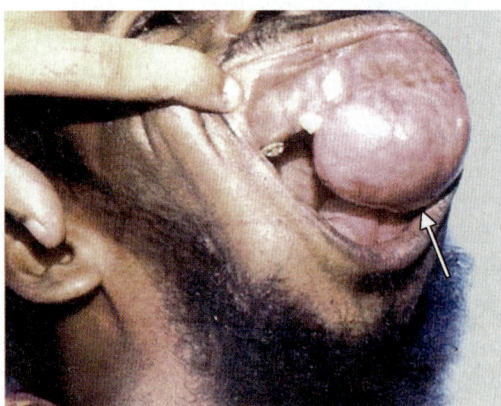

Fig. 2.51: Aggressive ossifying fibroma of maxilla.

- The tumor is normally slow growing and gradual increase in its size causes facial deformity.
- Expansion and distortion of the cortical plates and displacement of the regional teeth are often seen.
- Pain and paresthesia generally do not occur in case of central ossifying fibroma.
- Although most of the lesions follow a simple benign course, some lesions especially those affecting the children may be rapidly growing and locally aggressive in nature (Fig. 2.53). The fast growing lesion produce a massive swelling, and are often

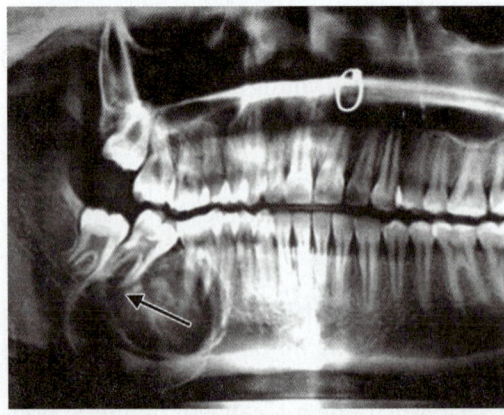 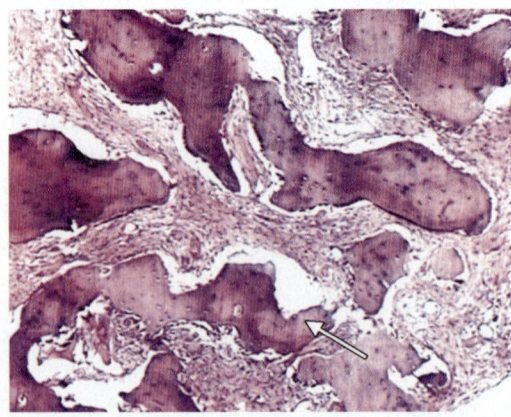

Fig. 2.52: Central ossifying fibromas—early stage.

Fig. 2.53: Photomicrograph of central ossifying fibroma—low power.

referred to as "aggressive ossifying fibromas" and they cause severe disfigurement of the face.

Radiographic Features
- Radiographically, central ossifying fibroma presents a well-defined, mostly unilocular or sometimes multilocular radiolucent area with clearly demarcated borders.
- Expansion of the cortical plates and a smooth, downward bowing expansion of the lower border of the mandible are commonly observed.
- The lesion often extends between the roots of the teeth and causes root divergence and displacement of teeth. Root resorption may sometimes occur.
- In the earlier stages, the lesion is small and is almost completely radiolucent.
- As the lesion enlarges multiple, small radiopaque areas gradually appear within it.
- In the more mature stages of the disease, large radiopaque masses are seen within the lesion that almost completely fill up the area with only a thin rim of radiolucency separating the lesion from the surrounding normal bone.
- In ossifying fibroma, the neoplasm does not blend with the surrounding normal bone, rather it is always demarcated from it by a thin zone of fibrous tissue capsule.

Macroscopic Features
The cut surface of central ossifying fibroma often exhibits a whitish-yellow mass, with variable consistency and the tissue always has a gritty surface.

Histopathology
Histologically central ossifying fibromas reveal the following features:
- A highly cellular fibroblastic stroma with the presence of delicate collagen fibers, which are arranged in a typical "whorled pattern".

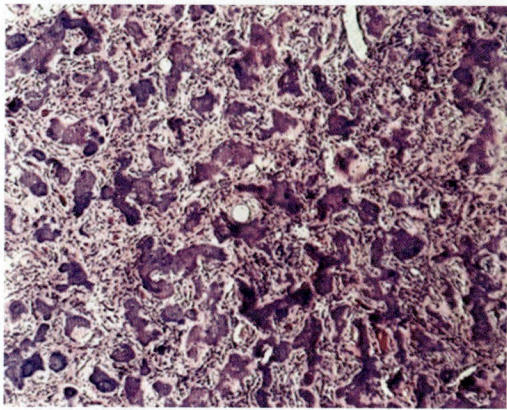

Fig. 2.54: Photomicrograph of ossifying fibroma with "psammoma bodies".

- The lesion is well-demarcated from the normal bone by a thin zone of fibrous capsule.
- Numerous blood capillaries run across in stroma although intralesional major hemorrhage is rarely seen.
- In early lesions, the fibrous elements often predominate and there can be presence of multiple small foci of osteoid trabeculae of variable size and shape, the osteoids at this stage are poorly calcified.
- In more mature stages of the disease, osteoid tissues within the lesion increase in size, as small individual osteoid trabeculae fuse together and give rise to large irregular calcified masses.
- Besides osteoids, there may be presence of mature bone as well as poorly cellular, basophilic spherules that resemble cementum.
- Psammoma bodies are concentric lamellated calcified structures, which are sometimes present in ossifying fibromas; such lesions are known as "psammomatoid" type ossifying fibroma (Fig. 2.54).
- In central ossifying fibroma various types of calcified materials are seen such as osteoids, bone and cementum like spherules this structural pattern typically differs from fibrous dysplasia as the later exhibits a more uniform pattern of osseous differentiation (Figs. 2.55A and B).

Ossifying fibroma	Cementifying fibroma
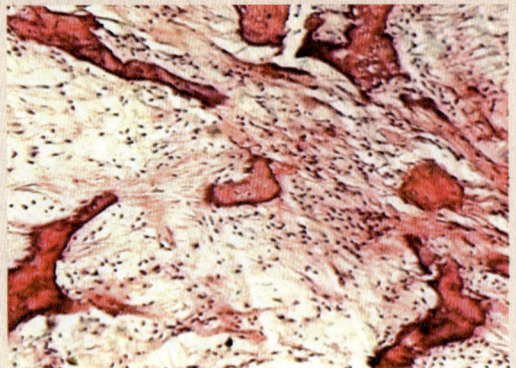	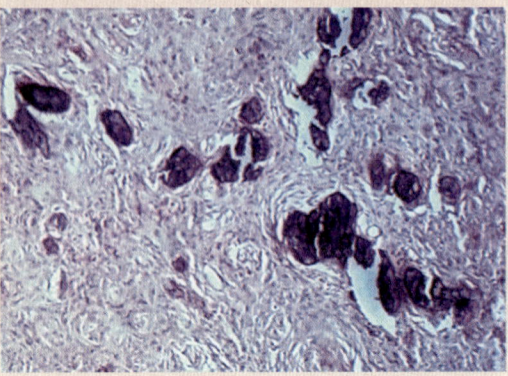
• The bony trabeculae are often lightly stained • The trabeculae are relatively larger in size and elongated in shape.	• The cemental trabeculae are more deeply stained • The trabeculae are relatively smaller in size and round in shape.

Figs. 2.55A and B: Distinction between ossifying and cementifying fibromas.

Differential Diagnosis
- Fibrous dysplasia of bone
- Desmoplastic fibroma
- Central giant cell granuloma
- Myxoma
- Schwannoma

Treatment
Surgical enucleation is the treatment of choice and can be easily accomplished in smaller lesions. The aggressive lesions of central ossifying fibroma may require radical treatments like resection and bone grafting, especially in cases of repeated recurrences.

GIANT CELLS

Definition of giant cells: Giant cells are very large, multinucleated, modified macrophages, which may be formed by coalescence of mononuclear cells or by nuclear division without cytoplasmic division of monocytes, particularly in response to the presence of a foreign body. Both giant cells and macrophages express similar antigenic marker; and many of the giant cells have osteoclastic behavior.

PERIPHERAL GIANT CELL GRANULOMA

Definition
Peripheral giant cell granuloma (PGCG) is the most common of all the giant cell lesions, which arise from the tooth bearing areas of the jaw and they typically appear as a purplish-red nodules on the gingiva (Box 2.14).

Box 2.14	Common giant cell lesions of oral cavity.
	• Peripheral giant cell granuloma • Central giant cell granuloma • Brown tumor of hyperparathyroidism • Giant cell tumor of bone (osteoclastoma) • Cherubism • Fibrous dysplasia of bone • Aneurysmal bone cyst • Solitary bone cyst • Hodgkin's lymphoma • Fibrous histiocytoma • Calcifying epithelial odontogenic cyst • Tuberculosis • Sarcoidosis • Langerhans cells disease • Eosinophilic granuloma

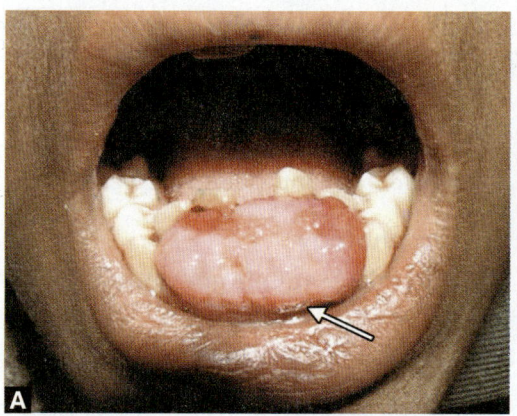 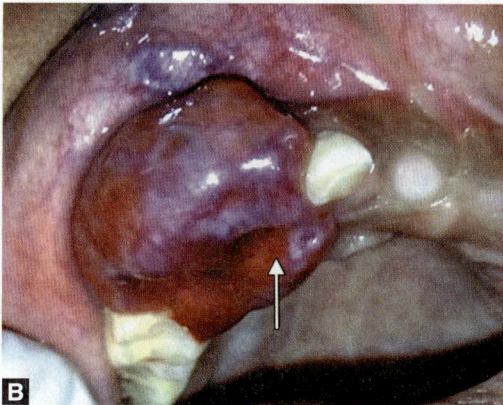

Figs. 2.56A and B: Peripheral giant cell granuloma.

Origin

The lesion probably develops from the connective tissue of the periosteum of jaw bone or from the periodontal ligament tissue.

Etiology

The etiology of peripheral giant cell granuloma is unknown; these lesions probably develop due to exaggerated response of the gingival tissue local irritation.

Clinical Features

- *Age*: The lesion usually arises either during the mixed dentition period or during the 3rd and 4th decade of life
- *Sex*: Definite predilection for females (M:F—3:1).
- *Site*: From the interdental papilla in dentulous patients. Sometimes, it can also develop from the edentulous alveolar ridge. Mandible is more frequently affected than maxilla.

Clinical Presentation (Figs. 2.56A and B)

- Peripheral giant cell granuloma clinically appears as a small, exophytic, well-circumscribed, pedunculated lesion on the gingival surface.
- The lesion is usually painless, firm and lobulated and the surface is either smooth or granular.
- Most lesions of peripheral giant cell granulomas measure less than 2 cm in diameter, however larger lesions are also occasionally seen.
- The color of the lesion varies from purplish-red to dark-red and the overlying epithelium is often ulcerated.
- Some of the lesions could be firm in consistency and these are often relatively pale in appearance.
- There can be bleeding from the surface of the lesion either spontaneously or upon provocation with an instrument.
- Careful examination of the lesion reveals multiple, small areas of hemosiderin pigmentation on the surface of the lesion.
- Since the lesion develops and descends from the deeper periodontium, it may increase the space between the affected teeth.
- In some cases the lesion may develop with an "hour-glass" shape and in such cases the waist of the lesion is located between the teeth and the lobulated extremities projecting both buccally and lingually.
- Clinically, peripheral giant cell granuloma often looks very similar to pyogenic granuloma, however, peripheral giant cell granulomas are more firm in consistency and are bluish-purple in color, whereas pyogenic granulomas are much softer in consistency and are more reddish in color.

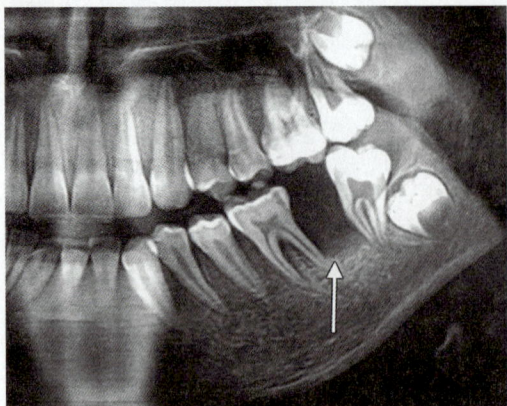

Fig. 2.57: Radiograph of peripheral giant cell granuloma showing "peripheral cuffing of bone" with displacement of teeth.

Radiographic Features

Peripheral giant cell granuloma has the potential to erode the underlying alveolar bone and on radiograph this type lesion is often known as "peripheral cuffing" of bone (Fig. 2.57).

Macroscopic Features (Fig. 2.58)

- Macroscopically, peripheral giant cell granuloma appears as a lobulated, firm growth having a pedunculated base.
- The cut surface of the lesion often presents a homogeneous, reddish-brown, granulomatous tissue.
- Some lesions may exhibit a peripheral brownish zone that is interrupted by pale radiating streaks.
- The surface epithelium is often ulcerated and there is also presence of several pigmented spots (blood pigments).

Histopathology

Peripheral giant cell granuloma usually presents the following histologic features (Fig. 2.59):
- The overlying covering epithelium is mostly ulcerated with areas of hemorrhage.
- The underlying connective tissue stroma reveals numerous proliferating fibroblasts, blood capillaries and multiple multinucleated giant cells, which are scattered throughout the lesion.
- The entire lesion is situated within the subepithelial connective tissue of gingiva and is separated from the overlying epithelium by a thin rim of fibrous septa.
- The fibroblasts present in the hypercellular stroma are mostly plump ovoid or spindle shaped and they contain oval shaped nuclei.
- The giant cells are often larger in size and contain only few to several dozens nuclei, (more number of nuclei in individual giant cells as compared to that of true giant cell tumors).

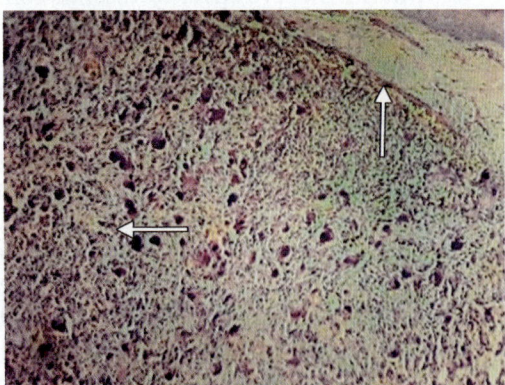

Fig. 2.58: Photomicrograph of peripheral giant cell granulomas (low power).

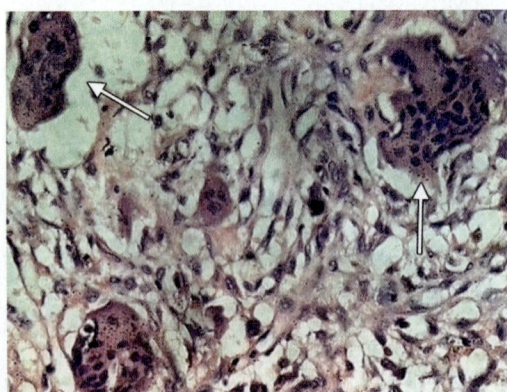

Fig. 2.59: Photomicrograph of peripheral giant cell granuloma with typical giant cells in high power.

- The nuclei within the giant cells can either be large vesicular in nature or they can be small, pyknotic type of nuclei.
- Interestingly, the giant cells in this lesion often tend to aggregate or assemble around the blood capillaries and in few cases, they can be even found within the lumen of the capillaries.
- Often there is little chronic inflammatory cell infiltration.
- Areas of hemorrhage and hemosiderin pigments are often present within the connective tissue stroma.
- Sometimes foci of osteoids or even mature bone tissue may be present within the stroma, especially near the periphery.

Key Points of Peripheral Giant Cell Granuloma

- Most common giant cell lesions of the oral cavity arise from the tooth bearing areas of jaw.
- More commonly seen in females and the lesion often presents small, lobulated, purplish-red colored, pedunculated growth with occasional surface ulcerations and bleeding, etc.
- Lesions are exophytic, mostly painless, grow in the gingival area in a typical "hour glass" pattern, pressure from the growing lesions may create gap between teeth.
- The radiograph reveals "peripheral cuffing" in the bone.
- Histologically, the lesion exhibits overlying thin ulcerated epithelium and the underlying connective tissue shows proliferating fibroblasts, numerous blood capillaries and multiple multinucleated giant cells, etc.
- The giant cells are large and they tend to group around the blood capillaries.

Differential Diagnosis
- Pyogenic granuloma
- Fibroepithelial polyp
- Peripheral ossifying fibroma
- Fibroma
- Traumatic neuroma.

Treatment
By surgical excision with curettage.

CENTRAL GIANT CELL GRANULOMA

Definition
Central giant cell granuloma is a relatively common benign intraosseous destructive giant cell lesion, which often affects the anterior part of the jawbone.

Lesions similar to central giant cell granulomas can occur in relation to the long bones as well and they often follow an aggressive course. Central giant cell granuloma is often confused with giant cell tumor of bone (osteoclastoma), however, it should be noted that giant cell granuloma is a reactive lesion, whereas giant cell tumor is a neoplastic condition of the bone. Moreover osteoclastomas are very rarely seen within the jawbones.

Clinical Features
- *Age*: This lesion usually occurs among young adults (mostly below the age of 30).
- *Sex*: Female predilection (female to male ratio is 2:1).
- *Site*:
  - Central giant cell granulomas affect mandible more often (nearly 70% cases) than maxilla. The lesions occur mostly in the body of the mandible anterior to the first molar area (in the zone where previously the deciduous teeth existed).
  - Most of the lesions develop in the tooth bearing areas of jaw and some lesions may even cross the midline of the mandibular bone.

Presentation (Figs. 2.60A and B)
- Most of the central giant cell granulomas are asymptomatic lesions and are discovered incidentally during routine radiographic examinations.
- Other lesions produce small, slow enlarging and bony hard swelling of the jaw, with expansion of the cortical plates.
- Some lesions produce pain and paresthesia in the jaw.

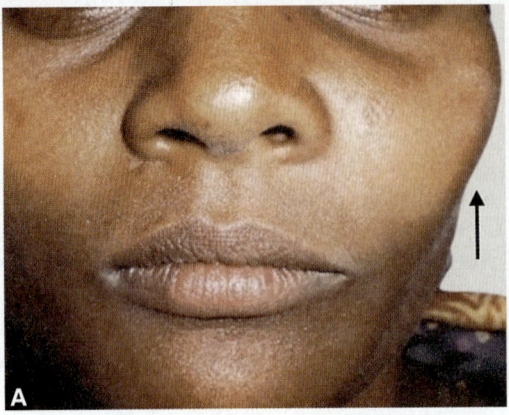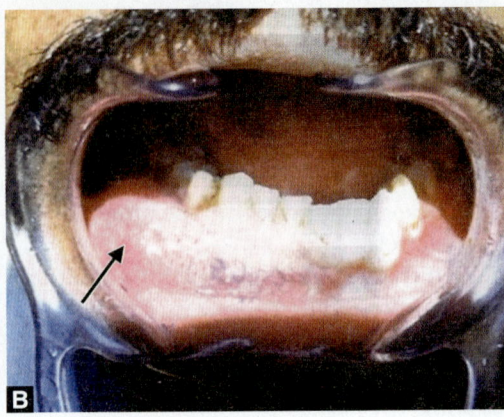

Figs. 2.60A and B: Central giant cell granuloma causing: (A and B) Swelling of left maxilla, and of right mandible.

- The lesion causes expansion and distortion of both buccal and lingual cortical plates and often there is displacement or mobility of the regional teeth.
- Some lesions may cause perforation of the cortical plate and as a result of this the intrabony lesions may protrude outside jawbone as a flat-based, dome-shaped, soft, purplish nodule over the alveolar ridge.
- Central giant cell granulomas sometimes follow an aggressive course and in such cases they produce a fast enlarging, large, painful swelling in the jaw, with anesthesia or paresthesia in the region.
- Larger lesions often cause loosening or displacement of teeth in the jaw and root resorptions and are found to be often crossing the midline.
- The teeth in the affected region are always vital.

Radiological Features (Fig. 2.61)

- Radiographically the lesion produces a well delineated, multilocular radiolucent area in the jaw, with a "soap-bubble" appearance.
- The margin of the lesion is usually scalloped and well-demarcated, but it is always non-corticated.

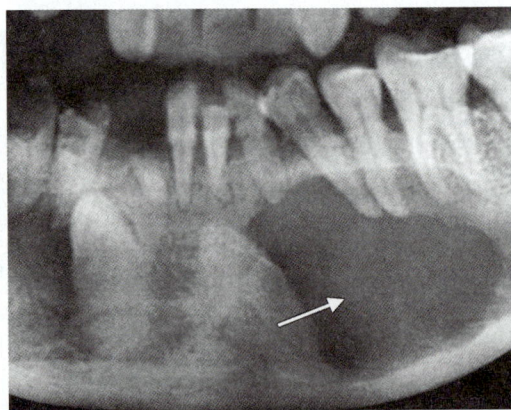

Fig. 2.61: Radiograph of central giant cell granuloma.

- Sometimes central giant cell granulomas can be unilocular and they produce "drop-shaped" radiolucencies in the jawbone and such lesions often resemble cysts.
- Expansion and distortion of the cortical plates are common and in some cases there may be perforation of the cortical plate.
- Resorption of roots of the nearby teeth or divergence of roots is common feature of this lesion.

Histopathology (Figs. 2.62 and 2.63)

- Histologically, central giant cell granuloma exhibits a lobulated mass of fibrovascular

Benign and Malignant Neoplasms of the Oral Cavity

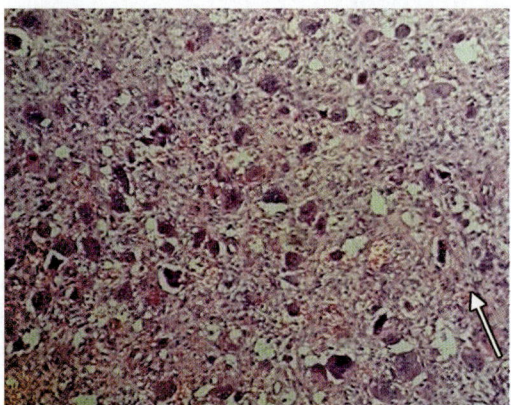

Fig. 2.62: Photomicrograph of central giant cell granuloma (low power).

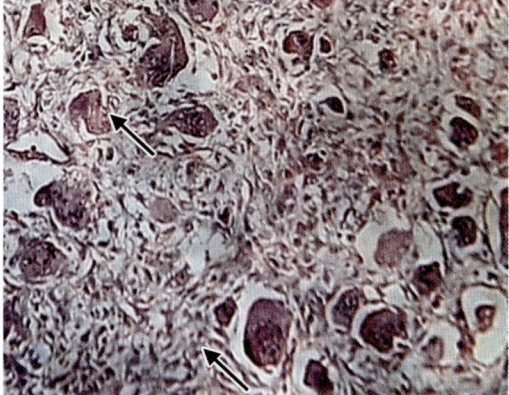

Fig. 2.63: Photomicrograph of central giant cell granuloma (high power).

connective tissue, consisting of numerous proliferating ovoid or spindle shaped stromal cells and variable amount of interlacing collagen fibers (Table 2.11).

- Multiple multinucleated giant cells of varying size are dispersed throughout the fibrous tissue stroma, where numerous small blood capillaries are also found.
- Sometimes giant cells may assemble in great numbers in a focal area of the tumor.
- Several areas of hemorrhage and hemosiderin pigmentation are also evident.
- Giant cells are often found around the blood capillaries or near the areas of hemorrhage.
- In central giant cell granuloma, the small giant cells usually contain about five nuclei, however the larger giant cells of the same lesion may contain as many as 20 or more nuclei.
- The stromal cells are plump and spindle-shaped and these cells often exhibit frequent mitosis.
- Small foci of osteoids or oven normal bone are often found near the periphery of the lesion.

Key Points of Central Giant Cell Granuloma

❖ This is a central jaw lesion, which causes bony hard swelling with expansion of the bone.
❖ The disease is a type of reactive lesion and not a truly neoplastic one.
❖ Although some lesions are aggressive in nature but it is generally a slow enlarging and painless condition.
❖ Expansion of the bone occurs with occasional cortical perforation, tooth mobility and root resorptions.
❖ Radiograph reveals multilocular, well-defined jaw lesions with a "soap-bubble" appearance; present generally anterior to the first molar regions, some lesions are typically "drop-shaped".

Table 2.11: Histological distinction between central giant cell granuloma and giant cell tumor of bone.

Central giant cell granuloma	Giant cell tumor of bone
• Giant cells are of variable size, some cells are large while others are small	• Giant cells are of uniform size and most cells are large
• Average size of the giant cells are smaller than those seen in giant cell tumor	• Average size of the giant cells are larger than those of granuloma
• Giant cells are often haphazardly distributed; somewhere giant cells are more and in other areas they are less	• Giant cells are uniformly distributed throughout the lesion
• Areas of hemorrhage are common	• Hemorrhagic areas are less often present
• Inflammatory cells are more in numbers	• Less number of inflammatory cells are seen

> - Histologically, the lesion shows proliferating spindle shaped stromal cells in a fibrovascular connective tissue stroma, which characteristically contains multiple multinucleated giant cells.
> - Hemorrhage and hemosiderin pigmentations are often seen in tumor.

- There may be little amount of chronic inflammatory cell infiltration in the connective tissue stroma.
- Central giant cell granuloma and giant cell tumor of bone one often confused histologically, but the fact is that in central giant cell granuloma the giant cells are relatively less in number and are very irregularly distributed throughout the lesion.
- Whereas, in giant cell tumor of bone (osteoclastoma), the number of giant cells are more in number and they are evenly distributed throughout the stroma.

Pathogenesis

The exact etiopathogenesis of central giant cell granuloma is not known:
- According to some investigators, central giant cell granuloma develops as a reparative process in response to the intrabony hemorrhage or inflammation.
- Some other scientists believe that central giant cell granuloma is a truly neoplastic condition.
- According to other investigators, the lesion occurs as a developmental anomaly and its pathogenesis is similar to that of aneurysmal bone cyst.

Differential Diagnosis

In the differential diagnosis of central giant cell granuloma following lesions should be included:
- Brown tumor of hyperparathyroidism
- Giant cell tumor of bone
- Ameloblastoma
- Aneurysmal bone cyst
- Central odontogenic fibroma
- Fibrous dysplasia
- Cherubism
- Odontogenic keratocyst
- Calcifying epithelial odontogenic cyst
- Osteoblastoma.
- Myxoma.

Note: It is often difficult to differentiate between central giant cell granuloma and brown tumor of hyperparathyroidism on the basis of clinical, radiological and histopathological features. For this reason biochemical analysis of blood is always necessary. Normally the raised serum calcium and serum alkaline phosphatase level along with depressed serum phosphate levels confirm the diagnosis of hyperparathyroidism. However, in cases of central giant cell granuloma the above mentioned biochemical changes in the blood is not observed.

Treatment

Surgical excision and thorough curettage.

BENIGN FIBROUS HISTIOCYTOMA

Definition

Benign fibrous histiocytoma is a locally aggressive benign neoplasm of fibroblasts with a propensity to differentiate into histiocytes. These tumors actually arise from the facultative fibroblasts, which are mesenchymal cells that have potential to differentiate into both fibroblasts and histiocytes.

Clinical Features

- *Age*: These tumors usually arise in the middle aged and older adults.
- *Sex*: Male people are more prone to develop this lesion as compared to females.
- *Site*: Oral soft tissues such as tongue, buccal mucosa, vestibule, palate and jawbones, etc.

Clinical Presentation

- Benign fibrous histiocytoma clinically produces a nodular, soft or firm, nontender swelling of varying size (Fig. 2.64).

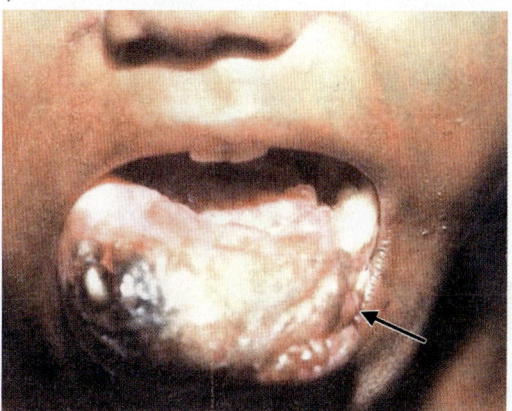

Fig. 2.64: Benign fibrous histiocytoma of mandible.

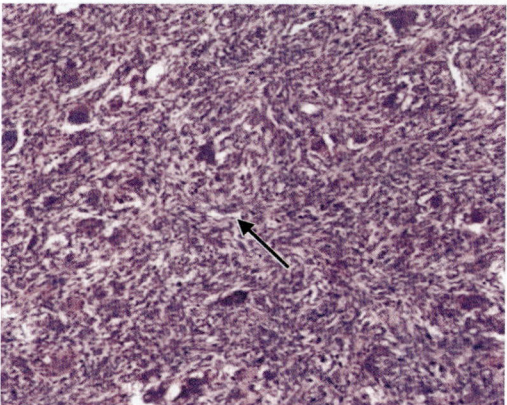

Fig. 2.65: Photomicrograph of benign fibrous histiocytoma.

- Intrabony lesions produce expansile swelling with displacement of the regional teeth.
- The size of the tumor varies between few millimeters to several centimeters in size.
- The superficial lesions are generally smaller in size, while the deep tissue lesions tend to be larger in size.

Radiographic Finding
Bony lesions produce unilocular or multilocular radiolucent areas with ill-defined border.

Macroscopy
Macroscopically benign fibrous histiocytoma presents a lobulated, fleshy mass, which is firm in consistency.

Histopathology (Fig. 2.65)
- Histologically, the tumor presents actively proliferating fibroblasts and histiocytes, which are often arranged in short interlacing fascicles.
- The fibrous histiocytoma is poorly demarcated from surrounding tissues and is separated from overlying mucosa by a zone of fibrovascular connective tissue (grenz zone).
- The fibroblasts are elongated and spindle-shaped with vesicular nuclei, and these cells synthesize mature collagens.
- The histiocytes are large cells with oval nuclei and have a very thin cytoplasm.
- The tumor cells often exhibit a characteristic "storiform" pattern of arrangement, as it resembles the irregular, whorled appearance of a typical "straw-mat".
- Mitotic figures are uncommon in the tumor cells, however there may be presence of few "Touton type" multinucleated giant cells.

Treatment
Local excision.

MYXOMA

Definition
Myxomas are true neoplasms, which are made up of tissues that often resemble primitive mesenchyme. The lesions are benign and do not metastasize, although they frequently infiltrate into the adjacent tissues.

Clinical Features
- *Age*: It can occur at any age.
- *Sex*: There is no definite sex predilection.
- *Site*: Oral submucosal area, salivary gland and jawbones.

Presentation
Soft tissue myxomas are rare lesion and they usually produce a nondescript, firm, nodular growth of varying size.

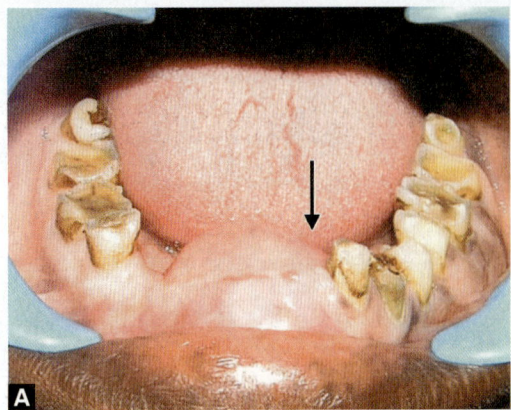
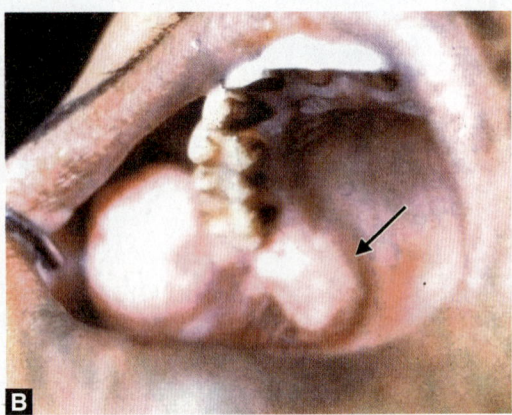

Figs. 2.66A and B: Myxoma of (A) anterior mandible and (B) of maxilla.

Bony myxomas produce aggressive swelling with expansion and destruction of the cortical plates; since the lesion infiltrates locally it causes loss of alveolar bone resulting in mobility and displacement of the regional teeth (Figs. 2.66 and 2.67).

Histopathology (Fig. 2.68)

- The lesion is composed of a loose textured tissue containing delicate reticulin fibers and mucoid material.
- Within the loosely arranged tissue, stellate-shaped cells are sparsely distributed.
- Some myxomas exhibit increased vascularity and are named as "angiomyxomas".

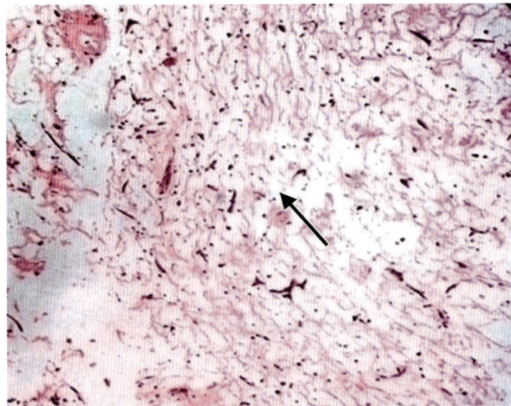

Fig. 2.68: Photomicrograph of myxoma.

- The tumor is not encapsulated and can invade into the surrounding tissues.

Treatment

Since myxomas are locally aggressive neoplasms, radical surgery is often recommended for their treatment.

■ NODULAR FASCIITIS

Definition

Nodular or pseudosarcomatous fasciitis is a localized benign lesion, which is composed of fibroblasts and myofibroblasts and is often clinically mistaken for malignancy.

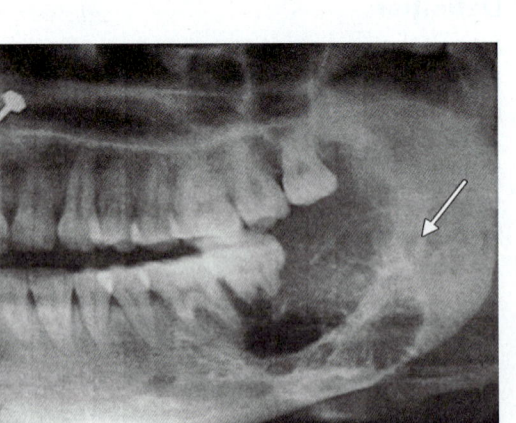

Fig. 2.67: Myxoma producing a typical "tennis racket" like radiolucency in left mandibular molar region.

Clinical Features

This lesion occurs more commonly in the extremities. About 15–20% lesions appear in the head and neck region including the oral cavity.
- *Age*: 3rd, 4th and 4th decade of life.
- *Sex*: Both sexes can be affected, but there is a male predominance.
- *Site*: Buccal mucosa, skin of the face, tongue, alveolar mucosa, parotid gland and submucosa overlying the mandible and zygoma.

Presentation

- Clinically, nodular fasciitis presents a rapidly growing, firm, submucosal mass, the rate of growth is sometimes so fast that clinically malignancy is often suspected.
- The lesion is usually measuring less than 5 cm in diameter and it can be partially encapsulated.
- Most of the lesions produce pain and tenderness upon palpation.
- Although the onset is very rapid, however the growth potential of this neoplasm is limited.
- These are benign lesions and if left untreated they regress spontaneously.

Histopathology

- Microscopically nodular fasciitis exhibits spindle or stellate-shaped cells with vesicular nuclei, which are arranged in a fascicular or swirled pattern.
- Hypercellularity, cellular pleomorphism and multiple mitotic activities are often seen.
- Tissue spaces are often filled with extracellular mucin, which have a myxoid appearance.
- Multiple multinucleated giant cells may be present in some lesions.
- Nodular fasciitis is often histologically confused with fibrosarcoma.
- However, the individual cell nuclei are monomorphic and uniform in appearance, thereby indicates a nonmalignant condition.

Differential Diagnosis

- Fibrous histiocytoma
- Fibromatosis
- Neurofibroma
- Fibrosarcoma.

Treatment

Local excision. Recurrence is uncommon.

BENIGN NEOPLASM OF ADIPOSE TISSUE ORIGIN

LIPOMA

Definition

Lipoma is a benign neoplasm of adipose tissue origin and is composed of mature fat cells (lipoblasts).

However, the metabolism of lipoma is completely independent of normal body fat.

Clinical Features

- *Age*: Most of the lesions occur in adults above 40 years of age and are rarely seen in children.
- *Sex*: Both sexes are almost equally affected.
- *Site*: Intraoral lipomas generally arise from the superficial connective tissue and few lesions develop within the deep tissues of cheek and buccal vestibule. Tongue, lips, floor of the mouth and salivary glands are also sometimes affected.

Presentation

- Clinically, lipoma presents a relatively well defined, very soft, frequently movable lump, within the underlying connective tissue (Fig. 2.69).
- Lipomas are smooth surfaced, nodular, pedunculated or sessile lesions.
- These are painless lesions and on palpation often there is a cyst-like feeling.
- Fibrolipoma is a variant of lipoma, which feels firm on palpation.
- The superficial lipomas usually appear yellow in color and they exhibit a smooth

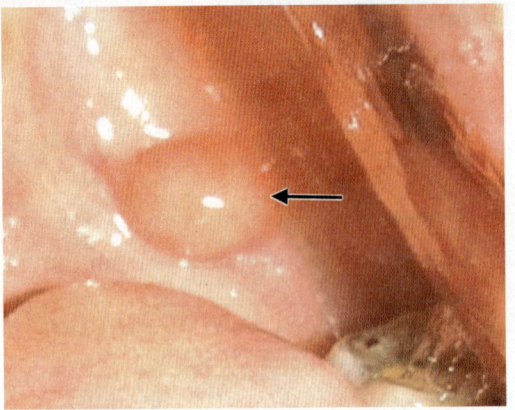

Fig. 2.69: Lipoma on the buccal mucosa.

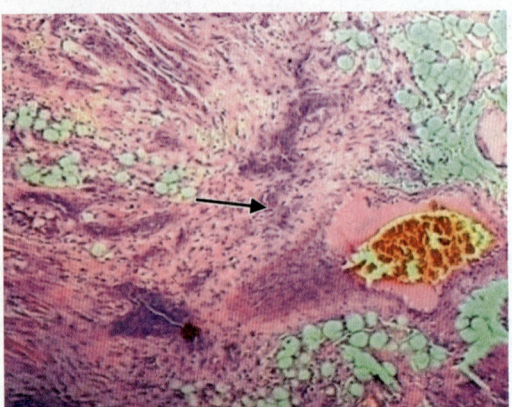

Fig. 2.71: Photomicrograph of angiolipoma showing vascular tissue proliferation in lipoma.

overlying surface. However, the deep lesions of lipoma often appear pink in color.
- Lipomas are mostly asymptomatic lesions and they measure about below 3 cm in diameter in most instances.

Macroscopic Appearance

Macroscopically lipoma appears as a soft, yellow, lobulated mass, which floats in aqueous solutions such as formalin fixatives.

Histopathology (Figs. 2.70 and 2.71)

- Histologically, lipomas present well-circumscribed areas of proliferating mature fat cells (adipocytes) within a loose areolar tissue stroma.
- Individual tumor cells are round and vacuolated with clear cytoplasm and centrally placed nuclei.
- In most of the lesions, lobules of fat cells are often separated at places by fibrous tissue septa.
- Occasionally, lipomas may contain benign lipoblasts; these are multinucleated cells with nuclei arranged in a "floret" pattern. These cells often produce a 'soap-bubble' appearance due to the presence of intracytoplasmic vacuoles.
- In some lipomas, myxomatous, fibrous, angiomatous, osseous or cartilaginous tissues may be present in addition to the fat cells, these cells develop as a result of metaplastic change in the tumor cells of lipoma.

Histologic Variants of Lipoma

- *Fibrolipoma*: Characterized by a significant fibrous component intermixed with the lobules of fat cells.
- *Angiolipoma*: Consists of an admixture of mature fat and numerous small blood vessels.
- *Spindle cell lipoma*: Demonstrates variable amounts of uniform appearing spindle cells in conjunction with a more typical lipomatous component.
- *Osteolipoma*: Characterized by formation of bone within the tumor.

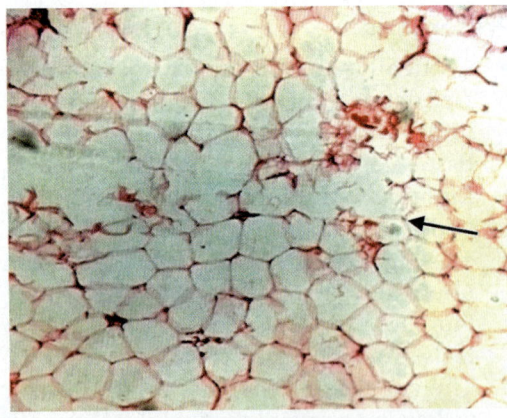

Fig. 2.70: Photomicrograph of lipoma.

Benign and Malignant Neoplasms of the Oral Cavity

Table 2.12: Differences between hemangioma and vascular malformation.

Hemangiomas	Vascular malformations
• Not present at birth • True neoplasms with active proliferation of endothelial cells • Regress in size with age • Size of the lesion does not increase with age, not affected by hormonal influence • Responds to steroid therapy • Mast cells count increased • No nerve seen within the tumor	• Present at birth • Congenital malformations of vascular tissues but no change in endothelial cell cycle • Stable lesions, present throughout life • Increase with age of the patient, accelerated growth during pregnancy and puberty (hormonal influence) • Do not respond to steroid therapy • Normal mast cell count • Nerves may be present in the vicinity

- *Myxoid lipoma*: Some spindle cell lipomas exhibit a mucoid background.
- *Pleomorphic lipomas*: These are characterized by presence of spindle-shaped cells along with bizarre, hyperchromatic giant cells.
- *Intramuscular (infiltrating) lipomas*: These are more deeply situated and have an infiltrative growth pattern that extends between skeletal muscle bundles.
- *Sialolipoma*: It was coined to describe tumors that secondarily entrap salivary gland tissue.

Treatment

Simple surgical excision.

BENIGN NEOPLASM OF VASCULAR TISSUE ORIGIN

HEMANGIOMA

Definition

There are two common vascular abnormalities often encountered, one is a pure neoplasm (hemangioma) and the other one is called a "vascular malformation"; these lesions differ in their pathogenesis and biologic behavior. Hemangiomas are relatively common benign proliferative lesions of vascular tissue origin, which may be present either at birth or may arise during early childhood.

Hemangiomas exhibit neoplastic proliferation of vascular tissue that often closely resembles the normal vessels.

Vascular malformations are congenital malformations of vascular tissues, made up of morphologically altered tortuous vessels.

The differences between hemangiomas and vascular malformations are given in Table 2.12.

Clinical Features

- *Age*: Being the commonest neoplasm of infancy, most hemangiomas are present either at birth or they arise at an early age.
- *Sex*: It is seen more commonly among females.
- *Site*: About 60% lesions occur in the head and neck region. Intraorally hemangiomas frequently occur over the facial skin, tongue, lips, buccal mucosa and palate, etc. It can also develop within the jaw bones as a central lesion. Hemangiomas sometimes develop intramuscularly or within the salivary glands.

Growth Pattern

Hemangiomas appear as pale macules with a thread-like telangiectasia over the skin and mucous membrane. During the first few weeks of life, there is rapid growth of the lesion and these are fully recognizable at about 8 weeks of life.

Hemangiomas of Skin and Mucous Membrane (Figs. 2.72 to 2.74)

- Hemangiomas of the oral mucosa are usually raised, localized, slow growing, painless, multinodular or flat lesions. The

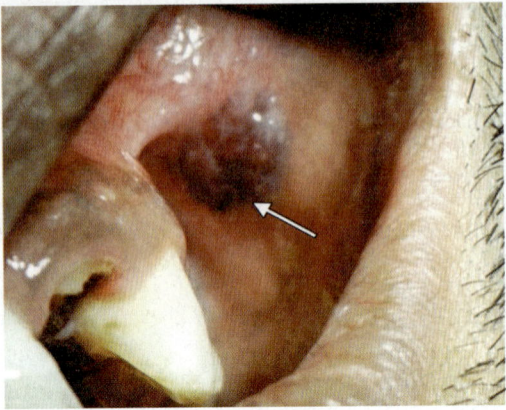

Fig. 2.72: Hemangioma of cheek.

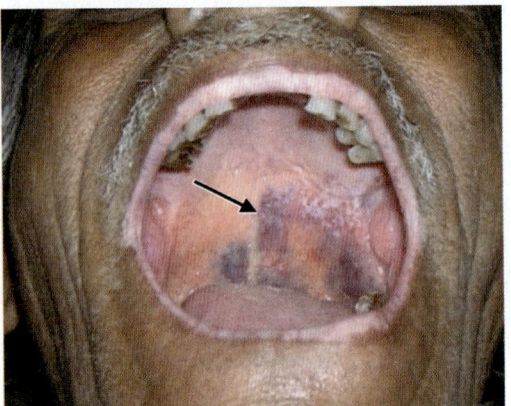

Fig. 2.73: Vascular malformation of palate.

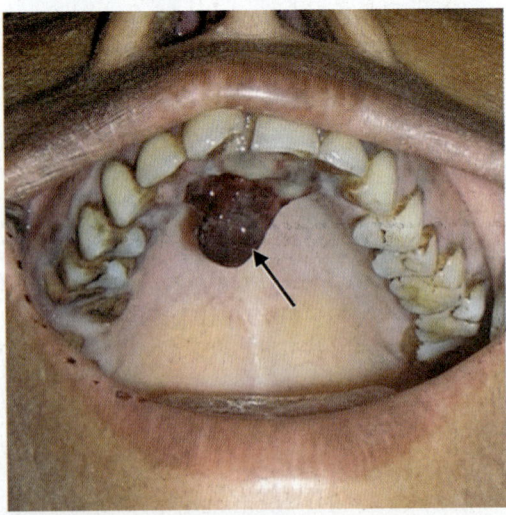

Fig. 2.74: Hemangioma of the hard palate.

deeper lesions appear as slightly raised mass with only a bluish hue.
- The color of the lesion ranges from distinctly red to blue or to purple colors.
- After the initial development some of these lesions enlarge continuously while others become static and make no further progress. The mature lesions generally appear dull purple in color.
- Moreover, some lesions of hemangiomas can even resolve slowly and finally disappear completely.
- When a hemangioma lesion is compressed with the help of a glass microscopic slide, it blanches (reddish color disappears) because the erythrocytes are pushed out of the vascular channels due to pressure. However, once the pressure is released, its reddish appearance returns back due to refilling of the tumor vessels with blood.
- When a hemangioma is connected with a large blood vessel, "bruits" can be heard during auscultation with a stethoscope.
- On palpation hemangioma is always soft, compressible and pulsatile.
- Trauma or laceration to the covering skin or mucosa often causes excessive uncontrolled bleeding from the lesion.
- Larger lesions in the neck and laryngeal region may cause airway obstructions.

Strawberry Hemangiomas

Sometimes, the bright red bosselated lesions of the skin occur which are called "strawberry hemangiomas"; commonly seen on the facial skin of small children.

Intramuscular Hemangioma

- Hemangiomas can frequently occur within skeletal muscles and in the orofacial region, masseter and orbicularis oris muscles are often affected.
- Muscular hemangiomas commonly produce diffuse, pulsatile swelling with occasional pain.

- During examination, the lesion can be moved across the long axis of the muscle, but it cannot be moved along it.

Port-wine Stain (Figs. 2.75 and 2.76)

- Port-wine stain is a unique type of hemangioma (mostly capillary type), which is often encountered over the face.
- The lesion is characterized by a diffuse, purplish macule with irregular borders and is sharply demarcated from the normal skin.
- Port-wine stains sometime exhibit nodular elevations.
- The lesion is unilateral in distribution and it often appears to follow the course of the first, second or the third divisions of the trigeminal nerve.
- A specific syndrome called "Sturge–Weber" syndrome is sometimes identified, which includes unilateral port-wine stain of the face, intracranial hemangiomas and epilepsy.
- Intracranial hemangiomas may produce calcifications within the walls of the meningeal vessels, which lead to a unique radiographic appearance of parallel radiopaque lines, and this have been termed as "tramline" calcifications.

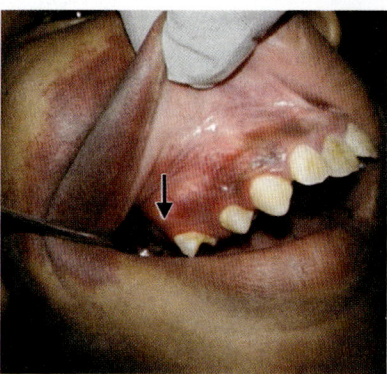

Fig. 2.76: Port-wine stain with oral lesions.

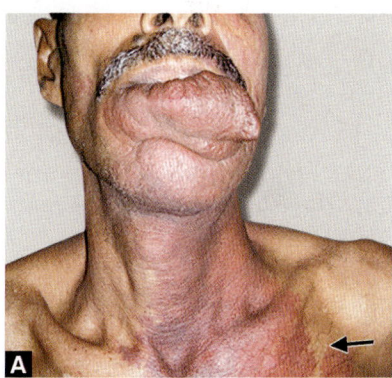
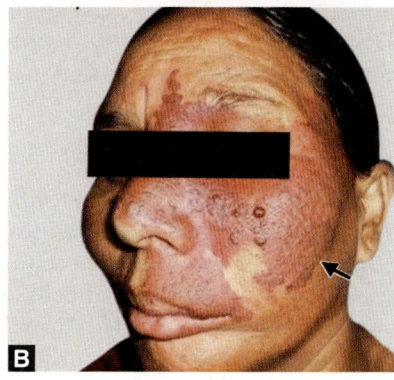

Figs. 2.75A and B: Port-wine stain.

Central Hemangiomas (Intraosseous)

Central hemangiomas represent benign vascular proliferation within the bone.
- Central hemangiomas most commonly affect the vertebrae and skull. Among the jawbones, mandible is affected more often than maxilla.
- These lesions usually occur in the 2nd decade of life and females are affected about 2–3 times more frequently than males.
- Clinically central hemangioma often presents a slow enlarging, occasionally painful, non-tendered, expansile jaw swelling.
- Long-standing lesions may cause severe erosion in the bone and thereby make the affected bone pulsatile, thin and compressible.
- There can be considerable amount of expansion of the affected bone, however bruits are not usually detected in these lesions.

- Loosening of teeth and sometimes spontaneous bleeding from the gingival crevice of the regional teeth can occur.
- Central hemangiomas may produce a throbbing pain in the bone and anesthesia or paresthesia of the affected part of the jaw.

Radiographic Appearance of Central Hemangiomas

Radiographically hemangiomas of the jaw bone usually present multilocular radiolucent area, with a typical "soap-bubble" appearance. It may also produce a "sun ray" appearance occasionally.

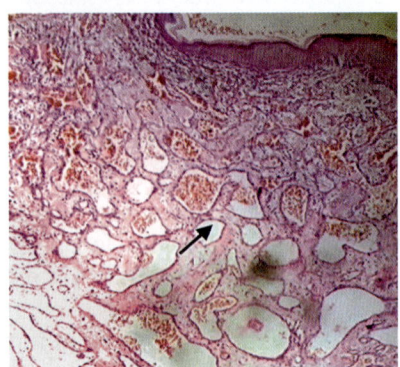

Fig. 2.77: Photomicrograph of capillary hemangioma—low power.

Macroscopic Findings

- Macroscopically hemangiomas can be either diffuse or circumscribed lesions. The teeth in the affected areas may be loose and often there is bleeding from the gingival crevices of these teeth.
- Although the teeth are mobile, their extraction may result in severe hemorrhage.

Histopathology

There are several histologic types of hemangiomas found in the oral cavity, among them two very common types are: (1) capillary hemangioma and (2) cavernous hemangioma.

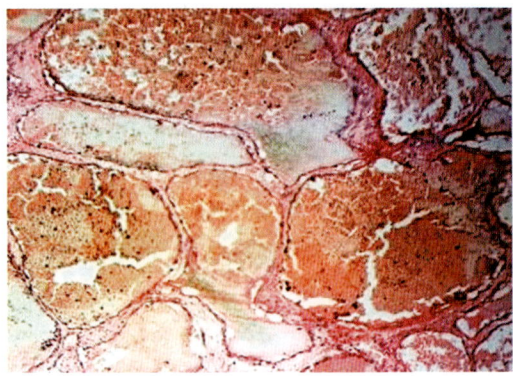

Fig. 2.78: Photomicrograph of cavernous hemangioma.

Capillary Hemangioma (Fig. 2.77)

- Capillary hemangiomas are histologically characterized by numerous, minute, small, endothelial-lined capillaries in the lesion, which are densely packed with erythrocytes.
- The cells of the endothelial lining are usually single layered and are supported by a connective tissue stroma.
- These cells (endothelial) are well-formed, spindle shaped or slightly elongated and plump.
- Although, well-formed capillaries are mainly present throughout the lesion, there may be some foci of proliferating endothelial cells, which form small aggregates or rosettes.
- Capillary hemangioma often histologically resembles pyogenic granuloma, however, presence of certain features like intercellular edema and chronic inflammatory cell infiltration, etc. are very common in pyogenic granuloma but are rare in case of capillary hemangioma.

Cavernous Hemangiomas (Fig. 2.78)

- Cavernous hemangiomas histologically reveal large, irregularly shaped, dilated, blood vessels or sinusoids; lined by single layer of flattened endothelial cells, which contain large aggregates of erythrocytes.
- These blood-pooled sinuses are often intercommunicating with one another.

- These sinuses are of variable caliber and they usually lack a muscular coat on their walls.
- A mature fibrous connective tissue stroma often separates one sinus from the other.
- Large areas of hemorrhage and hemosiderin pigmentation are often seen within the cavernous hemangioma lesions.
- However, inflammatory cell infiltration is very rare unless the lesion is secondarily infected or traumatized.

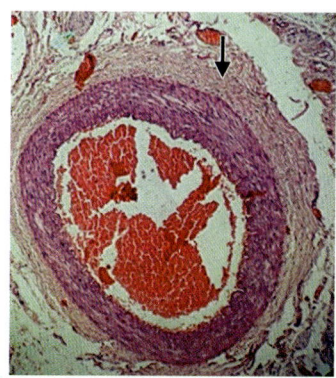

Fig. 2.79: Vascular malformation showing an abnormally large vessel along with nerves in the surrounding tissue.

Key Points of Hemangioma

- Hemangiomas are benign vascular tissue neoplasms arising from the vascular tissue which generally occur during infancy.
- These are commonly seen over the face, tongue, palate, cheek, muscles and bones including the jawbones.
- Lesion of the soft tissue presents painless, soft, fluctuant swelling with a typical red or blue or purple color.
- Soft tissue lesions are characteristically pulsatile and "bruits" can be heard during auscultation with a stethoscope, if the lesion is associated with a large vessel.
- Hemangiomas sometimes produce "port-wine stain" lesions over the facial skin, which are diffuse, purple, macules with irregular borders and are sharply demarcated from the normal skin.
- Moreover strawberry hemangiomas also develop on the facial skin, which are bright red, bosselated lesions.
- Intramuscular lesions of hemangioma produce diffuse, firm, movable swelling with occasional history of pain.
- Intraosseous lesions cause slow enlarging, painless, bony hard swelling of the jaw with loosening of teeth. They produce multilocular radiolucency in the bone with a typical "soap-bubble" appearance on radiograph.
- Hemangiomas have two main histological patterns: capillary type—which exhibits numerous, proliferating young blood capillaries, lined by single layer of spindle-shaped endothelial cells. The other important type is cavernous hemangioma, which exhibits few large, dilated, blood filled sinuses of irregular size, lined by a single layer of flat endothelial cells.
- Treatment of hemangioma is difficult and is done by local excision for smaller lesions; however larger lesions are excised surgically after pretreatment with sclerosing agents.

Histology of Other Forms of Hemangiomas

Port-wine Stain

- The "port-wine stain" lesions are composed of numerous, microvascular channels, similar to capillary hemangiomas.
- However, these vessels are often separated from one another by a mature fibrous tissue stroma (Fig. 2.79).

Central Hemangiomas

- Central hemangiomas are histologically similar to the cavernous type, although tumors of capillary variety may also occur.
- The vascular spaces are usually few and far between and there is presence of a relatively thick connective tissue stroma.
- Sometimes areas of osteoid or mature oven bone formation can also be seen in the lesion.

Differential Diagnosis

- Pyogenic granuloma
- Mucoceles
- Kaposi's sarcoma
- Salivary gland neoplasm
- Inflammatory hyperplasia of the tissue.

Treatment

- Local excision is the treatment of choice in small lesions.

Table 2.13: Outline of diagnosis in hemangiomas.

From clinical point of view	• Color of the lesion—bright red or bluish-red • Pulsation—often present • Auscultation—bruits can be heard during auscultation of the lesion with a stethoscope
Radiography	Intraosseous or central hemangiomas present multilocular radiolucency with "soap-bubble" appearance
Imaging	Doppler angiography. Contrast time-lapse angiography
Histopathology	Capillary and cavernous types

- Larger lesions are treated by excision after pretreatment of the lesion with repeated injections of sclerosing agents; which cause damage to the vessels and induce fibrosis, thereby making surgical excision safer.
- Hemangiomas in children may be left untreated until puberty, anticipating their spontaneous regression.

The outline of diagnosis in hemangiomas is given Table 2.13.

BENIGN NEOPLASM OF LYMPHATIC VESSELS

LYMPHANGIOMA

Definition

Lymphangiomas are uncommon benign, cavernous or cystic neoplasms composed of dilated lymphatic vessels. These are very common in the head and neck region; many lesions are present at birth and others occur during the first few years of life. They may occur either as a focal superficial lesion within the oral cavity or may develop as deep seated, massive, diffuse lesions of the neck, which are called cystic hygromas (Table 2.14).

Clinical Features

- *Age*: Most of the lesions are present at birth or they can arise during childhood (90% lesions occur within 2 years of age).
- *Sex*: There is no sex predilection.
- *Site*: Intraoral lesions predominantly affect the tongue and besides this, they can sometimes occur in relation to the palate, buccal mucosa, gingiva and lip, etc.

Lymphangiomas of the neck are referred to as "cystic hygromas".

Presentation (Figs. 2.80 and 2.81)

- Intraoral lesions predominantly occur on the tongue, present irregular nodularity on the dorsum of tongue many gray and pink grape-like, projections.
- The projections make the tongue surface "pebbly" (bosselated) and sometimes the superficial tumor resembles "frog-eggs" or "tapioca-pudding".
- The color of the lesion is usually pale and it is often lighter (translucent) than the color of the surrounding normal mucosa, however on few occasions lymphangiomas may sometimes produce a "red-blue" discoloration of the surface. Sometimes few black spots may be seen on the surface of the lesion, which indicate focal areas of hemorrhage.
- Some intraoral lymphangiomas produce deep-seated lesions and they often present diffuse, soft, painless, submucosal lumps. When such deep-seated lesions of tongue become extensive they cause macroglossia.

Table 2.14: Types of lymphangioma.

Capillary lymphangioma	Containing numerous small lymphatic capillaries
Cavernous lymphangioma	Containing large dilated lymphatic vessels
Cystic hygroma	Massive diffuse lesion of neck, containing macroscopic cyst like spaces of lymphatic vessels

Benign and Malignant Neoplasms of the Oral Cavity

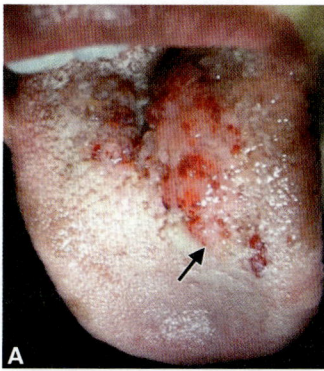

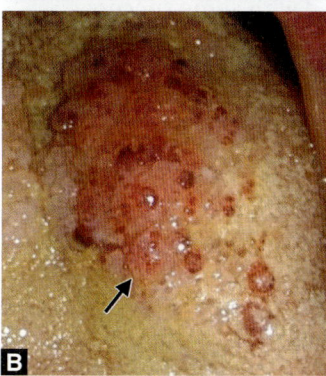

Figs. 2.80A and B: (A) Lymphangioma of tongue; (B) The tumor showing "pebbly surface with many vesicle-like blebs".

- On palpation, lymphangiomas often produce a typical "crepitate sound", which occurs due to sudden movement of the intralesional lymphatic fluids from one part of the lesion to the other because of the pressure from palpation (crepitations).
- A lymphangioma may suddenly increase in size due to intralesional hemorrhage and in such cases the tumor looks purple in color.
- Lymphangioma in the lip often produce diffuse, painless swelling with difficulty in lip closure.
- Oral lesions may gradually enlarge into a moderate size and then remain static or may even regress spontaneously.

CYSTIC HYGROMA

Cystic hygromas are unusually large lymphangiomas, which are massive in size and contain extensively dilated lymphatic vessels. They mostly occur in the first or second year of life are seen in the lateral neck (posterior triangle) or submandibular region or in the floor of mouth (Fig. 2.82).

- Clinically, these lesions present massive, "pendulous", fluctuant swelling on the lateral neck, measuring about several centimeters in diameter.
- Cystic hygromas sometimes cause severe disfigurement and few lesions may cause dysphagia and respiratory distress.
- Unlike intraoral lymphangiomas, the cystic hygromas do not regress spontaneously.
- Patients with Down's or Turner's syndrome often have a tendency to develop cystic hygromas.

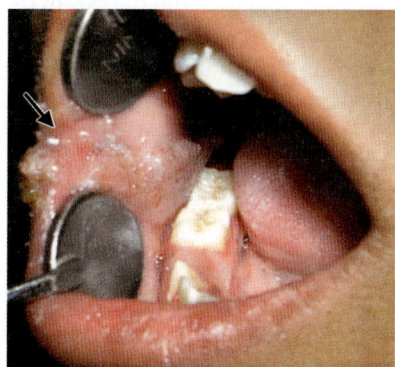

Fig. 2.81: Lymphangioma of the commissure.

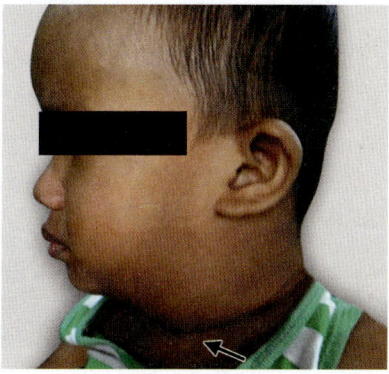

Fig. 2.82: Cystic hygroma.

Macroscopy

The tumor exhibits a multicystic or spongy mass, the cut section shows multiple cavities containing watery or milky fluid.

Histopathology (Fig. 2.83)

- Histologically, lymphangioma presents numerous proliferating, thin walled, markedly dilated lymphatic vessels of different size, which are lined by flattened endothelial cells.
- The lumens of the lymphatic vessels contain an eosinophilic or pinkish proteinaceous coagulum (results from fixation of lymph) with occasional presence of erythrocytes and lymphocytes in it. Some lumens can be empty or in few cases there can be interstitial fibrosis.
- Moreover, these lymphatic channels also about the overlying epithelium with no fibrous tissue stroma in between.
- The histologic appearance of cystic hygroma is similar to that of lymphangiomas of the oral cavity, however in cystic hygromas the lymphatic channels are often quite large and dilated (often have a cyst-like appearance).

Differential Diagnosis

- Hemangioma
- Mucocele
- Branchial cleft cyst

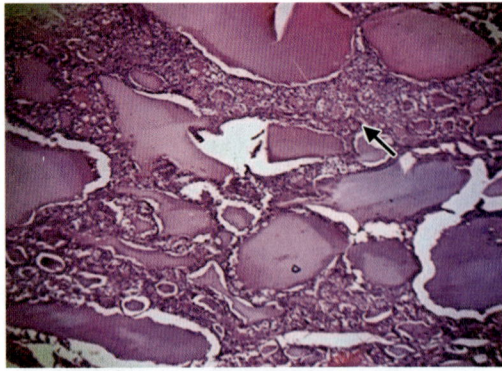

Fig 2.83: Photomicrograph of lymphangioma showing "pool of lymph".

- Sinus histiocytosis
- Lipoma
- Tuberculosis.

Treatment

- Many lesions of lymphangioma involute spontaneously during puberty.
- The persistent lesions are treated by surgical excision with careful dissection from the surrounding normal tissue.
- Sometimes, cryosurgery and laser surgery is used with some success.

BENIGN NEOPLASM OF BONE

OSTEOMA

Definition

Osteomas are benign neoplasms of bone (osseous tissue), which are consisting of either mature compact bone or cancellous bone. These neoplasms are almost exclusively found in the craniofacial region.

Types

Osteomas are of two types:
1. *Periosteal or exophytic osteoma*: Lesions arising peripherally from the outer surface of the bone.
2. *Endosteal or central osteoma*: Lesions arising centrally within the medullary region of bone.
    - Extraskeletal osteomas, typically located within muscle or the dermis of the skin osteoma cutis.
    - Common palatal tori, mandibular tori, and buccal exostoses are not considered to be osteomas, although they are histo-pathologically identical.

Clinical Features

- *Age*: 2nd to 5th decade of life.
- *Sex*: More frequent among females.
- *Site*: Osteomas occur either peripherally or centrally in relation to any bone of the cranium and the face.

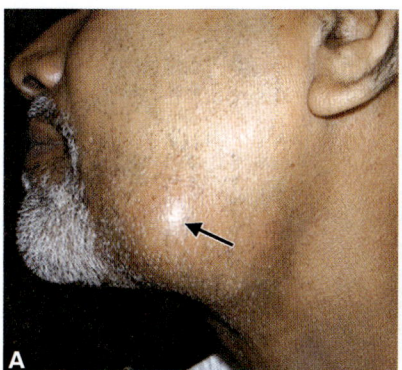
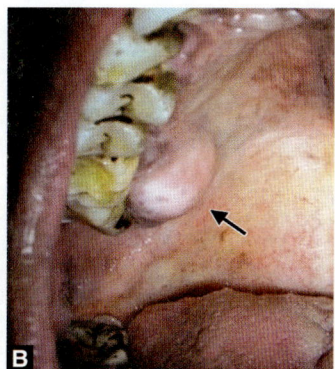

Figs. 2.84A and B: Osteoma of (A) mandible and (B) of maxilla.

Some lesions may arise from the soft tissues, e.g. tongue or buccal mucosa, etc.

Jawbones are often affected and interestingly osteomas often develop from those areas of the jaw from where tori usually do not arise. Body and condyle of the mandible in the molar region (lingual surface) is the most favored location of this tumor.

Presentation

- Osteoma often produces an asymptomatic, slow growing, nodular, exophytic, bony hard growth in the jaw (Figs. 2.84A and B).
- The lesion can be either solitary or multiple and the overlying skin or epithelium appears normal.
- Periosteal osteomas appear as polypoid or sessile masses on the bone surface, whereas endosteal osteomas may not be evident clinically unless they are large enough to cause expansion.
- Larger lesions of osteomas may cause facial deformity, with expansion of the cortical plates of bone and displacement of the regional teeth.
- Osteomas developing over the condyle of mandible often cause pain, decreased mouth opening, deviation of chin and derangement of occlusion, etc.
- Multiple osteomas often occur in association with Gardner syndrome, a hereditary condition with an autosomal dominant pattern.
- The syndrome also consists of multiple intestinal polyps with malignant potential, many unerupted normal or supernumerary teeth, epidermoid cyst and desmoid fibromas of skin.

Radiographic Features (Fig. 2.85)

Osteomas radiographically present well-circumscribed, solitary or multiple, round or oval, dense radiopacities in the bone. Larger lesions (endosteal type) cause expansion of the cortical plates and the peripheral outline or the border of the lesion is generally sclerotic.

Histopathology

Microscopically osteoma presents the following features (Fig. 2.86):
- The lesion is composed of dense cortical bone with a distinct lamellar pattern.

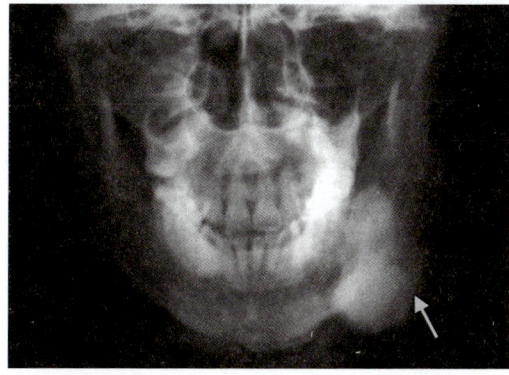

Fig. 2.85: Radiographic views of osteoma.

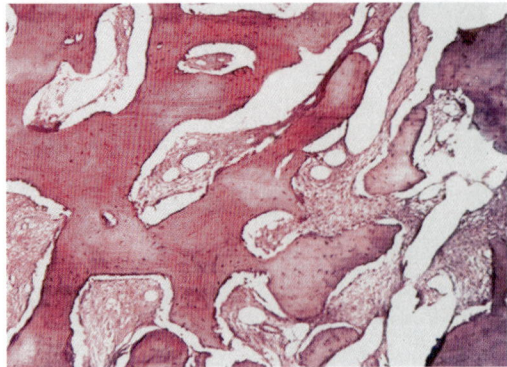

Fig. 2.86: Photomicrograph of osteoma.

- The cortical bone is sclerotic and relatively avascular.
- The medullary bone is denser than normal bone with reduced marrow spaces.
- The marrow spaces are composed of areolar fibrous tissue or adipose tissue.

Differential Diagnosis
- Odontomas
- Antrolith
- Exostoses
- Osteoblastoma
- Sclerotic cemental masses
- Focal sclerosing osteomyelitis.

Treatment
Surgical excision. Antral lesions are removed by Caldwell-Luc approach.

OSTEOID OSTEOMA/ OSTEOBLASTOMA

Definition
Osteoid osteomas and osteoblastomas are benign intraosseous neoplasms with almost similar clinical, radiographic and histologic features.

These lesions also share many common clinical and histological features with cementoblastoma as well, and therefore, all these lesions are considered to be the variants of a single disease entity.

Clinical Features
- Osteoid osteoma usually occurs among young patients, between the age of 10 years and 25 years.
- It arises more frequently among males than females.
- These lesions more commonly develop in the long bones and jaw lesions are very rare.
- Osteoid osteoma causes swelling of the bone with expansion of the cortical plates, most lesions measure about 1 cm in diameter.
- The lesion is almost always painful, especially when digital pressure is applied on it and the cause of the pain could be either due to the presence of numerous peripheral nerves in the tumor or due to the synthesis of prostaglandins by the tumor cells. The pain of osteoid osteoma is described as unrelenting and sharp, worse at night. Classically the pain is relieved by aspirin.
- After growing to the size of about 1 cm in diameter, the osteoid osteomas do not grow any further but it continues to remain painful.
- Osteoblastoma is another bony tumor that often causes expansion and distortion of the cortical plates of the jawbone, however its size is usually much bigger than that of the osteoid osteoma.
- Osteoblastoma clinically differs from osteoid osteoma by the fact that the former one is a progressively expansile lesion with a greater tendency to cause local bony expansion.
- These lesions often develop in mandible in the posterior region, most patients are below 30 years of age and the disease shows definite male predominance.
- The size of osteoblastoma is usually more than 1 cm in diameter (average is 2–4 cm) and it is also painful. However, the intensity of pain is much lesser as compared to the osteoid osteoma.

Radiological Features
- Radiographically osteoid osteoma presents a small, round or oval, well-defined,

radiolucent area that is surrounded by an area of increased radiodensity (reactive sclerosis). Rarely the lesion can be larger than 1 cm in diameter.
- The central area of radiolucency is often called the "nidus", which may sometimes exhibit some evidence of spotty calcifications.
- Osteoblastoma radiologically presents a well-defined, large, radiolucent area, containing patchy areas of mineralizations and it has a faint bony margin.
- Cementoblastoma is radiologically similar to osteoblastoma, but the former lesion always occurs in continuity with the root portion of a molar tooth.

Histopathology (Fig. 2.87)

- Histologically, both osteoid osteoma and osteoblastoma passes through several phases.
- Initially a small area of osteoblastic activity is seen, which is followed by a period of deposition of large osteoids.
- In the more mature stages the osteoids become well calcified.
- In osteoid osteoma, the "nidus" consists of an interlacing meshwork of bony trabeculae of variable size, within a vascular connective tissue stroma.
- Numerous osteoblasts are present and few osteoclasts are also seen in some areas.

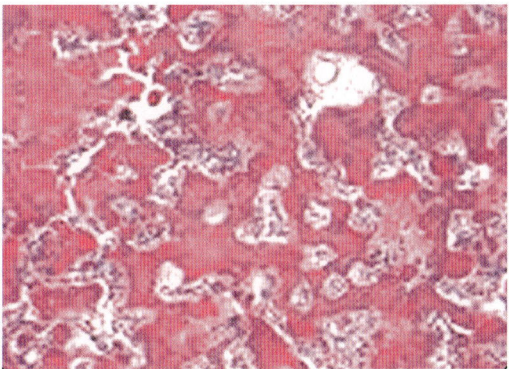

Fig. 2.87: Photomicrograph of osteoblastoma.

- Osteoblastoma is histologically very similar to the osteoid osteoma, however, the former lesion often exhibits an increased vascularity, a more uniform pattern of distribution of osteoid trabeculae and more number of osteoblast cells in the area. Unlike in osteoblastoma, neural staining techniques reveal many axons throughout an osteoid osteoma, which probably accounts for pain (the nidus). Levels of prostaglandin E2 are markedly elevated in the nidus; this is presumably the cause of pain and vasodilation.
- Moreover, there is no surrounding zone of reactive bone formation in osteoblastoma.

Differential Diagnosis

- Chronic nonsuppurative osteomyelitis
- Chronic sclerosing osteomyelitis
- Chronic bone abscess
- Central ossifying fibroma
- Central cementifying fibroma.

Treatment

Osteoid osteomas are often treated by surgical excision or curettage. Osteoblastoma is treated by large surgical en block resection.

BENIGN NEOPLASM OF CARTILAGE TISSUE

■ CHONDROMA

Definition

Chondromas are benign neoplasms of cartilaginous tissue origin and are consisting of mature chondrocytes. These are one of the very common neoplasms of the jawbone.

Clinical Features

- *Age*: Chondromas of the jawbone usually occur between the ages of 30–60 years. The highest incidence is seen in the 4th decade of life.
- *Sex*: Both sexes are almost equally affected.
- *Site*: Chondromas mostly arise from the vestigial cartilaginous rests present in

different parts of the jaw. The disease frequently affects the anterior part of maxilla and whenever the mandible is affected, the areas of preference will be the symphysis, premolar-molar area, the condyle and the coronoid process, etc. besides this, the nasal septum is also sometimes affected.

Presentation

- The neoplasm causes a slow enlarging, painless, bony hard swelling of the jawbone.
- Condylar tumors may cause pain, limited mouth opening, and deviation of the mandible from the midline.
- In some cases, the lesion shows an aggressive pattern of growth.
- Expansion and distortion of the cortical plates often occur and there can be mobility of the regional teeth.
- Chondromas are generally solitary tumors, however multiple chondromas can occur on rare occasions in association with some syndromes, e.g. Ollier's syndrome and Maffucci's syndrome, etc.

Radiographic Features

- Radiographically the chondroma typically appears as well-defined radiolucency with central opacification. Most cases arise within medullary bone (endochondromas), but some may arise just beneath the periosteum (periosteal chondromas).
- Most of the lesions cause resorption of roots of the adjacent teeth.

Histopathology

- The lesion consists of well-defined lobules of mature hyaline cartilage, containing multiple mature chondrocytes.
- The cartilage typically demonstrates well-formed lacunae containing small chondrocytes with pale cytoplasm and small, round nuclei; few tumor cells however have double nuclei.
- An intervening fibrous tissue septa is present, which separates the individual lobules of cartilage from one another.
- There are many areas of calcification within the lesion and moreover, there can be some areas of hemorrhage and tissue necrosis.

Differential Diagnosis

- Ossifying postsurgical bony defect
- Chronic osteomyelitis
- Osteogenic sarcoma
- Ossifying or cementifying fibroma
- Ossifying hematoma.

Treatment

Surgical excision.

■ BENIGN CHONDROBLASTOMA

Definition

Benign chondroblastomas are rare benign neoplasms arising from the epiphyseal ends of the long bones. Rarely these lesions can occur in the oral cavity.

Clinical Features

- *Age*: Most of the patients are below the age of 25 years.
- *Sex*: Male people are affected more often than females.
- *Site*: Intraoral benign chondroblastomas are usually rare and whenever they occur, mandibular condyle is the most favored site.

Clinical Presentation

- Benign chondroblastomas clinically present a relatively large, bony hard lesion, causing bulging of the jawbones.
- Displacement of the regional teeth often occurs.
- Pain may be present especially during palpation.

Radiographic Features

Radiographically benign chondroblastomas usually present a large radiolucent area in the bone, with ill-defined margins.

There can be presence of few radiopaque foci within the radiolucent zone.

Histopathology
- Histologically, benign chondroblastomas present a highly cellular structure consisting of numerous round or polyhedral "chondroblast-like" cells within a thin fibrous tissue stroma.
- Within the fibrous stroma, few areas of calcification are seen, besides this, there can be presence of multiple multinucleated giant cells.

Treatment
Surgical excision.

BENIGN NEOPLASM OF SMOOTH MUSCLES

LEIOMYOMA

Definition
Leiomyomas are benign neoplasms of the smooth muscle cells; which most commonly occur in the uterus, GI tract and skin. In the oral cavity, they are usually rare and are derived from the smooth muscle cells of the blood vessels.

Clinical Features
- *Age*: Leiomyomas usually occur among the middle-aged adults.
- *Sex*: Male predilection.
- *Site*: Intraorally, leiomyomas frequently occur in relation to the tongue, however other structures like palate, buccal mucosa and lips are also sometimes affected.

In addition to the common source of vascular smooth muscle cells, the pluripotential mesenchymal cells of the connective tissue may also give rise to these neoplasms.

Intraosseous leiomyomas may occur but are extremely rare and they mostly involve posterior part of mandible.

Presentation
- Clinically leiomyoma appears as a well-delineated, slow growing, painless, submucosal nodule.
- The surface of the lesion is usually smooth and is covered by a normal appearing non-ulcerated epithelium.
- The tumor often has a yellowish appearance, although the vascular type of leiomyoma can have a bluish hue.
- On palpation, the lesion feels firm and encapsulated, however the leiomyomas can be painful on rare occasions.
- Sometimes the lesion can be multinodular and whenever the neoplasm arises from the lip or the buccal mucosa, it is usually freely movable.
- The intraosseous leiomyoma of the jaw causes painless, bony hard swelling with expansion of the cortical plates.

Radiographic Feature
The intraosseous leiomyoma produces unilocular radiolucency in the jaw with sclerotic margins.

Histopathology
- Leiomyomas exhibit proliferation of spindle-shaped smooth muscle cells in solid sheets, the cells resemble fibroblasts.
- The cells usually evolve from blood vessels and are arranged in fascicles or in a "stream-like" fashion.
- The cells contain elongated, blunt-ended, pale nuclei, which often produce a "cigar-shaped" appearance.
- These spindle-shaped tumor cells also produce perivascular concentric laminations of parallel fascicles.
- In leiomyoma, the individual tumor cells lack distinct cell margins and because of this, the cytoplasm of one cell appears to be fused to the cytoplasm of the adjacent cells. The cells often reveal the presence of intracytoplasmic myofibrils.

Types

Histologically, leiomyomas are divided into three types:
1. Solid type
2. Vascular type
3. Epithelioid type.

Differential Diagnosis

- Fibroma
- Neurofibroma
- Myxoma
- Granular cell myoblastoma.

Special Investigation

Since the smooth muscle cells and the fibroblast cells both appear "pink" with routine hematoxylin and eosin stain, it is normally difficult to differentiate between leiomyoma from neurofibroma or fibroma. For this reason, special investigations are required.
- Masson's trichrome stain is used to differentiate between these two cells. With this special stain, the smooth muscle cells of leiomyoma appear "pink" while the collagenous structures of fibroblasts appear "blue or green."
- Mallory's phosphotungstic acid-hematoxylin stain helps to demonstrate myofibrils in leiomyoma.
- van-Gieson staining may also be used for this purpose, which stains the collagen fibers "red" and the smooth muscle fibers "yellow".

Treatment

Surgical excision including the surrounding normal tissue is the treatment of choice. Recurrence is usually rare.

BENIGN NEOPLASM OF STRIATED MUSCLE

■ RHABDOMYOMA

Definition

Rhabdomyomas are benign neoplasms of striated (skeletal) muscles and these are extremely rare lesions.

Rhabdomyomas of head and neck can be subclassified into two major categories: (1) adult rhabdomyomas (2) fetal rhabdomyomas.

Clinical Features

- *Age*: Peak age of occurrence is the 5th decade of life, however some cases have been reported at birth or during infancy.
- *Sex*: This lesion occurs more predominantly among males.
- *Site*: Rhabdomyomas of the oral cavity are often develop from base of the tongue, floor of the mouth and soft palate. Some lesions may also develop from the lip, larynx, pharynx and uvula, etc.

Adult rhabdomyomas: The most frequent sites are the pharynx, oral cavity and larynx; intraoral lesions are most common in the floor of the mouth, soft palate, and base of tongue.

Fetal rhabdomyomas: The most common locations are the face and periauricular region.

Presentation

- The neoplasm clinically presents a slow growing, well-circumscribed, painless mass.
- Some tumors can be "multinodular" with two or more nodules occurring at the same site.
- Some other lesions can be "multicentric" in nature and many occur at different locations at a time.
- The lesion is often deep-seated and the overlying tissue appears normal.
- Larger and untreated lesions in the pharyngeal or laryngeal region may sometimes cause airway obstructions.

Histopathology

- Microscopically, rhabdomyomas appear as sharply outlined, unencapsulated mass; consisting of large, round or oval striated muscle cells.
- These neoplastic cells have a granular eosinophilic cytoplasm and are rich in glycogen and glycoprotein.

- Multiple vacuoles are often present in the cell cytoplasm, which give rise to a spidery appearance to the cell.
- Irregular cross-striations are often seen and the cell nuclei are vesicular in nature.
- There can be presence of several multinucleated cells.
- Increased and abnormal mitotic activity is usually not seen.

Adult rhabdomyomas: The adult rhabdomyomas are composed of well-circumscribed lobules of large, polygonal cells, which exhibit abundant granular, eosinophilic cytoplasm. These cells often demonstrate peripheral vacuolization that results in a "spider web" appearance of the cytoplasm.

Fetal rhabdomyomas: The fetal rhabdomyoma has a less mature appearance and consists of a haphazard arrangement of spindle-shaped muscle cells that sometimes are found within a myxoid stroma.

Special Investigation

The diagnosis of rhabdomyoma can be confirmed by the electron microscopic demonstration of "myofibrils" in the tumor cells.

Differential Diagnosis

Rhabdomyomas should be differentiated clinically and histologically from the following lesions:
- Leiomyoma
- Granular cell myoblastoma
- Giant cell fibroma
- Neurofibroma.

Treatment

Surgical excision is the usually recommended treatment.

■ GRANULAR CELL TUMOR/ GRANULAR CELL MYOBLASTOMA

Definition

Granular cell tumors are benign neoplasm of soft tissue, which are composed of poorly defined plump granular cells. They can arise from different tissues like soft tissues (mostly tongue), skin, breast and lungs.

Origin

The true origin of this lesion is controversial. According to some investigators granular cells tumors arise from the striated muscle cells as a degenerative disease process. However other investigators believe that this neoplasm is of neural tissue (Schwann cell) origin as S-100 protein can be demonstrated from these tumor cells.

Clinical Features

- *Age*: Granular cell myoblastoma usually arises in the adult people between the ages of 30 years and 60 years, rare in children.
- *Sex*: Both sexes are affected with almost equal frequency. However, some investigators believe that this lesion has a female predilection.
- *Site*: More than 50% tumors develop in the head and neck region, intraorally tongue is most frequently affected, the other sites include—buccal mucosa, lips, floor of the mouth, gingiva, palate and uvula, etc.

Presentation

- The lesion clinically presents a slow enlarging, painless, well-circumscribed lump or mass on the dorsum of tongue, just beneath the covering epithelium.
- The size of the lesion is around 2 cm in diameter or less.
- On palpation, the neoplasm reveals a firm, nodular growth, which is nonmovable.
- The overlying covering epithelium usually appears normal and sometimes it exhibits a yellow or orange tinge.
- The covering epithelium at the site of the lesion may be atrophic with loss of papilla and hence it often presents a typical "leukoplakia-like" appearance.
- Multiple lesions sometimes can develop on the tongue.

- On rare occasions, granular cell myoblastomas could be very large in size and in such cases, they are often clinically mistaken as carcinomas.
- Midline lesions of granular cell myoblastoma over the tongue are also sometimes confused with median rhomboid glossitis.

Histopathology (Fig. 2.88)
- The unencapsulated neoplasm consists of diffuse sheets of large, oval or polygonal cells, with distinct cytoplasmic membrane.
- These neoplastic cells are often seem to merge with the muscle cells or they may be closely associated with peripheral myelinated nerves in other cases.
- The cell cytoplasms usually contain large number of discrete, punctate, eosinophilic granules [these granules stain positively with periodic acid Schiff (PAS)].
- The neoplastic cells sometimes also exhibit pale granular cytoplasm, however, the nucleus is always small and compact looking.
- The granular cells often extend upwardly toward the epithelium and are present between the rete pegs.
- Due to the presence of these cells, the overlying epithelium may exhibit an unusual proliferative response, which is often referred to as the "pseudoepitheliomatous hyperplasia".

- Pseudoepitheliomatous hyperplasia is characterized by elongated and branched rete pegs of the epithelium resembling the pattern of a neoplastic growth, especially SCC. The lesion is therefore confused as SCC on many occasions.

Differential Diagnosis
- Epidermoid carcinoma
- Neurofibroma
- Neurilemmoma
- Fibroma
- Salivary gland neoplasms.

Treatment
Surgical excision, prognosis is good.

BENIGN NEOPLASMS OF NEURAL TISSUE

NEURILEMMOMA (SCHWANNOMA)

Definition
Neurilemmomas are benign neoplasms derived from the Schwann cells. These cells are neuroectodermal in origin and they envelope the axons of the peripheral nerves in the form of a membrane. Bilateral schwannomas of the auditory vestibular nerve are a characteristic feature of the hereditary condition, neurofibromatosis type 2. Multiple schwannomas also occur in another genetic disorder known as schwannomatosis.

Clinical Features
- *Age*: The lesion usually arises before the age of 45 years (mostly seen in young and middle-aged adults).
- *Sex*: Females are affected more often than males.
- *Site*: Neurilemmomas can occur in relation to both the intracranial and the peripheral nerves.

    In case of peripheral nerve lesions, head and neck is a common site.

    Intraorally dorsum of the tongue is the most favored location. However other sites can

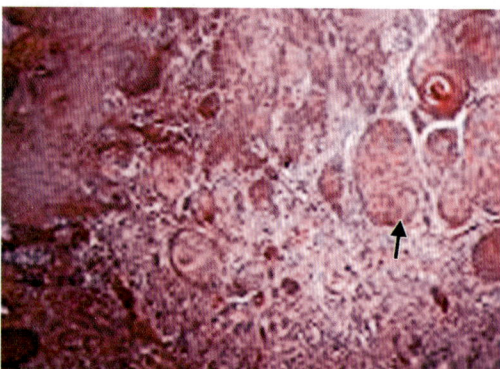

Fig. 2.88: Photomicrograph of granular cells tumor.

be affected, which include palate, floor of the mouth, buccal mucosa, gingiva and lips, etc.

Neurilemmomas often occur as central jaw lesions in relation to the inferior alveolar nerve; at the posterior part of mandible.

Presentation (Figs. 2.89A and B)

- Neurilemmoma clinically presents a slow enlarging, well-circumscribed, painless, nodule in the oral cavity.
- The lesion is smooth, firm, exophytic and often appears as a movable swelling beneath the mucosa.
- The size of the lesion greatly varies, and it ranges between few millimeters to several centimeters in diameter.
- These are painless and asymptomatic in most of the cases, however, some lesions can be tendered to palpation.
- Neurilemmoma typically develops in association with a nerve, and as the lesion enlarges the nerve is pushed toward the outer surface of the mass.
- Some lesions may grow at a faster pace with the development of pain and paresthesia. The later symptoms are more often associated with the intraosseous lesions.
- Sometimes small, lobulated, firm growths may occur in relation to the gingiva, which simulate the fibrous epulis.
- Central neurilemmoma of the jaw presents a well-demarcated, bony hard lesion that causes expansion of the cortical plates and sometimes displacement of the regional teeth.
- Intracranial neurilemmoma of the acoustic nerve is commonly referred to as "acoustic neuroma" and it often causes hearing loss.

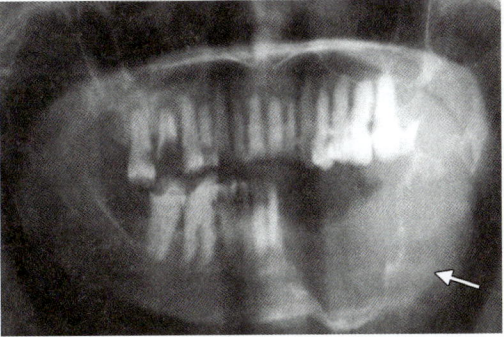

Fig. 2.90: Radiographic view of neurolemmoma showing multilocular radiolucency.

Radiographic Features (Fig. 2.90)

- Radiographically central neurilemmomas present well-defined, unilocular or multilocular radiolucent areas in the jawbone, with expansion and distortion of the cortical plates.
- Large lesions may cause extensive bone destruction with occasional perforation of the cortical plates.
- Lesions developing from the inferior alveolar nerve of mandible often cause enlargement of the mandibular canal.

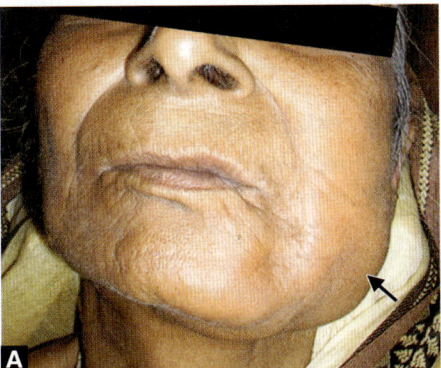
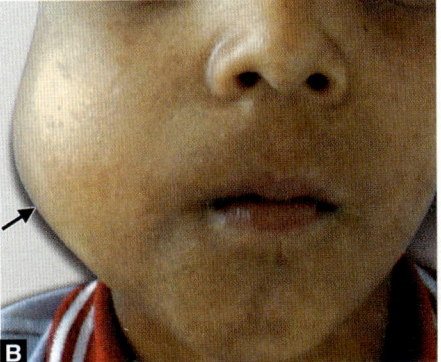

Figs. 2.89A and B: Neurilemmoma of mandible.

Macroscopy

The neoplasm presents a well-circumscribed, gray colored, encapsulated mass that is firm in consistency; it is always in touch with the nerve of its origin but never invading it and that makes the surgical excision much easier.

Histopathology

Histologically, neurilemmoma presents the following features (Figs. 2.91 and 2.92):
- Microscopically the lesion is comprised of an admixture of dense and loose areas, often referred to as Antoni A and Antoni B areas respectively.

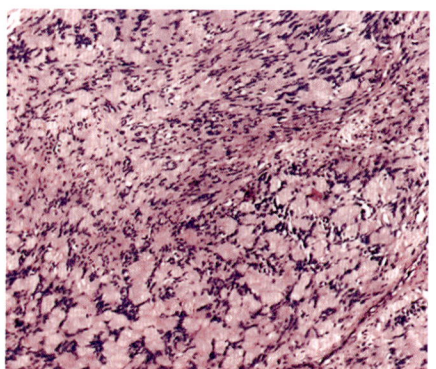

Fig. 2.91: Photomicrograph of neurilemmoma (low power).

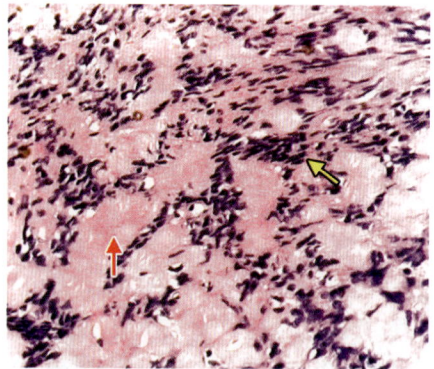

Fig. 2.92: Photomicrograph of neurilemmoma showing Schwann cells (yellow arrow) and "verocay bodies" (red arrow).

- The basic cellular constituents of the lesion are the proliferating spindle-shaped, neoplastic Schwann cells, which are typically arranged in a "palisading pattern". Individual tumor cells have prominent, elongated and wavy nuclei.
- The Antoni A areas are densely eosinophilic and highly cellular, which contain numerous spindle shaped Schwann cells. Here palisading of nuclei is common that is characterized by parallel rows of nuclei of Schwann cells with intervening "nuclear-free zones".
- Verocay bodies—the eosinophilic "nuclear-free zones" which are lying between the rows of palisading nuclei are called the verocay bodies. These are consisting of reduplicated basement membrane and cytoplasmic processes of tumor cells.
- The Antoni B areas are less cellular and less organized, they exhibits lack of typical palisading arrangement of the nuclei; the tumor cells here are randomly arranged within a loose myxomatous stroma with areas of microcyst formations.
- Normally in neurilemmoma, the "Antoni A tissue" forms multiple nodules, which are interspersed by Antoni B tissues.
- Sometimes, the cells of the Antoni B tissue are very large and hyperchromatic and hence are often confused with malignancy. However neurilemmomas in general have a very little tendency to undergo malignant transformation.
- The tumor cells will show a diffuse, positive immunohistochemical reaction for S-100 protein.

Differential Diagnosis

- Neurofibroma
- Fibroma
- Fibroepithelial polyp
- Leiomyoma
- Peripheral giant cell granuloma.

Treatment

Surgical excision.

NEUROFIBROMA

Definition

Neurofibromas are most common benign nerve sheath tumors arising from the perineural fibroblasts. These tumors are more heterogenous in composition than the schwannomas and here the neoplastic Schwann cells are often admixed with fibroblasts, mast cells and CD34+ spindle cells.

Neurofibroma may occur either as solitary lesion in the oral cavity or there may be multiple lesions in association with neurofibromatosis. *Multiple neurofibromatosis*: It is an autosomal dominant hereditary condition characterized by widespread overgrowth of nerve sheaths with formation of multiple neurofibromas on the skin and mucosa, along with "café-au-lait" pigmentation of the skin (Von Recklinghausen's disease).

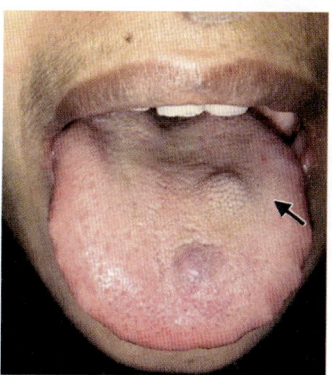

Fig. 2.93: Neurofibroma of tongue.

Origin

Neurofibromas arise from a mixture of cell types that include Schwann cells and the perineural fibroblasts.

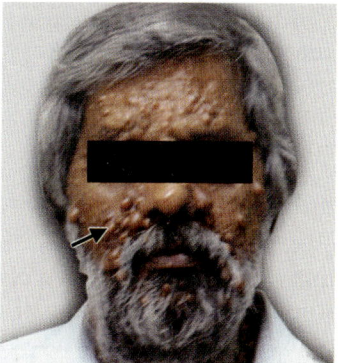

Fig. 2.94: Neurofibromatosis of skin.

Clinical Features

- *Age*: Neurofibromas may occur at any age, however most lesions are detected in young adults.
- *Sex*: Both sexes are equally affected.
- *Site*: Intraorally, solitary neurofibromas often arise from the tongue, buccal mucosa, vestibule and lips, etc. These lesions are very commonly seen over the skin surfaces and moreover sometimes they can occur as central jaw lesions as well (Fig. 2.93).

Presentation

- Clinically neurofibromas often present small, asymptomatic, soft or firm, submucosal mass often with a multilobulated surface.
- Lesions are well demarcated, freely movable mass below the skin or mucous membrane, and are almost always painless (Fig. 2.94).
- Neurofibromas may also occur as central jaw lesions in relation to the mandible or maxilla and in such cases, they often produce a slow growing, expansile, swelling of the jawbone.
- Pain and paresthesia are rarely present in these lesions.
- In multiple neurofibromatosis, the individual neurofibroma lesions are encountered over the skin and as well as the mucosal surfaces. Moreover, neurofibromas in relation to this disease may develop either as nodular lesions or as diffuse lesions.
- The nodular lesions vary in size from few millimeters to several centimeters in diameter, they are spherical in shape and often produce multiple, dome-shaped elevations of the skin.
- Their number varies from only few to several hundreds and in the oral cavity,

these lesions produce diffuse soft tissue overgrowths.
- The diffuse lesions can be quite "grotesque" with formation of pendulous masses, which may envelope an entire extremity.
- These lesions also produce massive flabby soft masses, which emanate from the neck or involve the subcutaneous tissue of the face and scalp.
- Another classic feature of neurofibromatosis is the presence of one or more, large, diffuse, macular brown pigmentations of the skin, which are known as the "café-au-lait" spots. Rarely these café-au-lait spots can be visible on the oral mucosa.
- In the oral cavity, neurofibromatosis causes macrognathia, macroglossia and deformity of the mandible, sphenoid bone, and the sigmoid notch, etc.

Radiographic Features

Radiographically neurofibroma of the jawbone usually produces a relatively well-demarcated, unilocular or multilocular radiolucent area, with expansion of the cortical plates and divergence of roots of the regional teeth.

Histopathology (Figs. 2.95 and 2.96)

- Neurofibromas, whether they are occurring as solitary lesions or as a part of the disease

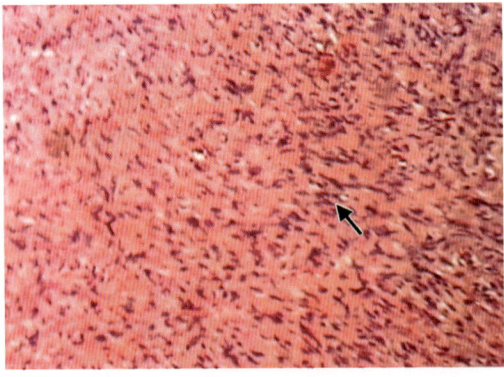

Fig. 2.95: Photomicrograph of neurofibroma—low power.

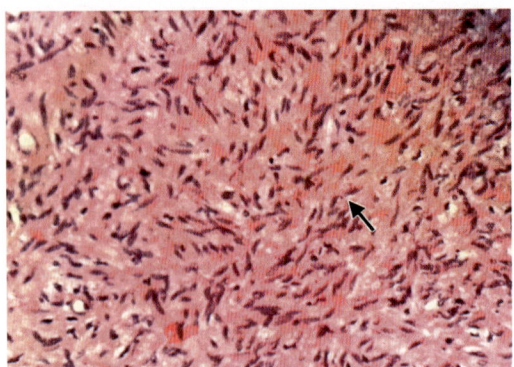

Fig. 2.96: Photomicrograph of neurofibroma—high power.

"multiple neurofibromatosis", histologically they produce similar appearances.
- Histologically, neurofibromas exhibit well-circumscribed areas of proliferating spindle-shaped cells, which often resemble fibroblasts (neurofibroblasts).
- These cells are often haphazardly arranged in interlacing bundles and the tumor cells have typical wavy nuclei.
- The neoplastic elements in neurofibroma fail to exhibit any specific well-organized cellular orientation pattern as seen in neurilemmoma, however, the ground substance sometimes produce a myxoid appearance.
- Large numbers of mast cells are sometimes found within the tumor tissue and are of diagnostic importance.
- The "café-au-lait" pigmentations microscopically reveal basilar melanosis without any proliferation of melanocytes.
- Immunohistochemically, the tumor cells show a scattered, positive reaction for S-100 protein.

Treatment

Solitary neurofibromas are treated by surgical excision.
Neurofibromatosis is not treated since surgical intervention may trigger the malignant potential of the individual lesions.

Table 2.15: Common differences between neurilemmoma and neurofibroma.

S. No.	Differential features	Neurilemmoma	Neurofibroma
1.	Relationship to the nerve of origin	Develops as an eccentric mass around the nerve	Occurs as a fusiform mass involving the whole nerve
2.	Circumscription	Often encapsulated	Encased within the nerve
3.	Cellular organization of tumor cells	More homogenous	Often heterogenous
4.	Order of arrangement of cells	Highly organized	Often disorganized
5.	Nuclear palisading	Present	Absent
6.	Myxoid stroma	Rarely seen	Often present
7.	Vascular prominence within the tumor	Commonly seen	Less common
8.	Xanthoma cells	Often present	Generally absent
9.	S-100 protein	Most cells positive	Few cell positive
10.	Chances of developing multiple tumors	Rare	Multiple lesions often develop in association with neurofibromatosis
11.	Presence of CD34 cells	Absent	Present
12.	Neurofilament	Absent	Present

The common differences between neurilemmoma and neurofibroma are given in Table 2.15.

MELANOTIC NEUROECTODERMAL TUMOR OF INFANCY

Definition

Neuroectodermal tumor of infancy is a rare benign, pigmented neoplasm of the jawbone, which is derived from the primitive neural crest cells.

Clinical Features

- *Age*: The lesion occurs mainly in infants before the age of 6 months; some lesions are present at birth (the usual range of age being 1–3 months) (Fig. 2.97).
- *Sex*: Both sexes are equally affected.
- *Site*: Majority of the neoplasms arise from the anterior part of maxilla, however mandible is also sometimes affected (about 25% cases).

Rarely the lesion may develop from extraoral sites like—shoulders, scapula, mediastinum and anterior fontanel, etc.

Presentation

- Neuroectodermal tumor of infancy clinically presents a fast enlarging swelling of the jawbone with expansion and distortion of the cortical plates.
- The swelling often cases elevation of the lip and facial asymmetry.
- Destruction of the underlying bone often causes displacement of developing teeth in the jaw.
- Pain and tenderness is usually not present.
- The surface of the lesion may exhibit a brown or black pigmentation.

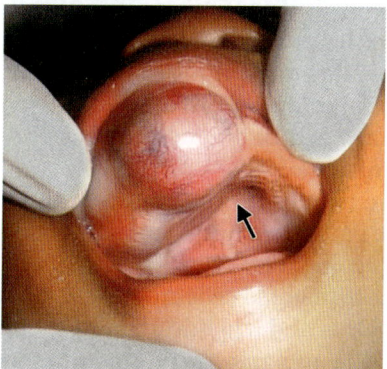

Fig. 2.97: Neuroectodermal tumor of infancy.

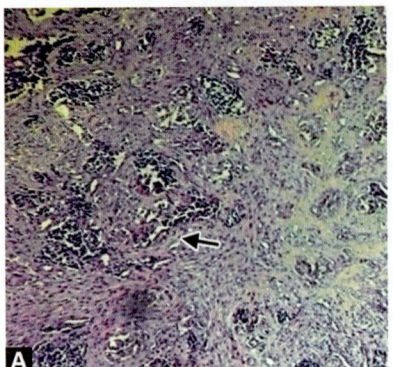 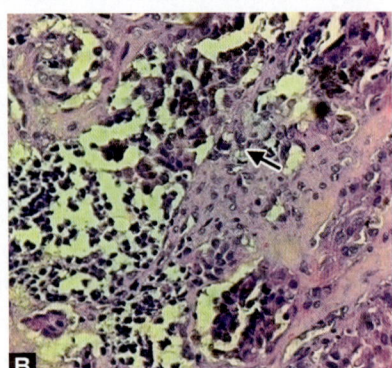

Figs. 2.98A and B: Photomicrograph of neuroectodermal tumor of infancy in (A) Low power; (B) High power.

Radiographic Features

- Radiographically neuroectodermal tumor of infancy often exhibits a well-defined radioluceny in the jaw that often resembles a cyst.
- The lesion often causes displacement of the developing tooth buds.
- Bone destruction is sometimes associated with bone formation (osteogenesis) and such lesions often radiographically exhibit a typical "sun-ray" appearance.

Macroscopic Appearance

The cut surface of the lesion exhibits a typical "slate-blue" or "grayish-black" appearance. In some cases, there may be presence of some "grayish-white" streaks in the lesion.

Histopathology (Figs. 2.98A and B)

- The lesion is composed of two types of cells—the pigmented cells and the nonpigmented cells, both of which are found within a dense connective tissue stroma.
- The neoplastic cells often proliferate in the patterns of nests or tubules or alveolar structures, etc.
- The pigmented cells are large with an open nucleus and a lightly staining cytoplasm, which occasionally contains coarse melanin granules.
- These cells are flattened or cuboidal in shape with large, pale nuclei and are often arranged in large masses.
- The nonpigmented cells are small with dark, dense nuclei and a scanty cytoplasm and they often resemble lymphocytes.
- These unpigmented cells are arranged in clusters within the connective tissue stroma.

Special Investigations

Patients with neuroectodermal tumor of infancy generally have high urinary levels of vanillylmandelic acid and this observation is suggestive of the neuroectodermal origin of the neoplasm.

Treatment

Surgical excision with thorough curettage.

TRAUMATIC NEUROMA

Definition

It is a reactive proliferation of Schwann cells after transection or other damage of a nerve bundle. These lesions arise subsequent to tooth extraction or other surgical procedures.

Clinical Features

- *Site*: It can at any location but are most common in mental foramen area, tongue, lower

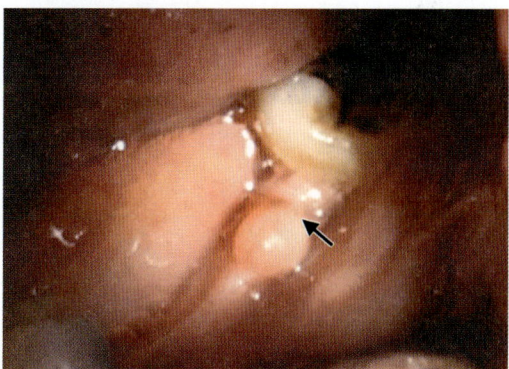

Fig. 2.99: Traumatic neuroma: From inferior alveolar nerve.

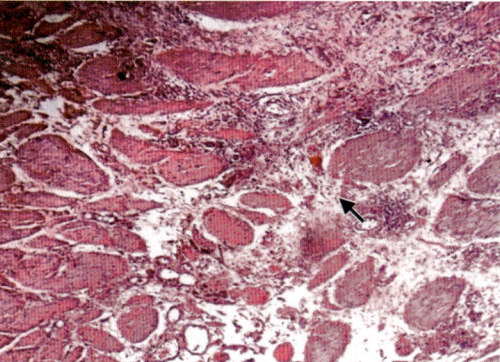

Fig. 2.100: Photomicrograph of traumatic neuroma.

lip, and the alveolar ridge in edentulous area (Fig. 2.99).
- *Clinical presentation*: They are smooth-surfaced, nonulcerated nodules or swelling on mucosa, slow growing and seldom reaches a size greater than a centimeter in diameter.
- It can be painful. This pain can be intermittent or constant and ranges from mild tenderness to severe radiating pain.
- Burning sensation may occur.
- Anesthesia or dysesthesia may occur.

Histopathologic Features
- Microscopic examination of traumatic neuromas shows haphazard proliferation of mature, myelinated and unmyelinated nerve (Fig. 2.100).
- The connective tissue stroma shows densely arranged collagen or myxomatous in nature.

Treatment
Surgical excision.

NEOPLASM OF THE MIXED TISSUE

TERATOMA

Teratoma is a tumor with tissue or organ components resembling normal derivatives of more than one germ layer and such tissues are not native to the site where the tumor developed.

Hamartoma: It is a benign focal tumor-like growth or malformation, composed of tissue elements normally native to that site but is growing in a disorganized manner.

Features of Teratoma (Fig. 2.101)
- The tumor contains mature or immature cells of tissues derived from more than one germ-cell layer and sometimes all the three.
- It originates from totipotential cells such as those normally present in ovary and testis and abnormally present in sequestrated midline embryonic rests.
- The cells have capacity to differentiate into any of the cell types found in the adult body.

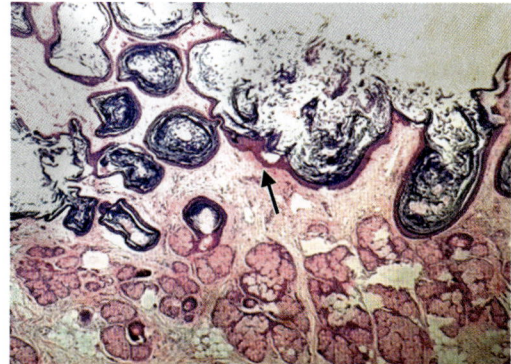

Fig. 2.101: Photomicrograph of teratoma of oral cavity showing sebaceous glands and hair follicles—low power.

- It may give rise to neoplasms, which might contain bits of bone, epithelium, muscle, fat, nerve and other tissues.

MALIGNANT NEOPLASMS OF MESENCHYMAL TISSUE

■ FIBROSARCOMA

Definition

Fibrosarcomas are malignant neoplasms of the fibroblast cells, which often exhibit an aggressive and destructive behavior.

Two main types of fibrosarcoma of bone exist, primary and secondary.
1. *Primary fibrosarcoma*: Primary fibrosarcoma is a fibroblastic malignancy that produces variable amounts of collagen. It is central, arising within the medullary canal, or peripheral arising from the periosteum.
2. *Secondary fibrosarcoma*: Arising from a preexisting lesion or after radiotherapy to an area of bone or soft tissue. This is more aggressive tumor with poor prognosis.

   May arise from preexisting lesions, such as fibrous dysplasia, chronic osteomyelitis, bone infarcts, Paget's disease and in previously irradiated areas of bone.

Clinical Features

- *Age*: The neoplasm can occur at any age, but most commonly affects the young adults and children.
- *Sex*: Both sexes are almost equally affected.
- *Site*:
  – Intraorally fibrosarcomas commonly arise from the cheek, tongue, gingiva, palate, floor of the mouth, maxillary sinus and other paranasal sinuses and the pharynx, etc.
  – Intraosseous lesions, which occur either periosteally, or endosteally, frequently involve the jawbones.
  – Among the jaw lesions, mandible is affected far more commonly than maxilla (*See* Figs. 2.94 and 2.95).

Clinical Presentation (Figs. 2.102 to 2.104)

- In the initial stages, fibrosarcoma mostly remains symptomatic and the condition often resembles a benign fibrous overgrowth.

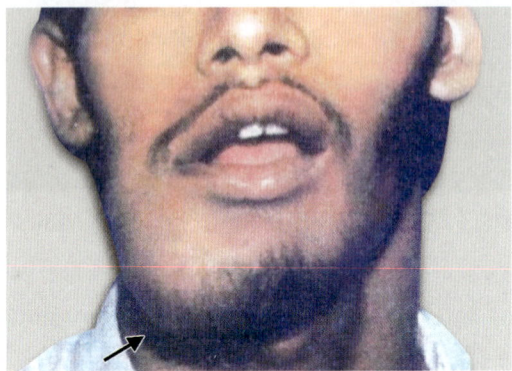

Fig. 2.102: Fibrosarcoma developing in mandible.

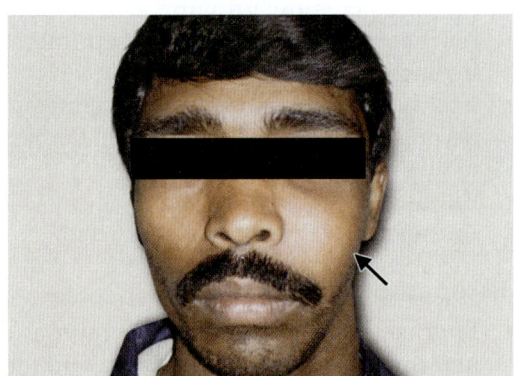

Fig. 2.103: Fibrosarcoma of maxilla.

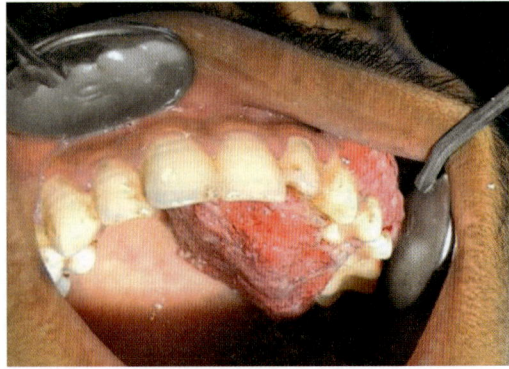

Fig. 2.104: Fibrosarcoma of maxilla (intraoral).

- In the later stages, the lesion becomes fast enlarging and within a short span of time, it gives rise to a large, painful, bulky, lobulated "fleshy" mass.
- The surface of the lesion is smooth and it often becomes ulcerated due to trauma.
- Pain and secondary infections are also common.
- The neoplasm is usually firm in consistency and it is often indurated with the surrounding normal tissue.
- Intrabony lesions of fibrosarcoma often produce severe swelling and destruction of the affected bone with loosening and exfoliation of the regional teeth.
- Pain, anesthesia or paresthesia in the affected region is often present.
- Lesions developing in the maxillary sinus or other paranasal sinus regions often produce obstructive symptoms and epistaxis.
- The patients are usually severely ill and exhibit marked deterioration of their general health.

Radiographic Features
- Fibrosarcoma of the jawbone radiographically produces a sharply defined radiolucent area with severe destruction of bone.
- Expansion and marked thinning of cortical bone, displacement of teeth and resorption of roots, etc. are common.

Histopathology (Fig. 2.105)
Microscopically, fibrosarcoma reveals the following features:
- Active proliferation of numerous spindle shaped, malignant fibroblast cells within the connective tissue stroma.
- The malignant fibroblast cells often have a "tadpole" like appearance and most of the cells in fibrosarcoma are well differentiated.
- Individual tumor cells contain large, uniformly stained, elongated hyperchromatic nuclei and a thin scanty cytoplasm.

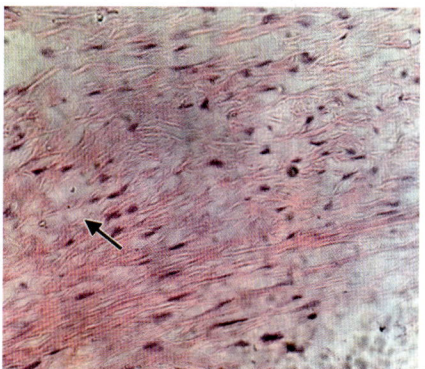

Fig. 2.105: Photomicrograph of fibrosarcoma (high power).

- Normally, there is a "streaming fashion" of proliferation of the malignant fibroblast cells in the connective tissue.
- Synthesis of collagen is very minimum and often the collagen bundles are arranged in a typical "Herringbone" pattern.
- The mitotic activity is very minimum in the "well-differentiated" lesions of fibrosarcoma, however the rate of mitotic activity gradually increases with more and more poorly differentiated lesions.
- In poorly differentiated fibrosarcomas, the individual malignant fibroblast cells appear large, plump, round or oval, and these cells synthesize very little collagen.
- In many cases, the tumor cells exhibit abnormal mitotic activity in the form of "biradiate" or "triradiate" mitosis, etc.
- Multinucleated giant cells are rarely seen in high grade fibrosarcoma.

There are several histologic grades of fibrosarcomas:
- Well-differentiated fibrosarcoma
- Intermediate grade fibrosarcoma
- High-grade fibrosarcoma
- Sclerosing epithelioid fibrosarcoma
- Anaplastic form of fibrosarcoma.

In the anaplastic form of fibrosarcoma, the tumor cellularity is markedly increased, mitotic figures become numerous and there can be even presence of few malignant giant cells.

Distant metastasis is rare but local infiltration to the adjacent tissues is very common in fibrosarcoma.

Differential Diagnosis
- Malignant fibrous histiocytoma
- Rhabdomyosarcoma
- Liposarcoma
- Neurogenic sarcoma
- Nodular fasciitis.

Treatment
Radical surgical excision and chemotherapy is the treatment of choice. Radiotherapy is not effective. Prognosis is good because metastasis occurs only in few cases.

MALIGNANT FIBROUS HISTIOCYTOMA

Definition
Malignant fibrous histiocytomas (MFH) are a group of aggressive malignant neoplasms, arising from the undifferentiated mesenchymal cells that differentiate along both fibroblastic and histiocytic pathways.

Clinical Features
- *Age*: The disease predominantly affects the people of relatively older age group.
- *Sex*: Both sexes are almost equally affected.
- *Site*: Malignant fibrous histiocytomas are slightly uncommon neoplasm in the oral cavity. Whenever, they occur intraorally, they can be found in the maxillary antrum, tongue, buccal mucosa and maxillary or the mandibular bones, etc.

Presentation
- The neoplasm clinically presents a fast expanding, exophytic, lobulated and ulcerated growth in the oral cavity (Fig. 2.106).
- Malignant fibrous histiocytomas often have a "fleshy" appearance and thus they clinically resemble the fibrosarcomas.
- Pain and surface ulceration may or may not be present.

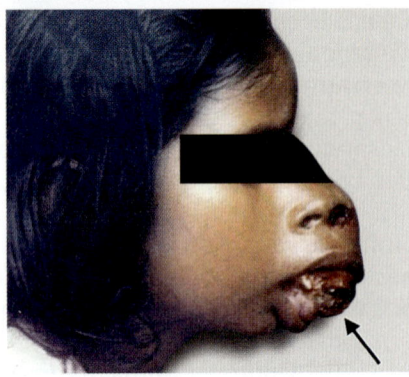

Fig. 2.106: Malignant fibrous histiocytoma causing massive swelling of the maxilla.

- Pain, hemorrhage, anesthesia or paresthesia of the neighboring structures is commonly seen.
- Intraosseous lesions often produce large, painful, expansile growth in the jawbone with mobility or spontaneous exfoliation of the regional teeth.

Radiographic Features
- Malignant fibrous histiocytoma radiographically presents a large, multilocular radiolucent area in the jawbone, with severe expansion and distortion of the cortical plates.
- Destruction of inter-radicular bone and perforation of the cortical plates occur quite frequently.
- On rare occasions, pathological fractures of the bone can be seen.

Histopathology (Fig. 2.107)
- Histologically, the neoplasm reveals actively proliferating, numerous polyhedral or oval-shaped malignant histiocytes and many spindle-shaped malignant fibroblast cells.
- Short fascicles of malignant cells are often arranged in a typical "cart-wheel" or "storiform" pattern.
- The classic pattern is the one most frequently encountered in head and neck

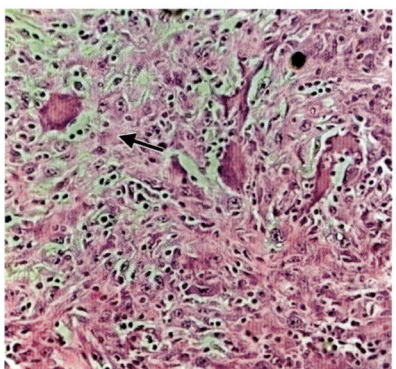
Fig. 2.107: Photomicrograph of malignant fibrous histiocytoma—low power.

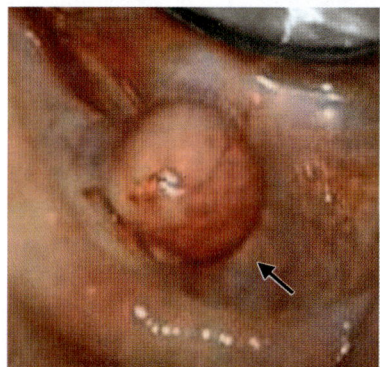
Fig. 2.108: Liposarcoma in floor of mouth with vascular prominence on the surface of the lesion.

sites and is often referred to as the storiform pleomorphic MFH.
- The histiocytic cells have either abundant eosinophilic cytoplasm or pale foamy cytoplasm, and cell membranes are not easily visualized.
- In many cases, there can be presence of multiple multinucleated "touton type" giant cells and in addition to these, few large foam cells are also found.

Treatment
Wide surgical excision coupled with radiotherapy and chemotherapy.

LIPOSARCOMA

Definition
Liposarcomas are malignant neoplasms derived from cells that differentiate along adipose tissue lines and show some evidence of fat synthesis. This is the second most common soft tissue sarcoma of the adults.

The most recent WHO classification of soft tissue tumors recognizes five categories of liposarcomas:
1. Well-differentiated, which includes the adipocytes, sclerosing, and inflammatory subtypes
2. Dedifferentiated
3. Myxoid
4. Round cell
5. Pleomorphic.

Clinical Features
- *Age*: The peak age of occurrence is between 40 years and 60 years.
- *Sex*: Male people are affected more often than females.
- *Site*: In the oral cavity, the lesions frequently develop from tongue and buccal mucosa (Fig. 2.108); the other common sites include the soft palate, floor of the mouth and the maxilla or the mandible, etc.

Presentation
- These are externally rare neoplasms especially in the oral cavity. In the head and neck region, they are more often encountered in the deep tissues of the neck.
- Clinically liposarcomas produce relatively slow growing, occasionally painful, submucosal masses.
- Lesions are mostly poorly demarcated and lobulated in nature, and are soft or firm in consistency.
- The overlying epithelium may be either normal or yellow in color.
- These neoplasms are sometimes so soft and fluctuant that they can be clinically mistaken for a large cyst.

- Liposarcomas more often arise as "de novo" lesions rather than through malignant transformation of a preexisting lipoma.

Histopathology (Fig. 2.109)

- Histologically, liposarcomas are more cellular lesions than lipomas and they consist of multiple numbers of foamy and "fat-containing" malignant lipoblast cells.
- Many cells with "signet-ring" appearance (vacuolated cytoplasm) are also found in these neoplasms.
- The nuclei in the tumor cells are prominently displaced to the side of a large vacuole.
- Some liposarcomas are composed of poorly-differentiated round cells, with only focal evidence of cytoplasmic vacuolization.
- In some cases, there can be presence of irregularly shaped giant cells having foamy cytoplasms.
- In liposarcoma, the malignant lipoblast cells often produce large amount of fat within the tumor and this often leads to a myxoid appearance of the lesion.
- There are five histologic types of liposarcomas—namely the myxoid type, round cell type, well-differentiated type, dedifferentiated type and the pleomorphic type.

Treatment

Radical surgery and radiotherapy.

■ HEMANGIOENDOTHELIOMA

Definition

Hemangioendothelioma is a malignant angiomatous neoplasm of mesenchymal tissue origin, which is derived from the endothelial cells of the blood vessels or lymphatic vessels.

There are in fact three distinct neoplasms, which are categorized as angiosarcomas and these are named as hemangioendothelioma, hemangiopericytoma and the Kaposi's sarcoma.

The hemangioendothelioma and hemangiopericytoma are "quasi-malignant" neoplasms of vascular endothelium and vascular pericytes respectively.

Clinical Features

- *Age*: Hemangioendotheliomas are more commonly seen in children and young adults.
- *Sex*: Females are affected more often than males with a ratio of about (2:1).
- *Sites*: Oral lesions are rare and they may arise from the lips, palate, gingiva and tongue, etc. The neoplasm can also occur as central jaw lesions in relation to either maxilla or mandible (Fig. 2.110).

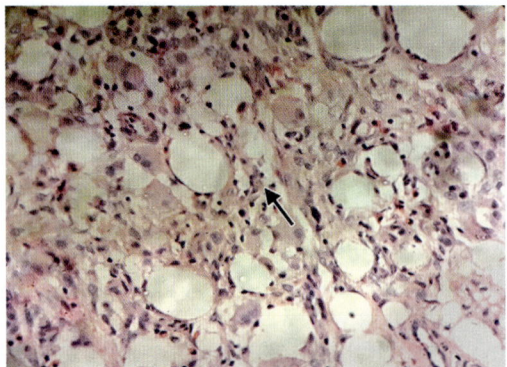

Fig. 2.109: Photomicrograph of liposarcoma (high power).

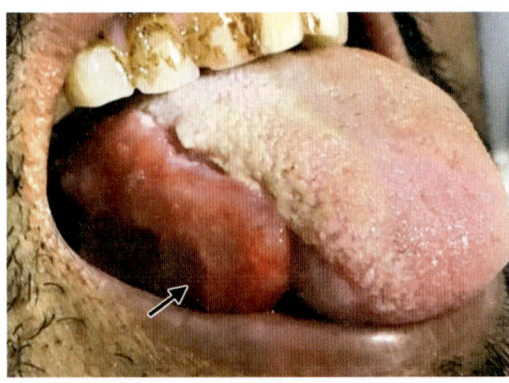

Fig. 2.110: Hemangioendothelioma.

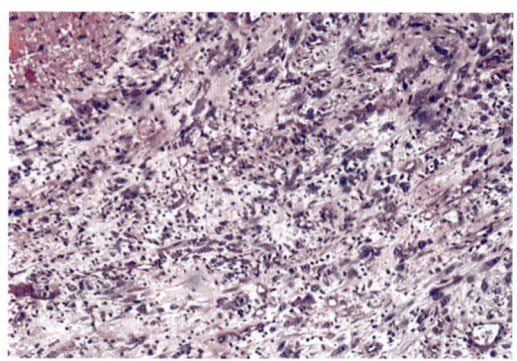

Fig. 2.111: Photomicrograph of hemangioendothelioma.

Presentation

- Hemangioendothelioma clinically presents a fast enlarging, localized, painful, nodular swelling.
- The lesion often shows surface ulceration, moreover, paresthesia or anesthesia of the affected area is also common.
- Hemangioendothelioma sometimes clinically exhibit hemangioma-like appearance and in such cases the neoplasm appears as flat or slightly raised lesion, with a dark-red or bluish-red surface.
- The central jaw lesions usually produce expansile, destructive growths with swelling, pain and cortical expansion, etc.

Histopathology (Fig. 2.111)

- Hemangioendotheliomas often a poorly circumscribed lesion that exhibits biphasic proliferation of venous or capillary vessels; microscopically it presents neoplastic proliferation of malignant endothelial cells with variable degrees of individual cell differentiation.
- The cells are pleomorphic, large, polyhedral or slightly flattened with a faint cytoplasmic outline.
- The nuclei are hyperchromatic, round and contain several minute nucleoli.

Treatment

Surgical excision and radiotherapy.

HEMANGIOPERICYTOMA

Definition

Hemangiopericytomas are malignant neoplasms arising from the pericytes around the blood vessels (these are contractile cells that along with their interlacing processes form a network around the outer aspect of the capillary walls).

Clinical Features

- *Age*: The neoplasm can occur at any age, however majority of the lesions arise before the age of 50 years.
- *Sex*: Both sexes are affected with almost equal frequency.
- *Site*: Tongue, lips, floor of the mouth, gingiva and jawbones, etc. (Figs. 2.112A and B).

Presentation

- Hemangiopericytoma clinically presents a slow enlarging, painless, well-circumscribed growth (Fig. 2.113).
- It is often firm in consistency and the surface is usually nodular.
- There may–may not be any reddish appearance in the lesion, which could be indicative of its vascular origin. However, the superficial lesions may have vascular prominence and pigmentations.
- Some neoplasms can be fast enlarging and they produce large, painful, nodular swellings with surface ulceration.
- Central jaw lesions may produce large, expansile, painful growths of the jawbone with mobility or exfoliation of the regional teeth.

Histopathology (Fig. 2.114)

Histologically, the neoplasm reveals the following features:
- There will be multiple number of normal appearing, "capillary-like" tubules lined by a single layer of flattened endothelial cells.
- The capillary-like tubules are bordered on their outer aspect by some densely or

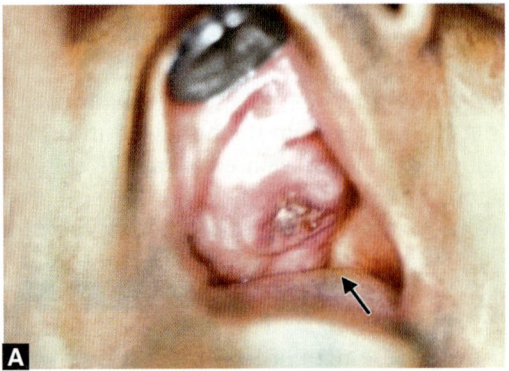
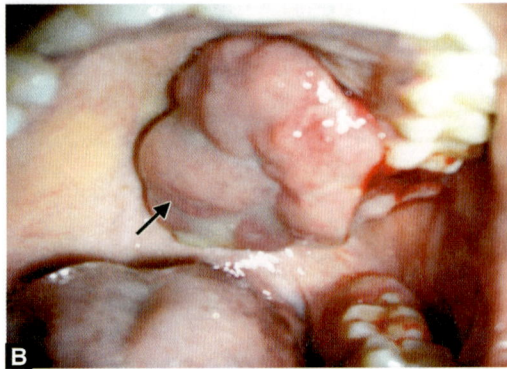

Figs. 2.112A and B: Hemangiopericytoma of the palate (two images).

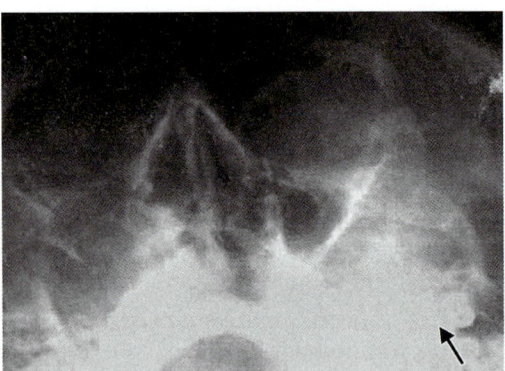

Fig. 2.113: Hemangiopericytoma of palate causing invasion into the left maxillary antrum.

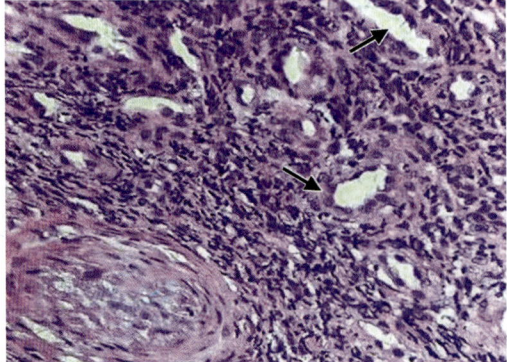

Fig. 2.114: Photomicrograph of hemangiopericytoma.

loosely packed cells, which are showing plump nuclei and indistinct cytoplasm.
- These cells at the periphery of the capillaries are malignant pericytes and they often exhibit cellular pleomorphism, nuclear hyperchromatism and increased abnormal mitotic activity, etc.
- The malignant pericytes are often spindle shaped and these cells are often haphazardly arranged within the tumor.
- The blood vessels often exhibit irregular branching and therefore produce a typical "stag-horn" or "antler-like" appearance.

Differential Diagnosis
- Hemangioma
- Kaposi's sarcoma
- Glomus tumor.

Treatment
Surgical excision is the treatment of choice, the lesion is radioresistant.

KAPOSI'S SARCOMA

Definition (Figs. 2.115 and 2.116)
Kaposi's sarcoma is a malignant neoplasm arising from the endothelial cells of the blood capillaries and it is considered to be the commonest sarcoma of the angiomatous tissue.

Clinical Types of Kaposi's Sarcoma
Four clinical types recognized, which are as follows:
1. Classic
2. Endemic (African)
3. Iatrogenic (transplant associated)
4. Epidemic (AIDS related).

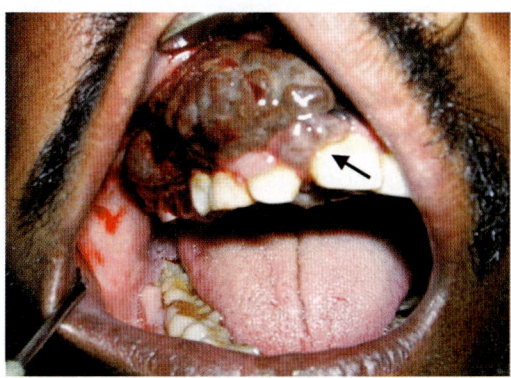

Fig. 2.115: Kaposi's sarcoma of gingiva.

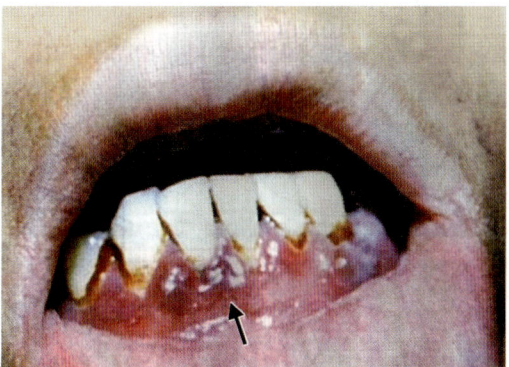

Fig. 2.116: Gingival lesion in Kaposi's sarcoma.

Endemic Kaposi's Sarcoma

Kaposi's sarcoma was first reported by Moritz Kaposi in 1872 and it was described as a rare endemic disease among elderly persons of Central European or Mediterranean origin. The endemic form of the disease is also seen among the children and young black Africans.

The endemic Kaposi's sarcoma usually affects the skin and the lymph nodes; and it rarely affects the viscera.

Epidemic Kaposi's Sarcoma

- Kaposi's sarcoma has really become an epidemic since 1981, as large numbers of cases are being reported in association with patients suffering from AIDS.
- The AIDS-associated Kaposi's sarcomas affect skin, lymph nodes, bone and viscera (especially the GI tract), etc.
- AIDS patients with history of homosexuality develop Kaposi's sarcoma very frequently.
- According to some investigators, Kaposi's sarcoma occurs in association with cytomegalovirus (CMV) infection as well.

Etiology

The following factors are believed to "triggers" the initiation of Kaposi's sarcoma:
- Genetic predisposition
- Infection by HIV or CMV
- Immunosuppression
- Environmental factors.

Clinical Features

In Kaposi's sarcoma, oral lesions are seen in about 10% cases and these are mostly seen in the palate. Other intraoral sites, which may be involved, are the maxillary gingiva and tongue, etc.

Kaposi's sarcoma is usually present in three different clinical stages, namely—(1) the patch stage, (2) the plaque stage and (3) the nodular stage.

- *Patch stage*: Patch stage is the initial stage of the disease and during this a pink, red or purple macule appears over the oral mucosa.
- *Plaque stage*: Patch stage is actually continued into the plaque stage with time and during this stage, the lesion appears as a large, raised, violaceous plaque.
- *Nodular stage*: It is the last stage of the disease and is characterized by the occurrence of multiple nodular lesions on the skin or the mucosa.

Histopathology (Fig. 2.117)

The microscopic features of Kaposi's sarcoma vary depending upon the clinical stage of the disease:

Patch Stage

During the "Patch Stage", Kaposi's sarcoma histologically shows multiple dilated, irregular blood vessels, which are lined by normal appearing endothelial cells.

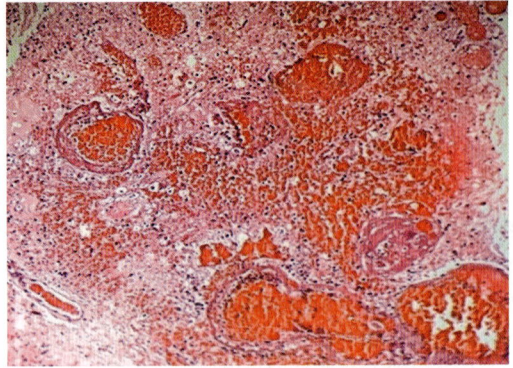

Fig. 2.117: Photomicrograph Kaposi's sarcoma.

Plaque Stage

The "Plaque stage" histologically shows many dilated, jagged, vascular channels, lined by "spindle-type" cells. Similar looking cells are also present as perivascular aggregates.

In between the vascular structures, RBCs, macrophages, plasma cells, lymphocytes and hemosiderin pigments, etc. are often present.

Nodular Stage

Microscopically, nodular lesion of Kaposi's sarcoma consists of sheets of spindle-shaped cells in a background of scattered blood vessels and "slit-like" spaces containing RBC.

Marked hemorrhage, hemosiderin pigmentation, lymphocyte and macrophage infiltrations are also commonly seen.

Differential Diagnosis

- Pyogenic granuloma
- Hemangioma
- Angiosarcoma.

Treatment

Kaposi's sarcomas are treated by radiotherapy and chemotherapy, surgery is a difficult proposition since the disease is often multicentric. Intralesional injection of vinblastine is used to control individual lesions.

■ EWING'S SARCOMA/EWING'S TUMOR (ENDOTHELIAL MYELOMA, ROUND CELL SARCOMA)

Definition

Ewing's sarcoma is a highly malignant, distinctive primary neoplasm of bone, characterized by primitive round cells without obvious differentiation. The tumor is named after James Ewing who first reported it in 1921.

- Ewing's sarcoma is the third most common primary malignant bone tumor after osteosarcoma and chondrosarcoma.
- Moreover Ewing's sarcomas the second most common primary malignant bone tumor in pediatric patients after osteosarcoma.

Examples of Common Round Cell Tumors

- Lymphoma
- Ewing sarcoma
- Small cell osteosarcoma
- Neuroblastoma
- Alveolar rhabdomyosarcoma
- Langerhans cell histiocytosis
- Burkitt's lymphoma
- Multiple myeloma.

Histogenesis

The exact cell of origin of Ewing's sarcoma is not known, however, it is generally believed that the lesion arises from either the endothelial cells of the blood vessels within the bone or from the undifferentiated reticuloendothelial cells. Recent investigators believe that Ewing's sarcoma is neuroectodermal in origin.

Clinical Features (Figs. 2.118A to C)

- *Incidence*: Ewing's sarcomas constitute about 10% of all the malignant bone tumors.
- *Age*: The neoplasm usually occurs in children and young adults, between the ages of 5 years and 25 years. 80% patients are below 20 years of age.
- *Race*: Majority of the people are whites; black people are rarely affected.

Benign and Malignant Neoplasms of the Oral Cavity

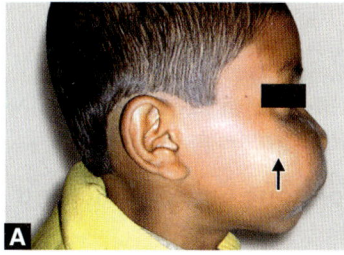 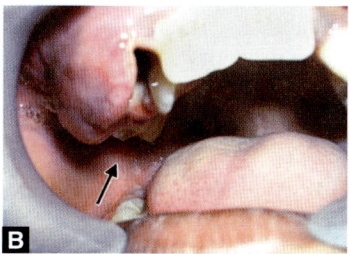 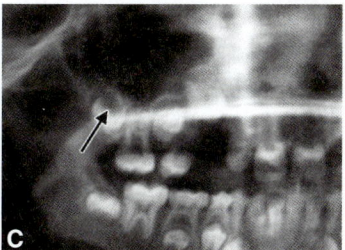

Figs. 2.118A to C: (A) Ewing's sarcoma of maxilla causing massive swelling; (B) Intraoral lesion of the patient; (C) Ewing's sarcoma of maxilla, radiograph showing large destructive lesion.

- *Sex*: There is a slight male predominance seen in the disease (M:F ratio 60:40)
- *Site*: The disease is mostly encountered in the long bones of the lower extremity, e.g. femur and pelvic bones, etc. Among the jaw lesions, mandible is affected more often than the maxilla.

Jaw lesions of Ewing's sarcoma are sometimes metastatic in origin and in such cases long bones are the primary sites of the neoplasm.

Presentation

- The tumor causes rapid swelling in the affected part of the bone, which is often associated with severe pain.
- The initial symptoms of Ewing's sarcoma are very similar to that of osteomyelitis and care should be taken in this regard while making the diagnosis.
- Expansion of the jawbone with paresthesia or anesthesia of the area can be frequently seen.
- Sometimes, the tumor perforates the cortical plate of the bone and protrudes as a soft tissue mass overlying the affected area of bone.
- Unexplained loosening of the tooth is a very common feature of Ewing's sarcoma.
- In the later stages, the neoplasm develops surface ulceration.
- Patients with Ewing's sarcoma may develop moderate fever, leukocytosis, anemia and raised ESR, etc. These symptoms often indicate a poor prognosis of the disease.

Radiographic Features

- Radiographically Ewing's sarcoma usually presents a radiolucent area in the bone with ill-defined margins (Fig. 2.119).
- Expansion and distortion of the cortical bones often occur along with widespread destruction of the alveolar bone.
- In this disease, the periosteum of the bone characteristically exhibits lamellar layering (an osteophytic reaction), which is known as onion-skin appearance. Onion skin radiographic appearance is present in both Ewing's sarcoma, Garre's osteomyelitis.

Macroscopic Features

The tumor mass is usually located within the medullary cavity and it invades the cortex, periosteum and the soft tissue. The tissue is soft, tan-white in color and frequently exhibits areas of hemorrhage and necrosis.

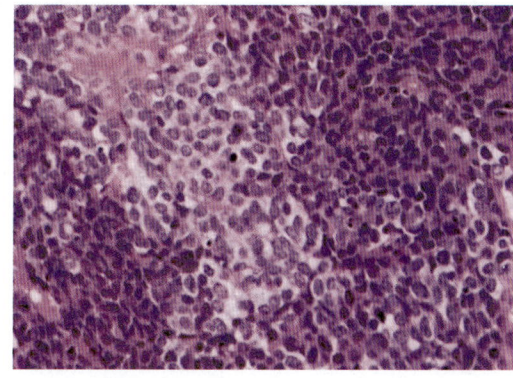

Fig. 2.119: Photomicrograph of Ewing's sarcoma.

Histopathology (Fig. 2.119)

- Microscopically Ewing's sarcoma presents sheets or lobules of uniform, small round cells, which slightly larger and more closely packed than lymphocytes.
- The individual malignant round cell has a large hyperchromatic nucleus, with scant cytoplasm that appears white due to higher glycogen content.
- Besides the typical small round cells, there may be another group cells present in Ewing's sarcoma, which are larger and have finely granular nuclei with faint ill-defined cytoplasms.
- The sheets or lobules of neoplastic cells are often separated from one another by a thin fibrous band, containing small blood vessels and chronic inflammatory cells.
- There may be presence of "Homer-Wright rosettes" in some tumors, which appear as round groupings of cells with a central fibrillary core.
- Increased mitotic activity with areas of tissue necrosis and hemorrhage are also commonly observed in Ewing's sarcoma.

Differential Diagnosis

- Neuroectodermal tumor of infancy
- Embryonal rhabdomyosarcoma
- Garre's osteomyelitis
- Lymphoma
- Metastatic carcinoma
- Neuroblastoma
- Leukemia
- Myeloma
- Mesenchymal chondrosarcoma
- Small cell osteosarcoma.

STAGING SYSTEM FOR BONE CANCER INCLUDING EWING TUMOR: BY AMERICAN JOINT COMMITTEE ON CANCER (AJCC)

It also involves the TNM factors (but the values are different from those used in squamous cell carcinoma) plus a new factor G (grade of tumor) is used here.

- T-size of primary tumor
- N-lymph node involvement
- M-distant metastasis
- G-grade of the tumor (Low grade: good prognosis, High grade: poor prognosis).

T-Categories of Bone Cancer including Ewing Tumors

T0: No evidence of primary tumor
T1: Tumor size less 8 cm (about 3 inches) in diameter
T2: Tumor size more than 8 cm in diameter
T3: Tumor involving more than one site in the same bone.

N-Categories of Bone Cancer including Ewing Tumors

N0: No spread to regional nodes
N1: Tumor spreading to regional nodes.

M-Categories of Bone Cancer including Ewing Tumors

M0: No distant metastasis
M1a: Metastasis only in the lung
M1b: Metastasis in other sites also.

G-Categories of Bone Cancer including Ewing Tumors

GX: Grade of tumor cannot be assessed
G1-G2: Low grade
G3-G4: High grade
(*All Ewins tumors are considered G4*).

STAGES

Stage IA: T1, N0, M0, G1 to G2 (or GX)
Stage IB: T2, N0, M0, G1 to G2 (or GX)
Stage IIA: T1, N0, M0, G3 to G4
Stage IIB: T2, N0, M0, G3 to G4
Stage III: T3, N0, M0, G3 to G4
Stage IVA: Any T, N0, M1a, any G
Stage IVB (either of the two) : Any T, N1, any M, any G, or: Any T, any N, M1b, any G

Treatment

Radiotherapy and multidrug chemotherapy; surgery is occasionally attempted, 5-year survival rate is only 10%.

Benign and Malignant Neoplasms of the Oral Cavity

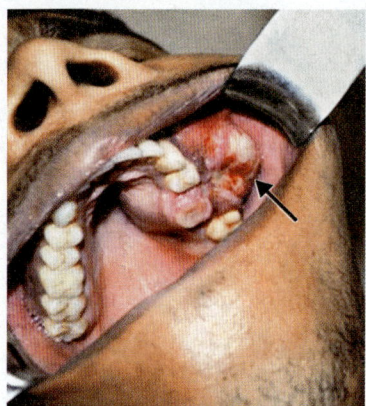

Fig. 2.120: Chondrosarcoma.

■ CHONDROSARCOMA

Definition

Chondrosarcomas are malignant neoplasms of bone, in which the neoplastic cells exclusively produce abnormal cartilage tissue but no osteoids or bone. It is the second most common primary malignant neoplasm arising from bone (Fig. 2.120).

Histogenesis

Chondrosarcomas may be of two types:
1. *Primary chondrosarcoma*: Lesion arising directly from the bone as a malignant neoplasm.
2. *Secondary chondrosarcomas*: Lesion arising from the preexisting benign cartilaginous neoplasms such as chondromas or osteochondromas, etc.
- Besides this, chondrosarcomas may also arise from other preexisting bony diseases like—Paget's disease of bone, Ollier's disease (multiple enchondromatosis) and Maffucci syndrome (multiple enchondromatosis, hemangiomas and fibromas).
- In the jawbone, nearly all chondrosarcomas arise as de novo malignant lesions.
- It is also important to note that malignant cartilaginous tissue neoplasms are far more common in the jaw bones, as compared to their benign counterparts.

Clinical Features

- *Age*: Most patients of chondrosarcomas are above 40 years of age.
- *Sex*: It is more commonly seen among males (M:F ratio 2:1).
- *Site*: Bones of the axial skeleton, e.g. pelvic bones, femur, humerus, ribs, scapula and sternum are commonly affected.

In the jawbones, chondrosarcomas develop less frequently in maxilla as compared to the osteosarcomas and these are mostly confined to the anterior part, where pre-exiting nasal cartilage is present.

In the mandible, the disease mostly occurs in the posterior region, at the site of the embryonically derived Meckel's cartilage. Besides this, mandibular lesions may also develop from the symphysis, coronoid or the condylar processes. Few lesions may occur in relation to the nasal septum and the paranasal sinuses.

Presentation

- The most common symptom of chondrosarcoma is dull bone pain, which may continue for months and typically the pain worsens at night.
- With further enlargement, the lesion produces severe expansile swelling and tenderness in the area and facial asymmetry; loosening of teeth, anesthesia or paresthesia are also common.
- Many patients may die of extensive local tissue destruction.
- The edentulous patients may feel poor fitting of the artificial dentures due to swelling of the jaw caused by the tumor.
- Chondrosarcomas occurring in the anterior maxilla may produce nasal obstruction, epistaxis, photophobia, visual loss and breathing difficulties, etc.

Periosteal chondrosarcoma (juxtacortical lesions): Tumors arising from the outer surface of bone, may be from the periosteal tissue.

Radiographic Features (Fig. 2.121)

- Radiographically chondrosarcoma appears as an expansile "moth-eaten"

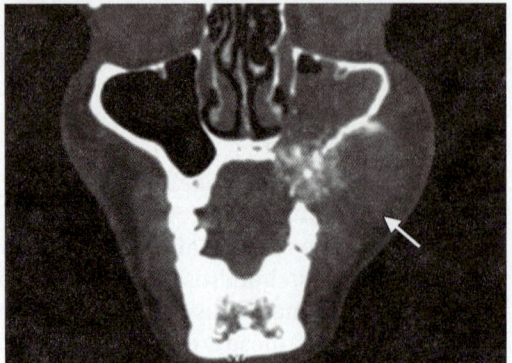

Fig. 2.121: Radiograph of chondrosarcoma of left maxilla showing "sun-burst" appearance.

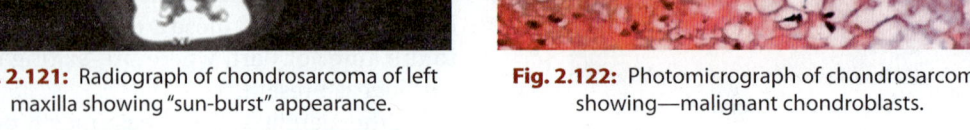

Fig. 2.122: Photomicrograph of chondrosarcoma showing—malignant chondroblasts.

radiolucent area in the bone with ill-defined borders.
- Within the radiolucent area, multiple flecks or blotchy areas of radiopacities are found, which occur due to endochondral mineralization of multiple hyaline cartilage.
- These intratumor mineralizations are often known as "popcorn" calcifications; which typically shows "rings and arcs" that resemble popped corn kernels.
- Widening of the periodontal ligament space of the adjoining teeth may be present with occasional root resorptions.
- Peripheral osteogenic reaction may sometimes produce the typical "sun-ray" appearance, as often seen in osteosarcomas.

Histopathology (Fig. 2.122)

The microscopic appearance of chondrosarcoma is highly variable.
- Some lesions are well-differentiated and resemble benign cartilaginous neoplasms, whereas, other lesions could be anaplastic in nature and are composed of spindle-shaped malignant chondrocytes, with little or no evidence of cartilage formation.
- In well-differentiated lesions, typical lacuna formation is seen within the chondroid matrix; the chondroid tissue penetrates the host bony trabeculae.
- The neoplastic cells of chondrosarcoma are pleomorphic and hyperchromatic, and many of them contain multiple nuclei. (Binuclear cells are very common).
- Most of the neoplastic cells in these highly cellular malignant lesions tend to surround an abnormal cartilage.
- Calcification and ossification often occur within the cartilage matrix.

The hallmark feature in the histological distinction between chondrosarcoma and osteosarcoma is that bone formation never occurs in chondrosarcoma (forms only cartilage within the tumor) but osteosarcomas can produce both bones as well as cartilage within the tumor.

Variants of Chondrosarcoma (Table 2.16)

- Clear cell chondrosarcoma is a low-grade variant.
- The malignant cells have large clear cytoplasm and distinct cytoplasmic border; moreover, numerous osteoclast type giant cells and intralesional reactive bone formation is also seen (because of that, this variant is often confused with osteosarcoma).
- Dedifferentiated chondrosarcoma is defined as a low-grade chondrosarcoma, also having a high-grade component, the later does not produce cartilage.
- Myxoid chondrosarcoma is characterized by a proliferation of cells with clear,

Benign and Malignant Neoplasms of the Oral Cavity

Table 2.16: Histological grading of chondrosarcoma.

Grade I	This variant exhibits less cellularity and less nuclear atypia with presence of calcification. The tumor often resembles a "chondroma"
Grade II	The grade II variant shows increased cellularity and nuclear atypia. The cartilage matrix is myxoid in nature
Grade III	This variant of chondrosarcoma exhibits extreme cellularity due to increased rate of mitosis; often with presence of pleomorphic anaplastic cells. There is little or no sign of calcification.

vacuolated, or eosinophilic cytoplasm within a background of mucoid material (Fig. 2.123).
- Mesenchymal chondrosarcoma is composed of islands of well-differentiated hyaline cartilage surrounded by sheets of small round bluish cells (this variant is often confused with Ewing's sarcoma).

Treatment
Wide surgical excision is the only viable treatment. Radiotherapy and chemotherapy are not effective. Prognosis of chondrosarcoma is poorer as compared to the osteosarcoma.

Mesenchymal Chondrosarcoma

Definition

Mesenchymal chondrosarcoma is a highly malignant variant of the conventional chondrosarcoma and it occurs more commonly from the jawbone and extraskeletal soft tissues (Fig. 2.124).

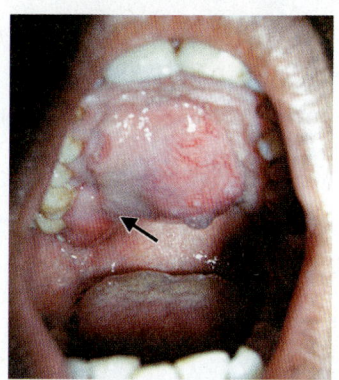

Fig. 2.124: Mesenchymal chondrosarcoma.

Clinical Features
- *Age*: This lesion often affects the younger people, usually in the 2nd and 3rd decade of life.
- *Sex*: Males and females are almost equally affected.
- *Site*: Unlike the conventional chondrosarcomas, these lesions affect the jawbones more frequently. 25–30% tumors occur in relation to the soft tissues rather than bone.

Presentation

Mesenchymal chondrosarcomas present rapidly developing swelling and pain in the affected area of bone. The clinical nature of the tumor is much aggressive than that of the conventional chondrosarcoma (Figs. 2.125 to 2.127).

Radiological Findings (Figs. 2.128A and B)

Radiographically, the tumor presents well-circumscribed radiolucency with ill-defined borders, foci of calcification may be seen within the lesion.

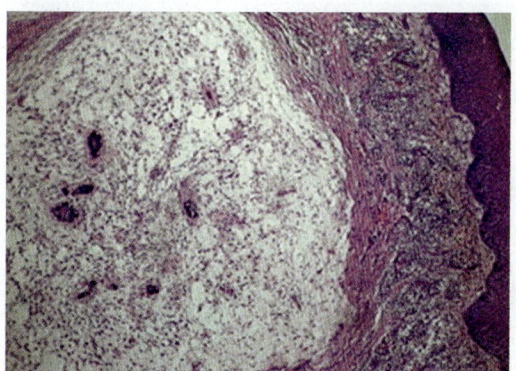

Fig. 2.123: Photomicrograph of myxoid chondrosarcoma.

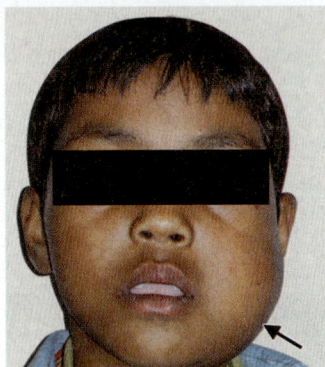

Fig. 2.125: Osteosarcoma of mandible.

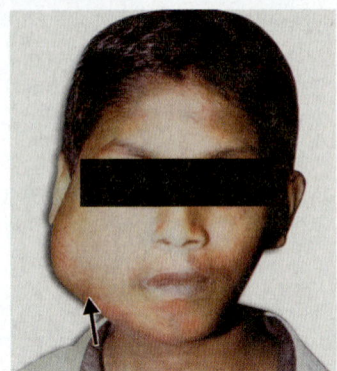

Fig. 2.127: Osteosarcoma of the jaw.

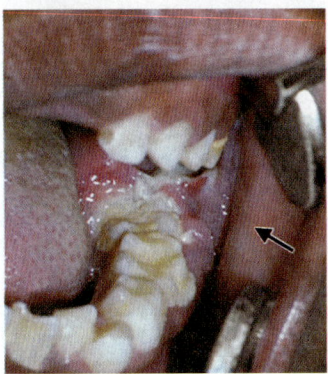

Fig. 2.126: Intraoral view of osteosarcoma of lower jaw.

Histopathology

- Microscopically mesenchymal chondrosarcoma shows sheets of proliferating round or oval-shaped malignant chondrocytes, interspersed by small islands of well-differentiated cartilages.
- Increased abnormal mitosis and cellular pleomorphism, etc. are rare.
- Sometimes, the cartilage tissue within the tumor shows calcification and metaplastic bone formation.
- A typical branching vascular pattern is seen in the soft tissue variant of the disease.

Differential Diagnosis

- Ewing's sarcoma
- Lymphoma
- Hemangiopericytoma
- Metastatic small cell carcinoma.

Treatment

Surgery is the best treatment. Prognosis is usually poor.

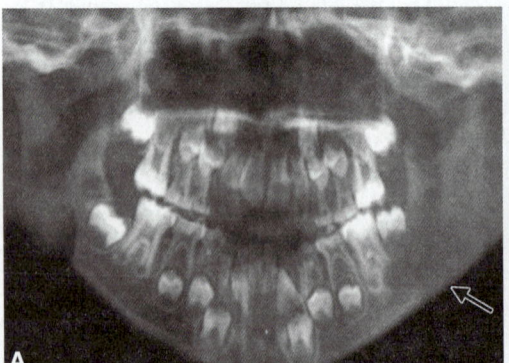
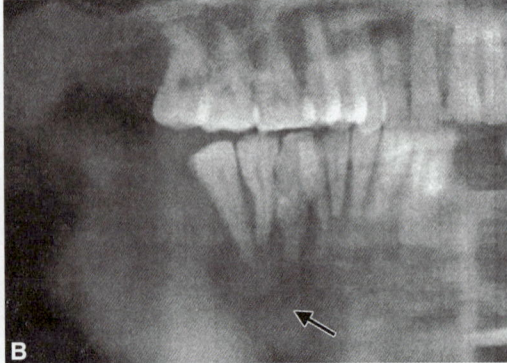

Figs. 2.128A and B: Radiograph of osteosarcoma showing: (A) Severe bone destruction, and (B) Bone formation within the lesion.

OSTEOSARCOMA

Definition

Osteosarcoma is a common highly malignant primary neoplasm arising from the bone and beside plasma cell myeloma, it is the most common primary bone tumor. The neoplastic cells in osteosarcoma characteristically exhibit the ability to produce osteoids or immature bone within the tumor.

Etiology

The exact etiology is not known, many patients give a history of previous trauma to the particular area of bone wherefrom the tumor has developed later. In many cases, radiotherapy to preexisting bony diseases may cause development of this tumor and such bony lesions are as follows:
- Paget's disease of bone
- Fibrous dysplasia
- Giant cell tumor of bone
- Osteochondroma
- Bone infarct
- Chronic osteomyelitis
- Osteogenesis imperfecta.

Types of Osteosarcoma

The osteosarcomas may be of various types and these are as follows:

According to Location of the Lesion
- Medullary osteosarcoma
- Periosteal osteosarcoma
- Parosteal osteosarcoma (arising from the external surface of bone)
- Soft tissue osteosarcoma (extraskeletal).

According to the Radiological Characteristics
- Early osteolytic type of osteosarcoma
- Osteoblastic type of osteosarcoma
- Mixed type.

According to the Tumor Histology
- Osteoblastic type of osteosarcoma
- Chondroblastic type of osteosarcoma
- Fibroblastic type of osteosarcoma
- Telangiectatic type of osteosarcoma
- Small cell type
- Giant cell type.

Clinical Features of Osteosarcoma

Osteosarcomas account for about 20% of all sarcomatous lesions occurring in the body and about 5% of them occur in the jawbones.
- *Age*: The tumor has bimodal age distribution (i.e. the maximum number of cases occurs between 10 years and 20 years of age and above 50 years of age). However the jaw lesions particularly occur at the mean age of about 34 years (1–2 decades later than the other skeletal osteosarcomas).
- *Sex*: Males are affected more frequently than females.
- *Site*: The tumor most commonly involves the long bones, e.g. lower end of the femur, upper end of the tibia, humerus and fibula, etc.

In the jawbones, maxilla is slightly more commonly affected than mandible. The lesions of the upper jaw frequently involve the alveolar ridge area, the antrum and sometimes the palate.

The mandibular lesions on the other hand commonly involve the symphysis, the angle and the ramus area, as well as the temporomandibular joint.

Extraskeletal (soft tissue) osteosarcomas occur rarely in the oral cavity and they may involve the tongue and the lip.

Clinical Presentation

Clinically, osteosarcomas may present the following features.
- A very fast enlarging, firm, painful swelling of the jaw, causing expansion and distortion of the cortical plates (Fig. 2.129).
- Severe facial deformity and difficulty in taking food due to restricted jaw movements.
- Displacement and loosening of the regional teeth are often seen and sometimes the pain arising from the tumor can mimic toothache.
- The mandibular tumors (Fig. 2.130) frequently cause paresthesia or numbness of the lower lip and the chin regions, which

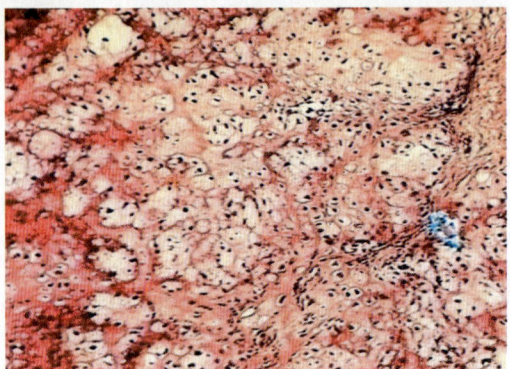

Fig. 2.129: Photomicrograph of classic osteosarcoma showing—malignant osteoblasts.

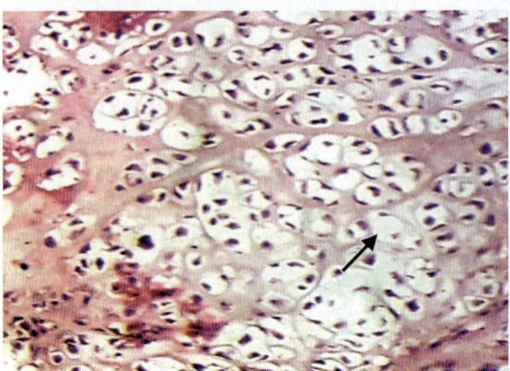

Fig. 2.131: Photomicrographs of osteoblastic osteosarcoma (high power).

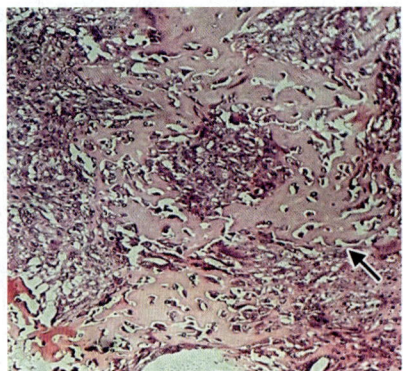

Fig. 2.130: Photomicrograph of osteoblastic osteosarcoma with varying degrees of ossification.

may be due to the involvement of inferior alveolar and mental nerves.
- The maxillary lesions cause paresthesia of the infraorbital nerve, epistaxis, nasal obstruction, loosening of teeth and pressure sensation in the eyes, etc.
- The overlying skin or mucosa often appears red and inflamed, and careful examination may reveal a vascular prominence in the area.
- Ulceration, hemorrhage, pathological fracture of bone, etc. are the commonly associated features.
- Jaw lesions are usually not associated with any past history of trauma or any preexisting bony diseases.

- Some lesions of osteosarcomas are slow growing and are present for long durations before diagnosis.

Radiological Features (Fig. 2.131)

The radiological features of the osteosarcomas are highly variable.
- In osteolytic type of osteosarcoma, the lesion commonly presents a large, irregular, radiolucent area in the bone with a typical "moth-eaten" appearance.
- Expansion, destruction and perforation of the cortical plates are also commonly seen (Fig. 2.132).
- Few lesions cause resorption of roots of the teeth often causes tapered narrowing of the teeth and hence, it is called "spiking resorption".
- The osteoblastic type of osteosarcomas commonly exhibit multiple, irregular foci of radiopacities within the large radiolucent zone. Due to the deposition of newly formed bony trabeculae within the tumor.
- In osteoblastic type of osteosarcoma, there may be deposition of new bone on the surface of the lesion in a "radiating fashion" and on radiographs, it may produce a typical "sun-ray" or a "sunburst" appearance at the periphery (best seen in standard occlusal radiographs) (Box 2.15).

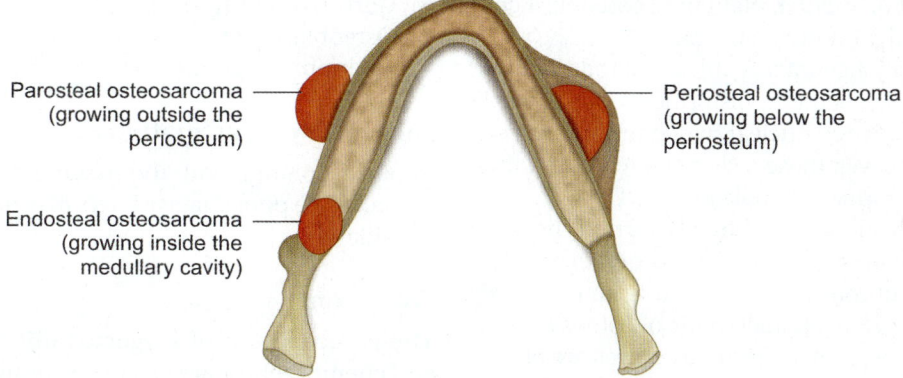

Fig. 2.132: Types of osteosarcomas as per their sites of origin.

Box 2.15	Lesions which may have "sun-ray" appearance.

- Osteosarcoma
- Chondrosarcoma
- Central hemangioma
- Complex odontoma.

Key Points of Osteosarcoma

❖ It is the common primary malignant neoplasm of bone, with unique clinical, radiological and histological characteristics.
❖ Predominantly affects children and clinically the disease causes very fast enlarging bony swelling with facial asymmetry.
❖ Pain, swelling of the jaw, mobility and displacement of teeth are the general complaints. Sometimes, the pain mimics toothache.
❖ Anesthesia and paresthesia of the affected area are also common.
❖ Maxillary lesions may cause pain, swelling, pressure sensation in the eye and epistaxis, etc.
❖ Radiograph reveals "moth-eaten" radiolucency with multiple small radiopaque foci within it, deposition of new bone on the surface of the lesion in a radiating fashion often produces a "sun-ray" appearance. Besides this, symmetric widening of periodontal ligament space is also commonly seen.
❖ Microscopically, osteosarcoma reveals neoplastic proliferation of spindle or oval-shaped malignant osteoblast cells with production of osteoids or newly formed bone within the lesion.
❖ There may be chondroblastic, fibroblastic or telangiectatic variant of osteosarcomas.

- As there is new bone formation below the periosteum at the outer margin of the jaw, it often causes lifting or elevation of the periosteum and this phenomenon is often known as Codman's triangle.
- Early osteosarcomas are characterized by localized, symmetric widening of the periodontal ligament space around the regional teeth. This phenomenon occurs as a result of invasion of the tumor cells into the periodontal ligament space and subsequent destruction of the supporting alveolar bone.
- Loss of supporting bone often causes displacement of the regional teeth.
- Many lesions osteosarcoma radiologically present the evidence of pathological fractures.
- In contrast to the conventional radiographic pictures, few larger lesions of osteosarcomas may produce only little radiographic changes in the affected part of bone.
- Chest radiographs are mandatory since early lung metastasis is common in case of osteosarcoma.

Macroscopy

The tumor shows a bulky mass made up of gritty, gray-white tissue which fills up the medullary spaces; it is often showing areas of hemorrhage and cystic degenerations.

Histopathology

- There will be presence of numerous, actively proliferating, spindle-shaped,

oval or angular, malignant osteoblast cells within a cellular stroma.
- The malignant osteoblast cells often exhibit cellular pleomorphism, increased abnormal mitosis and nuclear hyperchromatism, etc. Moreover, these cells are often larger than the normal osteoblasts.
- Multiple areas of newly formed bone or osteoid tissues are often present within the fibrous stroma and it is an extremely important characteristic of osteosarcoma.
- The osteoid areas or structures are always bordered at the periphery by the malignant tumor cells.
- Increased mitotic activity may be seen in few lesions, making the tumor an extremely cellular one, with minimum or no tumor bone formations. Histologically, this form of osteosarcoma often resembles the fibrosarcoma.
- In the chondroblastic variants of osteosarcoma, the malignant tumor cells produce large amount of cartilaginous tissues within the tumor, with little or no bone tissue formation. These variants are commonly seen in the oral cavity and they often have a better prognosis.
- Osteosarcomas in few cases may be extremely vascular in nature and exhibit multiple numbers of large, poorly formed, blood vessels within stroma. These types of lesions are known as telangiectatic type of osteosarcomas.
- Well-differentiated osteosarcomas often exhibit minimum cellular atypia with abundant bone formations, such lesions are sometimes confused with fibrous dysplasia of bone.
- On rare occasions, there may be presence of giant cells in osteosarcoma.

Differential Diagnosis

- Chondrosarcoma
- Fibrosarcoma
- Fracture callus
- Organized hematoma
- Garre's osteomyelitis
- Osteoblastoma
- Eosinophilic granuloma.

Laboratory Investigations

In osteosarcoma, both the tissue and the serum alkaline phosphatase levels may be raised considerably.

Treatment

The combination of surgery, radiotherapy and chemotherapy are usually recommended in the treatment of osteosarcoma. Prognosis is usually poor due to early metastasis of the tumor cells to the lung, brain and other areas. The average 5-year survival rate is only 10–20%.

Majority of the patients in osteosarcoma die of uncontrolled local spread of the tumor cells.

Parosteal (Juxtacortical) Osteosarcoma

This uncommon variant of osteosarcoma develops from the external surface of bone, the lesion produces a lobulated nodule attached to the cortex by a stalk. There is no elevation of the periosteum and no peripheral bone formation or regeneration. The tumor microscopically presents many well-formed bony trabeculae in a fibrocellular stroma. This tumor does not show the same degree of cellular pleomorphism as seen in case of the endosteal variety. It grows slowly and metastasizes late, and thereby has a much better prognosis.

Periosteal Osteosarcoma (Fig. 2.133)

Periosteal osteosarcomas are sessile lesions, which arise from the outer cortex of the affected bone and cause elevation of the overlying periosteum. There are also significant periosteal new bone formations and formation of Codman's triangle; this type of osteosarcomas is more aggressive in nature.

The common differences between osteosarcoma and Ewing's sarcoma are given in Table 2.17.

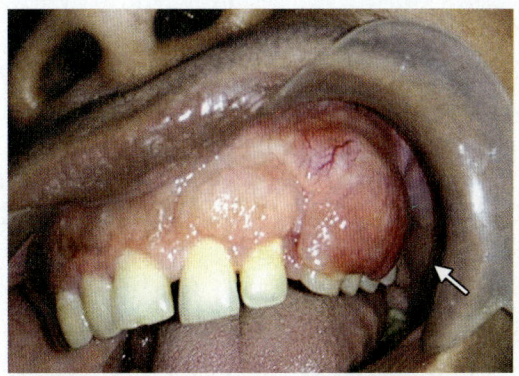

Fig. 2.133: Periosteal osteosarcoma of maxilla.

LYMPHOMAS

Definition

Lymphomas are malignant neoplasms of the cells native to the lymphoid tissue (i.e. lymphocytes, histiocytes and their precursors and derivatives). Unlike leukemias lymphomas are solid tumors, although lymphocytic lymphomas can be accompanied by lymphocytic leukemias as well. Lymphomas arise from T-lymphocytes, B-lymphocytes and occasionally from the histiocytes, however majority of the lesions arise from B cells.

Two broad groups of lymphomas have been recognized: (1) Hodgkin's lymphoma, and (2) non-Hodgkin's lymphoma. Although, diseases arise from the lymphoid tissue, the Hodgkin's lymphoma differs from the non-Hodgkin's lymphoma by the presence of Reed-Sternberg giant cells and an increased number of non-neoplastic inflammatory cells which frequently outnumber the neoplastic cells (Reed-Sternberg giant cells) in the former lesion.

Risk Factors for the Development of Lymphoma

- Age—although the disease occurs both in children and adults, but it is more common above 60 years of age.
- Family history—several members of the same family can be affected.
- Immunosuppressive treatment.
- Infections such as HIV/AIDS, Epstein Barr virus infection, Hepatitis C and *Helicobacter pylori* infections.
- Radiation therapy
- Cytotoxic drug therapy
- Rheumatoid arthritis
- Sjögren's syndrome
- Benign lymphoepithelial lesions.

Classification of Lymphomas

The WHO Classification, published in 2001 and updated in 2008 is the latest classification of lymphoma and is based upon the foundations laid within the "Revised European-American Lymphoma Classification" (REAL). This system attempts to group lymphomas by cell type (i.e. the normal cell type that most resembles the tumor) (Table 2.18). There are three large groups: the B cell, T cell, and natural killer cell tumors.

Table 2.17: Common differences between osteosarcoma and Ewing's sarcoma.

	Osteosarcoma	Ewing's sarcoma
Age	Children or older adults above 50 years	Children (mostly second decade)
Race	All	Mostly white
Sex	Slight male predilection	Second decade of life
Predisposing factors	Trauma, retinoblastoma, radiation, fibro-osseous lesions	None
Typical radiographic finding	"Sun ray" or "sun-burst" appearance	"Onion-skin" appearance
Change in jaw tumors	Widening of periodontal ligament spaces	Absent
Microscopic appearance of tumor cells	Spindle-shaped, oval or angular cells	Sheets or lobules of uniform, small round cells
Osteoid formation by tumor cells	Common	None
Prognosis	Relatively better	Poorer than osteosarcoma

Table 2.18: World Health Organization (WHO) classification of lymphomas.

Mature B cell neoplasms	• Chronic lymphocytic leukemia/small lymphocytic lymphoma
	• B-cell prolymphocytic leukemia
	• Lymphoplasmacytic lymphoma (such as Waldenström macroglobulinemia)
	• Splenic marginal zone lymphoma
	• Plasma cell neoplasms:
	   – Plasma cell myeloma
	   – Plasmacytoma
	   – Monoclonal immunoglobulin deposition diseases
	   – Heavy chain diseases
	• Extranodal marginal zone B cell lymphoma, also called MALT lymphoma
	• Nodal marginal zone B cell lymphoma (NMZL)
	• Follicular lymphoma
	• Mantle cell lymphoma
	• Diffuse large B cell lymphoma
	• Mediastinal (thymic) large B cell lymphoma
	• Intravascular large B cell lymphoma
	• Primary effusion lymphoma
	• Burkitt lymphoma/leukemia

Mature T cell and natural killer (NK) cell neoplasms	• T cell prolymphocytic leukemia
	• T cell large granular lymphocytic leukemia
	• Aggressive NK cell leukemia
	• Adult T cell leukemia/lymphoma
	• Extranodal NK/T cell lymphoma, nasal type
	• Enteropathy-type T cell lymphoma
	• Hepatosplenic T cell lymphoma
	• Blastic NK cell lymphoma
	• Mycosis fungoides/Sezary syndrome
	• Primary cutaneous CD30-positive T cell lymphoproliferative disorders
	   – Primary cutaneous anaplastic large cell lymphoma
	   – Lymphomatoid papulosis
	• Angioimmunoblastic T cell lymphoma
	• Peripheral T cell lymphoma, unspecified
	• Anaplastic large cell lymphoma

Hodgkin lymphoma	• Classical Hodgkin lymphomas:
	   – Nodular sclerosis
	   – Mixed cellularity
	   – Lymphocyte-rich
	   – Lymphocyte depleted or not depleted
	• Nodular lymphocyte-predominant Hodgkin lymphoma

Non-Hodgkin's Lymphoma

Non-Hodgkin's lymphomas (NHL) are a diverse and complex group of malignancies arising from the lymphoreticular system. The disease occurs more frequently in the oral cavity as compared to the Hodgkin's lymphomas and the oral NHL lesions frequently exhibit involvement of the extranodal tissues. Recent literatures also suggest a high incidence of these tumors among AIDS patients.

Clinical Features of Non-Hodgkin's Lymphoma

- *Age*: Middle-aged or elderly persons are commonly affected.
- *Sex*: Slightly more common among males.

- *Site*: In the head and neck region the most common site for non-Hodgkin's lymphoma is the lymphoid tissue of Waldeyer's ring. The other common intraoral sites are the hard palate, buccal vestibule, tongue, floor of the mouth, gingival, retromolar areas, tonsils and maxillary or mandibular bones.

Clinical Presentation (Figs. 2.134 to 2.137)

Clinically, NHL presents the usual features of a sarcomatous lesion.
- The patients may develop some constitutional symptoms like fever of unknown origin, fatigue, night sweats, pruritus, malaise, anorexia, dyspnea and weight loss, etc. along with generalized lymphadenopathy and abdominal pain, etc.

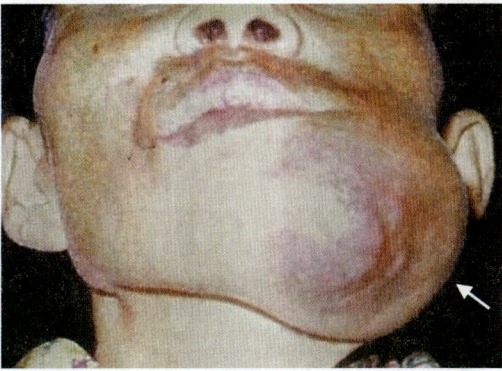

Fig. 2.136: Non-Hodgkin's lymphoma of mandible. (erythema of the skin overlying the tumor).

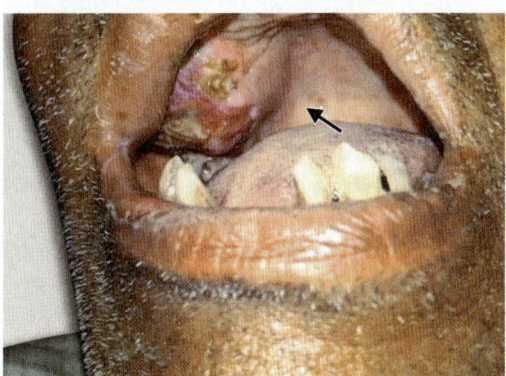

Fig. 2.137: Non-Hodgkin's lymphoma of maxilla.

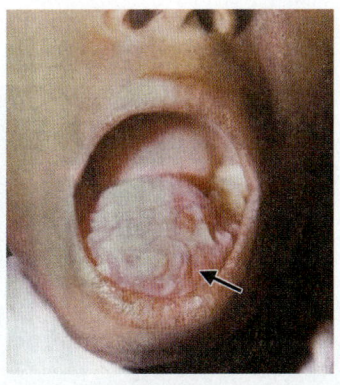

Fig. 2.134: Non-Hodgkin's lymphoma of mandible.

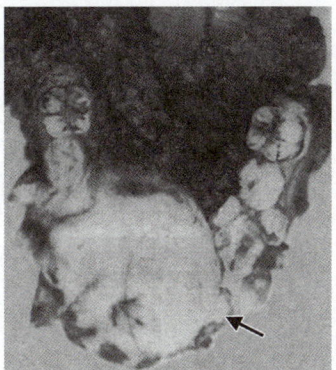

Fig. 2.135: Resected mandible of the same patient after surgery (of Figure 2.134).

- Oral non-Hodgkin's lymphomas frequently occur in association with HIV/AIDS.
- The nodal lesions produce slow enlarging, non-tendered, freely movable swellings of long duration (6 months or above) and as the disease progresses more and more number of lymph nodes get involved.
- The high grade tumors show more rapid growth (Table 2.19).
- The affected lymph nodes become firm or rubbery in consistency and they often get fixed or matted together, and gradually the lesion invades directly into the adjacent tissue structures.
- In the oral cavity, the soft tissue lesions are characterized by fast enlarging, diffuse,

Table 2.19: Staging system of non-Hodgkin's lymphoma (NHL)*.

Stage I	Localized disease; single lymph node region or single organ
Stage II	Two or more lymph node regions on the same side of the diaphragm
Stage III	Two or more lymph node regions above and below the diaphragm
Stage IV	Widespread disease; multiple organs, with or without lymph node involvement

*Both nodal as well as non-nodal tissue involvement is seen in NHL, high grade tumors often exhibit rapid growth and extensive spread in the body. Higher stage (as mentioned here) means more serious nature of the disease.

- exophytic, non-tendered, soft or firm swellings with boggy consistency.
- Misfitting dentures are common complaints for older individuals and it occurs due to gradual expansion of the jawbone.
- The overlying surface epithelium appears red or purplish and inflamed, and extensive tissue necrosis often causes ulceration, bleeding and superadded candidal infections, etc.
- In the later stages of the disease, multiple lymph node groups are enlarged, e.g. meningeal and axillary, etc. along with hepatosplenomegaly.
- Nasopharyngeal lymphoma is a multifocal destructive disease, which frequently produces swelling and ulceration of the palate.
- Non-Hodgkin's lymphomas are the second most common malignancy in AIDS patients after Kaposi's sarcoma.
- Intrabony lesion of the jaw initially produces vague pain and discomfort which mimics toothache, with further progression of the disease a large, expansile swelling develops in the jaw with pain, paresthesia and mobility of the regional teeth.
- Swelling of the gingiva and palate are common, and pathological fracture of the involved bone is also seen in some cases.
- The jaw lesions of the NHL occur either as central jaw lesions (called the primary lymphoma of bone) or they involve the jawbones secondarily as an extension from the nearby soft tissue lesions.
- The untreated central jaw lesions may cause perforation of the cortical plates and protrude outside the bone as a nontendered, lobulated soft tissue lump.

Radiology (Fig. 2.138)

Radiographically non-Hodgkin's lymphoma of bone reveals the presence of a diffuse, large, irregular or "ragged" area of radiolucency with expansion and destruction of the cortical bone. The regional teeth appear to be "floating" inside the radiolucent zone.

Histopathology (Figs. 2.139 to 2.141)

- Histologically, NHL is characterized by monotonous proliferation of malignant

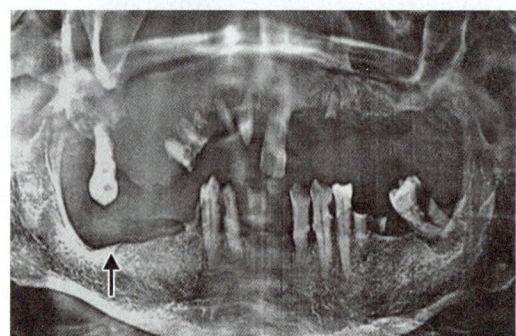

Fig. 2.138: Non-Hodgkin's lymphoma of mandible.

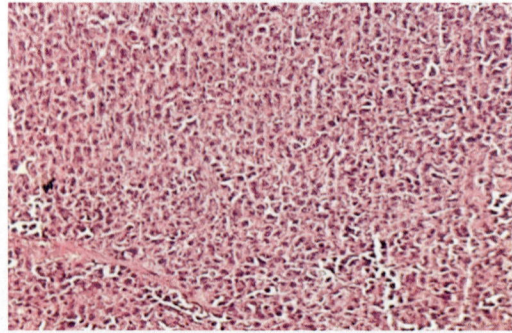

Fig. 2.139: Non-Hodgkin's lymphoma—diffuse large cell type (low power).

Benign and Malignant Neoplasms of the Oral Cavity

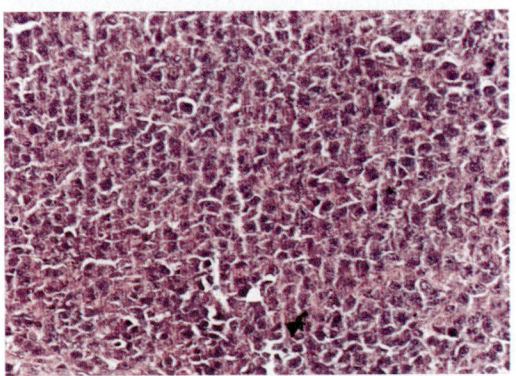

Fig. 2.140: Non-Hodgkin's lymphoma—more square type cells in high power.

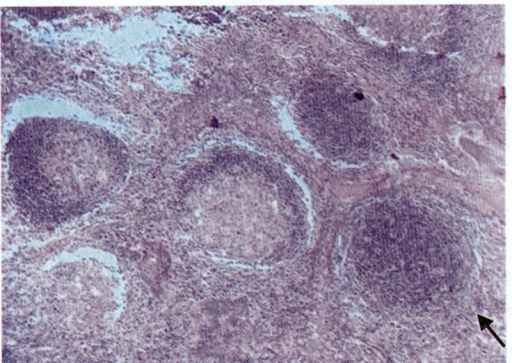

Fig. 2.141: Photomicrograph of Non-Hodgkin's lymphoma (follicular type).

lymphocytes with varying degrees of differentiation.
- The malignant cells in NHL may be small in size and uniform in shape, and they can be readily recognized as lymphocytes. In other instances, the tumor cells may be very large and immature in appearance and they often resemble histiocytes.
- The tumor cells in NHL exhibits a mixture of two types of malignant lymphocytes, which are known as centroblasts and centrocytes.
- *Centroblasts*: These are large non-cleaved follicular center cells with vesiculated nuclei and pale staining cytoplasm.
- *Centrocytes*: These are small non-cleaved follicular center cells with denser, more hyperchromatic nuclei and scant cytoplasm.
- Most cells are relatively uniform in size and they proliferate in broad sheets and generally there is no evidence of tissue necrosis or hemorrhage in the tumor
- Oral tumors mostly have cells of B-cell lineage with "diffuse large cell type" being the most common.

These malignant cells, whether large or small, are mostly arranged in two distinct patterns: (1) *follicular pattern*, and (2) *diffuse pattern*.

Follicular pattern: In this pattern of NHL, the tumor cells (both large or small) tend to aggregate in large follicles, which are separated from one another by very thin connective tissue septa.

Diffuse pattern: The tumor cell in this pattern exhibit diffuse proliferation within the connective tissue, with no evidence of follicle formation.

The tumors are further categorized according to their cell types (small cell type or large cell type) and according to the cell arrangements (follicular or diffuse).

Accordingly some tumors may be diffuse large cell type (very common in oral cavity) or diffuse small cell type; in higher magnification, the large malignant lymphocyte cells often look square shaped.

Key Points of Non-Hodgkin's Lymphoma

- Non-Hodgkin's lymphoma is a relatively common malignant neoplasm of the lymphoreticular system.
- It occurs in the oral cavity more often than the Hodgkin's lymphoma, the other important variant of lymphoma.
- It also commonly occurs in AIDS patients.
- Non-Hodgkin's lymphomas affect the lymph nodes as well as the extranodal sites, the orofacial structures commonly affected include palate, cheek, tongue and jaws, etc.
- The nodal lesions produce slow enlarging swelling of the affected node with fixation.
- The extranodal lesions often produce fast enlarging, gross painful swelling with ulceration and super-added candidal infection, etc.

- Whenever the jaw bone is involved, it radiographically shows multilocular radiolucency with irregular border and displacement of teeth.
- Histologically, non-Hodgkin's lymphoma presents neoplastic proliferations of uniform looking lymphocytes in diffuse sheets with minimum intervening connective tissue stroma.
- Sometimes the neoplastic cells, which resemble lymphocytes or histiocyte, tend to aggregate in large clusters.
- Special investigations like immunohistochemistry and DNA-hybridization, etc. are often done for confirmation of diagnosis of these lesions.
- T cell marker CD 2, 3, 4, 7, 8.
- B cell marker CD 10, 19, 20, 21, 22.
- NK cell marker 16, 56.
- Chemotherapy provides the best result in the treatment of non-Hodgkin's lymphoma.

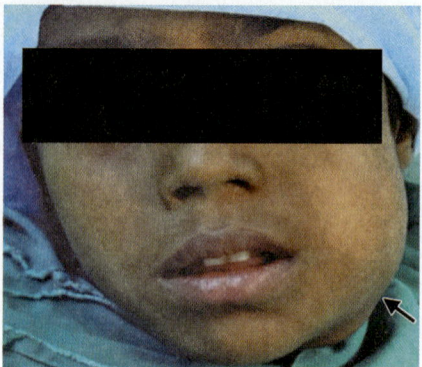

Fig. 2.142: Burkitt's lymphoma.

Special Investigations
- DNA-hybridization study reveals Epstein-Barr virus DNA in the malignant B-lymphocytes.
- Bone marrow biopsy
- Liver biopsy
- Laparotomy
- Bone scan
- Liver scan
- Blood picture
- CT-scan
- Bone marrow biopsy
- Immunohistochemistry—monoclonal nature of the malignant lymphocytes can be recognized by the production of kappa and lambda light chains only.

Treatment
Chemotherapy is the most successful treatment modality in lymphomas. However, radical surgery and radiotherapy are also commonly done. The overall 5-year survival rate is about 30%.

Burkitt's Lymphoma

Definition
Burkitt's lymphoma is an uncommon, highly aggressive form Non-Hodgkin's lymphoma (B-lymphocytic origin), which occurs commonly among the African children. This tumor is believed to be caused by the Epstein-Barr virus and the disease frequently occurs in areas of malaria endemic. The tumor was first reported by Denis Burkitt (a surgeon) in 1958. Burkitt's lymphoma is one of the fastest growing malignancies in humans, with a very high growth fraction.

Clinical Features (Figs. 2.142 and 2.143)
- *Age*: Burkitt's lymphoma occurs commonly at the age of about 1–3 years.
- *Sex*: More commonly seen among male children.
- *Site*: The tumor predominantly involves the extra nodal areas. Maxilla and mandible

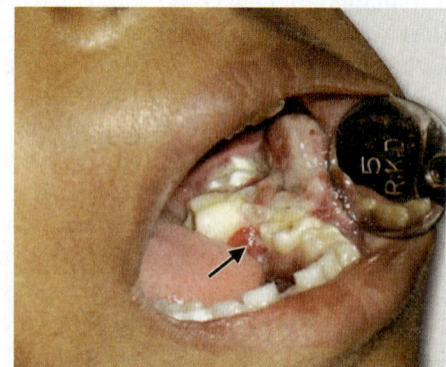

Fig. 2.143: Burkitt's lymphoma intraoral view of the same patient (in Figure 2.142).

are the most frequently affected sites in the head and neck region, however maxilla is more frequently affected than mandible. The lesion can also develop from the other visceral organs like ovary, kidney, liver and endocrine glands, etc.

Pathogenesis

It has been observed that Burkitt's lymphomas occur commonly in the geographic areas, where the malarial infections are very common.

The most accepted explanation for this phenomenon is that acute malarial infections cause reactive lymphoid hyperplasia and as a result body's control over the proliferation of "Epstein-Barr virus specific B lymphocytes" is lost. This results in an increased abnormal neoplastic proliferation of B-lymphocytes, leading to the development of Burkitt's lymphoma.

Chromosomal abnormality is believed to be the most important factor in the development of Burkitt's lymphoma. In this neoplasm, translocation of a portion of chromosome 8 to chromosome 2, 14 and 22 is often observed, which results in over expression of the *C-myc oncogene*. Overexpression of *C-myc oncogene*, which is a DNA-binding transcription protein results in the activation of cell cycling in B lymphocytes.

Types of Burkitt's Lymphoma

Burkitt's lymphoma is generally divided into three forms:
1. *Endemic form (African type)*: This is the most common type and is seen in children in equatorial Africa. Almost all cases are associated with Epstein-Barr virus infection.
2. *Non-endemic or sporadic (non-African) form*: Burkitt's lymphoma is very uncommon outside Africa, hence it is called the sporadic form. About 20% cases are associated with Epstein-Barr virus infection.
3. *Immunodeficiency associated form*: Occurs in adults with HIV infection or organ transplant patients undergoing immunosuppressive drug therapy.

According to WHO Burkitt's lymphomas are classified into three types:
1. Classic Burkitt's lymphoma
2. Burkitt's lymphoma with plasmacytoid proliferations
3. A typical Burkitt's/Burkitt-like lymphoma.

Clinical Features of Burkitt's Lymphoma

- The earliest sign of the disease is characterized by rapid painless expansile swelling of the jaws with loosening of teeth, it starts from the posterior part of the jaw and gradually moves to the anterior area.
- Within a short span of time the lesion produces gross deformity of the face and proptosis of the eyeball.
- The nature of the swelling is usually massive, painless and uniform, and it often causes facial asymmetry.
- The mucosa overlying the tumor is often ulcerated and there can be areas of hemorrhage.
- Toothache itself is a frequent complaint among these patients (especially adults), which occurs due to the invasion and damage of dental pulp by tumor cells.
- The tumor cells frequently involve the mental and the infraorbital nerves, damage to these nerves often leads to paresthesia or anesthesia of the related structures. Paraplegia in the facial region is also common
- Peripheral lymphadenopathy is uncommon in Burkitt's lymphomas.
- Advanced lesions of Burkitt's lymphoma produce massive expansion of the jaw with displacement of teeth, derangement of the dental arch and malocclusion, etc.
- As the tumor mass increases in size, it causes massive enlargement of the gingiva or the alveolar process in the jaw, as a result many deciduous or even permanent teeth are pushed out of their socket and some of which may exfoliate prematurely.
- Sometimes, the tumor is so large that it may fill up the entire oral cavity, in such cases a large tumor mass often protrudes

outside the mouth, which contains many rootless teeth.
- Some tumors cause perforation of the cortical plates of jawbone and in such cases, a soft tissue lump often protrudes from these perforated openings.
- Abdominal swelling is also common in Burkitt's lymphomas and the tumor cells frequently invade the kidney and the ovary, etc.
- In AIDS patients, Burkitt's lymphoma often produces a soft nodular mass in the palate, which has severe hemorrhagic tendency. Such lesions frequently resemble the Kaposi's sarcoma.
- Involvement of the maxillary antrum is common and these patients often have epistaxis and pressure in the eyeball.

Radiological Features

- Radiographically, Burkitt's lymphoma presents a large, irregular radiolucent area in the bone with a ragged "moth-eaten" appearance.
- In the initial stages of the disease, there are multiple small radiolucent foci seen in the jaw, these small lesions coalesce together with time to form a large, massive defect in the bone.
- The earliest sign of the disease is the loss of lamina dura and enlargement of the crypt of the developing tooth, which occur due to involvement of the dental papilla by the tumor cells.
- Tooth displacement and root resorption are common.
- Some lesions cause blurring of the shadow of maxillary antrum.
- Widening of the periodontal ligament space occurs due to invasion of the tumor cells in the area.
- Pathological fracture of the bone is seen in few cases.

Histopathology (Figs. 2.144 and 2.145)

- Histologically, Burkitt's lymphoma is characterized by monotonous proliferation of small, non-cleaved B-lymphocytes in diffuse sheets.

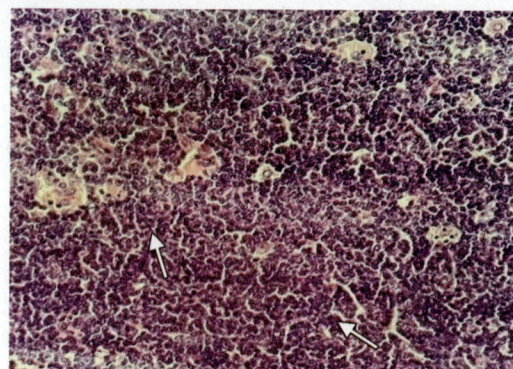

Fig. 2.144: Photomicrograph of Burkitt's lymphoma (low power) showing a typical "starry sky" appearance.

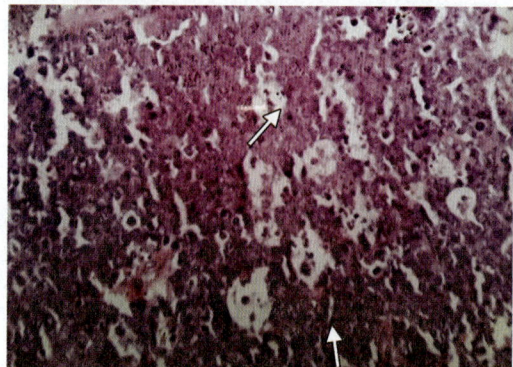

Fig. 2.145: Photomicrograph of Burkitt's lymphoma (high power).

- These malignant lymphocytes often have large round nuclei with prominent nuclear membrane, moreover they also exhibit stippled nucleoplasm, prominent nucleoli and minimal cytoplasm.
- Each nucleus is surrounded by a cytoplasm, which gives the sheets of neoplastic cells a syncytial appearance.
- The mitotic activity is abundant and this tumor probably shows the fastest rate of cell multiplication among all malignant lesions (each cell doubles itself in just 24 hours).
- Numerous macrophages with abundant clear cytoplasm containing cellular debris are usually found scattered uniformly throughout the tumor and this often gives

rise to a very characteristic "starry-sky" appearance.
- In starry-sky appearance the "white stars" are produced by macrophages (due to their clear large cytoplasms) and the vast "darkness of the night" is produced by the darkly stained or hyperchromatic nuclei of the malignant lymphocytes.
- The malignant cells often invade into the periodontal ligament tissue and some cells can even invade into the dental pulp.
- Few multinucleated giant cells may also be seen within the tumors.

Treatment

Chemotherapy gives the best response in Burkitt's lymphoma, of course surgery and radiotherapy are the other therapeutic options.

Hodgkin's Lymphoma

Definition

Hodgkin's lymphoma (HL) is an extremely rare lymphoproliferative disorder characterized by the presence of Reed-Sternberg giant cells (RS cells) in the tumor, these RS cells are modified malignant lymphocytes and they are the chief malignant cells of this tumor. A large number of non-neoplastic inflammatory cells are always present in this tumor, which often outnumber the neoplastic components, i.e. RS cells. The disease mostly affects the lymphoid (nodal) tissues and seldom affects the non-nodal tissues like the oral cavity; in most of the cases, oral structures are involved secondarily due to the extension of the cervical lymph node tumors (Box 2.16).

Clinical Features

- *Age*: The disease commonly occurs between the age of 15 years and 35 years, although it can occur at a higher frequency in the later part of life (beyond 55 years).
- *Sex*: Slight male predilection is seen.
- *Site*: The tumor occurs more commonly from the lymphoid tissues of the cervical chain of lymph nodes and the tonsils, extranodal areas in the oral cavity like the submucosa, maxilla and mandible, etc. are also affected in few cases. Axillary and inguinal nodes may also be involved.

Clinical Presentation (Fig. 2.146)

- Persistent generalized lymphadenopathy is the most important feature of Hodgkin's lymphoma (HL) and the enlarged lymph nodes are nontendered, firm and rubbery in consistency.
- In the initial stages of the disease, the affected lymph nodes are freely movable, however as the disease progresses, the nodes become matted and fixed to the surrounding tissues.
- Generalized weakness, pain in the abdomen and back, weight loss, low grade episodic fever and night sweats are the initial systemic complaints.
- Patients also have persistent cough, dyspnea due to pressure in the trachea, anorexia, itching of the skin (pruritus).
- Edema of the extremities due to progressive venous obstructions, obstructive

Box 2.16	Risk factors of Hodgkin's lymphoma.

- *Age*: Mostly between 15 and 35 years or above 55 years
- *Family history*: Very significant
- *Gender*: More in males
- *Past history of Epstein–Barr virus infection*: Especially infectious mononucleosis

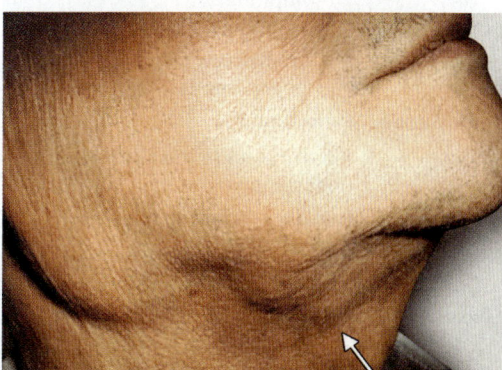

Fig. 2.146: Hodgkin's lymphoma of submandibular lymph node.

jaundice, plural or pericardial effusion and hemoptysis or melena, etc. are the other constitutional symptoms.

- In untreated cases, the disease spreads from one lymph node to the other and eventually spreads to several vital organs such as spleen, liver, lung and bone marrow, etc.
- As the disease involves the liver and spleen, hepatosplenomegaly soon develops, and it is a common feature of Hodgkin's lymphoma.
- Oral lesions of Hodgkin's lymphoma are rare and mostly present large submucosal swellings with ulceration, pain, paresthesia, etc.
- Although, primary oral lesions do occur in Hodgkin's lymphoma but in most of the cases oral lesions in this disease develop as a result of dissemination of the tumor cells into the oral soft tissues or jaw bones from the cervical areas (Table 2.20).

> **Key Points of Hodgkin's Lymphoma**
> - Hodgkin's lymphoma (HL) is an extremely rare malignant neoplasm of lymphoid tissue characterized by the presence of Reed-Sternberg giant cells in the tumor.
> - The disease causes persistent generalized lymphadenopathy and the involved nodes are nontendered, firm and rubbery in consistency.
> - The constitutional symptoms are very significant in this disease and they include generalized weakness, pain in the abdomen and back, weight loss, generalized pruritus (itching), low grade episodic fever and night sweats, etc.
> - Histologically, Hodgkin's lymphoma is characterized by the proliferation of malignant lymphoid cells and non-neoplastic inflammatory cells, including lymphocytes, macrophages, plasma cells and eosinophils, etc.
> - "Reed-Sternberg giant cells" (RS cells) with two mirror image nuclei, that often creates an "owl eye" appearance are the chief malignant cells of the tumor.
> - Radiotherapy and chemotherapy are the common modes of treatment, prognosis is often poor.

Table 2.20: Major systemic changes in Hodgkin's lymphoma (HL).

Constitutional	• Fever • Night sweats • Unexplained weight loss—more than 10% loss of body weight in 6 months • Asymptomatic-HL may also occur without any constitutional symptoms
Blood	• Anemia • Thrombocytopenia • Hypercalcemia
Bone marrow	Pancytopenia
Skin	Inflammatory lesion like erythema nodosum
Lymph nodes	Painless lymphadenopathy
Brain	• Cerebellar degeneration • Limbic encephalitis
Spleen	Often enlarged
Liver	Sometimes enlarged

Histopathology (Fig. 2.147)

- In Hodgkin's lymphoma, the involved lymph nodes are histologically characterized by the presence of malignant lymphoid cells and non-neoplastic inflammatory cells, including lymphocytes, macrophages, plasma cells and eosinophils, etc.
- The chief malignant cells of this tumor are the "Reed-Sternberg giant cells" (RS cells); these are morphologically altered

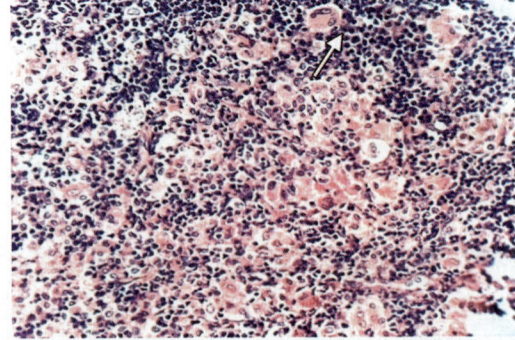

Fig. 2.147: Photomicrograph of Hodgkin's lymphoma showing "Reed–Sternberg" giant cells.

malignant lymphocytes characteristically having two or more nuclei in its cytoplasm. In many cases these RS cell may have two mirror image nuclei, each containing a large acidophilic nucleolus surrounded by a distinctive clear zone; together they impart an "owl-eye" appearance.

Histological Types of Hodgkin's Lymphoma (Table 2.21)

There are four recognized histologic types of Hodgkin's disease.

1. *Lymphocyte predominant*: Characterized by abundant lymphocytes, few plasma cells with occasional RS cells. This type carries the most favorable prognosis.
2. *Mixed cellularity*: Characterized by lymphocytes, plasma cells, eosinophils and easily identifiable RS cells.
3. *Lymphocytes depletion*: This type shows sparse lymphocytes and stromal cells, with areas of fibrosis and highly malignant bizarre RS cells. This type carries the poorest prognosis.
4. *Nodular sclerosis*: Characterized by bands of collagen, subdividing the tumor cells into many small islands within the lymph node.

Table 2.21: Staging system of Hodgkin's lymphoma (HL)*.

Stage I	Involvement of single lymph node region or single extranodal site (Ie)
Stage II	Involvement of two or more nodes on the same side of diaphragm or with contagious extranodal site (IIe)
Stage III	Involvement of both sides of diaphragm or with spleen (IIIs), or contagious extranodal site (IIIe)
Stage IV	Diffuse involvement of extra nodal sites with/or nodal disease

*The disease primarily involves the nodal tissue (lymph node) and whenever there is involvement of extranodal areas, it indicates more serious nature of the disease with poor prognosis.

Common extralymphatic (outside lymph nodes) sites involved in Hodgkin's lymphoma:
- Thymus
- Spleen
- Waldeyer's ring
- Appendix
- Payer's patches.

Laboratory Investigations

- Biopsy of the lymph nodes to see the characteristic histopathologic findings.
- Complete blood count.
- Chest X-ray and tomography.
- Radiographic skeletal survey.
- Technetium bone scans.
- Liver function test and scan.
- Bone marrow biopsy.
- Lymphangiogram to see the size of the node.
- Laparotomy to see the extent of the disease.

Treatment

By chemotherapy and radiotherapy. The overall prognosis is good and 5-year survival rate is about 80%.

The differences between Hodgkin's and non-Hodgkin's lymphoma are given in Table 2.22.

■ MULTIPLE MYELOMA

Definition

Multiple myeloma represents a malignant disease of the plasma cells, which develops in the bone marrow and is characterized by excessive proliferation of terminally differentiated B lymphocytes or plasma cells. The name "multiple myeloma" is given to the disease since it develops from several parts of the body (wherever bone marrow is present, e.g. pelvis, spine, ribs, etc.). The clinical manifestations caused by multiple myeloma could be due to (Box 2.17):

1. Uncontrolled proliferation of neoplastic plasma cells, which infiltrate into the bone as well as the soft tissues.
2. Production of abnormal immunoglobulins (monoclonal) by the neoplastic plasma cells.

Table 2.22: Difference between Hodgkin's lymphoma and non-Hodgkin's lymphoma.

Hodgkin's lymphoma	Non-Hodgkin's (NH) lymphoma
• Hodgkin's lymphoma classically originates from accessible lymphoid tissue, e.g. cervical, axillary, inguinal regions • Classically arises from lymph node; does not develop from non-nodal tissue • Hodgkin's lymphoma spread in an orderly fashion and predictable fashion into the contagious tissues • Usually diagnosed in the early stage • Predictable response to the treatment • Have lots of nonspecific clinical symptoms in the advanced stage • The most important histopathological difference is presence of Reed–Sternberg cell • Histologically non-specific inflammatory cells outnumber the malignant cells	• Non-Hodgkin's lymphoma may originate from accessible tissue or deep tissue, e.g. may originate from Waldeyer's ring, gastrointestinal system and bone • 30% of NH originates from extranodal tissue • NH spread in a disorderly and unpredictable fashion • Usually diagnosed in relatively advanced stage • Unpredictable response to treatment • Nonspecific clinical features are less common in NHL • Reed–Sternberg cell absent • Histologically non-specific inflammatory cells outnumber the malignant cells

Box 2.17 List of common symptoms in multiple myeloma.

- Bone pain typically in the back and thorax
- Generalized weakness
- Anemia and bleeding tendency
- Neuropathies
- Spinal cord compression
- Hypercalcemia
- Pathologic fracture of bone
- Infection due to disturbed immune function
- Renal failure

Flowchart 2.2: Outline of pathogenesis of multiple myeloma.

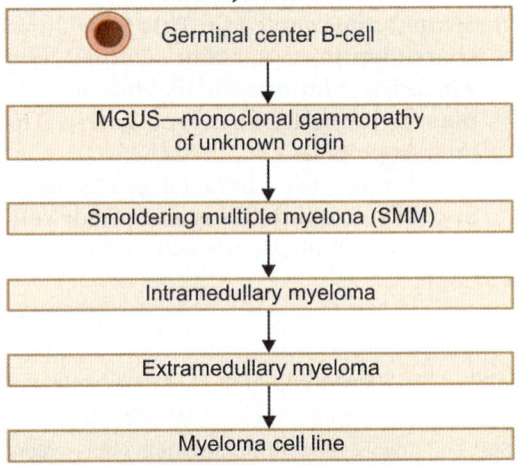

The outline of pathogenesis of multiple myeloma is given in Flowchart 2.2.

Clinical Features of Multiple Myeloma

- *Age*: 40 to 70 years.
- *Sex*: Both sexes are equally affected.
- *Race*: Black people are affected twice as often as the whites.
- *Site*: Bones anywhere in the skeleton can be affected and among the jawbones, mandible is more frequently affected than maxilla.

Mandibular lesions are often multiple and they commonly occur over the molar-ramus region or the angle. In some cases, the lesion can occur in relation to the gingival tissue.

Clinical Presentation

- Severe deep bone pain and tenderness are the most common and characteristic early symptoms, these symptoms often increase as then patient moves.
- When the disease affects the mandibular bone it causes early development of numbness in the lips or chin.
- Patients also suffer from nausea, vomiting and marked anemia, etc.
- Increased bleeding tendency with petechial hemorrhage in the skin and mucous

membrane due to severe fall in the number of platelets.
- There are also increased chances of renal complications as the kidney is overburdened by the excess and abnormal protein production in the body by the neoplastic plasma cells.
- In multiple myeloma, jaw lesions occur in about 15% cases, initially these jaw lesions produce pain that often simulates toothache.
- The jaw lesions in advanced stages, produce fast enlarging, painful swelling, with expansion and destruction of the bone.
- Severe bone destruction may lead to the "egg-shell cracking" or pathological fractures.
- The regional teeth in the jaw are usually mobile due to weakness of the bone and as a result malocclusion often develops.
- Extraction of teeth in these patients usually causes severe uncontrolled hemorrhage and delayed wound healing.
- Multiple myelomas sometimes cause immunosuppression and thereby increase the risk of secondary infection, in the oral cavity; this often results in candidiasis and oral hairy leukoplakia.
- Production of abnormal proteins such as amyloids occur in multiple myeloma, deposition of amyloids in the form of nodular swellings may occur in various parts of the body as well as the oral cavity; in the tongue such deposits often cause macroglossia.
- Metastatic calcification of the oral and other soft tissues may occur due to hypercalcemia secondary to tumor related osteolysis.

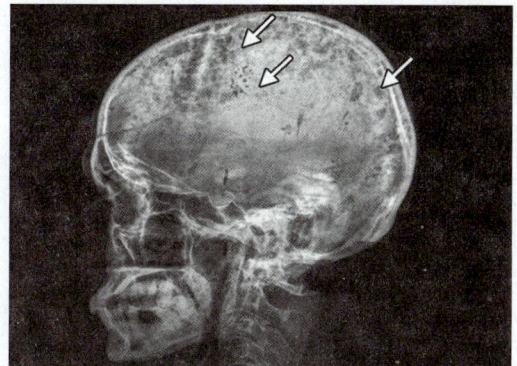

Fig. 2.148: Multiple myeloma producing several "punched-out", circular radiolucencies in the skull.

The New International Myeloma Working Group (IMWG) criteria for multiple myeloma diagnosis are given in Table 2.23.

Radiological Features
(Fig. 2.148, Box 2.18)

In multiple myeloma, the radiograph shows numerous well-defined, punched-out radiolucencies with no peripheral bone reaction. The lesions commonly involve the skull, vertebrae, ribs and jaw bones. Diffuse radiolucency in case of multiple myeloma may be seen occasionally.

Histopathology (Figs. 2.149A and B)

- The lesion is histologically characterized by diffuse sheets of closely packed, monotonous, round or oval cells, which often resemble the typical plasma cells.

Table 2.23: New International Myeloma Working Group (IMWG) criteria for multiple myeloma diagnosis*.

Biomarkers of malignancy	CRAB features
• Clonal bone marrow plasma cells ≥60% • Involved: Uninvolved sFLC ratio ≥100 • >1 focal lesion on MRI studies	• Hypercalcemia—serum calcium >11.5 mg/dL • Renal insufficiency -serum creatinine >1.73 mmol/dL or eGFR ≤40 ml/min • Anemia—normocytic normochromic with Hb% <10 g/dL • Bone lesions—lytic lesion, severe osteopenia or pathologic fracture

*Clonal bone marrow plasma cells ≥10% or biopsy-proven bony or extramedullary plasmacytoma and one or more of the CRAB features and myeloma defining events.

Box 2.18 Laboratory investigations for multiple myeloma.

- Routine hemogram shows anemia, neutropenia, thrombocytopenia and greatly raised ESR
- Most of the multiple myeloma patients exhibit hyperglobulinemia, with reversal of the serum albumin-globulin ratio.
- There will be an abnormal increase in the production of light chain proteins (known as Bence–Jones protein) by the tumor cells as a result the serum protein level may become very high (measuring up to 8–16 g%)
- Presence of *Bence–Jones protein in urine* is also reported in (30–50%) patients of multiple myeloma and it is one of the most important hallmarks in the diagnosis of the disease
- Serum and urinal protein immunoelectrophoresis is done to detect these abnormal proteins in multiple myeloma
- The Bence–Jones protein coagulates when the urine is heated to the temperature of 42°C to 60°C, it disappears when the urine is boiled and finally it reappears again as the urine is cooled
- Occasionally, the Bence–Jones protein in urine can also be present in patients with *polycythemia or leukemia*. However, the absence of this protein also does not rule out the presence of multiple myeloma in a patient
- Biopsy of the bone marrow in multiple myeloma patients exhibits the presence of at least 10% atypical plasma cells in the total marrow cell population

- Among these neoplastic plasma cells, some are well-differentiated while the rests are poorly differentiated.
- The cells eccentrically placed nuclei and they often exhibit chromatin clumping in a typical "cart-wheel" or a "checker-board" pattern.
- Mitotic figures may be high in few cases, with occasional presence of binucleated or multinucleated cells.
- These neoplastic plasma cells often invade and destroy the normal tissues of the body.
- Deposition of amyloids may be seen in the tissue beneath the plasma cells, which appear as homogenous, eosinophilic acellular areas.

Key Points of Multiple Myeloma

- Multiple myelomas represent a group of malignant diseases of plasma cells, which infiltrate the bone and soft tissues.
- The tumor consists of terminally differentiated B-lymphocytes or plasma cells.
- Production of abnormal immunoglobulins (monoclonal) by these neoplastic plasma cells is also another important feature of the disease.
- Clinically, it presents severe, deep bone pain and tenderness; often there is early development of numbness in the lips or chin.
- Increased bleeding tendency with petechial hemorrhage, occasional uncontrolled hemorrhage and delayed wound healing, etc. are the other important features of the disease.
- Radiograph shows numerous well-defined, punched-out radiolucencies in the affected bone. Severe bone destruction may even lead to the "egg-shell cracking" or pathological fractures.
- Presence of Bence-Jones protein in urine is an important feature of multiple myeloma.
- Histology reveals diffuse sheets of closely packed monotonous, round or oval cells, which often resemble the typical plasma cells.
- Chemotherapy is mostly given but the disease is fatal.

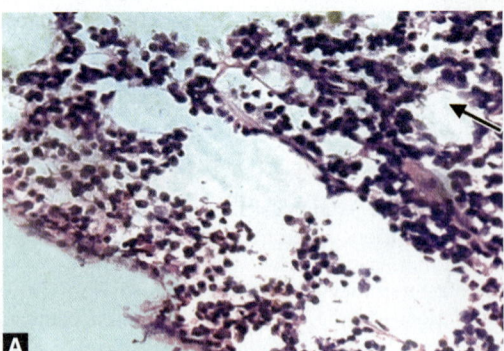
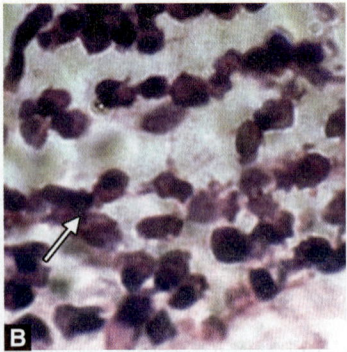

Figs. 2.149A and B: (A) Photomicrograph of multiple myeloma showing proliferation of numerous plasma cells; (B) Photomicrograph of typical plasma cells in multiple myeloma (high power).

Treatment

Chemotherapy is mostly given but the disease is fatal.

■ SOLITARY PLASMACYTOMA

Solitary plasmacytoma is a unifocal, monoclonal, neoplastic proliferation of plasma cells that often arises within an extranodal site, especially the bone. Rarely the tumor may develop in the soft tissue (often in the upper air passages) and such tumors are called "extramedullary plasmacytoma". This lesion is believed to be the least aggressive variant of the large group of plasma cell neoplasms including the multiple myeloma; although solitary plasmacytoma may ultimately transform into multiple myeloma.

Clinical Features

- *Age*: Adults are generally affected (average age 55 years).
- *Sex*: More common in males (ratio is 3:1)
- *Site*: Mostly affects the bone, sometimes soft tissue lesions (extramedullary plasmacytomas) occur in the tongue, nasopharynx, parotids and paranasal sinuses, etc.

Presentation (Fig. 2.150)

- Solitary plasmacytomas commonly cause swelling of the affected bone with pain and tenderness.
- Some lesions are asymptomatic.
- Soft tissue lesions produce well-circumscribed, painless, soft nodule in the affected organ.
- Systemic complications like anemia or renal failure, etc. are generally absent in solitary plasmacytoma.
- About 50% lesions of solitary plasmacytomas turn into multiple myelomas over time.

Radiographic Findings

Radiographically solitary plasmacytoma produces well-defined, unilocular radiolucency in the bone with no sclerotic reaction at the margin.

Histopathology (Fig. 2.151)

Histopathologic appearance of solitary plasmacytoma is same as multiple myeloma, it exhibits sheets of proliferating neoplastic plasma cells with varying degrees of differentiation.

Laboratory Investigation

- Bence-Jones protein is present but very little in amount as compared to multiple myelomas.
- Atypical plasma cells are not found in the bone marrow.

Treatment

By radiotherapy.

■ LEIOMYOSARCOMA

Leiomyosarcomas are malignant neoplasms of the smooth muscle cell origin.

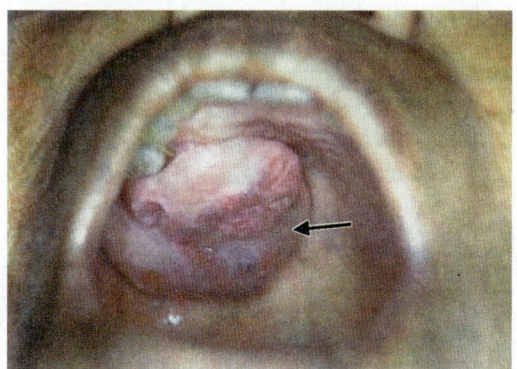

Fig. 2.150: Solitary plasmacytoma of the palate.

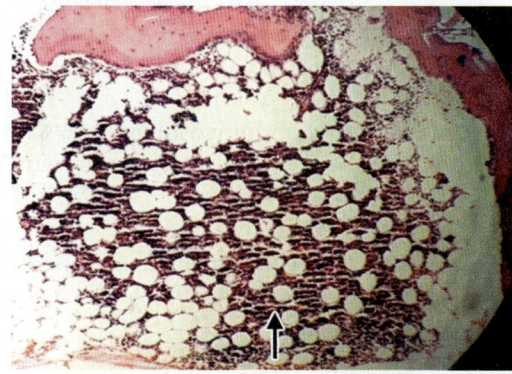

Fig. 2.151: Photomicrograph of solitary plasmacytoma.

Clinical Features

Oral lesions of leiomyomas are rare, whenever they occur the lesions involve the jawbones. Clinically the lesions produce fast enlarging swelling of the affected tissue with development of a soft or firm lobulated mass, which can be painful.

Histopathology

Histologically, leiomyomas present neoplastic proliferation of spindle-shaped malignant smooth muscle cells in fascicles. The malignant cells often have blunt ended or cigar shaped nuclei and abundant eosinophilic cytoplasm. Some tumor cells are round and somewhat epithelioid in shape.

Treatment

Combination of surgery, radiotherapy and chemotherapy.

■ RHABDOMYOSARCOMA

Definition

It is a malignant neoplasm developing from the striated (skeletal) muscle cells. It is the most common soft tissue sarcoma among children head, and neck area is the most frequent site.

Types

Rhabdomyosarcomas are histologically categorized into three variants:
1. Embryonal rhabdomyosarcoma (60–70%)—occurs in children up to 10 years of age.
2. Alveolar rhabdomyosarcoma (20–30%)—occurs between 10 years and 25 years of age.
3. Pleomorphic rhabdomyosarcoma (5% or less)—occurs at the age of about 40 years.

Clinical Features

- *Age*: Most of these tumors arise during childhood, some lesions occur in teenagers or young adults.
- *Sex*: Both sexes are equally affected.

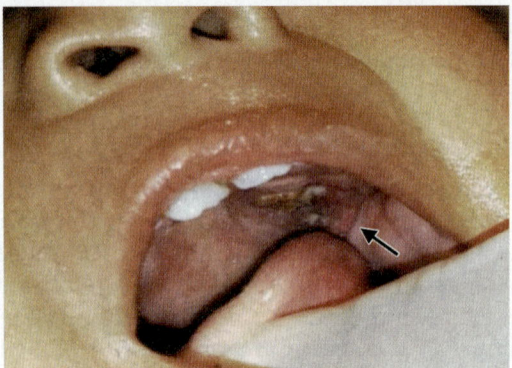

Fig. 2.152: Rhabdomyosarcoma of the palate.

- *Site*: The embryonal and the alveolar types predominantly affect the head and neck region.

Presentation (Fig. 2.152)

- Rhabdomyosarcomas usually are rapidly growing lesions, which cause swelling, pain and extensive tissue damage.
- These lesions are indurated, fixed and are often ulcerated.
- Some exophytic lesions produce polypoid growths that resemble "cluster of grapes".
- Lesions of the maxillary sinus may often break the sinus wall and invade into the oral cavity.

Histopathology (Figs. 2.153A and B)

Microscopically, rhabdomyosarcomas are composed of malignant rhabdomyoblasts.
- Embryonal rhabdomyosarcoma—histologically this variant is characterized by small round cells with monotonous looking hyperchromatic nuclei.
- Alveolar rhabdomyosarcoma—histologically it is characterized by rounds cells, which assume a pattern similar to the lung alveoli.
- Pleomorphic rhabdomyosarcoma—this variant is the more differentiated form and it exhibits primitive muscle fiber formation. The cells are having extremely pleomorphic nuclei and many prominent

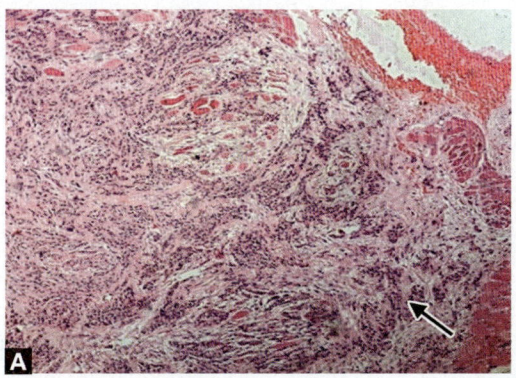
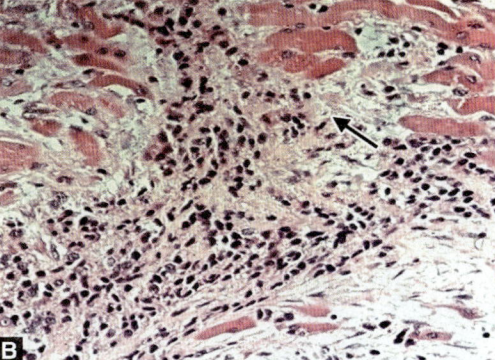

Figs. 2.153A and B: Photomicrograph of embryonal rhabdomyosarcoma: (A) Low power; (B) High power.

nucleoli. The cell cytoplasms are brightly eosinophilic and many of these cells reveal cross-striations.

Treatment

Surgery, radiotherapy and chemotherapy. All the variants have a poor prognosis.

■ NEUROGENIC SARCOMA

Definition

Neurogenic sarcomas are malignant neoplasms of perineural fibroblast or Schwann cells with a poor prognosis.

Origin

The disease can occur either from the preexisting neurofibromatosis lesions or as *de novo* lesions.

Clinical Features

- Neurogenic sarcomas mostly occur in young adults, common intraoral sites are mandible, lips and buccal mucosa, etc.
- The disease produces rapidly growing, non-compressible exophytic masses, which cause paresthesia of the lower lip and expansion of the mandible (Figs. 2.154 and 2.155).
- Lesions are often painful, indurated and nonmovable.
- Intrabony lesions often cause severe expansion and destruction of jaw with mobility of the regional teeth.

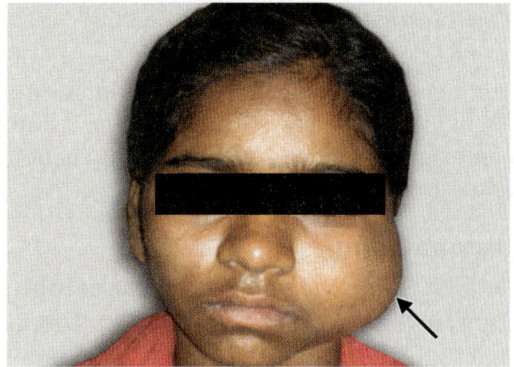

Fig. 2.154: Neurogenic sarcoma of jaw.

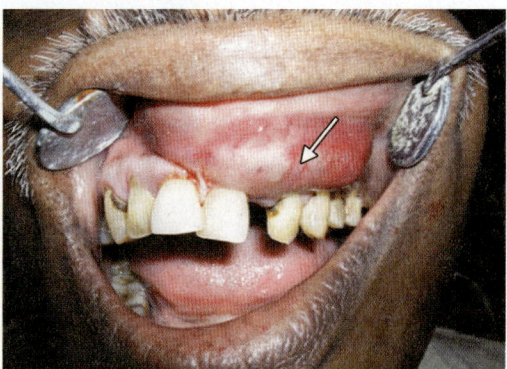

Fig. 2.155: Neurogenic sarcoma of maxilla.

- The tumor often occurs inside the mandibular canal, in association with the mandibular nerve.

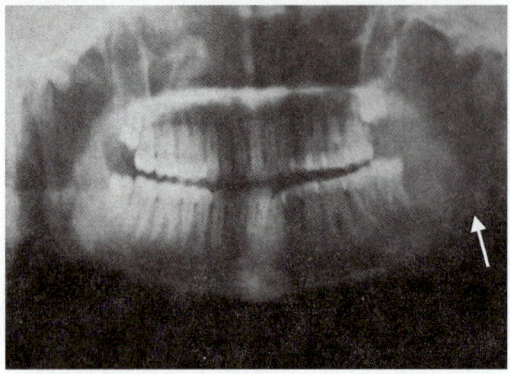

Fig. 2.156: X-ray neurogenic sarcoma of mandible.

Radiological Features (Fig. 2.156)

Radiologically, neurogenic sarcomas may produce a small area of fusiform widening of the mandibular canal. However, some lesions may even cause large area of bone destruction. Root resorption is uncommon.

Histopathology (Fig. 2.157)

- Histologically the neoplasm exhibits numerous fascicles of spindle-shaped cells with variable number of mitotic figures.
- The tumor cells often resemble to those of fibrosarcoma, however neurogenic sarcoma cells are more irregular in shape and have "comma" shaped wavy nuclei.
- The nuclei are often pleomorphic and hyperchromatic.
- The fascicles often exhibit some resemblance to the "Antoni-A" type of tissue with palisading nuclei.
- Neoplastic cells often spread along the course of the involved nerve.

Treatment

Surgical excision, radiotherapy and chemotherapy.

■ METASTATIC TUMORS OF THE JAWS

Metastatic tumors are the most common type of skeletal malignancy, easily outnumbering any form of primary bone cancer.

In adults, the majority of the skeletal metastases originate from the primary lesions of
- Prostate
- Breast
- Kidney
- Lung.

In children, the metastatic lesions predominantly arise from the
- Neuroblastoma
- Osteosarcoma
- Ewing's sarcoma
- Rhabdomyosarcoma.

Clinical Features (Fig. 2.158)

- Metastatic tumors can develop from both soft as well as hard tissues of the oral cavity, however the jawbones are particularly targeted more often than the soft tissues.

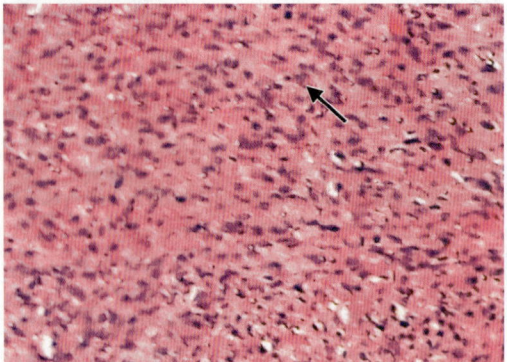

Fig. 2.157: Photomicrograph of neurogenic sarcoma.

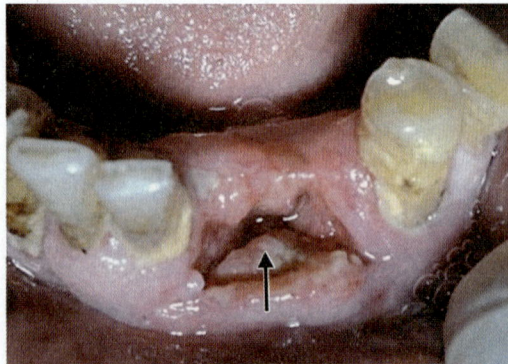

Fig. 2.158: Metastatic tumor of mandible.

- These lesions occur mostly in older individuals and more than 80% metastatic jaw tumors involve the mandible.
- Interestingly, jaw metastasis often indicates that the primary lesion has widely disseminated in the entire body.
- Sarcomas of both bone and soft tissue origin can metastasize into the jaws.
- Jaw metastasis predominantly occurs from primary tumors located in the breast, lung, prostate, thyroid and kidney, etc.
- More precisely tumors from the breast metastasize into the maxillary or mandibular bones, while the tumors from the lung often metastasize into the oral soft tissues.
- The metastatic jaw lesion mostly causes pain, swelling, expansion of the cortical plates, paresthesia or anesthesia of the region, loosing of teeth and pathological fractures of the bone, etc.
- Metastatic tumor of mandible with involvement of the inferior alveolar nerve may produce "numb chin syndrome", which is characterized by unexplained loss of sensation in the lower lip and chin.
- A metastatic lesion is often detected at the site of a recently extracted tooth, where the lesion presents either a non-healing ulcer or a nodular soft tissue mass protruding from the socket.
- Some metastatic lesions are asymptomatic and are discovered accidentally; in about 20–30% cases, these tumors are the first indication of the disease.

Radiography

- Radiographs often reveal osteolytic or sometimes osteoblastic areas in the jaw with hazy outlines.
- The bony defects may also appear either as a cyst or as a "moth-eaten" defect, severe loss of alveolar bone results in widening of the periodontal ligament space.
- Metastatic jaw tumors are sometimes discovered during thorough examination of a nonhealing extraction socket.

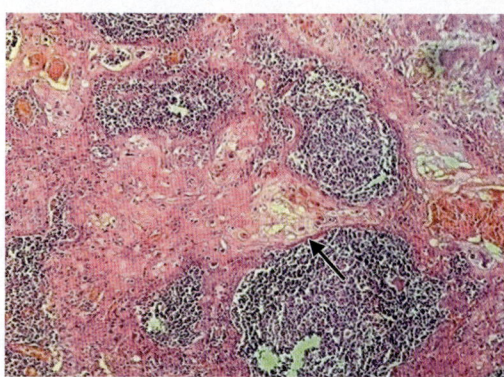

Fig. 2.159: Photomicrograph of metastatic tumor.

Histopathology (Fig. 2.159)

- Any primary carcinoma or sarcoma can metastasize in the jaws, however adenocarcinomas are the most common histologic type of tumors, which metastasize into the jawbones.
- The metastatic lesions often histologically resemble the primary lesions and these are mostly poorly differentiated in nature. Making the diagnosis of a metastatic lesion and locating its primary site of origin is a challenging job.

Investigations

- Total hemogram
- X-ray of the involved area
- Total skeletal survey
- CT scan
- MRI.

Treatment

Treatment of metastatic as well as the primary tumor (if accessible) is to be done at a time by surgery, radiotherapy or chemotherapy. These tumors often carry a grave prognosis and average survival time is less than year.

BIBLIOGRAPHY

1. Abby LM, Page DC, Sawyer DR. The clinical and histopathologic features of a series of 464 oral squamous papillomas. Oral Surg Oral Med Oral Pathol. 1980;49:419-28.

2. Adair FE, Pack GT, Farrior JH. Lipomas. Am J Can. 1932;16:1104-20.
3. Ajagbe HA, Daramola JO, Junaid TA. Chondrosarcoma of the jaw: review of 14 cases. J Oral Maxillofac Surg. 1985;43:763-6.
4. Albert S, Child M. Familial cancer in the general population. Cancer. 1977;40:1674-9.
5. Alexiou C, Kau RJ, Dietzfelbinger H, et al. Extramedullary plasmacytoma: tumor occurrence and therapeutic concepts. Cancer. 1999;85 (11):2305-14.
6. Allan CJ, Soule EH. Osteogenic sarcoma of the somatic soft tissues. Cancer. 1971;27:1121.
7. Allen CM, Kapoor N. Verruciform xanthoma in a bone marrow transplant recipient. Oral Surg Oral Med Oral Pathol. 1993;75(5):591-4.
8. Almadori G, Bussu F, Galli J, et al. Serum folate and homocysteine levels in head and neck squamous cell carcinoma. Cancer. 2002;94:1006-11.
9. Al-Nafussi AI, Azzopardi JG, Salm R. Verruciform xanthoma of the skin. Histopathology. 1985;9(2): 245-52.
10. American Cancer Society. Guidelines on diet, nutrition, and cancer prevention: reducing the risk of cancer with healthy food choices and physical activity. CA Cancer J Clin. 1996;46:325-41.
11. Anderson DL. Cause and prevention of lip cancer. J Can Dent Assoc.1971;37:138-42.
12. Angervall L, Kindblom LG, Nielsen JM, et al. Hemangiopericytoma. A clinical copathologic, angiographic and microangiographic study. Cancer. 1978;42:2412.
13. Arafat A, Ellis GO, Andian JC. Ewing's sarcoma of the jaws. Oral Surg Oral Med Oral Pathol. 1983;55:589-96.
14. Auclair PL, Cuenin P, Kratochvil FJ, et al. A clinical and histomorphologic comparison of the central giant cell granuloma and the giant cell tumor. Oral Surg Oral Med Oral Pathol. 1988;66:197-208.
15. Baker F, Ainsworth SR, Dye JT, et al. Health risks associated with cigar smoking. JAMA. 2000;284:735-40.
16. Barnard NA, Scully C, Everson JAW. Oral cancer development in patients with oral lichen planus. J Oral Pathol Med. 1993;22:421-4.
17. Basic Dental Research Unit. Early detection of oral cancer and precancerous lesions, 2nd edition. Bombay: Tata Institute of Fundamental Research;1981.
18. Batsakis JG, Regezi JA. Solomon AR, et al. The pathology of head and neck tumors: mucosal melanomas, part 13. Head Neck Surg. 1982;4:404.
19. Baumgartner JC, Stanley HR, Salomone JL. Peripheral ossifying fibroma. J Endod. 1991;17:182-5.
20. Beltran J, Simon DC, Levy M. Aneurysmal bone cysts: MR imaging at 1.5 T. Radiology. 1986;158(3):689-90.
21. Berquist TH, Ehman RL, King BF, et al. Value of MR imaging in differentiating benign from malignant soft-tissue masses: study of 95 lesions. Am J Roentgenol. 1990;155(6):1251-5.
22. Bharucha EK, Mehta MJ. Multicentric carcinoma of the oral cavity. Ind J Surg. 1976;38:421-8.
23. Bhaskar SN, Beasley JD III, Cutright DE. Inflammatory papillary hyperplasia of the oral mucosa: report of 341 cases. J Am Dent Assoc. 1970;81:949-52.
24. Bielamowicz S, Dauer MS, Chang B, et al. Noncutaneous benign fibrous histiocytoma of the head and neck. Otolaryngol Head Neck Sur. 1995;113:140-6.
25. Bill AH Jr, Summer DS. A unified concept of lymphangioma and cystic hygroma. Surg Gynecol Obstet. 1965;120:79-86.
26. Bras J, Batsakis JG, Luna MA. Malignant fibrous histiocytoma of the oral soft tissues. Oral Surg Oral Med Oral Pathol. 1987;64:57-67.
27. Brockband J. Hemangiopericytoma of the oral cavity, report of cases and review of literature. J Oral Surg. 1977;37:659-69.
28. Burkhardt A. Advanced method in the evaluation of premalignant lesions and carcinoma of the oral mucosa. J Oral Pathol. 1985;14:751-8.
29. Calle EE, Rodriquez C, Jacobs EJ, et al. The American Cancer Society cancer prevention study II nutrition cohort. Cancer. 2002;94:2490-501.
30. Calmettes C, Ponder BA, Fischer JA, et al. Early diagnosis of the multiple endocrine neoplasia type 2 syndrome: consensus statement. Eur J Clin Invest. 1992;22:755-60.
31. Campbell JA. Where does dentistry stand on radiation? J Calif Dent Assoc. 1986;14:17-20.
32. Capanna R, Allbisinni U, Picci P. Aneurysmal bone cyst of the spine. J Bone Joint Surg Am. 1985;67(4):527-31.
33. Capanna R, Van Horn JR, Baigini R. Aneurysmal bone cyst of the sacrum. Skeletal Radiol. 1989;18(2):109-13.

34. Casino AJ, Sciubba JJ, Ohri GL, et al. Oral-facial manifestations of the multiple endocrine neoplasia syndrome. Oral Surg. 1981;51:516.
35. Chainani-Wu N, Silverman S Jr, Lozada-Nur F, et al. Orallichen planus: patient profile, disease progression and treatment responses. J Am Dent Assoc. 2001;132:901-9.
36. Chambers PW, Schwinn CP. Chordoma. A clinicopathologic study of metastasis. Am J Clin Pathol. 1979;72:765-76.
37. Chan JK, Hui PK, Ng CS, et al. Epithelioid hemangioma (angiolymphoid hyperplasia with eosinophilia) and Kimura's disease in Chinese. Histopathol. 1989;15:557-4.
38. Chen S, Miller AS. Neurofibroma and Schwannoma of the oral cavity. Oral Surg Oral Med Oral Pathol. 1979;47:522-8.
39. Cheng KP. Ophthalmological manifestations of Sturge-Weber Syndrome. In: Brodensteiner JB, Roach ES (Eds). Mt. Freedom, New Jersey: Sturge-Weber Foundation; 1999. pp. 17-26.
40. Chretien PB. The effects of smoking on immunocompetence. Laryngoscope. 1978;88: 11-3.
41. Christen AG. Tobacco cessation, the dental profession, and the role of dental education. J Dent Educ. 2001;65:368-74.
42. Clark JL, Unni KK, Dahlin DC, et al. Osteosarcoma of the jaw. Cancer. 1983;51:2311-6.
43. Clausen F, Poulsen H. Metastatic carcinoma to the jaws. Acta Pathol Microbiol Scand. 1963;57:361.
44. Clemmesen J. The alleged association between artificial fluoridation of water supplies and cancer: a review. Bull World Health Organ. 1983;61:871-3.
45. Corio RL, Lewis DM. Intraoral rhabdomyomas. Oral Surg Oral Med Oral Pathol. 1979;48:525-31.
46. Dahnert W. Bone soft-tissue disorders. In: Radiology Review Manual, 2nd edition. Philadelphia: Lippincott/Williams and Wilkins; 1993. pp. 31-2.
47. Day GL, Blot WJ. Second primary tumors in patients with oral cancer. Cancer. 1992;70:14-9.
48. Dayan D, Buchner A, Spirer S. Bone formation in peripheral giant cell granuloma. J Periodontol. 1990;61(7):444-6.
49. De Santos LA, Jing BS. Ewing's sarcoma of the jaws. Br J Radiol.1978;51:682-7.
50. De Vito MA, Tom, LW, Bogan TV, et al. Desmoplastic fibroma of the mandible. Ear Nose Throat J. 1989;68:553-6.
51. Diller L. Rhabdomyosarcoma and other soft tissue sarcomas of childhood. Curr Opin Oncol. 1992;4:689-95.
52. Dimopoulos MA, Goldstein J, Fuller L, et al. Curability of solitary bone plasmacytoma. J Clin Oncol. 1992;10(4):587-90.
53. Doll R, Payne P, Waterhouse J. Cancer incidence in five countries. Berlin: Springer-Verlag; 1966.
54. Edwards BK, Howe HL, Ries LA, et al. Annual report to the nation on the status of cancer, 1973–1999, featuring implications of age and aging on U.S. cancer burden. Cancer. 2002;94:2766-92.
55. Elazy RP, Dutx W. Myxomas of the paroral-oral soft tissue. Oral Surg. 1978;45:246.
56. Elder D, Elenitsas R, Jaworsky C, et al. Lever's Histopathology of the skin, 8th edition. Philadelphia: Lippincott-Raven; 1997.
57. Ellis GL, Corio RL. Spindle cell carcinoma of the oral cavity. A clinicopathologic assessment of fifty-nine cases. Oral Surg Oral Med Oral Pathol. 1980;50:523-33.
58. Eversole LR. Central benign and malignant neural neoplasms of the jaws. J Oral Maxillofac Surg. 1969;47:60-4.
59. Faughnan ME, Hyl RH, Nanthakumar K, et al. Screening in hereditary hemorrhagic telangiectasia patients. Chest. 2000;118(2):566-7.
60. Field JK. Oncogenes and tumor-suppressor genes in squamous cell carcinoma of the head and neck. Oral Oncol. 1992;28B:67-76.
61. Fletcher C. Diagnostic histopathology of tumors. London: Churchill Livingstone; 2000.
62. Fletcher CD, McKee PH. Sarcomas—a clinicopathologic guide with particular reference to cutaneous manifestations: III: angiosarcoma. Clin Exp Dermatol. 1985;10(4):332-49.
63. Forastiere A, Koch W, Trotti A, et al. Head and neck cancer. N Engl J Med. 2001;345:1890-900.
64. Frazell EL, Lucas JC Jr. Cancer of the tongue. Report of the management of 1554 patients. Cancer. 1962;15:1085-99.
65. Fuhr AH, Krough JA. Congenital epulis of the newborn: Centennial review of the literature and a report of a case. J Oral Maxillofac Surg. 1972;30:30.
66. Gandagule VN, Agarwal S. Oral and pharyngeal cancer in Madhya Pradesh. J Ind Med Assoc. 1969;53:582-5.
67. Gardner DG. The peripheral odontogenic fibroma: an attempt at clarification. Oral Surg. 1982;54(1):40-8.

68. Geothalas PL, Harrison EJ Jr, Devine KD. Verrucous carcinoma of the oral cavity. Am J Surg. 1963;106:845-51.
69. Giansanti JS, Waldron CA. Peripheral giant cell granuloma: review of 720 cases. J Oral Maxillofac Surg. 1969;27(10):787-91.
70. Going RE, Hsu SC, Pollack RL, et al. Sugar and fluoride content of various forms of tobacco. J Am Dent Assoc. 1980;100:27-33.
71. Goldberg MH, Nemarich AN, Danielson P. Lymphangioma of the tongue: medical and surgical therapy. J Oral Surg. 1977;35:841-4.
72. Gonzalez YM, de Nardin A, Grossi SG, et al. Serum cotinine levels, smoking and periodontal attachment loss. J Dent Res. 1996;75:796-802.
73. Gordon RS. From the NIH—Human wart virus found in many papillomas. JAMA. 1980;244:2041.
74. Gorsky M, Silverman S Jr. Denture wearing and oral cancer. J Prosthet Dent. 1984;52:164-6.
75. Gorsky M, Silverman S Jr. Tobacco use in patients with head and neck carcinomas: habit changes and second primary oral/pharyngeal cancers in patients from San Francisco. Cancer J. 1994;7:78-80.
76. Granstein RD, Sober AJ. Current concepts in ultraviolet carcinogenesis. Proc Soc Exp Biol Med. 1982;170:115.
77. Greene GW Jr, Natiella JR, Spring PN. Osteoid osteoma of jaws. Oral Surgery. Oral Med Oral Pathol. 1968;26:342-51.
78. Gupta PC, Mehta FS, Pindborg JJ, et al. Intervention study for primary prevention of oral cancer among 36000 Indian tobacco users. Lancet. 1986;ii:1235-9.
79. Gupta PC, Pinborg JJ, Mehta FS. Comparison of carcinogenicity of betel quid with and without tobacco: an epidemiological review. Ecol Dis. 1982;1:213-9.
80. Harsany DL, Ross J, Fee WE Jr. Follicular lymphoid hyperplasia of the hard palate simulating lymphoma. Otolaryngol Head Neck Surg. 1980;88:349.
81. Harty LC, Caporaso NE, Hayes RB, et al. Alcohol dehydrogenase-3 genotype and risk of oral cavity and pharyngeal cancers. J Natl Cancer Inst. 1997;89:1698-705.
82. Heber D, Byerly LO, Chi J, et al. Pathophysiology of malnutrition in the adult cancer patient. Cancer. 1986;58:1867-73.
83. Herron GS, Rouse RV, Kosek JC, et al. Benign lymphangioendothelioma. J Am Acad Dermatol. 1994;31:362-8.
84. Hirayama T. An epidemiological study of oral and pharyngeal cancer in Central and South East Asia. Bull WHO. 1966;34:41-69.
85. Hoffman D, Djordjevic MV, Fan J, et al. Five leading U.S. commercial brands of moist snuff in 1994: assessment of carcinogenic N-nitrosamines. J Natl Cancer Inst. 1995;87:1862-9.
86. Houston GD. The giant cell fibroma. A review of 464 cases. Oral Surg Oral Med Oral Pathol. 1982;53:582-7.
87. International Agency for Research on Cancer. Tobacco smoking, IARC monographs on the evaluation of the carcinogenic risk of chemicals to human, no. 38. Lyon: IARC; 1986.
88. Isaacson PG. Lymphoma of mucosa associated lymphoid tissue (malt) histopathology 1990;16:617-9.
89. Jayant K. Statistical appraisal of the association of smoking and chewing habits to oral and pharyngeal cancers. Ind J Can. 1977;14:293-9.
90. Johnson NW. Histological and histochemical studies of oral cancer. Int Dent J. 1977;27:25-34.
91. Jones AS, Morar P, Phillips DE, et al. Second primary tumors in patients with head and neck squamous cell carcinoma. Cancer. 1995;75:1343-53.
92. Jones RB. Tobacco or oral health: past progress, impending challenge. J Am Dent Assoc. 2000;131:1130-45.
93. Jussawalla DJ, Jain DK. Cancer incidence in grater Bombay 1970–1972. Three yearly reports. Bombay: The Indian Cancer Society; 1976.
94. Kadin MW, Bensch KG. On the origin of Ewing's tumor. Cancer. 1971;27:257-73.
95. Keller AZ. Alcohol, tobacco and age factors in the relative frequency of cancer among males with and without liver cirrhosis. Am J Epidemiol. 1977;106:194-202.
96. Kelly DE, Harrigan WF. Leiomyoma of the tongue: report of a case. J Oral Surg. 1977;35:316-8.
97. Khanolkar VR. Oral cancer in India. Acta Unio Internationalis Contra Cancrum. 1959;15:67-77.
98. Khnna JN, Khanapurkar CR. Bilateral vascular lesion of the tongue, hemangioma and lymphangioma. J Ind Dent Assoc. 1979;51:139-41.
99. Lewin F, Norell SE, Johansson H, et al. Smoking tobacco, oral snuff, and alcohol in the etiology of squamous cell carcinoma of the head and neck. Cancer. 1998;82:1367-75.
100. Liversedge RL. Oral malignant melanoma. Br J Oral Surg. 1975;13:2777-86.

101. Lucas RB. Pathology of tumours of the oral tissues, 4th edition. Edinburgh: Churchill Livingstone; 1984.
102. Lupulescu AP. Hormones, vitamins, and growth factors in cancer treatment and prevention. Cancer. 1996;78:2264-80.
103. Mahboubi E. The epidemiology of oral cavity, pharyngeal and esophageal cancer outside of North America and Western Europe. Cancer. 1977;40:1879-86.
104. Malaowalla AM, Silverman S Jr, Mani NJ, et al. Oral cancer in 57,518 industrial workers of Gujarat, India: a prevalence and follow up study. Cancer. 1976;37:1882-6.
105. Mashberg A, Garfinkel L, Harris S. Alcohol as a primary risk factor in oral squamous cell carcinoma. Cancer J Clin. 1981;31:146-55.
106. Mashberg A. Erythroplasia: the earliest sign of asymptomatic oral cancer. J Am Dental Assoc. 1978;96:615-20.
107. McNelis FL, Pai VT. Malignant lymphoma of the head and neck. Laryngoscope. 1969;79:1076-87.
108. Mehta FS, Pindborg JJ, Gupta PC, et al. Epidemiologic and Histologic study of Oral cancer and Leukoplakia among 50915 villagers in India. Cancer. 1969;24:832-49.
109. Mehta FS. Report on investigations of oral cancer and precancerous conditions in Indian rural populations 1966-1969. Copenhagen: Munksgard; 1971.
110. Melrose RJ, Abrams AM. Juvenile fibromatosis affecting the jaws. Report of three cases. Oral Surg Oral Med Oral Pathol. 1980;49:317-24.
111. Miller EC, Miller JA. Carcinogens and mutagens that may occur in foods. Cancer. 1986;58: 1795-803.
112. Minkow B, Laufer D, Gutman D. Treatment of oral hemangiomas with local sclerosing agents. Int J Oral Surg.1979;8:18-21.
113. Mirvish SS. Effects of vitamins C and E on N-nitroso compound formation, carcinogenesis and cancer. Cancer. 1986;58:1842-50.
114. Myers JN, Elkins T, Roberts D, et al. Squamous cell carcinoma of the tongue in young adults: increasing incidence and factors that predict treatment outcomes. Otolaryngol Head Neck Surg. 2000;122:44-51.
115. Naik R, Kamath AS. Granular cell tumor: a clinicopathological study. Indian J Pathol Microbial. 1993;36:227-32.
116. National Cancer Institute. Changing adolescent smoking prevalence. Where it is and why. Smoking and tobacco control monograph no. 14. Bethesda: National Cancer Institute; 2001.
117. National Cancer Institute. Risks associated with smoking cigarettes with low machine-measured yields of tar and nicotine. Smoking and tobacco control monograph no. 13. Bethesda: National Cancer Institute; 2001.
118. O'Driscoll PM. The oral manifestations of multiple neurofibromatosis. Br J Oral Surg. 1965;3:22-31.
119. Petridou E, Zavras AI, Lefatzis D, et al. The role of diet and specific micronutrients in the etiology of oral carcinoma. Cancer. 2002;94:2981-8.
120. Pindborg JJ. Atlas of diseases of the oral mucosa, 4th edition. Copenhagen: Munksgaard; 1985.
121. Pitman KT, Johnson JT, Wagner RL, et al. Cancer of the tongue in patients less than forty. Head Neck. 2000;22:297-302.
122. Reade PC, Radden BG. Oral fibrosarcoma. Oral Surg Oral Med Oral Pathol. 1966;22:217-25.
123. Regezi J, Hayward JR, Pickens TN. Superficial melanomas of oral mucous membranes. Oral Surg Oral Med Oral Pathol. 1978;45:730-40.
124. Rigotti NA. Clinical practice. Treatment of tobacco use and dependence. N Engl J Med. 2002;346:506-12.
125. Robertson PB, Derouen TA, Ernster V, et al. Smokeless tobacco use: how it affects the performance of major league baseball players. J Am Dent Assoc. 1995;126:1115-24.
126. Sadeghi EM, Sauk JJ. Liposarcoma of the oral cavity: Clinical tissue culture, and ultra structure study of a case. J Oral Pathol. 1982;11:263-75.
127. Safai B, Johnson KG, Myskowski PL. The natural history of Kaposi's sarcoma in the acquired immunodeficiency syndrome. Ann Int Med. 1985;103:744-50.
128. Schantz SP, Yu GP. Head and neck cancer incidence trends in young Americans, 1973-1997, with a special analysis for tongue cancer. Arch Otolaryngol Head Neck Surg. 2002;128:268-74.
129. Schwartz LH, Ozahin M, Zhang GN, et al. Synchronous and metachronous head and neck carcinomas. Cancer. 1994;74:1933-8.
130. Scully C. Oncogenes, onco-suppressors, carcinogenesis and oral cancer. Br Dental J. 1992;173:53-9.
131. Scully C. Oral precancer: preventive and medical approaches to management. Oral Oncol. 1995;31B:16-26.

132. Scully C. The immunology of cancer of the head and neck with particular reference to oral cancer. Oral Surg Oral Med Oral Pathol. 1982;53:157-69.
133. Scully C. Virus and oral squamous cell carcinoma. Oral Oncol. 1992;28B:57-9.
134. Searles GE, Markman S, Yazdi HM. Primary oral Kaposi's sarcoma of the hard palate. J Am Acad Dermatol. 1990;23(Pt1): 518-9.
135. Shafer WG. Oral carcinoma in situ. Oral Surg Oral Med Oral Pathol.1975;39:227-38.
136. Shiboski CH, Shiboski SC, Silverman S Jr. Trends in oral cancer rates in the United States, 1973-1996. Community Dent Oral Epidemiol. 2000;28:249-56.
137. Shimizu S, Hasimoto H, Enjoji M. Nodular fasciitis: an analysis of 250 cases. Pathology. 1984;16:161-6.
138. Silverman S Jr, Gorsky M, Lozada-Nur F, et al. A prospective study of findings and management in 214 patients with oral lichen planus. Oral Surg Oral Med Oral Pathol. 1991;72:665-70.
139. Silverman S Jr, Thompson JS. Serum zinc and copper in oral/oropharyngeal carcinoma. A study of seventy-five patients. Oral Surg Oral Med Oral Pathol. 1984;57:34-6.
140. Silverman S Jr. Demographics and occurrence of oral and pharyngeal cancers: the outcomes, the trends, the challenge. J Am Dent Assoc. 2001;132:7S-11S.
141. Stevens RG, Jones DY, Micozzi MS, et al. Body iron stores and the risk of cancer. N Engl J Med. 1988;319:1047-52.
142. Tepperman BS, Fitzpatrick PJ. Second respiratory and upper digestive tract cancers after oral cancer. Lancet. 1981;2:547-9.
143. Thun MJ, Peto R, Lopez AD, et al. Alcohol consumption and mortality among middle-aged and elderly U.S. adults. N Engl J Med. 1997;337:1705-14.
144. Underhill TE, Kimura K, Chilvarguer I, et al. Radiobiologic risk estimation from dental radiology. Part II. Cancer incidence and fatality. Oral Surg Oral Med Oral Pathol. 1988;66:261-7.
145. Vincent SD, Fotos PG, Baker KA, et al. Oral lichen planus: the clinical, historical and therapeutic features of 100 cases. Oral Surg Oral Med Oral Pathol. 1990;70:165-71.
146. Waxman H. The future of the global tobacco treaty negotiations. N Engl J Med. 2002;346:936-8.
147. Werning JT. Nodular fasciitis of the orofacial region. Oral Surg Oral Med Oral Pathol. 1979;48:441-6.
148. White SC, Frey NW. An estimation of somatic hazards to the United States population from dental radiology. Oral Surg Oral Med Oral Pathol. 1977;43:152-9.
149. Wright BA, Wright JM, Binnie WH. Oral cancer: clinical and pathological considerations. Boca Raton: CRC Press; 1988.
150. Wynder EL, Mushinski MH, Spivak JC. Tobacco and alcohol consumption in relation to the development of multiple primary cancers. Cancer. 1977;40:1872-8.
151. Yamamoto E, Shibuya H, Yoshimura R, et al. Site specific dependency of second primary cancer in early stage head and neck squamous cell carcinoma. Cancer. 2002;94:2007-14.
152. Ziober BL, Silverman S Jr, Kramer RH. Adhesive mechanisms regulating invasion and metastasis in oral cancer. Crit Rev Oral Biol Med. 2001;12:499-510.

CHAPTER 3

Oral Precancerous Lesions and Conditions

INTRODUCTION

Oral cancers are sometimes preceded by some clinically visible lesions, which are noncancerous to begin with and have therefore been termed as "precancers". However, it is widely understood that neither do all the precancerous lesions progress to cancer, nor all cancers necessarily originate from such lesions.

According to the World Health Organization (WHO), the oral precancerous state is divided into two broad groups: (1) precancerous lesions and (2) precancerous conditions.

PRECANCEROUS LESION

A precancerous lesion is defined as "a morphologically altered tissue in which cancer is more likely to occur than in its apparently normal counterpart"—WHO 1978.

Leukoplakia, erythroplakia, stomatitis nicotina, chronic candidiasis, etc. are the common examples of precancerous lesions found in the oral cavity.

PRECANCEROUS CONDITION

A precancerous condition is defined as "the generalized state of the body, which is associated with a significantly increased risk of cancer"—WHO 1978.

Oral submucous fibrosis (OSF), sideropenic dysphagia (mucosal atrophy with chronic iron deficiency anemia), syphilis, oral lichen planus, etc. fall into this category.

[WHO in 2005 proposed a new concept of *Potentially Malignant Disorders* (PMDs) which

---

Box 3.1   Precancerous lesions and conditions.

Precancerous lesions:
- Erythroplakia
- Stomatitis nicotina
- Chronic candidiasis
- Leukoplakia

Precancerous conditions:
- Syphilis
- Oral lichen planus
- Oral submucous fibrosis
- Sideropenic dysphagia

---

was defined as *the risk of malignancy being present in a lesion or condition either at time of initial diagnosis or at a future date*].

Examples of precancerous lesions and conditions have been shown in Box 3.1.

It is important to note that all these precancerous lesions and conditions mentioned earlier, produce a wide variety of clinical and histopathological features, but the most important criteria for evaluating their malignant potential is the microscopic study of "epithelial dysplasia". It has been reported by a large number of investigators that the "dysplastic" lesions carry a risk of malignant transformation, which is nearly 15 times higher than the nondysplastic lesions.

LEUKOPLAKIA

Definition

Leukoplakia can be defined as a "white patch" or "plaque" in the oral cavity, which cannot be scraped off or stripped off easily and moreover, which cannot be characterized clinically or pathologically as any other disease"—WHO 1978.

This definition was revised 5 years later at the International Conference and the new definition states that "leukoplakia is a white patch or plaque in the oral cavity, which cannot be scraped off or stripped off easily and which cannot be characterized clinically or pathologically as any other disease and it is not associated with any physical or chemical agents except the use of tobacco".

Recent definition of leukoplakia: Oral leukoplakia has recently been redefined as "a predominantly white lesion of the oral mucosa that cannot be characterized as any other definable lesion; some oral leukoplakia will transform into cancer" (Axell T 1996).

Preleukoplakia

Preleukoplakia is defined as a low grade or very mild reaction of the oral mucosa, appearing as a gray or grayish-white, but never completely white area with a slightly lobular pattern and with indistinct borders blending into the adjacent normal mucosa (Fig. 3.1) (Pindborg et al. 1968).

Etiology of Leukoplakia

The exact etiology of leukoplakia is unknown but a large number of factors have been implicated for their occurrence, which are known as the "predisposing" factors. The common predisposing factors for leukoplakia are tobacco, alcohol, candidiasis, dietary deficiency, syphilis, viral infections, hormonal imbalance, chronic irritation, galvanism, and actinic radiation, etc.

Among these, tobacco is considered to be the single most important factor (Box 3.2).

Box 3.2	Etiological factors of leukoplakia.
• Tobacco (in smoking and smokeless forms)
• Alcohol
• Candidiasis
• Dietary deficiency
• Syphilis
• Viral infections
• Hormonal imbalance
• Chronic irritation
• Actinic radiation
• Galvanism

Tobacco

- It is used by large number of people in various forms, such as smoking and chewing:
  - *Smoking form of tobacco*—of cigarettes, cigars, pipe, and bidis (country made cigarettes).
  - *Chewing form of tobacco*—tobacco chewing (e.g. Gutkha and Jarda, etc.), "Pan" chewing (a mixture of betel leaf, lime, betel-nuts, and tobacco), snuff dipping, etc.
- It has been confirmed that the people those who use tobacco in any form, develop leukoplakia more often than the people those who do not use them.
- Furthermore, the leukoplakic lesions regress significantly more often when the tobacco habits are discontinued.
- It is believed that during smoking a significantly large amount of tobacco end products are produced in the oral cavity, these products in association with the heat, (generated during smoking) cause severe irritation to the oral mucous membrane

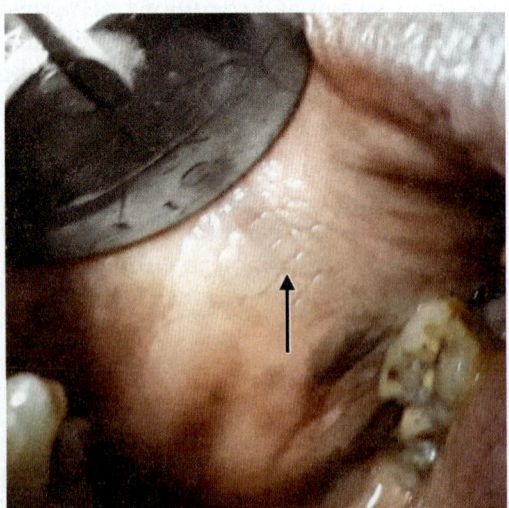

Fig. 3.1: Preleukoplakia of the buccal mucosa.

> **Box 3.3** Classification of oral mucosal lesions on different types of tobacco habits.
>
> *Predominantly associated with smoking*:
> - Leukoedema
> - Leukokeratosis nicotina palati
> - Palatal erythema
> - Central papillary atrophy of tongue
>
> *Predominantly associated with chewing*:
> - Pan chewers lesion
> - Oral lichen planus-like lesion
> - Oral submucous fibrosis
>
> *Associated with smoking and chewing (mixed habit)*:
> - Leukoplakia and preleukoplakia
> - Oral lichen planus
> - Oral squamous carcinomas

and finally results in the development of leukoplakia.
- An important observation in this regard is the higher rate of occurrence of leukoplakia among the "*reserve smokers*" (those who keep the burning end of the cigarettes inside the mouth).
- Finally, it is important to note that the risk of development of leukoplakia in a person depends upon the frequency and duration of the tobacco habits, and the age and sex of the person concerned (Box 3.3 and Fig. 3.2).

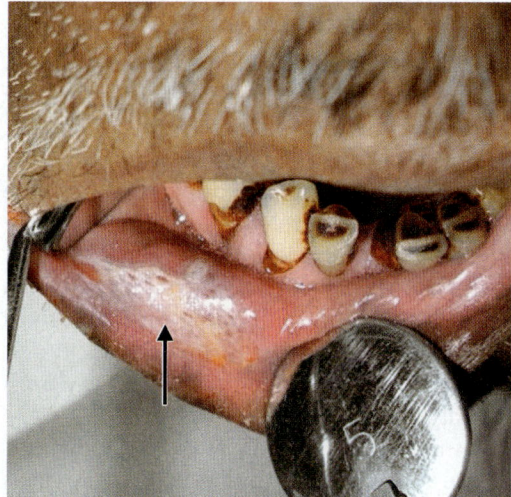

Fig. 3.2: Leukoplakia in "khaini" chewing.

Alcohol

Alcohol itself is not an important risk factor for leukoplakia but many people may develop leukoplakia who consume alcohol as well as use tobacco in some form. Therefore, it is believed that the synergistic effect of tobacco and alcohol, both, increase the risk of leukoplakia more often than in cases where a single habit is practiced.

Candidiasis

Chronic candidal infections are often associated with leukoplakia; however, it is not very clear whether the fungi are directly responsible for the initiation of the disease or they are only producing secondary infections in a pre-existing leukoplakia. However, it has been observed that the *Candida*-associated leukoplakias develop more epithelial dysplasia than the noncandidal lesions.

Dietary Deficiency

Deficiency of vitamin A causes metaplasia and hyperkeratinization of the epithelium, which may eventually result in the development of leukoplakia. Deficiency of vitamin B complexes may also cause leukoplakic changes in the oral mucosa, but the exact pathogenesis is not clear.

Syphilis

In the older literatures, syphilis was considered to be a very important predisposing factor for the development of leukoplakia, especially the tertiary stage of the disease, which presents mucous patches over the tongue and buccal mucosa.

Viral Infections

Experimental studies indicate that, oral mucosal infections caused by the herpes virus hominis type I [herpes simplex virus (HSV)–I] and human papilloma virus (HPV) may have some role in the development of leukoplakia.

Hormonal Imbalance

Imbalance or dysfunctions of both male and female sex hormones may induce some

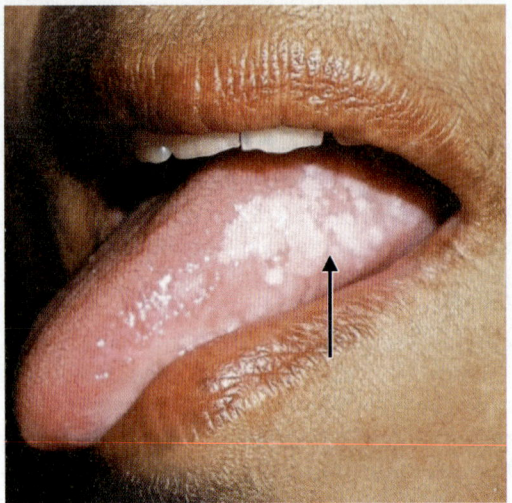

Fig. 3.3: Leukoplakia of tongue due to chronic irritation.

keratogenic changes in the oral epithelium and these changes may ultimately lead to the development of leukoplakia.

Chronic Irritation
Chronic irritation to the mucosa by ill-fitting dentures, sharp cuspal edges of teeth, hot or spicy foods, etc. may cause leukoplakia (Fig. 3.3).

Actinic Radiation
Actinic or solar radiation may bring about some hyperkeratotic changes in the oral mucosa, especially the lip mucosa and this can be a predisposing factor for leukoplakia in rare cases.

Galvanism
Galvanic reactions may occur in the oral cavity when there is difference in the electrical potential between two dissimilar metallic restorations. These reactions often lead to the development of leukoplakia in the oral mucosa.

Clinical Features of Leukoplakia
- *Age*: Usually, the lesion occurs in the fourth, fifth, sixth, and seventh decade of life. Only about 5% lesions occur below the age of 30 years.
- *Sex*: Leukoplakia occurs more often in males than females. However, this trend is changing very fast due to the gradual increase in the tobacco-related habits among females, with subsequent increase in the incidence of leukoplakia among them.
- *Site*: Buccal mucosa and commissural areas are the most frequently affected sites (*See* Fig. 3.2), followed by alveolar ridge, tongue, lips, hard and soft palate, floor of the mouth, gingiva, etc. Multiple areas of involvement may be seen in few cases.

Clinical Presentation
- Oral leukoplakias often present solitary or multiple "white patches". They can be nonpalpable, faintly translucent, white areas over the mucosa.
- Many lesions can be thick, fissured, indurated or papillomatous in nature.
- The size of the lesion may vary from a small, well-localized patch measuring about few millimeter in diameter to a diffuse large lesion, covering a wide mucosal surface.
- The surface of the lesion may be smooth or finely wrinkled or even rough on palpation, and the lesion cannot be removed by scraping.
- The lesions are usually white or grayish or yellowish-white in color and in some cases, due to the heavy use of tobacco, they may take a brownish-yellow color.
- Some lesions may exhibit a pumice-like surface, which occurs due to the presence of multiple discrete keratotic striae on the surface of these lesions.
- Leukoplakia of the floor of the mouth sometimes has an ebbing-tide pattern of appearance.
- The thickness of the patch may vary from only faint to considerably thick.
- In most of the cases, leukoplakia lesions are asymptomatic; however, in some cases they may cause pain, a feeling of thickness, burning sensations, etc.

Clinical Classification of Leukoplakia (Box 3.4)

Homogenous Leukoplakia

It clinically presents extensive white patch having uniformly smooth, flat or corrugated surface with an irregular margin. These lesions usually maintain a relatively consistent pattern throughout the clinical course (Figs. 3.4 and 3.5).
- These lesions are mostly associated with the oral use of snuff.
- They can be either nonelevated or slightly elevated and the margin is not well-demarcated from the surrounding normal epithelium.

Nonhomogenous Leukoplakia

It is defined as predominantly white or white-red lesion that may be irregularly flat, nodular or exophytic. The term nonhomogenous is applicable to the aspect of both color (a mixed white and red lesion) and texture (exophytic, papillary or verrucous) of the lesion.

Homogenous Ulcerative Leukoplakia

It clinically exhibits either predominantly white or mixed red and white lesions, in which there is a central ulceration (Fig. 3.6).

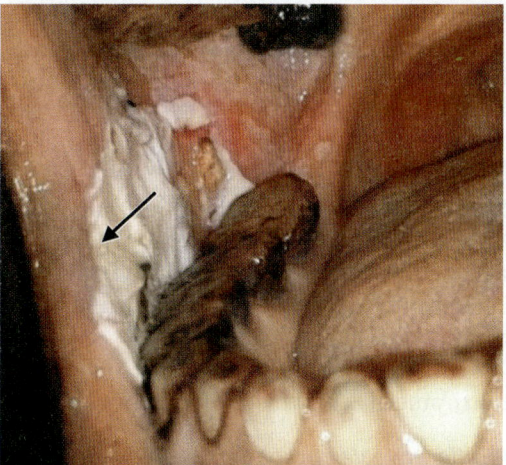

Fig. 3.4: Homogenous leukoplakia-I.

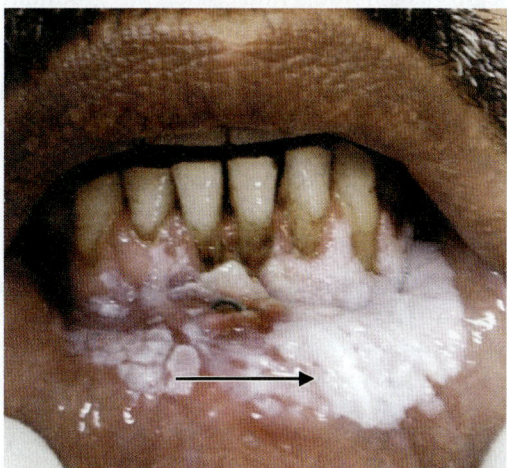

Fig. 3.5: Homogenous leukoplakia-III.

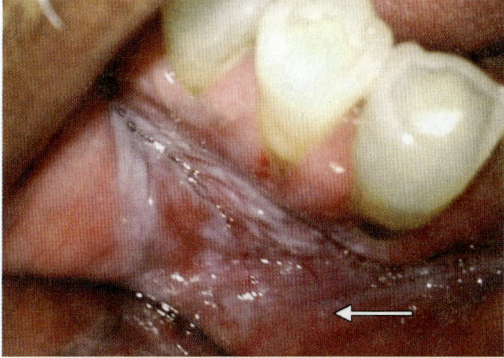

Fig. 3.6: Homogenous ulcerative leukoplakia of vestibule.

Box 3.4 Classification of leukoplakia.

Clinical Classification of Leukoplakia (WHO 1980):
- Homogenous leukoplakia: Lesions which are uniformly white
- Nonhomogenous leukoplakia: Lesions in which part of the lesion is white and rest of the area is red.

Alternate clinical classification of leukoplakia with subdivisions:
- Homogenous leukoplakia: (A) Smooth, (B) Furrowed (Fissured), and (C) Ulcerated
- Nonhomogenous: Nodulospeckled.

Final shape of the above classification with inclusion of three different subdivisions:
1. Homogenous: Smooth and fissured
2. Homogenous: Ulcerated
3. Nonhomogenous: Nodulospeckled.

Adapted from Community Dentistry and Oral Epidemiology. 1980;8:1-26.

- The ulcerated center of the lesion appears red and it may have a yellowish fibrin coating.
- White patches are seen at the periphery of these lesions.

Nodulospeckled Leukoplakia

It clinically presents mixed red and white lesions; the mucosa is entirely red within which multiple small, slightly raised, rounded, keratotic nodules or granules are seen scattered throughout (Fig. 3.7).

This variety of leukoplakia often carries the maximum risk of malignant transformation.

Proliferative Verrucous Leukoplakia

It is a special type of leukoplakia, which begins as a homogenous patch but gradually turns to an exophytic, diffuse or multifocal, progressive and irreversible lesion. Recognized as a particularly aggressive form of oral idiopathic leukoplakia that has a considerable morbidity and a strong potential for malignant transformation.

Verrucous Hyperplasia

This is a forerunner of verrucous carcinoma and the transition is so consistent that the hyperplasia, once diagnosed, should be treated like verrucous carcinoma.

Proliferative verrucous leukoplakia and verrucous hyperplasia (VH) are two related oral mucosal lesions. The terms, however, are not clinically or pathologically interchangeable. The term PVL is preferably a clinical one, but the diagnosis of VH, on the other hand, must be made histologically.

Histopathology

Under microscope leukoplakia generally presents hyperorthokeratinization or hyperparakeratinization or both, with or without the presence of epithelial dysplasia (Figs. 3.8 and 3.9).

- Keratinization pattern
- Thickness of the epithelium
- Changes in the cellular layers

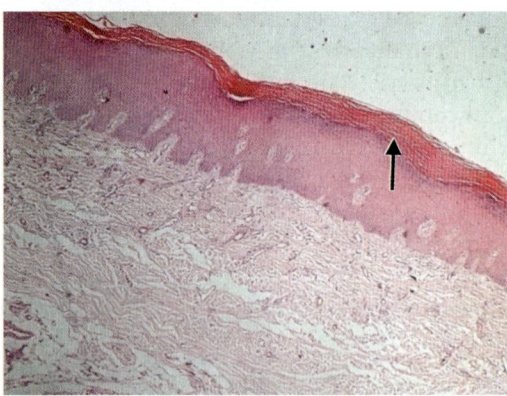

Fig. 3.8: Hyperorthokeratinized epithelium with no nuclear remnant in keratin.

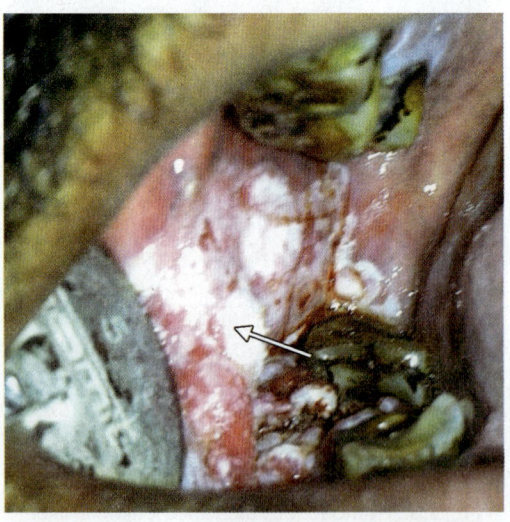

Fig. 3.7: Nodulospeckled leukoplakia of the cheek.

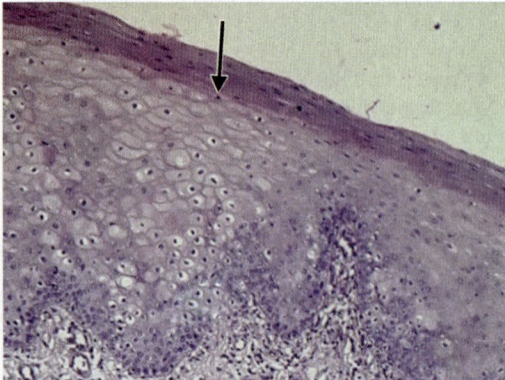

Fig. 3.9: Hyperparakeratinized epithelium showing "pyknotic nuclei" with keratin.

- Alterations in the underlying connective tissue stroma.

Histopathology of Leukoplakia in Detail

Changes in the Keratinization Pattern

Keratin is a strong natural fibrous protein that is present on the surface of skin and epithelium for protection (*it is also the main structural constituent of hair, feathers, claws, and horns of animals*). Cells which are capable of producing keratin are called the "*keratinocytes*"; keratin is of two types—*orthokeratin and parakeratin*.

Orthokeratin: It is the pure form of homogenous keratin, which does not contain any nuclear remnants (pyknotic nuclei) in its structure.

Parakeratin: It is the other type of keratin, in which nuclear remnants or pyknotic nuclei are present.

(In normal keratinized epithelium, an optimum thickness of keratin is present on the surface but in nonkeratinized mucosa there is no keratin present on the surface).

Hyperkeratinization: It represents a dual condition:
- An abnormal increase in the thickness of keratin layer in an epithelium that is normally keratinized (it can be either orthokeratin or parakeratin or both).
- Formation of keratin in an epithelium, which is normally nonkeratinized.

Hyperorthokeratinization: Refers to an abnormal increase in the thickness of orthokeratin layer in a keratinized epithelium or some degree of orthokeratinization in a nonkeratinized epithelium.

Hyperparakeratinization: It is an abnormal condition characterized by an abnormal increase in the thickness of parakeratin layer in a keratinized epithelium or some degree of parakeratinization in a nonkeratinized epithelium. Epithelial dysplasia is more frequently associated with hyperparakeratinized lesions.

(In some leukoplakias both hyperorthokeratinization and hyperparakeratinization may be seen).

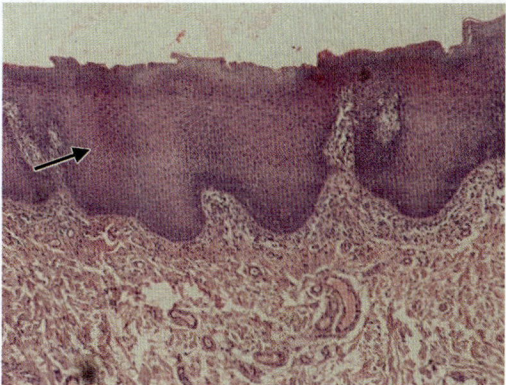

Fig. 3.10: Epithelial hyperplasia with cellular atypia.

Changes in the Thickness of Epithelium

In leukoplakia the thickness of the epithelium is often altered and it occurs in the form of epithelial atrophy or epithelial hyperplasia or acanthosis, etc.

Hyperplasia: An increase in the thickness of any tissue due to increase in the number of cells; in leukoplakia it is seen mostly in the spinous cell layer (acanthosis) and in basal and parabasal layer (basal cell hyperplasia) (Fig. 3.10).

Acanthosis: An abnormal increase in the thickness of stratum spinosum of the epithelium is called acanthosis. In leukoplakia, acanthosis often causes elongation, thickening, and blunting of the rete pegs.

Changes in the Cellular Layer

In any precancer and particularly in leukoplakia a variety of *architectural and cytological changes* take place which are collectively called "*epithelial dysplasia*". The only cytological changes are referred to as "*cellular atypia*".

Dysplasia (dys-abnormal, plasia-formation): Dysplasia refers to the spectrum changes in the epithelial tissue, which combines both architectural disturbance as well as cytological atypia. The term "squamous intraepithelial neoplasia" (SIN) is used synonymously with dysplasia. Epithelial dysplasia is the hallmark in the histological changes in leukoplakia and

> **Box 3.5** Features of epithelial dysplasia.
>
> ***Cytological changes of dysplasia (atypia) in the epithelium:***
> - Anisonucleosis—variation in the size of nuclei in different cells
> - Anisocytosis abnormal variation in individual cell size
> - Cellular pleomorphism—abnormal variation in cell shape
> - Nuclear pleomorphism (altered size and shape of cell nuclei)
> - Nuclear hyperchromatism (deeply stained nuclei, which are abnormally large for the size of the cell)
> - Increased nuclear–cytoplasmic ratio (from 1:4 to 1:1, at the expense of the cytoplasmic volume)
> - Atypical mitotic figures (mitosis is not only more abundant but it can be seen in unusual locations within the epithelium rather than the usual basal layer)
> - Increased number and size of nucleoli
> - Poikilocarynosis (division of nucleus without division of cytoplasm)
>
> ***Architectural changes of dysplasia in the epithelium:***
> - Irregular epithelial stratification (cells are disorderly arranged with loss of usual order of organization of cell layers in epithelium)
> - Loss of polarity of basal cells (basal cells could unusually be found in any suprabasal layers)
> - More than one layer of cells having basaloid appearance
> - Drop-shaped rete pegs with basal cell hyperplasia
> - Individual cell keratinization or dyskeratosis (premature keratinization of single cells)
> - Keratin pearls within the rete pegs
> - Increased number of mitotic figures (accelerated pace of cell division)
> - Presence of mitotic activity even in the superficial half of the epithelium
> - Dyskeratosis (abnormal expression of keratin production)
> - Diminished intercellular adherence

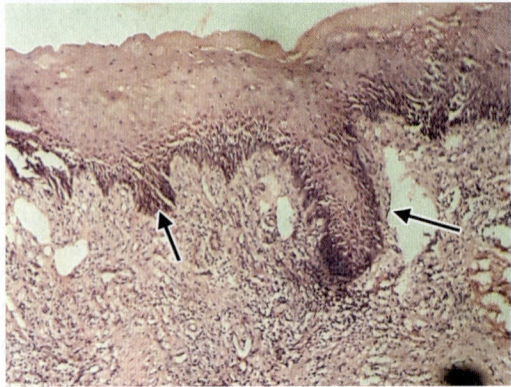

Fig. 3.11: Photomicrograph of severe dysplasia with "drop-shaped" rete pegs and basilar hyperplasia.

other PMDs and its presence is an important indicator of the precancerous nature of the disease (Box 3.5 and Fig. 3.11).

Some of the important features of epithelial dysplasia:

- Increased nuclear–cytoplasmic ratio (size of nucleus increases but size of cytoplasm remains unchanged; so the cytoplasmic space is gradually filled by the enlarging nucleus; in normal epithelial cells the ratio is 1:4 and in dysplastic cells the ratio changes to 1:1).
- Loss of polarity of basal cells: Basal cells can be found above their normal position in the more superficial parts of the epithelium.
- Increased number of mitotic figures (few abnormal mitosis may also be present)
- Presence of mitotic activity even in the superficial half of the epithelium (normally, it is seen in the basal layer)
- *Individual cell keratinization:* Cell loses its nucleus and the cytoplasm is filled with keratin.
- Dyskeratosis (abnormal expression of keratin production in the superficial as well as in the deep layers of epithelium).

Histological classification of dysplasia and related changes (WHO-2005) (Fig. 3.12):
- Squamous cell hyperplasia
- Mild dysplasia
- Moderate dysplasia
- Severe dysplasia
- Carcinoma in situ.

Grades of epithelial dysplasia: Depending upon the degree and the extent to which the dysplastic changes have developed in a lesion of leukoplakia, epithelial dysplasias may be divided into three categories, namely—

1. *Mild epithelial dysplasia:* Architectural disturbances are limited to the lower third of the epithelium accompanied by the cytological criteria (Figs. 3.13A and B).
2. *Moderate epithelial dysplasia:* Architectural disturbances extending into the middle third of the epithelium, accompanied by increased cellular atypia (Figs. 3.14A and B).
3. *Severe epithelial dysplasia:* It may have two variants (Figs. 3.15A and B)—
    i. Architectural disturbances are greater than two-thirds of the epithelium with associated cellular atypia.
    ii. Architectural disturbances are in the middle third of the epithelium but the degree of cellular atypia is much higher than what is seen in moderate dysplasia.

Although malignant transformation can occur in both dysplastic as well as nondysplastic lesions, however more severe dysplasia in a lesion means it is associated with a greater

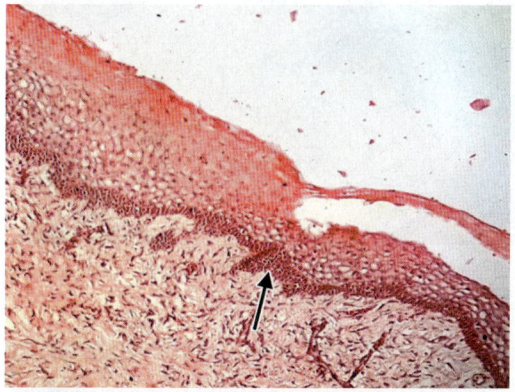

Fig. 3.12: Basilar hyperplasia of the epithelium.

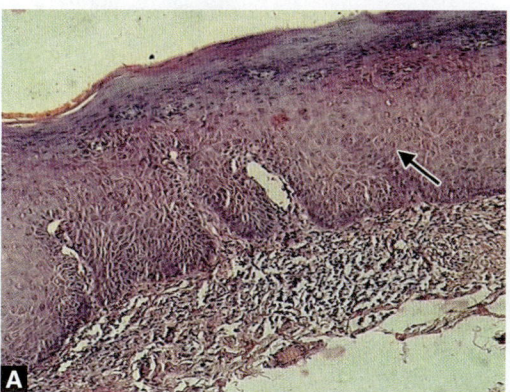
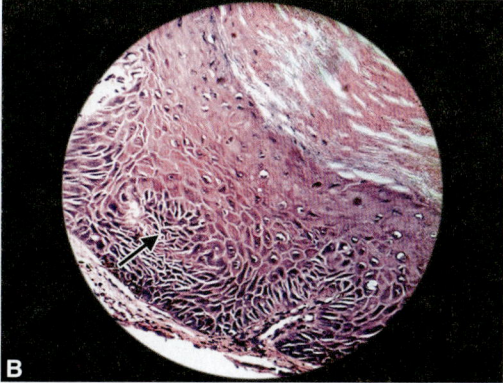

Figs. 3.13A and B: Photomicrograph showing mild epithelial dysplasia.

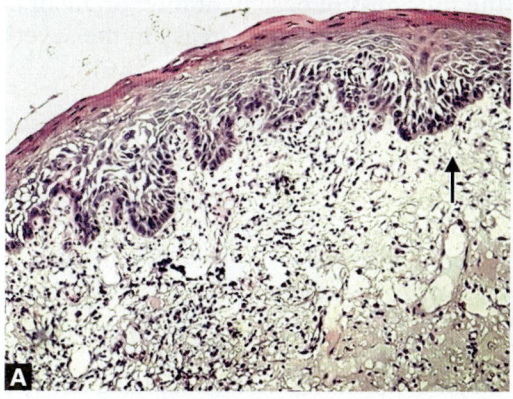
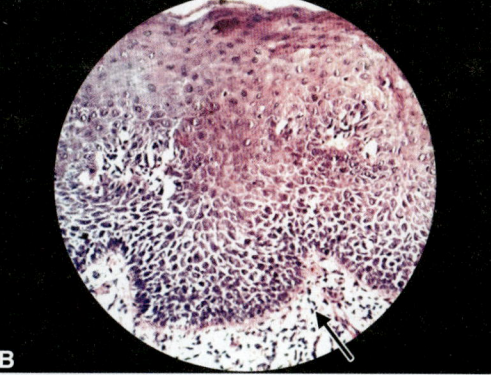

Figs. 3.14A and B: Photomicrograph showing moderate epithelial dysplasia.

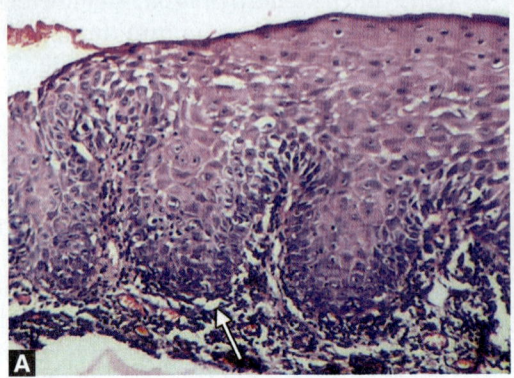 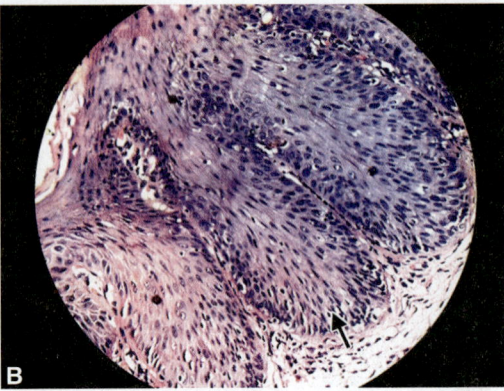

Figs. 3.15A and B: (A) Photomicrograph showing severe epithelial dysplasia with drop-shaped rete pegs; (B) Photomicrograph showing drop-shaped rete pegs.

likelihood of progression to malignancy. Similarly mild dysplasia in a lesion means it carries a relatively lesser chance of undergoing malignant transformation.

Carcinoma in situ: It refers to the condition, in which malignant transformation has occurred in the epithelium but invasion is not present.

However the dysplastic changes in a lesion are reversible and the degrees of epithelial dysplasia in a lesion may change with time. If the predisposing factors are removed, the dysplastic lesions can turn back toward normal (Box 3.6).

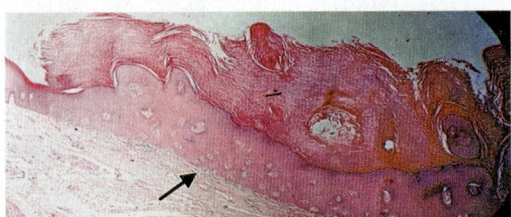

Fig. 3.16: Photomicrograph of proliferative verrucous leukoplakia.

Candidal hyphae: Histologic sections of leukoplakia often reveal the presence of candidal hyphae in the epithelium. The Candida-associated leukoplakias may have an increased tendency for malignant transformation.

Reduction in thickness of basement membrane: In leukoplakia, there is a gradual reduction in the thickness of basement membrane of the epithelium, with the increase in the severity of the epithelial dysplasia (Fig. 3.16).

Changes in the Underlying Connective Tissue

Chronic inflammatory cell infiltration: In leukoplakia, there are often variable degrees of destruction of the collagen fibers and moreover chronic inflammatory cell infiltration is also present in the underlying connective tissue stroma.

Staging System for Oral Leukoplakia

Staging system for oral leukoplakia has been shown in Boxes 3.7 and 3.8.

Box 3.6 | Factors determining the degree of epithelial dysplasia in leukoplakia.

- Age and sex of the individual having precancerous lesion in the mouth
- Frequency and duration of oral habits
- Types of oral habits (tobacco, alcohol, and snuff)
- Types of tobacco used and mode of consumption (smoking, chewing or others)
- Any synergism (combination) of multiple habits or not
- Location of the lesion in the oral cavity (lips, tongue, and floor of the mouth)
- Presence or absence of secondary infections (candidiasis, syphilis, human papillomavirus or herpes simplex virus)
- Systemic health of the individual (hormonal factors or nutritional status)

Oral Precancerous Lesions and Conditions

Box 3.7 A modified classification and staging system for oral leukoplakia—by Van der Waal et al. 2000 (on the basis of size of the leukoplakia lesion and presence or absence of epithelial dysplasia).

L—size of leukoplakia:
- L1: Size of leukoplakia is <2 cm
- L2: Size of leukoplakia is 2–4 cm
- L3: Size of leukoplakia is >4 cm
- Lx: Size of leukoplakia is not specified.

P—pathology of the lesion:
- P0: No epithelial dysplasia
- P1: Distinct epithelial dysplasia
- Px: Dysplasia not specified in pathology report

Box 3.8 Oral leukoplakia staging system of leukoplakia.

- Stage I: L1 P0
- Stage II: L2 P0
- Stage III: L3 P0 or L1 L2 P1
- Stage IV: L3 P1

Special Investigations in Leukoplakia

In leukoplakia, the presence of epithelial dysplasia and the malignant transformation potential of the lesion cannot always be assessed properly with the help of simple histopathology alone. In such cases, special investigative techniques should be employed which are as follows:
- Histochemistry
- Enzyme histochemistry
- Immunohistochemistry
- Exfoliative cytology
- Cell proliferation study
- Stereological techniques
- DNA histograms
- In vitro testing of living tissue.

Differential Diagnosis of Leukoplakia

- Lichen planus
- Candidiasis
- Frictional keratosis
- Verrucous carcinoma
- White sponge nevus
- Chemical burns
- Discoid lupus erythematosus
- Leukoedema
- Syphilitic patches.

Key Points of Leukoplakia

- Leukoplakia is a common precancerous lesion of the oral cavity.
- It appears as a "white patch" or "plaque" in the oral mucosa, which cannot be scraped off or stripped off easily and more over, which cannot be characterized clinically or pathologically as any other disease.
- Clinically, it presents well-defined solitary or multiple "white patches". They can be nonpalpable, faintly translucent, white areas over the mucosa.
- The surface of the lesion may be smooth or finely wrinkled or even rough.
- The lesions are usually white or grayish or yellowish-white in color.
- Clinically, leukoplakias are divided into three types—(1) homogenous leukoplakia, (2) ulcerative leukoplakia, and (3) nodular or speckled leukoplakia.
- Under microscope, leukoplakia generally presents hyperorthokeratinization or hyperparakeratinization or both, with or without the presence of epithelial dysplasia.
- The epithelial dysplasia may be of mild, moderate, and severe types.
- The overall malignant transformation rate of leukoplakia is about 3–6%.
- Treatment includes surgical excision of the lesion or cryosurgery along with stoppage of all oral habits.

Malignant Transformation in Leukoplakia

According to WHO, the overall malignant transformation rate of leukoplakia is about 3–6% and such transformations in leukoplakia leads to squamous cell carcinoma.

Criteria for Malignant Transformations in Leukoplakia

The malignant potentiality of a leukoplakia lesion also depends upon several factors like the age and sex of the patient, type and duration of habits, frequency of habit, site of the lesion, clinical type of leukoplakia, degree of dysplasia in the lesion, promptness in carrying out treatment, etc.

Individual Criteria

- *Clinical type of leukoplakia:* The speckled or nodular leukoplakias show the highest rate of malignant transformation, while the homogenous leukoplakias have the

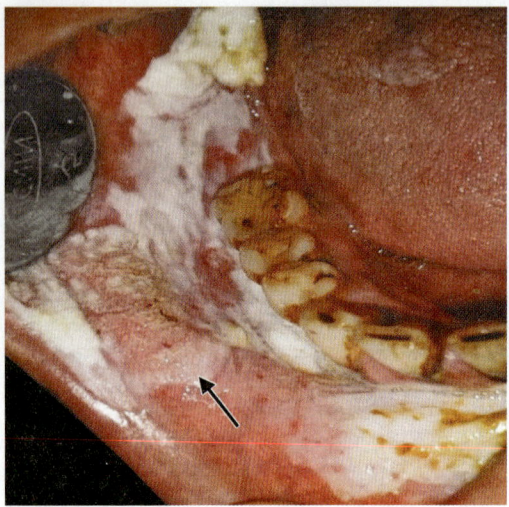

Fig. 3.17: Leukoplakia turning into squamous cell carcinoma.

least chance undergoing of malignant transformation (Fig. 3.17).
- *Degree of epithelial dysplasia:* Moreover, leukoplakias with severe or moderate dysplasia have more risk of malignant transformation as compared to mildly dysplastic or nondysplastic lesions.
- *Age of the patient:* Risk of malignant transformation increases with older age.
- *Gender or sex:* Women have higher risks of malignant transformation from leukoplakia than men.
- *Site of the lesion:* Leukoplakias of floor of the mouth and ventral surface of tongue carry the highest risk.
- *Promptness of treatment:* Untreated lesions of longer durations have more risk.

Treatment of Leukoplakia

Treatment includes stoppage of all oral habits, surgical excision of the lesion, cryosurgery, CO_2 laser surgery, and administration of heavy doses of vitamin A and antioxidants.

Antioxidants

These are chemical agents, which prevent oxidative biomembrane damage (free radical injury) of cells and tissues. Free radical injury is among the important causes of cancer.

■ TOBACCO POUCH KERATOSIS

Highly keratinized lesions develop on the oral mucosa in people with the habit of keeping tobacco in the mouth for long durations. It develops mostly in heavily addicted "Khaini" or "pan" chewers and the lesion often consists of thick brownish black encrustation in the buccal or labial mucosa at the site of placement of the tobacco quid. It could be scraped off with a piece of gauze (Fig. 3.18).

The lesions cause diffuse or focal whitening of the oral mucosa or there may be "slate-blue" or gray pigmentation.

Histologically the epithelium may be hyperplastic or atrophic and it exhibits pale staining parakeratin-like surface layers of epithelium, containing round nuclear remnants, ballooning and vacuolated cells, and epithelial hyperplasia. There is no dysplasia as such in most cases but these lesions do have premalignant potential (Fig. 3.19).

■ ORAL HAIRY LEUKOPLAKIA

Definition

Oral hairy leukoplakia is a human immunodeficiency virus (HIV)–associated mucosal disorder and is considered as a reliable marker for the presence of HIV virus in the body and

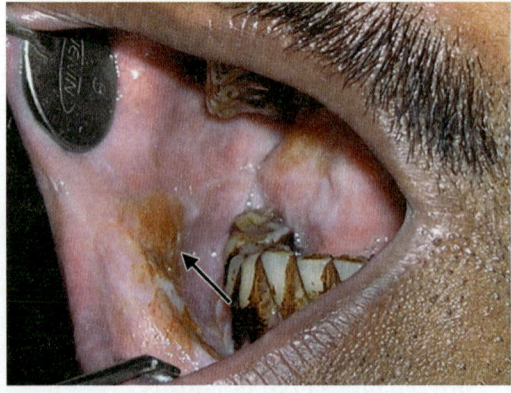

Fig. 3.18: Tobacco pouch keratosis of buccal vestibule.

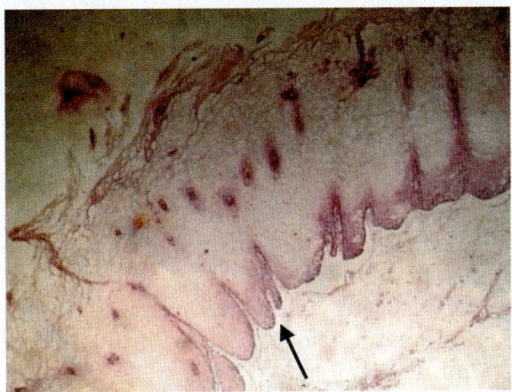

Fig. 3.19: Tobacco pouch keratosis histology: Low power.

is also a precursor of full blown acquired immunodeficiency syndrome (AIDS).

It is most commonly seen in homosexual men with HIV infection. The condition probably occurs due to opportunistic infections by the Epstein–Barr virus in immunosuppressed individuals.

Clinical Features

- Clinically, oral hairy leukoplakias occur as white patchy lesions, which are most frequently seen on the lateral borders and adjacent ventral surfaces of the tongue. However, it can also occur on the floor of the mouth, buccal or labial mucosa and palate, etc.
- The lesions often appear as painless, slightly raised, white plaques with vertically corrugated, irregular surface.
- There is often presence of numerous linear vertical folds or projections on the surface of the lesion and sometimes these projections are so marked that they may resemble "hairs" (hence, the name hairy leukoplakia has been coined).
- There is no evidence of malignant transformation in this form of leukoplakia.

Histopathology

- Microscopy reveals acanthosis and hyperparakeratosis of the epithelium with verruciform, hair-like surface projections. The parakeratin layer is often colonized by candidal organisms.
- Immediately below the parakeratotic layer there is a zone of vacuolated and enlarged keratinocytes, which exhibit intensely basophilic and pyknotic nuclei with perinuclear clearing. These cells are called "koilocytes" or "balloon cells".
- No dysplastic changes are seen in oral hairy leukoplakia and neither there is evidence of any malignant transformation.

Differential Diagnosis

- Chronic candidiasis
- Lichen planus
- White sponge nevus
- Geographic tongue
- Verrucous leukoplakia
- Chronic tongue biting habits.

Special Investigation

The particles of Epstein–Barr virus or the viral antigens can be demonstrated in the koilocyte cell nuclei with the help of immunohistochemistry.

Treatment

No treatment is separately required for hairy leukoplakia; it may resolve spontaneously or subsides following antiviral drug therapy with acyclovir.

■ LEUKOEDEMA

Definition

Leukoedema is an alteration of the oral epithelium characterized by intracellular accumulation of fluid (edema) within the spinous cell layer.

Etiology

The etiology of leukoedema is not known. According to many investigators, the condition is a variation of normal epithelium rather than a disease.

Clinical Features

- Leukoedema more commonly occurs among black population; age of occurrence is about 45 years.

- The oral mucosa exhibits an asymptomatic, diffuse, translucent, grayish-white area with a filmy appearance.
- It is commonly seen on the buccal mucosa (often bilaterally) near the occlusal plane.
- The affected mucosa may be wrinkled or corrugated in extreme cases.
- When the mucosa is stretched, the lesion often disappears or is greatly decreased (Figs. 3.20A and B).

Histopathology

- Histologically, leukoedema is characterized by thickening of the epithelium with mild degree of parakeratosis and acanthosis.
- Within the spinous cell layer, large amount of intracytoplasmic fluid and glycogen often accumulate, which results in enlarged spinous cells with pyknotic nuclei and clear cytoplasm.

Treatment

No treatment is necessary.

CARCINOMA IN SITU

Definition

Carcinoma in situ is a preinvasive, intraepithelial malignancy of the skin, oral and glandular mucosa; it is localized, laterally spreading lesion, which does not break the basement membrane and therefore no invasion takes place. The lesion is considered to be the earliest stage of conventional squamous cell carcinoma; however the mucosal lesions often resemble leukoplakia in all respects.

It exhibits the following important changes in the epithelium:
- Most severe stage of epithelial dysplasia
- Involvement of the entire thickness of epithelium
- No dyskeratosis
- An intact basement membrane.

Clinical Features

- *Age:* Elderly
- *Sex:* More common among males than females.

Presentation

- Clinically, the lesions may appear either as white plaques or as ulcerated, eroded or reddened areas over the oral mucosa.
- The common sites of occurrence of these lesions are the floor of the mouth, tongue or lips, etc.

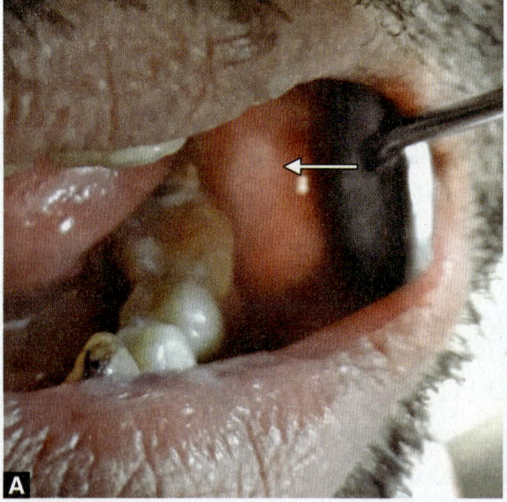
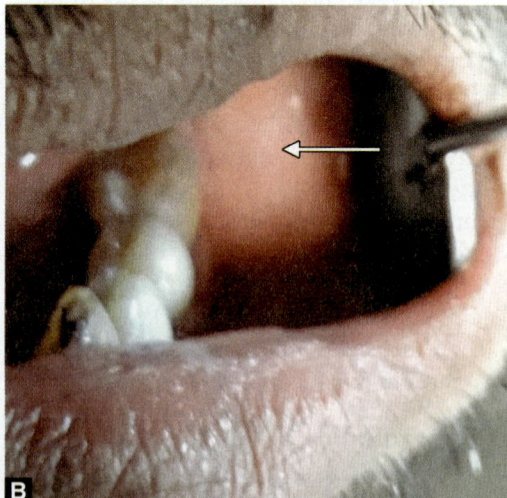

Figs. 3.20A and B: (A) White lesion of leukoedema on the cheek; (B) Lesion not visible as the mucosa is stretched.

- Cytologically, carcinoma in situ is similar to squamous cell carcinoma except that architecturally the epithelial basement membrane is intact and no invasion of the dysplastic cells into the underlying connective tissue has occurred.

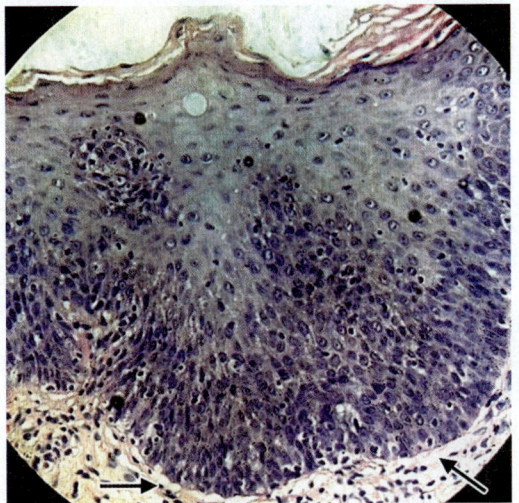

Fig. 3.21: Photomicrograph of carcinoma in situ showing severe dysplasia in all layers and intact basement membrane.

> **Key Points of Carcinoma In Situ**
> - Carcinoma in situ is the most severe stage of epithelial dysplasia and is also called laterally spreading, intraepithelial type of superficial carcinoma.
> - The dysplastic process involves the entire thickness of the epithelium; however, the basement membrane remains intact.
> - It commonly develops in the floor of the mouth, tongue, lips, etc.
> - Histologically, the epithelium is generally hyperplastic or sometimes it can be atrophic.
> - The lesion often characteristically exhibits loss of orientation and loss of polarity of the dysplastic epithelial cells.
> - Since the basement membrane is intact, there is no invasion of the neoplastic cells into the underlying connective tissue.

- The lesion may sometimes clinically appearing either as leukoplakia or erythroplakia.

Histopathology (Fig. 3.21)

- Histologically, hyperkeratosis may or may not be present on the surface of the lesion and if it is present, it will usually be the hyperparakeratosis.
- The epithelium is generally hyperplastic or sometimes it can be atrophic.
- The features like individual cell keratinization and keratin pearl formation, etc. are exceedingly rare.
- In fact, if keratin pearls are found, invasive carcinoma should be suspected rather than carcinoma in situ.
- One of the most consistent features of carcinoma in situ is the loss of orientation and loss of polarity of the dysplastic epithelial cells.
- A sharp line of division between the normal and the dysplastic epithelium is always present, which extends from the surface up to the connective tissue.
- Basement membrane of epithelium always remains intact.

Treatment

Treatment is done by surgery, radiotherapy, electrocautery, etc. The untreated cases will eventually transform into invasive squamous cell carcinoma.

■ ERYTHROPLAKIA

Erythroplakia is a clinical term, which refers to "a red patch or plaque in the oral mucosa, which cannot be rubbed off and cannot be characterized clinically or pathologically as any other condition and which has no apparent cause" (WHO 1978).

It was first reported by Queyrat in 1911 as a red, velvety lesion on the mucosa of the glans penis of elderly males. Oral erythroplakias represent the most severe type among all oral precancerous lesions and histologically, these lesions almost always exhibit dysplastic changes. Malignant potential of erythroplakia is almost 17 times more than that of leukoplakia.

Etiology

The exact etiology is not known. However, excessive use of tobacco (cigarette or bidi smoking) and heavy drinking of alcohol are believed to be responsible for the disease.

Clinical Features

- *Prevalence rate:* About 0.09% in USA and 0.02% in India.
- *Age:* Fifth, sixth, and seventh decade of life.
- *Sex:* Males and females are almost equally affected.
- *Site:* Floor of the mouth and retromolar areas are most frequently involved. The other intraoral sites are buccal mucosa, gingiva, tongue (ventral and lateral surfaces), soft palate, etc.

The gingiva and alveolar ridge lesions are more frequently seen among females. Multiple lesions may be present in some cases.

Presentation

Clinically, erythroplakia appears as a small or extensive, red, velvety lesion with clearly defined margins. The red color is due to vascular submucosal tissue shining through nonkeratinized mucosa of the oral cavity. Although the redness is not always a prominent feature of this disease since the color may not be uniformly present in all parts of the lesion.

Clinical Types

Erythroplakia clinically presents three distinctive patterns, which are described here.

Homogenous Erythroplakia

This type of lesion appears as uniform, brightly red, velvety, soft areas on the oral mucosa, with an irregular but well-defined margin.

Erythroplakia Interspersed with Patches of Leukoplakia

In this type of erythroplakia, there is presence of multiple, irregular erythematous areas in the oral epithelium and along with that few white leukoplakic patches are also present (Fig. 3.22).

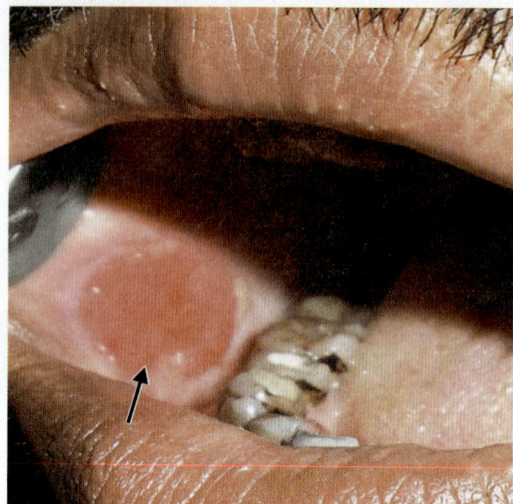

Fig. 3.22: Erythroplakia of the cheek.

Speckled Erythroplakia

These lesions are similar to the speckled leukoplakias of the oral cavity and are characterized by the presence of soft, irregular, raised, erythematous areas in the epithelium with a granular surface. There are some tiny, focal white plaques distributed all over the red surface.

Histopathology

- Erythroplakia should be viewed with high degree of alert, since most of the lesions (80–90%) exhibit features of invasive epidermoid carcinoma or carcinoma in situ or at least severe epithelial dysplasia (Fig. 3.23).
- The areas which clinically appear red histologically exhibit atrophy of the epithelium with reduction in the keratin production. Moreover, there is also an increase in the vascularity of the submucosal connective tissue.
- The underlying connective tissue shows intense chronic inflammatory cell infiltration.

Differential Diagnosis

- Erosive lichen planus
- Early squamous cell carcinoma
- Atrophic candidiasis

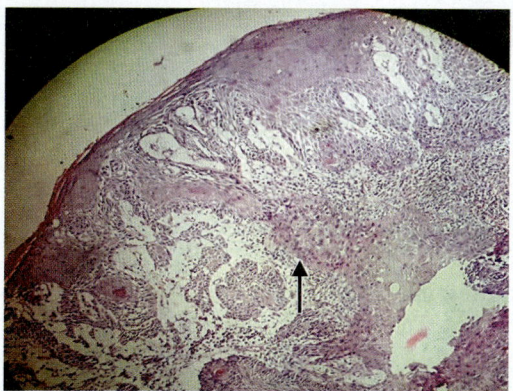

Fig. 3.23: Photomicrograph of erythroplakia showing severe dysplasia and areas of early invasive carcinoma.

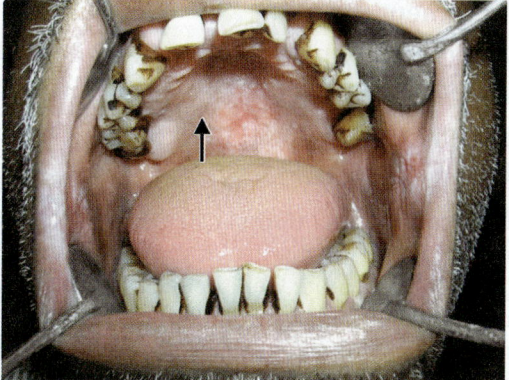

Fig. 3.24: Leukoplakia of cheek bilaterally with stomatitis nicotina.

- Kaposi's sarcoma
- Contact allergy
- Palatal erythema due to heavy smoking.

Treatment

Deep and wide surgical excision of the lesion and regular follow-up examinations are mandatory.

STOMATITIS NICOTINA

Definition

Stomatitis nicotina (smoker's keratosis) is a tobacco-related keratosis of the oral mucosa and is commonly seen in the palate of the excessive pipe or cigar smokers (Fig. 3.24).

Clinical Features

- Majority of the patients are male and only few cases occur in heavy cigarette smokers.
- The condition affects both hard and the soft palates.
- The disease represents two separate abnormalities simultaneously; one is the hyperkeratosis of the epithelium and the other is the inflammatory swelling of the palatal mucous glands.
- Initially, the areas of palatal mucosa exposed to the tobacco smoke become inflamed and red; and later on the areas become white due to increased thickening and hyperkeratosis.
- Hyperkeratosis causes obstruction to the ducts of the underlying minor salivary glands, which then become inflamed and red.
- Classically, there is whitening of palatal mucosa with tessellated plaque formation; within which the inflamed salivary duct openings appear as few red, dot-like areas surrounded by elevated, white keratotic rings.

Histopathology

- The histopathology of stomatitis nicotina shows hyperorthokeratosis and acanthosis of the surface epithelium.
- The palatal mucous glands are inflamed and there is often dilatation of the ducts.
- The keratinization process may extend down into the palatal salivary gland ducts, besides that, the ductal epithelium may also exhibit squamous metaplasia.
- Sometimes, there is partial or complete atrophy of the minor salivary glands of the palate.
- Moderate degree of inflammatory cell infiltration is seen in the palatal connective tissue and there may be even interstitial inflammation in the palatal minor salivary glands.
- Dysplastic changes are rare and so are the risks of malignant transformation in stomatitis nicotina.

Treatment

Complete stoppage of all oral habits and observation.

ORAL SUBMUCOUS FIBROSIS

Definition

Oral submucous fibrosis is a chronic, progressive scarring disease of the oral mucosa; characterized by juxtaepithelial inflammatory reaction followed by a fibroelastic transformation of the lamina propria leading to mucosal atrophy, rigidity, and trismus. Excessive collagen synthesis along with lack of collagen degradation is the hallmark of the disease (Fig. 3.25).

It is the most predominant precancerous condition involving oral cavity, oropharynx, nasopharynx, and esophagus. OSF mostly affects the people of Indian subcontinent and the Southeast Asian origin; it was first reported by Schwartz (1952) in the name of "Atrophia idiopathica (tropica) mucosae oris". The present name OSF was coined by Dr Joshi from Bombay in the year 1953.

Epidemiology

The disease is more common among the people of Southeast Asian countries—especially the Indians, Bangladeshis, Nepalese, Burmese, Vietnamese—South Africans, etc. The extreme climatic conditions in these regions and adherence of the people to more spicy foods, is believed to be the main reason behind the higher incidence of the disease. OSF may undergo malignant transformation and develop squamous cell carcinoma in the mouth.

Box 3.9	Etiology of oral submucous fibrosis.

Local factors:
- Chilies
- Areca nut (major factor)

Systemic factors:
- Nutritional deficiency
- Genetic predisposition
- Autoimmunity

Etiology (Box 3.9)

- *Excessive "areca nut" (Supari) chewing*: (*The whole fruit with the skin or husk is called "areca-nut" and the inner kernel or seed obtained after removing husk is called the "betel-nut"*). Excessive chewing of areca nut either alone or in combination with betel leaf, lime, tobacco, etc. is a common practice among the people of Indian subcontinent. Consumption of areca nut increases the possibility of submucous fibrosis because it contains chemical substances like *arecoline, arecaidine, guvacine, guvacoline*, etc. (arecoline is the strongest one). These chemicals cause stimulation of the fibroblast cells of the lamina propria and produce excessive amount of collagen, which eventually results in the development of submucosal fibrosis with rigidity of oral mucosa in OSF (Figs. 3.26 and 3.27).

Other Important Etiologic Factors in OSF

- *Excessive consumptions of red chilies*: Chilies contain an active ingredient called "capsaicin" that produces hypersensitivity reactions in the oral mucosa, such type reactions induce increased collagen synthesis and might cause OSF.
- *Nutritional deficiency*: Deficiency of vitamin A, B complex, C, etc. as well as the deficiency of iron and zinc in the diet.

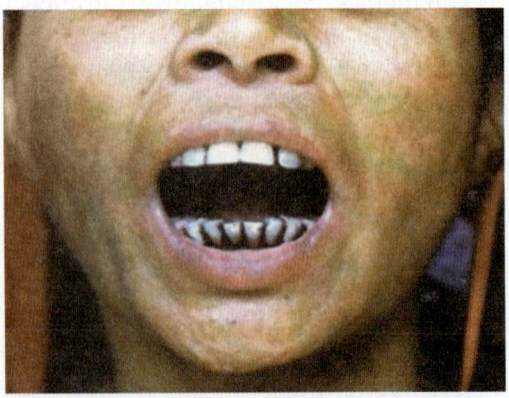

Fig. 3.25: Oral submucous fibrosis with restricted mouth opening.

Oral Precancerous Lesions and Conditions

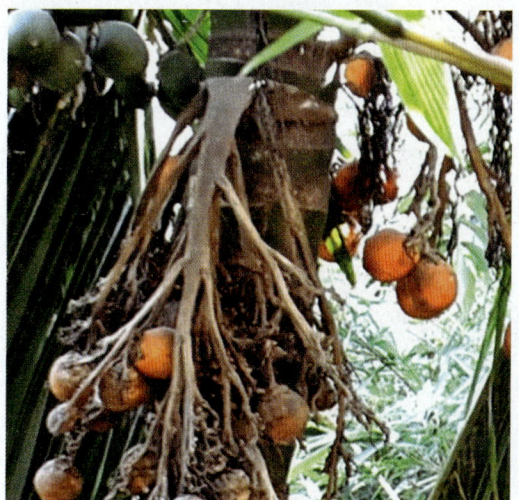

Fig. 3.26: Areca nut or supari (it is the whole fruit with skin).

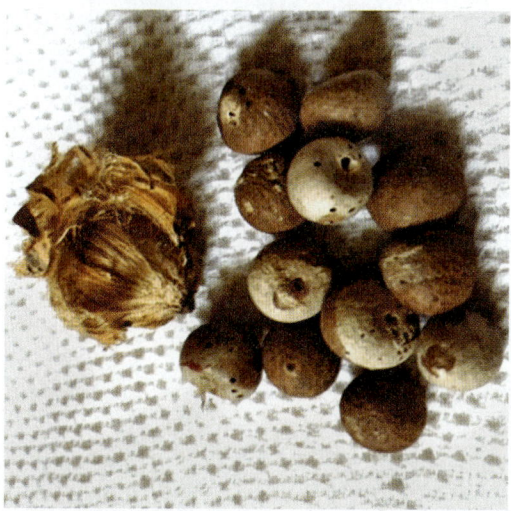

Fig. 3.27: Betel nut (it is the seed after husking the skin).

- *Immunological factors*: According to some investigators, OSF exhibits increased number of eosinophils both in the circulation as well as in the tissue.
- *Genetic factors:* Some people are genetically more susceptible to this disease.
- *Protracted tobacco use:* Excessive use of chewable tobacco.
- *Deficiency of micronutrients:* Patients with deficiency of selenium, zinc, chromium, and other trace elements may fail to prevent the free radical injury in the body and can therefore develop OSF.

Pathogenesis (Flowchart 3.1)

- Chewing of areca nut causes release of its alkaloids (e.g. arecoline, arecaidine, guvacine, guvacoline, etc.) in the mouth, which cause stimulation of the fibroblasts cells in the lamina propria of the oral epithelium.
- Stimulation of fibroblasts results in excess synthesis of collagen.
- New phenotypes of fibroblasts form which are capable of producing more collagen than the normal fibroblasts.

Cross-linking of collagen molecules occur, with the help of copper and tannin, both coming from areca nut; this alteration makes the collagen more stable and is resistant to degradation than normal collagen molecules. (*Copper is the component of enzyme lysyl oxidase that increases the cross-linking of collagen triple helix, making it more resistant to degradation*).

- Initially more number of type-III collagens form, (are more elastic in nature) but later on, there is an increase in the formation of type-I collagen, which are more stable and resistant to degradation.
- Finally due to increased collagen synthesis along with decreased collagen degradation, huge amount of collagen fibers accumulate in the submucosa and the condition is known as oral submucous fibrosis.
- *Degeneration of muscle fibers in OSF:* Continuous chewing of areca nut demands more nutritional supply to the muscles, but in OSF the glucose and oxygen supply to the muscle is often reduced since the feeding vessels to the muscles are constricted due to perivascular fibrosis. Muscular overactivity and lack of nutritional supply eventually results in atrophy and degeneration of its fibers.

Flowchart 3.1: Step by step events in the pathogenesis of oral submucous fibrosis.

```
                          Chewing of areca nut
       ┌──────────────┬──────────────┬──────────────┐
       ▼              ▼              ▼              ▼
Release of areca   Flavonoids     Copper      Constant chewing
nut alkaloids in
mouth (Arecoline,
Arecaidine,
Guvacine, and
Guvacoline)
       │              │              │              │
       ▼              ▼              ▼              │
   Arecoline    Tannin and    High amount           │
       │        Catechin      of soluble            │
       ▼                      copper in saliva      │
  Hydrolysis                                        │
  [enhanced by                                      │
  addition of                                       │
  slaked lime,                                      │
  Ca(OH)2]                                          │
       │              │              │              │
       ▼              ▼              ▼              │
   Arecaidine   Guvacine     Inhibition of   Increased
                Guvacoline   Collagenase     lysyl oxidase
       │                     enzyme          activity
       ▼                                                   Muscular
  Chemical injury                                          overactivity
  to the mucosa                                            and contracture
  with juxtaepithelial
  inflammation
       │                          │              │
       ▼                          ▼              ▼
  Stimulation of fibroblasts    Reduced       Insoluble
  and proliferation of          breakdown     collagen
  fibroblast phenotype with     of collagen
  increased ability to
  synthesize collagen
       │
       ▼
  Increased synthesis of
  collagen in lamina propria
       │
       ▼
                  Oral submucous fibrosis
       │
       ▼
  Juxtaepithelial hyalinization
       │
       ▼
  Perivascular fibrosis → Reduced tissue vascularity → Depletion of glycogen
                              │                              │
                              ▼                              ▼
                        Muscle fibrosis  ←  Muscle fatigue and degeneration
                              │
                              ▼
                           Trismus
```

Clinical Features

- *Age:* 20–40 years of age
- *Sex:* Females are affected more often than males
- *Site:* In submucous fibrosis, fibrotic changes are frequently seen in the buccal mucosa, retromolar area, uvula, soft palate, palatal fauces, tongue, lips, pharynx, esophagus, etc.

It is believed that the disease initiates from the posterior part of the oral cavity and then it gradually spreads to the anterior locations.

Presentation

Features of Early Oral Submucous Fibrosis

- The onset of the disease is either insidious or it may develop gradually over a period of 2–5 years.
- Initially, the patient complains of burning sensations in the mouth, particularly during taking hot and spicy foods.
- This is often accompanied or followed by the formation of multiple vesicles over the oral mucosa.
- There can be either excessive salivation or decreased salivation (xerostomia).

Oral Precancerous Lesions and Conditions

- Defective gustatory (taste) sensations while taking foods.
- In the early stages of OSF, palpation of the mucosa elicits a typical "wet-leathery" feeling and also there is feeling of pain in the areas where fibrotic bands are appearing.
- Early OSF also presents many petechial spots (vascular response to areca nut) over the mucosal surfaces.

Features of Advanced Oral Submucous Fibrosis

- As the disease progresses, blanching (white marble-like appearance) the oral mucosa develops; palate and faucial pillars are affected first in majority of the cases; however in other cases buccal mucosa and the lips are affected first (Figs. 3.28 and 3.29).
- Fibrous bands begin to appear in the mouth; some of these bands are "vertical" (which are seen in the buccal mucosa) and some are "circular bands" seen around the mouth orifice.
- The most incredible change in OSF is gradual stiffening of the oral mucosa with loss of tissue resiliency; fibrosis of the pterygomandibular region often leads to difficulty in mouth opening or "trismus".
- Fibrosis of the soft palate often causes it's restricted movements; also there will be deviation or shrinkage of the uvula (the uvula often has "bud-like" or "Hockey-stick" like appearance). Soft palate also reveals several fibrous bands, which radiate from the pterygomandibular raphe to the anterior faucial pillars.
- Fibrosis involves faucial pillars which make them thick and short.
- Because of stiffness of the lips and the tongue, patients are unable to blow whistles or even blow out a candle.
- The stiffened oral mucosa in OSF may occasionally exhibit leukoplakic or erythroplakic patches.
- In advanced cases of OSF, the fibrosis extends on the deeper organs like esophagus

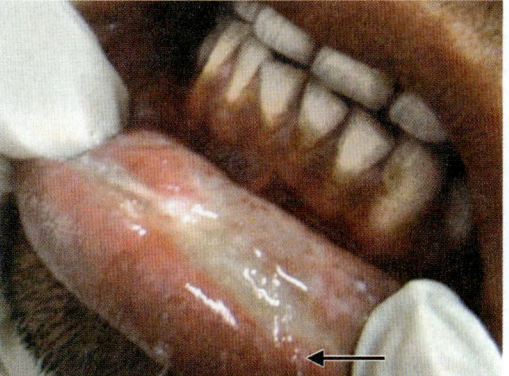

Fig. 3.29: Blanched appearance of labial fibrous bands in buccal mucosa.

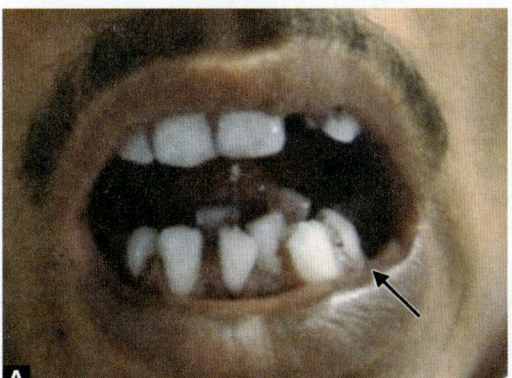
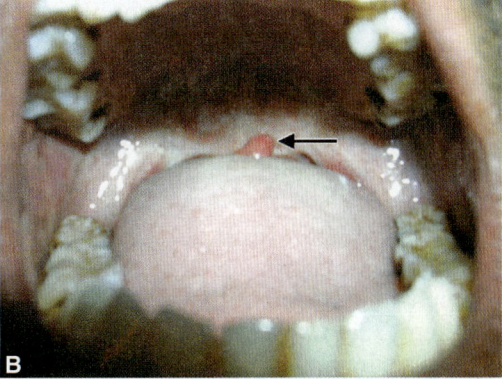

Figs. 3.28A and B: (A) Oral submucous fibrosis causing difficulty in mouth opening and (B) Blanching of oral mucosa with shrunken uvula.

and oropharynx, which causes difficulty in deglutition (dysphagia).
- Compression of the Eustachian tube by fibrosis may cause deafness and also there may be referred pain in the ear.
- There is change in the tone of voice due to vocal cord involvement; involvement of nasopharynx by the disease often causes nasal intonation of voice.
- Fibrosis causes stiffness in the tongue with restriction in its movements; loss of papillae (depapillation) and glossitis is other important feature of OSF.
- Fibrosis results in circumoral fibrotic bands with thinning and stiffening of the lips (microchelia).
- Areas of hypo- or hyperpigmentations are seen in the oral mucosa along with loss of stippling of the gingiva.
- Floor of the mouth becomes blanched and it gives a leathery feeling during palpation.

Histopathology

In OSF major histopathologic changes are observed in two areas—*epithelium* and the *connective tissue stroma*.

Epithelial Changes

- The changes occurring in the epithelium in OSF are secondary to the changes in the connective tissue (submucosa); epithelium in the early stages may remain normal but gradually it becomes atrophic with flattening of rete pegs.
- There may be increased keratinization, intracellular edema, appearance of "signet cells" (cells with large cytoplasmic vacuole) and cellular atypia, and dysplasia in rare cases.
- Excess collagen in underlying lamina propria causes upward pressure, resulting in atrophy and flattening of rete pegs (Fig. 3.30).
- The epithelium shows loss of pigmentation because the melanocytes are surrounded by dense collagen and therefore fail to release melanin.

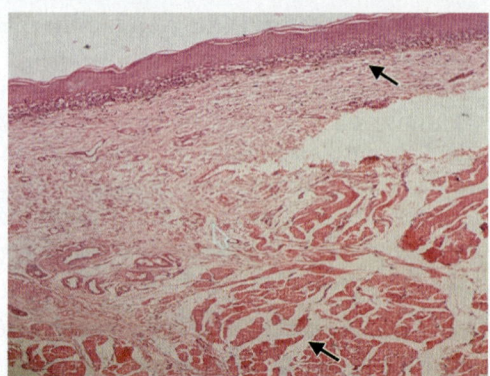

Fig. 3.30: Oral submucous fibrosis with atrophy of mucosa, flattening of rete pegs, and fibrosis of the lamina propria (low power).

Connective Tissue Changes

- *Initial stage:* Initially there will be juxta-epithelial inflammation with marked edema in the lamina propria; proliferation of plump fibroblasts, dilatation of blood vessels, and inflammatory cell infiltration by polymorphonuclear neutrophils (PMN) and few eosinophils. Collagens at this stage are fine and fibrillar in nature.
- *Early stage:* Thickening of the collagen bundles is seen with early hyalinization, a number of fibroblasts are slightly reduced, early vasoconstriction in blood vessels, and nature of inflammatory cells shift to lymphocytes, plasma cells, and eosinophils (Fig. 3.31).

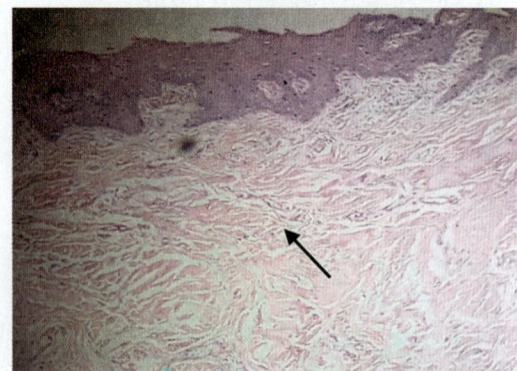

Fig. 3.31: Oral submucous fibrosis with excessive collagen formation with reduced vascularity.

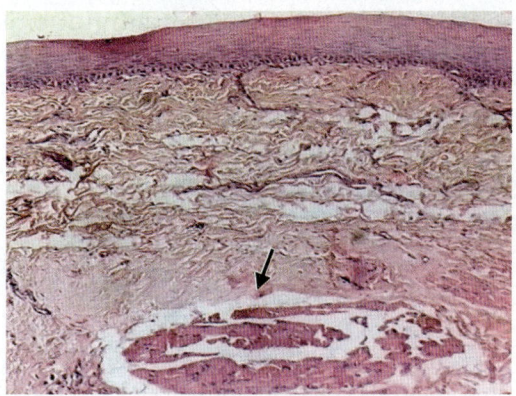

Fig. 3.32: Photomicrograph of oral submucous fibrosis showing muscle degeneration.

- *Moderately advanced stage:* More thickening of collagen bundles with amorphous changes (homogenization) at the juxtaepithelial region; fibroblasts are much less in number and they are no longer plump, they become compressed with elongated nuclei and scanty cytoplasm. Blood vessels are constricted with sign of perivascular fibrosis.
- *Advanced stage*: Collagen is completely hyalinized (hyalinization of collagen indicates the advanced stage of the disease) and seen as a smooth sheet instead of separate bundles; complete loss of cellularity and vascularity, degeneration of the muscle fibers, and few lymphocytic cell infiltration (Fig. 3.32).
- Degeneration of the muscle fibers due to lack of nutritional supply (owing to perivascular fibrosis) is also another important finding in the disease.
- Chronic inflammatory cell (lymphocyte, plasma cell, etc.) infiltration in the connective tissue is commonly seen.
- The malignant transformation rate of OSF is about 4.5–7.6%.

Laboratory Investigations

- Raised erythrocyte sedimentation rate
- Anemia
- Eosinophilia
- Hypergammaglobulinemia
- Increased serum alkaline phosphatase levels
- Alteration in the zinc and iron ratio in the tissue as well as in the blood
- Decreased serum vitamin A levels
- Scanning and transmission electron microscopy.

Staging of Oral Submucous Fibrosis

Based on Clinical Findings

Pindborg JJ 1989:
- *Stage I—(stomatitis and vesiculations):* Oral mucosa shows erythema with presence of vesicles, ulcers, and petechiae.
- *Stage II—Stage of fibrosis:* Fibrosis in healing vesicles and ulcers; blanching, palpable bands, mottled marble-like appearance of mucosa.
- *Stage III—Stage of sequelae and complication*: Fibrosis with additional presence of leukoplakia, erythroplakia, and speech and hearing impairment.

Functional staging—(Chandramani More et al. 2011):
- *M1:* Interincisal mouth opening up to or more than 35 mm
- *M2:* Interincisal mouth opening between 25 mm and 35 mm
- *M3:* Interincisal mouth opening between 15 mm and 25 mm
- *M4:* Interincisal mouth opening less than 15 mm.

Haider SM (2000):
- *Clinical stage:*
    - Stage I: Faucial bands only
    - Stage II: Faucial and buccal bands
    - Stage III: Faucial, buccal, and labial bands
- *Functional stage*:
    - Stage I: Mouth opening more than or equal to 20 mm
    - Stage II: Mouth opening 11–19 mm
    - Stage III: Mouth opening less than 10 mm.

Prakash R et al. (based on morphologic variants of soft palate):
- *Type 1*: Leaf shaped
- *Type 2*: Rat tail shaped
- *Type 3*: Butt shaped
- *Type 4*: Straight line
- *Type 5*: Deformed "S" shaped
- *Type 6*: Crook shaped.

Treatment
Stoppage of all habits, grinding and rounding of sharp cuspal edge of teeth, and routine extraction of all third molars are the preliminary steps in the treatment plan.

The definitive treatment of OSF includes intralesional injections of collagenase, corticosteroids, fibrinolysins, etc.

Systemic administration of steroids is also done in severe cases.

Biopsy is mandatory before treatment and if the dysplastic features are present in the epithelium, steroids should be avoided from the treatment schedules.

SIDEROPENIC DYSPHAGIA

Definition
Sideropenic dysphagia or Paterson–Brown–Kelly syndrome (or Plummer–Vinson syndrome) occurs primarily due to chronic iron deficiency and this disease is often associated with a high risk of cancer of the oral cavity and the aerodigestive tract.

Clinical Features
- Sideropenic dysphagia is found more often among the middle aged females.
- Difficulty in swallowing is a common problem, which occurs as a result of formation of esophageal webs.
- Angular cheilosis, mucosal pallor with atrophy, and a depapillated, smooth, glossy tongue are frequently present.

Investigations
- Examination of blood reveals the presence of severe iron deficiency anemia.
- Histological examination of oral and aerodigestive tract mucosa often exhibits mucosal atrophy and increased mitotic activity.

Sideropenic Dysphagia and Oral Cancer
- Sideropenic dysphagia is often associated with an increased risk of cancer.
- Malignant transformation of sideropenic dysphagia leads to the development of squamous cell carcinoma.

LICHEN PLANUS

Definition
The term *lichen* in Greek means "tree moss" and *planus* in Latin means "flat". Lichen planus is a unique, inflammatory chronic mucocutaneous disease, which probably arises due to an abnormal immunological reaction. The disease frequently affects skin, mucous membrane, nails, and hair; and it produces various clinical types of lesions (Fig. 3.33). Moreover, this disease has some tendency to undergo malignant transformation.

Etiopathogenesis
The exact etiologic factors causing lichen planus are unknown; however psychological stress often aggravates the condition (Flowchart 3.2).

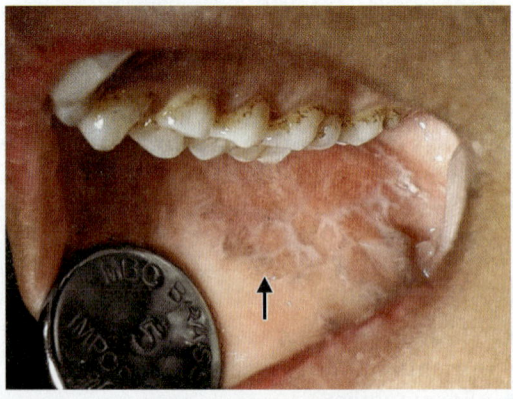

Fig. 3.33: Lichen planus.

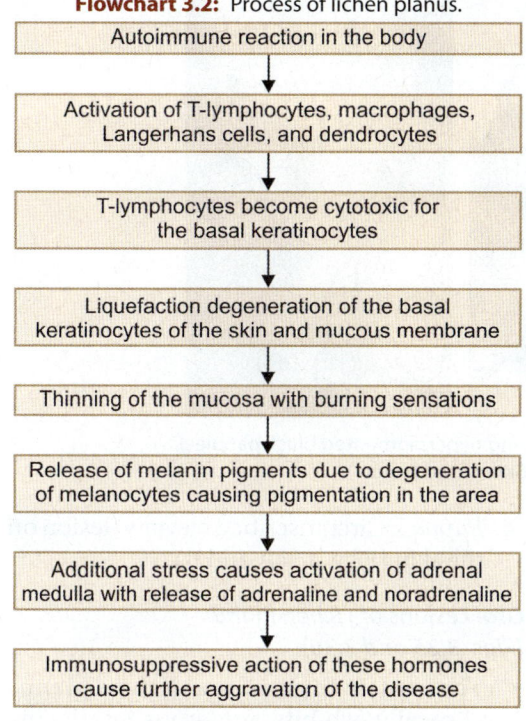

Flowchart 3.2: Process of lichen planus.

Clinical Features

- *Incidence:* Lichen planus is a common skin disease and it occurs in about 1% of the population. The cutaneous lesions alone occur in about 35% cases, the mucosal lesions alone occur in about 25% cases; however, 40% patients exhibit both mucosal and cutaneous lesions together.
- *Age*: Lichen planus occurs among the middle aged or elderly people. Rarely, it can affect children.
- *Sex*: Both sexes can be affected but there is often a predilection for females (65%).
- *Site*: Lichen planus can involve several areas of the body and important among those areas or sites are as follows:
  - *Cutaneous lesions*: Lichen planus of the skin usually involves (A) flexor surface of the wrist and forearms, (B) inner aspect of the knee and thigh, (C) upper part of the trunk, (D) scalp, nail beds, genitalia, etc.
  - *Oral lesions*: Oral lesion of lichen planus commonly occurs on the mucosal surfaces of the buccal mucosa, vestibule, tongue, lips, gingiva, etc. Palate and floor of the mouth are the least affected sites.

In many cases, oral lesions develop bilaterally.

Presentation

Cutaneous Lesions of Lichen Planus

- The cutaneous lesions of lichen planus clinically present itchy, erythematous or violaceous, flat-topped papules, which coalesce focally to form plaques. These lesions often occur in a bilaterally symmetrical pattern.
- A network of white lines or dots often overlies the papules, which are known as "Wickham striae" and they make a clinically highlighting effect in the lesion.
- Lichen planus lesions have often dark-brown color due to release of melanin into the dermis as the basal cell layer is undergone liquefaction degeneration.

- It is believed that an abnormal recognition and expression of basal keratinocytes of the epithelium as foreign antigens by the Langerhans cells, induces an autoimmune reaction in the body, which results in the initiation of this disease.
- Initially, Langerhans cells recognize an antigen, which is similar to the antigens on the epithelial keratinocytes of the susceptible patient with certain classes of major histocompatibility antigens.
- Thereafter, during the processing of antigens and subsequent stimulation of the T-lymphocytes by the Langerhans cells, some lymphocytes which are cytotoxic to the epithelial keratinocytes are produced.
- These cytotoxic T-lymphocytes accumulate in the sub-basilar connective tissue region of the epithelium and interact with the basal keratinocytes and eventually cause "liquefaction degeneration" of these cells.

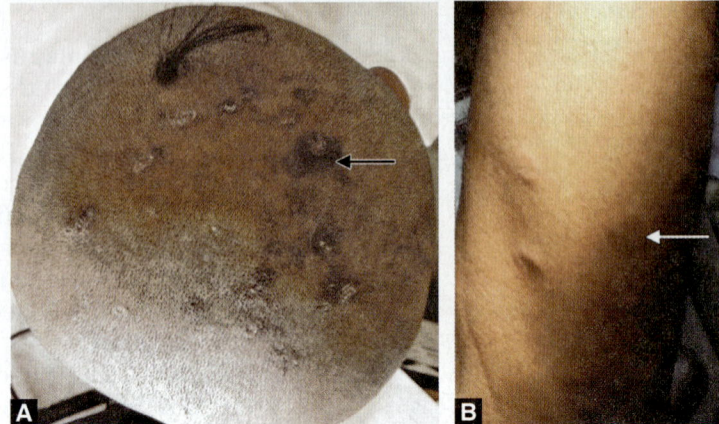

Figs. 3.34A and B: Lichen planus (showing hyperpigmented black papules) (A) On the scalp; (B) Skin of the hand.

- Koebner phenomenon: Development of lichen planus lesions in a linear pattern along the scratch marks or line of trauma; it often occurs as the patient scratches around the preexisting skin lesions because of the itching sensation (pruritus).

The characteristic "4 Ps" of cutaneous (skin) lichen planus lesions:
1. *Pruritic*: Lesion that causes itching
2. *Purple*: Lesion having a color intermediate between red and blue
3. *Polygonal*: Flat-shaped lesions with many sides
4. *Papules*: Circumscribed elevated lesion on the skin (Figs. 3.34A and B).

Oral Lesions of Lichen Planus (Figs. 3.35 and 3.36)

- The classic form of oral lichen planus clinically exhibits numerous interlacing white keratotic lines, which often produce a typical "*lace-like*" or reticular pattern against an erythematous of the oral mucosa. Another common pattern shows numerous small "ring-like" arrangements of the keratotic lines on the mucosa and is called the "*annular*" pattern.

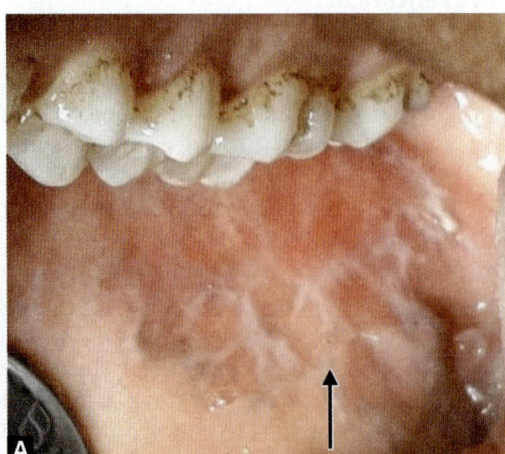
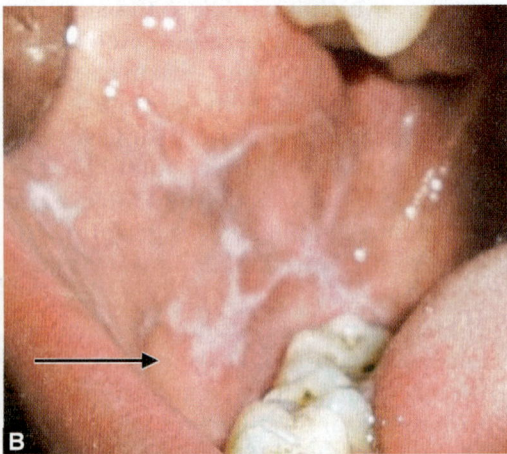

Figs. 3.35A and B: Lichen planus of the cheek showing white patch and typical "radiating striae".

Oral Precancerous Lesions and Conditions

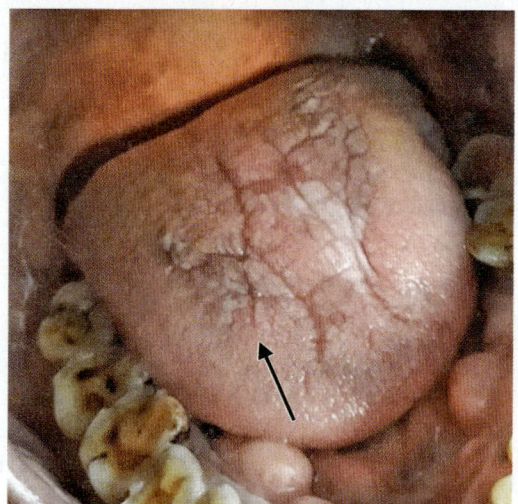

Fig. 3.36: Ulcerative lichen planus of tongue.

- A tiny white elevated dot like structure is frequently present at the point of intersection of the white lines, which is known as "striae of Wickham".
- Posterior part of buccal mucosa is the most frequent site (often bilaterally); tongue is the second most common site (especially the lateral aspect of the dorsum and occasionally the mid-dorsum), gingiva (mostly the atrophic type) and lips. The undersurface of the tongue, floor of mouth, and palate are rarely affected.
- Oral lesions are generally asymptomatic, although few lesions can cause pain and burning sensation while taking hot or spicy foods.
- In some cases, patients with lichen planus may also simultaneously have other mucosal lesions like submucous fibrosis, leukoplakia, etc. in the oral cavity.

Clinical Types of Lichen Planus

Papular Form or Type

It is seen in the initial of the disease and it shows multiple small white dots and minute white papules on the mucosa. The papules gradually enlarge to form the reticular, annular or plaque type.

Reticular Type (Net-like)

Reticular type of lichen planus is the most common type (occurs in about 70% cases).
- It usually consists of numerous raised, fine, snowy-white lines or striae, which radiate and crisscross to produce a "net-like" or "spider web-like" (reticular) appearance. The lines are usually wavy and nonelevated.
- At the periphery of the striae there is erythematous zone reflecting subepithelial inflammation in the mucosa.
- Reticular lichen planus most commonly occurs on the buccal mucosa (bilaterally) and buccal vestibule.

Erosive Type

- The erosive form of lichen planus exhibits shallow irregular areas of epithelial destructions.
- Clinically, the lesion presents a mixture of erythematous, ulcerated, and white areas, which are often covered with a yellowish-white pseudomembranous coating.
- There can also be atrophic erythematous areas with central ulceration.
- A faint white zone resembling radiating striae is frequently seen at the junction where the erosive area meets with the normal epithelium.
- Most of the lesions develop on the buccal mucosa and the vestibule.
- When the epithelial atrophy and ulcerations are confined only to the gingival area, the condition is referred to as "desquamative gingivitis".
- Patients with erosive lichen planus often complain of severe pain and burning sensation in the mouth, at the time of taking hot or spicy foods or during taking alcoholic beverages.

Ulcerative Type

Ulcerative form is a subtype of erosive lichen planus and it shows fibrin-coated ulcers on the mucosa surrounded by an erythematous zone, frequently exhibiting peripheral radiating striae (Fig. 3.37).

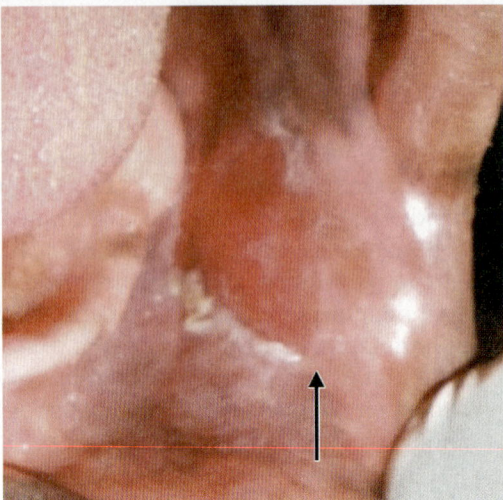

Fig. 3.37: Ulcerative lichen planus on the buccal mucosa.

Plaque Type (Fig. 3.38)

- The plaque type of lichen planus clinically presents several homogenous, well demarcated, white plaques but not always surrounded by striae.
- The plaques are irregular in shape, raised or flattened and are most commonly seen on the dorsal surface of the tongue.
- Several plaques may fuse together to form larger white patches similar to leukoplakia.

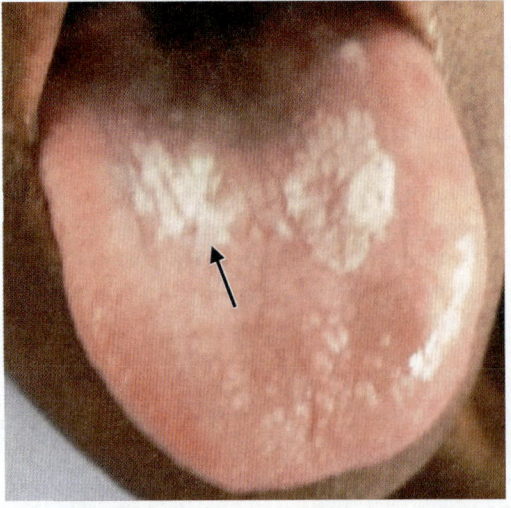

Fig. 3.38: Plaque type of lichen planus.

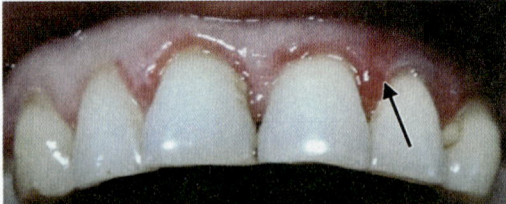

Fig. 3.39: Atrophic lichen planus of the gingiva.

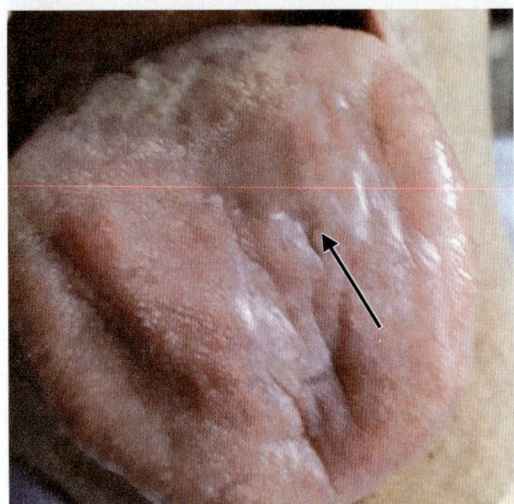

Fig. 3.40: Atrophic lichen planus of tongue.

Atrophic Type (Figs. 3.39 and 3.40)

- Atrophic lichen planus often clinically presents smooth, poorly defined, homogenous erythematous areas on the oral mucosa, with or without the presence of peripheral radiating striae.

Bullous Type

- It is a rare form of lichen planus and is characterized by the formation of large vesicle or bullae (size ranges between 4 mm and 2 cm in diameter) on the oral mucosa.
- The lesions usually develop within an erythematous base and they rupture to leave painful ulcers on the mucosal surface (Fig. 3.41).

Differential Diagnosis

- Leukoplakia
- Lichenoid reaction

Oral Precancerous Lesions and Conditions

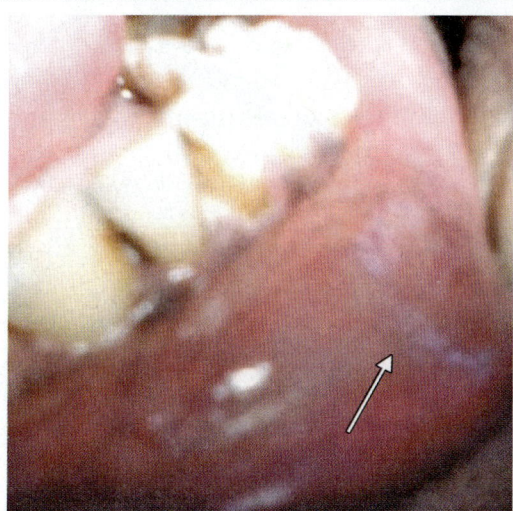

Fig. 3.41: Bullous lichen planus of the lip.

- Candidiasis
- Mucous membrane pemphigoid
- Discoid lupus erythematosus
- Syphilis
- Graft versus host reaction
- Dermatitis herpetiformis
- Atrophic glossitis.

Key Points of Lichen Planus

❖ Lichen planus is a common skin disease, which often affects the mucous membrane and the disease arises probably due to some immunological abnormality.
❖ Oral lichen planus clinically exhibits numerous interlacing white keratotic lines, which often produce a typical "lace-like" pattern, against an erythematous base.
❖ A tiny white elevated dot-like structure is frequently present at the point of intersection of the white lines, which is known as "striae of Wickham".
❖ Oral lesions are generally asymptomatic, although few lesions can cause pain and burning sensations while taking hot or spicy foods.
❖ Clinically, lichen planus has several types, which include reticular, erosive, bullous, ulcerative, plaque, atrophic, etc.
❖ Histologically, the disease presents hyperortho- or hyperparakeratinization of the epithelium with thickening of the granular cell layer and acanthosis.
❖ Characteristic findings of the disease are the necrosis and liquefaction degeneration of the basal cell layer of the epithelium, which bring the spinous cell layer of epithelium directly in contact with the connective tissue.

❖ Thick "band-like" infiltration of chronic inflammatory cells (predominantly lymphocytes) occurs in the juxtaepithelial region.
❖ Local and systemic steroid therapy is the main treatment.

Histopathology

Microscopically, lichen planus often reveals the following features (Fig. 3.42):

- The overlying surface epithelium exhibits hyperorthokeratinization or hyperparakeratinization or both.
- Thickening of the granular cell layer.
- One of the most important histologic features of lichen planus is the presence of "necrosis and liquefaction (hydropic) degeneration" of the basal cell layer of the epithelium.
- Due to the liquefaction degeneration of the basal cell layer, the epithelium becomes thin and the spinous cell layer often comes in direct contact with the underlying connective tissue.
- As a result liquefaction degeneration of the basal cell layer, the rete pegs are shortened and pointed which often create an angulated "zigzag" contour of the dermal-epidermal junction ("saw-tooth" appearance) (Figs. 3.43A and B). This appearance is more commonly seen in the skin lesions.

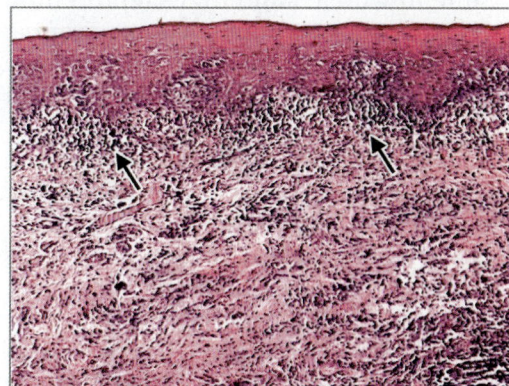

Fig. 3.42: Photomicrograph of lichen planus showing "liquefaction degeneration" of the basal cells, "band-like" infiltration of the lymphocytes and Max-Joseph space (arrow).

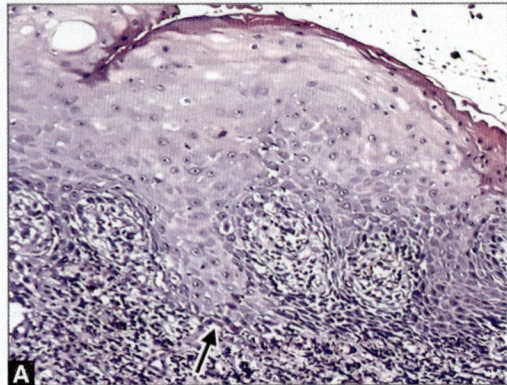

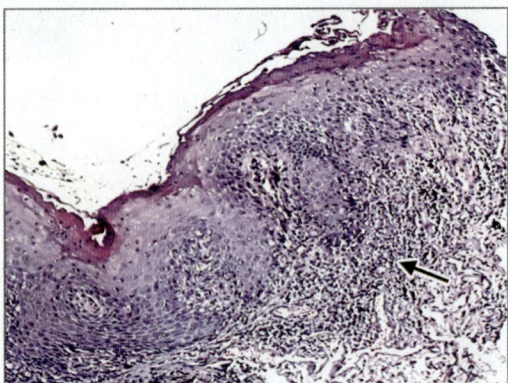

Fig. 3.44: Photomicrograph showing dysplastic changes in lichen planus.

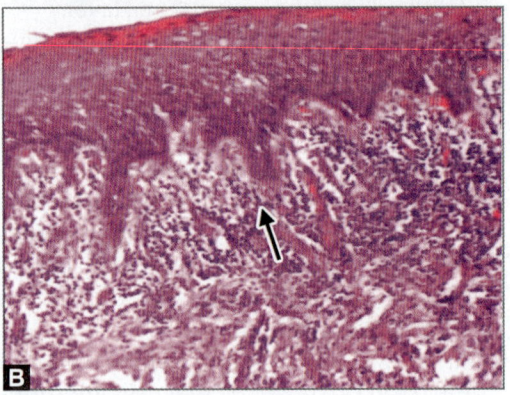

Figs. 3.43A and B: Photomicrograph of lichen planus showing (A) "liquefaction degeneration" of the basal cells (arrow) in high power and (B) "saw-tooth" rete pegs.

- In lichen planus, the affected epithelium exhibits dysplastic changes in about 4% cases, out of which about 0.3–10% cases may undergo malignant transformation (Fig. 3.44).

Special Investigations

- Direct immunofluorescent test demonstrates deposition of fibrinogen along the basement membrane of the epithelium with vertical extensions into the immediate underlying connective tissue (Fig. 3.45).

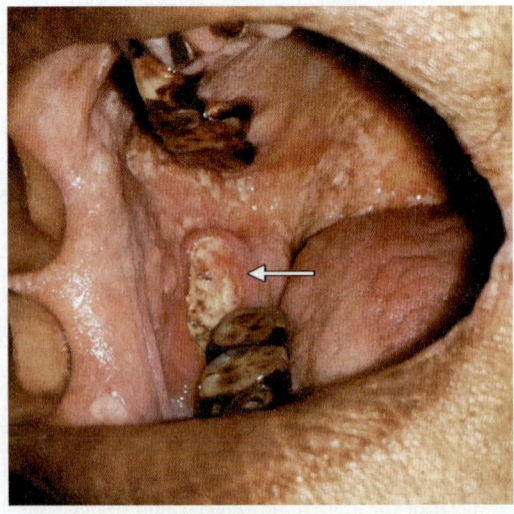

Fig. 3.45: Erosive lichen planus turning into carcinoma.

- Loss of desmosomal attachments occurs due to which, sometimes, epithelium gets separated from the lamina propria, creating small spaces at the interface between the two; these spaces are called "Max Joseph spaces".
- Another important histologic feature is "thick, band-like" infiltration of lymphocytes in the juxtaepithelial region.
- Later on these chronic inflammatory cells may often extend into the middle or upper layer of the epithelium.
- A nucleate, necrotic (dead basal keratinocytes) may become incorporated in the inflamed connective tissue as round or ovoid, amorphous, eosinophilic bodies, which are known as "civatte bodies".

- Immunohistochemical study by using the antibody to S100 protein indicates an increase in the Langerhans cells in the mid-layers of the epithelium.
- Antinuclear antibody (ANA) test.
- Immunoglobulin assay.
- PAS staining.

Treatment

Small lesions of lichen planus are treated well with topical steroids, e.g. fluocinonide.

In more resistant cases, systemic administration of methylprednisolone is effective either alone or in combination with topical steroids.

Intralesional injections of steroid have been used with some degree of success but are often not well tolerated by the patient.

Patient's psychological balance must be restored.

■ LICHENOID REACTIONS

Lichenoid reactions are mucocutaneous lesions that look similar to lichen planus and it is often clinically difficult to differentiate between the two (Fig. 3.46). These lesions are triggered by some topical or systemic agents, especially due to mucosal contact with some dental materials, e.g. metal restorations or acrylic resins, other drugs, etc. Therefore direct contact with an offending agent is the cause of lichenoid reactions, while autoimmunity is the most likely cause of lichen planus. White striae are present but interestingly they do not crisscross as seen in lichen planus (Box 3.10).

Clinically, lichenoid reaction presents the similar white mucosal lesion in the mouth like lichen planus; but here the white, wavy, parallel, nonelevated striae on the mucosa do not crisscross (as seen in lichen planus) and moreover often there is presence of an offending agent (e.g. metal restoration) in the mouth close to the lesion.

The condition resolves automatically after the offending agent is removed.

Box 3.10	Important features of lichenoid reactions.

- Presence of a metal or other restorations in the vicinity of the lesion
- White striae present but they do not crisscross as in lichen planus.

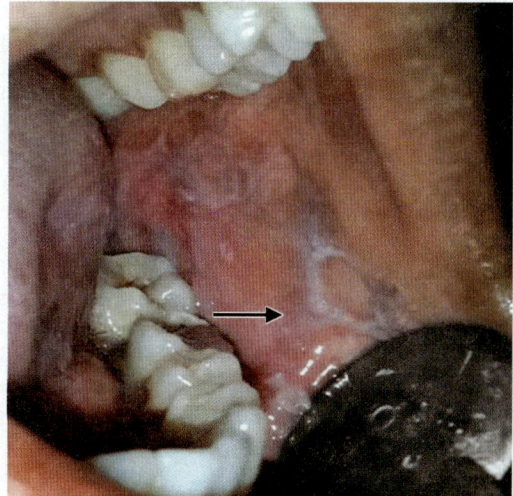

Fig. 3.46: Lichenoid reaction in the buccal mucosa following an amalgam.

BIBLIOGRAPHY

1. Andreasen JO. Oral lichen planus. 1. A clinical evaluation of 115 cases. Oral Surg Oral Med Oral Pathol. 1968;25(1):31-42.
2. Andreasen JO. Oral lichen planus. II. A histological evaluation of ninety-seven cases. Oral Surg Oral Med Oral Pathol. 1968;25:158-66.
3. Axell T. A prevalence study of oral mucosal lesions in an adult Swedish population. Odontol Revy Suppl. 1976;36:1-103.
4. Batsakis JG, Suarez P, Fl-Naggar AK. Proliferative verrucous leukoplakia and its related lesions. Review Oral Oncology. 1999;35:354-9.
5. Bhonsle RB, Murti PR, Daftary DK, et al. An oral lesion in tobacco-lime users in Maharashtra, India. J Oral Pathol. 1979;8(1):47-52.
6. Bonoczy J, Rigo O. Comparative cytologic and histologic studies in oral leucoplakia. Acta Cytol. 1976;20(4):308-12.
7. Bonoczy J. Follow-up studies in oral leukoplakia. J Maxillofac Surg. 1977;5(1):69-75.
8. Bonoczy J. Oral leucoplakia. Budapest: Akademiai Kiado; 1982.

9. Brown RS, Bottomley WK, et al. A retrospective evaluation of 193 patients with oral lichen planus. J Oral Pathol Med. 1993;22:69-72.
10. Burkhardt A. Advanced methods in the evaluation of premalignant lesions and carcinoma of the oral mucous. J Oral Pathol. 1985;14:751-8.
11. Eversole LR. Oral mucosal disorders of the keratinization process. In: Millard HD, Mason DK (Eds). World Work Shop on Oral Medicine. Chicago: Year Book Medical Publishers; 1989. pp. 95-9.
12. Eveson JW. Oral premalignancy. Cancer Survey. 1983;2:403-24.
13. Gupta PC, Hamner JE, Murti PR (Eds). Control of Tobacco-related Cancers and Other Diseases. Bombay: Oxford University Press; 1992.
14. Gupta PC. Epidemiologic study of the association between alcohol habits and oral leukoplakia. Community Dent Oral Epidemiol. 1984;12:47-50.
15. Joshi SG. Submucous fibrosis of the palate. Indian J Otolaryngol. 1953;4:1-4.
16. Kini MG, Rao KVS. The problem of cancer. Indian Medical Gazette. 1973;72:677-9.
17. Kramer IR, El-labban N, Lee KW. The clinical features and risk of malignant transformation in sublingual keratosis. Br Dent J. 1978;144:171-80.
18. Kramer IR, Pindborg JJ, Bezroukov V, et al. Guide to epidemiology and diagnosis of oral mucosal diseases and conditions. World Health Organization. Community Dent Oral Epidemiol. 1980;8:1-26.
19. Lahner T. Quantitative assessment of lymphocytes and plasma cells in leukoplakia, candidiasis, and lichen planus. J Dent Res. 1971;50:1661-5.
20. Lal D. Diffuse oral submucous fibrosis. J All India Dent Assoc. 1953;26:1-3.
21. Pinborg JJ. Fibrous dysplasia or fibro-osteoma. Acta Radiol. 1951;36:196.
22. Pindborg JJ, Chawla TN, Srivastava AN, et al. Clinical aspects of oral submucous fibrosis Acta Odontol Scand. 1964;22:6
23. Pindborg JJ, Chawla TN, Srivastava AN, et al. Epithelial changes in oral submucous fibrosis Acta Odontol Scand. 1965;23:277.
24. Pindborg JJ, Jolst O, Renstrup G, et al. Studies in oral leukoplakia: a report on the period prevalence of malignant transformation in leukoplakia based on a follow-up study of 248 patients. J Am Dent Assoc. 1968;76(4):767-71.
25. Pindborg JJ, Mehta FS, Daftary DK. Incidence of oral cancer among 30,000 villagers in India in a 7-year follow-up study of oral precancerous lesions. Community Dent Oral Epidemiol. 1975;3(2):86-8.
26. Pindborg JJ, Mehta FS, Gupta PC, et al. Prevalence of oral submucous fibrosis among 50,915 Indian villagers. Br J Cancer. 1968;22:6
27. Pindborg JJ, Reibel J, Roed-Petersen B, et al. Tobacco-induced changes in oral leukoplakic epithelium cancer. 1980;45:2330.
28. Pindborg JJ, Renstrup G, Poulsen HE, et al. Studies in oral leukoplakias. Acta Odontol Scand. 1963;21:4
29. Pindborg JJ, Sirsat SM. Oral submucous fibrosis. Oral Surg. 1966;22:764.
30. Pindborg JJ, Zachariah J. Frequency of oral submucous fibrosis among 100 South Indians with oral cancer bull. WHO. 1965;32:750.
31. Pindborg JJ. Diseases of the skin. In: Jones JH, Mason DK (Eds). Oral Manifestations of Systemic Disease, 2nd edition. London: WB Saunders; 1990;pp. 537-92.
32. Platkajs MA. A clinicopathologic study of oral leukoplakia with emphasis on the keratinisation pattern. J Can Dent Assoc. 1979;3:107.
33. Praetorius-Clausen F. Historadiographic study of oral leukoplakias. Scand J Dent Res. 1970;78:479.
34. Rajendran R. Oral submucous fibrosis: etiology, pathogenesis and future research - Review. Bulletin WHO 1994,72:985.
35. Silverman S Jr, Renstrup G, Pindborg JJ. Studies in oral leukoplakias. III. Effects of vitamin a comparing clinical, histopathologic, cytologic, and hematologic responses. Acta Odontol Scand. 1963;21:271-92.
36. Silverman S, Gorsky M, Lozada F. Oral Leukoplakia and malignant transformation. A follow-up of 2157 patients. Cancer. 1984;53:563-8.
37. Smith C, Pindborg JJ. Histological grading of oral epithelial atypia by the use of photographic Standards. World Health Organization's International Reference Centre for Oral Precancerous Conditions, Copenhagen, 1969.
38. Smith C. Carcinoma in situ. Hum Pathol. 1978;9:373.
39. van der Waal I, Schepman KR, van der Meij EH, et al. Oral leukoplakia: a clinicopathological review. Oral Oncol. 1997;33(5):291-301.

CHAPTER 4

Diseases of the Salivary Glands

■ INTRODUCTION

Oral cavity normally has a moist environment and it is because of the continuous production and secretion of saliva in the mouth by the salivary glands. Salivary glands comprise of three paired major glands namely the parotids, the submandibular, and the sublingual glands. Besides these major glands, there are numerous minor salivary glands (their number may be up to 300) present in almost every part of the oral cavity especially in the hard and soft palate, tongue, lip and buccal mucosa, except the gingiva. These minor glands are also found in the oropharynx, paranasal sinuses, sinonasal tracts, and the upper respiratory tracts, etc. The secretion of saliva is essential for the normal health and function of the mouth; the functional unit of salivary gland is the secretory acini, salivary ducts, and the myoepithelial cells.

The functional unit of salivary glands is the secretory acinus (plural is acini) and the secretory products of the salivary gland may be of three types—serous, mucous, and mixed. The nature of secretion in different glands is listed below—

Major salivary glands:
- Parotid is an almost purely serous gland.
- Submandibular is a mixed gland but predominantly serous.
- Sublingual is also a mixed gland but predominantly mucous type.

The minor salivary glands may also have different characters:

- Minor salivary glands of the ventral tongue, palate, and retromolar area are predominantly mucous in nature.
- Minor glands of the lateral aspect of tongue, lips, and buccal mucosa are seromucous type.
- Minor glands related to the circumvallate papillae (von Ebner's glands) are serous type.

The serous acini are made up of wedge-shaped secretory glandular epithelial cells having their nuclei located at the base and the cytoplasm contains densely basophilic, periodic acid–Schiff (PAS)-positive zymogen granules. The main secretion of serous acini is amylase.

The secretory cells of mucous acini also have basally placed nuclei and they have clear vacuolated cytoplasm.

The salivary duct system: Once the saliva is produced by the acinar cells, it is collected in a lumen at the center of each acini; from there it flows through a duct called "intercalated duct" (lined by a single layer of cuboidal cells with large centrally placed nuclei; these cells have some secretory function).

At its end, the intercalated duct joins with the much larger "striated duct" (lined by tall columnar cells with eosinophilic cytoplasm) and this striated duct is the primary site for sodium reabsorption and potassium secretion.

Striated duct joins with the excretory duct (lined by pseudostratified columnar epithelial cells and few mucous cells), which finally drains into the main collecting duct of the salivary gland.

The myoepithelial cells (also called "basket cells") form the basal cell layer of the glandular epithelium; these are stellate-shaped cells with long dendritic processes that embrace the secretory acini and also surround the intercalated ducts. The myoepithelial cells have contractile property (as they contain smooth muscle actin and myosin) and by their contraction they help in expelling the salivary secretions from the acini and also through the intercalated duct. Myoepithelial cells can also act as epithelial progenitor cells.

Disorders of salivary gland function, which affect the composition and secretion of saliva, predispose to many oral diseases. Salivary gland diseases are broadly divided into two categories—non-neoplastic disease and neoplastic disease.

CLASSIFICATION OF SALIVARY GLAND DISEASES (TABLE 4.1)

Non-Neoplastic Disorders

Developmental Anomalies
- Aplasia (agenesis) of the salivary gland
- Hypoplasia
- Aberrant salivary gland
- Atresia
- Accessory ducts
- Diverticuli
- Lingual mandibular salivary gland depression.

Reactive Lesions
- Mucous retention cyst
- Mucous extravasation cyst
- Sialolithiasis
- Postradiation sialadenitis
- Chronic sclerosing sialometaplasia.

Infective Lesions

Bacterial sialadenitis:
- Acute
- Chronic
- Recurrent.

Viral sialadenitis:
- Mumps
- Cytomegalic inclusion disease.

Immune-mediated diseases:
- Mikulicz's disease
- Sjögren's syndrome.

Miscellaneous Diseases
- Heerfordt syndrome
- Sialosis
- Ptyalism and aptyalism
- HIV-associated salivary gland disease.

Neoplastic Disorders (Table 4.1)

Classification: Thackray and Sobin, 1972.

Epithelial Tissue Neoplasms

Adenomas:
- Pleomorphic adenoma (mixed tumor)
- Monomorphic adenoma
- Adenolymphoma (Warthin's tumor)
- Oxyphilic adenoma.

Other types:
- Mucoepidermoid tumor
- Acinic cell tumor
- Carcinomas
- Adenoid cystic carcinoma
- Adenocarcinoma
- Epidermoid carcinoma
- Undifferentiated carcinoma
- Carcinoma in pleomorphic adenoma (malignant mixed tumor).

Connective Tissue Neoplasms
- Fibroma
- Fibrosarcoma
- Lipoma
- Neurilemmoma
- Hemangioma
- Melanoma
- Lymphoma.

DEVELOPMENTAL ANOMALIES OF THE SALIVARY GLAND

Aplasia or Agenesis of the Salivary Gland

Definition

Congenital absence of the salivary glands (both major and minor glands) due to complete failure of their development or genesis is called salivary gland aplasia.

Diseases of the Salivary Glands

Table 4.1: WHO histological classification of tumors of the salivary glands.

Malignant epithelial tumors	• Acinic cell carcinoma 8550/3 • Mucoepidermoid carcinoma 8430/3 • Adenoid cystic carcinoma 8200/3 • Polymorphous low-grade adenocarcinoma 8525/3 • Epithelial–myoepithelial carcinoma 8562/3 • Clear cell carcinoma, not otherwise specified 8310/3 • Basal cell adenocarcinoma 8147/3 • Sebaceous carcinoma 8410/3 • Sebaceous lymphadenocarcinoma 8410/3 • Cystadenocarcinoma 8440/3 • Low-grade cribriform cystadenocarcinoma • Mucinous adenocarcinoma 8480/3 • Oncocytic carcinoma 8290/3 • Salivary duct carcinoma 8500/3 • Adenocarcinoma, not otherwise specified 8140/3 • Myoepithelial carcinoma 8982/3 • Carcinoma ex pleomorphic adenoma 8941/3 • Carcinosarcoma 8980/3 • Metastasizing pleomorphic adenoma 8940/1 • Squamous cell carcinoma 8070/3 • Small cell carcinoma 8041/3 • Large cell carcinoma 8012/3 • Lymphoepithelial carcinoma 8082/3 • Sialoblastoma
Benign epithelial tumors	• Pleomorphic adenoma 8940/0 • Myoepithelioma 8982/0 • Basal cell adenoma 8147/0 • Warthin tumor 8561/0 • Oncocytoma 8290/0 • Canalicular adenoma 8149/0 • Sebaceous adenoma 8410/0 • Lymphadenoma • Sebaceous 8410/0 • Nonsebaceous 8410/0 • Ductal papillomas • Inverted ductal papilloma 8503/0 • Intraductal papilloma 8503/0 • Sialadenoma papilliferum 8406/0 • Cystadenoma 8440/0
Soft tissue tumors	Hemangioma 9120/0
Hematolymphoid tumors	• Hodgkin lymphoma • Diffuse large B-cell lymphoma 9680/3 • Extranodal marginal zone B-cell lymphoma 9699/3
Secondary tumors	

Clinical Features

- It is an exceptionally rare anomaly in which either a single gland or multiple glands can be involved either unilaterally or bilaterally.
- In some patients, salivary gland aplasia may occur alone, however in other patients this condition is associated with some congenital facial malformations.
- Aplasia of the major salivary gland commonly produces xerostomia (dryness of mouth), due to lack of production of saliva in the oral cavity.

- Congenital aplasia of the salivary glands may be associated with hereditary ectodermal dysplasia, mandibulofacial dysostosis, congenital aplasia of the lacrimal glands, and hemifacial microstomia, etc.

Treatment

Patients with congenital salivary gland aplasia will require continuous dental supervision and administration of systemic or topical fluorides to prevent dental caries.

Hypoplasia of the Salivary Glands

Relative underdevelopment of the salivary gland is known as salivary gland hypoplasia. Hypoplasia of the salivary glands may occur either due to their congenital absence or due to atrophy of the gland secondary to lack of neuromuscular stimulations.

Salivary gland hypoplasia is often associated with Melkersson–Rosenthal syndrome, which consists of cheilitis granulomatosa, facial paralysis, and fissured tongue.

Ectopic Salivary Glands (Aberrant)

Definition

The occurrence of normal salivary gland tissue in anatomically unusual locations is known as salivary gland ectopia and such glands are known as ectopic salivary glands.

- Sometimes, the salivary gland tissue may be present within the body of the mandible.
- Majority of the Stafne bone cysts and the intraosseous salivary gland tissue within the body of the mandible may occur as part of the phenomenon called lingual mandibular salivary gland depressions.
- Ectopic salivary gland tissues may be found in the gingiva and where it produces a tumor-like mass, which is known as gingival salivary gland choristoma.
- Sometimes, the ectopic salivary gland tissue may occur within the masseter muscle. Moreover, ectopic salivary glands can also be found in the upper portion of the neck in the region of branchial cleft.
- Pathological conditions, like sialolithiasis, neoplasms, and cysts, etc., which commonly affect the normal salivary gland can also involve the ectopic salivary gland tissues.

Common Locations of Ectopic Salivary Glands

The ectopic salivary glands are often found in the following locations:
- Mandibular body
- Gingiva
- Masseter muscle
- Upper portion of neck near the branchial cleft.

Atresia

Atresia of the salivary gland excretory ducts refers to the congenital absence or narrowing of excretory duct system.

Atresia is an extremely rare condition, which may produce severe xerostomia. It can also result in the formation of retention cyst of the salivary gland.

Accessory Ducts

Accessory salivary ducts are relatively common developmental malformations, which can occur in relation to any gland, though it is seen more often in association with the parotids. The accessory parotid ducts are usually found either above or below the normal Stensen duct.

Diverticuli

Diverticuli refer to the small pouches or outpocketings of the ductal system of major salivary glands and is predominantly found in relation to parotids. Diverticuli may produce recurrent swellings and acute sialadenitis due to retention of saliva in those areas where the pouches are present along the course of the duct. Diverticuli can be diagnosed by sialogram.

■ REACTIVE LESIONS OF THE SALIVARY GLAND

Salivary Gland Cysts

Mucous retention cyst and mucous extravasation cysts are discussed in the chapter of "Cysts of the Oral Regions".

Sialolithiasis

Definition

Sialolithiasis is a pathological condition, characterized by the presence of one or more calcified stones (sialoliths) within the salivary gland itself or within its duct.

Pathogenesis

- The exact mechanism of formation of sialolith is not known. It is generally believed that initially a small and soft nidus forms within the salivary gland or its duct, due to some unknown reason.
- The nidus is made up of mucin, protein, bacteria, and desquamated epithelial cells.
- Once a small nidus forms, it allows concentric lamellar crystallizations to occur due to the precipitation of calcium salts.
- The sialolith increases in size with time as layer after layer of salts become deposited, just like growth rings in a tree.
- It is important to note that the formation of sialolith is more common in relation to the submandibular gland and its ducts (about 70–90% cases).

The reasons why sioliths form more in relation to the submandibular salivary glands:

- Multiple sharp bends or curvatures in the Wharton's duct
- More viscous nature of saliva of this gland
- Higher calcium levels in saliva of this gland
- Dependent position of the gland often increases the chance of stasis of saliva.

Clinical Features

- *Age*: Sialolithiasis usually occurs among the middle-aged adults, however some cases are reported in children.
- *Sex*: There appears to be a slight predilection for males.
- *Sites*: Majority (70%) of the sialoliths form within the excretory ducts of the submandibular gland and sometimes they

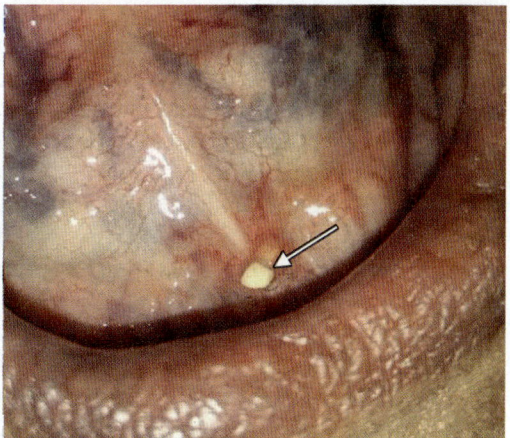

Fig. 4.1: Sialolith in the left submandibular duct.

may occur within the substance of the submandibular gland itself (Fig. 4.1).

The parotid gland is the next most commonly involved gland (about 23% cases), while the sublingual and the minor salivary glands are affected in about 4% of cases.

Sialoliths of the minor salivary glands most often develop within the glands of the upper lip or buccal mucosa.

Clinical Presentation

- In many cases, sialoliths do not produce any symptoms and are detected only on routine radiographic examination.
- The chief complaints are intermittent pain, discomfort, and recurrent submandibular swellings especially during meals (as the taste and smell of the food increase the salivary secretion).
- The pain occurs due to occlusion of the salivary gland duct by the sialolith, resulting in retention of saliva in the blocked portion of the duct.
- The pain can be felt like a pulling, drawing or a stinging sensation in mild cases due to partial obstruction of the duct by the sialolith.
- However, swelling increases and the pain can be very severe and stabbing type when there is complete obstruction of the duct.

- Clinically symptoms are more obviously felt when the patient takes any sour food or when direct stimulation of salivary secretion is done with a lemon drop candy.
- The affected glands become enlarged and firm but are still movable.
- The stone or the sialolith in the submandibular gland duct can often be palpated by bimanual palpation with finger of both hands.
- Small sialoliths may sometimes be seen at the duct orifices.
- Chronic obstruction by the sialolith eventually leads to chronic sclerosing sialadenitis.
- Sialoliths usually form unilaterally, however bilateral cases are sometimes reported.
- Multiple stones may develop within ductal branches throughout the gland and long standing lesions may result in complete calcification of the entire gland.
- Involvement of the submandibular gland often produces unilateral glandular enlargement medial to the inferior border of the mandible. The swelling is often firm and tender on palpation.
- Secondary infection causes pain, swelling, and formation of sinus tracts or fistulas. Ulcerations in the area may also develop in chronic cases.
- Parotid stone often causes firm swelling over the ramus of the mandible. The swelling also increases during meals.
- Minor salivary gland stone formation occurs commonly in the upper lip and buccal mucosa. Clinically, these lesions produce palpable, hard, and movable nodule within the submucosa.
- Sialoliths do not cause xerostomia since they involve only one or two glands.

Diagnosis of Sialolithiasis

Radiography
- Submandibular sialolithiasis are easily detected by mandibular standard occlusal radiographs which typically disclose the presence of calcification in the floor of the mouth.
- When a sialolith is located within the submandibular gland, a lateral jaw film may be helpful in detecting its exact location.
- A panoramic radiograph usually detects parotid stones.
- If only branches of the submandibular gland duct are affected, a posterior occlusal film, submentovertex, and sometimes a lateral jaw film may be required.

Sialography: Sialography refers to the method by which detection of salivary stones within the gland or its duct is done by giving a retrograde injection of a radiopaque dye within the duct system and obtaining a radiograph thereafter in order to see the size and distribution of the sialolith.

Ultrasonography and CT scan: Diagnostic sialendoscopy also can be a valuable tool in the evaluation and diagnosis of ductal obstructions. In this technique, a miniaturized endoscope is inserted into the duct orifice, allowing visualization of the ductal system for any stones, strictures, or adhesions.

Macroscopic Appearance of Sialolith

- On gross examination, sialoliths appear as round or oval, rough or smooth solid masses, which vary considerably in their size.
- These stones are heavily calcified and are often multinodular, although some stones are found in small aggregates.
- The color of the stone is usually yellowish or yellowish-white.

Composition of Sialolith

Following are the general constituents of a sialolith:
Calcium phosphate: 75%
Calcium carbonates: 12%
Soluble salt: 5%
Organic matter: 5%
Water: 3%

Histopathology

- Microscopically, the salivary stone is acellular and amorphous and when

Diseases of the Salivary Glands

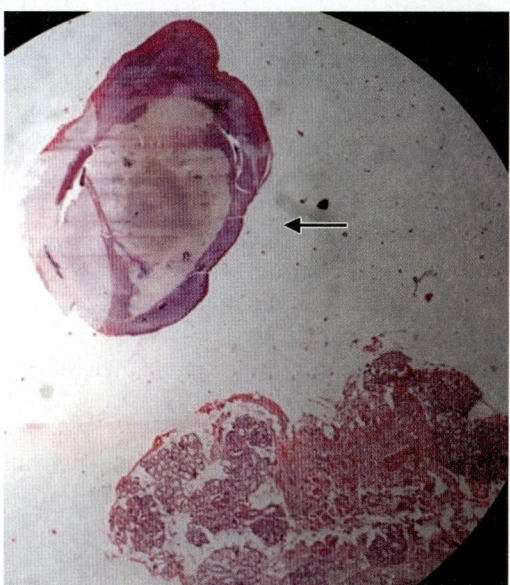

Fig. 4.2: The excised salivary gland along with the sialolith.

decalcified, it presents concentric laminations of amorphous basophilic matrix (Fig. 4.2).
- The outer margin may exhibit aggregates of microbial colonies.
- The ductal lining which surrounds the stone shows oncocytic, squamous and/or mucous metaplasia of varying degree.
- As a result of the metaplastic change, the ductal lining of the gland is often changed into a stratified squamous type of epithelium, which contains numerous mucous goblet cells.
- The rest of the gland tissue shows varying degrees of acinar degeneration and intense mononuclear cell infiltration.

Differential Diagnosis
- Endemic parotitis
- Salivary gland neoplasm
- Mesenchymal neoplasm
- Hypervitaminosis-A
- Calcification of lymph node in chronic long-standing tuberculosis.

> **Key Points of Sialolithiasis**
> - Sialolithiasis is a pathological condition characterized by formation of calcified stones (sialoliths) within the salivary gland or within its duct.
> - It occurs more commonly in relation to the submandibular gland and its ducts.
> - The sialolith causes occlusion of the salivary gland duct resulting in retention of saliva which results in intermittent pain, discomfort, and recurrent swelling of the affected gland.
> - Pain and discomfort occurs especially during meals (as the taste and smell of the food increase the salivary secretion).
> - Moreover, the symptoms become more severe when the patient takes any sour food or when direct stimulation of salivary secretion is done with a lemon drop candy.
> - The sialolith can be palpated by bimanual palpation with finger of both hands.
> - Untreated cases may cause secondary infections in the affected gland which produce pain, ulcerations, swelling, and formation of sinus tracts or fistulas, etc.
> - The sialolith can be easily detected by mandibular standard occlusal radiographs or by sialography.
> - Structurally, the sialolith is acellular and amorphous and it contains about 75% calcium phosphate.
> - Surgical removal of the stone is the treatment of choice.

Treatment
- Small stones in the distal parts of the duct can be removed through the orifice by digital manipulation only.
- Whenever, digital maneuvers fail, surgical removal of the stone is indicated.
- Lithotripsy sometimes can be used as a noninvasive technique for disintegrating large sialoliths.
- Whenever the conditions like intraglandular stones, multiple stones in a single gland or diffuse glandular calcification, etc. occur in association with pain, indurations, and chronic lack of function, removal of the stone along with the gland (sialoadenectomy) should be recommended.
- Minor salivary gland stones are treated by simple surgical excision.

It is important to remember that stones may occur secondarily in association with neoplasms such as acinic cell carcinoma and mucoepidermoid carcinoma and other condition such as HIV infection).

Postradiation Sialadenitis

Radiation-induced sialadenitis is a common complication of radiotherapy in the head and neck region.
- The severity of damage of the salivary gland tissue is usually directly proportional to the doses of radiation.
- When the dose of radiation is not very high, it may cause reversible damage to the salivary gland tissue and therefore some degree of salivary function may return after several months.
  However, in cases of very high dose of radiation, irreversible damage generally occurs in the salivary gland tissue and in such cases the gland acini are replaced by fibrous tissue with complete loss of function of the gland.
- Serous acini of the salivary gland are more susceptible to radiation damage than the mucous acini.

Chronic Sclerosing Sialadenitis

Definition

Chronic sclerosing sialadenitis can be defined as chronic inflammation of the salivary gland tissue resulting in degeneration and subsequent replacement of acini by fibrous tissue.

Etiology

- Autoimmune disease
- Systemic and metabolic disorders
- Direct trauma
- Infection
- Occlusion of the duct by calculi
- Compression of the gland or duct by neoplasms
- Salivary glands cysts
- Radiation therapy
- Medication and drugs.

Clinical Features

- The affected salivary gland may be either the major glands or the minor glands.
- There may be presence of sialolith in the gland or there can be mucous extravasations within the gland tissue.
- The affected gland is often enlarged either due to accumulation of saliva in the duct or due to inflammatory change.

Histopathology

- There will be progressive destruction of the salivary gland acinar cells, as a result of both apoptosis and necrosis.
- There is chronic inflammatory cell infiltration in the gland comprising of lymphocytes and plasma cells.
- Once the acini are lost, the gland parenchyma undergoes progressive sclerosis or fibrosis.
- In chronic sclerosing sialadenitis, the ductal elements often remain unaffected.

Treatment

- Etiologic factors should be removed.
- If the gland parenchyma is completely destroyed, sialoadenectomy should be done.
- Artificial saliva should be prescribed.

Necrotizing Sialometaplasia

Definition

Necrotizing sialometaplasia is a spontaneous disease of unknown etiology, characterized by necrosis of minor salivary glands of the palate along with the surface epithelium and the underlying connective tissue.

Predisposing Factors

- Odontogenic infections
- Traumatic injury
- Ill-fitting dentures
- Tumor in the adjacent areas
- Chronic throat infections.

Pathogenesis

- Many investigators believe that necrotizing sialometaplasia occurs due to infarction of the tissue, although the underlying cause of the infarction is unknown. Some people have reported about initiation of the disease following a local palatal anesthetic injection.

- It is also associated with long-term intubation complicated by herpetic infection of the trachea, sickle cell disease, and chronic vomiting, etc.

Clinical Features
- *Age*: The disease often occurs in adults and the mean age is about 47 years, although this disease affects women at a much younger age.
- *Sex*: It occurs in males more often than the females.
- *Site*: Mostly the palate is affected at the region of the junction between hard and soft palate.

In some rare cases, the disease can occur in other gland bearing oral mucosal sites. Parotid gland is occasionally affected.

Clinical Presentation
- Necrotizing sialometaplasia initially presents one or two nonulcerated swellings on the palate with pain and paresthesia, etc.
- Later on, one or two deep-seated, punched-out ulcerations characteristically develop over the hard or the soft palate.
- The deeply excavating ulcers do not have any raised or rolled borders.
- The ulcer measures about 2–3 cm in diameter and at the base, there is presence of few gray, granular lobules representing the necrosed minor salivary glands.
- The lesions heal spontaneously usually within 1–3 months.

Histopathology
The histologic features of necrotizing sialometaplasia are characteristic and highly specific:
- The base of the ulcer shows absence of epithelium, which is replaced by necrotic debris and eosinophilic fibrinous materials.
- The minor salivary gland tissues, which are present below the necrotic debris, exhibit features of coagulation necrosis.
- The salivary acinar cells show absence of nuclei; these cells are distended and often appear pale and basophilic.
- The cytoplasmic borders of the necrotic acinar cells remain intact and despite the cell damage, the lobular architecture of the salivary gland is often maintained.
- In the zone of necrosis, accumulated mucin is often seen and also there is presence of numerous scattered neutrophils and foamy histiocytes.
- The salivary epithelium adjacent to the necrotic zone shows squamous metaplasia with loss of normal acinar morphology.
- These metaplastic foci often appear as round or oval epithelial islands.
- The microscopic appearance of necrotizing sialometaplasia is to some extent similar to that of the mucoepidermoid carcinoma.

Differential Diagnosis
- Mucoepidermoid carcinoma
- Squamous cell carcinoma
- Adenocarcinoma
- Tuberculous ulcer
- Syphilitic ulcer
- Traumatic ulcer
- Chemical burns.

Treatment
Once the diagnosis is confirmed, no treatment is required and the lesion heals spontaneously in about 1–3 months time.

INFECTIVE LESIONS (SIALADENITIS)
Bacterial Sialadenitis (Fig. 4.3)
Acute Bacterial Sialadenitis
Acute bacterial sialadenitis is an uncommon disease, which frequently affects the parotid gland. Therefore, the disease can be synonymous to "acute parotitis or acute suppurative parotitis". In some cases, the condition can affect the submandibular salivary gland also.

Causative organisms:
- Acute parotitis is mostly caused by *Streptococcus pyogenes* and *Staphylococcus aureus*.
- Less commonly *Hemophilus* and bacterioid groups may be involved.

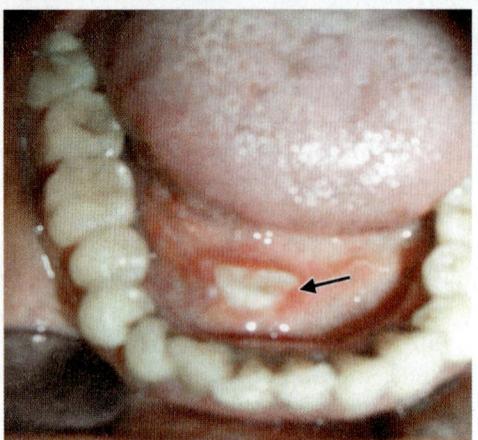

Fig. 4.3: Sialadenitis.

Route of spread of infection: Infection is usually of ascending type and the bacteria reach the gland via the Stensen duct.

Predisposing factors:
- Previous major surgery (especially abdominal surgery)
- Diabetes
- Malignancy
- Prematurely born infants
- Sjögren's syndrome
- Immunocompromised patients.

Clinical features:
- Sudden onset of painful swelling in the pre-auricular region.
- The parotid gland may be involved either unilaterally or bilaterally.
- The constitutional symptoms like fever, malaise, and redness of the skin overlying the parotid are often present.
- Many patients complain of trismus and difficulty in swallowing.
- Intraorally, the parotid papilla may be inflamed and often pus or exudates may be expressed from the duct opening.

Treatment: Drainage and antibiotic therapy, management of pre-existing systemic diseases is essential.

Chronic Bacterial Sialadenitis

Definition: Chronic bacterial sialadenitis is a nonspecific inflammatory disease of the salivary gland secondary to duct obstruction or low-grade sustained ascending infection.

Clinical features:
- The condition occurs in adults as well as in children and it more frequently affects the parotid gland, usually unilaterally.
- Recurrent tendered swelling of the affected gland is a common feature.
- The duct orifice may be inflamed and in case of acute exacerbation, there can be purulent discharge from it.

Recurrent Parotitis

Recurrent parotitis is a rare condition, which affects both children and adults.

Clinical features:
- The condition may occur either unilaterally or bilaterally.
- Recurrent painful swelling of the affected gland.
- Discharge of pus from the duct orifice.
- Several conditions may resolve spontaneously.

IMMUNE-MEDIATED DISEASE

Mikulicz's Disease

Definition

Mikulicz's disease is a progressive autoimmune disease of the salivary gland characterized by replacement of gland acini by dense infiltrates of T lymphocytes along with squamous metaplasia of the ductal epithelium.

It is a localized benign lymphoepithelial lesion, which frequently involves the parotid and lacrimal glands. According to many investigators, the disease is closely related to Sjögren's syndrome.

Etiology

The exact etiology of the disease is not known, some people believe that genetic abnormality or defective cell-mediated immunity probably causes the disease.

Clinical Features

- *Age*: Middle-aged or elderly adults
- *Sex*: Male predilection.

- *Site*: Parotid, submandibular, and lacrimal glands.

Presentation

- There is often unilateral or bilateral diffuse swelling of the involved glands.
- The swelling is soft, movable, and painless. It frequently measures about few centimeters in diameter.
- The disease can be associated with xerostomia, which is sometimes very severe.
- The onset of the disease is often marked with fever, upper respiratory tract infection, and any other oral or orofacial infections, etc.
- Sometimes, Mikulicz's disease can be a manifestation of Sjögren's syndrome or AIDS.
- However, Mikulicz's disease should not be confused with Mikulicz's syndrome, which refers to parotid and lacrimal gland enlargements accompanied by the enlargement of lymph nodes. The Mikulicz's syndrome may represent some generalized specific diseases, e.g. lymphomas or tuberculosis, etc.

Histopathology

- Histologically, Mikulicz's disease is characterized by replacement of the salivary gland acini by benign infiltration of lymphocytes and squamous metaplasia of the ductal epithelium.
- There is presence of several myoepithelial islands or epimyoepithelial islands that represent persisting salivary gland ducts in which the epithelial lining has undergone extensive proliferation.

Treatment

Moderate doses of steroid (20–30 mg prednisolone daily) may help to control the disease.

Sjögren's Syndrome

Definition

Sjögren's syndrome is a multisystem immune-mediated chronic inflammatory disease, characterized by lymphocytic infiltration and acinar destruction of salivary and lacrimal glands, with a marked predilection for women.

Pathogenesis

Although, exact etiopathogenesis of Sjögren's syndrome is not known, it is strongly believed that the disease is an autoimmune disorder. Rheumatoid factors, which are associated with many autoimmune disorders, are frequently present in Sjögren's syndrome. Presence of serum antinuclear antibodies (ANA), e.g. anti-Sjögren's syndrome-A (anti-SSA) and anti-Sjögren's syndrome-B (anti-SSB), also further increases the probability of this disease. Viruses such as Epstein–Barr virus (EBV) or human T-cell lymphotropic virus, may play a pathogenetic role in Sjögren syndrome.

Clinical Features

Incidence rate: Sjögren's syndrome occurs in 0.5–1% of the population.
- *Age*: Middle-aged adults.
- *Sex*: Strong predilection for females (M:F ratio is about 20:80).

Sjögren's syndrome is generally classified into two groups:

Primary Sjögren's syndrome (Box 4.1)
- When the disease affects only salivary and lacrimal glands without other coexisting systemic autoimmune diseases, it is called primary Sjögren's syndrome.
- Primary Sjögren's syndrome is also referred to as "sicca syndrome" in which dry mouth

---

Box 4.1   San Diego Criteria for Sjögren's Syndrome

Primary Sjögren's syndrome
- Symptoms and objectives signs of ocular dryness:
  - Schirmer's test less than 8 mm wetting per 5 minutes
  - Positive Rose Bengal staining of cornea or conjunctiva to demonstrate keratoconjunctivitis sicca.
- Symptoms and objectives signs of dry mouth:
  - Decreased parotid flow rate using Lashley cups or other methods,
  - Abnormal findings from biopsy of minor salivary gland.
- Serologic evidence of a systemic autoimmunity
  - Elevated rheumatoid factor > 1.320.

(xerostomia) and dry eyes (xerophthalmia or keratoconjunctivitis sicca) are the principal features.

Secondary Sjögren's syndrome
Secondary Sjögren's syndrome characteristically have xerostomia, xerophthalmia, and an associated autoimmune connective tissue disease, usually the rheumatoid arthritis. The associated disease could also be any of the following:
- Lupus erythematosus
- Systemic sclerosis
- Primary biliary cirrhosis
- Periarteritis nodosa
- Polymyositis
- Dermatomyositis or macroglobulinemia, etc.

Clinical Presentation (Table 4.2)
- The most common symptoms of Sjögren's syndrome are xerostomia, xerophthalmia, and arthralgia (pain in the joints) (Table 4.2).
- The primary Sjögren's syndrome produces more severe oral and ocular changes than the secondary Sjögren's syndrome.
- Severe tiredness and fatigue are the important features of the disease with depression in few cases and most of the patients may sleep for about 10–15 hours in a day.
- Xerostomia or dryness of mouth often causes soreness of mouth with difficulty in eating, swallowing, and talking, etc.
- The saliva appears frothy and there can be disturbance of taste sensation and associated oral candidiasis. Some patients develop angular cheilitis as well.
- Oral mucosa appears red, dry, tendered, smooth, and glazed and often there is a "parchment-like appearance" of the mucosa.
- Patients often feel difficulty in wearing dentures with increased susceptibility to secondary infections in the oral mucosa.
- Xerostomia and recurrent candidiasis affects the tongue and the dorsum of the tongue reveals red and atrophic mucosa with varying degrees of fissuring and labulations on the surface ("cobble-stone" appearance).
- Moreover, development of rapidly progressive dental caries (typically in the cervical areas of teeth) is also common.
- The "sicca syndrome" (sicca means "dry") produces a gritty, burning sensation in the eye. Patients may feel like there is a foreign body inside the eye, which is causing blurred vision and itching pain in the eye.
- In case of Sjögren's syndrome, parotid glands are persistently enlarged, often

Table 4.2: List of general signs and symptoms in Sjögren's syndrome.

Eye	• Conjunctivitis • Dry eyes • Corneal ulceration
Oral	• Xerostomia • Burning mouth • High caries index • Oral ulcerations • Difficulty in chewing and speech • Disturbed taste sensations • Candidiasis
Neurological (central)	• Poor concentration • Brain fog
Neurological (peripheral)	Neuropathy (numbness and tingling of extremities)
Skin	• Dry skin, vasculitis • Raynaud's phenomenon
Digestive system	• Stomach upset • Gastroparesis • Autoimmune pancreatitis
Throat	• Dysphagia • Heartburn • Reflux esophagitis
Respiratory	• Recurrent bronchitis • Pneumonia
Muscle and joints	• Arthritis • Muscle pain
Sino nasal system	• Dry nose • Epistaxis • Sinusitis
Hepatic system	• Disturbed liver function • Autoimmune hepatitis • Biliary cirrhosis
Genital	• Dryness of genital mucosa.

bilaterally and the swelling is usually painless.
- However, in case the parotid swelling is due to suppurative parotitis and not Sjögren's syndrome, then the affected gland will be hot on palpation, tendered, and the overlying skin will be red and inflamed.
- Although parotid gland is predominantly affected, sometimes submandibular or minor glands can also be affected.
- Enlargement of lacrimal glands is rare.
- Sjögren's syndrome is associated with an increased risk of development of extrasalivary malignant lymphoma.
- Patients may have dryness of the nasal, pharyngeal, and laryngeal mucosa.

Histopathology

Histologically, Sjögren's syndrome reveals the following features (Figs. 4.4 and 4.5):
- Initially, there is infiltration of lymphocytes in the intralobular ducts of the involved salivary gland, which gradually replaces the entire lobule.
- The infiltration is accompanied by atrophy of the salivary gland acini and proliferation of the ductal epithelial cells.
- The hyperplasia of the ductal epithelium eventually obliterates the ductal lumen and this leads to the formation of discrete islands of epithelial tissue, which are known as the myoepithelial islands.
- In the fully developed lesions, the entire glandular tissue is replaced by multiple myoepithelial islands, which are surrounded by proliferating lymphoid tissue.

Investigations in Sjögren's Syndrome

- *Biopsy*: Labial salivary gland biopsy is a helpful investigative method in establishing the diagnosis of Sjögren's syndrome.
- *Sialography*: In Sjögren's syndrome, sialography often produces a "snow-storm" or "cherry tree in blossom"-like appearance.
- *Scintigraphy*: Salivary scintiscanning using [Tc-pertechnetate] reveals reduced uptake of the isotope in Sjögren's syndrome. Although the normal salivary gland tissue usually shows an increased uptake of the said isotope.
- *Staining*: The keratoconjunctivitis sicca is characterized by corneal keratotic lesions, which stain pink when "rose bengal" dye is used (Rose bengal is a sodium salt containing stain, which is commonly used in eye drops to stain damaged conjunctival and corneal cells).

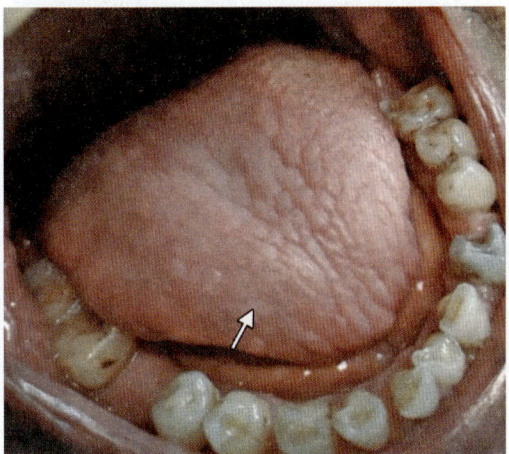

Fig. 4.4: Sjögren's syndrome showing dry mouth and "cobble stone" appearance of tongue

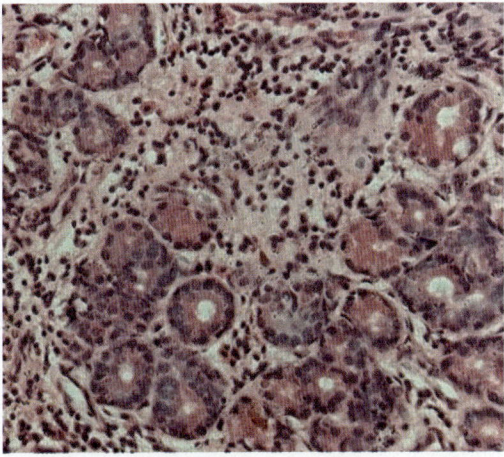

Fig. 4.5: Photomicrograph of Sjögren's syndrome: showing autoimmune damage to salivary gland tissue with metaplasia of ductal epithelium.

- *Schirmer test*: The reduced lacrimal flow rate in Sjögren's syndrome is measured by this test. A strip of filter paper is placed in between the eye and the eyelid to determine the degree of tearing, which should be measured in millimeter. When the flow is reduced to less than 5 mm in a 5-minute sample period, the patient should be considered positive for Sjögren's syndrome.

Key Points of Sjögren's Syndrome

- Sjögren's syndrome is a multisystem immune-mediated chronic inflammatory disease of the salivary and lacrimal glands which predominantly affects women.
- The disease occurs in two forms—primary and secondary:
  - When the disease affects only salivary and lacrimal glands without other coexisting systemic autoimmune diseases, it is called primary Sjögren's syndrome.
  - Secondary Sjögren's syndrome affects salivary and lacrimal glands and it is also characteristically associated with autoimmune connective tissue disease, usually the rheumatoid arthritis.
- Although, exact etiopathogenesis of Sjögren's syndrome is not known, it is strongly believed that the disease is an *autoimmune* disorder.
- Primary Sjögren's syndrome is also referred to as "*sicca syndrome*" in which dry mouth (xerostomia) and dry eyes (xerophthalmia or keratoconjunctivitis sicca) are the principal features.
- Severe tiredness and fatigue are the important features of the disease with depression.
- Secondary Sjögren's syndrome has all the above features and in addition has rheumatic arthritis and systemic lupus erythematosus (SLE), etc. the former disease causes severe joint pain.
- Histologically the disease is characterized by lymphocytic infiltration and acinar destruction of salivary and lacrimal glands.

Specific laboratory tests:
- Raised ESR
- Diminished total salivary flow rate
- Hypergammaglobulinemia—elevated levels of certain immunoglobuline in blood serum.
- Positive serologic test for rheumatoid factors.
- *Immunohistochemistry* detects the presence of antinuclear antibodies ANA (anti-SSA and anti-SSB) in the serum of large number of patients.

Treatment

- Use of artificial saliva
- Use of systemic steroids
- Antibiotic eye drops
- Antifungal drugs to treat secondary candidiasis.

Prognosis

Patients with Sjögren's syndrome have a lifetime risk for lymphoma of 5–15%.

MISCELLANEOUS DISORDERS OF SALIVARY GLAND

Heerfordt's Syndrome

The Heerfordt's syndrome or uveoparotitis is a rare syndrome and is characterized by the following features:
- Swelling of the parotid gland
- Fever
- Paralysis of the facial nerve.

Sialosis

Definition

Sialosis or sialadenosis is a condition characterized by bilateral, recurrent, noninflammatory, non-neoplastic swelling of the salivary glands.

Etiology

Sialosis occurs probably due to the following reasons:
- Disturbance in the neurosecretory control
- Hormonal disturbance such as thyroid insufficiency
- Administration of certain sympathomimetic drugs
- Malnutrition
- Liver cirrhosis or chronic alcoholism
- Mucoviscidosis
- Diabetes mellitus
- Bulimia
- Pregnancy
- Idiopathic.

Clinical Features

- It frequently affects the parotid and occasionally the submandibular salivary gland.

Diseases of the Salivary Glands

- The swelling may cause little pain and discomfort. However, in some cases the condition may produce severe pain.

Histopathology
- Hypertrophy of the serous acinar cells, which may be up to twice the normal size.
- The cytoplasm may be packed with secretory granules.
- Edema of the interstitial connective tissue.
- Lipomatosis may occur in the gland.

Treatment
No treatment is generally required. Elimination of the causative systematic factors is usually enough. However, in case of severe pain in the affected gland, surgical excision of the gland may be necessary.

Ptyalism (Excessive Salivation)

Definition
Ptyalism is an abnormal condition characterized by increased secretion of saliva in the mouth.

Etiology of Ptyalism (Hypersecretion of Saliva)
- Metal poisoning
- Abnormal neurosecretory stimulation.
- Acute necrotizing ulcerative gingivitis
- General stomatitis
- Aphthous ulcer
- Psychological factor
- Following oral examination procedure
- Major surgery in the oral cavity
- Improper swallowing due to any cause
- Insertion of new prosthesis in the mouth
- Idiopathic

Aptyalism (Xerostomia or Dry Mouth)

Aptyalism is the pathological condition characterized by a decrease or complete cessation of secretion of saliva, causing dryness of mouth (Tables 4.3 and 4.4).

Common Effects of Xerostomia
In xerostomia, several oral diseases develop due to the following reasons:

Table 4.3: Causes of xerostomia.

Temporary causes	• Playing or outdoor activity for long time on a hot day • Psychological disorders, e.g. anxiety and depression • Consumption of alcohol and smoking • Sialadenitis • Medications like—atropine, antihistaminics, bronchodilators, diuretics, and antidepressants • Impaired fluid intake • Dehydration due to diarrhea or vomiting and hemorrhage • Lack of mastication • Mouth breathing
Permanent causes	• Aplasia of salivary glands (hereditary ectodermal dysplasia) • Artesia of salivary glands • Radiotherapy in the head or neck region (destruction of gland acini and reduced vascularity) • Sjögren's syndrome • Diabetes mellitus and diabetes insipidus • Vitamin deficiency (A and B complex) • Sarcoidosis, HIV-associated salivary gland disease, amyloidosis • Pernicious and iron deficiency anemia • Graft-versus-host reaction • Parkinson's disease • Defective secretomotor stimulations and aging

Table 4.4: Common medications causing xerostomia.

• Anticholinergics • Antihistaminics • Antipsychotic drugs • Antihypertensives • Antidepressants	• Atropine • Scopolamine • Diphenhydramine • Chlorpheniramine • Phenothiazine derivatives • Haloperidol • Reserpine • Methyldopa • Chlorothiazide • Furosemide • Calcium channel blockers • Amitriptyline

1. Decreased oral pH with increased accumulation of plaque.
2. Increased trauma and irritation due to dryness of mucosa.

3. Decreased remineralization of tooth enamel by saliva.
4. Increased periodontal diseases.
5. Increased susceptibility to opportunistic infections in mouth.

Clinical Features of Xerostomia

- *General symptoms*:
  - Soreness, burning or pain sensations in the mouth.
  - Difficulty in taking foods (especially dry and crispy foods, e.g. cereals and crackers) as it causes irritation and burning sensation.
- *Problems in oral mucosa*:
  - Erythematous changes in the oral mucosa
  - Cracking, fissuring and occasional ulceration of mucosa
  - Candidiasis
  - Red spots over the mucosal surfaces of tongue, hard and soft palate
- *Tongue problems*:
  - Due to dry sticky oral mucosa, tongue always sticks to the palate.
  - Atrophy of the tongue papilla with cracking, fissuring, and occasional ulceration of the surface.
- *Symptoms in lips*:
  - "Lipstick sign" is positive for women (lipstick always sticks to the upper front teeth).
  - Inflammation and fissuring of the lips (chelitis).
- *Throat problems*:
  - Constant sore throat and there is difficulty in swallowing.
  - Hoarseness of voice and speech difficulty.
- *Change in saliva and salivary gland*:
  - Parotid swelling with sialadenitis
  - Little or no pool of saliva in the floor of the mouth.
  - Whatever saliva is present it looks stringy, ropy or foamy.
- *Tooth and gum problems*:
  - Increase in the incidence of dental caries due to lack of protective action of saliva.
  - Increased incidences of periodontal disease with gum bleeding.
  - Early tooth loss in adults.
  - Difficulty in wearing artificial prosthesis.
- *Miscellaneous problems*:
  - Taste disorder (dysgeusia) and burning tongue (glossodynia).
  - Increased need to drink water especially at night.
  - Difficulty in maintaining proper oral hygiene and persistent halitosis.
  - Dry nasal passage.

Diagnosis of Xerostomia

- Patients history.
- Clinical features in the mouth.
- Sialometry—detects the salivary flow rate; salivary flow rate can be increased by giving the patient some citrus materials to chew. Generally the resting or unstimulated salivary flow rate is about—0.3–0.5 mL/minute, while the stimulated salivary flow rate is about 1–2 mL/minute, values below 0.1 mL/minute are considered xerostomia.
- Sialography—imaging techniques to detect stones or other mass inside the gland.
- Salivary scintigraphy—helps in assessing salivary gland function.
- Biopsy—helps to detect cellular changes in the gland.

Treatment

- Removal of local or systemic causes
- Frequent sipping of sugarless fluids
- Chewing xylitol containing gums
- Regular use of artificial saliva (carboxymethyl cellulose containing saliva)
- Antifungal drugs
- Avoidance of antihistaminic and decongestant drugs.

NEOPLASM OF THE SALIVARY GLANDS

The salivary gland neoplasms are relatively uncommon entities and they comprise about 3% of all neoplastic disorders of the human body. These neoplasms may be derived from salivary epithelium (parenchymal) or the supportive connective tissues stroma (mesenchymal).

The epithelial tissue neoplasms are more prevalent among adults whereas the mesenchymal tissue neoplasms are more often encountered among children.

The overall incidence rate of salivary gland neoplasms among general population is about 1–3% per 100,000 people. However, the people of Inuit and parts of Scotland exhibit a slight to tenfold increase in the prevalence rate of these lesions (Table 4.5).

About 70% of the neoplasms are derived from the major glands and the rests are developing from the minor glands. Among the major gland neoplasms, 90% occur in the parotid gland and about 10% occur in the submandibular gland, however the sublingual gland lesions are exceptionally rare.

More than 50% of minor salivary gland neoplasms occur in the palate, about 20% lesions develop in the upper lip, and lower lip lesions are rare. Malignant variety of salivary gland neoplasms occur far more frequently in relation to the minor glands.

On rare occasion, salivary gland neoplasms may occur as central jaw lesions (mainly in relation to mandible) and in such cases, the neoplasms can be derived from either the ectopic entrapped salivary glands or from mucous metaplasia in the lining of the odontogenic jaw cyst (Table 4.6).

Pleomorphic Adenoma

Definition

Pleomorphic adenoma or benign mixed tumor is the most common neoplasm of the salivary glands, which is histologically characterized by complex intermingling of epithelial components and the mesenchymal areas. The neoplastic cells exhibit differentiation of epithelial cells (luminal), myoepithelial cells (albuminal) as well as a very characteristic stromal tissue comprising of chondroid, myxoid, osseous, and myxochondroid elements.

The complexity and diversity of appearance of this neoplasm account for the term "pleomorphic", however the term does not imply cellular pleomorphism.

Origin

According to the multicellular theory, these tumors originate from intercalated duct cells and myoepithelial cells of the salivary glands. There is molecular evidence using human androgen receptor gene (HUMARA) that the epithelial and stromal cells in pleomorphic adenoma arise from the same origin.

Table 4.5: Genetic abnormalities in different salivary gland neoplasms.

Neoplasm	Underlying genetic defect
Pleomorphic adenoma	*PLAG-1* and *HMGI-C* genes Chromosomes 3p21, 8q12 and 12q13-15 rearrangements
Mucoepidermoid tumor and adenocarcinoma	Over-expression of *HER-2* gene
Adenoid cystic carcinoma and Carcinoma ex pleomorphic adenoma	Molecular alterations in 12q, 6q, and 8q
Warthin's tumor and mucoepidermoid tumor	Translocations of chromosomes 11q21 and 19p13

Table 4.6: Relative frequency of benign and malignant tumors in different salivary glands.

Gland type	Overall incidence of tumors	Benign tumors	Malignant tumors
Parotid gland	Above 80%	80%	20%
Submandibular gland	Only 15%	50%	50%
Sublingual and minor glands	Only 5%	30%	70%

Hubner and his associates have postulated that the myoepithelial cell is responsible for the morphologic diversity of the tumor, including the production of the fibrous, mucinous, chondroid, and osseous areas.

Regezi and Batsakis postulates that the intercalated duct reserve cell can differentiate into ductal and myoepithelial cells and the latter, in turn, can undergo mesenchymal metaplasia, since they inherently have smooth muscle like properties.

Clinical Features

- *Age*: Pleomorphic adenomas can occur at any age but they develop more frequently in the 5th and 6th decade of life (mean age is 40 years), 10% cases occur in children.
- *Sex*: More common among females than males (60:40).
- *Site*: It accounts for 60–65% of all neoplasms of the parotid, 50% of submandibular, and 25% of sublingual gland. Approximately 45% of minor gland lesions are pleomorphic adenomas and intraorally palate (posterolateral aspect) is the most frequent site for their development (55% intraseally). Minor gland neoplasms may also occur in upper lip (25%) and cheek (10%) and 10% lesions occur in other oropharyngeal sites.

Parotid tumors usually arise within the superficial lobe, especially its lower pole, but 10% may occur in the deep lobe or from an accessory parotid gland.

Pleomorphic adenomas may also arise from the heterotopic salivary gland tissue in cervical lymph node; soft tissue of the neck, upper and lower limbs, axilla, and trunk; mandible; lung; breast, lacrimal gland, ear and mediastinum, etc.

Pleomorphic adenomas are the most common salivary tumors showing metachronous or synchronous association with other salivary neoplasms, especially with Warthin's tumors, in the same or other glands.

Clinical Presentation (Figs. 4.6 and 4.7)

- Pleomorphic adenoma usually produces a slow growing, painless, well-delineated,

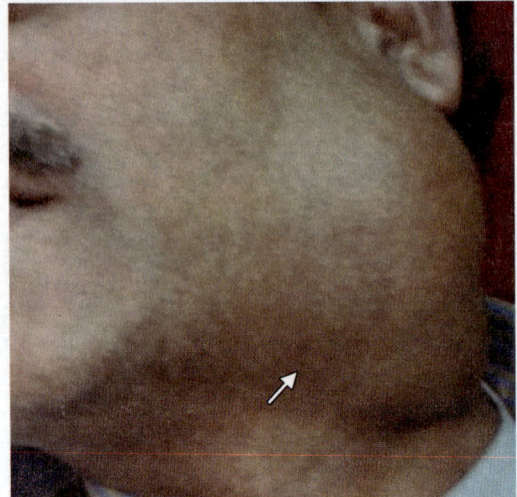

Fig. 4.6: Pleomorphic adenoma of the parotid gland.

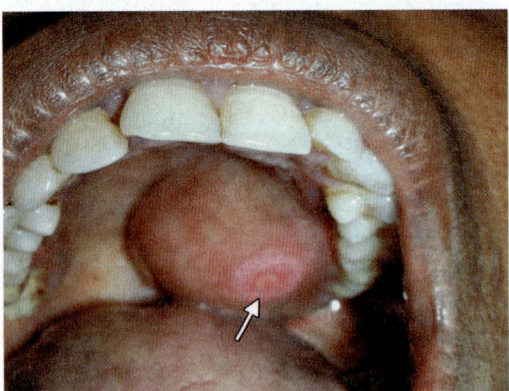

Fig. 4.7: Pleomorphic adenoma of minor salivary glands of palate.

and nodular exophytic growth of the affected salivary gland.
- These lesions take several years to grow to a size of 1 inch in diameter.
- The neoplasm is usually solitary but sometimes there can be multiple lesions (multinodular) especially in case of recurrent lesions.
- The surface of the lesion is mostly nonulcerated, smooth and lobulated, and generally there is no pain.
- Anesthesia or paresthesia of the facial nerve in benign pleomorphic adenomas is rare.

- The neoplasm is usually soft or rubbery in consistency and since it is not fixed to the overlying or the underlying tissues the tumor is always freely movable. However, the larger tumors are relatively less movable as compared to the smaller lesions.
- Some lesions can be present for many years and assume massive size and the overlying skin or mucosa is generally intact.
- The parotid gland lesions are usually superficial and often arise in the superficial lobe as a small mass overlying the angle of mandible or anterior to the external ear.
- Neoplasms arising from the deep lobe of parotid may not always be detected as a facial mass, since these may protrude into the lateral wall of the oropharynx.
- Sometimes the lesion can be multinodular and they can assume an enormous size, especially the longstanding lesions.
- The minor gland neoplasms in the oral cavity frequently exhibit smooth surfaced, soft or slightly firm, dome-shaped nodular swellings on the hard or soft palate without any ulceration on the surface.
- The junction of the hard and soft palate unilaterally is the most common site, and here the tumors are often fixed to the underlying mucoperiosteum.
- The palatal neoplasms are usually firm in consistency and are less movable due to the tough nature of the palatal mucosa, these lesions sometimes exhibit surface ulceration especially when traumatized.
- Large intraoral lesions are often associated with disturbance in speech and mastication, etc.
- In the buccal mucosa or the lip, pleomorphic adenoma presents small, painless, well-defined, and movable nodular lesion with intact overlying mucosa.
- Malignant transformation is uncommon in pleomorphic adenomas but may occur on rare occasions.

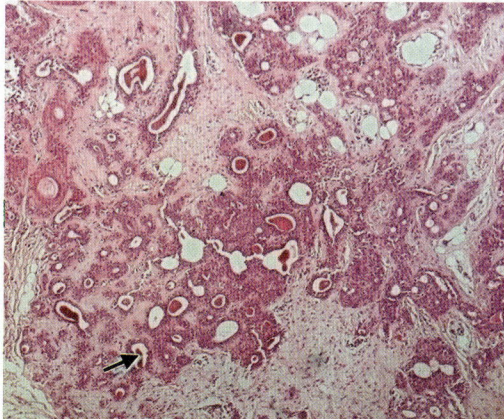

Fig. 4.8: Photomicrograph of Pleomorphic adenoma showing ductal proliferation and stroma

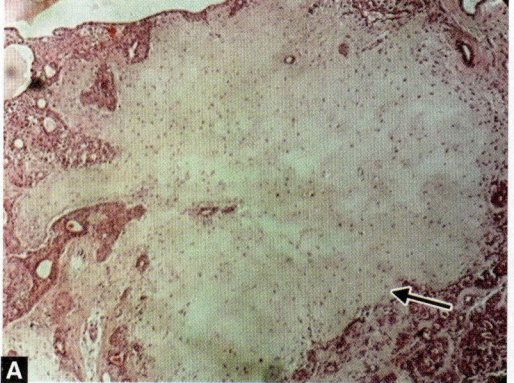
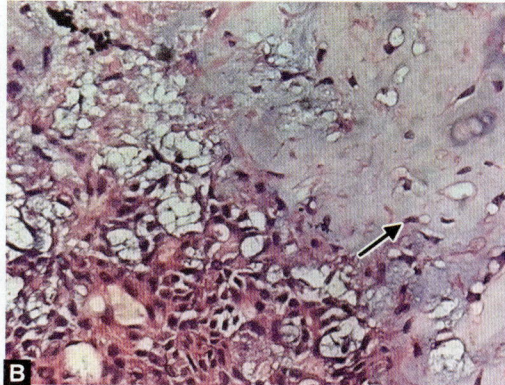

Figs. 4.9A and B: (A) Photomicrograph of pleomorphic adenoma (high power); (B) Myxochondroid stroma of the tumor.

Macroscopic Findings

- Macroscopically, pleomorphic adenoma appears as a well-circumscribed, lobulated, globular mass, which is surrounded by a capsule of variable thickness or completeness.
- On palpation, these lesions feel like rubbery, resilient masses with bosselated surface.
- The cut surface shows a variegated appearance with presence of few hemorrhagic or cystic areas. The tumor sometimes causes compression of the surrounding capsule.
- Isolated nodules of the neoplasm may sometimes be seen within or even outside the capsule.

Histopathology (Figs. 4.8 and 4.9)

- The microscopic appearance of pleomorphic adenoma is highly variable because of the diverse (pleomorphic) nature of the epithelial and the mesenchymal tissue components of the neoplasm.
- The neoplasm often exhibits proliferation of well-differentiated glandular, basophilic epithelial cells in the form of diffuse sheets or cords, ducts or clusters, etc.
- The neoplastic epithelial cells are polygonal, spindle or stellate-shaped and they have a tendency to form duct-like structures.
- The most common microscopic feature is the presence of several duct-like structures of varying size, shape, and number widely distributed within the lesions.
- Histologically, each duct-like structure exhibits an inner row of cuboidal or columnar cells and an outer row of spindle-shaped myoepithelial cells. At the center of each duct-like structure, there is often presence of either clear or brightly eosinophilic, PAS-positive material (epithelial mucin).
- The myoepithelial cells of the tumor often appear cuboidal, flattened or spindle-shaped; they gradually merge into the surrounding connective tissue stroma. Moreover, these cells sometimes constitute the bulk of the neoplastic tissues and in such cases the neoplasm may have a "fibroma-like" appearance.
- Neoplastic myoepithelial cells sometimes proliferate to form a thick, ill-defined sheath around the salivary gland ducts or in other cases these cells become swollen or hydropic to, appear cartilage-like cells (chondroid change).
- In some lesions of pleomorphic adenoma, the epithelial cells may be ovoid-shaped, having concentric nuclei and abundant hyaline cytoplasm; these cells often produce a plasmacytoid appearance in the neoplasm.
- The ductal epithelial cells in pleomorphic adenoma often show "squamous metaplasia" and sometimes there may be even formation of keratin pearls by these metaplastic epithelial cells (Fig. 4.10).
- The connective tissue is often made up of loose, chondromyxoid, hyalinized stroma, which often characteristically exhibits metaplastic changes that result in the formation of mucoid, myxoid, chondroid, and even osseous tissues. The mitotic activity is rare in the tumor cells.
- Such diverse variety of mesenchymal tissues is formed within the tumor due to the pluripotential nature of the myoepithelial cells.

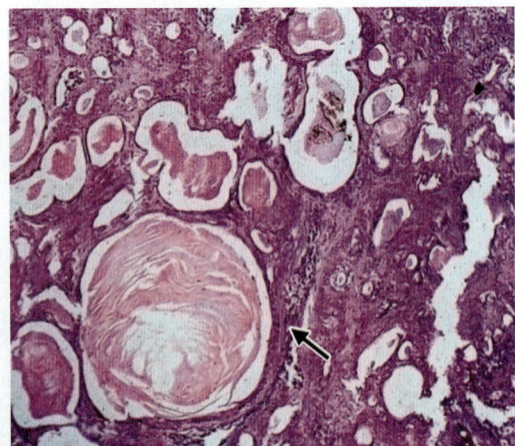

Fig. 4.10: Photomicrograph of pleomorphic adenoma. showing (A) squamous metaplasia of the tumor cells.

Diseases of the Salivary Glands

- The fibrous in nature of the stroma is often consisting of either delicate network or of dense bundles of collagen fibers, which may undergo hyalinization to form a structureless, homogeneous material.
  - In myxoid areas, strands or clumps of epithelial cells are seen widely separated and surrounded by mucoid material.
- Sometimes fibromyxoid appearance of the stroma is seen with abundant elastic tissues.
- The chondroid areas of the stroma exhibit isolated, rounded epithelial cells lying in lacunae within the mucoid material.
- The mucoid materials in myxochondroid areas are composed of glycosaminoglycans and consist mainly of chondroitin sulfates.
- Fat cells are frequently seen in the stroma of pleomorphic adenoma, particularly in minor glands. Tumors that have a lipomatous stromal component of 90% or more have been called "lipomatous" pleomorphic adenoma.
- The presence of capsule is also not a consistent finding in pleomorphic adenoma and sometimes extracapsular stellate cell nests are found.
- Histologically, benign lesions may sometimes cause metastasis and such lesions are known as "metastasizing benign pleomorphic adenomas".
- Malignant transformations can occur (less than 1% cases), usually in neoplasms, which have been present from many years.

Box 4.2	Histological types of pleomorphic adenoma
Foote and Frazell (1954) categorized the tumor into the following types: • Principally myxoid • Myxoid and cellular components present in equal proportion • Predominantly cellular • Extremely cellular.	

Differential Diagnosis

- Polymorphous low grade adenocarcinoma
- Adenoid cystic carcinoma
- Warthin's tumor
- Oncocytoma
- Adenocarcinoma
- Squamous cell carcinoma
- Mucoepidermoid carcinoma
- Fibroma
- Lipoma
- Chondroma
- Myxoma.

Special Investigation

Fine-needle aspiration cytology (FNAC): Aspiration cytology can be helpful in making the diagnosis of pleomorphic adenomas.

MRI: Magnetic resonance imaging is a reliable diagnostic method in determining the extent of the disease present in major glands.

Special stain: Special stains may be used for the detection and differentiation of specific tissue components, e.g. myxoid, osseous or chondroid tissues of the neoplasm.

Immunohistochemistry: Immunohistological analysis may provide important information regarding the biological and histological nature of tissues present in this neoplasm. The luminal cells of pleomorphic adenoma are positive for cytokeratins 3, 6, 10, 11, 13, and 16, whereas the neoplastic myoepithelial cells are irregularly positive for cytokeratins 13, 14, and 16 and pancytokeratin. The neoplastic myoepithelial cells are positive for vimentin.

Treatment

Complete surgical removal of the small lesion is generally curative.

For parotid lesions, surgical excision (lobectomy or gland extirpation) is the frequent choice. Recurrence rate is less than 2%, facial nerve palsy and the auriculotemporal syndrome may be the common complications occurring following surgical intervention in the neoplasms of the parotid gland.

Monomorphic Adenoma

Definition

Monomorphic adenomas are a group of rare benign salivary neoplasms, characterized by proliferation of a single epithelial cell type that has a distinctive architectural pattern.

Monomorphic adenomas do not exhibit the wide cellular diversities, which are normally encountered in pleomorphic adenomas.

Types of Monomorphic Adenomas

- Basal cell adenoma
- Canalicular adenoma
- Sebaceous adenoma
- Glycogen rich adenoma
- Clear cell adenoma.

Among the different types of monomorphic adenomas, basal cell adenoma is the most common type, moreover only the basal cell adenomas and the canalicular adenomas exhibit distinct clinicopathologic characters.

Clinical Features of Different Monomorphic Adenomas

The monomorphic adenomas are generally slow growing, encapsulated lesions, similar to pleomorphic adenomas, however they have a much lower tendency for recurrence after treatment.

Basal Cell Adenoma

- This monomorphic adenoma commonly occurs almost exclusively in adults (mostly in the 6th decade of life) and more frequently seen among females.
- More than 80% lesions arise in the major salivary glands.
- The lesion involves parotid in about 75% cases, where it develops mostly from the superficial lobe.
- Twenty percent of the lesions are seen in the oral cavity and intraoral lesions commonly arise from the upper lip and buccal mucosa (Fig. 4.11).
- Clinically, basal cell adenomas present slow enlarging, firm, encapsulated, and freely movable lesions and they usually measure less than 3 cm in maximum diameter.
- On palpation, these lesions are firmer than pleomorphic adenomas and have a smooth surface.

Canalicular Adenoma

- Canalicular adenomas usually occur in the 7th decade of life and are rarely seen among children.
- Like other adenomas, these are also more prevalent among females.
- It occurs almost exclusively in the minor salivary glands.
- Minor salivary glands of the upper lip are the most frequent sites of development of this neoplasm (75% cases), followed by buccal mucosa (25% cases), however involvement of the major gland is rare.
- Canalicular adenomas clinically appear as small, painless, and movable encapsulated lesions being covered by a smooth intact epithelium.
- The color of the overlying mucosa is generally normal, however in some cases the covering epithelium may have a slight bluish tinge and thus it can be mistaken for a mucocele (although, mucoceles are rare in upper lip).
- Capsule may or may not be present and there can be multifocal growth on some occasions.

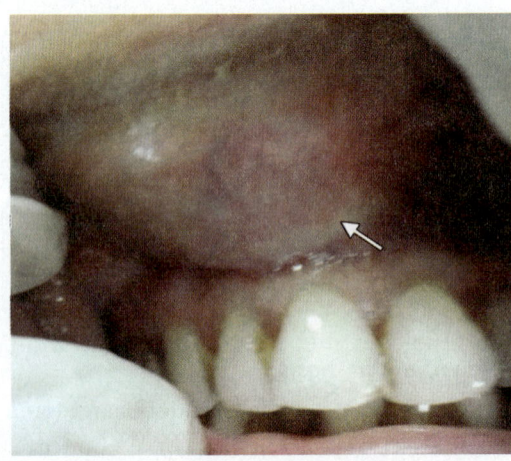

Fig. 4.11: Monomorphic adenomas lip.

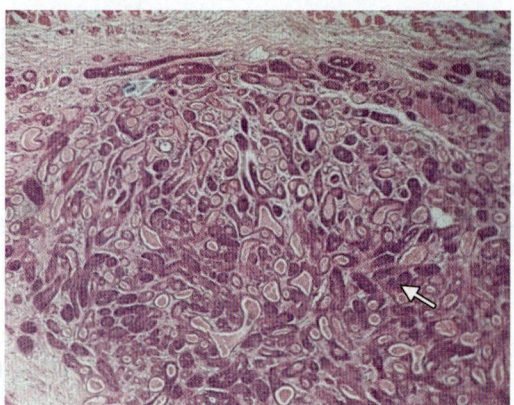

Fig. 4.12: Photomicrograph of basal cell adenoma.

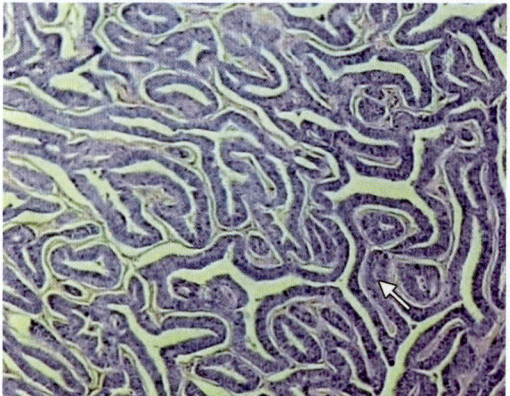

Fig. 4.13: Photomicrograph of monomorphic adenoma (canalicular type).

Histopathology

Basal cell adenoma
- Basal cell adenomas histologically present clusters of proliferating neoplastic glandular epithelial cells in the form of oval-shaped nests (Fig. 4.12).
- The outermost layer of cells, which surround each cell nest are cuboidal type, while the inner core of cells are uniform in size and resemble basal cells of the stratified squamous epithelium.
- The lesion is usually surrounded by a well-defined fibrous capsule.
- The individual, small, well-defined cell nests often resemble basal cell carcinoma of skin.
- In some lesions, there may be proliferation of basaloid cells in diffuse sheets within which keratin pearl formation may be seen.

On the basis of their microscopic appearance, basal cell adenomas are divided into four subtypes—solid type, trabecular type, tubular type, and membranous type.

Solid type: In solid type of basal cell adenoma, the neoplastic cells proliferate in solid sheets.

Trabecular type: This pattern of basal cell adenoma exhibits elongated, anastomosing cords of basal cells, which are surrounded by mature connective tissue stroma.

Tubular type:
- In this pattern, nests of basal cells often surround a duct-like structure.
- The ducts are filled with homogeneous eosinophilic material and are lined by cuboidal epithelial cells.

Membranous type: This type of basal cell adenomas exhibit islands of neoplastic basaloid cells surrounded by a hyalinized basal lamina.

Canalicular adenoma: Canalicular adenomas are histologically characterized by numerous anatomizing networks of cuboidal and columnar cells, which give the impression of multiple, interconnecting canals and hence the term canalicular has been given (Fig. 4.13).

Treatment

Monomorphic adenomas are mostly non-aggressive lesions and are treated by surgical excision along with little bit of surrounding normal tissue. Recurrence is extremely uncommon.

Myoepithelioma

These are rare salivary gland neoplasms and they account for only 1.5% of all salivary gland tumors.

Clinical Features
- *Age*: Mostly occurs in the 5th and 6th decade of life.
- *Sex*: More common in females.
- *Site*: Mostly occurs in relation to parotids (40%) followed by palatal minor glands (21%).

Clinical Presentation

Slow growing, painless mass, the parotid lesions never cause facial nerve palsies and the palatal lesions never ulcerate.

Macroscopic Findings

Myoepitheliomas macroscopically appear as well-circumscribed, frequently encapsulated growths, with features similar to pleomorphic adenomas except the absence of grossly myxoid or chondroid areas. The lesions have solid, tan-yellow, and glistening surface.

Histopathology

Microscopically, myoepitheliomas exhibit three distinct patterns:
1. *Spindle cell pattern*: It is the most common histologic type and consists of proliferating spindle-shaped neoplastic cells having eosinophilic cytoplasms. The neoplastic cells are often arranged in diffuse sheets or in interlacing fascicles. Myoepitheliomas are hypercellular lesions although there is limited mucoid or myxoid stroma present in them.
2. *Plasmacytoid pattern*: Microscopically this pattern reveals group of round cells with eccentric nuclei and eosinophilic cytoplasm. The neoplastic cells proliferate either as closely packed sheets of round cells or in group of cells separated by a loose myxoid stroma.
3. *Combination pattern*: This type exhibits the combined features of both plasmacytoid and solid patterns.

Malignant counterpart of this tumor is known as myoepithelial carcinoma or malignant myoepithelioma; it is a high grade malignancy and often occurs in the preexisting pleomorphic adenomas.

Oncocytoma (Oxyphilic Adenoma)

Definition

Oncocytomas are rare benign salivary gland neoplasms occurring primarily in the parotid and are composed of clusters of large eosinophilic granular cells (oncocytes). Oncocyte is an epithelial cell characterized by an excessive amount of mitochondria resulting in an abundant acidophilic granular cytoplasm.

Clinical Features

- Oncocytoma accounts for about 1% of all the salivary gland neoplasms.
- They usually occur among older individuals, in their 8th decade of life.
- There is definite female predilection.
- Superficial lobe of the parotid is the most favored location. Minor salivary glands are rarely affected.
- Clinically the tumor often produces slow enlarging, painless, uninodular or sometimes multinodular, movable swelling anterior to the ear or over the ramus of the mandible.

Histopathology

- Histologically, oncocytoma exhibits proliferation of numerous polygonal or cuboidal oncocytes, showing prominent eosinophilic and granular cytoplasm with compact nuclei.
- These neoplastic cells are often arranged in organoid or acinar pattern.
- Some oncocytomas exhibit organoid cell clusters, which form solid cords or "doughnut-shaped" cellular configurations.
- The cluster of neoplastic cells stain intensely eosinophilic and are surrounded by a fine vascular stroma.
- The individual neoplastic cell of the cluster exhibits a copious amount of granular cytoplasm with centrally placed small, pyknotic nuclei.
- A malignant variety of this neoplasm is also reported and is called "malignant oncocytoma".

Differential Diagnosis

- Adenolymphoma
- Pleomorphic adenoma
- Enlarged parotid lymph node.

Treatment

Surgical excision by lobectomy.

Warthin's Tumor (Papillary Cystadenoma Lymphomatosum/ Adenolymphoma)

Warthin's tumor is a benign salivary gland neoplasm with limited growth potential. It is primarily occurring in the parotid and is composed of cystic spaces with intraluminar projections lined by double layer of cells. The tumor also contains abundant lymphoid tissue in the stroma.

Warthin's tumor was first reported by Albrecht and Arzt in the year 1910 and later described by Warthin in 1929. It is the second most frequent tumor arising in the parotid gland after pleomorphic adenoma.

Pathogenesis

The pathogenesis of Warthin's tumor is debatable mainly because of the presence of lymphoid tissue components in its stroma. Some investigators propose that the tumor develops as a result of neoplastic proliferation of ectopic salivary gland tissues, which are situated within the intraparotid or paraparotid lymph nodes.

Other investigators believe that neoplastic proliferation of the salivary gland epithelial cells initiates a secondary reactive response in the lymphoid tissue of the stroma.

Clinical Features

- *Age*: The neoplasm is commonly seen among elderly people between the ages of 50 years and 70 years.
- *Sex*: It is more prevalent among males (M:F—5:1).
- *Site*: Warthin's tumor occurs almost exclusively in relation to the parotid gland (mostly tail of the parotid) (Figs. 4.14A and B). It comprises of about 20% of all parotid gland neoplasms. The lesion rarely occurs in other major or minor glands.

Presentation

- Warthin's tumor clinically presents a slow enlarging, well-circumscribed, soft, painless swelling in the parotid gland.
- It is usually well-encapsulated, movable and consistently found over the angle of the mandible in the superficial lobe of parotid.
- The maximum size of the lesion could be up to 2–4 cm in diameter.
- In some cases Warthin's tumor may develop in association with pleomorphic adenomas in the parotid.
- Warthin's tumors produce a compressible and doughy feeling upon palpation and they are usually not fixed to the adjacent tissues.

Macroscopic Appearance

- Cut section of a "fresh" specimen of Warthin's tumor exhibits exudation of

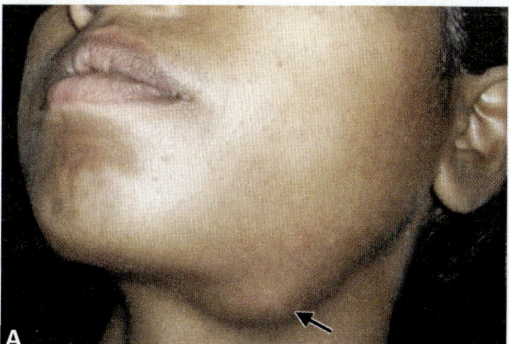 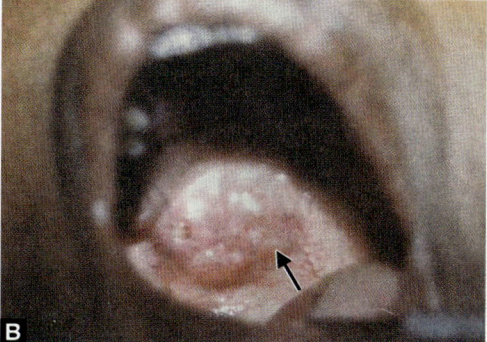

Figs. 4.14A and B: Warthin's tumor of (A) parotid gland; (B) Palate.

watery or sometimes chocolate-colored fluid from the tissue.
- Macroscopically the neoplasm also exhibits multiple confluent cystic spaces and variable amount of lymphoid tissue with follicles.
- A dense fibrous capsule surrounds the neoplasm.

Histopathology (Figs. 4.15 and 4.16)

Microscopically, Warthin's tumor presents the following features:
- There is presence of multiple cystic spaces, which are lined by pseudostratified tall columnar epithelial cells having distinct eosinophilic cytoplasm (columnar oncocytes).
- The epithelial cells are arranged in a double-layered pattern with the nuclei oriented in the basilar area of the bottom row and in the superior aspect of the upper row.
- The inner luminal layer consists of tall columnar cells with centrally placed, palisaded, and slightly hyperchromatic nuclei. Beneath this is a second layer of cuboidal or polygonal cells with more vesicular nuclei.
- The epithelial cells cover papillary folds, which extend into the cystic spaces.
- The papillary folds are supported by large amounts of lymphoid tissue with scattered germinal centers.
- The cystic lumens are often filled with a homogeneous eosinophilic material.
- In some lesions, mucous goblet cells are interspersed within the neoplastic pseudostratified epithelial cells.

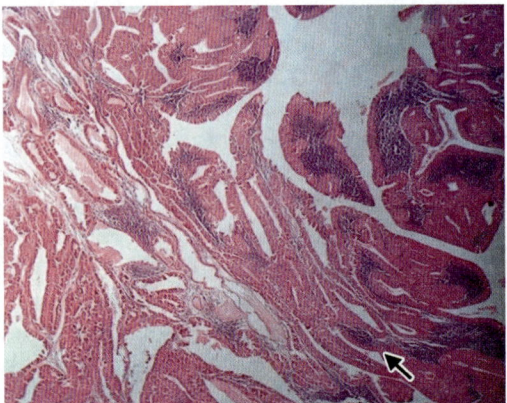

Fig. 4.15: Photomicrograph of Warthin's tumor.

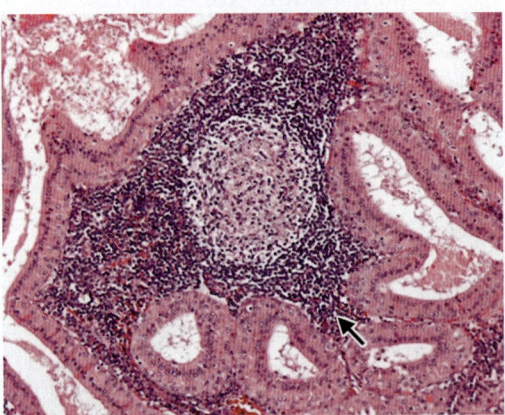

Fig. 4.16: Photomicrograph of Warthin's tumor. Showing lymphoid elements.

Differential Diagnosis

- Pleomorphic adenoma
- Oncocytoma
- Enlarged parotid lymph node
- Mucoepidermoid tumor
- Lipoma
- Mucous retention cyst
- Malignant lymphoma.

Treatment

Simple surgical enucleation.

MALIGNANT SALIVARY GLAND NEOPLASMS

Malignant Pleomorphic Adenoma (Mixed Tumor)

Malignant pleomorphic adenoma (mixed tumor) is a relatively uncommon malignant tumor of salivary gland and it accounts for 3% of all salivary glands tumors.

Malignant mixed tumors are broadly divided into two groups:
1. Carcinoma ex-pleomorphic adenoma
2. De-novo type.

Carcinoma ex-pleomorphic adenoma: This lesion is developing as a result of malignant transformation in a preexisting benign pleomorphic adenoma (occurs in about 2–7% cases). Diagnosis requires the identification of benign tumor in the tissue sample.

- It is ranked as 6th most common malignant salivary gland tumor after mucoepidermoid carcinoma, adenocarcinoma, acinic cell carcinoma, polymorphous low grade adenocarcinoma, and adenoid cystic carcinoma.
- **Based on the pattern of growth, carcinoma ex-pleomorphic adenoma can be divided into three subcategories:**
  - *Invasive*: Shows malignant cells penetrating greater than 1.5 mm from the tumor capsule into adjacent tissue.
  - *Minimally invasive*: Show extracapsular invasion that measures 1.5 mm or less.
  - *Noninvasive*: Discovered as a small malignant focus within the center of an encapsulated pleomorphic adenoma but without violation of the tumor capsule.
  - *De-novo type*: A tumor in the salivary gland, which is malignant from the very beginning. The latter type often shows malignant change in both the epithelium and the connective tissue components of the salivary gland, and therefore it is called "carcinosarcoma". These lesions carry a much poorer prognosis than the other.
    - The carcinosarcoma is a biphasic tumor.
    - It demonstrates both carcinomatous and sarcomatous areas.

Clinical Features (Figs. 4.17 and to 4.18)

- Malignant mixed tumor usually occurs at the age of around 60 years and it most frequently involves the parotid. Besides that submandibular, sublingual, and minor gland of the palate, lips paranasal sinuses and nasopharynx may be affected.
- The tumor occurs more frequently among males.
- Majority of the patients have a benign mixed tumor for about 15–20 years and that few of them may undergo malignant transformation.
- In case of *de novo* lesions, small innocuous looking tumor may eventually show severe malignant change.

Symptoms Indicating Malignant Transformation in a Preexisting Pleomorphic Adenoma

- Very rapid growth in the recent time, within 3–6 months
- Severe pain

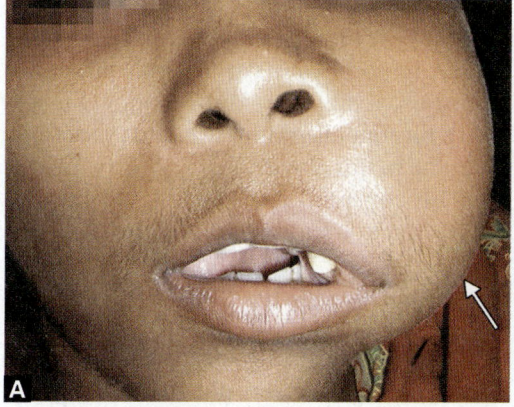 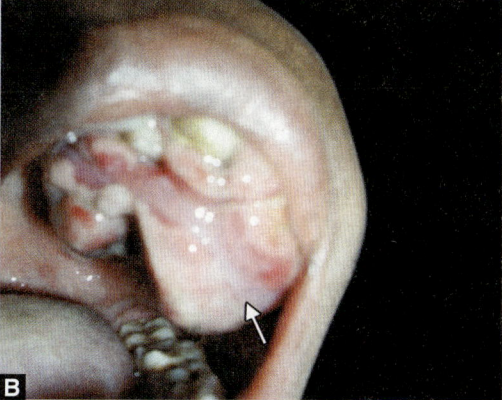

Figs. 4.17A and B: Malignant mixed tumor of palate.

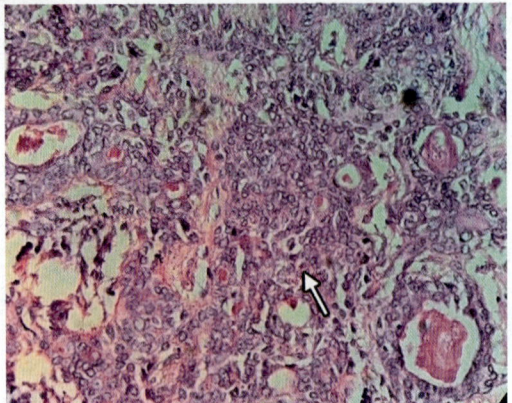

Fig. 4.18: Photomicrograph of malignant mixed tumor (high power).

- Anesthesia or paresthesia of the facial nerve
- Fixation of the tumor to the overlying skin or underlying muscle or bone
- Non-healing ulcer on the overlying skin and mucous membrane
- Hemorrhage
- Regional lymphadenopathy
- Secondary candidal infection on the superficial ulcerated surface.

HISTOPATHOLOGY

- Microscopically, bulk of the tumor appears benign, but there are small areas of cytologically altered malignant glandular epithelial cells found within the lesion.
- These malignant cells often cause invasion into the surrounding normal tissue.
- Malignant transformation in a benign tumor results in the development of adenocarcinoma, undifferentiated carcinoma or epidermoid carcinoma, etc.
- During histopathological evaluation in a suspected malignant mixed tumor, the following histological changes should be checked cautiously:
  - Destructive infiltrative growth pattern
  - Marked cytologic atypia with abnormal mitotic activity
  - Cellular pleomorphism and nuclear hyperchromatism
  - Areas of micronecrosis
  - Hemorrhage
  - Excessive hyalinization
  - Dystrophic calcification
  - Vascular permeation or perineural invasion.
- Malignant mixed tumor, the entity should only be recognized if there is histological evidence of benign pleomorphic adenoma tissues in the lesions.

Treatment

Extensive surgery followed by radiotherapy and chemotherapy. Prognosis is mostly poor.
- 5-year survival rate is—55% approximately
- 10-year survival rate is—30% approximately.

Adenoid Cystic Carcinoma (Cylindroma)

Adenoid cystic carcinoma is a malignant neoplasm arising from the glandular epithelium of either major or minor salivary glands. It has profound tendency to invade into the perineural lymphatic spaces.

The cylindromas were first reported by Bilroth in 1856, Spies first used the term adenoid cystic carcinoma in 1930.

Clinical Features

Incidence: Adenoid cystic carcinoma accounts for about 6% of all parotid tumors and 30% of minor salivary gland tumors.
Age: The tumor frequently occurs at the age of 50–70 years.
Sex: Slightly more prevalent among females.
Site: Adenoid cystic carcinomas affect both major as well as the minor glands, however these tumors affect minor glands more often than the major glands.

The common sites for development of this lesion in minor glands are the palate and tongue.

In the major gland category, it cylindroma, although it also frequently affects parotid.

Besides this, the lesions also develop from the lacrimal glands, esophagus, and glands of the paranasal sinuses, etc.

Diseases of the Salivary Glands

Presentation (Figs. 4.19 and 4.20)

- The lesion often produces a relatively slow enlarging growth, with frequent surface ulcerations.
- Parotid tumors produce asymptomatic subcutaneous mass anterior to or below the external ear.
- Since this tumor has a propensity to surround nerve trunk, parotid lesions often surround and invade the facial nerve sheath. Besides facial nerve, adenoid cystic carcinomas frequently invade the lingual and the hypoglossal nerves.
- Pain is very common feature in this tumor and severe neurological signs like anesthesia, paresthesia or palsy frequently develop.
- Often there is fixation and induration of the tumor to the underlying structures along with local invasion.
- Submandibular gland tumors become quite large before patients notice it.
- Palatal lesions are often accompanied by toothache, loosening of teeth, and delayed healing of the socket in case the tooth is extracted.
- Tumor developing in association with minor glands of palate produces a nodular growth, resembling an eccentric node with an ulcerated surface.
- Palatal paresthesia may be present due to involvement of greater palatine nerve.
- Extensive bone involvement may occur in few cases.

Histopathology (Figs. 4.21 to 4.25)

- The adenoid cystic carcinoma is composed of a mixture of myoepithelial cells and ductal

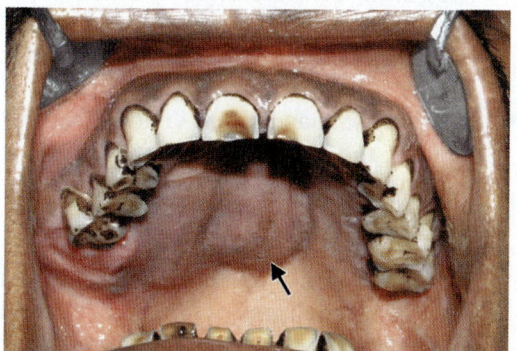

Fig. 4.19: Adenoid cystic carcinoma of palate.

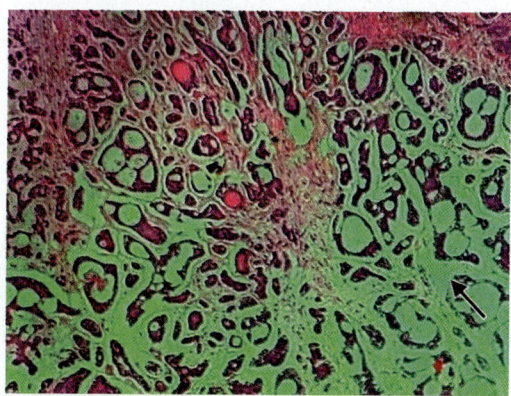

Fig. 4.21: Photomicrograph of typical adenoid cystic carcinoma.

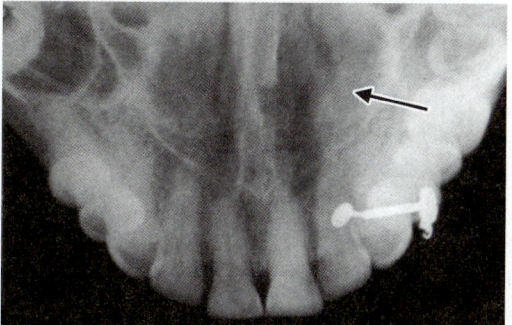

Fig. 4.20: Adenoid cystic carcinoma causing destruction of palate.

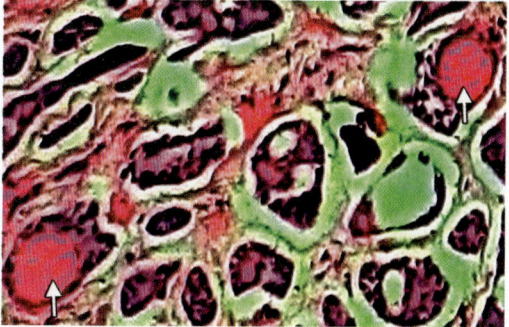

Fig. 4.22: Photomicrograph showing "swiss-cheese" pattern in adenoid cystic carcinoma.

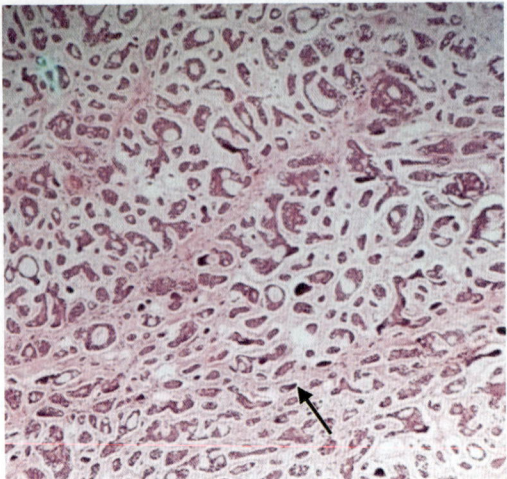

Fig. 4.23: Photomicrograph of adenoid cystic carcinoma showing cribriform pattern.

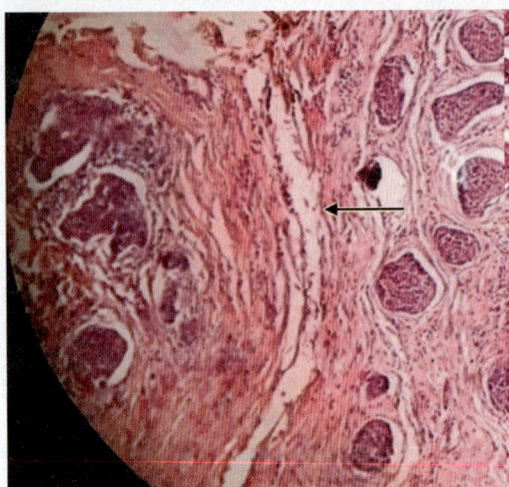

Fig. 4.25: Adenoid cystic carcinoma showing perineural invasion.

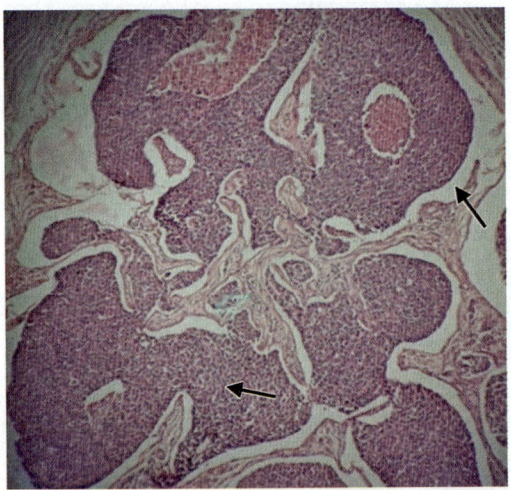

Fig. 4.24: Photomicrograph of adenoid cystic carcinoma showing a solid pattern.

cells that can have a varied arrangement; histologically it is characterized by the presence of numerous small, darkly staining, polygonal or cuboidal cells of uniform size.
- These cells often resemble basal cells of the oral epithelium and they have hyperchromatic nuclei and minimum mitotic activity.
- Double layer of tumor cells are often arranged in a duct-like or "cylinder-like"

pattern that contains an eosinophilic coagulum at the center and this often gives rise to a classic "Swiss-cheese" appearance of the adenoid cystic carcinoma.
- Microcystic spaces often divide the gland lobules; the tumor cells which are lining the microcysts are not well-polarized as seen in case of true ductal cells.
- The stromal connective tissue of the tumor is hyalinized which surrounds and segregates small groups of tumor cells and thus forms the structural pattern of many cylinders (from this the name "cylindroma" has evolved).

Histologically, adenoid cystic carcinomas have three subtypes:
1. Cribriform pattern
2. Solid pattern
3. Tubular pattern.

Cribriform pattern: It is the most classical histologic pattern of adenoid cystic carcinoma. Here the neoplastic epithelial components consist of small, uniform, and polygonal cells with basophilic cytoplasms. This pattern is characterized by proliferating mass of epithelial cells being penetrated by numerous cylindrical spaces and thereby producing a "cribriform" appearance.

Solid pattern: In this pattern, the tumor cells proliferate to form solid masses with areas of central necrosis.

Tubular pattern: In this pattern, the tumor cells exhibit less stratification and they proliferate as small tubular units with a single central lumen.

- Besides these usual patterns, some lesions consist of solid nests of basal cells and resemble basal cell carcinoma or basal cell adenoma.
- Some tumors even show scanty amount of tumor cells being dispersed in an abundant hyalinized stroma. These cells often exhibit hyperchromatism and pleomorphism and an increased mitotic activity.
- *Perineural invasion*: One of the most striking features of adenoid cystic carcinoma is the spread of the tumor cells via the perineural or intraneural spaces. This phenomenon is known as "neurotrophism" and it occurs in about 80% cases of this tumor.
- Besides the perineural invasions, the tumor cells often make intravascular or perivascular invasions in the surrounding tissue, thus distal metastasis occurs via the hematologic spread of the tumor cells to the bone and lung, etc.

Differential Diagnosis

- Pleomorphic adenoma
- Monomorphic adenoma
- Mucoepidermoid carcinoma
- Adenocarcinoma
- Acinic cell tumor
- Basal cell carcinoma.

Treatment

By wide surgical excision. Postsurgical radiotherapy is effective since the tumor cells are radiosensitive. Short-term prognosis is good but long-term prognosis is grave.

Mucoepidermoid Tumor

Mucoepidermoid tumor is an unusual type of malignant salivary gland neoplasm, which

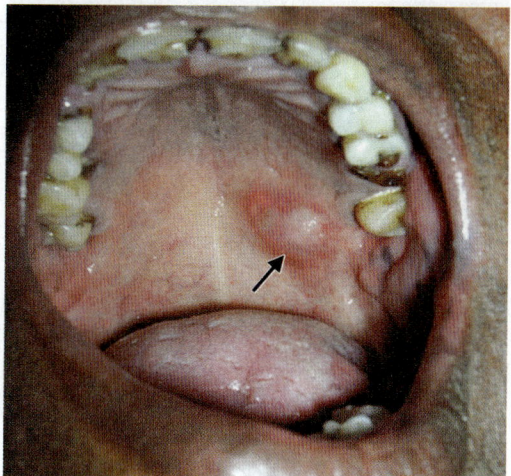

Fig. 4.26: Mucoepidermoid tumor with a typical "cyst-like" appearance and another tumor showing.

exhibits varying degree of aggressiveness. According to the multicellular theory, the mucoepidermoid tumors arise from the excretory duct cells of the salivary gland (Fig. 4.26).

- It is the most common malignant neoplasm observed in the major and minor salivary glands.
- It is the most common malignant salivary gland tumor in children.

Clinical Features

- *Age*: The tumor usually occurs at the age of 30 to 50 years (sometimes in children also).
- *Sex*: There is a slight female predilection.
- *Site*: The tumor frequently involves the parotid and the minor salivary glands of the palate (most common intra-oral site), lips, buccal mucosa, tongue and retromolar areas, etc.

Presentation

- The tumor mostly produces a slow growing and painless swelling that often has a cystic feeling.
- It often clinically resembles the pleomorphic adenoma.
- In many cases, rapid growth of the tumor with pain, hemorrhage, ulceration, and paresthesia, etc. may occur (Fig. 4.27).

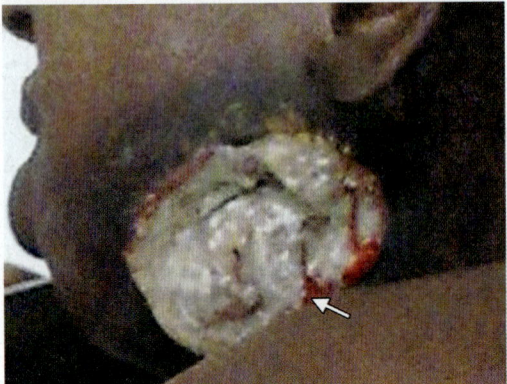

Fig. 4.27: Mucoepidermoid tumor of parotid with large, external ulcer.

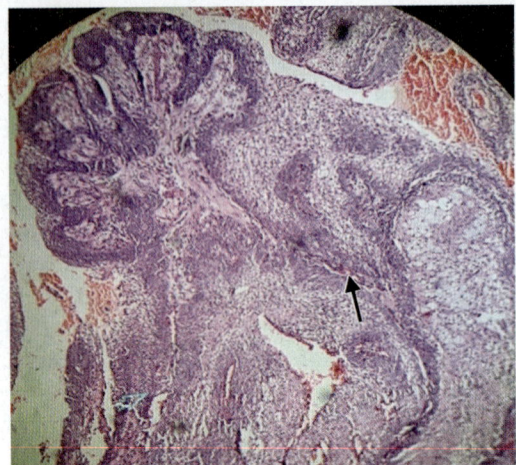

Fig. 4.28: Photomicrograph of mucoepidermoid tumor high power.

- Facial nerve paralysis sometimes occurs in relation to parotid lesions.
- Low-grade tumors are often fluctuant in nature while the high-grade tumors are firm and are fixed to the adjacent tissues.
- Low-grade tumors clinically appear as non-ulcerated, often fluctuant growths with a slight bluish color, these tumors contain several cystic structures and are often confused with mucoceles.
- The tumor of high-grade malignancy grows rapidly and does produce pain as an early symptom. Facial nerve paralysis is frequent in parotid tumors.

Radiographic Features

Mucoepidermoid tumor may also develop as a central jaw lesion especially in mandible and such intraosseous lesions may develop either from the ectopic intra-bony salivary glands or from the metaplastic lining epithelium of the odontogenic cysts. Radiographically, these lesions produce unilocular or multilocular radiolucent areas in the jawbone.

Histopathology (Figs. 4.28 and 4.29)

Histologically this unencapsulated tumor consists of three distinct types of cells: (1) large pale mucous secreting cells, (2) epidermoid cells, and (3) intermediate type of cells (these cells can differentiate into either of the two cells mentioned earlier).

According to the distribution of these cell types, the mucoepidermoid tumor is divided into two grades.

Histopathologic grades of different malignant salivary gland tumors are described in Table 4.7.

Well-Differentiated or Low-Grade Tumor

- This tumor consists mainly of mucous-secreting cells and epidermoid cells with no evidence of cellular pleomorphism.
- Cells of either type may predominate in a mucoepidermoid tumor, if the mucous cells predominate, the tumor tends to become cystic type and if the epidermoid cells predominate then the tumor becomes solid type. The solid tumors are often more aggressive in nature than the cystic type.
- The mucous cells frequently line many "cyst-like" spaces within the tumor in single or double layers.
- The epidermoid cells either line the cysts or they form solid sheets or strands and thereby give the impression of an epidermoid carcinoma, although the keratinization is minimum.
- Discharge of mucous in the cyst causes distension and even rupture of the cyst and this often results in hemorrhage,

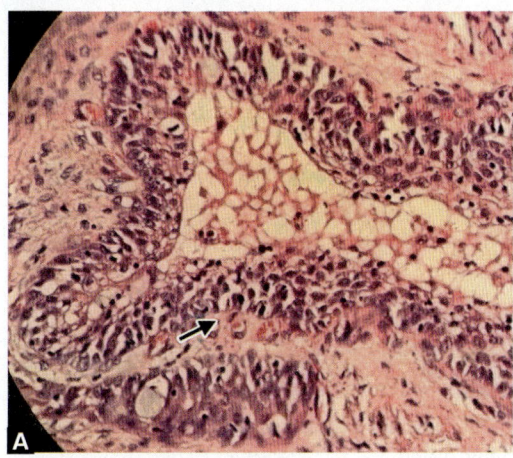 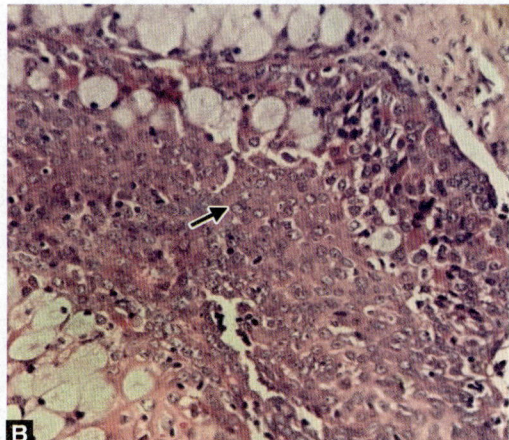

Figs. 4.29A and B: Photomicrograph of mucoepidermoid tumor showing (A) Mucous cells and (B) Epidermoid cell.

inflammation, fibrosis, and foreign body type giant cell reaction in the stroma.
- The tumor islands and the cystic areas are demarcated by a mature fibrous stroma.
- The intermediate cells lack true squamous differentiation and are smaller than the other two types.
- These polygonal cells have dark nuclei and pale eosinophilic cytoplasm. In some cases bone formation is seen in mucoepidermoid tumor.

Intermediate Grade

Tumors have solid areas of epidermoid cells or squamous cells with intermediate basaloid cells. Cyst formation is seen but is less prominent than that observed in low-grade tumors. All cell types are present, but intermediate cells predominate.

Poorly Differentiated or High-Grade Tumor (Figs. 4.30A and B)

- These lesions consist mainly of solid proliferations of epidermoid and intermediate cells; these cells often exhibit cellular pleomorphism, nuclear hyperchromatism, and infiltrative growth into the surrounding tissue and the lymph nodes.
- The low-grade lesions often appear to advance on a broad "pushing front" and these lesions are very aggressive in nature.
- Cystic spaces are not prominent and sometimes it is difficult to distinguish these tumors from the squamous cell carcinomas.
- The cells are often poorly differentiated and they often exhibit highly infiltrative growth.
- A clear cell variant of the mucoepidermoid tumor exists, which often shows sheets of

Table 4.7: "Histopathologic Grades" of different malignant salivary gland tumors.

Tumors	Common grade
Carcinoma ex pleomorphic adenoma	Generally high grade
Adenocarcinoma	Generally high grade
Adenoid cystic carcinoma	Generally high grade
High-grade mucoepidermoid tumor	Generally high grade
Squamous cell carcinoma	Generally high grade
Acinic cell carcinoma	Generally low grade
Low-grade mucoepidermoid tumor	Generally low grade

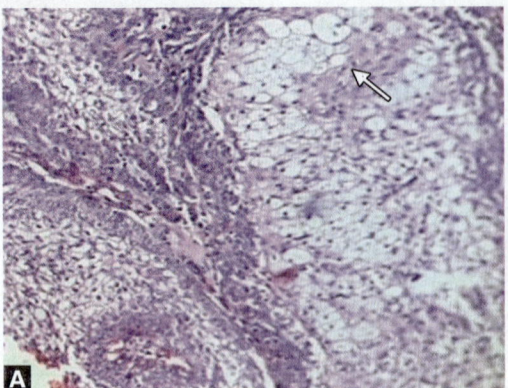 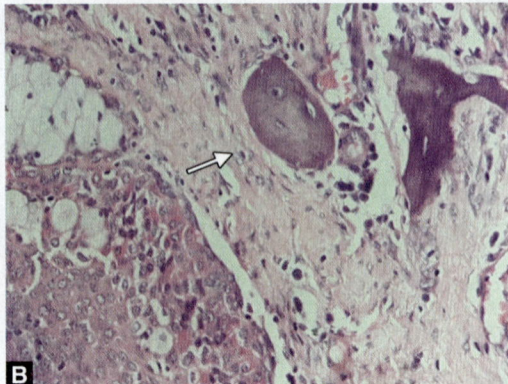

Figs. 4.30A and B: Photomicrograph of mucoepidermoid tumor: (A) Clear cell variant; and (B) Intra-tumor calcification in same lesion.

clear vacuolated cells that do not stain for mucin and these cells gradually merge with the squamous epithelial cells.

Differential Diagnosis
- Pleomorphic adenoma
- Adenocarcinoma
- Squamous cell carcinoma
- Metastatic carcinoma.

Treatment
By surgical excision and radiotherapy. The overall 5-year survival rate is 70% (for high grade it is 80%). In low-grade tumors local recurrence is seen in about 10% cases.

Acinic Cell Carcinoma

Acinic cell carcinomas (ACCs) are malignant neoplasms of the salivary gland, in which at least some of the neoplastic cells demonstrate serous acinar cell differentiation, which are characterized by cytoplasmic zymogen granules. Besides the principal acinar cells, the tumor also exhibits ductal epithelial cells as its component. According to the multicellular theory these tumors originate from the cells of the salivary gland acini.

Clinical Features (Fig. 4.31)
- The tumor chiefly occurs among middle-age or elderly persons, with a slight predilection for females.

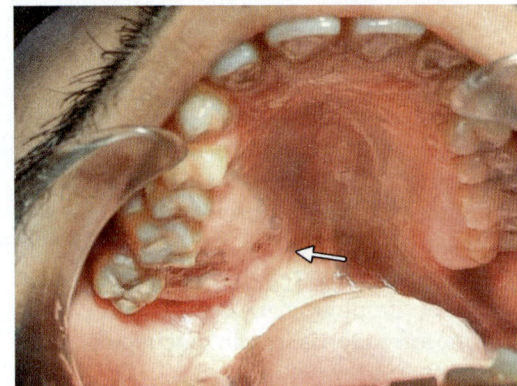

Fig. 4.31: Acinic cell tumor of the palate.

- Parotid is most frequently affected in as many as 90% cases and about 17% cases occur from the minor salivary glands; it is rarely seen in submandibular glands.
- After mucoepidermoid carcinoma, acinic cell tumor is the second most common malignant salivary gland neoplasm occurring in childhood.
- Acinic cell tumor is the third most bilateral salivary gland tumor after Warthin tumor and pleomorphic adenoma.
- The lesion presents a well-defined, slow growing, painless, firm, and movable swelling that often resembles pleomorphic adenoma.
- The size of the lesion is usually about 3 cm in diameter, the overlying skin or

epithelium is intact and few lesions can be fluctuant in nature due to the presence of intralesional cystic spaces.
- Rarely intraoral lesions of acinic cell tumor may occur on the lip or cheek region and they present well-defined, firm, painless, and submucosal nodular growths.

Histopathology
- Histologically the tumor is well-circumscribed and sometimes may even appear encapsulated, and consists of either serous or mucous acinar cells of the salivary gland.
- The malignant cells are large, round or polyhedral in shape and have granular basophilic cytoplasm (PAS-positive zymogen-type secretory granules) and dark eccentrically placed nuclei.
- These cells are often arranged in acinus-like clusters and they often resemble the serous acinar cells of the salivary gland.
- The cell cytoplasms may be vacuolated or sometimes entirely clear (Fig. 4.32).
- These tumor cells may also be arranged in sheets or solid or cystic or even papillary cystic patterns within a lymphoid stroma.
- Acinic cell tumor is nonencapsulated and it often shows either a "pushing-margin" type or a definite infiltrative pattern of growth.

- Four growth patterns—(1) solid; (2) papillary cystic; (3) follicular, and (4) microcystic. In general, one pattern predominates, although combinations can occur.

Differential Diagnosis
- Pleomorphic adenoma
- Mucoepidermoid tumor
- Sialadenitis
- Stromal tumor
- Enlarged lymph nodes.

Treatment
By wide local excision or superficial parotidectomy. 5-year survival rate is seen in about 75% cases.

Adenocarcinoma
Adenocarcinomas are rare but aggressive neoplasms of the salivary gland; occur more commonly in relation to intraoral minor salivary glands and are less common in the parotid, however some lesions may develop from the preexisting pleomorphic adenomas (Figs. 4.33 and 4.34).

Clinical Presentation
- The majority of the patients are in their sixth decade of life and females are more likely to suffer.
- Initially the tumor presents a slow growing, firm, and painless mass with no surface ulceration.

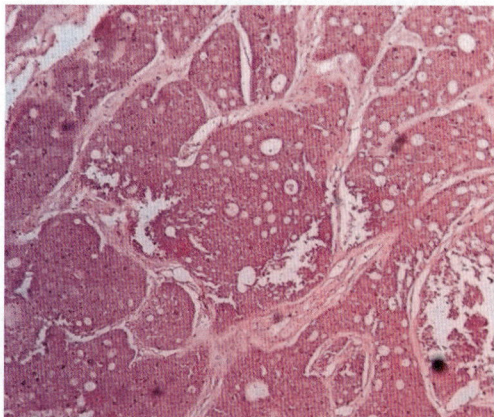

Fig. 4.32: Photomicrograph of acinic cell tumor (high power).

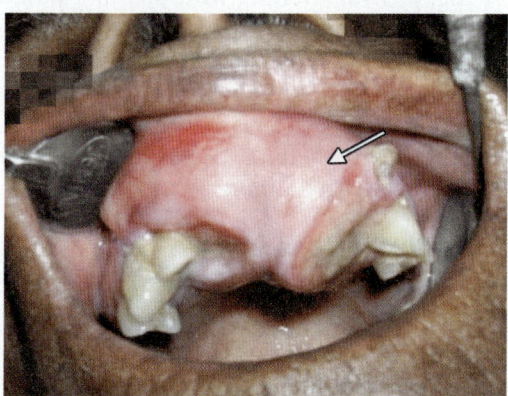

Fig. 4.33: Adenocarcinoma of maxilla.

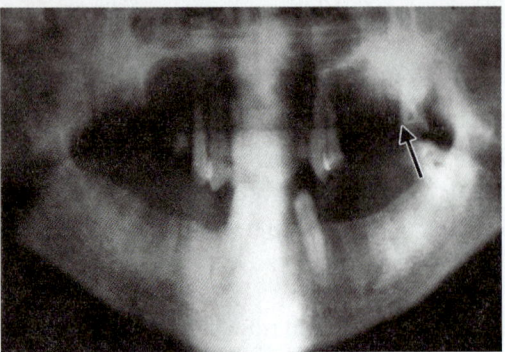

Fig. 4.34: Radiograph of adenocarcinoma showing destruction of the maxillary bone.

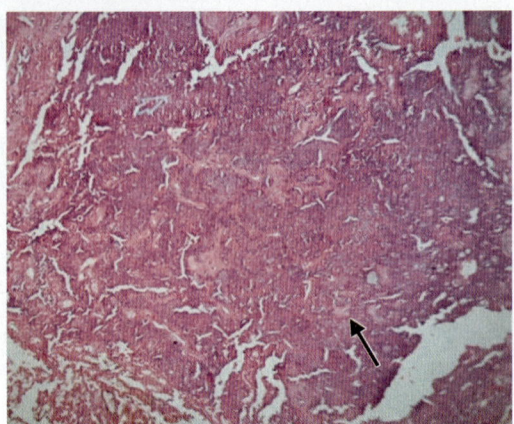

Fig. 4.36: Photomicrograph of polymorphous low-grade adenocarcinoma (PLGA), low power.

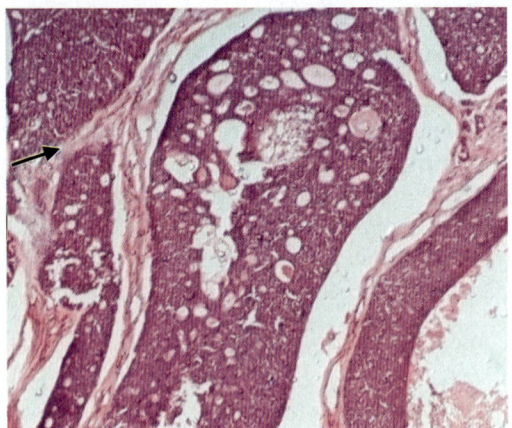

Fig. 4.35: Photomicrograph of adenocarcinoma.

- Later on the tumor develops a fast enlarging, painful swelling with ulceration and paresthesia, etc.
- Palate is the most common intraoral site, followed by lips and tongue.
- The palatal lesions are often fixed to the adjacent tissues and they usually measure about 3 cm in diameter.

Histopathology (Figs. 4.35 and 4.36)

- Microscopy reveals numerous proliferating malignant ductal epithelial cells with areas of hemorrhage and necrosis.
- At the periphery of the lesion, the tumor cells are arranged in parallel arrays of elongated tubular formations and thereby producing an "*onion-skin*" appearance.
- Some tumors produce many cyst-like spaces, containing large quantity of mucous and in few cases papillary in-growths into the cystic spaces are also seen.
- The tumor cells often invade into the surrounding normal tissues.

Treatment

Wide surgical excision. Prognosis is usually poor.

TNM CLASSIFICATION OF CARCINOMAS OF THE SALIVARY GLANDS

T–Primary Tumor

TX: primary tumor cannot be assessed
T0: no evidence of primary tumor
T1: tumor 2 cm or less in greatest dimension without extraparenchymal extension
T2: tumor more than 2 cm but less than 4 cm in greatest dimension without extraparenchymal extension
T3: tumor more than 4 cm and/or tumor with extraparenchymal extension
T4a: tumor invades skin, mandible, ear canal, or facial nerve

T4b: tumor invades base of skull, pterygoid plates, or encases external carotid artery.

N–Regional (Cervical) Lymph Nodes

NX: regional lymph nodes cannot be assessed
N0: no regional node metastasis
N1: metastasis in a single ipsilateral node, 3 cm or less in greatest dimension
N2: has categories:
N2a: metastasis in a single ipsilateral node, more than 3 cm but not more than 6 cm in greatest dimension
N2b: metastasis in multiple ipsilateral nodes, none more than 6 cm in greatest dimension
N2c: metastasis in bilateral or contralateral nodes, none more than 6 cm in greatest dimension.
N3: metastasis in a lymph node more than 6 cm in greatest dimension.

(*Note*: Midline nodes are considered ipsilateral nodes)

M–Distant Metastasis

MX: distant metastasis cannot be assessed
M0: no distant metastasis
M1: distant metastasis.

The Stage Grouping

The stage grouping for the classification of carcinomas of the salivary glands is described in Table 4.8.

Table 4.8: The stage grouping.

Stage			
Stage I	T1	N0	M0
Stage II	T2	N0	M0
Stage III	T3	N0	M0
	T1, T2, T3	N1	M0
Stage IV A	T1, T2, T3	N2	M0
	T4a	N0, N1, N2	M0
Stage IV B	T4b	Any N	M0
	Any T	N3	M0
Stage IV C	Any T	Any N	M1

BIBLIOGRAPHY

1. Abbodanzo SL. Extranodal marginal-zone B-cell lymphoma of the salivary gland. Ann Diagn Pathol. 2001;5(4):246-54.
2. Abrams AM, Melrose RJ, Howell FV. Necrotizing sialometaplasia. A disease simulating malignancy. Cancer. 1973;32:130-5.
3. Allenspach EJ, Maillard I, Aster JC, et al. Notch signalling in cancer. Cancer Biol Ther. 2002;1(5):466-76.
4. Atkinson JC, Fox PC. Sjogren's syndrome: oral and dental considerations. J Am Dent Assoc. 1993;124:74-6,78-82,84-6.
5. Attie JN, Sciubba JJ. Tumors of major and minor salivary glands: clinical and pathologic features. Curr Probl Surg. 1981;18:65-155.
6. Baker SR, Malone B. Salivary gland malignancies in children. Cancer. 1985;55:1730-6.
7. Batsakis JG, Brannon RB, Scuibba JJ. Monomorphic adenomas of major salivary glands: a histologic study of 96 tumors. Clin Otolaryngol. 1981;6:129-43.
8. Batsakis JG, Luna MA. Undifferentiated carcinomas of salivary glands. Ann Otol Rhinol Laryngol. 1991;100:82-4.
9. Batsakis JG. Primary squamous cell carcinomas of major salivary glands. Ann Otol Rhinol Laryngol. 1983;92:97-8.
10. Batsakis JG. Salivary gland neoplasias: an outcome of modified morphogenesis and cytodifferentiation. Oral Surg Oral Med Oral Pathol. 1980;49:229-32.
11. Batsakis JG. The lymphoepithelial lesion and Sjogren's syndrome. Head and Neck Surgery. 1982;5:150-63.
12. Bodner L, Azaz B. Submandibular sialolithiasis in children. J Oral Maxillofac Surg. 1982;40:551-4.
13. Brandwein MS, Ferlito A, Bradley PJ, et al. Diagnosis and classification of salivary neoplasms: pathologic challenges and relevance to clinical outcomes. Acta Otolaryngol. 2002;122(7):758-64.
14. Brannon RB, Sciubba JJ, Giulani M. Ductal papillomas of salivary gland origin: A report of 19 cases and a review of the literature. Oral Surg Oral Med Oral Pathol Oral Radiol Endod. 2001;92:68-77.
15. Brill SJ, Gilfillan RF. Acute parotitis associated with influenza type A: a report of twelve cases. N Engl J Med. 1977;296:1391-2.

16. Brookstone MS, Huvos AG. Central mucoepidermoid tumors of the jaws. Oral Surg. 1975;40:631.
17. Buchner A, Screebny LM. Enlargement of salivary glands. Review of the literature. Oral Surg Oral Med Oral Pathol. 1972;34:209-22.
18. Burke JS. Waldeyer's ring, sinonasal region, salivary gland, thyroid gland, central nervous system, and other extranodal lymphomas and lymphoid hyperplasias. In: Knowles DM (Ed). Neoplastic Hematopathology. Baltimore, Md: Williams & Wilkins; 1992. pp. 1047-79.
19. Chang A, Harawi SJ. Oncocytes, oncocytosis and oncocytic tumors. Pathol Annu. 1992;27(pt-1): 263-304.
20. Cho KJ, Kim YI. Monomorphic adenomas of the salivary glands: a clinico-pathologic study of 12 cases with immunohistochemical observation. Path Res Pract. 1989;184:614-20.
21. Daniels TE, Fox PC. Salivary and oral components of Sjogren's syndrome. Rheum Dis Clin North Am. 1992;18:517-38.
22. David C, Augusto F. Basaloid tumors of the salivary glands Ann Diagn Pathol. 2002;6(6): 364-72.
23. Donohue WB, Bolden TE. Tuberculosis of the salivary glands: a collective review. Oral Surg Oral Med Oral Pathol. 1961;14:576-88.
24. Evans HL, Batsakis JG. Polymorphous low grade adenocarcinoma of minor salivary glands. Cancer. 1984;53:935-42.
25. Eveson JW, Cawson RA. Warthin's tumor (cystadenolymphoma) of salivary glands: a clinicopathological investigation of 278 cases. Oral Surg. 1986;61:256-62.
26. Fowler CB, Brannon RB. Subacute necrotizing sialadenitis: report of 7 cases and a review of the literature. Oral Surg Oral Med Oral Pathol Oral Radiol Endod. 2000;89(5):600-9.
27. Fox PC. Bacterial infections of salivary glands. Curr Opin Dent. 1991;1:411-4.
28. Friedrich RE, Bleckmann V. Adenoid cystic carcinoma of salivary and lacrimal gland origin: localization, classification, clinical pathological correlation, treatment results and long-term follow-up control in 84 patients. Anticancer Res. 2003;23(2A):931-40.
29. Gardner DG, Bell MEA, Wesley RK, et al. Acinic cell tumors of minor salivary glands. Oral Surg. 1980;50:545.
30. Gleeson MJ, Bennett MH, Cawson RA. Lymphomas of salivary glands. Cancer. 1986; 58(3):699-704.
31. Gnepp DR. Malignant mixed tumors of the salivary glands: a review. Pathol Annu. 1993;28 (pt-1):279-328.
32. Goldblatt LI, Ellis GL. Salivary gland tumors of the tongue: analysis of 55 new cases and review of the literature. Cancer. 1987;60:74-81.
33. Gomes AP, Sobral AP, Loducca SV, et al. Sialadenoma papilliferum: immuno-histochemical study. Int J Oral Maxillofac Surg. 2004;33(6):621-4.
34. Hansen J, Fikentscher R, Roseburg R. Schirmer test of lacrimation. Its clinical importance. Arch Otolaryngol. 1975;101:293-5.
35. Hornick JL, Fletcher CD. Cutaneous myoepithelioma: a clinicopathologic and immunohistochemical study of 14 cases. Hum Pathol. 2004;35(1):14-24.
36. Hunter RM, Davis BW, Gray GF, et al. Primary malignant tumors of salivary gland origin: a 52-years review. Am Surg. 1983;49:82-9.
37. Isacsson G, Shear M. Intraoral salivary gland tumors: a retrospective study of 201 cases. J Oral Pathol. 1983;12:57-62.
38. Jensen JL. Idiopathic diseases. In: Ellis GL, Auclair PL, Gnepp DR (Eds). Surgical Pathology of the Salivary Glands. Philadelphia: WB Saunders Co; 1991. pp. 60-82.
39. Leonetti JP, Marzo SJ, Petruzzelli GJ. Recurrent pleomorphic adenoma of the parotid gland. Otolaryngol Head Neck Surg. 2004;131(2):65-6.
40. Leung AKC. Benign Lymphoepithelial Lesion. NORD Guide to Rare Disorders. Philadelphia, PA: Lippincott Williams & Wilkins; 2003.
41. Leung SY, Chung LP, Yuen ST, et al. Lympho-epithelial carcinoma of the salivary gland: in situ detection of Epstein-Barr virus. J Clin Pathol. 1995;48(11):1022-7.
42. Lewis JE, Olsen KD, Weiland LH. Acinic cell carcinoma. Clinicopathologic review. Cancer. 1991;67(1):172-9.
43. Loughran DH, Smith LG. Infectious disorders of the parotid gland. N J Med. 1988;85:311-4.
44. Lowry TR, Heichel DJ. Pleomorphic adenoma of the hard palate. Otolaryngol Head Neck Surg. 2004;131(5):793.
45. Luna MA, Batsakis JG, el-Naggar AK. Salivary gland tumors in children. Ann Otol Rhinol Laryngol. 1991;100:869-71.

46. Machado de Sousa SO, Soares de Araújo N, Corrêa L, et al. Immunohistochemical aspects of basal cell adenoma and canalicular adenoma of salivary glands. Oral Oncology. 2001;37(4):365-8.
47. Mintz GA, Abrams AM, Melrose RJ. Monomorphic adenomas of the major and minor salivary glands. Report of 21 cases and review of the literature. Oral Surg Oral Med Oral Pathol. 1982;53:375-86.
48. Noel S, Brozna JP. Epithelial-myoepithelial carcinoma of salivary gland with metastasis to lung: report of a case and review of the literature. Head Neck. 1992;14(5):401-6.
49. Perez-Ordonez B. Selected topics in salivary gland tumor pathology. Curr Diag Pathol. 2003;96(6):355-65.
50. Piattelli A, Iezzi G, Rubini C, et al. Intraductal papilloma of the palate. Report of a case. Oral Oncol. 2002;38:398-400.
51. Potdar GG, Paymaster JC. Tumors of minor salivary glands. Oral Surg Oral Med Oral Pathol. 1969;28:310-9.
52. Romagosa V, Bella MR, Truchero C, et al. Necrotizing sialometaplasia (adenometaplasia) of the trachea. Histopathology. 1992;21(3):280-2.
53. Rosai J. Major and minor salivary glands. In: Rosai J (Ed). Ackerman's surgical pathology, 8th edition. St. Louis, Mo: Mosby; 1996. pp. 815-56.
54. Savera AT, Sloman A, Huvos AG, et al. Myoepithelial carcinoma of the salivary glands: a clinicopathologic study of 25 patients. Am J Surg Pathol. 2000;24(6):761-74.
55. Schiodt M. HIV associated salivary gland disease: a review. Oral Surg Oral Med Oral Pathol. 1992;73:164-7.
56. Seifert G, Donath K. Multiple tumors of the salivary glands-terminology and nomenclature Oral Oncol. 1996;32:3-7.
57. Seifert G, Sobin LH. The World Health Organization's Histological Classification of Salivary Gland Tumors: a commentary on the second edition. Cancer. 1992;70:379-85.
58. Seifert G. Histopathology of malignant salivary gland tumors. Eur J Cancer B Oral Oncol. 1992;28B:49-56.
59. St. Clair EW. New developments in Sjogren's syndrome. Curr Opin Rheumatol. 1993;5: 604-12.
60. Thackray AC, Sobin LJ. Histological typing of salivary gland tumors. World Health Organization. Geneva; 1972.
61. Tonon G, Modi S, Wu L, et al. t(11:19)(q21;p13) translocation in mucoepidermoid carcinoma creates a novel fusion product that disrupts a Notch signaling pathway. Nat Genet. 2003;33(2):208-13.
62. Tortoledo ME, Luna MA, Batsakis JG. Carcinomas ex-pleomorphic adenoma and malignant mixed tumors. Arch Otolaryngol. 1984;110: 172-6.
63. Tsurumi K, Kamiya H, Yokoi M, et al. Papillary oncocytic cystadenoma of palatal minor salivary gland: a case report. J Oral Maxillofac Surg. 2003;61(5):631-3.
64. Weiss SW, Goldblum JR. Enzinger and Weiss's Soft Tissue Tumors, 4th edition. St. Louis, MO: Mosby; 2001.
65. Wenig BM. Necrotizing sialometaplasia of the larynx. A report of two cases and a review of the literature. Am J Clin Pathol. 1995;103(5): 609-13.
66. Zschoch H. Mucus gland infarct with squamous epithelial metaplasia in the lung. A rare site of so-called necrotizing sialometaplasia. Pathologe. 1992;13(1):45-8.

CHAPTER 5

Odontogenic Neoplasms

■ DEFINITION

Odontogenic neoplasms are a complex group of lesions derived from the dental formative tissues or their remnants (tissues associated with the development of tooth and its supporting structures). The constituent tissues in each of these neoplasms can resemble the various tissues found during normal odontogenesis, from inception of the tooth germ to tooth eruption.

The tooth formation or odontogenesis begins in the 6th week intrauterine life and it originates from the oral epithelium covering the maxillary and mandibular alveolar processes. During the initial period "bud-like" swellings appear from the basal layer of the oral epithelium at specific locations, where individual teeth are to be formed in future.

The development of tooth occurs in the following stages:
- *Stage of formation of dental lamina:* The epithelial bud elongates in the form of a solid "tube-like" structure that projects into the underlying connective tissue and this process is known as "elongation". The elongated epithelial structure is called the "dental lamina", from which the future tooth develops.
- *Cap stage:* Once the appropriate depth is achieved, the basal layer at the tip of the dental lamina thickens and forms a concavity.
- *Early bell stage:* The cap shaped structure enlarges as odontogenesis proceeds and within few days the bottom layer of the epithelium (inner enamel epithelium) separates from the top layer (outer enamel epithelium). The intervening zone is composed of loosely arranged "star-shaped" epithelial cells called stellate reticulum cells. During this stage elongation of the periphery of the epithelial structure occurs, which gives shape of the crown of the individual teeth.
- *Late bell stage (formation of dental papilla):* During this stage the cells of the inner enamel epithelium becomes elongated and palisaded, the nuclei of these cells are often elongated away for the basement membrane and these cells are called "presecretory ameloblasts".

These presecretory ameloblasts induce the undifferentiated cells of the adjacent dental papilla to differentiate into presecretory odontoblasts. The later group of cells aligns in a palisaded manner adjacent to the basement membrane opposite the pre-secretory ameloblasts. Once the ameloblasts become mature the odontoblasts are stimulated to secrete dentin matrix, which in turn initiates the deposition of enamel matrix on the opposite side of the basement membrane.

■ FORMATION OF DENTAL PAPILLA

During the early bell stage the mesoderm immediately adjacent to the inner enamel epithelium proliferates and forms a zone of embryonic and myxomatous connective tissue called "dental papilla". It may be further induced to form dentin or pulp tissues.

DENTAL FOLLICLE

During early bell stage an outer zone of dense and fibrous connective tissue forms, which encapsulates the developing of tooth bud and is known as the "dental follicle". The dental follicle encloses the developing tooth until it erupts into the oral cavity.

After eruption of the tooth the coronal portion of the dental follicle becomes part of the connective tissue of the free gingival margin.

Likewise the radicular part of the follicle eventually becomes the periodontal ligament, which separates the cementum from the alveolar bone.

FORMATION OF ROOT

After formation of the tooth crown the outer enamel epithelium elongates and forms a thin, transient membrane called the "epithelial root sheath of Hertwig" which determines the shape and length of the roots of the individual teeth. During root formation, initially the dentin is formed. This newly formed dentin stimulates the adjacent dental follicle to differentiate into cementoblasts. The cementoblast cells form a calcified layer over the root dentin, which is known cementum. Cementum serves to anchor the periodontal ligament and collagen of the dental follicle to the tooth root.

Once the process of odontogenesis is completed, the dental lamina leaves behind some cell remnants in the connective tissue, which are called the "cell rests of Serres". Similarly, the remnants of the epithelial root sheath of Hertwig also remain within the periodontal ligament and are known as "cell rests of Malassez". These cellular remnants play important role in the development of various odontogenic tumors.

Classification of Odontogenic Tumors (Modified WHO Classification)

A. Benign
I. Odontogenic epithelium without odontogenic ectomesenchyme
   - Ameloblastoma
   - Squamous odontogenic tumor
   - Calcifying epithelial odontogenic tumor (Pindborg tumor)
   - Adenomatoid odontogenic tumor

II. Odontogenic epithelium with odontogenic ectomesenchyme with or without hard tissue formation
   - Ameloblastic fibroma
   - Ameloblastic fibrodentinoma
   - Ameloblastic fibro-odontoma
   - Odontoameloblastoma
   - Calcifying odontogenic cyst
   - Complex odontoma
   - Compound odontoma

III. Odontogenic ectomesenchyme without included odontogenic epithelium
   - Compound odontoma
   - Odontogenic fibroma
   - Myxoma
   - Cementoblastoma (benign cementoblastoma, true cementoma).

B. Malignant
I. Odontogenic carcinomas
   - Malignant ameloblastoma
   - Primary intraosseous carcinoma
   - Clear cell odontogenic carcinoma.

II. Odontogenic sarcomas
   - Ameloblastic fibrosarcoma
   - Ameloblastic fibro-odontosarcoma
   - Ameloblastic fibrodentinosarcoma.

NEOPLASMS OF DEBATABLE ORIGIN

- Melanotic neuroectodermal tumor of infancy
- Congenital gingival granular cell tumor (congenital epulis).

AMELOBLASTOMA

DEFINITION

Ameloblastoma is a benign locally aggressive neoplasm arising from the odontogenic epithelium and it is the most common odontogenic neoplasm of the oral cavity.

Ameloblastoma the word has evolved from the early English words—"Amel" meaning enamel, and "blastos"—meaning germ.

- It was first recognized by Cusack in 1827 and it was named "adamantinoma" in 1885 by Luis-Charles Malassez. It was finally renamed as "ameloblastoma" in 1934 by Ivey and Churchill. It has been described very aptly by Robinson as benign tumor that is usually unicentric, nonfunctional, intermittent in growth, anatomically benign and clinically persistent.
- Ameloblastoma is the most common odontogenic neoplasm in India.

ETIOLOGY

Exactly not known, however the following factors may predispose the formation of ameloblastoma:
- Trauma
- Infection
- Previous inflammation
- Extraction of tooth
- Dietary factors
- Viral infection.

HISTOGENESIS OF AMELOBLASTOMA

Ameloblastoma develops from the odontogenic epithelial cells or their remnants but the exact cell of its origin is not very clearly known. According to different investigators, the possible cells or tissues from where ameloblastomas may arise are as follows:
- Enamel organ of the developing tooth germ
- Cell rest of Serres (remnants of dental lamina)
- Epithelial lining of the odontogenic cysts, especially the dentigerous cyst
- The basal cell layer of the oral epithelium (rarely)
- Reduced enamel epithelium
- Cell rest of Malassez.

CLINICAL FEATURES

- *Incidence:* Approximately 1% among all oral tumors and 18% of all odontogenic tumors are ameloblastomas.
- *Age:* 2nd, 3rd, 4th and 5th decade of life, the mean age of occurrence is about 32 years.

This lesion occurs more commonly in blacks than whites. Women are generally 4 years younger than men when the tumor is first noticed.
- *Sex:* Males are affected more often than females. Tumor size is usually larger in women.
- *Site:* Ameloblastoma in most of the cases involve the mandible (80%), especially in the molar-ramus area (70%), although some lesions may develop in the premolar (20%) or symphysis (10%) regions.

Maxillary tumors also commonly involve its posterior part and the lesions often have a tendency to invade into the antrum (15%) or the nasal floor.

Extraosseous or peripheral ameloblastomas can rarely occur mostly in relation to the gingiva.

Types of Ameloblastoma
- Unicystic ameloblastoma
- Multicystic ameloblastoma
- Peripheral ameloblastoma
- Malignant ameloblastoma.

CLINICAL PRESENTATION (FIGS. 5.1A TO C; BOX 5.1)

- Clinically ameloblastoma presents a slow enlarging, painless, ovoid or fusiform, bony hard swelling of the jaw.
- The lesion causes expansion and distortion of the cortical plates of the jawbone and displacement of the regional teeth, and these are often leading to gross facial asymmetry (Fig. 5.1B).
- Pain, paresthesia and mobility of the regional teeth may be present only in few cases.
- Most of the patients report with a typical long time history of presence of an "abscess" or a "cyst" in the jaw bone that was operated on several occasions but has recurred after each attempt.
- Larger lesions often cause severe thinning of the cortical plates, which often result in "fluctuations" in the affected area.

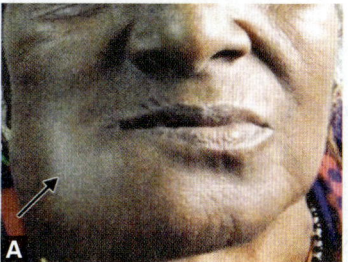 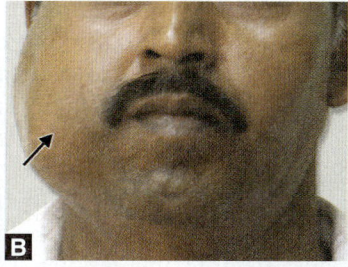 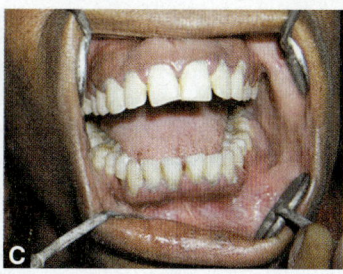

Figs. 5.1A to C: (A and B) Ameloblastoma of mandible causing large expansile swelling. (C) Ameloblastoma of mandible intraoral swelling.

- In case of extreme cortical thinning, the affected bone might crack during palpation or under digital pressure and the phenomenon is called "egg shell crackling".
- In ameloblastoma, the thin and weak bone at the site of the tumor may get easily fractured with minimum trauma or while chewing only and this type of bone damage is called "pathological fracture".
- The mucosa overlying the tumor appears normal and the regional teeth are usually vital.
- In some cases, smaller lesions may remain asymptomatic and are detected incidentally during routine radiographic examinations.
- Many untreated lesions may reach to an enormous size with time and cause extensive deformity of the jaws and face (Fig. 5.2).
- Sometimes larger lesions may perforate the cortical plate and protrude outside the bone as a nodular soft tissue mass; however it should be noted that cortical perforation is a rare entity in ameloblastoma, interestingly in case the tumor perforates the bone ameloblastic carcinoma should be suspected rather than simple ameloblastoma.
- Maxillary tumors can invade into the maxillary air sinus and extend further up to the orbit or the nasopharynx and thereby leading to pressure sensation in the eyeball or nasal obstruction, etc.
- Some of the lesions may progress to ethmoidal air sinuses or even up to the cranial base.
- Extraosseous ameloblastoma often produces a small, nodular growth in the gingiva.

Box 5.1 Lesions which may cause perforation of cortical plates of bone.

- Central giant cell granuloma
- Ameloblastoma
- Odontogenic keratocyst (OKC)
- Squamous cell carcinoma
- Osteosarcoma
- Non-Hodgkin's lymphoma
- Burkitt's lymphoma
- Aneurysmal bone cyst
- Calcifying epithelial odontogenic cyst (COC)
- Primary intra-alveolar carcinoma
- Neurilemmoma
- Desmoplastic fibroma
- Pindborg's tumor
- Acute suppurative osteomyelitis

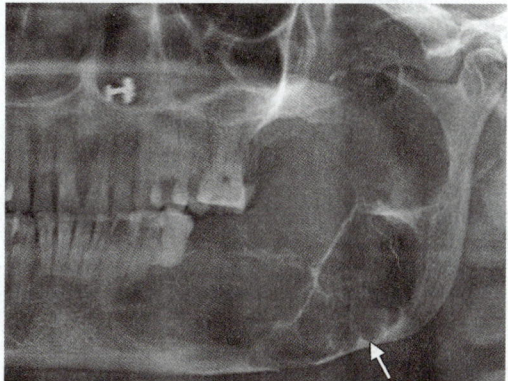

Fig. 5.2: Radiograph of ameloblastoma showing multilocular radiolucency with expansion and thinning of cortical plates.

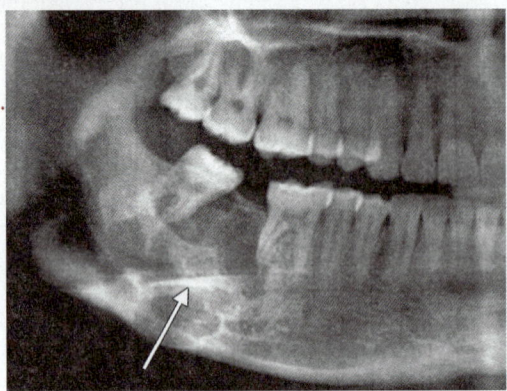

Fig. 5.3: Radiograph of ameloblastoma producing typical "honey-comb" appearance.

- Desmoplastic ameloblastoma is a special variant, which unlike other lesions of ameloblastoma develops from the anterior part of the jaw, especially maxilla.

RADIOLOGICAL FEATURES

- Radiographically ameloblastoma usually presents a well-defined, multilocular, radiolucent area in the bone with a typical "honey-comb" or "soap-bubble" appearance (Fig. 5.3, Box 5.2). Few lesions can be unilocular too.
- For multilocular lesions, when the loculations are large the appearance will be "soap-bubble" type and when the loculations are small the appearance will be "honey-comb" type.
- In radiograph, the lesion typically exhibits an irregular and "scalloped" margin.
- The larger lesions often cause expansion, thinning and distortion of buccal and lingual cortical plates of the jawbone.

Box 5.2	Lesions producing "soap-bubble" radiographic appearance.

- Ameloblastoma
- Odontogenic keratocyst (OKC)
- Central giant cell granuloma
- Central hemangioma
- Cherubism

Note: Histologically tumor cells of lipoma and liposarcoma often resemble "soap-bubbles".

- Although ameloblastoma causes severe thinning of the bone but perforation of the cortical plate is not common in them.
- In many cases the weak and thin bone at the tumor site may exhibit pathological fractures.
- Resorption of roots of the adjoining normal teeth is often seen in rapidly growing lesions.
- Ameloblastoma can cause expansion of the lower border of mandible.
- As the neoplasm progresses, it sometimes become associated with an impacted tooth (mostly the third molars) and in such cases the lesion may resemble a dentigerous cyst.
- Desmoplastic ameloblastoma presents a mixed radiolucent and radiopaque appearance, thus often resemble a fibro-osseous lesion. It happens due to osseous metaplasia within the connective tissue (tumor cells, however do not produce any calcification in the lesion) (Fig. 5.4).

DIFFERENTIAL DIAGNOSIS

- Odontogenic keratocyst
- Dentigerous cyst
- Central giant cell granuloma
- Central hemangioma
- Aneurysmal bone cyst

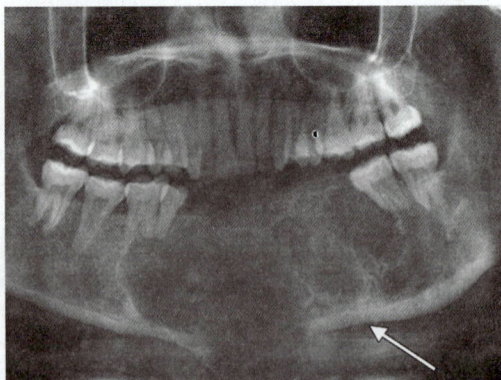

Fig. 5.4: Root resorption and bone destruction in ameloblastoma with expansion of lower border of mandible.

- Pindborg's tumor
- Fibromyxoma.

MACROSCOPIC FEATURES

- On naked eye examination the tumor presents a cylindrical or fusiform swelling, which expands the bone so severely that it can be broken by digital pressure (egg-shell crackling).
- Pathological fracture is common but perforation of the cortical plate is uncommon.
- Cut section of ameloblastoma often appears as a "grayish-white" or "grayish-yellow" mass, which contains some "cyst-like" spaces. However no calcified tissue is usually found within the tumor.
- Some lesions are made up entirely of solid tissue mass although most of them have some cystic spaces of varying sizes within them.
- Some intratumor cysts are large and contain either a straw colored fluid or a semisolid gelatinous material.
- Sometimes, one or two teeth may be present within the lesion.

HISTOPATHOLOGICAL FEATURES

Histologically ameloblastoma shows neoplastic proliferation of odontogenic epithelial cells (ameloblast-like cells), which are arranged in different characteristic patterns within the tumor.

Histologically ameloblastomas present two distinct patterns: (1) Plexiform and (2) Follicular pattern, besides these two there are few other relatively uncommon histological patterns, namely the acanthomatous pattern, basal cell pattern, granular cell pattern and desmoplastic pattern, etc.

PLEXIFORM AMELOBLASTOMA (FIG. 5.5)

- In this variant of ameloblastoma the neoplastic odontogenic epithelial cells proliferate in the form of "long continuous anastomosing strands or cords" hence the term plexiform has been given.
- This pattern of neoplastic cell proliferation is also often called a "fish-net like" pattern (Fig. 5.5).
- The peripheral layer of cells of the epithelial cords are tall columnar in nature and they often resemble the ameloblasts.
- Reverse polarization of the nuclei of these bordering cells is indistinct.
- The triangular shaped cells situated at the center portion of the strands often resemble the stellate reticulum cells, while the cells located between the columnar cells and the stellate reticulum cells often resemble the stratum intermedium.
- The intervening connective tissue stroma is usually loose and vascular with minimum cellularity. There may cyst formation within the stroma in some cases (Fig. 5.6).

FOLLICULAR AMELOBLASTOMA (FIG. 5.7)

- In follicular type, the neoplastic odontogenic epithelial cells proliferate in the form

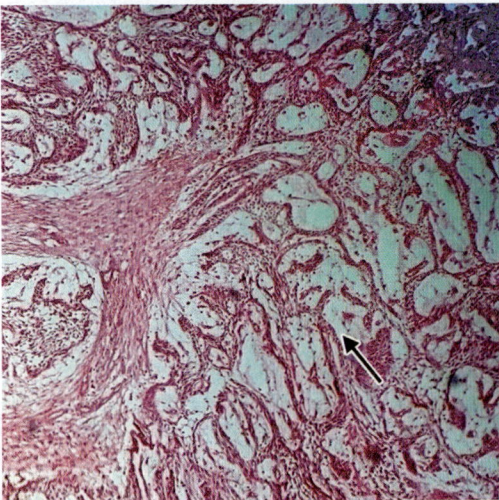

Fig. 5.5: Photomicrograph of plexiform ameloblastoma producing a typical "fish-net" pattern of neoplastic cell proliferation.

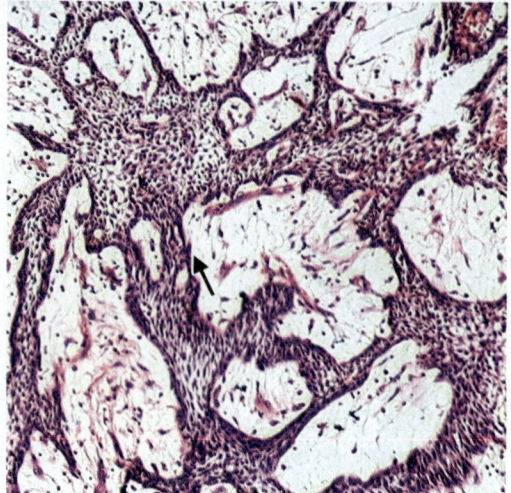

Fig. 5.6: Photomicrograph of plexiform ameloblastomas (high power).

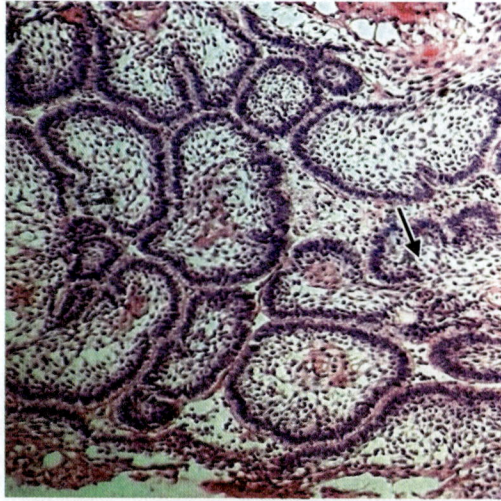

Fig. 5.7: Photomicrograph of follicular ameloblastoma (low power).

of multiple, discrete follicles or islands within the fibrous connective tissue stroma.
- Each follicle-like structure is bordered on the periphery by a single layer of tall columnar cells resembling ameloblasts. These cells have well-defined nuclei, which are situated away from the basement membrane on the opposite pole, this type of nuclear positioning is called "reverse polarization".
- Sometimes these peripheral cells bordering the follicles are cuboidal in nature and resemble basal cells.
- The cells located at the center of the follicles are loosely arranged and are star shaped or triangular in shape; these cells are widely separated from one another but appear to be interconnected and they often resemble stellate reticulum cells (normally seen in the bell stage of odontogenesis).
- While the cells located in between the peripheral and the central group of cells, appear as the stratum intermedium.
- Occasionally, a distinctive zone of hyalinization is seen surrounding the follicles.
- Microcyst formation is often observed inside these follicles and the cysts sometimes may be large enough to occupy the entire inner part of the follicles (Figs. 5.8 and 5.9).
- The intervening connective tissue stroma is delicate in nature and it consists chiefly of collagen bundles, fibroblasts and blood vessels, etc.
- Extraosseous ameloblastomas also exhibit follicular structures as seen in the conventional intraosseous ameloblastomas, however the lining cells are often basaloid in nature.

Possible reason why no hard tissue (enamel) forms in ameloblastoma: The developing enamel organ demonstrates three types: (1) ameloblasts, (2) stellate reticulum, and (3) stratum intermedium. The tumor cells seen within ameloblastoma mimic ameloblasts and stellate reticulum but fail to exhibit significant areas that resemble stratum intermedium. This missing portion of the enamel organ is thought to be responsible for the inability of the ameloblastoma to demonstrate enamel formation.

OTHER HISTOLOGICAL PATTERNS OF AMELOBLASTOMA

Besides the plexiform and the follicular patterns, some other histological types of

Odontogenic Neoplasms

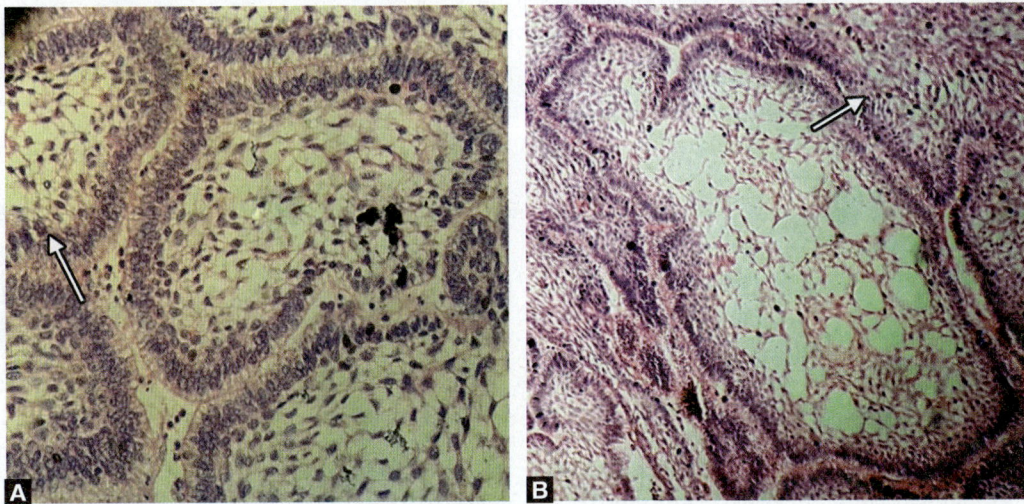

Figs. 5.8A and B: (A) Photomicrograph of follicular ameloblastoma (high power) showing tall columnar cells at the periphery of the follicle and stellate reticulum-like cells at the center; (B) Microcyst formation within the follicle.

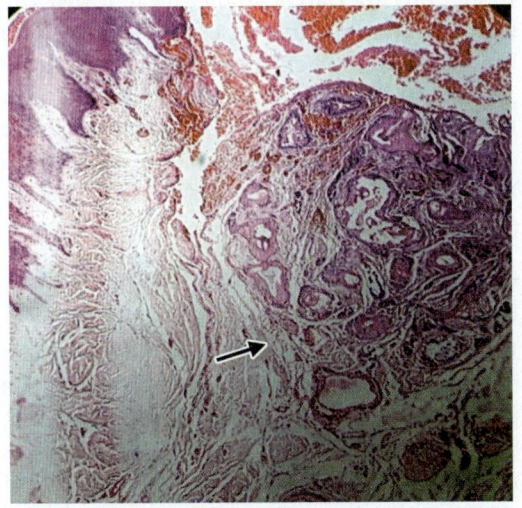

Fig. 5.9: Photomicrograph showing peripheral (soft tissue) ameloblastoma.

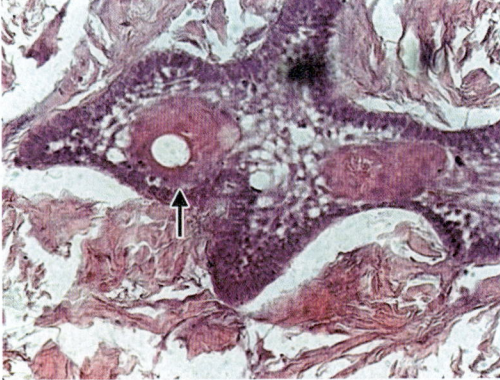

Fig. 5.10: Photomicrograph of squamous metaplasia (high power).

ameloblastomas can occur and they are as discussed here.

Acanthomatous Ameloblastoma

It occurs mostly in relation to follicular ameloblastoma and in this type, the stellate reticulum-like cells at the center of the follicles undergo squamous metaplasia (Fig. 5.10).

Sometimes, the neoplastic epithelial cells can even produce "keratin pearls". Within the follicles the neoplastic cells may exhibit individual cell keratinization. Metaplasia does not indicate any aggressive nature of the tumor. If extensive keratin pearl formation is noted within the islands, the variant can be named as keratoameloblastoma.

Granular Cell Ameloblastoma

This type also structurally resembles follicular ameloblastoma and the cytoplasm

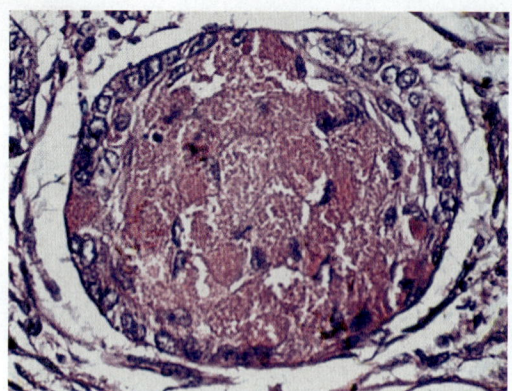

Fig. 5.11: Photomicrograph of ameloblastoma (granular cell type).

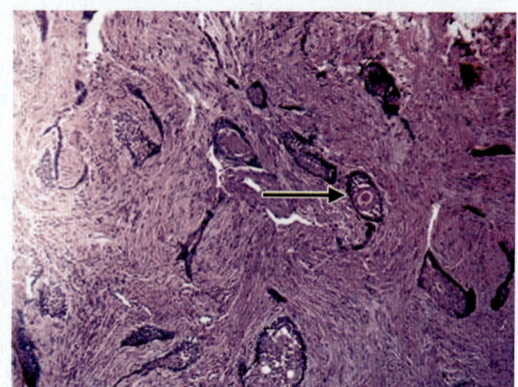

Fig. 5.13: Photomicrograph of desmoplastic ameloblastoma.

of the stellate reticulum-like cells and even the ameloblast-like cells appear swollen and the cells are often densely packed with multiple, coarse, eosinophilic granules (Fig. 5.11).

Histologically this lesion often resembles "granular cell myoblastoma".

Basal Cell Type of Ameloblastoma (Fig. 5.12)

This lesion shows excessive proliferation of uniform looking basaloid cells in several nests, with the absence of stellate reticulum or other centrally located cells. The cells bordering the nests are cuboidal in shape rather than columnar type and these tumors often resemble basal cell carcinomas.

Desmoplastic Type of Ameloblastoma

In this type the epithelial islands or the strands are small in size and the cells are cuboidal in shape and are darkly stained (Fig. 5.13). The tall columnar ameloblast-like cells are scanty in this lesion. The cells of the epithelial components are widely separated by dense fibrous tissue and the neoplastic cells often infiltrate into the surrounding trabecular bone. Formation of metaplastic osteoid trabecular (osteoplasia) may be present.

Hemangiomatous Ameloblastoma (Fig. 5.14)

It is a rare variant of ameloblastoma, in which neoplastic odontogenic epithelial cells proliferate either in the firm of anastomosing chords or numerous discrete follicles; besides that the stromal tissue shows prominent vascular components comprising of blood filled spaces of varying sizes.

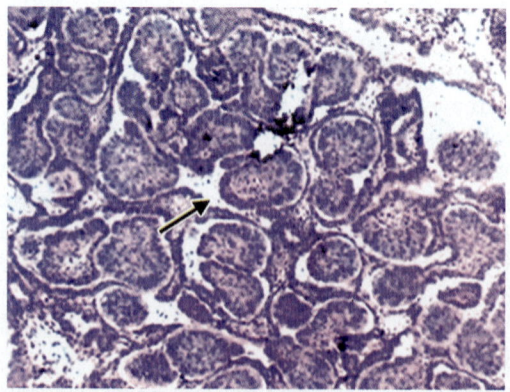

Fig. 5.12: Photomicrograph of basal cell type of ameloblastoma.

> ### Key Points of Ameloblastoma
> ❖ Ameloblastoma is the most common odontogenic neoplasm of the oral cavity and it is a benign locally aggressive tumor arising from the odontogenic epithelium.
> ❖ It occurs between 2nd and 5th decade of life, more often in males.
> ❖ Ameloblastoma in most of the cases involve the mandible especially in the molar-ramus area, maxillary bone is also commonly affected by the disease.

- Clinically, ameloblastoma produces slow enlarging, painless, ovoid or fusiform, bony hard swelling of the jaw.
- Some lesions cause expansion and distortion of the cortical plates of the jawbone, pain, paresthesia, displacement and mobility of the regional teeth and gross facial asymmetry.
- Untreated lesions cause extensive destruction and thinning of bone, leading to "egg-shell" crackling and pathological fracture, etc.
- Radiographically ameloblastoma usually presents a well-defined, multilocular, radiolucent area in the bone with a typical "honey-comb" or "soap-bubble" appearance. The border of the lesion is often scalloped.
- Histologically, the tumor shows neoplastic proliferation of odontogenic epithelial cells (ameloblast-like cells) in plexiform or follicular patterns.
- In plexiform pattern, the neoplastic odontogenic epithelial cells proliferate in the form of long continuous anastomosing strands cords.
- In follicular pattern, the neoplastic odontogenic epithelial cells proliferate in the form of multiple, discrete follicles or islands.
- Treatment is done by surgical enucleation of the tumor and through curettage.

Treatment

Surgical enucleation of the tumor and thorough curettage of the surrounding bone. Recurrence is common. Sometimes, radical surgical approach may have to be adopted in cases of repeated recurrences. Some tumors may cause distant metastasis also.

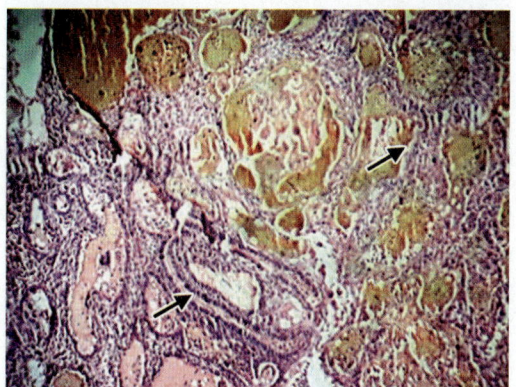

Fig. 5.14: Photomicrograph of hemangiomatous ameloblastoma.

UNICYSTIC AMELOBLASTOMA

Unicystic ameloblastoma is separate entity from conventional ameloblastoma, it constitutes about 10–15% of all intraosseous ameloblastomas.

■ ORIGIN

The tumor arises either as a de novo lesion or it develops due to neoplastic transformation of the preexisting cystic epithelium.

Clinical Features

- *Age:* Young people are mostly affected (2nd decade of life).
- *Site:* Mandible is predominantly involved.

■ CLINICAL PRESENTATION (FIGS. 5.15A AND B)

Unicystic ameloblastoma produces painless swelling of the jaw with expansion of the cortical plates and disturbance in occlusion, etc. Some lesions can be asymptomatic.

■ RADIOGRAPHIC FINDING

The lesion often exhibits a well-circumscribed, large unilocular, radiolucent area in the bone that often surrounds the crown of an impacted 3rd molar tooth (Fig. 5.16).

In some instances, the radiolucent area may have scalloped margins.

■ HISTOPATHOLOGY

Histologically, unicystic ameloblastomas reveals neoplastic proliferation of tall columnar cells, resembling ameloblasts; the hallmark feature of the tumor is the cystification within the lesion. With presence of a prominent epithelial lining (Fig. 5.17).

The cyst lining has basal cells that are columnar or cuboidal in nature and exhibit reverse polarity. Besides the lining, the stroma presents variable amount of neoplastic cells either in follicular or in plexiform pattern.

There are three distinct types of unicystic ameloblastoma—(1) luminal type, (2) intraluminal type, and (3) mural type.

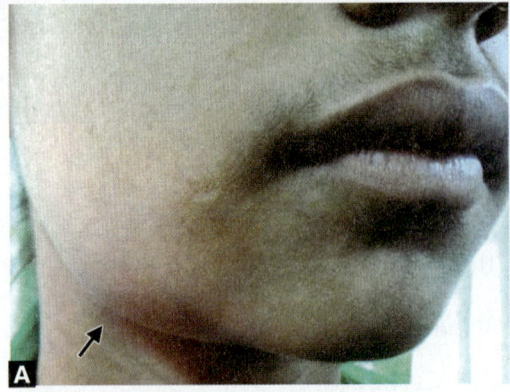
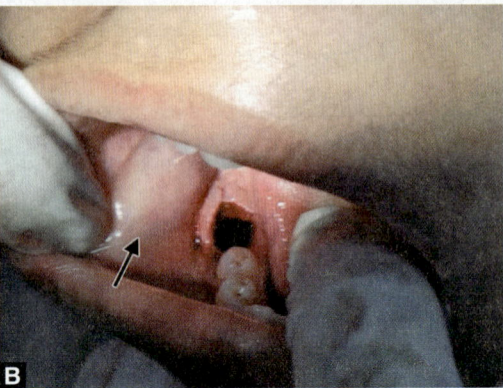

Figs. 5.15A and B: (A) Unicystic ameloblastoma of mandible; (B) Intraoral lesion of the same patient.

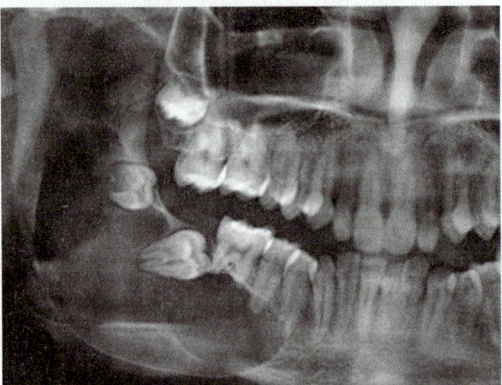

Fig. 5.16: Radiograph of unicystic ameloblastoma of mandible.

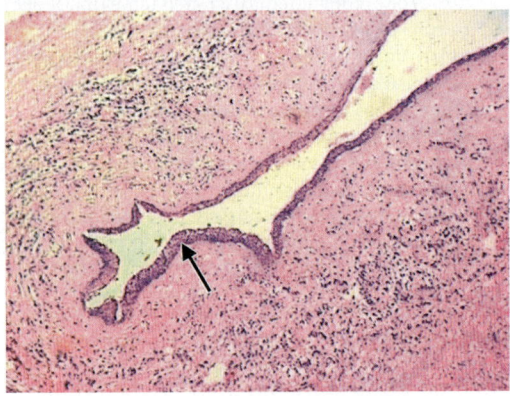

Fig. 5.17: Photomicrograph of unicystic ameloblastoma (low power).

Luminal Unicystic Ameloblastoma

This type of unicystic ameloblastoma shows localized excess cell growth on the luminal surface of the cyst (Fig. 5.18).

Intraluminal Unicystic Ameloblastoma

This type of lesion produces several nodular growths; which project from the cyst lining into the cystic lumen (Fig. 5.19).

Mural Unicystic Ameloblastoma

In this lesion the neoplastic cells instead of projecting inside the cystic lumen infiltrates into the connective tissue wall of the cyst capsule.

The differences between unicystic ameloblastoma and a normal cyst are given in Table 5.1.

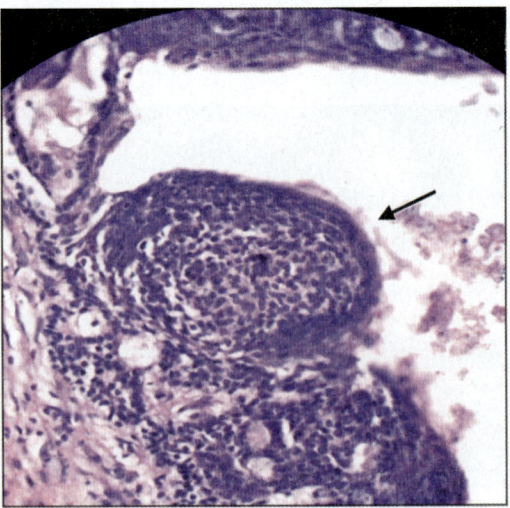

Fig. 5.18: Photomicrograph of luminal unicystic ameloblastoma.

Odontogenic Neoplasms

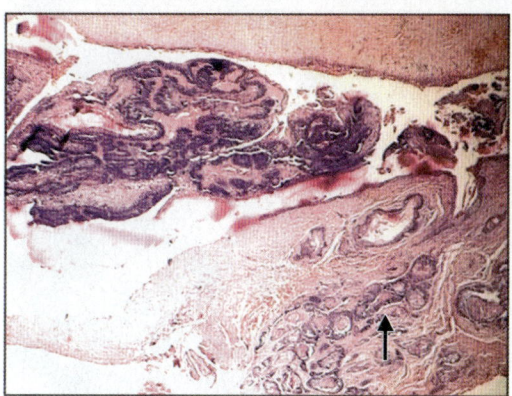

Fig. 5.19: Photomicrograph of (A) Intraluminal; (B) Mural unicystic ameloblastoma.

DIFFERENTIAL DIAGNOSIS

- Dentigerous cyst
- Calcifying epithelial odontogenic cyst (COC)
- Adenomatoid odontogenic cyst (AOT)

Treatment

Enucleation and curettage, recurrence rate is low as compared to the conventional ameloblastomas.

ADENOMATOID ODONTOGENIC TUMOR

DEFINITION

The adenomatoid odontogenic tumor is a relatively uncommon, well-circumscribed, odontogenic neoplasm characterized by the formation of multiple "ducts-like" structures by the neoplastic epithelial cells.

The name "adenomatoid" has been given to the neoplasm because histologically numerous duct-like structures are often interspersed throughout the lesion, which gives a glandular or adenomatoid appearance to it.

ORIGIN

The tumor probably arises from the reduced enamel epithelium, during the presecretory phase of enamel organ development. Some other investigators believe that it develops from either the dental lamina associated with the gubernacular cord or from a preexisting dentigerous cyst.

CLINICAL FEATURES

- *Age:* The tumor usually occurs in the younger age (e.g. 2nd and 3rd decade of life).
- *Sex:* Females are more commonly affected in comparison to the males, with a ratio of 2:1.
- *Site:* The lesion most typically occurs in the maxillary anterior region (upper lateral incisor-canine area). Sometimes it can occur in the premolar region. Rarely does it involve the mandible in the angle-ramus area. In about 70% cases, the neoplasms occur in association with an unerupted tooth. Some lesions develop extraorally in relation to the gingiva.

Table 5.1: Differences between unicystic ameloblastoma and a normal cyst.

	Unicystic ameloblastoma	*Cyst*
- Rate of growth	Fast as it is a tumor	Slow growth rate
- Cortical reaction	Bicortical swelling	Often unicortical swelling
- Margin	Often scalloped and noncorticated	Smooth and corticated
- Internal structures	Structures like tooth, etc. are displaced due to the growing tumor mass	Less chance of displacement
- Degree of bone expansion and thinning	More	Relatively less
- Risk of pathological fracture	More	Less
- Recurrence	More	Relatively less
- Histopathological features (confirmatory)	Exhibits ameloblastoma	Reveals cyst

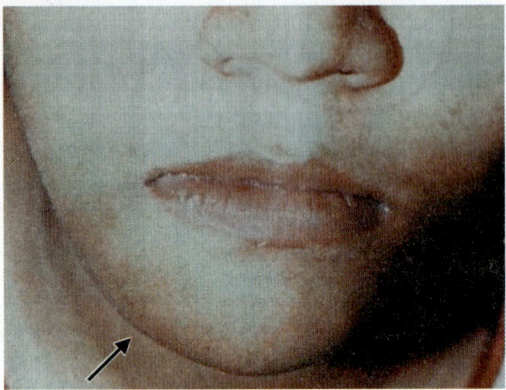

Fig. 5.20: Adenomatoid odontogenic tumor (AOT) of mandible with swelling on the right side.

CLINICAL PRESENTATION

- The tumor usually presents a slow enlarging, small, bony hard swelling in the maxillary anterior region (Fig. 5.20). Most AOTs are relatively small and they seldom exceed 3 cm in greatest diameter.
- The lesion often causes elevation of the upper lip on the involved side (Fig. 5.21).
- Displacement of the regional teeth, mild pain and expansion of the cortical bones are usually present (Fig. 5.22).
- If the lesion is very large it may cause severe expansion of the bone, which may sometimes elicit fluctuations.
- Many lesions are asymptomatic in nature.

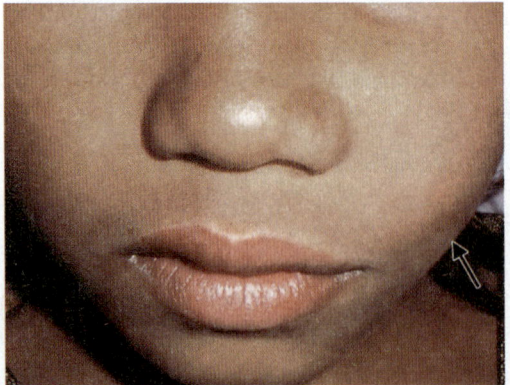

Fig. 5.21: Adenomatoid odontogenic tumor (AOT) causing swelling on the upper canine regions.

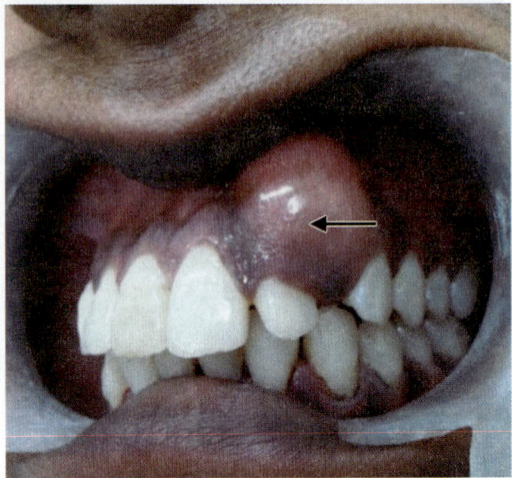

Fig. 5.22: Adenomatoid odontogenic tumor (AOT) with swelling in the anterior maxilla.

- Occasionally, adenomatoid odontogenic tumor may occur extraosseously in the anterior maxillary gingiva.

RADIOLOGICAL FEATURES

- Radiographically, adenomatoid odontogenic tumor presents a well-circumscribed, unilocular, radiolucent area, which often encloses a tooth or tooth-like structure (mostly maxillary canine) (Fig. 5.23).
- Multiple small, radiopaque foci of varying radiodensity may be present inside the lesion and the finding is known as "snowflake" calcifications.
- Some lesions may present unilocular, well-defined radiolucencies between the roots of the erupted teeth and they do not enclose any tooth.
- Expansion and distortion of the cortical plates and displacement of the roots of the adjacent teeth are sometimes seen.
- Orbital and maxillary sinus encroachments have been reported.
- Gingival lesions may cause slight erosion of the underlying alveolar bone cortex.
- The border of the lesion is not well corticated which distinguish it from a cystic lesion and moreover AOT consistently engulfs

Odontogenic Neoplasms

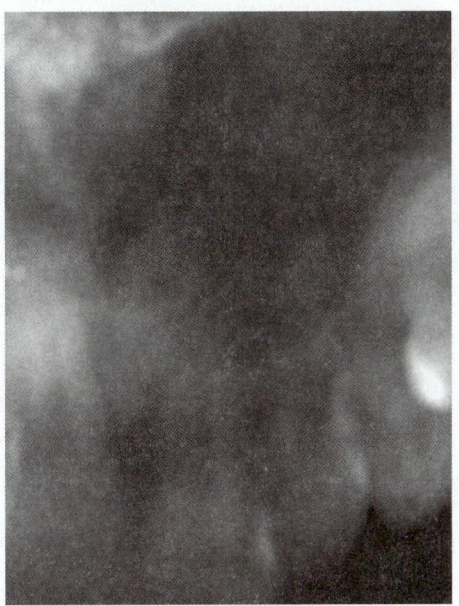

Fig. 5.23: Radiologically adenomatoid odontogenic tumor (AOT) producing a unilocular radiolucent lesion enclosing a tooth.

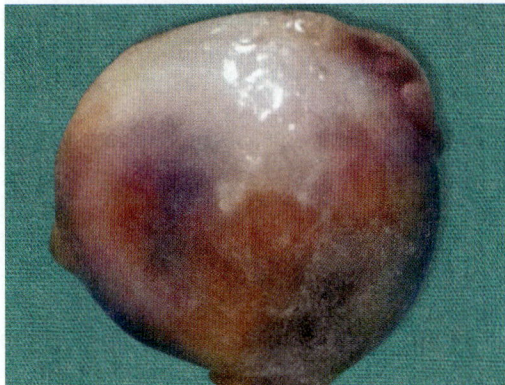

Fig. 5.24: Enucleated specimen of adenomatoid odontogenic tumor (AOT).

the impacted tooth including its root. This feature differentiates adenomatoid odontogenic tumor from dentigerous cyst since the later lesion encloses only the crown portion of an impacted tooth.

MACROSCOPIC FEATURES

Macroscopically the AOT is a well-defined lesion that is usually surrounded by a thick, fibrous capsule (Fig. 5.24). When the lesion is bisected, the central portion of the tumor may be essentially solid or may show varying degrees of cystic changes.

DIFFERENTIAL DIAGNOSIS

- Dentigerous cyst
- Globulomaxillary cyst
- Lateral periodontal cyst
- Odontome
- Unicystic ameloblastoma
- Ossifying or cementifying fibroma
- Calcifying epithelial odontogenic tumor
- Calcifying epithelial odontogenic cyst.

HISTOPATHOLOGICAL FEATURES

- Microscopically, adenomatoid odontogenic tumor reveals spindle shaped, neoplastic odontogenic epithelial cells proliferating in multiple "duct-like" patterns, within a thin but well-vascularized stroma (Fig. 5.25).
- The presence of these duct-like or tubular structures is very characteristic, which often give the lesion an adenomatoid or

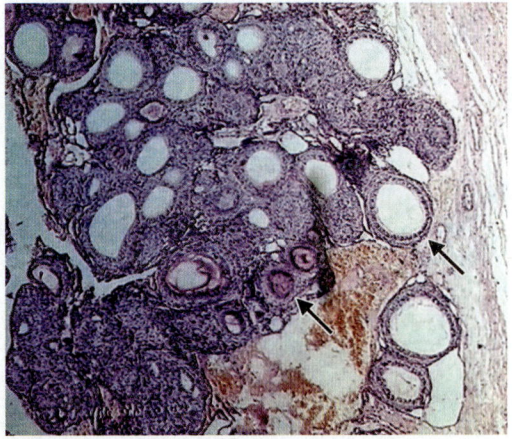

Fig. 5.25: Photomicrograph of adenomatoid odontogenic tumor (AOT) showing duct-like proliferation of tumor cells with areas of calcification and the surrounding capsule.

glandular appearance. However, no actual glandular element is found in this tumor.
- Each duct-like structure exhibits a central space, which is bordered on the periphery by a single layer of tall columnar cells resembling ameloblasts or preameloblasts.
- Nuclei of these ameloblast-like cells are often polarized away from the central space; Moreover sometimes these bordering cells can be cuboidal in nature.
- These duct like or microcyst lumina are frequently lined by an eosinophilic rim of varying thickness (the so called hyaline ring).
- The lumen of the duct-like structures is generally filled with a homogenous eosinophilic coagulum (mostly amyloids); although some lumens can be empty (Fig. 5.26).
- Small foci of calcifications are often seen scattered throughout the lesion (sometimes even larger masses are found). This type of calcification within the lesion probably indicates an abortive attempt toward formation of enamel, dentin or cementum by the tumor cells.

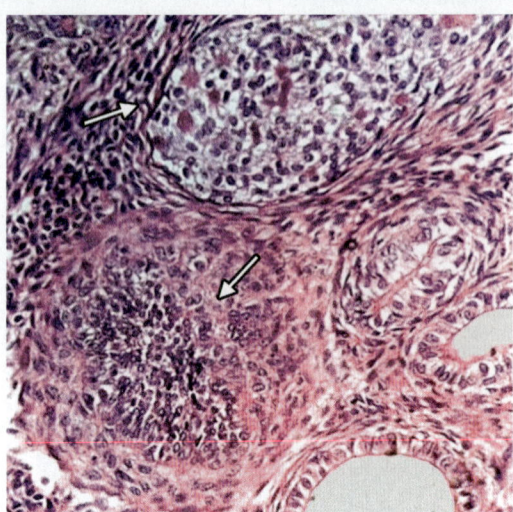

Fig. 5.27: Adenomatoid odontogenic tumor (AOT): Solid proliferation with no ductal areas.

- In some cases, the neoplastic cells are arranged in solid nests, sheets or *rosette-like pattern* (refers to a circular cluster of cells of same size radiating from a center and resembling the petals of a rose), and these cells sometimes may even fill up the entire lumen of some of the ducts (Fig. 5.27).
- The neoplasm is almost always well-encapsulated. Occurrence of a hyaline, dysplastic material or calcified osteodentin may be found in AOTs. It is likely the result of a metaplastic process.

Treatment

By surgical enucleation. The associated tooth has to be removed and recurrence is rare.

CALCIFYING EPITHELIAL ODONTOGENIC TUMOR (CEOT)/ PINDBORG'S TUMOR

Calcifying epithelial odontogenic tumor (CEOT) is a locally invasive epithelial neoplasm, characterized by the development of intraepithelial structures, probably of an amyloid-like nature, which may be liberated

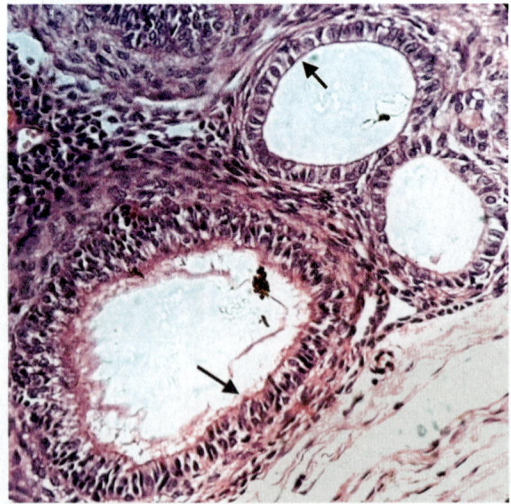

Fig. 5.26: Photomicrograph of adenomatoid odontogenic tumor (AOT, high power) duct-like structure showing peripheral tall columnar cells and eosinophilic enameloid material.

as cells breakdown—WHO (1992). It is also known as Pindborg tumor (named after Prof JJ Pindborg, who first reported it).

ORIGIN

The lesion arises from either the cells of the stratum intermedium of the enamel organ or the reduced enamel epithelium or even the remnants of the dental lamina.

Its biologic behavior of CEOT that it has similarity with ameloblastoma as both tumors cause bone destruction and expansion. However, it differs from ameloblastoma by the fact that it is less aggressive, composed of spherical cells and not the ameloblast-like cells as seen in ameloblastoma. Moreover calcifying epithelial odontogenic tumor always contains some calcified materials within it mass, which is never seen in ameloblastoma (Some investigators mention it as calcifying ameloblastoma).

CLINICAL FEATURES

- *Incidence rate:* The calcifying epithelial odontogenic tumor constitutes about 1% of all odontogenic neoplasms.
- *Age:* The tumor commonly occurs in middle-aged adults (mean age 40 years).
- *Sex:* Both sexes are almost equally affected.
- *Site:* The mandible (two-thirds number of cases) is involved more often than the maxilla (one-third number of cases), the molar region is the most common site of occurrence followed by the premolar region. Rarely the tumor develops extraosseously from the gingiva as peripheral lesions. In about 50% cases the neoplasms are associated with impacted teeth.

CLINICAL PRESENTATION (FIGS. 5.28A AND B)

- The tumor usually presents a slow enlarging, painless swelling of the jaw with expansion and distortion of the cortical plates.
- Most of the tumors occur in the mandibular molar/premolar region and nearly half of the lesions have an impacted or unerupted tooth inside them.
- The swelling is usually bony hard and clinically it can be either well defined or diffuse in nature.
- Displacement of regional teeth, with derangement of occlusion and facial asymmetry, etc. are commonly present.
- Pain, paresthesia and other related symptoms may develop on rare occasions, and few lesions may be even completely asymptomatic.
- Large maxillary lesions may invade into the antrum or the nasal floor.
- Extraosseous or peripheral lesions may cause nonspecific, sessile, superficial soft tissue swellings of gingiva.

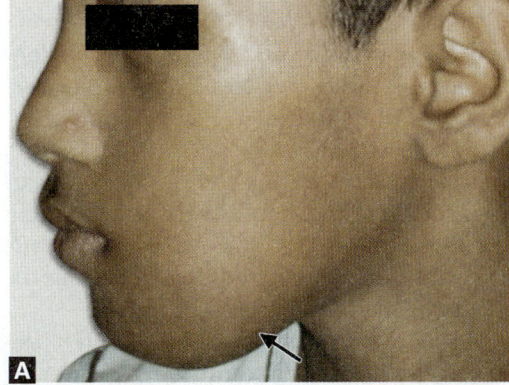
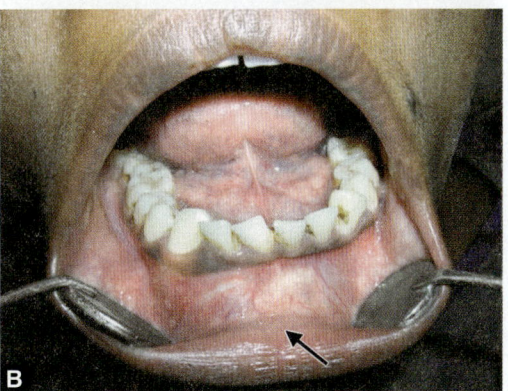

Figs. 5.28A and B: (A) Calcifying epithelial odontogenic tumor (CEOT) causing large mandibular swelling; (B) Intraoral view of the same patient.

RADIOLOGICAL FEATURES

- Radiographically calcifying epithelial odontogenic tumor usually presents a well-defined, multilocular (rarely unilocular) radiolucent area in the jaw.
- Calcifications within the tumor is a characteristic finding and radiographically it often exhibits multiple, small, radiopaque foci of varying radiodensity within the tumor (Fig. 5.29).
- Calcified areas within the tumor often produces a typical "driven snow" appearance; moreover, some tumors produce radiolucent lesion with "smoky dense" areas.
- The border of the lesion is often scalloped and the lesion frequently causes expansion and destruction of the cortical plates of jawbones.
- In approximately half of the cases, an unerupted tooth (mostly mandibular third molar) may be seen within the tumor (Fig. 5.30).
- Perforation of the cortical plates, pathological fractures and root resorptions, etc. are seen in few cases.
- Peripheral (extraosseous) lesions sometimes cause superficial "cupped out" erosion of the cortical bone.

DIFFERENTIAL DIAGNOSIS

- Calcifying epithelial odontogenic cyst
- Adenomatoid odontogenic tumor

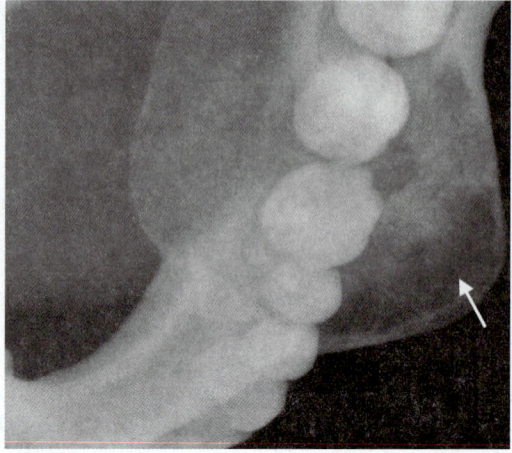

Fig. 5.30: Radiograph of calcifying epithelial odontogenic tumor (CEOT) showing calcification within the tumor.

- Poorly differentiated carcinoma
- Ameloblastoma
- Ameloblastic fibro-odontome
- Dentigerous cyst
- Central ossifying or cementifying fibroma.

HISTOPATHOLOGICAL FEATURES (FIGS. 5.31 AND 5.32)

- Histologically, the tumor reveals sheets, islands or strands of closely packed, polyhedral epithelial cells, in a noninflamed fibrous connective tissue stroma.

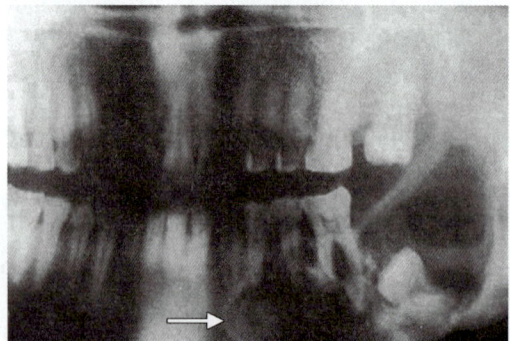

Fig. 5.29: Calcifying epithelial odontogenic tumor (CEOT) producing a large radiolucent area containing multiple radiopaque foci.

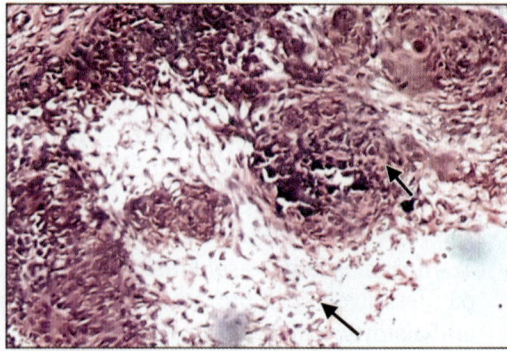

Fig. 5.31: Photomicrograph of calcifying epithelial odontogenic tumor (CEOT) showing polyhedral tumor cells with areas of calcifications.

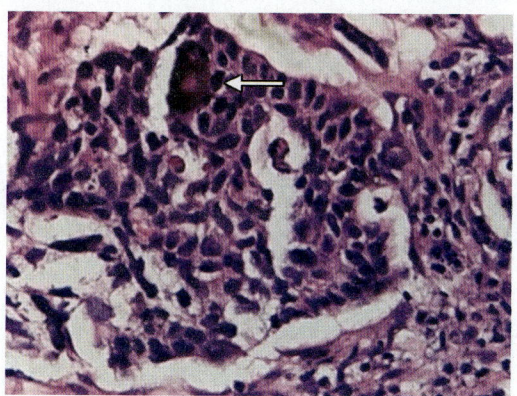

Fig. 5.32: Photomicrograph of calcifying epithelial odontogenic tumor (CEOT, high power).

- Some tumors exhibit excessive cellularity and contain very little calcified mass within the tumor whereas other tumors may have diffuse large calcified areas with only small islands or nests of epithelial cells.
- In few tumors large numbers of "clear cell" are found and because of this, the tumor often resembles the clear cell variant of mucoepidermoid tumor.
- Calcifying epithelial odontogenic tumor is nonencapsulated lesion and sometimes it is locally aggressive in nature.

- Sometimes the neoplastic cells may have a "cribriform" arrangement and they enclose areas of hyalinized stoma.
- The tumor cells have homogeneous eosinophilic cytoplasm and contain large oval-shaped nuclei and prominent nucleoli.
- Nuclei exhibit considerable variation in size and shape; few cells have multiple nuclei or a single bizarre giant hyperchromatic nucleus (the latter is not indicative of malignancy since mitotic activity is rare).
- Prominent intercellular bridges and distinct cell boundaries are characteristically seen in the tumor.
- The tumor cells produce a homogenous, amorphous, hyaline material, which is believed to be *amyloid* or amyloid-like and take positive staining with "Congo red" and fluorescence with Thioflavin T.
- These amyloid-like materials calcify in a concentrically lamellated *"tree ring"* pattern (these rings also called *Liesegang rings*).
- One of the most distinctive histological characteristics of CEOT is the presence of several of these calcified bodies or masses within the lesion.
- Sometimes individual calcified structures are fused together to form a large complex mass within the tissue.
- Non-calcifying variants also occur and are more common in extraosseous tumors.

Key Points of Calcifying Epithelial Odontogenic Tumor

- Calcifying epithelial odontogenic tumor is a locally aggressive, benign odontogenic tumor, whose biologic behavior is similar to that of ameloblastoma.
- The tumor predominantly affects posterior part of the jaws, and clinically produces slow enlarging, painless swelling with expansion and distortion of the cortical plates.
- Radiographically, calcifying epithelial odontogenic tumor presents a well-defined, multilocular radiolucent area, which contains multiple, small, radiopaque calcified foci of varying radiodensity.
- This type of calcification within the tumor often produces a typical "driven snow" appearance.
- Histologically, the tumor reveals sheets or islands of closely packed, polyhedral epithelial cells, in a noninflamed connective tissue stroma.
- The neoplastic cells have hyperchromatic nuclei and prominent intercellular bridges.
- Several calcified substances and amyloids are characteristically present in the lesion.
- Surgical enucleation is the treatment of choice.

Treatment

By surgical enucleation. Incomplete removal of the lesion is likely to be followed by recurrences.

DENTINOGENIC GHOST-CELL TUMOR

It is a variant of calcifying epithelial odontogenic cyst (COC) but the cells here do not form the cyst lining but they proliferate diffusely into the stroma like a tumor; the behavior of the lesions is similar to ameloblastoma or odontoma.

286 Essentials of Oral Pathology

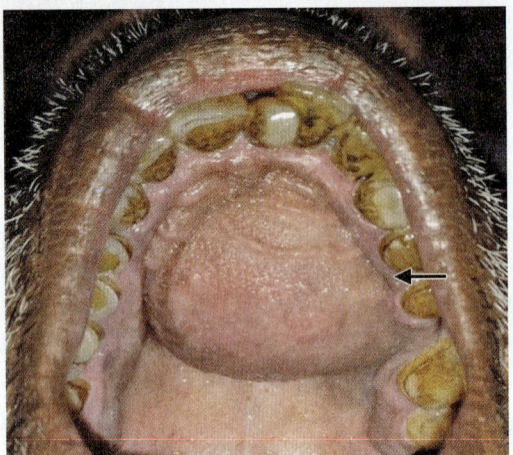

Fig. 5.33: Dentinogenic ghost-cell tumor of maxilla.

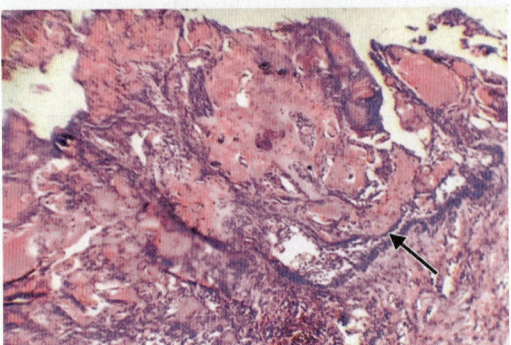

Fig. 5.34: Photomicrograph of dentinogenic ghost-cell tumor of maxilla.

Intraosseous jaw tumors are more common, however peripheral lesions may develop mostly from the gingiva (Fig. 5.33).

The tumor produces expansile jaw swelling with displacement of teeth and facial asymmetry, etc.

Radiograph shows radiolucency in the jawbone with variable amounts of radiopacities within the lesion.

Histologically the lesion presents neoplastic proliferation of odontogenic epithelial cells with formation some homogenous eosinophilic amyloid-like material and few round or ovoid shaped calcified tissues (mostly *dentinoid* materials) along with the presence of many ghost cells (Fig. 5.34).

SQUAMOUS ODONTOGENIC TUMOR/ BENIGN EPITHELIAL ODONTOGENIC TUMOR

■ DEFINITION

Squamous odontogenic tumors are rare, sometimes multifocal, potentially aggressive neoplasms derived from the odontogenic epithelium.

■ ORIGIN

This neoplasm was first reported in the year 1975 and it probably originates from the following tissue remnants found on the lateral root surfaces of the erupted teeth:
- Remnants of dental lamina.
- Cell rests of Malassez
- Periodontal ligament that is associated with the lateral root surface of an erupted tooth.

■ CLINICAL FEATURES

- *Age:* It occurs more commonly among young adults.
- *Sex:* Female predilection.
- *Site:* Maxillary incisor-canine area and mandibular molar area.

■ PRESENTATION

- Initially, there can be a painless swelling on the gingival areas of the jaw with mobility and looseness of the regional teeth (Fig. 5.35).
- Intraosseous lesions are usually small and slow enlarging.
- There can be local tenderness in the area upon palpation.
- Many lesions are asymptomatic and are discovered incidentally during radiographic examinations.

■ RADIOGRAPHIC FEATURES (FIG. 5.36)

- Radiographically, squamous odontogenic tumor presents a well-circumscribed, often semilunar or triangular shaped, unilocular radiolucent area with sclerotic border.

Odontogenic Neoplasms

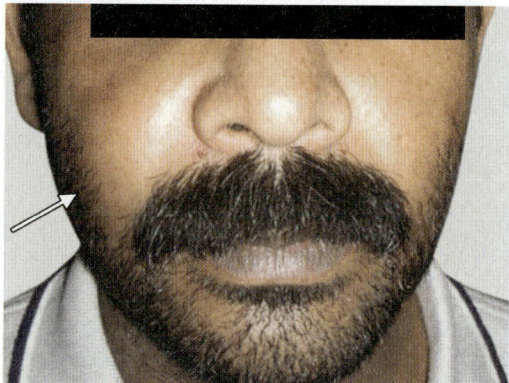

Fig. 5.35: Squamous odontogenic tumor of right maxilla.

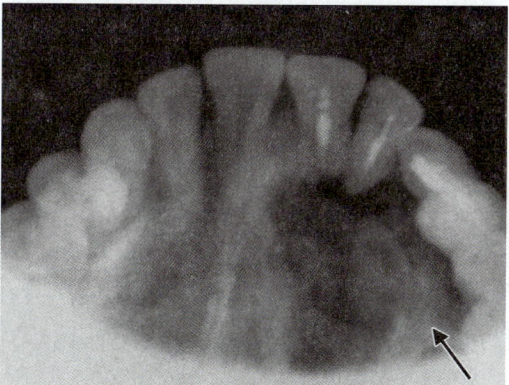

Fig. 5.36: Radiograph of squamous odontogenic tumor.

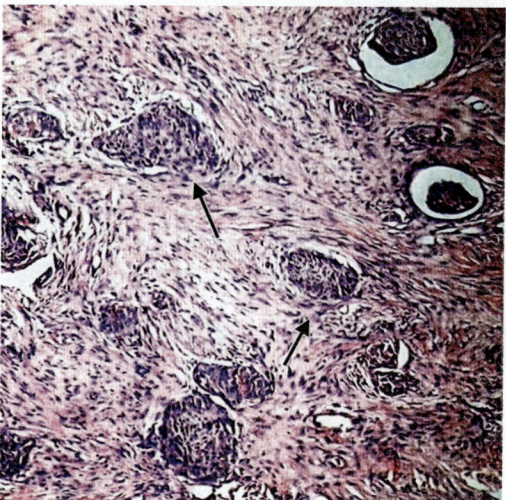

Fig. 5.37: Photomicrograph of squamous odontogenic tumor.

- These lesions are interspersed between contagious teeth near their roots.
- Some lesions can be multilocular.
- Resorptions of root are usually absent.
- Most of the time lesions are small that seldom exceed 1.5 cm in greatest diameter.

HISTOPATHOLOGY

- Microscopically, squamous odontogenic tumor presents irregularly-shaped, islands of well-differentiated squamous epithelium in a mature fibrous connective tissue stroma (Fig. 5.37).
- The islands can be of round or oval in shape and there is absence of peripheral palisaded or polarized basal cells.
- Individual cell keratinization is often seen in this tumor, moreover focal areas keratin or parakeratin formation by the neoplastic epithelial cells is also sometimes noticed.
- The basal cell layer in squamous odontogenic tumor is usually made up of inactive looking cuboidal cells.
- The remaining epithelial cells of the islands are composed of mature intermediate type of cells with prominent desmosomal bridges.
- Many epithelial islands reveal central areas of microcyst formations.
- Some of the epithelial islands contain spherical or irregularly shaped calcified structures, indicating dystrophic calcifications within the tumor and globular, hyaline, eosinophilic structures within the islands which are not amyloid.
- Similar calcifications can also be found within the connective tissue stroma as well.
- Although the tumor is benign, the tumor cells sometimes invade into the adjacent tissues (it is more often seen in maxillary tumors).
- The fibrous stroma of the tumor is simply mature bundles of collagen fibers.

- Squamous odontogenic tumor may be confused with well differentiated squamous cell carcinoma; however, the islands in squamous odontogenic tumor are well defined, and the cells lack variation in cell size, shape and nuclear staining and mitotic figures that are characteristically seen in squamous cell carcinoma. Significant keratin formation also is not typical.

DIFFERENTIAL DIAGNOSIS
- Acanthomatous ameloblastoma
- Lateral periodontal cyst
- Squamous cell carcinoma
- Central ossifying or cementifying fibroma
- Histiocytosis-X
- Collateral type of keratocyst.

Treatment
Surgical enucleation with thorough curettage.

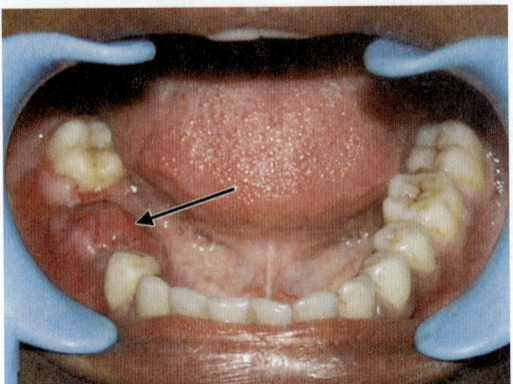

Fig. 5.38: Ameloblastic fibroma of mandible.

AMELOBLASTIC FIBROMA

Ameloblastic fibroma is a true benign odontogenic tumor in which both the epithelial and the mesenchymal elements are neoplastic (in ameloblastoma only the epithelium is neoplastic).

CLINICAL FEATURES
- *Age:* It occurs usually below the age of 20 years (average age 14 years).
- *Sex:* More often in males than females.
- *Site:* Mandibular posterior (premolar-molar) region is the most common site, maxillary tumors are usually rare.

CLINICAL PRESENTATION (FIG. 5.38)
- A slow growing, painless, bony hard swelling of the jaw.
- Few lesions can be completely asymptomatic and discovered accidentally during routine examinations.
- There may be mobility of the regional teeth, with obvious facial asymmetry.

- The tumor develops predominantly above the impacted or unerupted molar teeth as a pericoronal lesion.

RADIOLOGICAL FEATURES (FIG. 5.39)
On radiograph, the tumor usually presents a well-defined, unilocular or multilocular radiolucent area that often resembles ameloblastoma or dentigerous cyst. Lesions are well corticated and they vary considerably in size.

HISTOPATHOLOGICAL FEATURES (FIG. 5.40)
- Ameloblastic fibroma histologically consists of neoplastic epithelial as well as mesenchymal components of odontogenic tissue.

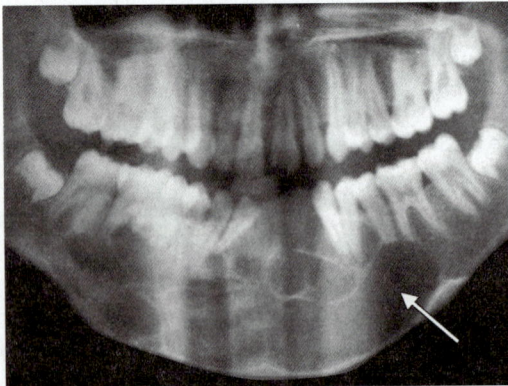

Fig. 5.39: Radiograph of ameloblastic fibroma.

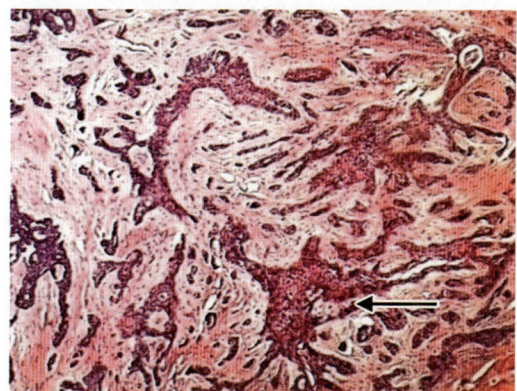

Fig. 5.40: Photomicrograph of ameloblastic fibroma showing neoplastic proliferation of epithelial cells.

- The epithelial components of the tumor consist of multiple sharply defined, strands, islands or narrow cords.
- Sometimes the tumor cells exhibit a "mushroom" type proliferation within a loose connective tissue stroma.
- The epithelial cords may be as thin as only few cells thickness, the epithelial islands are small and discrete, and they resemble the follicular stage of a developing enamel organ.
- The epithelial components are circumscribed by a basal membrane and at the periphery these are bordered by tall columnar cells resembling ameloblasts.
- The cells, which are located at the center of the islands or strands, resemble the stellate reticulum cells.
- Although the epithelial components of this neoplasm resemble ameloblastoma but the stellate cells are much less abundant and cyst formation is rare.
- There may be a narrow cell free zone of hyaline connective tissue bordering the epithelial component.
- The mesenchymal component of the tumor consists of plump stellate or ovoid cells with a loose fibroblastic stroma that often resembles the dental papilla of the developing tooth.

Treatment

By surgical excision with thorough curettage of the bone, recurrence is uncommon. Rarely ameloblastic fibroma may undergo malignant transformation to develop ameloblastic fibrosarcoma.

AMELOBLASTIC FIBRO-ODONTOME

It is a benign neoplasm of odontogenic origin and is characterized by the presence of combined features of ameloblastic fibroma along with the presence of calcified enamel or dentin-like tissues.

CLINICAL FEATURES

- *Age:* Children and young adults (mean age 8–12 years).
- *Sex:* No predilection.
- *Site:* Posterior region of jaw, more common in mandible.

CLINICAL PRESENTATION

- Most of the lesions are asymptomatic.
- Lesions are often associated with an impacted or missing tooth (Fig. 5.41).
- Larger lesions cause progressive, painless swelling of the jaw with expansion of the cortical plates.
- Untreated lesions can result in severe facial deformity.

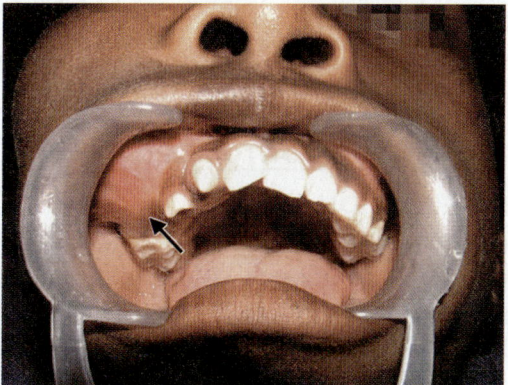

Fig. 5.41: Ameloblastic fibro-odontome.

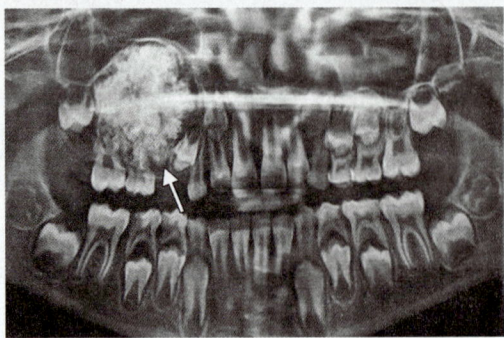

Fig. 5.42: Radiograph of ameloblastic fibro-odontome.

RADIOLOGICAL APPEARANCE

Radiographs show unilocular radiolucent area (rarely multilocular) containing multiple radiopaque foci having radiodensity similar to that of tooth. Sometimes, a solid conglomerated mass is seen inside the lesion (Fig. 5.42).

HISTOPATHOLOGY

- Histologically the tumor exhibits neoplastic odontogenic epithelial cells proliferating in the form of small discrete islands or narrow cords as may be seen in ameloblastic fibromas.
- Connective tissue stroma is loose, primitive looking and it often resembles the dental papilla.
- Multiple calcified foci of enamel and dentin matrix are found near the epithelial components.

TREATMENT

Surgical excision and curettage; prognosis is excellent and chance of recurrence is rare.

ODONTOMES

DEFINITION

Odontomes are a group of common hamartomatous odontogenic lesions with limited growth potential. These lesions are capable of producing normal appearing enamel, dentin, cementum and pulp, etc. in an unorganized fashion.

The tumor probably occurs during the development of teeth at a point after the stage of histodifferentiation but prior to the stage of morphodifferentiation.

TYPES

Two types of odontomes are commonly recognized:
1. Compound odontome, and
2. Complex odontome (both these lesions are closely related malformation).

Compound odontome: Compound odontome presents localized collections of numerous small, discrete, tooth-like structures. Most odontogenic tissues in compound odontome bear superficial anatomical resemblance to normal teeth.

Complex odontome: It consists of a completely disorganized and diffuse mass of odontogenic tissue with haphazardly arranged enamel, dentin and cementum.

CLINICAL FEATURES

- *Frequency:* Odontomes represent about 7% of all odontogenic neoplasms.
- *Age:* These lesions usually occur among children or young adults (preferably in their 2nd decade of life).
- *Sex:* Both sexes are almost equally affected or there may be a slight male predominance.
- *Site:* Maxilla is more commonly affected than the mandible. Odontomes are most commonly seen in the pericoronal area of the permanent teeth.

Compound odontomes usually involve the anterior part of the maxilla (intercanine area).

Complex odontomes often involve the posterior (premolar-molar) region of the jaw and are slightly more common in mandible. Some lesions may occur extraosseously in the gingival soft tissues.

CLINICAL PRESENTATION

- Odontomes generally produce small, asymptomatic lesions, which are detected incidentally.

Odontogenic Neoplasms

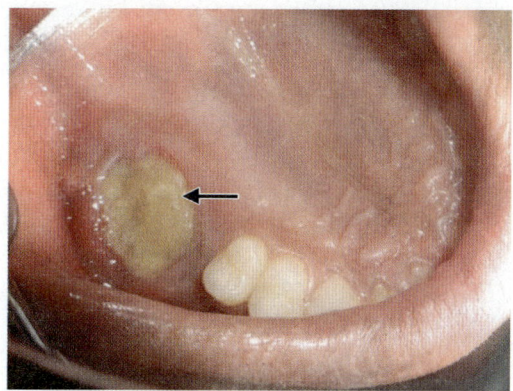

Fig. 5.43: Odontome of mandible.

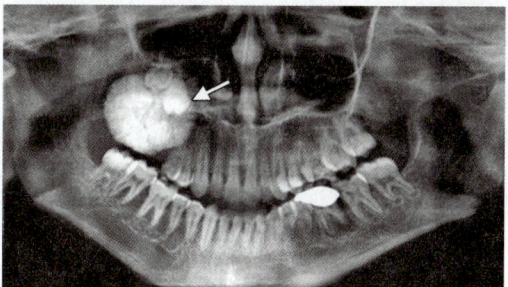

Fig. 5.44: Compound odontome.

- The lesions vary in size greatly, it can be as small as a tooth or it may be as large as 6 cm in diameter.
- In few cases, they may produce large, bony hard swellings of the jaw, with expansion of the cortical plates and displacement of the regional teeth (Fig. 5.43).
- A tooth may be often missing from the dental arch as the odontome can block the eruption path of the tooth.
- The lesions are often associated either with an impacted tooth or a retained deciduous tooth.
- If the odontomes are located high in the alveolus, they may tend to erupt in the oral cavity by resorbing the overlying bone and as a result there may be pain, inflammation, ulceration or fistula formation, etc.
- Some odontomes may exhibit cyst formation around the tumor mass (mostly dentigerous cyst).

RADIOLOGICAL FEATURES

Odontomes usually produce pericoronal radiolucencies with well-defined and well-corticated borders. A developing odontome may look completely radiolucent as the calcified elements do not form in the initial stages.

The compound odontome: The compound odontomes radiographically appear as numerous, small, miniature teeth or tooth-like structures, which are projecting from a single focus (Fig. 5.44).

- Apparently they look like "a bag of teeth" and are commonly located between the roots of the erupted permanent teeth or above the crown of an impacted tooth.

The complex odontome: The complex odontomes radiographically appears as round or oval or "sunburst-like", conglomerated radiopaque mass within the jawbone (Fig. 5.45).

- They do not produce any morphologically identifiable tooth or tooth-like structures.
- Both types of odontomes are usually surrounded by a thin radiolucent zone at their periphery, which represents the capsule.

DIFFERENTIAL DIAGNOSIS

- Calcifying epithelial odontogenic tumor (CEOT)
- Ameloblastic fibrodentinoma
- Ameloblastic fibro-odontome
- Osteoma

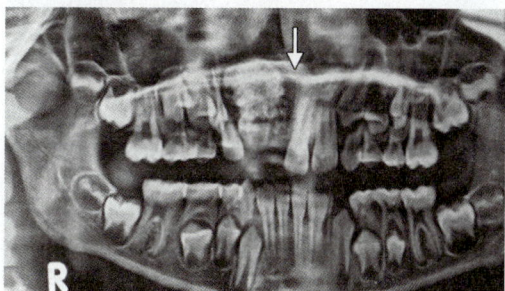

Fig. 5.45: Complex odontome.

- Odontoameloblastoma
- Focal sclerosing osteomyelitis.

HISTOPATHOLOGY

- Fully developed compound odontome histologically reveals the presence of an encapsulated mass of multiple separate denticles, embedded in a fibrous tissue stroma (Fig. 5.46).
- Morphologically most of the denticles do not resemble the tooth of the normal dentition.
- The number of denticles in a compound odontome varies from as few as 2–3 or as many as 20–30.
- Histologically, the fully developed complex odontome presents an irregularly arranged but well-formed mass of enamel, dentin, cementum and pulp, etc. which is surrounded by a fibrous tissue capsule (Fig. 5.47).
- The dentinal tissue lies in direct contact with a connective tissue that resembles dental pulp.
- Most of the enamel tissues are fully calcified and on decalcified sections, they appear as small clefts or circular empty spaces.
- If the enamel is not fully calcified then the empty spaces contain fibrillar enamel matrix or immature enamel.

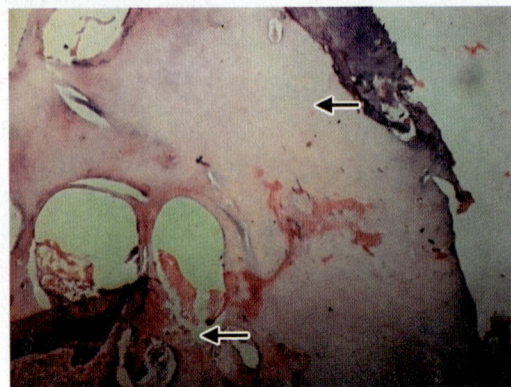

Fig. 5.47: Photomicrograph of odontome (complex).

- A thin layer of cementum may be present about the periphery of the tumor.
- Small islands of epithelial ghost cells are seen in the tumor, which are remnants of the odontogenic epithelium.

TREATMENT

By surgical enucleation. Recurrence is rare.

Key Points of Odontomes

- ❖ Odontomes are benign hamartomatous odontogenic lesions, capable of producing normal appearing enamel, dentin, cementum and pulp, etc. in an unorganized fashion.
- ❖ Two types of odontomes are found—*compound odontome and complex odontome.*
- ❖ Compound odontomes usually involve the anterior part of the maxilla (intercanine area).
- ❖ Complex odontomes often involve the posterior (premolar-molar) region of the jaw.
- ❖ Clinically, small odontomes produce painless, asymptomatic lesions, which are detected incidentally.
- ❖ The larger lesions however can be as large as 6 cm in diameter and they cause expansion and distortion of cortical plates, displacement of teeth and malocclusion, etc.
- ❖ Odontomes are often associated either with an impacted tooth or a retained deciduous tooth.
- ❖ The compound odontomes radiographically appear as numerous, small, miniature teeth or tooth-like structures, projecting from a single focus and thus apparently look like *"a bag of teeth".*
- ❖ The complex odontomes radiographically appear as round or oval or "sunburst-like", conglomerated radiopaque mass within the jawbone.

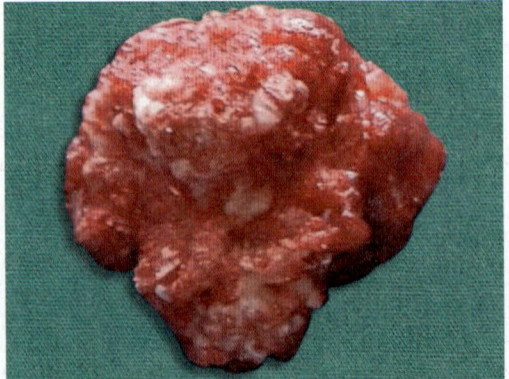

Fig. 5.46: Excised specimen of complex odontome.

- ❖ Fully developed compound odontome histologically presents an encapsulated mass of multiple separate denticles, embedded in a fibrous tissue stroma.
- ❖ Histologically, fully developed complex odontome presents an irregularly arranged mass of well-formed enamel, dentin, cementum and pulp, etc.
- ❖ Treatment is done by surgical enucleation.

ODONTOGENIC FIBROMA

DEFINITION

Odontogenic fibroma is a rare benign neoplasm derived from connective tissue of odontogenic origin and it can be either a peripheral lesion or a central (intraosseous) lesion. At present the term odontogenic fibroma is applied to two histological types of lesions: (1) the epithelium–poor type (formerly termed simple type), and (2) the epithelium–rich type (formerly termed complex or WHO–type).

PERIPHERAL ODONTOGENIC FIBROMA

DEFINITION

Peripheral odontogenic fibroma is the most common form of the disease, which develops extraosseously from the tooth bearing areas of the jaw.

ORIGIN

The lesion probably arises from the overlying gingival epithelium or the cell rests of the dental lamina.

CLINICAL FEATURES

- Peripheral odontogenic fibroma clinically appears as a slow enlarging, exophytic, well-circumscribed, sessile growth of the gingiva.
- The lesion is usually firm in consistency, it is painless and the overlying epithelium is of normal color.
- Most of the lesions occur on the facial gingiva and their size ranges between 0.5 cm and 1.5 cm in diameter.
- Epithelium, which result from trauma.
- Interdental lesions may cause separation of the teeth.
- Consistency of the lesion often varies, since lesions may occur with ossification or without ossification.
- Since peripheral odontogenic fibromas are small lesions and they occur extraosseously within the gingiva.
- However in certain cases saucerization of the cortical bone or widening of the periodontal ligament space.
- Numerous foci of small radiopaque masses are sometimes found within few lesions which indicate calcifications within the tumor.

HISTOPATHOLOGY

- Histologically peripheral odontogenic fibroma reveals a mass of dense connective tissue with few spindle-shaped fibroblasts, which is separated from the adjacent normal loose connective tissue.
- Surface epithelium shows long, slender rete-pegs projecting deep into the connective tissue.
- Small islands of odontogenic epithelium are present near the rete-pegs or deep within the connective tissue.
- Epithelial islands often contain few clear cells.
- Areas of hyalinized tissue with calcification can be present within the lesion.

DIFFERENTIAL DIAGNOSIS

- Peripheral ossifying fibroma
- Peripheral giant cell granuloma
- True fibroma
- Neurofibroma
- Fibroepithelial polyp.

TREATMENT

Surgical excision.

CENTRAL ODONTOGENIC FIBROMA

DEFINITION

Central odontogenic fibroma is a relatively uncommon odontogenic neoplasm arising within the jawbone.

CLINICAL FEATURES

- *Age:* Wide age range (mean age is 20 years).
- *Sex:* Female predilection is seen.
- *Site:* It occurs more often in relation to mandible than maxilla. Maxillary lesions mostly occur anterior to the first molar tooth. Mandibular lesions generally occur in the posterior part (Fig. 5.48).
- Central odontogenic fibroma produces a slow enlarging, non-descript, painless swelling of the jaw.
- Cortical expansion is often minimum.

RADIOGRAPHIC FEATURES (FIG. 5.49)

- Radiographically, the lesion presents a well-circumscribed, rounded, unilocular radiolucent area in the jaw.
- Some lesions are multilocular with sclerotic borders.
- Lesions often contain several small radiopaque flecks of varying radiodensity.
- Resorption of roots of the adjoining teeth is often seen in this tumor.

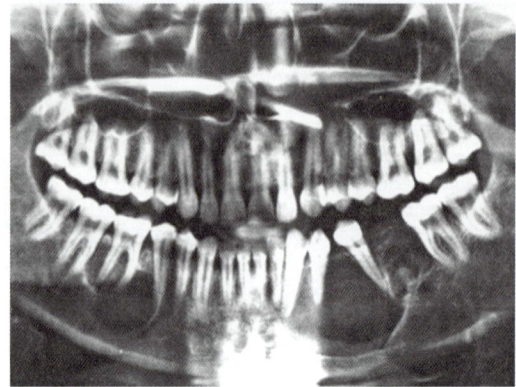

Fig. 5.49: Odontogenic fibroma mandible producing a large irregular radiolucent area containing numerous radiopaque foci.

HISTOLOGICAL PRESENTATION

- Histologically central odontogenic fibroma presents a cellular connective tissue, containing numerous thin strands of odontogenic epithelium (Fig. 5.50).
- The epithelial component closely resembles dental lamina and it often contains some clear cells.
- The connective tissue exhibits stellate fibroblast cells, which are often arranged in "whorled" pattern.

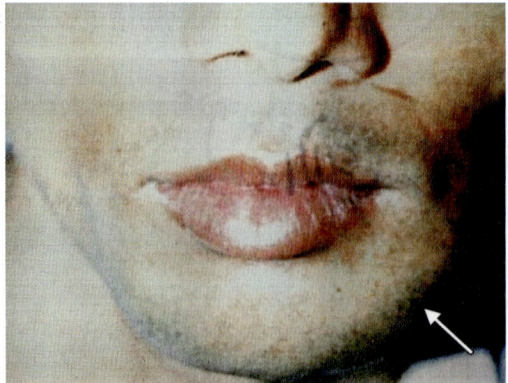

Fig. 5.48: Central odontogenic fibroma of left mandible.

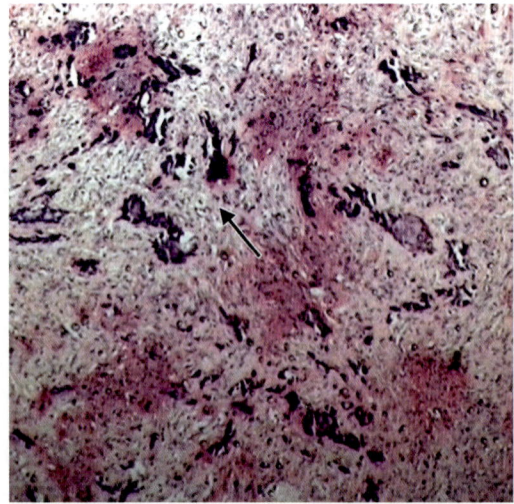

Fig. 5.50: Photomicrograph of odontogenic fibroma.

- Areas of spherical or diffuse calcifications are often present in the lesion.
- Some lesions may contain giant cells.

DIFFERENTIAL DIAGNOSIS
- Calcifying epithelial odontogenic tumor (CEOT)
- Ameloblastoma
- Cementifying fibroma
- Calcifying epithelial odontogenic cyst
- Central giant cell granuloma.

TREATMENT
Surgical excision and curettage.

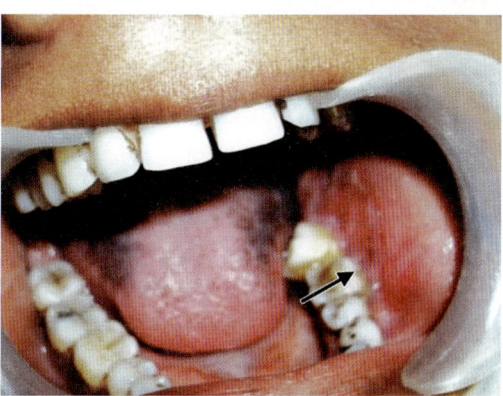

Fig. 5.51: Odontogenic myxoma producing a large swelling of left-sided mandible.

ODONTOGENIC MYXOMA

DEFINITION
Odontogenic myxomas are aggressive, intraosseous neoplasms derived from embryonic odontogenic mesenchyme. It is characterized by stellate and spindle-shaped cells embedded in an abundant myxoid or mucoid extracellular matrix.

ORIGIN
Odontogenic myxomas probably arise from the dental papilla or follicular mesenchyme.

CLINICAL FEATURES
- *Age:* Young and middle aged adults.
- *Sex:* Both sexes are equally affected.
- *Site:*
  - Nearly all lesions are found in the tooth bearing areas of maxillary and mandibular bone.
  - Mandibular lesions are commonly found in the premolar-molar area. Some lesions may be found in the ramus of mandible or other non-tooth bearing areas.

PRESENTATION
- Odontogenic myxomas are slow growing but locally aggressive lesions, which often cause painless swellings in the jaw (Fig. 5.51).
- Sometimes they cause displacement of the regional teeth.
- Maxillary lesions can perforate the bone and spread into the sinus. Afterwards they can cross the midline septa and invade into the opposing sinus cavity.
- Mandibular lesions also often extend into the ramus area.
- Few lesions are asymptomatic and are detected only during routine radiographic examinations.

RADIOGRAPHIC FEATURES
- The lesions often produce multilocular radiolucency with a "soap-bubble" or "honey comb" appearance in the bone.
- Thin and extremely delicate septa of residual bone are often seen to course through the radiolucent area.
- These wispy trabeculae of thin bones are often arranged at right angles to one another and thus they produce a "spider-web" like or "tennis racket" like appearance.
- Displacement of teeth is common and often there is root resorption in the adjacent teeth.
- Border of the lesion is mostly ill-defined, irregular and scalloped.
- Smaller lesions of myxoma often appear as unilocular nonspecific radiolucent areas in the jawbone.

MACROSCOPIC APPEARANCE

On naked eye examination the tumor appears as a loose gelatinous mass of tissue.

HISTOLOGICAL PRESENTATION (FIG. 5.52)

- Microscopically, odontogenic myxomas present widely separated, undifferentiated, spindle or angular or stellate shaped cells with long fine anastomosing processes.
- These cells are dispersed in a loose mucoid, non-fibrillar, basophilic ground substance.
- There is often presence of focal areas of delicate immature collagen fibrillar strands and as a whole the ground substance represents a myxomatous tissue.
- The myxomatous tissue often invades widely into the surrounding normal bony trabeculae.
- Oval shaped islands of odontogenic epithelial cell rests are sometimes present within the lesion.
- Some lesions may also have areas of calcification.

DIFFERENTIAL DIAGNOSIS

- Central giant cell granuloma
- Aneurysmal bone cyst
- Chondromyxoid fibroma
- Ameloblastoma
- Calcifying epithelial odontogenic tumor
- Hyperparathyroidism
- Central neurilemmoma.

TREATMENT

Since myxomas consist of a grossly gelatinous or mucoid material, which often penetrate the surrounding trabecular spaces of bone, surgical excision of the lesion and curettage is not always successful and hence resection of the jaw should be done in larger lesions.

PERIAPICAL CEMENTAL DYSPLASIA (CEMENTOMA)

Cementoma is a relatively uncommon odontogenic neoplasm, occurring in relation to the periapical bone and cementum at the root apex of vital teeth.

CLINICAL FEATURES

- *Age:* Usually third and fourth decade of life.
- *Sex:* Females are affected far more commonly than males.
- *Site:* Mostly in relation to the mandibular anterior teeth, maxillary teeth are also affected in some cases.

CLINICAL PRESENTATIONS

The lesions are mostly asymptomatic and are detected only during routine radiographic examinations. These are usually small and multiple in number and the associated teeth are always vital (Fig. 5.53).

RADIOLOGICAL FEATURES

The radiographic appearance of cementoma varies in different stages of the disease.
- In the initial osteolytic stage, the lesion presents a small, well-defined, radiolucent area near the apex of the involved tooth.

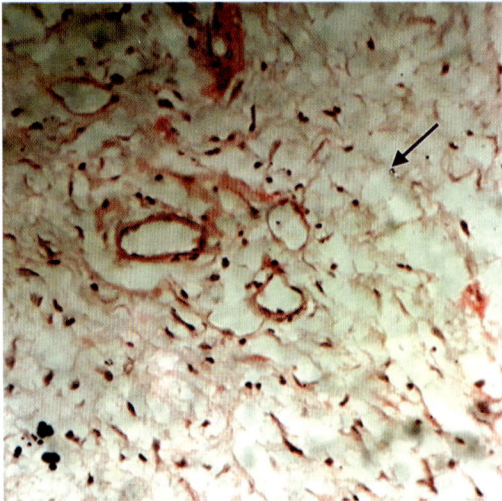

Fig. 5.52: Photomicrograph of odontogenic myxoma.

Odontogenic Neoplasms

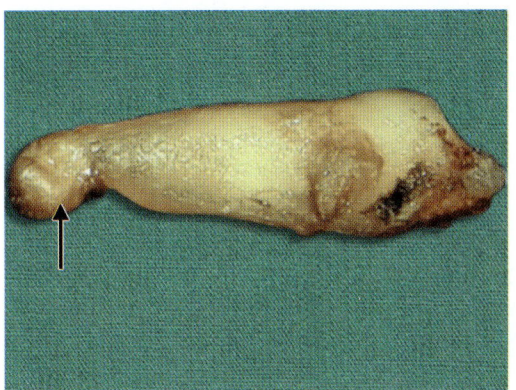

Fig. 5.53: Cementoma.

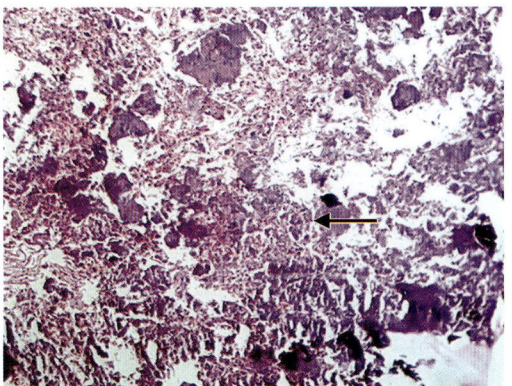

Fig. 5.54: Cementoma showing discrete cemental masses in the periapical area.

The radiolucency is always found to be in continuation with the periodontal ligament space.
- In the second or the cementoblastic stage, the lesion appears as a radiolucent area containing multiple small radiopaque foci.
- In the third or the mature stage, cementoma presents a well-defined radiopaque mass at the root apex, being surrounded by a thin radiolucent zone.

HISTOPATHOLOGY
- In the initial stage of the disease, the cemental tissue at the apex of the involved teeth as well as the periapical alveolar bone are destroyed and are replaced by a fibrous connective tissue (Fig. 5.54).
- During the cementoblastic stage, small amorphous masses of immature cementum form within the fibrous tissue stroma.
- In the mature stage of cementoma, the entire fibrous tissue is replaced by a large mass of mature cemental tissue at the apex of the teeth.

DIFFERENTIAL DIAGNOSIS
- Periapical granuloma
- Periapical cyst
- Condensing osteitis
- Bony artifacts.

TREATMENT
No treatment is required for cementoma, periodic observation and time-to-time vitality test of the involved teeth are to be done.

CENTRAL CEMENTIFYING FIBROMA
These are benign mesenchymal tissue neoplasm of the odontogenic origin characterized by formation of cemental tissue within a fibrous connective stroma (Fig. 5.55A). The tumor clinically and radiographically often resembles the ossifying fibroma (Fig. 5.55B); however histologically the lesion clearly shows presence of cemental tissue or both cemental as well as osseous elements (Fig. 5.56). The cemental tissues in the tumor are characteristically more hematoxyphilic and are more often round or oval in shape; while the osseous elements are more eosinophilic in nature and they form elongated trabeculae.

FAMILIAL GIGANTIFORM CEMENTOMA

DEFINITION
Familial gigantiform cementoma is a rare benign condition, which appears to represent a dysplastic or hamartomatous malformation of the cementum forming tissues.

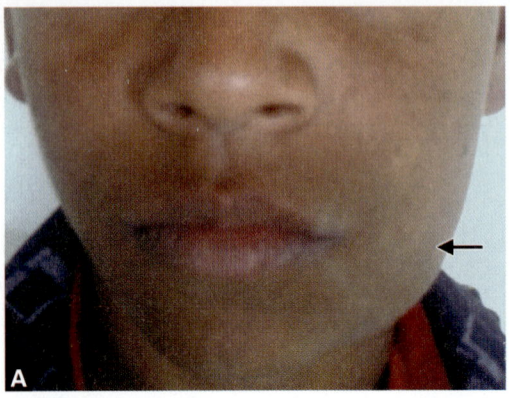
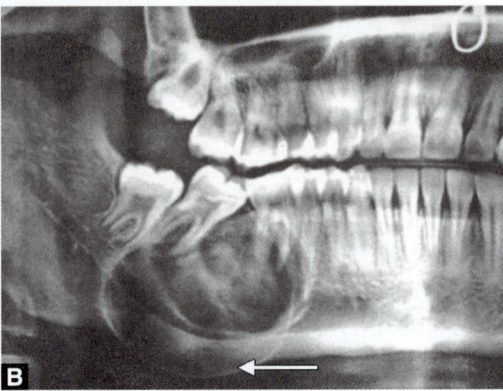

Figs. 5.55A and B: (A) Central cementifying fibroma of mandible; (B) X-ray showing calcified tissues within the same tumor.

ORIGIN

The disease often shows a familial tendency for occurrence.

CLINICAL FEATURES

- *Age:* The condition develops during childhood.
- *Sex:* Females are affected more often than males.
- *Site*
  - Both jaws are affected and it can be bilateral.
  - Initially familial gigantiform cementoma presents slow growing painless expansile jaw swelling.
- Multiple lesions often develop simultaneously at different sites involving all the four quadrants of the jaw.
- Lager lesions cause obvious facial asymmetry.

RADIOGRAPHIC FEATURES

- Radiograph reveals a large, sometimes massive expansile lesion of the jaw with well-defined margins.
- The lesion presents features of mixed radiolucency and radiopacity, however, it becomes more radiopaque with time.

HISTOLOGICAL PRESENTATION

- Histologically, the lesion presents a loose vascular tissue stroma consisting of delicate collagen fibers and numerous monomorphic fibroblasts.
- Large irregular masses of dense mineralized tissue resembling acellular cementum are scattered throughout the stroma.
- Small ovoid calcifications are also common.

DIFFERENTIAL DIAGNOSIS

- Florid osseous dysplasia
- Garre's osteomyelitis
- Paget's disease of bone.

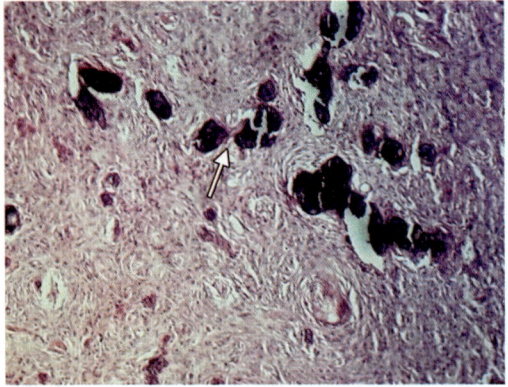

Fig. 5.56: Cementifying fibroma.

TREATMENT

Surgical recontouring of bone.

CEMENTOBLASTOMA

Cementoblastoma is a rare benign odontogenic neoplasm arising from the cementoblast cells. The tumor develops as an irregular rounded mass in continuity with the apical cemental layer of a vital molar or premolar tooth.

CLINICAL FEATURES

- *Age:* Usually second and third decade of life (Peak age of incidence is about 19 years).
- *Sex:* Seen more frequently among males.
- *Site:* Mandible is affected more often (75% cases) than the maxilla and posterior part of the jaw is usually the site of choice.

ORIGIN

Cementoblastoma or "true cementoma" is a true neoplasm of the cemental tissue. It arises from the cementoblast cells of the cemental layer of the apical third of a vital tooth.

CLINICAL PRESENTATION

- Cementoblastoma often produces a slow enlarging, bony hard swelling of the jaw that only rarely causes expansion of the jaw and displacement of the regional teeth (Fig. 5.57).
- Both buccal and lingual cortical plates are expanded uniformly.
- In most of the cases, low-grade intermittent pain may be present, which is felt more often, when the area is palpated.
- The lesion is often attached to the apical third of a vital premolar or molar tooth. Mandibular first molar is predominantly involved (50% cases).
- A dull sound is produced when percussion is done in the involved tooth; vitality of the tooth remains intact.

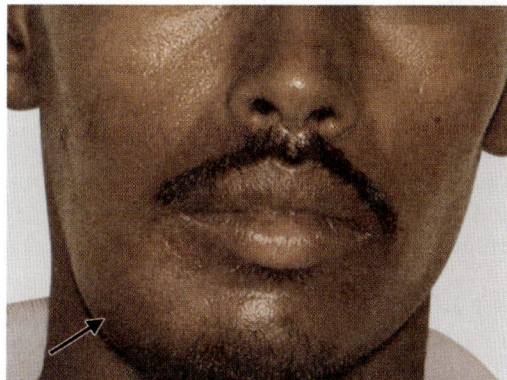

Fig. 5.57: Benign cementoblastoma of right side of mandible.

RADIOLOGICAL FEATURES (FIG. 5.58)

- Radiographically the tumor often presents a well-defined, large, dense, radiopaque mass that is often attached to one or more vital tooth roots. The early lesions may be radiolucent.
- Resorption and subsequent fusion of the tumor to the roots of the tooth often make them (roots) completely obscured, when seen in the radiograph.
- Loss of root outline and obliteration of the periodontal ligament space are common findings.
- The lesion is surrounded by a thin zone of radiolucency at the periphery.

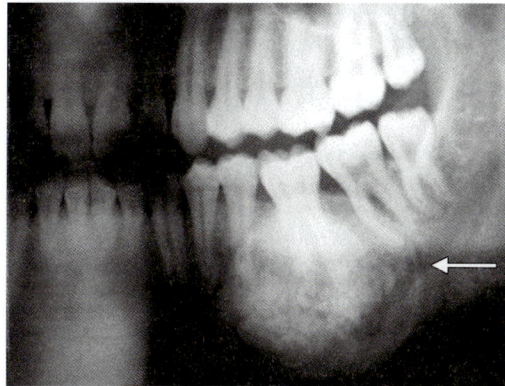

Fig. 5.58: Radiograph of benign cementoblastoma.

- Roots adjacent to the growing lesion often exhibit resorption of their apical third.

■ MACROSCOPY

The tumor consists of a rounded or nodular mass attached to one or more tooth roots and is surrounded by a gray to tan layer of irregular soft tissue.

■ HISTOPATHOLOGY (FIG. 5.59)

- Histologically, cementoblastoma presents a large mass of amorphous cemental tissue that often shows irregularly placed lacunae.
- The lesion also shows the presence of multiple basophilic reversal lines.
- On histologic sections, the tumor characteristically shows its fusion with the roots of the tooth.
- A fibrovascular connective tissue stroma is present between the individual mineralized trabeculae.
- Individual trabeculae are often bordered at the periphery by cementoblast or cementoblast-like cells.
- The periodontal ligament that is adjacent to the normal cementum becomes integrated with capsule and separates the neoplasm from the surrounding normal bone.
- The peripheral area of the lesion is relatively acellular while the central zone is composed of a highly mineralized tissue with intervening areas of loose, very cellular tissue with increased vascularity.
- Multinucleated cells are present in large numbers in the central area and are associated with active resorption.

■ DIFFERENTIAL DIAGNOSIS

- Osteoblastoma
- Osteoid osteoma
- Paget's disease of bone
- Osteosarcoma
- Focal sclerosing osteomyelitis.

■ TREATMENT

By surgical excision.

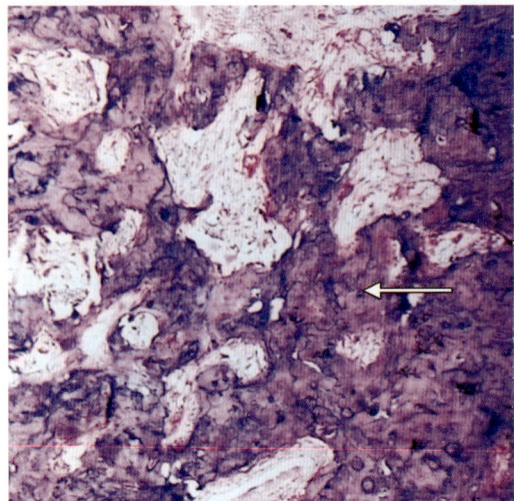

Fig. 5.59: Photomicrograph of cementoblastoma.

MALIGNANT ODONTOGENIC NEOPLASMS

■ MALIGNANT AMELOBLASTOMA

Definition

Malignant ameloblastomas are lesions with the histological features of common ameloblastoma in which metastasis has occurred. In many cases, these lesions are recurrent, although metastasis can occur from a primary lesion. Metastasis usually occurs to the distant regional lymph nodes; however, metastasis to other distant sites, e.g. lung and extragnathic bones can also occur.

In all the cases malignant ameloblastoma lesions appear cytologically benign.

■ AMELOBLASTIC CARCINOMA

Definition

Ameloblastic carcinoma is a true malignant neoplasm of odontogenic epithelial tissue, in which the epithelial components of the lesion are cytologically malignant (Fig. 5.60).

These lesions are clinically more aggressive and metastasis occurs very often. The lesions can affect both maxilla and mandible (Fig. 5.61).

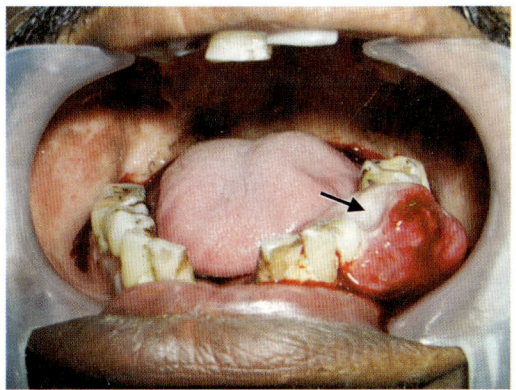

Fig. 5.60: Ameloblastic carcinoma.

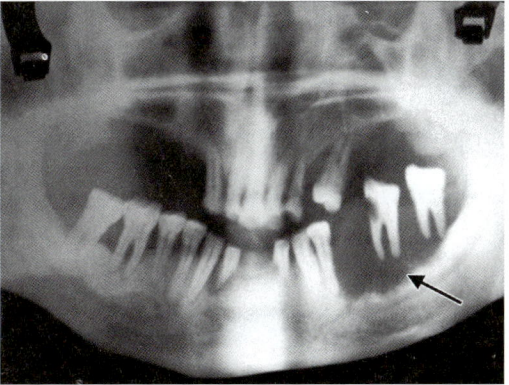

Fig. 5.61: Radiograph of ameloblastic carcinoma.

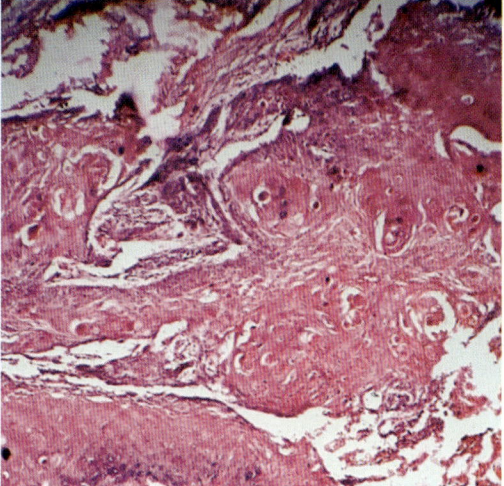

Fig. 5.62: Photomicrograph of ameloblastic carcinoma.

Cytologically the epithelial components of the lesion exhibit cellular pleomorphism and nuclear hyperchromatism. Some of the ameloblastomas exhibit basilar hyperplasia and an increased mitotic index but these findings are probably insufficient to permit a diagnosis of ameloblastic carcinoma in the absence of nuclear pleomorphism, perineural invasion, or other histologic evidence of malignancy (Fig. 5.62).

Radical surgical intervention should be undertaken.

■ ODONTOGENIC CARCINOMA

Definition

These are aggressive and destructive intraosseous lesions consisting of poorly differentiated epithelial cells and clear cells in a pattern that is reminiscent of early odontogenesis.

■ CLINICAL FEATURES

- *Age:* About 50 years.
- *Sex:* More prevalent among females.
- *Site:* These are uncommon lesions, which can affect both maxilla and mandible.

Clinical feature is not pathognomonic, there can be large swelling of the jaw with expansion of the cortical plates. Mobility of the teeth is very common.

■ RADIOGRAPHIC FEATURES

Radiographically, the neoplasm appears as a diffuse radiolucent area with a "honey comb" appearance. Considerable amount of bone destruction is often evident.

■ HISTOPATHOLOGY

The lesion is composed of islands or strands of clear cells, which are scattered throughout the fibrous tissue stroma. The clear cells are glycogen rich. The nonclear cells often resemble cells of dental lamina. The epithelial components are often surrounded by a zone of myxomatous connective tissue.

The cellular features of malignancy in the epithelial cells are minimum.

TREATMENT

Radical surgical excision.

ODONTOGENIC SARCOMAS

Odontogenic sarcomas are exceedingly rare lesions occurring in maxilla and mandible. The histological features exhibit a fibrosarcoma like appearance. The epithelial components are non-neoplastic in nature and there may be presence of few dental hard tissues.

CLEAR CELL ODONTOGENIC CARCINOMA

Definition

Clear cell odontogenic tumor is a locally aggressive, rare odontogenic neoplasm of epithelial cell origin. It is characterized by sheets and islands of vacuolated and clear cells.

CLINICAL FEATURES

- *Age:* Above 50 years of age.
- *Sex:* More prevalent among females.
- *Site:* Both maxilla and mandible can be affected but the most frequently affected site is the mandible.

CLINICAL PRESENTATION

Clinical features are not pathognomonic and both jaws can be affected by the tumor. Clinically there can be mild pain and swelling of the jawbone with expansion of the cortical plates and mobility of the teeth.

RADIOLOGICAL FINDING

The tumor produces irregular radiolucent area in the bone with a ragged border. Root resorption may occur.

HISTOLOGICAL PRESENTATION

- Histologically this neoplasm is poorly circumscribed and it consists of sheets of odontogenic epithelial cells with clear cytoplasms and centrally placed nuclei. These cells are glycogen rich and are distributed throughout a fibrous connective tissue stroma.
- Dark staining basaloid cells with scant eosinophilic cytoplasm may be seen.
- In addition, ameloblastomatous islands with palisaded peripheral cells may be observed.

Differential Diagnosis

- Salivary gland tumors
- Melanotic tumors
- Metastatic renal cell carcinoma
- Clear cell variant of calcifying epithelial odontogenic tumor.

TREATMENT

Surgical excision and curettage.

PRIMARY INTRA-ALVEOLAR CARCINOMA

Refer Chapter 2 (Neoplasms of neural tissue).

BIBLIOGRAPHY

1. Abdelsayed RA, Eversole LR, Singh BS, et al. Gigantiform cementoma: clinicopathologic presentation of 3 cases. Oral Surg Oral Med Oral Pathol Oral Radiol Endod. 2001;91:438-44.
2. Abiko Y, Murata M, Ito Y, et al. Immunohistochemical localization of amelogenin in human odontogenic tumors, using a polyclonal antibody against bovine amelogenin. Med Electron Microsc. 2001;34(3):185-9.
3. Adekeye EO. Ameloblastoma of the jaws: a survey of 109 Nigerian patients. J Oral Surg. 1980;38:36-41.
4. Ajagbe HA, Daramola JO, Junaid TA, et al. Adenomatoid odontogenic tumor in a black African population: report of thirteen cases. J Oral Maxillofac Surg. 1985;43:683-7.
5. Altini M, Hille JJ, Buchner A. Plexiform granular cell odontogenic tumor. Oral Surg Oral Med Oral Pathol. 1986;61:163-7.
6. Altini M, Thompson SH, Lownie JF, et al Ameloblastic sarcoma of the mandible. J Oral Maxillofac Surg. 1985;43:789-94.

7. Ameerally P, McGurk M, Shaheen O. Atypical ameloblastoma: report of 3 cases and a review of the literature. Br. J Oral Maxillofac Surg. 1996;34(3):235-9.
8. Anand SV, Davey WW, Cohen B. Tumors of the jaw in West Africa. A review of 256 patients. Br J Surg. 1967;54:901-17.
9. August M, Faquin W, Troulis M, et al. Clear cell odontogenic carcinoma. Evaluation of reported cases. J Oral Maxillofac Surg. 2003;61:580-685.
10. Baden E, Moskow BS, Moskow R. Odontogenic gingival epithelial hamartoma. J Oral Surg 1968;26:702-14.
11. Badger JV, Gardner DG. The relationship of adamantinomatous craniopharyngioma to ghost cell ameloblastoma of the jaws: a histopathologic and immunohistochemical study. J Oral Pathol Med. 1997;26:349-55.
12. Barker BF. Odontogenic myxoma. Semin Diagn Pathol. 1999;16:297-301.
13. Baker WR, Swift JQ. Ameloblastic fibro-odontoma of the anterior maxilla: report of a case. Oral Surg Oral Med Oral Pathol. 1993;76:294-7.
14. Baroni C, Farneti M, Stea S, et al. Ameloblastic fibroma and impacted mandibular first molar: a case report. Oral Surg Oral Med Oral Pathol. 1992;73:548-9.
15. Barrett AW, Morgan M, Ramsay AD, et al. A clinicopathologic and immunohistochemical analysis of melanotic neuroectodermal tumor of infancy. Oral Surg Oral Med Oral Pathol Oral Radiol Endod. 2002;93:688-98.
16. Barron RP, Kainulainen VT, Forrest CR, et al. Tuberous sclerosis: clinicopathologic features and review of the literature. J Craniomaxillofac Surg. 2002;30:361-6.
17. Barros RE, Dominguez FV, Cabrini RL. Myxoma of the jaws. Oral Surg Oral Med Oral Pathol. 1969;27: 225-36.
18. Basu MK, Matthews JB, Sear AJ, et al. Calcifying epithelial odontogenic tumor: a case showing features of malignancy. J Oral Pathol. 1984;13:310-9.
19. Batsakis JG, Clearly KR. Squamous odontogenic tumor. Ann Oral Rhinol Laryngol. 1993;102:823-4.
20. Becker J, Reichart PA, Schuppan D, et al. Ectomesenchyme of ameloblastic fibroma reveals a characteristic distribution of extracellular matrix proteins. J Oral Pathol Med. 1992;21:156-9.
21. Brannon RB, Fowler CB, Carpenter WM, et al. Cementoblastoma: an innocuous neoplasm? A clinicopathologic study of 44 cases and review of the literature with special emphasis on recurrence. Oral Surg Oral Med Oral Pathol Oral Radiol Endod. 2002;93:311-20.
22. Brannon RB, Goode K, Eversole LR, et al. The central granular cell odontogenic tumor: report of 5 new cases. Oral Surg Oral Med Oral Pathol Oral Radiol Endod. 2002;94:614-21.
23. Braunshtein E, Vered M, Taicher S, et al. Clear cell odontogenic carcinoma and clear cell ameloblastoma. A single clinicopathologic entity? A new case and comparative analysis of the literature. J Oral Maxillofac Surg. 2003;61:1004-10.
24. Breuer W, Geisel O, Linke RP, et al. Light microscopic, ultra structural and immunohistochemical examination of two calcifying epithelial odontogenic tumors in a dog and a cat. Vet Pathol. 1994;31:415-20.
25. Browne RM, Gough NG. Malignant change in the epithelium lining odontogenic cysts. Cancer. 1972;29:1199-207.
26. Buchner A, Sciubba JJ. Peripheral epithelial odontogenic tumors: a review. Oral Surg Oral Med Oral Pathol. 1987;63:688-97.
27. Budnick S. Compound and complex odontomas. Oral Surg Oral Med Oral Pathol. 1976;42:501-6.
28. Calvo N, Alonso D, Prieto M, et al. Central odontogenic fibroma granular cell variant: a case report and review of the literature. J Oral Maxillofac Surg. 2002;60:1192-4.
29. Cannon JS, Keller EE, Dahlin DC. Gigantiform cementoma: report of two cases (mother and son). J Oral Surg. 1980;38:187-95.
30. Carinci F, Francioso F, Piattelli A, et al. Genetic expression profiling of six odontogenic tumors. J Dent Res. 2003;82(7):551-7.
31. Carr MM. Compound odontoma: case report and brief review. Oral Dent. 1990;67:24-6.
32. Cataldo E, Giunta JL. A clinicopathological presentation ameloblastic fibroma. T Mass Dent Soc. 1984;33:158.
33. Ciment LM, Ciment AJ. Malignant ameloblastoma metastatic to the lungs 29 years after primary resection: a case report. Chest. 2002;121(4):1359-61.

34. Corio RL, Goldblatt LI, Edwards, PA, et al. Ameloblastic carcinoma: a clinicopathologic study and assessment of eight cases. Oral Surg Oral Med Oral Pathol. 1987;64:570-6.
35. Cuestas-Carnero RB, Gendelman H. Odontogenic Myxoma: a report of a case. J Oral Maxillifac Surg. 1988; 46:705-9.
36. Dal-Cin PD, Sciot R, Fossion E, et al. Chromosome abnormalities in cementifying fibroma. Cancer Genet Cytogenet. 1993;71:170-2.
37. Daley TD, Wysocki GP. Peripheral odontogenic fibroma. Oral Surg Oral Med Oral Pathol. 1994;78:329-36.
38. Dhir K, Sciubba J, Tufano RP. Case report. Ameloblastic carcinoma of the maxilla. Oral Oncol. 2003:39:736-41.
39. Doyle JL, Lamster IB, Baden E. Odontogenic fibroma of the complex (WHO) type: report of six cases. J Oral Maxillofac Surg. 1985;43:666-74.
40. Dunlap CL. Odontogenic fibroma. Semin Diagn Pathol. 1999;16:293-6.
41. Eisenberg EM, Murthy AS, Vawter GF, et al. Odontogenic neoplasms in Wister rats treated with N-methylnitrosourea. Oral Surg Oral Med Oral Pathol. 1983;55:481-6.
42. El-Mofty SK. Psammomatoid and trabecular juvenile ossifying fibroma of the craniofacial skeleton: two distinct clinicopathologic entities. Oral Surg Oral Med Oral Pathol Oral Radiol Endod. 2002;93:296-304.
43. Elzay RP. Primary intraosseous carcinoma of the jaws. Review and update of odontogenic carcinomas. Oral Surg Oral Med Oral Pathol. 1982;54:299-303.
44. Eversole LR, Leider AS, Hansen LS. Ameloblastomas with pronounced desmoplasia. J Oral Maxillofac Surg. 1984;42(11):735-40.
45. Eversole LR. Malignant epithelial odontogenic tumors. Semin Diagn Pathol. 1999;16: 317-24.
46. Eversole LR, Duffey DC, Powell NB. Clear cell odontogenic carcinoma. A clinicopathologic analysis. Arch Otolaryngol Head Neck Surg. 1995;121:685-9.
47. Gardener DG. Peripheral ameloblastoma. Cancer. 1977;39:1625-33.
48. Gardener DG. The central odontogenic fibroma: an attempt al clarification. Oral Surg. Oral Med Oral Pathol. 1980;50:425-32.
49. Gardner DG. Some current concepts on the pathology of ameloblastomas. Oral Surg Oral Med Oral Pathol Oral Radiol Endod. 1996;82(6):660-9.
50. Geist SM, Mallon HL. Adenomatoid odontogenic tumor: report of an unusually large lesion in the mandible. J Oral Maxillofac Surg. 1995;53(6):714-7.
51. Goldblatt LI, Brannon RB, Ellis GL. Squamous odontogenic tumor. Oral Surg Oral Med and Oral Pathol. 1982;54:187-96.
52. Gorlin RJ, Chaudhry AP, Pindborg JJ. Odontogenic tumors. Classification, histopathology, and clinical behavior in man and domesticated animals. Cancer. 1961;14:73-101.
53. Hansen LS, Eversole LR, Green TL, et al. Clear cell odontogenic tumor—a new histological variant with aggressive potential. Head Neck Surg. 1985;8:115-23.
54. Hensen LS, Ficarra G. Mixed odontogenic tumors: an analysis of 23 new cases. Head Neck Surg. 1988;10:330-43.
55. Hopper TL, Sadeghi EM, Pricco DF. Squamous odontogenic tumor. Report of a case with multiple lesion. Oral Surg. Oral Med Oral Pathol. 1980;50:404-10.
56. Kramer IR, Pindborg JJ, Shear M. World Health Organization: International Histological Classification of Tumors Histological Typing of Odontogenic Tumors, 2nd edition. Verlag, Berlin: Springer; 1991.
57. Laughlin EH. Metastasizing ameloblastoma. Cancer. 1989;64:776-80.
58. Leider AS, Jonker IA, Cook HE. Multicentric familial squamous odontogenic tumor. Oral Surg Oral Med Oral Pathol. 1989;68:175-81.
59. Leider AS, Nelson JF, Trodahl JN. Ameloblastic fibrosarcoma of the jaws. Oral Surg Oral Med Oral Pathol. 1972;33:559-69.
60. Lucas RB. Pathology of tumors of the oral tissue, 4th edition. Edinburgh: Churchill Livingstone; 1984.
61. Maranda G, Gourgi M. Calcifying epithelial odontogenic tumor (Pindborg's tumor): review of the literature and case report. J Can Dent Assoc. 1986;52:1009-12.
62. Mehlisch DR, Dehlin DC, Masson JK. Ameloblastoma: a clinicopathologic report. J Oral Surg. 1972;30:9-22.
63. Mosadomi A. Odontogenic tumors in an African Population Analysis of twenty-nine cases seen over a 5-year period. Oral Surg Oral Med Oral Pathol. 1975;40:502-21.

64. Ord RA, Blanchaert Jr RH, Nikitakis NG, et al. Ameloblastoma in children. J Oral Maxillofac Surg. 2002;60(7):762-71.
65. Pradhan SA, Soman CS, Patel A. Well differentiated metastasizing ameloblastoma: report of a case with review if literature. Indian J Cancer. 1989; 26:255-9.
66. Reichert PA, Philipsen HP, Sonner S. Ameloblastoma: biological profile of 3677 cases. Oral Oncol Eur J Cancer. 1995;31B:86-99.
67. Sexby MS, Rippon JW, Sheron JE. Case report: squamous odontogenic tumor of the gingiva. J Periodontol. 1993;64:1250-2.
68. Slootweg PJ. Cementoblastoma and osteoblastoma: a comparison of histologic features. J Oral Pathol Med. 1992;21:385-9.
69. Slootweg PJ, Muller H. Malignant ameloblastoma of ameloblastic carcinoma: case report and review. J Oral Pathol Med. 1991;20:460-3.
70. Takeda Y, Suzuki A, Sekiyama S. Peripheral calcifying epithelial odontogenic tumor. Oral Surg Oral Med Oral Pathol. 1983;56:71-5.
71. Waldron CA, Small IA, Silverman H. Clear cell ameloblastoma and odontogenic carcinoma. J Oral Maxillofac Surg. 1985;43:707-17.

CHAPTER 6

Cysts of the Oral Region

DEFINITION

Cyst is a pathological cavity containing fluid, semifluid, or gas, which is usually lined by epithelium and is not formed by the accumulation of pus.

The above mentioned definition of the cyst requires some clarifications:

- *Pathological cavity:* Means any cystic lesion in the body must arise as a result of some pathological processes. Unlike the normal anatomical cavities in the body, e.g. gallbladder or plural cavity or pericardial cavity or urinary bladder, etc. which are also cyst like cavities but these are normal anatomical structures of the body. On the other hand, a cyst is not normal to the body but a pathological or a disease entity.
- *Contents of the cyst:* Generally cystic cavities are filled with a variety of materials. For example, the dentigerous, the radicular, the globulomaxillary cyst, etc. are normally filled with some fluid.

  The odontogenic keratocyst is usually filled with a thick and keratin-rich semifluid mass.

  On the contrary, some of the cysts like the solitary bone cyst or aneurysmal bone cyst, etc. are usually filled with gas.
- *Regarding cyst lining:* Most of the cystic cavities are lined by an epithelium, but the lining epithelium may be absent in few cysts, e.g. traumatic bone cyst or aneurysmal bone cyst or mucous extravasation cyst, etc.
  - *True cyst*: If the lining epithelium is present in a cyst, it is known as a true cyst.
  - *Pseudo or false cyst*: If the lining epithelium is absent in a cyst, it is called a false or pseudocyst.
- *Question of pus:* Unlike an abscess, a cyst is never formed by the accumulation of pus. However, in few cases, a cyst may be secondarily infected, resulting in the formation of pus within it. This type of abscess developing in a pre-existing cyst is known as "cyst abscess".

CLASSIFICATION OF CYSTS

Odontogenic (Table 6.1)

Developmental

- Gingival cyst of infants
- Odontogenic keratocyst (primordial cyst)
- Dentigerous (follicular) cyst
- Eruption cyst
- Lateral periodontal cyst
- Gingival cyst of adults
- Botryoid odontogenic cyst
- Glandular odontogenic (sialo-odontogenic) cyst
- Calcifying odontogenic cyst.

Inflammatory

- Radicular cyst—apical and lateral
- Residual cyst
- Paradental cyst and mandibular infected buccal cyst
- Inflammatory collateral cyst.

Table 6.1: Cell of origin of common odontogenic cysts.

Embryological structures	Cell rests	Cyst developing
Dental lamina	Cell rest of Serres	• Odontogenic keratocyst (OKC) • Lateral periodontal cyst • Gingival cyst of the adult • Dental lamina cyst of newborn • Sialo-odontogenic cyst
Enamel organ	Reduced enamel epithelium	• Dentigerous cyst • Eruption cyst • Paradental cyst
Epithelial root sheath of Hertwig	Cell rest of Malassez	• Radicular cyst • Residual cyst

Nonodontogenic
- Nasopalatine duct (incisive canal) cyst
- Nasolabial (nasoalveolar) cyst
- Midpalatal raphe cyst of infants
- Median palatine, median alveolar, and median mandibular cysts
- Globulomaxillary cyst.

Nonepithelial
- Solitary bone cyst (traumatic, simple, and hemorrhagic bone cyst)
- Aneurysmal bone cyst

Clinical Significance of Jaw Cysts
- Cystic lesions occur at a higher frequency in relation to the jawbones as compared to any other bone in the skeleton, because of the typical embryology of the facial skeleton and also because of the presence of teeth.
- The teeth are always associated with some epithelium or epithelial residues, which are potentially capable of forming a cyst.
- The widely varying clinical and biological behavior of different cystic lesions comprises a significant clinical problem in oral pathology.
- Jaw cysts generally present as well-defined radiolucent lesions, which may or may not be associated with erupted or unerupted teeth, or with other features such as expansions of the cortical bone and occlusal disharmony, etc. These features are not pathognomonic of a cyst and may be shared by other forms of cystic or noncystic pathology.

- The border of the lesion is mostly smooth, well delineated, and well corticated.
- Cystic lesions grow slowly in the jaw and displace the regional teeth but generally do not cause root resorptions. Therefore, a cystic lesion of the jaw should always be differentiated from other forms of pathology before any definitive treatment is done.
- Cystic fluids can be aspirated from the cysts and its biochemical nature among different cystic lesions.
- Moreover, different types of cysts must be clearly differentiated from one another during making the diagnosis, because the treatment protocols for various large cysts can vary significantly.
- Biologically, most of the cystic lesions of the jaw are slow growing and they maintain a relatively innocuous character for a considerable period of time.
- A fluctuant or compressible swelling often develops, if the cyst is present in the soft tissue or if the intrabony cyst has completely resorbed the overlying bone.
- However, few cystic lesions could cause severe bone destruction and involve a large part of the jaw without actually being noticed clinically during the initial stages, e.g. primordial cyst.
- A cyst may look bluish in color, if it is lying close to the overlying epithelial surface.
- Large cystic lesions eventually cause bone expansion and manifest with pain and discomfort in the jaw.
- Cystic lesions, especially the odontogenic cysts, may become infected, which can result in abscess formation and cellulites, etc.
- Rarely, large cysts may cause considerable amount of bone destruction and weaken the bone, which may result in pathological fracture.
- Cystic epithelium sometimes can undergo neoplastic changes and gives rise to the development of benign or malignant tumors.

Cysts Associated with the Maxillary Antrum
- Benign mucosal cyst of the maxillary antrum
- Postoperative maxillary cyst (surgical ciliated cyst of the maxilla).

Cyst of the Tissue of the Mouth, Face, and Neck
- Dermoid and epidermoid cysts
- Lymphoepithelial (branchial cleft) cyst
- Thyroglossal duct cyst
- Anterior median lingual cyst (intralingual cyst of foregut origin)

- Oral cysts with gastric or intestinal epithelium (oral alimentary tract cyst)
- Cystic hygroma
- Nasopharyngeal cysts
- Thymic cyst
- *Cysts of the salivary glands:* Mucous extravasation cyst, mucous retention cyst, and ranula
- *Parasitic cysts:* Hydatid cyst, cysticercus cellulosae, and trichinosis.

Cell Rests (Resting Cells)

After the process of tooth development (odontogenesis) is over, a large number of odontogenic epithelial cells (tooth formative cells) remain in a dormant state within the jawbones; these inactive cells are called "cell rests". In some abnormal situations, these cells again become reactivated and start to proliferate to form pathological lesions especially cysts. Characteristics of cell rests:

- Absence of mitotic activity
- Minimal metabolic activity
- Absence of developed Golgi complex.

ODONTOGENIC CYSTS (TABLE 6.2)

ODONTOGENIC KERATOCYST/ PRIMORDIAL CYST

Definition

Odontogenic keratocyst (OKC) is a common cystic lesion of the jaw, which arises from the remnants of the dental lamina; it has distinctive clinicopathological character and a higher tendency for recurrence after treatment. OKCs often have a more aggressive curse than any other cystic lesion of jaw; and for this reason, these are sometimes known as "benign cystic neoplasms".

There are three defining characters seen in OKCs—(1) epithelial lining not more than

Table 6.2: Differential diagnosis of major odontogenic cysts.

Name of the cyst	Major clinical features	Radiographic features	Histopathology
Odontogenic keratocyst	Aggressive type of cyst and highly destructive; spreads via medullary spaces, minimum bony expansion, high recurrence rate. Originates from cell rest of Serres, enamel organ of developing tooth, basal layer of oral epithelium	Multilocular soap–bubble radiolucency, may cross the midline of mandible (a rare feature of this cyst)	Keratinized, often corrugated cystic lining, presence of daughter cysts
Dentigerous cyst	Cyst enclosing the crown of an impacted tooth, slow growing and causes moderate painless expansion of the jaw, recurrence is rare Originates from reduced enamel epithelium	Unilocular radiolucency around the crown of impacted tooth	Thin nonkeratinized cystic lining, stroma looks like primitive odontogenic ectomesenchyme
Radicular cyst	Cyst developing at the root apex of a nonvital tooth, slow-growing inflammatory cyst, causes localized bone resorption, recurrence rare Originates from cell rest of Malassez	Unilocular well-defined radiolucency in relation to the root apex	Nonkeratinized thick lining, inflamed stroma, there may be presence of arcading pattern, Rushton and Russell bodies and cholesterol clefts

Contd...

Contd...

Name of the cyst	Major clinical features	Radiographic features	Histopathology
Residual cyst	It is actually a radicular cyst but the associated tooth is absent	Unilocular well-defined round radiolucency in the tooth bearing area of the jaw	Same as radicular cyst but less inflamed stroma and sign of progressive healing
Eruption cyst	Mucosal cyst overlying an erupting deciduous or permanent tooth. Presents a fluctuant and translucent swelling *Originates from the reduced enamel epithelial cells*	Small painless translucent swelling immediately above the erupting tooth	Same as dentigerous cyst
Gingival cyst of the adults	Cyst located in the gingival soft tissue and presents a soft, "dome-shaped" fluctuant, painless, swelling *Originates from cell rest of Serres*		Presents thin lining of flat or cuboidal cells having 2–3 cell layer thickness. Cystic epithelial cells exhibit pyknotic nuclei with perinuclear cytoplasmic vacuoles
Lateral periodontal cyst	Cyst arising from the lateral root surface of an erupted vital tooth. It is small, mostly asymptomatic and painless *Originates from the odontogenic epithelial cells rests present in the periodontal ligament tissue*	A "tear-drop" shaped radiolucency on the lateral aspect of the root	The cyst has a thin cystic lining made up of squamous or flattened cuboidal epithelial cells
Calcifying odontogenic cyst (COC)	An important cyst which is also considered as a tumor and it uniquely exhibits calcification within the cystic lumen. Presents an expansile jaw swelling with displacement of teeth *Originates from reduced enamel epithelium or remnants of odontogenic epithelium in the dental follicle, gingiva, or bone*	Multilocular radiolucency in the jaw containing numerous radiopaque foci	Moderately thick keratinized, cystic lining with presence of "ghost cells", amyloids and calcifications. Few lesions present satellite cyst and giant cells

10 cell layers in thickness; (2) palisading arrangement of basal cells; and (3) corrugated and keratinized epithelial lining.

This cyst often occurs as a solitary lesion in the angle of the mandible, however, in some cases multiple such cysts may occur in association with a syndrome called "nevoid basal cell carcinoma syndrome".

Pathogenesis

Odontogenic keratocyst arises mainly from the:
- Dental lamina or its remnants (cell rests of Serres).
- Primordium of the developing tooth germ or enamel organs.
- Sometimes from the basal layer of the oral epithelium.

It is mostly believed that the keratocyst develops due to the cystic degeneration of the cells of the stellate reticulum in a developing tooth germ (before its calcification starts). The daughter cysts, a common finding in this lesion, probably develop from the remnants of the dental lamina.

They are unique odontogenic lesions that have potential to behave aggressively,

| Box 6.1 | Odontogenic keratocyst (OKC) is a cyst or a tumor: World Health Organization (WHO) view changes. |

- 1971: Cyst odontogenic keratocyst
- 1992: Cyst "odontogenic keratocyst"
- 2005: Tumor "keratocystic odontogenic tumor"
- 2017: Cyst "odontogenic keratocyst"

that can reoccur, and can be associated with the nevoid basal cell carcinoma syndrome. Toller (1967) suggested that OKCs might be regarded as benign cystic neoplasms.

Nevoid basal cell carcinoma syndrome is a hereditary condition; and since OKCs develop in association with this syndrome, a strong correlation is believed to exist between genetic influence and the development of this cyst (Box 6.1).

Clinical Features

Incidence: Nearly 1% among all types of jaw cysts.
Age: Mostly second and third decade of life.
Sex: Males are affected slightly more often than females.
Site:
- Majority of the cases develop in relation to mandible (75%) as compared to maxilla.
- Among the mandibular lesions, 50% of the cases occur at the angle of the mandible, which extend for varying distances into the ascending ramus and the body of the mandible.
- Few cysts absolutely occur in the body of the mandible and some of these lesions can even cross the midline of the jaw.
- Maxillary lesions more frequently involve the anterior part of the jaw, however, some lesions can develop from the posterior region. Few lesions can even develop in relation to the maxillary air sinus.
- On rare occasions, this cyst may occur in the gingiva (extraosseous type).

Presentation

- In the initial stages (Figs. 6.1A and B) OKC does not produce any signs or symptoms

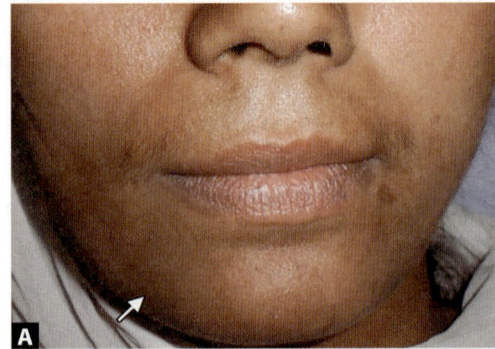
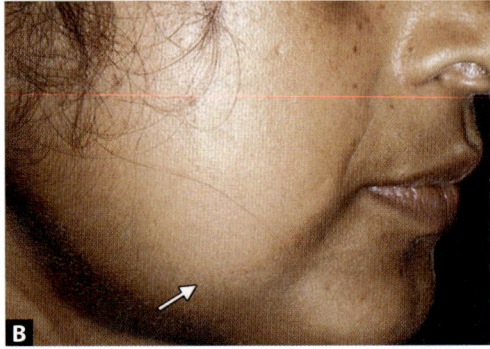

Figs. 6.1A and B: (A) Odontogenic keratocysts (OKC) causing expansion of right side of mandible; (B) Odontogenic keratocysts (OKC) causing swelling of anterior mandible.

and the lesion may be discovered only during routine radiographic examinations.
- Bony expansion is often minimum in OKC because in most of the cases, the cyst spreads via the medullary spaces of bone and as a result remarkable bony swelling is usually absent despite the cyst being very large in size.
- Some degree of bony expansion may be seen in about 60% cases of OKC; one-third of the maxillary lesions cause expansion of the buccal cortical plate, while expansion of the palatal cortical plate is rarely seen. Mandibular lesion exhibits buccal expansion in about 50% cases, while lingual expansion occurs in over 30% cases.
- Larger lesions of OKC however produce swelling of the jaw with facial asymmetry (Fig. 6.2); there may be pain in the jaw

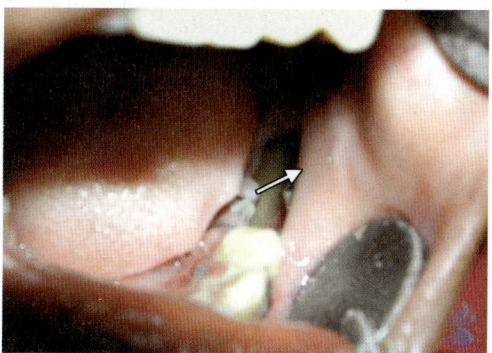

Fig. 6.2: Intraoral lesion in odontogenic keratocysts (OKC).

along with mobility and displacement of teeth.
- Some larger cysts can involve the entire ramus, condyle, and coronoid process of mandible without producing much clinically observable bony expansion.
- Larger OKCs of maxilla often involve the maxillary sinus, the orbit and the infra-temporal fossa, etc. such type of lesions may cause displacement or destruction of the orbital floor with protrusion of the eyeball.
- Even in few cases, larger cysts may remain asymptomatic until there is pathological fracture in the jaw; which results due to excessive expansion and thinning of the involved bone.
- There is often one tooth missing from the dental arch on clinical examination, which means that the cyst has developed from the developing tooth germ of that particular tooth.
- In some cases, completely extraosseous lesions may develop in relation to the gingiva.
- Some patients may have multiple OKCs in the jaw and it is often seen in "nevoid basal cell carcinoma syndrome" (Gorlin-Goltz syndrome) (Box 6.2).
- Paresthesia of the lower lip and teeth may be present occasionally; discharge of pus may be seen in case the cyst is secondarily infected.

Box 6.2	Nevoid basal cell carcinoma syndrome (Gorlin–Goltz syndrome).

Nevoid basal cell carcinoma syndrome is a hereditary disease and is inherited as an autosomal dominant trait. The features of this syndrome include the following:

A. *Cutaneous anomalies (Figs. 6.3 and 6.4)*:
  - Multiple basal cell carcinomas of skin
  - Epidermal cyst of the skin
  - Palmar and plantar keratosis
  - Dermal calcinosis

B. *Dental and osseous anomalies (Figs. 6.5 to 6.7)*:
  - Multiple odontogenic keratocyst
  - Frontal and parietal bossing with enlarged head circumference
  - Mild mandibular prognathism
  - Bifid ribs and abnormalities in vertebrae
  - Brachymetacarpalism.

C. *Ophthalmologic abnormalities*:
  - Ocular hypertelorism and broad nasal root
  - Dystopia canthorum (lateral displacement of the inner canthi of the eyes)
  - Congenital blindness and internal strabismus.

D. *Neurological anomalies*:
  - Mental retardation
  - Calcification of falx cerebri
  - Abnormal shape of sella turcica
  - Agenesis of corpus callosum
  - Congenital hydrocephalus
  - Occurrence of medulloblastomas

E. *Sexual abnormalities*:
  - Hypogonadism in males and ovarian tumors

F. *Other finding (Fig. 6.8)*:
  - Cleft lip and cleft palate in few cases.

Ehlers–Danlos syndrome is a hereditary disorder of connective tissue related to collagen metabolism. Rare occurrence of multiple OKCs has been reported in the syndrome.

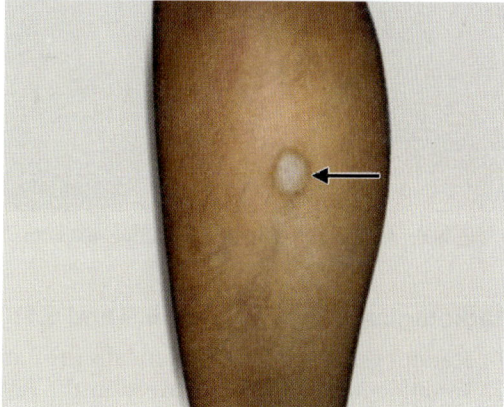

Fig. 6.3: Epidermoid cyst of skin.

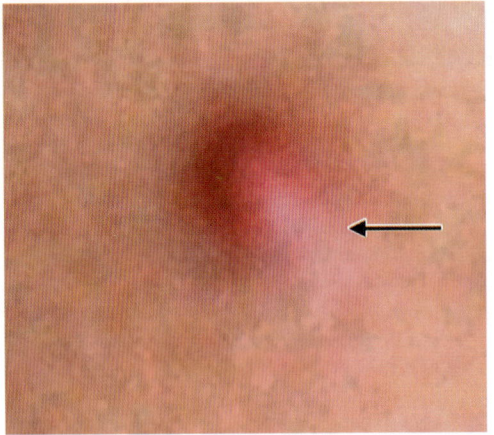

Fig. 6.4: Basal cell carcinoma of skin.

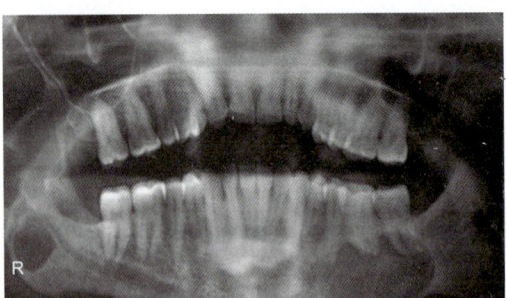

Fig. 6.5: Multiple odontogenic keratocysts in mandible.

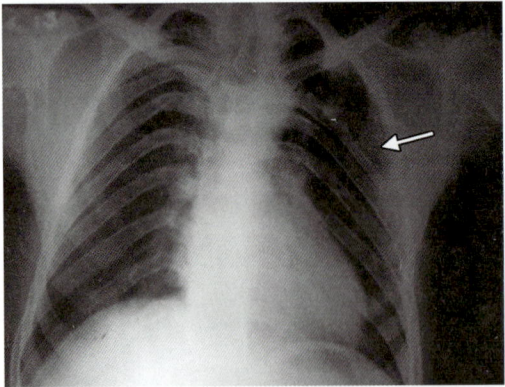

Fig. 6.6: Abnormally thin and defective ribs with missing ribs on left side.

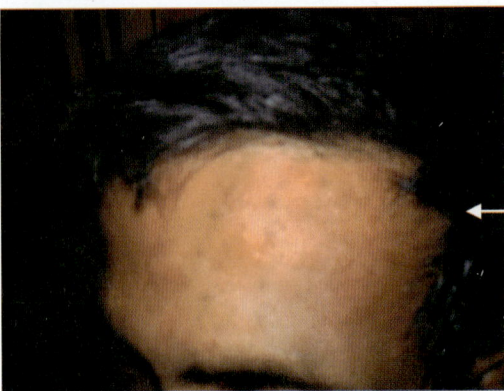

Fig. 6.7: Frontal bossing in Gorlin-Goltz syndrome.

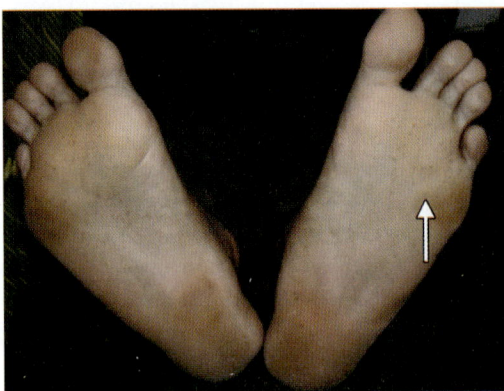

Fig. 6.8: Plantar (sole of feet) hyperkeratosis.

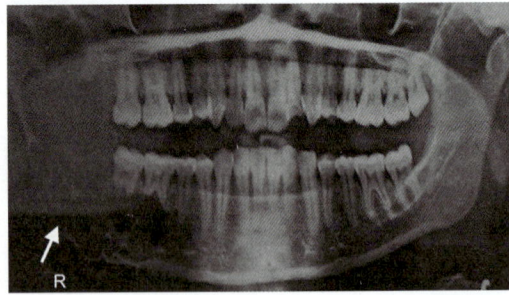

Fig. 6.9: Radiograph of odontogenic keratocyst (OKC) producing a multilocular radiolucency in jaw with "soap–bubble" appearance. Radiograph of OKC of mandible and crossing the midline.

Radiological Features (Figs. 6.9 and 6.10)

- Keratocysts often radiographically present multilocular radiolucent areas in the jaw with a typical "soap–bubble" appearance (generally representing a central cavity having satellite cyst).
- In many cases, the lesion can be unilocular with a well-corticated margin.

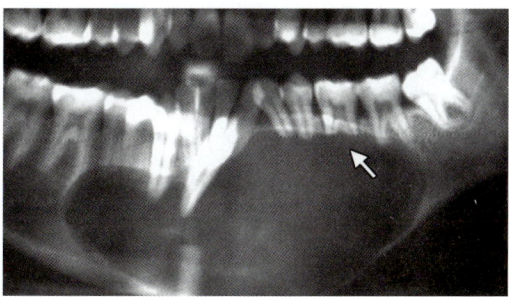

Fig. 6.10: Radiograph of odontogenic keratocyst (OKC) producing a multilocular radiolucent area in mandible with root resorption.

- Large mandibular cysts can spread from one side of the bone to the other side by crossing the midline; this is an important characteristic of OKC [other cyst that may cross the mandibular midline is glandular odontogenic cyst (GOC)].
- Sometimes the border of the cyst is smooth (slow-growing lesions) and sometimes it is scalloped (scalloping represents variation in the growth pattern of the cyst).
- Lesions in the angle of mandible often spread to the body as well as the ascending ramus up to the condyle and the coronoid process.
- Displacement of unerupted teeth and deflection of their roots are often seen.
- Sometimes multiple cysts may be seen in the jaw.
- Occasionally, there may be presence of an unerupted tooth in relation to the cyst.
- Some lesions cause pathological fracture or perforation of the cortical plates of the jaw (Box 6.3).
- Root resorption rarely occurs in association with OKCs.
- Expansion and distortion of the cortical plates are common and radiological size of the lesion is almost always significantly large than the clinical size of the lesion (Table 6.3; Figs. 6.11 and 6.12). (Clinically, the cyst appears much smaller than its actual size.)

Differential Diagnosis

- Ameloblastoma

| Box 6.3 | Common diseases causing pathological fracture of jawbone. |

- Ameloblastoma
- OKC
- Acute suppurative osteomyelitis
- Aneurysmal bone cyst
- Metastatic carcinoma
- Paget's disease of bone
- Hyperparathyroidism
- Multiple myeloma
- Squamous cell carcinoma (when invading bone)
- Diffuse scleroderma with resorption of mandible
- Dentigerous cyst
- Radicular cyst

Table 6.3: Radiological types of keratocyst.

Replacement type	When a keratocyst develops in place of a developing normal tooth, it is called the replacement type. In such cases, there will be absence of a normal tooth in the dental arch
Envelopmental type	When a cyst entirely encloses an impacted tooth within the bone, it is called the envelopmental type of keratocyst
Extraneous type	When a keratocyst develops away from the tooth bearing areas of the jaws, it is called extraneous type of keratocyst
Collateral type	When a cyst develops between the roots of a tooth, it is called collateral type of keratocyst

- Dentigerous cyst
- Aneurysmal bone cyst
- Odontogenic myxoma
- Stafne bone cyst
- Lateral periodontal cyst.

Macroscopic Findings of Keratocyst

- On naked eye examination, the OKC presents a cystic cavity, which is filled with a thick cheesy material (keratin debris).
- Some cysts are filled with a clear fluid.
- The cystic wall is thin, friable, collapsed, and folded; hence, it is very difficult to separate from the bone wall.

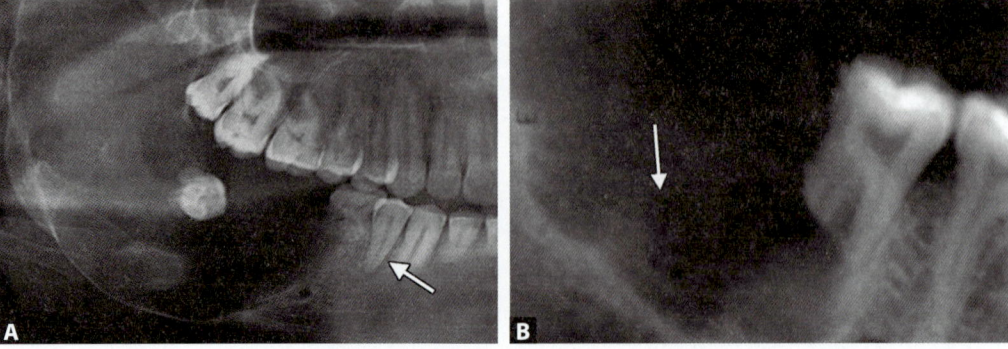

Figs. 6.11A and B: Radiograph of odontogenic keratocyst (OKC)—envelopmental type (A) and replacement type developing in place lower third molar (B).

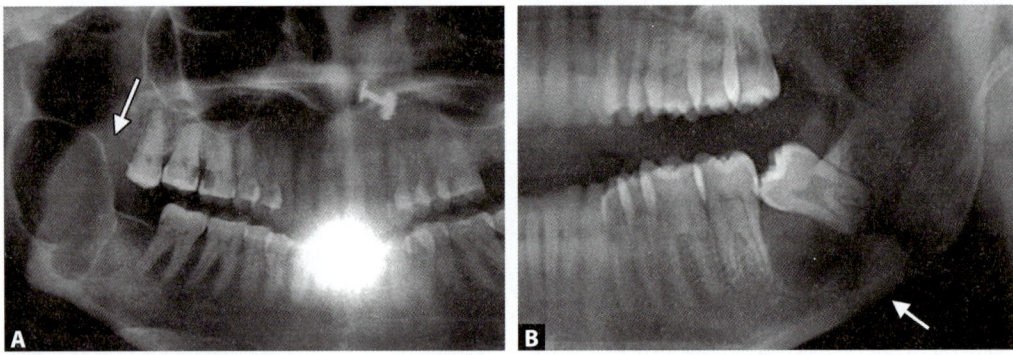

Figs. 6.12A and B: Radiograph of odontogenic keratocyst (OKC)—extraneous type (A) and collateral type (B).

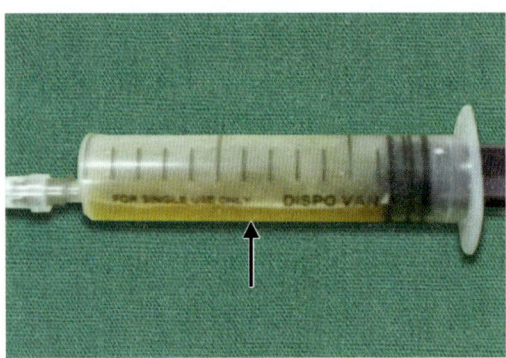

Fig. 6.13: Cystic fluid in odontogenic keratocysts (OKC).

Cystic Fluid (Fig. 6.13)

Aspiration of the cystic content reveals a straw colored fluid, which contains about 3.5 g% of soluble protein. Paper electrophoresis of the cystic fluid is useful in determining this protein level.

Paper electrophoresis

Electrophoretic analysis reveals that the cystic fluid of OKC has soluble protein levels, which is below 3–5 g per 100 mL whereas in cases of nonkeratinizing cysts, the level is about 5–11 g per 100 mL. It is, therefore, concluded that if the soluble protein level in a cyst is less than 4.5 g per 100 mL, it should be considered a keratocyst; and if the level is more than 5.0 g per 100 mL, it should be a nonkeratinizing cyst.

Histopathology (Figs. 6.14 to 6.16)

Histologically, OKC reveals the following features:
- The cyst is lined by a uniform looking keratinized epithelium of about 6–8 cell

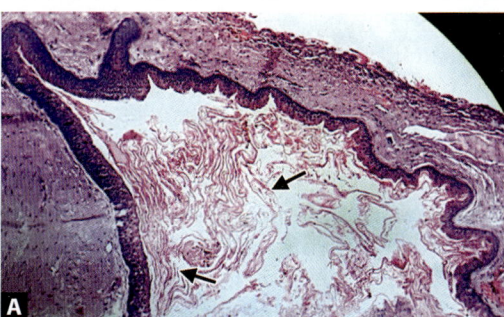
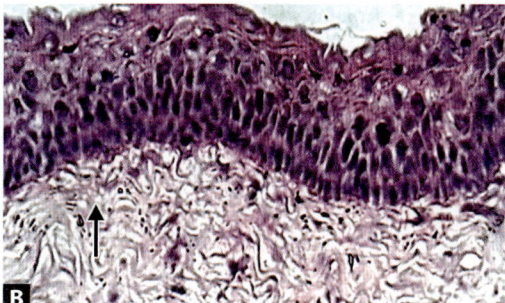

Figs. 6.14A and B: Photomicrograph showing "keratin flakes" in the lumen of odontogenic keratocysts (OKC) (A); and palisading arrangement of basal cells of the lining epithelium (B).

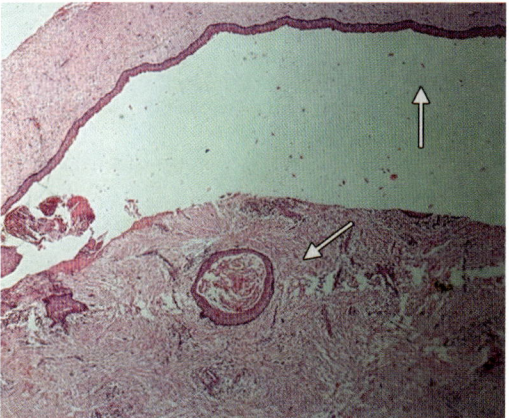

Fig. 6.15: Photomicrograph of odontogenic keratocyst (OKC) showing daughter cyst.

layers in thickness (epithelial thickness is never more than 10 cell layers).

- In about 80–90% cases, the cystic epithelium is keratinized and the epithelium is often flat and uniform in thickness with no rete-peg formations (unless secondarily infected).
- Majority of the OKCs (80–90% cases) exhibit parakeratinized lining and only few cysts can have orthokeratinized lining. Moreover, OKCs with parakeratinized lining have more aggressive behavior than the ones with orthokeratinized lining.
- Sometimes, both forms of keratinization (para and ortho) may be present in different parts of the lining of a single cyst. The parakeratinized cyst lining often have a typical corrugated or wrinkled appearance at the surface.
- The basal layer of the epithelium is made up of tall columnar cells or cuboidal cells; which exhibit a typical palisading arrangement. The prominent palisaded and polarized basal layer of cells in OKC

Odontogenic Keratocyst	Unicystic ameloblastoma
• Spinous layer is compact • Surface layer is corrugated • Palisading of basal cells is a prominent feature	• Spinous layer shows intercellular edema • Surface layer is nonkeratinized • Palisading of basal cells not so prominent

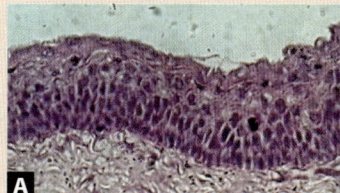
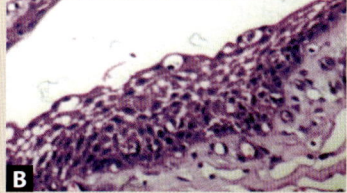

Figs. 6.16A and B: Differentiation between the lining of odontogenic keratocyst (OKC) and unicystic ameloblastoma.

have a characteristic "picket fence" or "tombstone" appearance.
- The lining epithelial cells contain intensely basophilic nuclei, which are often situated away from the basement membrane (reverse polarity of basal cell nuclei). Interestingly, reverse polarity of basal cell nuclei not seen in orthokeratinized OKC.
- Sometimes, the basal layer of the epithelium is made up of cuboidal cells.
- The orthokeratotic cysts often exhibit abundant orthokeratin formations and a well-defined granular layer.
- Mitotic activity is seen in both basal as well as suprabasal layers, but it is more frequent in suprabasal layers.
- Mitotic activity is higher in OKCs occurring in association with nevoid basal cell carcinoma syndrome.
- Large amounts of desquamated keratin are often found within the cystic lumen, which are called "keratin flakes".
- The cystic lining often shows a folded or corrugated appearance, which could be due to unequal growth pattern of the lining at different places.
- The junction between the cystic lining and the connective tissue capsule is weak and in many cases, the cystic epithelium may be detached from the underlying connective tissue.
- One of the most interesting histopathological features of OKC is the presence of multiple small microcysts within the cyst wall, which are known as "daughter cysts" or "satellite cysts".
- Besides "satellite cysts" the cyst wall may also contain many "solid nests" of proliferating epithelium.
- The fibrous capsule is usually thin with relatively few cells widely separated by stroma, usually devoid of inflammatory cells.
- In cases of intense secondary inflammation, the epithelial lining of the cyst often loses its characteristic cellular and architectural features and, therefore, looks like the lining of a radicular cyst.
- Sometimes area of ossification and calcification may be present, which represent dystrophic calcification caused by degeneration or foreign body reaction.
- The cystic epithelium of OKC sometimes shows dysplastic changes; and on rare occasions, the lining epithelium may undergo malignant transformation and develop squamous cell carcinoma.

Key Points of Odontogenic Keratocyst

- Odontogenic keratocyst is a common aggressive type of cystic lesion of the jaw; which arises from the remnants of the dental lamina.
- The cyst commonly occurs in 2nd and 3rd decade of life, and it frequently develops in mandible near the angle.
- Clinically, the smaller lesions are slow growing, painless, and asymptomatic; however, the larger lesions of OKC often produce extensive swelling of the jaw with facial asymmetry.
- Paresthesia in the jaw along with mobility and displacement of the teeth are frequently seen.
- On many occasions, a very large cyst can produce little bony expansion; because the cyst spreads via the medullary spaces of bone.
- Keratocysts often radiographically present multilocular radiolucent areas with typical "soap–bubble" appearance.
- Occasionally, the mandibular lesions cross the midline and extend from one side of body of mandible to the other side.
- Odontogenic keratocyst has four radiological types—(1) replacement type, (2) envelopmental type, (3) extraneous type, and (4) collateral type.
- The cystic fluid is generally straw colored and contains about 3.5 g% of soluble protein.
- Microscopically, the lesion presents a cystic cavity lined by a uniform looking keratinized stratified odontogenic epithelium having 6–8 cell layers thickness.
- The lining epithelium and connective tissue interface is flat and no rete-peg formation is seen in the lining epithelium of cyst.
- The cyst characteristically exhibits the presence of multiple small microcysts within the connective tissue wall; which are known as "daughter cysts" or "satellite cysts".
- Odontogenic keratocysts have a tremendous tendency for recurrence after treatment.
- Treatment is done by surgical enucleation; resection of jaw done in case of repeated recurrence.

Enlargement of Cyst (Box 6.4)

The OKC always tends to spread via the cancellous bone and the expansion of the cyst occurs through the following mechanisms.

Excessive Cell Proliferation

Peripheral cell division helps in encroachment of more and more space by the cyst and thus it expands; more or less all cysts enlarge in the same mechanism. However, since OKC develops from the preformative cells of dental lamina (not from cell rests), the lining epithelial cells of this cyst are more aggressive in terms of mitotic divisions. Such increased mitotic activity of the cystic epithelial cells may contribute to the greater expansion and more aggressive nature of this cyst.

Osmolarity of Cyst Fluid

- The average concentration of the cystic fluid is often higher than that of the blood serum or the tissue fluid in the surrounding area because the cystic fluid contains large amount of soluble proteins, e.g. albumin, globulin, fibrinogen, fibrin breakdown product, etc.
- Such proteins come either form the secretion of the cystic epithelial cells or as the breakdown product of the dying cells of the cyst lining.
- The osmotic difference between the two fluids increase in the osmotic pressure in the cyst, as it has the higher concentration; as a result more and more fluid from the surrounding tissue moves into the cystic lumen through the process of osmotic diffusion via the semipermeable cystic lining. The process increases the volume of the cystic fluid considerably, which exerts more pressure on the bony wall of the cyst resulting in its expansion.
- Moreover, the similar process of cyst expansion continues as the cystic fluid always maintains a higher osmolarity due to continuous incorporation of the cell break down proteins resulting from shedding of the older or dead cells of the cystic lining epithelium.

Hydrostatic Pressure

Hydrostatic pressure is the force exerted by any fluid on the walls of the container in which it is kept; in case of a cystic cavity, where the fluid volume keep on increasing (due to osmosis as well as transudation or exudation from the capsule), obviously creates pressure on the surrounding bony wall and thus causes resorption of the bone resulting in more and more expansion of the cyst. Goblet cells present in the cyst lining has the maximum secretory ability.

Bone resorbing activity

- Increased collagenase activity: This enzyme released by the lining cells causes destruction of collagen in the bone (collagenolysis) and results in increased bone resorption and subsequent expansion of the cyst.
- Inflammatory cells in the cyst capsule release lymphokines, e.g. osteoclast activating factor and interleukin-1, they cause stimulation of fibroblasts, subsequently, there is release of prostaglandins (PGE2 and PGE3) which are potent bone resorbing chemicals.
- Moreover, release of other agents like tumor necrosis factor, matrix metalloproteinase, and tenascin have also role in bone resorption and thereby expansion of cyst.

Box 6.4	Mechanism of cyst enlargement.

- Excessive cell proliferation
- Osmolarity of cystic fluid
- Hydrostatic pressure within the cyst
- Enzymatic mechanisms

Treatment

Treatment is done by either "surgical enucleation" or "marsupialization" of the cyst. The oral epithelium, which is overlying the cystic lesion, has to be excised to eliminate the pos-

| Box 6.5 | Main causes of recurrence in odontogenic keratocyst (OKC). |

- Satellite cyst
- New cyst formation
- Keratinization pattern
- Nature of cyst lining
- Basal layer of oral epithelium
- Conservative surgical approach

sibility of further recurrence (because some cysts may develop from the basal layer of the oral epithelium). Intraluminal injection of Carnoy's solution also has been used to free the cyst from bony wall, thereby allowing easier enucleation. Usually, the recurrence rate is very high in OKC; and in case of repeated recurrence of the cystic lesion, jaw resection is recommended (Box 6.5).

Causes of Recurrence in OKC

Odontogenic keratocysts may recur after treatment in about 60% cases, and the causes of this higher rate of recurrence are as follows:

- ***Satellite cyst:*** The satellite cyst or daughter cyst are common entities in OKCs and these small cysts often remain undetected within the tissue during treatment. The higher rate of recurrence in keratocysts could be due to the enlargement of the satellite cysts following treatment.
- ***New cyst formation:*** The cells of the OKC have an aggressive potential for multiplication (since these are preformative group of cells of the dental lamina) and this tendency may often cause formation of newer cysts in the jaw, which often appears to be a case of recurrence.

  Moreover, if any part of the cyst capsule remains within the bone during surgery, the retained part of the capsular tissue of the cyst (containing remnants of epithelial islands) may lead to recurrence due to multiplication and subsequent cystification of those epithelial remnants.
- ***Keratinization pattern of the cyst epithelium:*** OKCs, which have parakeratinized epithelium often have more possibility of recurrence.
- ***Corrugated nature of cyst lining:*** The lining of the OKC is thin and fragile and is often corrugated; due to these, it is very difficult to enucleate the entire lining of a large cyst during surgery.

  Moreover, the OKCs grow very fast; but as the bony expansion is too little, the size of the cyst is always smaller than what is expected; as a result, the cystic epithelium often folded. These narrow infoldings or finger-like projections extend deep into the cancellous bone up to a variable depth and during surgery these narrow infoldings are easily left behind, therefore increasing the risk recurrence.
- ***Basal layer of oral epithelium:*** New keratocysts may sometimes develop from the basal layer of oral epithelium.
- ***Conservative surgical approach:*** In an attempt to save a vital structure (a tooth, a nerve, or a blood vessel, etc.) adjacent to the cyst, sometimes conservative surgical approach is undertaken. This may result in incomplete removal of the cyst leading to recurrence.
- ***Association with Gorlin-Goltz syndrome:*** The OKCs associated with this syndrome have extreme tendency for recurrence.
- ***Aggressive nature of the cyst:*** OKCs often develop from preformative type of odontogenic cells and, hence, the nature of the cyst is more aggressive than those arising from the postformative cells, e.g. dentigerous or radicular cysts, etc. The aggressive growth pattern of OKC may contribute to its increased recurrence rate.

■ DENTIGEROUS CYST

Definition

Dentigerous cyst is a common odontogenic cystic lesion, which encloses the crown of an impacted tooth at its neck portion (*dentigerous* means tooth bearing). The cyst develops due to abnormal dilatation of the dental follicle around the crown of an unerupted tooth. This is the most common type of developmental odontogenic cyst, making up about 20% of all epithelium lined cysts of the jaws.

Pathogenesis

- Dentigerous cyst is derived from the cells of the reduced enamel epithelium, which surrounds the crown of the impacted or unerupted tooth.
- The cyst enlarges due to accumulation of fluid in-between the reduced enamel epithelium and the tooth crown.
- When the cyst develops around the crown of an impacted permanent tooth, periapical inflammation in the overlying deciduous tooth may be the triggering factor.
- A strong association is seen between failure of eruption of tooth and the development of dentigerous cyst. That is why, this cyst often develops in relation to lower third molars and the upper canines.
- Regardless of the size, dentigerous cyst always remains attached to the cervical margin (cementoenamel junction) of the involved tooth.
- The crown of the tooth is located within the lumen of the cyst, while the root remains outside (Flowchart 6.1).

Clinical Features

- *Incidence:* Incidence rate of dentigerous cyst is about 16% among all intraoral cysts.
- *Age:* Mostly second and third decade of life
- *Sex:* It is seen more commonly in males in comparison to females
- *Site:* This cyst occurs twice as common in mandible as in maxilla.

Mandibular third molar area is the most common site of occurrence of dentigerous cyst, although the maxillary canine, mandibular second premolar, and maxillary third molar areas are also commonly affected. The cyst also frequently occurs in relation to the supernumerary teeth or odontomes, etc.

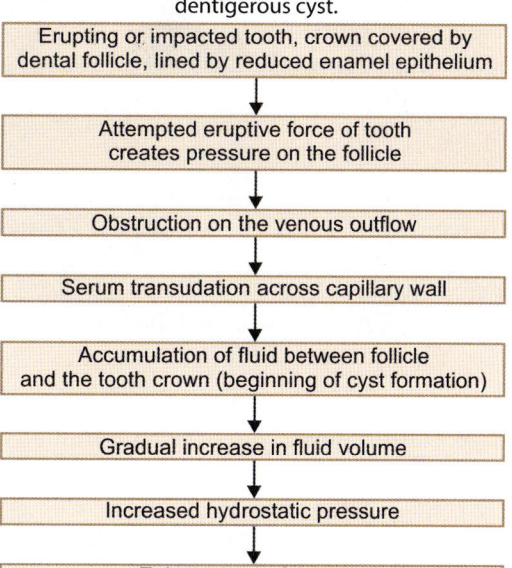

Flowchart 6.1: Outline of pathogenesis of dentigerous cyst.

Clinical Presentation (Figs. 6.17 and 6.18)

- In many cases, smaller cysts remain asymptomatic and are detected incidentally during the routine radiographic examinations.
- A cyst can also be found occasionally during radiographic examination of a retained deciduous tooth.
- Dentigerous cyst normally presents a slow enlarging bony hard swelling of the jaw with expansion of the cortical plates of bone.

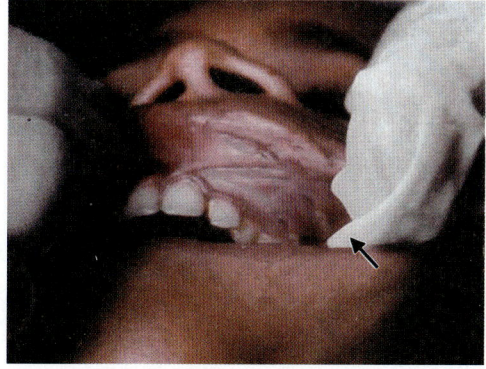

Fig. 6.17: Dentigerous cyst involving the left side of maxilla.

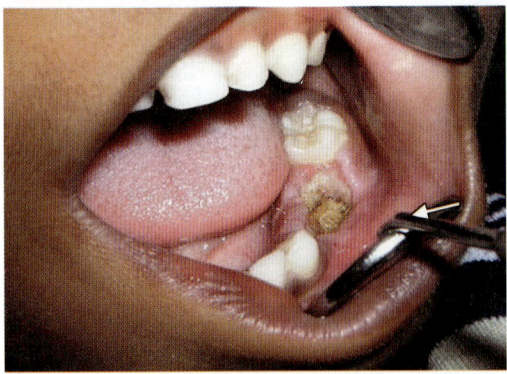

Fig. 6.18: Dentigerous cyst of mandible.

- Massive facial swelling, derangement of occlusion, development facial asymmetry, etc. are seen in extremely large lesions.
- Severe expansion of bone results in thinning of the cortical plates; and on palpation, the affected area of bone gives a "crepitus-like" sensation. Moreover, if the overlying bone is completely lost due to a growing cyst, "fluctuations" may be felt in the area.
- Occasionally, pain and accelerated swelling may be noticed, if the cyst gets secondarily infected.
- Paresthesia and anesthesia on the affected part of the jaw often develop. In few lesions, pathological fractures of the jawbone may occur.
- As the cyst develops around the crown of an impacted or embedded tooth, clinically often there is a missing tooth in the dental arch.

Radiological Features (Figs. 6.19A to C)

- Radiograph of dentigerous cyst reveals a well-defined and unilocular-rounded radiolucent area enclosing the crown of an impacted tooth. [Radiographic distinction between a small dentigerous cyst and an enlarged follicle around the crown of an unerupted tooth is difficult. For the lesion to be considered a cyst, some investigators believe that the radiolucent space surrounding the tooth crown should be at least 3–4 mm in diameter.]
- The tooth associated with the cyst is often displaced from its normal position in the jaw, e.g. the involved lower third molar is often pushed to the lower border of mandible or to the ramus area. Likewise, the upper tooth may be pushed to the maxillary sinus or to the floor of the orbit.
- Exceedingly large cysts may look multilocular due to the persistence of several residual bony trabeculae within the cystic space.
- Expansion and distortion of the cortical plates of bone occurs commonly and the periphery of the cyst is often bordered by well-corticated or sclerotic margin.
- The cyst occurs in association with an impacted tooth of regular series in the dentition or an impacted supernumerary tooth or even an odontome.
- Interestingly, the dentigerous cyst in most of the cases shows resorption of the roots of the neighboring erupted teeth. In long-standing lesions, the tooth which is

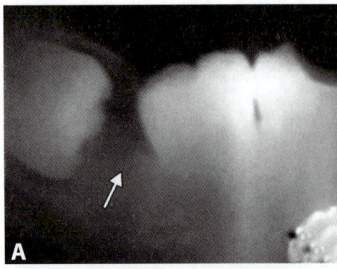
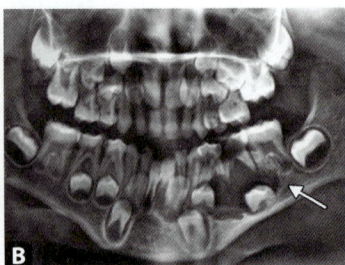
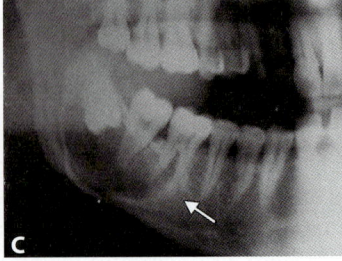

Figs. 6.19A to C: (A) Radiograph of a dentigerous cyst in the early stage; (B) Radiograph of dentigerous cyst of left mandible; and (C) The cyst on the right mandible.

enclosed within the cyst may also become resorbed.
- Chronically infected dentigerous cysts may have hazy or ill-defined borders.

Radiological Types of Dentigerous Cyst

On the basis of the position of tooth crown within the lumen of the cyst dentigerous cysts are divided into three types:
1. *Central type*: When the cystic cavity envelops or surrounds the crown of the impacted tooth symmetrically from all sides (Fig. 6.20). Hence, the tooth crown is positioned at the center of the lumen.
2. *Lateral type*: In this case, the cystic cavity is located on one side of the involved crown. It results from deflection of the dental follicle on one side of the crown during the eruption of the tooth. This type is mostly seen when the cyst develops in relation to a partially erupted and mesioangular type of mandibular third molar (Fig. 6.21).
3. *Circumferential type:* When the cystic cavity radiographically appears to enclose the entire tooth. This type of radiographic appearance is found when the impacted tooth is seen in a two-dimensional picture in the background of a very large cyst (although the cyst never encloses the tooth completely) (Fig. 6.22).

Cystic Fluid in Dentigerous Cyst

The cyst is usually filled with a straw-colored fluid that contains about 5 g% of soluble protein. Glycosaminoglycans (GAGs), predominantly hyaluronic acid, but also appreciable amounts of heparin and chondroitin 4-sulphates are present in fluids and walls of dentigerous cysts.

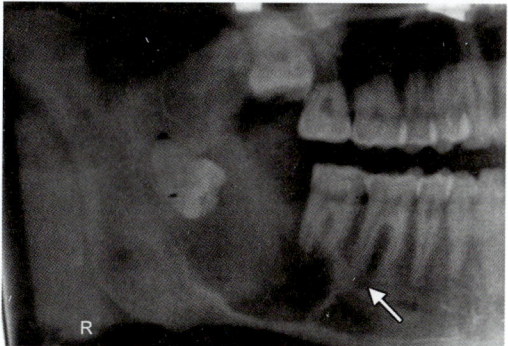

Fig. 6.20: X-ray of dentigerous cyst of "central type".

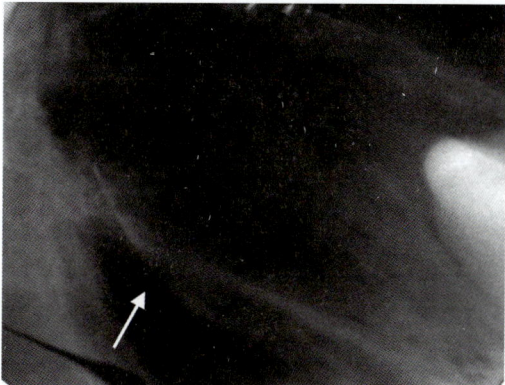

Fig. 6.21: X-ray of dentigerous cyst of "lateral type".

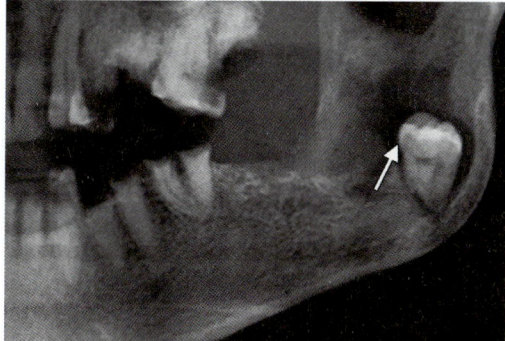

Fig. 6.22: X-ray of dentigerous cyst of "circumferential type".

Differential Diagnosis

- Adenomatoid odontogenic tumor (AOT)
- Odontogenic keratocyst
- Unilocular ameloblastoma
- Enlarged dental follicle
- Odontogenic keratocyst
- Ameloblastic fibro-odontome
- Ameloblastic fibroma
- Calcifying epithelial odontogenic cyst.

Histopathology (Figs. 6.23)

- Histologically, dentigerous cyst reveals the presence of a cystic cavity, which is lined by a thin layer of nonkeratinized, odontogenic epithelium (about 2–3 cell layer thickness). Thickness of the lining becomes more in case of inflammation.
- The cystic epithelium is generally nonkeratinized and the cells are usually flat or cuboidal in nature with uniform orientation of the cell layers.
- Cystic epithelium may undergo mucous metaplasia with development of mucous cells and ciliated epithelial cells in the lining.
- Sometimes, superficial layer of the cystic epithelium may be low columnar in nature and the cells partly resemble ameloblasts cells of the developing tooth germ.
- Nests, islands, and strands of odontogenic epithelium are sometimes seen within the capsule.
- Long-standing dentigerous cysts may occasionally exhibit areas of keratinization or dysplastic changes in the epithelial lining.
- The cyst lining is supported by a loosely arranged connective tissue stroma. (The stroma often resembles the odontogenic ectomesenchyme).
- Localized areas of "bud-like" proliferations of cystic epithelial cells may be seen in few areas of the cyst wall, which are known as "mural proliferations" and they indicate the neoplastic change in the cystic epithelium toward the development of "ameloblastoma" from the lining of the dentigerous cyst (Box 6.6).
- Besides ameloblastoma, many other tumors, e.g. AOT, squamous cell carcinoma, intraosseous mucoepidermoid carcinoma, etc. can develop from the dentigerous cyst lining (Box 6.7).
- Chronic inflammatory cell infiltration is rarely seen in the connective tissue stroma.
- Discontinuities in the epithelial lining may be seen due to secondary infections in the cyst and infected cyst lining may form rete-ridges (absent in noninfected lining).

Box 6.6 Vicker and Gorlin criteria for ameloblastoma.

Features in dentigerous cyst lining that might indicate the future development of ameloblastoma are:
- Hyperchromatism of the basal cell nuclei
- Palisading with polarization of basal cells
- Cytoplasmic vacuolization with intercellular spacing of the lining epithelium.

Box 6.7 List of potential complications in dentigerous cyst.

- Development of ameloblastoma and AOT
- Development of squamous cell carcinoma
- Development of mucoepidermoid carcinoma
- Conventional risk of recurrence, secondary infection, osteomyelitis, pathological fracture, etc.

Key Points of Dentigerous Cyst

- Dentigerous cyst is a common odontogenic cystic lesion, which encloses the crown of an impacted tooth at its neck portion.
- The cyst develops from the reduced enamel epithelium, which surrounds the crown of the impacted or unerupted tooth.
- Dentigerous cyst commonly develops from the mandibular third molar area. The other common sites include the maxillary canine, mandibular second premolar, and maxillary third molar areas, etc.
- Clinically, the cyst often presents a slow enlarging bony hard swelling of the jaw with expansion of the cortical plates of bone.
- Massive facial swelling, derangement of occlusion, development facial asymmetry, etc. are seen in extremely large lesions.

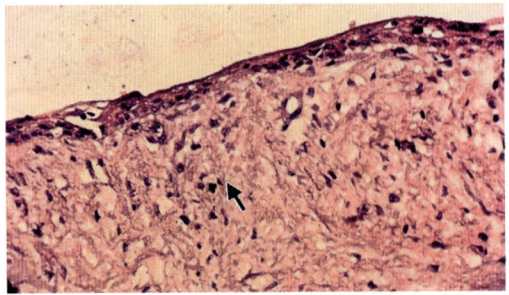

Fig. 6.23: Photomicrograph of dentigerous cyst (high power).

- Expansion and severe thinning of the bone may produce fluctuations in the area.
- Radiographically, the cyst reveals a well-defined unilocular-rounded radiolucent area enclosing the crown of an impacted tooth.
- Dentigerous cyst often exhibits resorption of roots of the adjoining teeth.
- The cyst has three radiological types—(1) central type, (2) lateral type, and (3) circumferential type.
- The cyst is usually filled with a straw-colored fluid that contains about 5 g% of soluble protein.
- Histologically, dentigerous cyst reveals the presence of a cystic cavity, which is lined by a thin, nonkeratinized epithelium of 2–3 cell layer thickness.
- The lining epithelium of the cyst is supported by a loosely arranged connective tissue stroma that resembles the odontogenic ectomesenchyme.
- Localized areas of "bud-like" proliferations of cystic epithelial cells may be seen in few areas of the cyst wall, which are known as "mural proliferations".
- Treatment is done by enucleation.

Enlargement

Excessive Cell Proliferation

Peripheral cell division helps in encroachment of more and more space by the cyst and thus it expands more or less; all cysts enlarge in the same mechanism. Since dentigerous cyst develops from the resting cells or postformative cells (reduced enamel epithelium), whose rate of proliferation is less, hence, this cyst expands slowly as compared to the OKC.

Osmolarity of Cyst Fluid

- The average concentration of the cystic fluid is often higher than that of the blood serum or the tissue fluid in the surrounding area because the cystic fluid contains large amount of soluble proteins, e.g. albumin, globulin, fibrinogen, and fibrin breakdown, etc.
- Such proteins come either form the secretion of the cystic epithelial cells or as the breakdown product of the dying cells of the cyst lining.
- The osmotic difference between the two fluids increase in the osmotic pressure in the cyst, as it has the higher concentration; as a result, more and more fluid from the surrounding tissue moves into the cystic lumen through the process of osmotic diffusion via the semipermeable cystic lining. The process increases the volume of the cystic fluid considerably, which exerts more pressure on the bony wall of the cyst resulting in its expansion.
- Moreover, the similar process of cyst expansion continues as the cystic fluid always maintains a higher osmolarity due to continuous incorporation of the cell break down proteins resulting from shedding of the older or dead cells of the cystic lining epithelium.

Hydrostatic Pressure

- Hydrostatic pressure is the force exerted by any fluid on the walls of the container in which it is kept; in case of a cystic cavity, where the fluid volume keep on increasing (due to osmosis as well as transudation or exudation from the capsule), obviously creates pressure on the surrounding bony wall and thus causes resorption of the bone resulting in more and more expansion of the cyst. Goblet cells present in the cyst lining have the maximum secretory ability.
- Dentigerous cysts release large amount of GAGs from its wall, which diffuse into the cystic fluid and increase its osmolality. This leads to increased internal hydrostatic pressure in the lumen and cause enlargement of the cyst.

Bone resorbing activity

- *Increased collagenase activity*: This enzyme released by the lining cells cause destruction of collagen in the bone (collagenolysis) and results in increased bone resorption and subsequent expansion of the cyst.
- Inflammatory cells in the cyst capsule release lymphokines, e.g. osteoclast-activating factor and interleukin-1, they cause stimulation of fibroblasts, subsequently, there is release of prostaglandins (PGE2 and PGE3), which are potent bone resorbing chemicals.

- Moreover, release of other agents like tumor necrosis factor, matrix metalloproteinase, tenascin have also role in bone resorption and thereby expansion of cyst.

Causes of Root Resorption in Dentigerous Cyst

The dentigerous cyst often shows resorption of root(s) of the adjacent normal teeth. The possible reasons for this could be the presence of reduced enamel epithelium in dentigerous cyst.
- During the normal physiological shedding of primary teeth, the reduced enamel epithelium actively participates in the root resorption of these deciduous teeth.
- This inherent tendency for root resorption may be retained by the cells of dentigerous cyst, which are also derived from the reduced enamel epithelium.
- The cystic epithelial cells release some chemicals substances, which can cause resorption of roots similar to that of the normal reduced enamel epithelial cells in a developing permanent tooth.

Treatment

Treatment of dentigerous cyst is done by "marsupialization" (if the involved tooth is to be preserved). In other cases, the treatment can be done by surgical enucleation of the cyst.

■ RADICULAR CYST

Definition

Radicular or periapical cyst is the most common odontogenic cystic lesion of inflammatory origin, which occurs in relation to the apex of a nonvital tooth.

In a radicular cyst, if the involved tooth is exfoliated or extracted and the cystic lesion remains within the bone, the condition is known as residual cyst.

Types (Figs. 6.24 and 6.25)

Types of radicular cyst according to their locations in relation to the associated nonvital tooth:
- *True radicular cyst:* When the cystic cavity is separated from the root apex by an

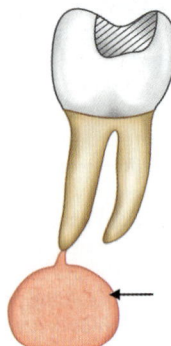

Fig. 6.24: True radicular cyst—cavity is little away from the root apex.

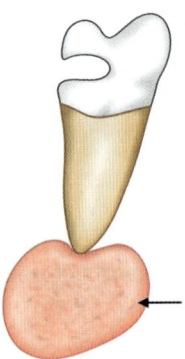

Fig. 6.25: Bay cyst—cavity is attached with the root apex.

intervening fibrous capsule, this cyst has a complete epithelial lining surrounding the lumen.
- *Bay cyst (pocket cyst):* This is a type of radicular cyst in which the root apex of the involved tooth projects into the cystic lumen and as a result the continuity of the cyst lining is lost at point of contact with the root apex.

Pathogenesis (Flowchart 6.2)

The radicular cyst develops due to the proliferation and subsequent cystic degeneration of the "epithelial cell rests of Malassez", in the periapical region of a nonvital tooth. The entire process of development of this cyst occurs in several phases.
- Phase of initiation
- Phase of proliferation

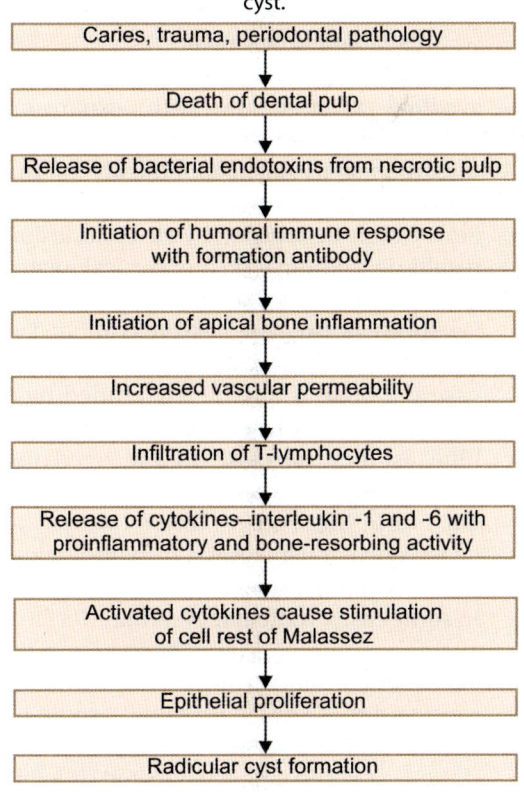

Flowchart 6.2: Outline of pathogenesis of radicular cyst.

- Phase of cystification
- Phase of enlargement.

Phase of Initiation

During this phase, the bacterial infection of the dental pulp or direct inflammatory effect of necrotic pulpal tissue, in a nonvital tooth causes stimulation of the "cell rest of Malassez", which are the remnants of Hertwig epithelial root sheath (HERS) present within the bone near the root apex of teeth.

Phase of Proliferation

The stimulation to the cell rests of Malassez leads to excessive and exuberant proliferation of these cells, which leads to the formation of a large mass or island of immature proliferating epithelial cells at the periapical region of the affected tooth.

During the cyst formation, both cell mediated and humoral immune reactions destroy the potential microorganisms, which are trying to enter into the periapical tissues. The activated T-cells play the major role in protecting the area from secondary infection and they keep the area sterile, thus facilitates in the development of cyst; otherwise infection in the area will form periapical abscess instead of periapical cyst.

Phase of Cystification

Once a large bulk of the cell rest of Malassez is produced, its peripheral cells get adequate nutritional supply, but its centrally located cells are often deprived of proper nutritional supply. As a result, the central or innermost group of cells undergoes ischemic liquefactive necrosis, while the peripheral group of cells survives. Moreover, large amount of stromal cells also die when they are surrounded by the proliferating epithelial cells. This eventually gives rise to the formation of a cavity and a peripheral lining of epithelial cells around it.

Mechanism of cystification by:
- Degeneration of central cells due to lack of nutrition and oxygen as the area is avascular.
- Necrosis of stromal cells when they become surrounded by the cystic epithelium from all sides.

Phase of Enlargement

Once a small cyst is formed, it enlarges gradually by the following mechanisms:
- Higher osmotic tension of the cystic fluid causes progressive increase in the amount of fluid inside its lumen and this causes increased internal hydrostatic tension within the cyst. The process results in cyst expansion due to resorption of the surrounding bone.
- The epithelial cells of the cystic lining release some bone resorbing factors like prostaglandins, collagenase, etc. which

destroy the bone and facilitate expansion of the cyst.

Clinical Features

- *Incidence:* Radicular cyst constitutes about 50% or more among all types of jaw cysts.
- *Age:* Mostly 3rd, 4th, and 5th decade of life.
- *Sex:* More common among males.
- *Site:* The cyst can occur in relation to any tooth of either jaw, but maxilla (60%) is usually more commonly affected than mandible (40%). The occurrences of more caries in the upper anterior teeth and the occasional presence of dens-in-dente in the upper lateral incisors are usually responsible for the higher incidence of this cyst in the maxilla.

Clinical Presentation (Figs. 6.26A and B)

- The involved tooth is always nonvital and it can be easily detected by the presence of caries, fractures, discolorations, etc. Moreover, the affected tooth does not respond to thermal or electric pulp testing.
- Radicular cyst may occur rarely in association with nonvital deciduous tooth (mostly molars).
- The cyst often causes localized and painless swelling in the area of affected tooth.
- The smaller cystic lesions are usually asymptomatic and are detected only when a radiograph is taken.
- The larger lesions produce bony hard swelling in the jaw with expansion and distortion of the cortical plates or disturbance in occlusion mostly of the regional teeth.
- Severe bone destruction by the cystic lesion results in thinning of the cortical plates and it may produce a "springiness" of the jawbone when digital pressure is applied.
- There may be presence of fluctuations in case the bone is completely eroded by a large cyst. These lesions clinically appear blue as they lie close to the overlying epithelium.
- On rare occasions, there may be occurrence of paresthesia or pathological fractures in the bone, etc.
- In some cases, radicular cysts may develop at the opening of a large accessory pulp canal on the lateral aspect of the tooth root; and these cysts are often termed as "lateral radicular cysts".
- If the cyst is secondarily infected, it leads to the formation of an abscess, which is called "cyst abscess".
- Multiple radicular cysts may develop in rare cases, when there are many nonvital teeth present in the mouth, e.g. multiple dense-in-dente or dentinogenesis imperfecta.

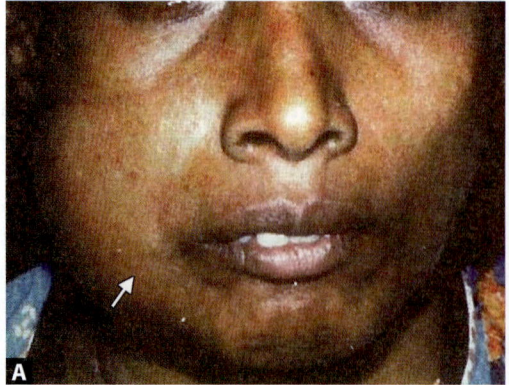 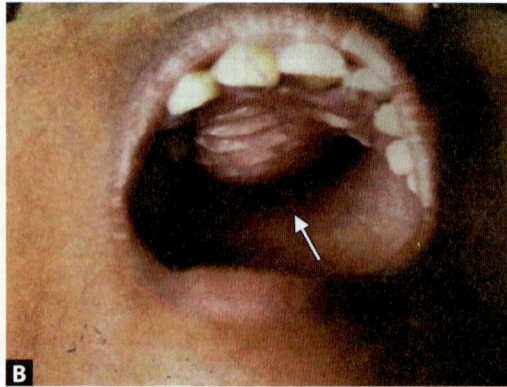

Figs. 6.26A and B: (A) Radicular cyst of mandible; (B) Radicular cyst of maxilla.

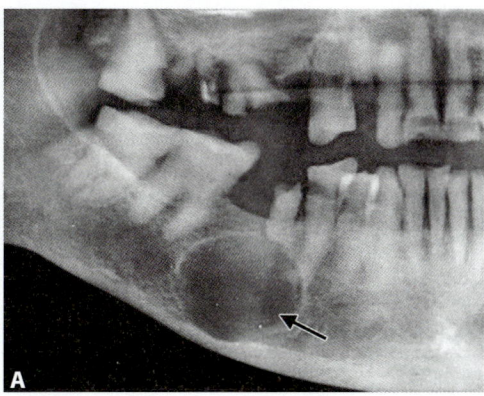
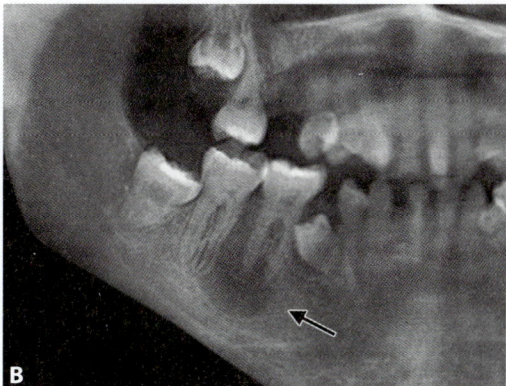

Figs. 6.27A and B: Radiograph of radicular cysts.

- A radicular cyst may persist in the jaw after the attached tooth has been extracted; such cyst is often called a **"residual cyst"**. These cysts frequently cause of swelling in the edentulous jaws and they regress slowly and spontaneously.

Radiological Features
(Figs. 6.27 and 6.28)

- On radiographs, radicular cysts present well-defined, unilocular, and round-shaped radiolucent areas of variable size (few millimeters to several centimeters in diameter).
- The cyst is always found in contact with the root apex of a nonvital tooth and it is bordered on the periphery by a well-corticated margin. The infected cysts often have hazy or an ill-defined border.
- The nonvital tooth with which the cyst is attached often have a large carious cavity or a fracture on the crown.
- The lateral radicular cysts appear as semicircular radiolucency on the lateral aspect of the root with loss of lamina dura.
- Root resorption is often seen in the associated nonvital tooth.
- Residual cyst appears as a round or oval radiolucent area in the alveolar ridge where from a tooth was extracted previously.

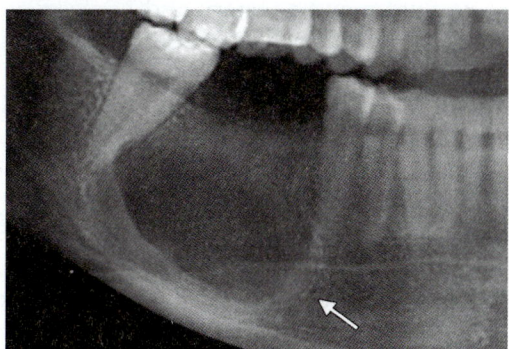

Fig. 6.28: Radiograph of residual cysts.

Macroscopic Appearance

- Macroscopic examination of radicular cyst reveals a round or ovoid soft tissue sack, which is attached to the root apex of a nonvital tooth.
- On cutting, a thin straw-colored fluid or a thick, paste like, yellow–brown coagulum is found within the lumen.
- Cholesterol crystals may be present within the cyst content, which appear as glistening particles.
- The cyst capsule is usually several millimeters thick and the internal luminal contour of the cyst may be smooth or corrugated.

Cystic Fluid

Aspiration of the cystic contents often reveals a straw-colored fluid, which may be

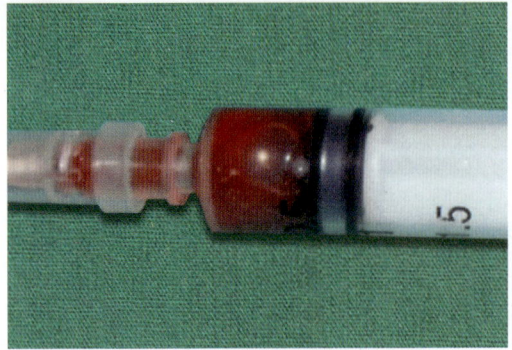

Fig. 6.29: Cystic fluid in radicular cyst.

sometimes blood-tinged. Sometimes, the cystic fluid may be watery and opalescent. The cystic fluid may also contain cholesterol crystals; which can be seen under microscope once a smear of the fluid is prepared (Fig. 6.29).

Paper electrophoresis indicates the presence of about 5 g% of soluble protein in it.

Histopathology (Figs. 6.30 to 6.32)

- Histologically, radicular cyst shows the presence of a cystic cavity, which is lined by a nonkeratinized and stratified squamous epithelium of about 6–20 cell layers thickness and the lining epithelium is backed by a well-vascularized and connective tissue stroma.
- Sometimes, discontinuities in the epithelial lining may be seen in the areas of inflammation.
- The lining epithelium often shows localized areas of increased cell proliferation and edema.
- The thickness of the lining is not same everywhere—in some areas, it is thin; while in some other areas, it is very thick. This entirely depends upon the presence of inflammatory stimulus within the cyst.
- Ciliated columnar epithelium or respiratory epithelium may also be present in radicular cyst on rare occasions due to metaplastic change in the cystic lining.
- Occasionally, there may be presence of mucous-secreting goblet cells in the

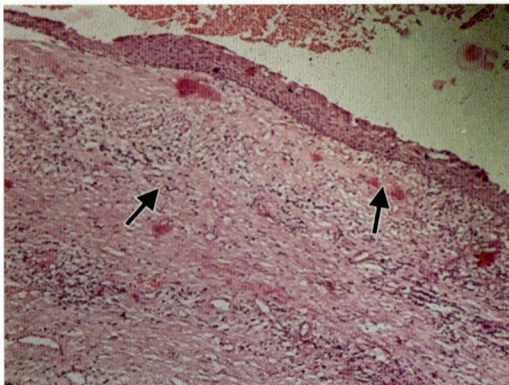

Fig. 6.30: Photomicrograph of radicular cysts (low power) showing lining epithelium and inflammatory cells in the capsule.

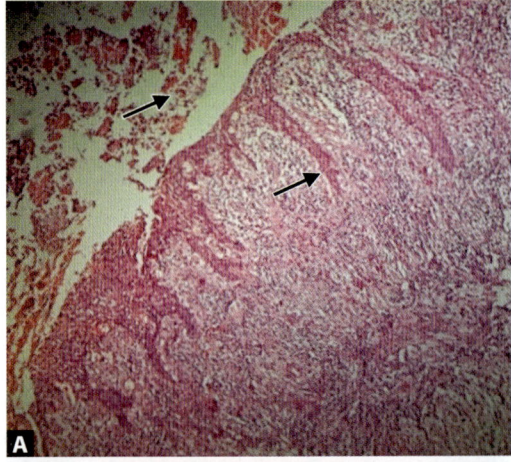

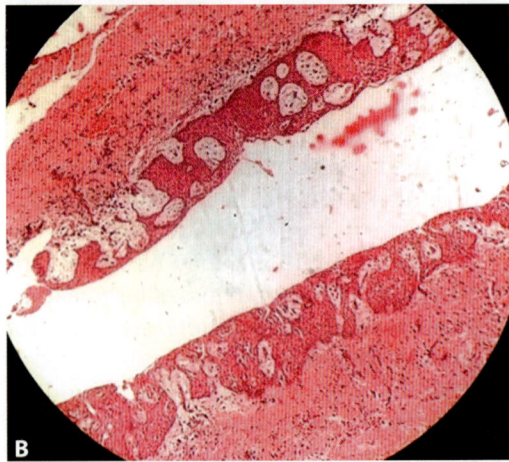

Figs. 6.31A and B: Photomicrograph of radicular cyst showing "arcading pattern" of the cystic epithelium.

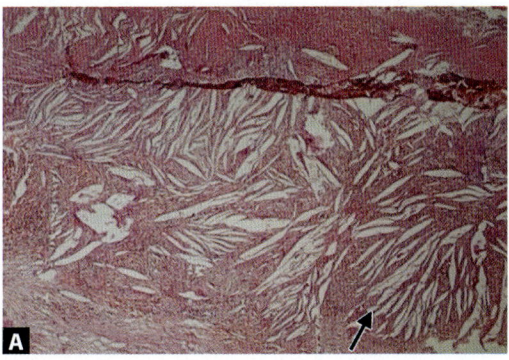 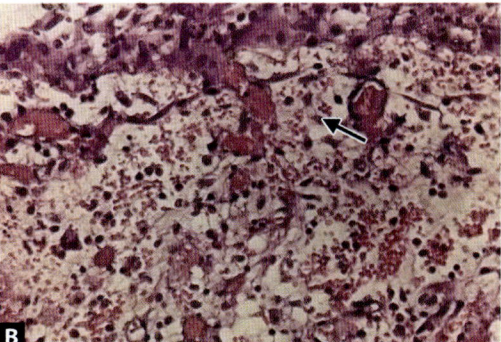

Figs. 6.32A and B: Photomicrograph of radicular cyst showing " (A) Cholesterol clefts"; and "(B) Russell bodies".

lining of the cyst (these cells form also as a result of metaplasia in the cystic lining).
- Focal or generalized keratinization may be seen in some cases in the cysts lining.
- The proliferating cystic epithelium may sometimes grow in a peculiar fashion, by enclosing or encircling a mass of connective tissue from all sides and this pattern of growth is called "arcading pattern".
- Presence of inflammatory cell infiltration and edema is often seen within the cystic lining.
- The cyst capsule is made up of vascular connective tissue, which is often infiltrated by chronic inflammatory cells (predominantly plasma cells).
- Multiple small, ribbon-shaped or needle-shaped, and cleft-like spaces are seen either in the cystic lumen or in the connective tissue capsule of the cyst; these are known as "cholesterol clefts". Normally, cholesterol is derived from breakdown of blood cells and is present in the cyst wall; only the cholesterol clefts are left out in the cyst, when cholesterol is dissolved during chemical processing of the tissue for sectioning.
- "Rushton bodies" or hyaline bodies appear as eosinophilic, straight or curved, rounded or irregular structures found within the cystic lining.
- "Russell bodies" may be present in the cyst; these are large, homogeneous, eosinophilic inclusion bodies found in the plasma cells, which are making excess immunoglobulines.
- The cystic epithelium may sometimes undergo malignant transformation.
- Multinucleated foreign body type of giant cells may be seen within the connective tissue.

Mechanisms of Enlargement of Cyst after Initial Development

- Cell proliferation
- Osmolarity of the cystic fluid
- Hydrostatic pressure within the cyst
- Bone resorption
- Growth in the form of arcading.

Excessive Cell Proliferation

Peripheral cell division helps in encroachment of more and more space by the cyst and thus it expands; more or less all cysts enlarge in the same mechanism.

Osmolarity of Cyst Fluid

- The average concentration of the cystic fluid is often higher than that of the blood serum or the tissue fluid in the surrounding area because the cystic fluid contains large amount of soluble proteins, e.g. albumin, globulin, fibrinogen, and fibrin breakdown, etc.
- Such proteins come either form the secretion of the cystic epithelial cells or as

the breakdown product of the dying cells of the cyst lining.
- The osmotic difference between the two fluids increases in the osmotic pressure in the cyst as it has the higher concentration; as a result, more and more fluid from the surrounding tissue moves into the cystic lumen through the process of osmotic diffusion via the semipermeable cystic lining. The process increases the volume of the cystic fluid considerably, which exerts more pressure on the bony wall of the cyst resulting in its expansion.
- Moreover, the similar process of cyst expansion continues as the cystic fluid always maintains a higher osmolarity due to continuous incorporation of the cell break down proteins resulting from shedding of the older or dead cells of the cystic lining epithelium.

Hydrostatic Pressure

Hydrostatic pressure is the force exerted by any fluid on the walls of the container in which it is kept; in case of a cystic cavity, where the fluid volume keep on increasing (due to osmosis as well as transudation or exudation from the capsule), obviously creates pressure on the surrounding bony wall and thus causes resorption of the bone resulting in more and more expansion of the cyst. Goblet cells present in the cyst lining has the maximum secretory ability.

Bone-resorbing Activity

- This is an inflammatory cyst, therefore inflammatory cell activity is very strong in this cyst; the cyst capsule releases lymphokines, e.g. osteoclast activating factor and interleukin-1, they cause stimulation of fibroblasts, subsequently there is release of prostaglandins (PGE2 and PGE3), which are potent bone-resorbing chemicals.
- Increased collagenase activity: This enzyme released by the lining cells causes destruction of collagen in the bone (collagenolysis) and results in increased bone resorption and subsequent expansion of the cyst.
- Moreover, release of other agents like tumor necrosis factor, matrix metalloproteinase, tenascin has also role in bone resorption and thereby expansion of cyst.

Arcading

It is the peculiar growth pattern of the proliferating cystic epithelium of the radicular cyst in which multiple narrow finger-like projections grow toward the connective tissue and encircle small mass of connective tissue. Cystic volume eventually increases as the encircled mass of connective tissue gets dissolved over the time.

> **Key Points of Radicular Cyst**
>
> ❖ Radicular or periapical cyst is the most common odontogenic cystic lesion of inflammatory origin, which occurs in relation to the apex of a nonvital tooth.
> ❖ The radicular cyst develops from the "epithelial cell rests of Malassez".
> ❖ Clinically smaller cystic lesions are usually asymptomatic and are detected only when a radiograph is taken.
> ❖ The larger lesions, however, produce a slow enlarging, bony hard swelling of the jaw with expansion and distortion of the cortical plates, displacement of teeth, malocclusion, etc.
> ❖ On radiograph, radicular cyst presents a well-defined, unilocular, and round-shaped radiolucent area at the root apex.
> ❖ The cystic fluid is often straw colored and contains about 5 g% of soluble protein.
> ❖ Histologically, radicular cyst presents of a cystic cavity lined by thick, nonkeratinized, and stratified squamous epithelium of about 6–20 cell layers thickness.
> ❖ The proliferating cystic epithelium may sometimes grow in a peculiar "arcading pattern".
> ❖ The cyst capsule is made up of vascular connective tissue, which is often infiltrated by many chronic inflammatory cells.

> - The cyst also contains many other important structures, e.g. cholesterol clefts, Russell body, Rushton body, etc.
> - Treatment is done by enucleation and marsupialization.
> - In radicular cyst, if the associated tooth is removed but the cyst remains inside the jaw, the condition is called "residual cyst".

Differential Diagnosis

- Periapical granuloma
- Central giant cell granuloma
- Periapical abscess
- Cementoma (Stage I)
- Traumatic bone cyst
- Bony artifact.

Scanning Electron Microscopy

- Scanning electron microscopy study of the inner surface of the radicular cyst shows that the surface epithelium is sometimes fairly smooth with shallow folding or ridges.
- Sometimes, it is irregular and ruffled.
- Irregular-shaped intraepithelial spaces are found, which can permit the penetration of white blood cell (WBC) or red blood cell (RBC).

Treatment

Small cysts are treated by root canal treatments of the affected teeth and apical curettage. The larger cysts are treated either by enucleation and marsupialization.

ERUPTION CYST (ERUPTION HEMATOMA)

Definition

Eruption cyst is an odontogenic cyst, which surrounds the crown of a tooth that has erupted through the bone, but not the soft tissue.

The eruption cyst develops due to the accumulation of fluid within the follicular space of an erupting tooth and hence can be called the soft tissue variant of dentigerous cyst.

Etiology

Unknown, but the presence of particularly dense fibrous tissue could be responsible.

Origin

The cyst is derived from the reduced enamel epithelial cells.

Clinical Features

- Clinically, the cyst presents a small, rounded, soft, and fluctuant swelling on the alveolar ridge, immediately superior to an erupting tooth.
- This soft tissue cyst is obviously common among the children and it can develop in relation to a deciduous or a permanent tooth.
- The lesion is most commonly associated with the deciduous mandibular central incisor first permanent molars, and deciduous maxillary incisors.
- The cyst contains either a clear fluid or a blood-tinged fluid and it often has a translucent hue.
- Masticatory trauma may induce hemorrhage within the cyst, which gives rise to the formation of "eruption hematoma" and the lesion often appears bluish-purple or red in color.

Histopathology

Histologically, the cyst is similar to the dentigerous cyst and exhibits a thin lining of nonkeratinized squamous epithelium.

The cyst may also have numerous epithelial ghost cells within the lumen of the cyst and these cells are derived from the exfoliating lining epithelial cell of the cyst. The underlying lamina propria shows a variable inflammatory cell infiltrate.

Treatment

No treatment is required for eruption cyst, as it disappears spontaneously once the tooth erupts into the oral cavity. Sometimes in long-standing lesions, the roof of the cyst is excised to allow the tooth to erupt in the oral cavity.

LATERAL PERIODONTAL CYST

Definition
The lateral periodontal cyst is an uncommon odontogenic cyst that develops on the lateral aspect or between the roots of erupted vital teeth. It is considered to be the intrabony counterpart of gingival cyst of adults.

This cyst is derived from the odontogenic epithelial remnants of the periodontal ligament tissue, e.g. cell rest of Malassez, reduced enamel epithelium, cell rests of Serres, etc.

Pathogenesis (Fig. 6.33)
The cyst develops initially over the occlusal surface of the associated tooth, before its eruption. Afterwards, as the tooth starts to erupt into the oral cavity, the cyst is gradually pushed down and it finally takes its position on the lateral wall of the root.

Clinical Features
- Lateral periodontal commonly occurs in adult males.
- Maxillary and mandibular anterior region is the common site; around 75–80% of cases occur in the mandibular premolar, canine, and lateral incisor area.
- Clinically, the lesion is mostly asymptomatic and detected during routine radiographic examinations.
- In few cases, there may be a small, painless soft tissue swelling within or just anterior to the interdental papillae.
- The overlying mucosa is generally normal in color, but in few cases, there may be a bluish discoloration.
- The tooth, with which the cyst is associated, is vital.
- The cyst is usually less than 1 cm in diameter and it never causes resorption of the root of the affected tooth.
- Rarely, it can cause cortical expansion.

Radiological Features (Fig. 6.34)
Radiographically, lateral periodontal cyst presents a small, well-defined, unilocular, and "teardrop-shaped" radiolucent area on the lateral aspect of the root (near the crest of the alveolar ridge). The lesion is often surrounded by a thin, delicately corticated margin at the periphery.

Differential Diagnosis
- Lateral periodontal abscess or granuloma
- Radicular cyst
- Early ameloblastoma
- Collateral type of primordial cyst
- Lateral dentigerous cyst
- Globulomaxillary cyst.

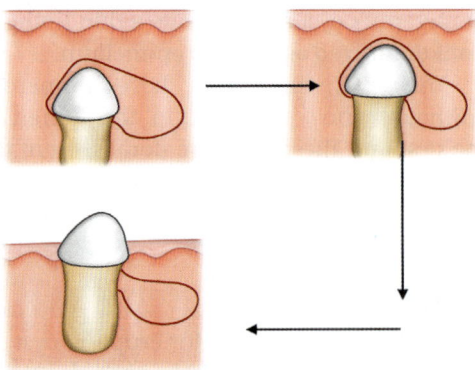

Fig. 6.33: Outline of the possible pathogenesis of lateral periodontal cyst.

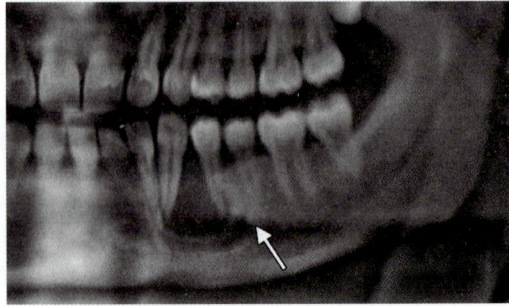

Fig. 6.34: Lateral periodontal cyst.

Histopathology

- Lateral periodontal cyst microscopically presents a small cystic cavity, backed by a thin and noninflamed connective tissue wall (Fig. 6.35).
- The lining of the cyst is made up of nonkeratinized stratified squamous or cuboidal epithelium of 2–3 cell layers thickness.
- The lining epithelial cells appear flattened and they often resemble the reduced enamel epithelial cells.
- Focal areas of plaque-like thickening of the lining epithelium may be seen, consisting of cluster of glycogen-rich, clear cells, with vacuolated cytoplasm.

Treatment

Treatment of lateral periodontal cyst is done by surgical excision along with the tooth. Sometimes, the related tooth can be saved, if healthy.

■ DENTAL LAMINA CYST (GINGIVAL CYST) OF THE NEWBORN

Definition

Gingival cysts of the newborn are multiple small, nodular, keratin-filled, and cystic

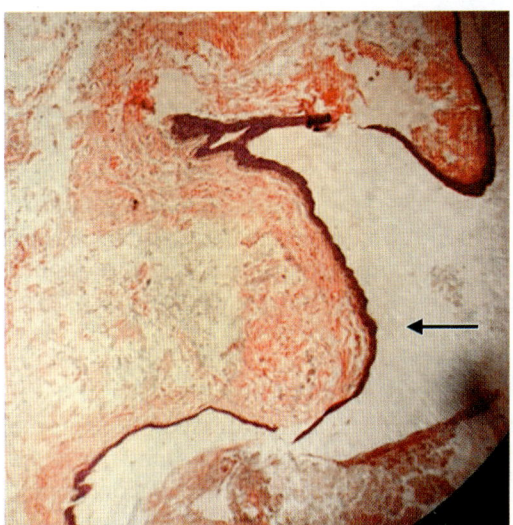

Fig. 6.35: Photomicrograph of lateral periodontal cyst.

Table 6.4: Gingival cysts of newborn.

Types of cyst	Location
Cysts of the dental lamina	Along the alveolar ridge
Epstein's pearls	Found linearly along the midpalatine raphe
Bohn's nodules	Along the junction of the hard and soft palate, and buccal and lingual aspects of alveolar ridge

lesions seen in the oral cavity of newborns or very young infants (from birth up to 3 months of age) (Table 6.4).

Depending upon their locations in the oral cavity, these cysts are divided into several types.

- **Cysts of the dental lamina:** These lesions are mostly found along the alveolar ridge and are odontogenic in origin (arising from the remnants of dental lamina).
- **Epstein's pearls:** These small creamy colored cystic lesions are found linearly along the midpalatine raphe and are probably derived from the epithelium, entrapped along the line of fusion of the palate during embryogenesis.
- **Bohn's nodules:** In this case, small cysts are usually found along the junction of the hard and soft palate and on the buccal and lingual aspects of alveolar ridge. These types of cysts are derived from remnants of the mucous glands.

Clinical Features (Fig. 6.36)

- All these types of cysts in the newborn usually appear as multiple, asymptomatic, small discrete, and white nodules, which develop in several parts of the oral cavity.
- Once formed, the dental lamina cysts may discharge the contents by fusion with the overlying alveolar mucosa or they may undergo spontaneous regression.
- The size of these cysts are very small and do not exceed 2–3 millimeters in maximum diameter.

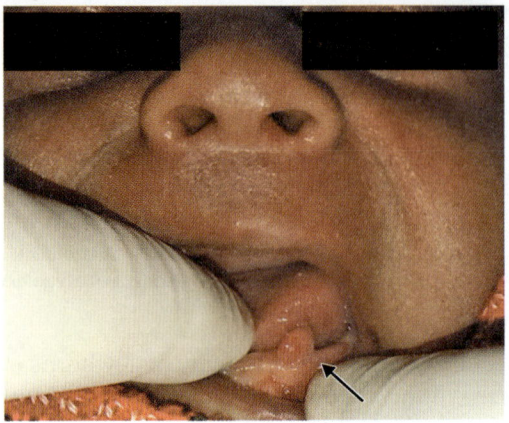

Fig. 6.36: Gingival cyst of the newborn.

- The gingival cysts of newborn involve the maxillary arch more often than mandibular arch.

Histopathology

Microscopic section exhibits a small keratin-filled cystic cavity, which is lined by a thin and stratified squamous epithelium, with a parakeratotic surface. The basal cells are flat, unlike those in the keratocyst. Epithelial-lined clefts may develop between the cyst and the surface oral epithelial.

Treatment

No treatment is required.

■ GINGIVAL CYSTS OF THE ADULT

Definition

Gingival cysts of the adult are small developmental odontogenic cysts of the gingival soft tissue. These are mostly derived from the cell rests of the dental lamina (cell rest of Serres).

Clinical Features

- *Age:* Fifth and sixth decade of life (after 40 years of age).
- *Sex:* It is more prevalent among females.
- *Site:* It is more common in relation to mandible in comparison to maxilla, particularly in the canine-premolar region. Facial side of the gingiva is more commonly affected.

Presentation

- The cyst is often small (less than 1 cm in diameter) located in the gingival tissue outside the bone.
- It clinically presents a firm but compressible, fluid-filled, and "dome-like" swelling on the mandibular or maxillary facial gingiva around the canine–premolar area.
- The swelling is often well circumscribed and it occurs in the attached gingiva or the interdental papilla.
- The surface of the lesion is smooth and is of the normal color of gingiva or bluish.
- The adjacent teeth are vital and the cyst is almost always vital.

Pathogenesis

The gingival cyst of adult arises from the cell rest of the dental lamina, interestingly, it is the same cell from which the lateral periodontal cyst also develops. For this reason, it is often believed that gingival cysts of adult and lateral periodontal cysts represent the extraosseous and intraosseous manifestations of the same entity.

Radiographic Findings

Since gingival cysts of adult are entirely extraosseous lesions, they do not reveal any radiographic change in the bone. However, in some cases, there may be a pressure-induced faint round superficial depression (cupping out) in the underlying alveolar bone, usually not detected on radiograph but is apparent when the cyst is excised.

Histopathology

- Histologically, gingival cysts of adult present a cystic cavity, which is lined by a thin epithelial lining made up of flat or cuboidal cells having 2–3 cell layer thickness.

- Many of the lining epithelial cells exhibit pyknotic nuclei with perinuclear cytoplasmic vacuoles.
- Layers of keratin may be present in the cystic lumen.
- Sometimes, localized areas of epithelial thickening (plaque) are observed in which the epithelial cells are arranged in a whorled manner.
- Like lateral periodontal cysts, some clear cells may also be present.

Treatment

Surgical enucleation.

SIALO-ODONTOGENIC CYSTS/ GLANDULAR ODONTOGENIC CYST

Definition

These are rare intraosseous odontogenic cysts, which often have an aggressive course. The lining epithelium of the cyst consists of cuboidal or columnar cells and at places squamous cells also. The cystic lining often have numerous mucus-secreting cells, which produce many "mucin pools" that appear as cyst-like spaces (lining crypts) within the thickness of the cystic epithelium. The presence of mucus-secreting cells and their ability to produce mucin are the hallmark feature of this cyst. Although the earlier name was sialo-odontogenic cyst, it was later on renamed as glandular odontogenic cyst (GOC) by the World Health Organization.

Origin

The cysts arise from the rests of dental lamina and are capable of glandular differentiation.

Clinical Features

- Sialo-odontogenic cysts are extremely rare and are usually seen among adults.
- There is no sex predilection.
- Mandible is more often affected than maxilla.
- Anterior part of the mandible is the most common site for the cyst.
- Clinically the sialo-odontogenic cysts appear as slow enlarging, asymptomatic, and central jaw lesions.
- Some aggressive lesions may attain a very large size and many of them cross the mandibular midline.
- Larger lesions often cause expansion and distortion of the cortical plates of bone, displacement of teeth; with pain and paresthesia of the affected area.

Radiographic Features

The radiographic appearances of sialo-odontogenic cysts are nonspecific; most of the cysts present unilocular or sometimes multilocular, radiolucent lesion with well-demarcated, sclerotic border.

Histopathology (Figs. 6.37 and 6.38)

Histologically, sialo-odontogenic cysts present the following features:
- The cyst is lined by a thin squamous epithelial lining, which may be of uniform thickness or there can be focal areas of thickening (plaque).
- Several small glandular structures or microcysts are found within the lining

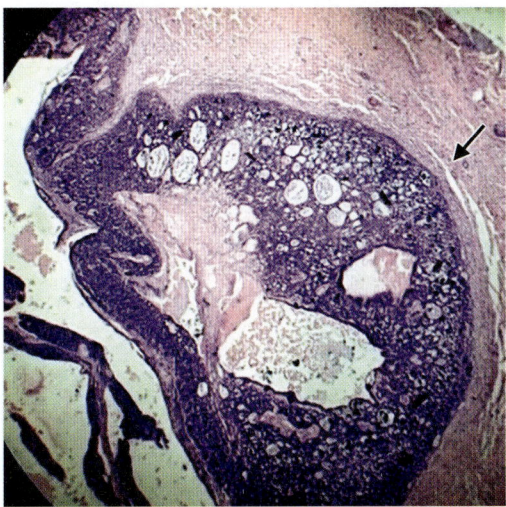

Fig. 6.37: Photomicrograph of glandular odontogenic cyst (low power).

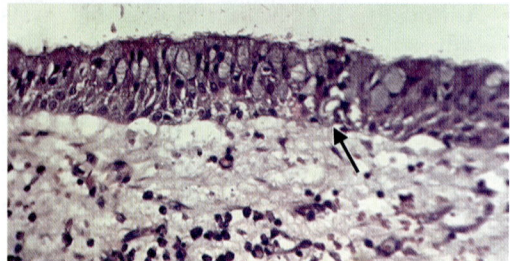

Fig. 6.38: Photomicrograph of glandular odontogenic cyst (high power).

epithelium, often containing mucicarmine-positive fluid.
- Organization of the glandular elements (occurs due to metaplasia of the cystic epithelium) may result in the formation of acinar-like clusters.
- There may be large collection of mucin in the cystic lumen.
- Occasionally, mucous cells resembling goblet cells of the intestinal mucosa are present.
- The superficial layer of the lining epithelium is made up of cuboidal or columnar cells, resulting in an uneven hobnail and sometimes papillary surface.
- Islands of odontogenic epithelium and even microcysts may be present in the connective tissue wall of the cyst.
- Irregular calcifications may be present in connective tissue wall.

Differential Diagnosis
- Odontogenic keratocyst
- Ameloblastoma
- Aneurysmal bone cyst
- Central giant cell granuloma
- Intraosseous mucoepidermoid tumor.

Treatment
Surgical excision, the cyst has a strong tendency to recur.

BOTRYOID ODONTOGENIC CYSTS
Definition
Botryoid odontogenic cysts are rare odontogenic cystic lesions, which resemble cluster of grapes. It is probably a variant of lateral periodontal cyst.

Pathogenesis
Botryoid odontogenic cyst is developing from a lateral periodontal cyst. There are numerous daughter microcysts, many of which also show epithelial plaques. These plaques may be pinched "off" to form granddaughter cysts.

Clinical Features
- Adults over 50 years of age are commonly affected and mandibular canine–premolar region is the most favorite site for this cyst.
- Clinically, the cyst presents a well-defined, painless, and expansile central jaw lesion.

Radiographic Finding
Radiographically, there can be presence of a unilocular or multilocular radiolucent area with well-corticated margin.

Histopathology (Fig. 6.39)
- Histologically, botryoid odontogenic cyst reveals multiple cystic cavities separated from one another by fine fibrous septa.
- The cystic cavities are lined by nonkeratinized cuboidal or squamous epithelium, which are of 1–2 cell layer thickness.

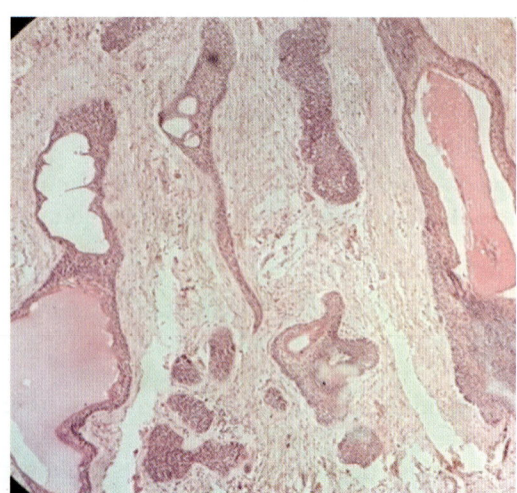

Fig. 6.39: Photomicrograph of botryoid odontogenic cyst.

- Focal areas of glycogen-containing clear cell clusters are often found along the lining.
- Sometimes bud-like proliferations of the lining epithelial cells protrude into the cystic lumen.

Treatment

Treatment by enucleation, this cyst has a strong tendency to recur.

■ CALCIFYING EPITHELIAL ODONTOGENIC CYST/GORLIN CYST

Calcifying epithelial odontogenic cyst (Gorlin cyst) is a relatively uncommon odontogenic cystic lesion of the jawbones; and in many instances, it is considered as a tumor. Important feature of this cyst is the formation of peculiar "ghost cells" and intracystic calcifications.

Clinical Features

- *Age:* Mostly the cyst develops in the second decade of life.
- *Sex:* Both sexes are equally affected.
- *Site:* Both jaws are affected but the most favored site is the mandibular premolar region. The other common sites of cyst are the anterior parts of maxilla and mandible, occasionally (soft tissue) extraosseous lesions develop from the gingiva too.

Clinical Presentation

- Clinically, the cyst presents a bony hard swelling of the jaw; the average size of the tumor is about 2–3 centimeters in diameter but sometimes it can be extensive (Figs. 6.40A and B).
- Expansion and distortion of cortical plates and displacement of regional teeth, etc. are usually common.
- Large bony lesions can cause perforation of the cortex.
- Extraosseous lesions produce circumscribed, sessile, or pedunculated gingival swelling; the associated tooth is vital.
- Pain is rarely present in the cyst and most of the smaller cysts are completely asymptomatic.
- Some cysts can develop in association with an odontome (Box 6.8).

Radiological Features (Fig. 6.41)

- Radiograph usually shows a unilocular radiolucent area with a typical cystic appearance; but sometimes, it can produce a multilocular radiolucency with well-corticated margin.
- Within the lesion, multiple small, irregular radiopaque calcified foci of varying radiodensity are often found. Sometimes, miniature tooth-like structures may also found within the cyst.

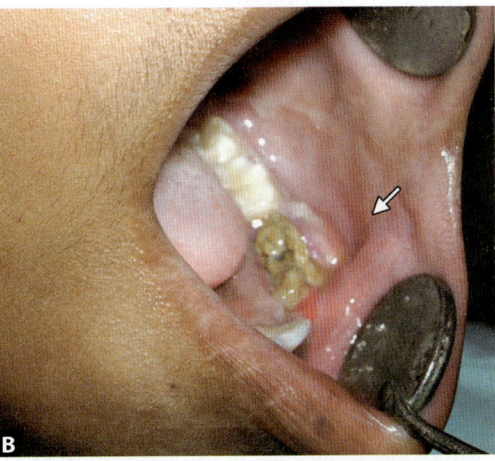

Figs. 6.40A and B: (A) Calcifying epithelial odontogenic cyst; (B) Intraoral view of the patient.

338 Essentials of Oral Pathology

> **Box 6.8** Classification of calcifying epithelial odontogenic cyst (COC).
>
> *Group 1: Simple cysts:* Calcifying odontogenic cyst
> *Group 2: Cysts associated with odontogenic hamartomas or benign neoplasm:* Calcifying cystic odontogenic tumors (CCOT)
> Following combination have been published:
> - CCOT associated with an odontome
> - CCOT associated with adenomatoid odontogenic tumor (AOT)
> - CCOT associated with ameloblastoma
> - CCOT associated with ameloblastic fibroma
> - CCOT associated with ameloblastic fibrodentinoma
> - CCOT associated with odontoameloblastoma
> - CCOT associated with odontogenic myxofibroma
>
> *Group 3: Solid benign odontogenic neoplasms with similar cell morphology to that in COC and with dentinoid formation:*
> - Dentinogenic ghost cell tumor
>
> *Group 4:* Malignant odontogenic neoplasms with features similar

(AOT: adenomatoid odontogenic tumor)

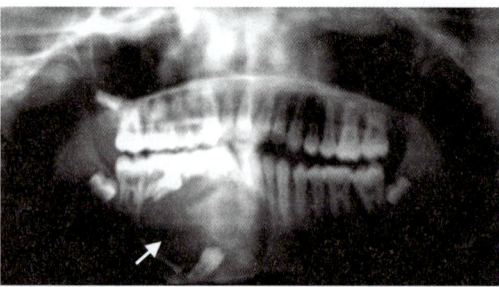

Fig. 6.41: Radiograph of calcifying epithelial odontogenic cyst.

- Some cysts may be associated with an unerupted tooth (mostly canines). Root resorption in the adjacent teeth is occasionally seen.
- The extraosseous lesion causes indentation on the overlying bone.
- Displacement of teeth is often seen. Resorption of the roots of adjacent teeth is a frequent finding.

Pathogenesis

The cyst probably develops from the reduced enamel epithelial cells or remnants of odontogenic epithelium in the dental follicle, gingiva, or bone.

Histopathology (Figs. 6.42 and 6.43)

- Microscopically calcifying epithelial odontogenic cyst presents a cystic cavity, lined by an odontogenic keratinized epithelium of about 6–8 cell layer thickness.
- The cystic epithelium in some areas is thick and these areas exhibit some cells, which closely resemble the stellate reticulum of the developing tooth germ.
- The basal cells of the lining epithelium are columnar or sometimes cuboidal in nature, and they often exhibit a palisading arrangement (these cells resemble ameloblasts). The overlying layer of loosely arranged epithelium may resemble the stellate reticulum of an ameloblastoma.
- The luminal surface epithelium often shows the presence of many "ghost cells", which are abnormally swollen epithelial cells with eosinophilic cytoplasm but devoid of nuclei. These cells gradually become paler, leaving only a faint outline, and hence are called ghost cells.
- The ghost cells often undergo calcification and for this reason there may be presence of multiple, small, and basophilic calcified bodies within the lumen of the cyst.

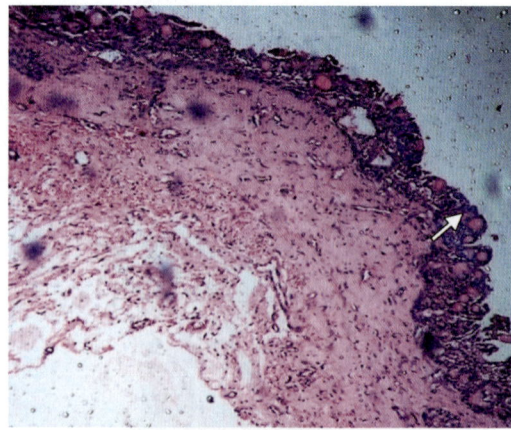

Fig. 6.42: Photomicrograph of calcifying epithelial odontogenic cyst (COC) (low power).

Cysts of the Oral Region

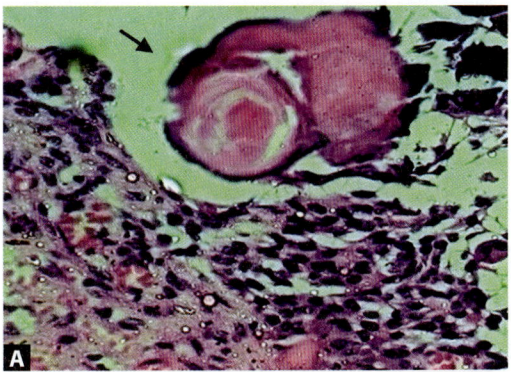

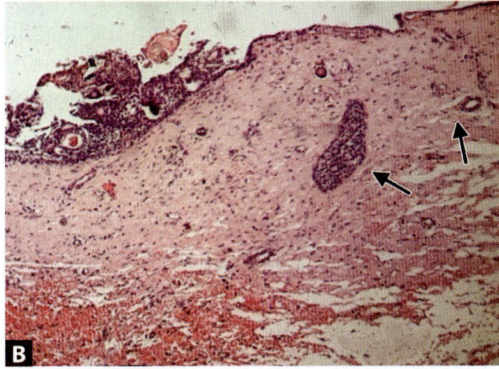

Figs. 6.43A and B: (A) Photomicrograph of "ghost cell" in calcifying epithelial odontogenic cyst (COC); (B) Showing daughter cyst in COC.

- The spinous cell layer of the cystic lining often resembles reduced enamel epithelium and the lining has the potential to induce formation of dysplastic dentin.
- The connective tissue capsule contains many "satellite" microcysts and in addition to this, there may be presence of multiple multinucleated giant cells.
- Sometimes, the cystic epithelial cells may proliferate in a solid sheets or islands and it is known as the "solid variant" of COC.
- Melanin pigmentation may be occasionally present in the cyst (Box 6.9).

Key Points of Calcifying Epithelial Odontogenic Cyst

- Calcifying epithelial odontogenic cyst (Gorlin cyst) is a relatively uncommon odontogenic cystic lesion of the jawbone.
- In many instances, it is considered as a tumor.

Box 6.9 Lesions in which ghost cells might be present.

Odontogenic lesions:
- Calcifying epithelial odontogenic cyst (COC)
- Calcifying epithelial odontogenic tumor (CEOT)
- Dentinogenic ghost cell tumor
- Odontomas
- Ameloblastoma
- AOT
- Odontogenic ghost cell carcinoma
- Ameloblastic fibroma
- Ameloblastic fibro-odontoma
- Eruption cyst

Nonodontogenic lesions:
- Pilomatricomas
- Craniopharyngioma

❖ The cyst probably develops from the reduced enamel epithelial cells or remnants of odontogenic epithelium.
❖ It frequently develops from the mandibular premolar region. Some lesions are extraosseous.
❖ Clinically, smaller lesions are asymptomatic. However, the larger lesions cause expansion and distortion of bone and displacement of regional teeth.
❖ Extraosseous lesions produce circumscribed, sessile, or pedunculated gingival swelling.
❖ Radiographically, the cyst presents unilocular or multilocular radiolucent area with well-corticated margin.
❖ Within the lesion, multiple small and irregular radiopaque calcified foci of varying radiodensity are often found.
❖ Histologically, calcifying epithelial odontogenic cyst presents a cystic cavity, lined by an odontogenic keratinized epithelium of about 6–8 cell layer thickness.
❖ The luminal surface epithelium often shows the presence of many "ghost cells".
❖ These are swollen, eosinophilic, abnormally keratinized cells devoid of nuclei; which gradually become paler, leaving only a faint outline, and hence are called ghost cells.
❖ The connective tissue capsule contains many "satellite" microcysts; and moreover, there may be presence of multiple multinucleated giant cells.

Differential Diagnosis

- Calcifying epithelial odontogenic tumor
- Adenomatoid odontogenic tumor
- Dentigerous cyst
- Ameloblastoma.

Treatment
By surgical enucleation.

■ PARADENTAL CYST

Definition
Paradental cyst is an inflammatory odontogenic cyst, which occurs on the root surface (near the cervical area) of an impacted or partially erupted vital tooth, usually the mandibular third molar.

Origin
The cysts arise due to inflammation in the adjacent periodontium of the involved tooth, which stimulates the cell rest of Malassez or the reduced enamel epithelium. After the odontogenic epithelial cells are stimulated, they undergo proliferation with subsequent cystification.

Clinical Features
- The cyst commonly occurs in males preferably in the third decade of life.
- It is commonly seen on the facial or distal aspect of a vital mandibular third molar tooth.
- In all the cases, the involved tooth had an associated history of pericoronitis.

Radiographic Features
Paradental cyst occurring on the distal aspect of the mandibular third molar presents a well-circumscribed radiolucent area.

Histopathology
Histologically, paradental cyst reveals a cystic cavity lined by hyperplastic and nonkeratinized squamous epithelium.
 Intense inflammatory reaction is seen in the capsule as well as in the epithelial lining.

Differential Diagnosis
- Radicular cyst
- Lateral dentigerous cyst
- Lateral periodontal cyst
- Simple pericoronitis
- Enlarged tooth follicle

Treatment
Surgical enucleation.

NONODONTOGENIC CYSTS

■ GLOBULOMAXILLARY CYST

Definition
Globulomaxillary cyst is a common type of developmental or fissural cyst that actually arises in the bone suture between the maxilla and premaxilla. Clinically, the usual location of the cyst is between maxillary lateral incisor and canine teeth.

Pathogenesis
Earlier, it was believed that the globulomaxillary cyst develops as a result of proliferation of the epithelium, entrapped along the line of fusion between the maxilla and premaxilla. But recently, this concept has been questioned by many investigators. The globulomaxillary cyst is now being considered as a variant of primordial cyst or lateral periodontal cyst.

Clinical Features (Figs. 6.44A and B)
- This cyst is usually asymptomatic and is detected during routine radiological examinations.
- It can cause pain and discomfort, etc. only when it is secondarily infected.
- On rare occasions, there may be a small swelling in-between the upper lateral incisor and canine teeth with elevation of the lip.
- The associated teeth are always vital.

Radiological Features
Radiograph reveals an inverted pear-shaped and radiolucent area between the roots of the upper lateral incisor and canine. It often causes divergence of the roots of these teeth (*See* Fig. 6.33).

Cysts of the Oral Region

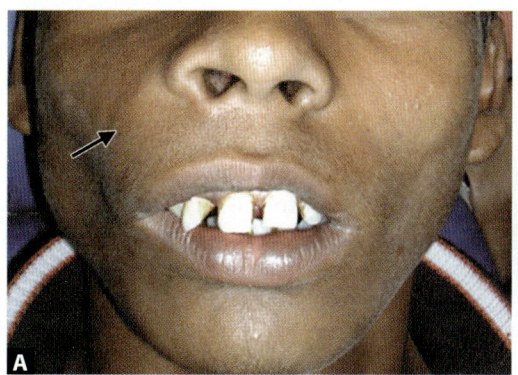
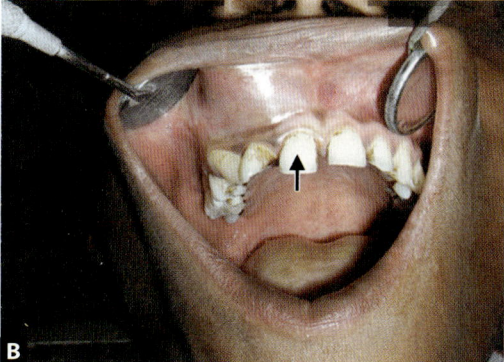

Figs. 6.44A and B: (A) Globulomaxillary cyst of right side; and (B) Intraoral view of the same patient.

Histopathology

Histologically, globulomaxillary cyst exhibits a cystic cavity, which is lined either by a stratified or pseudostratified ciliated columnar epithelium or by a thin squamous epithelium (Fig. 6.45).

The supporting connective tissue capsule often presents chronic inflammatory cell infiltration.

Treatment

By surgical excision, with preservation of the involved teeth.

■ NASOLABIAL CYST/NASOALVEOLAR CYST (KLESTADT'S CYST)

Definition

Nasolabial cysts are rare, soft tissue cysts arising on the upper lip deep into the nasolabial fold, just below the ala of the nose.

Origin

The possible origin of this lesion is from the lower part of the embryonic nasolacrimal duct. The other theory suggests that the cyst arises from the epithelial remnants entrapped at the line of fusion of maxillary, median nasal, and the lateral nasal processes during the development of face.

Clinical Features

- *Age:* 30–50 years

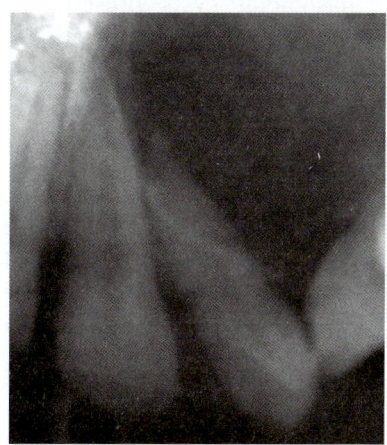

Fig. 6.45: Radiograph of globulomaxillary cyst.

- *Sex:* The cyst is commonly seen among the females (3:1 ratio).
- *Site:* Soft tissue of the anterior maxillary vestibule below the ala of the nose and deep in the nasolabial fold area.

Presentation

- The cyst produces a small and painless swelling in the upper lip lateral to the midline.
- The lesion often obliterates the nasolabial fold, raises the ala of the nose, and distorts the nostril on one side.
- Sometimes, it can be massive in size and therefore cause nasal obstruction and difficulty in wearing prosthesis.
- Sometimes, the cyst may project into the nasal floor and deviate the nasal vestibule.

- It is generally painless, unless secondarily infected. Some cysts may rupture spontaneously.

Radiological Finding

Because of its location entirely within the soft tissue, the cyst does not exhibit any radiographic change. However, sometimes it may produce focal pressure-induced resorption (saucerization) of the underlying bone.

Histopathology (Fig. 6.46)

- The nasolabial cysts present a small cystic lumen, which is supported by a connective tissue wall.
- The cyst is by a pseudostratified and nonciliated columnar epithelium with few goblet cells.
- Areas of cuboidal epithelium and squamous metaplasia are not unusual.
- Some cysts are lined by cuboidal or squamous epithelium.
- Small mucous glands may be present in the capsule.
- Inflammatory cell infiltration is usually absent in the capsule.

Treatment

Surgical excision is the recommended treatment and care should be taken, so that no ugly scar is formed on the lip. Recurrence is rare.

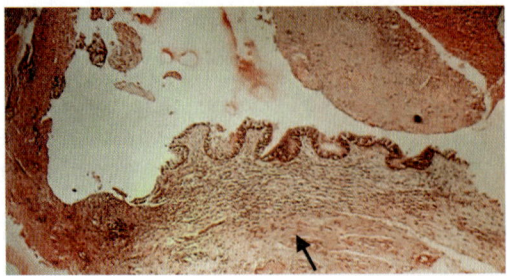

Fig. 6.46: Photomicrograph of nasolabial cyst.

NASOPALATINE DUCT CYST (INCISIVE CANAL CYST)

Definition

Nasopalatine duct cyst is a relatively common, nonodontogenic intraosseous, and cystic lesion arising within the nasopalatine duct or the incisive canal. On rare cases, the cyst may develop in the soft tissue, near the opening of the incisive canal on the palate.

Pathogenesis

This lesion is considered as a true developmental cyst; it arises usually due to proliferation and spontaneous cystic degeneration of the epithelial remnants remaining after closure of the embryonic nasopalatine duct. The initiating factors for the development of cyst may be trauma, inflammation, mucous retention in the nearby minor salivary glands, bacterial infection, etc.

Clinical Features

- *Incidence:* It is a common cyst and affects about 1% of the population.
- *Age:* Fourth, fifth, and sixth decade of life.
- *Sex:* Males are more commonly affected than females; the ratio being 4:1.

Clinical Presentation

- The cystic lesion clinically presents a small, painful, and fluctuant swelling in the midline of the anterior part of hard palate near the opening of the incisive foramen (Fig. 6.47). Occasionally, there can be a purulent or salty discharge from the lesion.
- Few cysts are asymptomatic and are detected by chance during routine radiographic examination.
- Some cysts often extend from palate onto the labial aspect of upper alveolar ridge and they make extensive labiopalatal swellings with typical through and

Cysts of the Oral Region

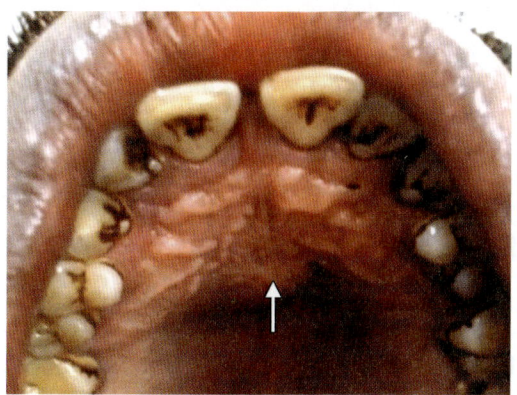

Fig. 6.47: Nasopalatine duct cysts.

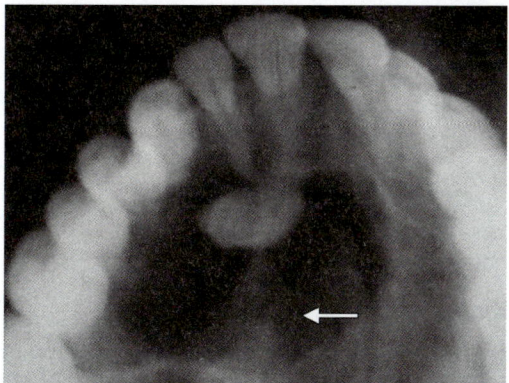

Fig. 6.48: Radiograph of nasopalatine duct cyst.

through "fluctuations" that can be elicited during bidigital palpation.
- The lesion often causes pressure sensation on the floor of the nose and displacement of the roots of upper central incisors and some patients complain of episodic swelling in the soft tissue between the upper central incisors.
- The regional teeth are always vital.

Radiology

- On radiograph, nasopalatine duct cyst presents a sharply demarcated symmetrical radiolucency in the midline of the anterior maxilla (Fig. 6.48).
- The most obvious presenting feature is a small round or heart-shaped radiolucent area between and apical to the roots of the upper central incisors in the midline.
- The typical heart shape of the cyst is found due to the radiographic superimposition of the nasal spine; the cyst often has a well-corticated border.
- Root resorption is rare and the cystic cavity does not come in contact with lamina dura of the upper incisor teeth.
- The cyst is sometimes confused with the incisive foramen and in such cases; a second radiograph should be taken at a different angle, which usually separates the incisive foramen and the nasopalatine duct cyst.
- The average size of nasopalatine duct cyst is 1–2.5 centimeter in diameter; whereas, the average size of incisive foramen is 6 millimeter in diameter only. Therefore, when there is a suspected lesion measuring about 6 millimeter or less and there is no clinical symptom; the diagnosis should be incisive foramen and not a cyst.
- In rare instances, a nasopalatine duct cyst may develop in the soft tissues of the incisive papilla area without any bony involvement. Such lesions often are called cysts of the incisive papillae, which often have a bluish color.

Key Points of Nasopalatine Duct Cyst

- Nasopalatine duct cyst is a nonodontogenic intraosseous cyst arising within the nasopalatine duct or the incisive canal.
- The lesion is considered as a true developmental cyst and it arises from the epithelial remnants remaining after closure of the embryonic nasopalatine duct.
- It clinically presents a small, painful, and fluctuant swelling in the midline of the anterior part of hard palate near the opening of the incisive foramen.
- Radiograph shows a small round or heart-shaped radiolucent area between and apical to the roots of the upper central incisors in the midline.

> - Histology reveals a cystic cavity and lined by the ciliated columnar or nonkeratinized stratified squamous epithelium.
> - The capsule is made up of densely collagenous fibrous connective tissue, which shows the presence of neurovascular bundles (nasopalatine as well as long sphenopalatine nerves and vessels).
> - The associated teeth are vital.
> - Surgical excision is the treatment.

Histopathology (Fig. 6.49)

- Histology reveals a cystic cavity, is lined by the ciliated columnar or nonkeratinized stratified squamous epithelium, and is backed by a connective tissue capsule.
- Sometimes, the lining epithelium can be made up of simple columnar or cuboidal epithelial cells; however in most cases, a mixed type of epithelial lining is seen in the cyst.
- Mucus secretory cells are commonly seen in the epithelial lining.
- The lining may be thick or thin and there can be presence of pigments in the lining.
- The capsule is made up of densely collagenous fibrous connective tissue, which shows the presence of neurovascular bundles (nasopalatine as well as long sphenopalatine nerves and vessels).

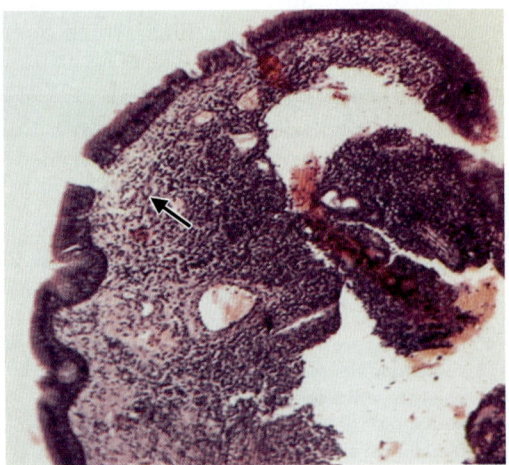

Fig. 6.49: Photomicrograph of nasopalatine duct cyst with the lining and the capsule with nerve and vessels.

- There may be chronic inflammatory cell infiltration in the cystic wall by lymphocytes, histiocytes, plasma cells, etc.

Treatment

By surgical excision.

SOLITARY BONE CYST (TRAUMATIC/HEMORRHAGIC BONE CYST)

Definition

Solitary or traumatic bone cyst represents a pseudocyst and it is characterized by a cavity in the bone, which is lined by a fibrous tissue wall and not by an epithelium.

It arises very frequently from mandible and rarely from maxilla; however, the overall incidence rate of this cyst is much higher in long bones.

Clinical Features

- *Age:* The cyst usually occurs among young people (between 10 years and 20 years) and these are uncommon after the age of 25 years.
- *Sex:* Females are more often affected than males (3:2).
- *Site:* Mandibular body, symphysis or ramus, and maxillary anterior regions are the common sites. Mandible is affected more often than maxilla and sometimes bilaterally.

Presentation

- In most of the cases, the cyst is asymptomatic and is detected accidentally during routine radiographic examinations.
- In other cases, it produces a painful and bony hard swelling of the jaw.
- Paresthesia of the lip, expansion of the cortical plates (mostly the buccal cortical plate of mandible), and displacement of the regional teeth are also common.
- Overlying teeth are vital.

Radiology

- Radiograph reveals an unilocular or rarely multilocular radiolucent area in the bone; with expansion and distortion of cortical plates.
- The radiographic size of the lesion is generally always bigger than the clinical size of the swelling.
- The cystic margin from the neighboring bone is well-demarcated.
- A prominent feature of the cyst is its tendency for scalloping in-between the roots of the teeth.
- Occlusal view shows radiolucency extending along the cancellous bone of the jaw.

Pathogenesis

The exact pathogenesis of solitary bone cyst is not clearly known, but it is believed that the condition develops due to trauma in the jawbone.

Investigators believe that following trauma to the bone and intrabony hemorrhage occur which generally undergo organization and repair. However, if the clot forming after hemorrhage does not organize properly or liquefaction occurs to the clot, then healing of the bony wound does not take place; and as a result, an intrabony cavity persists, which is later on called the solitary bone cyst.

Besides this trauma–hemorrhage theory, the other possible causes of development of solitary bone cyst include the following—local disturbance in bone growth, ischemic bone marrow defect, localized disturbed bone metabolism, and failure of venous drainage, etc.

Differential Diagnosis

- Aneurysmal bone cyst
- Central giant cell granuloma
- Ameloblastoma
- Calcifying epithelial odontogenic cyst
- Ameloblastic fibroma
- Central ossifying fibroma.

Macroscopy

Once the cystic cavity is opened, an empty space is found in the bone; which often contains very little blood, blood pigments, serous fluid, etc. A thin fibrous tissue membrane may line the cavity.

Histopathology

- Histology reveals a cystic cavity surrounded by a loose vascular connective tissue wall, but there is no epithelial lining (hence, it is called a false or pseudocyst).
- The connective tissue stroma is made up of fibrous tissue, showing areas of hemorrhage, hemosiderin pigmentation, bone resorption, etc.
- The cystic cavity often has a rough bony wall.
- Rarely, there can be features of myxoid deposition in the bone and/or presence of multinucleated giant cells.

Treatment

The treatment is done by surgical exploration of the cyst; it helps in causing further hemorrhage in the area with subsequent healing. Some lesions may resolve spontaneously.

■ STAFNE'S BONE CYST

It is developmental cyst of mandible usually in the third molar area.

Clinical Features

- Clinically, Stafney's bone cyst is a completely asymptomatic condition.
- It is almost exclusively seen among males.
- Usually seen in the mandibular third molar areas.

Radiographic Features (Fig. 6.50)

Radiographically, this relatively uncommon entity presents a unilocular, well-defined radiolucency typically located below the inferior alveolar canal in the region between the molars and the angle of mandible.

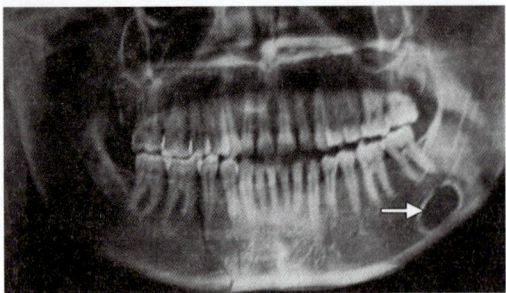

Fig. 6.50: Radiograph of Stafne's bone cyst.

Difference in the positions of Stafne's bone cyst and hemorrhagic bone cyst:
- Stafne's bone cyst—located below the inferior alveolar canal.
- Hemorrhagic bone cyst—lies above the inferior alveolar canal.

Differential Diagnosis

It is one of the few rare lesions, which involve the mandible below the inferior alveolar canal. Stafne's bone cyst should be differentially diagnosed from the following lesions:
- Metastatic carcinoma of the jaw
- Hemorrhagic bone cyst
- Salivary gland neoplasms.

■ TREATMENT

No treatment is required.

■ ANEURYSMAL BONE CYST

Definition

Aneurysmal bone cyst is an uncommon cystic lesion, which involves the bone anywhere in the body including the jaws and its clinical features are similar to that of central giant cell granuloma. It is an intraosseous accumulation of variable sized, blood-filled spaces surrounded by cellular fibrous connective tissue and reactive bone.

Because the lesion lacks an epithelial lining, it represents a pseudocyst rather than a true cyst.

Aneurysmal bone cysts may be classified as:
- Primary (i.e. arising de novo) or
- Secondary (arising in association with another bone lesion).

Clinical Features

Age: Usually second decade of life (10–19 years age group).
Sex: Females are more commonly affected.
Site: Mandibular molar–ramus area is most frequently affected, maxillary lesions also frequently involve the posterior region.

Clinical Presentation

- Aneurysmal bone cyst clinically presents a rapidly enlarging, diffuse, firm swelling of the jaw that often causes facial asymmetry.
- The swelling is painful and the affected area of the jaw may be pulsatile in some cases.
- Occasionally, severe expansion and thinning of the bone often result in "egg-shell crackling" and perforation of the cortical plates.
- Pathological fracture of the affected jawbone may occur in some patients.
- Accidental injury or perforation to the aneurysmal bone cyst may result in profuse bleeding.
- Paresthesia may be present on the affected side and regional teeth are often displaced, and resulting in derangement of occlusion. The displaced teeth are always vital.
- There may be difficulty in mouth opening, if the cyst causes impingement on the capsule of the temporomandibular joint.
- Maxillary lesions sometime invade into the paranasal sinuses and cause nasal bleeding, pressure sensation in the eye and nasal obstructions, etc.

Radiology

- Radiograph reveals a multilocular radiolucent area in the bone, with a typical "honeycomb" appearance.

- Border of the lesion can be either well demarcated or diffused.
- "Ballooning" expansion of the cortical plates, displacement of teeth, and resorption of the roots of the adjoining teeth are also commonly seen.
- A prominent feature of the cyst is the "blowout" bulging of the lower border of mandible.

Pathogenesis

Pathogenesis of aneurysmal bone cyst is controversial and it is believed that the cyst arises as a result of trauma with subsequent venous occlusion inside the bone.

It is also believed that the lesion occurs as a result of cystic transformation of a pre-existing pathology, especially the central giant cell granuloma.

Key Points of Aneurysmal Bone Cyst

- Aneurysmal bone cyst is an uncommon intraosseous, cystic lesion, which often affects the young individuals.
- It is believed to develop as a result of cystic transformation of a pre-existing central giant cell granuloma.
- Clinically, the cyst presents a rapidly enlarging, diffuse, firm, and painful swelling of the jaw that often causes facial asymmetry.
- Severe expansion and thinning of the bone often results in "egg–shell crackling" and perforation of the cortical plates.
- The affected area may be pulsatile and pathological fractures may occur.
- Radiograph reveals a multilocular radiolucent area in the bone, with a typical "honeycomb" appearance.
- Larger lesions cause "ballooning" expansion of the cortical plate and also "blowout" bulging of the lower border of mandible.
- Microscopically aneurysmal bone cyst presents multiple blood-filled spaces of varying size, which are lined by spindle-shaped cells or flat endothelial cells.
- Multiple multinucleated giant cells, scattered osteoids, areas of hemorrhage, and hemosiderin pigmentations are also seen.
- Treatment is done by surgical curettage.

Differential Diagnosis

- Fibrous dysplasia
- Intraosseous hemangioma
- Traumatic bone cyst
- Giant cell tumor of bone
- Osteoblastoma.

Macroscopy

An intact periosteum and a thin bony shell usually cover the cyst. However, the cortical bone is often perforated. The bony cavity is filled with vascular soft tissue containing blood-filled spaces. The intracystic tissue often looks like a blood-soaked sponge.

Aspiration

Aspiration often reveals fresh blood.

Histopathology

- Microscopically, aneurysmal bone cyst presents multiple blood-filled spaces of varying size, which are lined by many spindle-shaped cells or flat endothelial cells.
- Epithelial lining is absent in this cyst and the blood-filled intracystic spaces are separated from one another by loose connective tissue walls.
- Multiple multinucleated giant cells, scattered osteoids, areas of hemorrhage, hemosiderin pigmentations, etc. are commonly present in the hypercellular connective tissue stroma of the cyst.
- The cyst wall occasionally exhibits a lace-like pattern of calcification.

Treatment

By surgical curettage.

CYST OF THE SALIVARY GLAND

Cystic lesion developing from the salivary glands is commonly known as "mucoceles"; these lesions develop mostly in relation to the minor salivary glands and rarely in relation to the major salivary glands.

Mucoceles basically are of two types:
1. Mucous retention cyst
2. Mucous extravasation cyst.

Etiology and Pathogenesis

The mucous retention cyst develops as a result of obstruction to the duct of the minor or rarely major salivary glands; which leads to accumulation of saliva either within the gland or within its duct. More and more fluid accumulations cause increased intraluminal pressure in the gland itself or in the duct, which results in swelling. The retention cysts generally develop due to obstruction to the salivary gland ducts because of the following reasons—calculus formation, scarring, obstruction from mucin plug crushing of the duct (as a result of trauma), atresia (congenital absence of duct in the salivary gland), etc.

Mucous retention cyst is a true cyst, since it has a cystic epithelium made up of glandular epithelial cells of the salivary glands.

Mucous extravasation cyst, on the other hand, develops as a result of rupture of the salivary gland duct, which leads to spillage or extravasations of saliva into the connective tissue. Local trauma is believed to be the most important etiological factor in this cyst.

Clinical Features

- Mucoceles occur at any age; however, mucous extravasation cysts are more common among children, while the mucous retention cysts are more common among adults.
- Both sexes are almost equally affected.
- The cysts often affect minor glands, but on rare occasions, the major salivary glands can be affected.
- Mucoceles of minor glands predominantly affect the lower lip; however, the cheek, soft palate, floor of the mouth, tongue, etc. are also frequently involved (Figs. 6.51A and B).
- Cysts of the major glands predominantly affect the parotid; and these lesions clinically exhibit slow enlarging and painless soft swellings in the gland.
- Some swellings develop only during mealtime and are absent during the in-between periods.
- The superficial lesions appear as small, raised, vesicle-like, fluctuant areas measuring from few millimeters to few centimeters in diameter. The deep-seated lesions produce diffuse, relatively firm, and painless swellings in the oral cavity.
- The superficial lesions often have a bluish appearance; whereas, the deep-seated lesions do not exhibit any color change in the overlying mucosa.
- Lesions developing in the floor of the mouth near the submandibular duct area often have an amber color.
- Majority of the superficial lesions rupture within a short period of time and result pain, ulceration, secondary infection, etc. However, few lesions can survive for several days.
- The mucoceles often recur and the recurrent cysts tend to develop

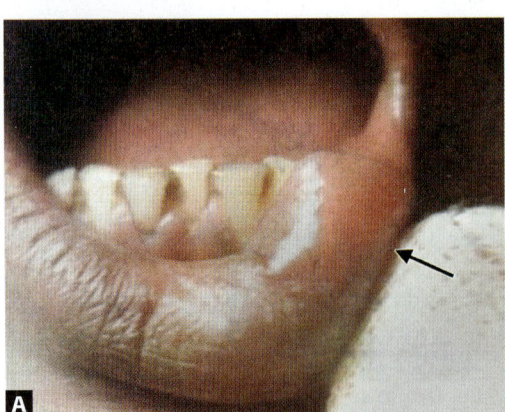
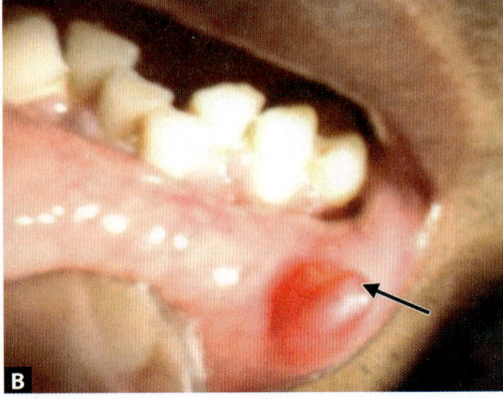

Figs. 6.51A and B: Mucoceles developing on the lower lip.

repeatedly at a particular location in the mouth.

Histopathology (Table 6.5)

Mucous Retention Cyst

Mucous retention cyst histologically presents a small cystic cavity, which is filled with mucous and is lined by flattened cuboidal or columnar epithelial cells of the salivary gland duct (Fig. 6.52). Sometimes, the cyst can be lined by an atrophic stratified squamous epithelium. The mucocele almost always have a minor salivary gland in its vicinity.

Mucous Extravasation Cyst (Fig. 6.53)

This lesion microscopically presents a cystic cavity in the connective tissue, which is filled with mucus but there is no lining epithelium present in this cyst.

Instead of a lining epithelium, the cystic cavity is often surrounded by a compressed connective tissue wall or a granulation tissue. The adjacent connective tissue stroma contains multiple macrophages, polymorphonuclear neutrophils, eosinophils, and especially large number of lymphocytes. Sometimes, ruptured salivary gland ducts may be seen under microscope.

Differential Diagnosis

- Salivary gland tumor
- Lipoma
- Fibroepithelial polyp
- Cysticercosis.

Treatment

Mucoceles are treated by surgical excision of the lesion along with the involved gland.

Table 6.5: Differences between mucous retention and mucous extravasation cyst.

Mucous retention cyst	Mucous extravasation cyst
• Mucous retention cyst develops as a result of obstruction to the duct of the minor salivary glands • It results due to accumulation of saliva either within the gland or within its duct • Mucous retention cysts are more common among adults • Mucous retention cyst has a cystic lining • Mucous retention cyst is a true cyst	• Extravasation cyst, on the other hand, develops as a result of rupture of the salivary gland duct • It occurs due to spillage or extravasations of saliva into the connective tissue • Mucous extravasation cysts are more common among children • Mucous extravasation cyst does not have any cystic lining • Mucous extravasation cyst is a false cyst

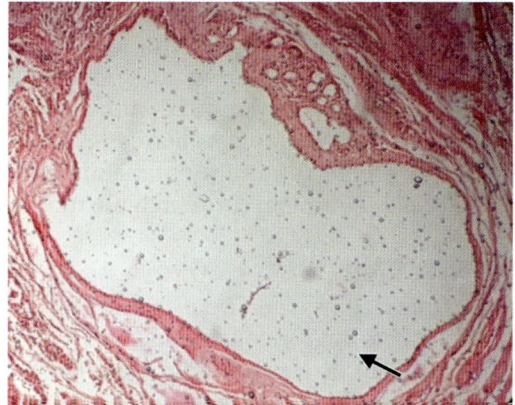

Fig. 6.52: Photomicrograph of mucous retention cyst.

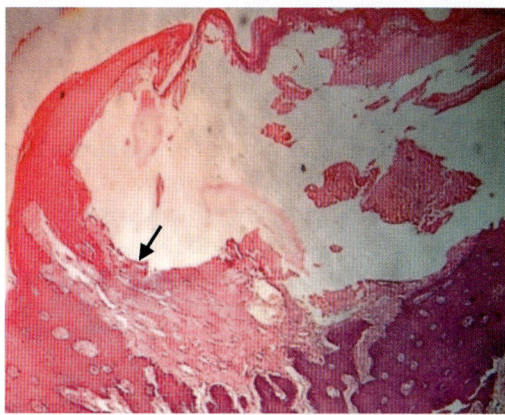

Fig. 6.53: Photomicrograph of mucous extravasation cyst.

RANULA

Definition

Ranula is a type of mucocele that typically causes a large and bluish fluctuant swelling in the floor of the mouth. The lesion occurs due to spillage of saliva from the sublingual salivary glands or rarely the submandibular gland or sometimes from the minor salivary glands.

The ranulas represent the extravasation cyst of the salivary glands. Unlike the submandibular gland, the sublingual gland produces a continuous flow of mucus even in the absence of neural stimulation, which accounts for its ability to produce a ranula after rupture of one of its multiple ducts.

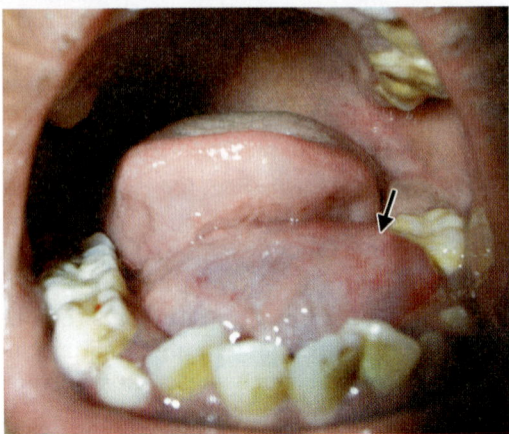

Fig. 6.54: Ranula.

> **Key Points of Ranula**
> - Ranula is a form of mucocele (mucous extravasation cyst) that typically causes a large and bluish fluctuant swelling in the floor of the mouth.
> - It occurs due to spillage of saliva from the sublingual salivary gland or rarely the submandibular gland.
> - Obstruction, compression, or perforation of the salivary gland duct is the likely causes of development of ranula.
> - Clinically ranula presents a dome-shaped, soft, fluctuant, and unilateral swelling in the floor of the mouth.
> - The ranulas typically have a bluish translucent appearance and clinically they often look like the "distended under belly of a large frog".
> - When the ranula herniates through the mylohyoid muscle and produces a swelling in the neck, it is called a "plunging" type of ranula.

Etiology

- Obstruction to the duct by calculus (sialolith) formation.
- Compression of the duct by trauma or a growing tumor in the vicinity.
- Perforation of the duct due to injury.
- Absence of the duct itself (atresia).
- Scar or stricture formation to the duct, especially after surgery.

Clinical Features

- Clinically "ranula" presents a dome-shaped, soft, fluctuant, and unilateral swelling in the floor of the mouth (Fig. 6.54).
- The lesion is generally very large (several centimeters in diameter), which often fills up the floor of the mouth and causes deviation of the tongue.
- The ranulas typically have a bluish translucent appearance and clinically they often look like the "distended under belly of a large frog" (in Latin the word "rana" means frog; for this the name "ranula" has been given to the cyst).
- If the lesion is a deep-seated one, the bluish coloration is usually absent.
- When the ranula herniates through the mylohyoid muscle and produces a swelling in the neck, it is called a "plunging" type of ranula.
- Ranulas are mostly located on either side of midline in the floor of the mouth; however in many cases, they can cross the midline of the floor of mouth and can even cause airway obstructions.
- Some ranulas rupture spontaneously and release their mucin content in the mouth.

Histopathology

The extravasation type of ranula microscopically presents large mucous-filled area, which is surrounded by a connective tissue wall or granulation tissue. Multiple foamy histiocytes are often present in the granulation tissue surrounding the cyst.

In many cases, sialoliths may be found within the salivary gland duct.

Differential Diagnosis
- Dermoid cyst
- Benign lymphoepithelial cyst
- Salivary gland tumors
- Cystic hygroma.

Treatment
Treatment is done by surgical excision or marsupialization.

The etiological factor has to be removed to eliminate the possibility of further recurrence. In case of repeated recurrences, the involved gland may have to be excised.

DERMOID CYST

Definition
It is a developmental cyst derived from remnants of embryonic skin. It is generally classified as a benign cystic form of teratoma. [Teratoma is a developmental tumor composed of tissue from more than one germ layer and sometimes all three—(1) ectoderm, (2) mesoderm, and (3) endoderm.]

Clinical Features
- *Age*: Children and young adults.
- *Sex*: Both sexes are equally affected.
- *Site*: Skin around the eyes, anterior upper neck, and floor of the mouth on the midline.

Presentation (Figs. 6.55A and B)
- A painless swelling, which often have a doughy or rubbery consistency.
- Dermoid cysts always develop on the midline of the floor of the mouth and thus they differ from ranulas, which develop on the lateral aspect of the midline.
- The cyst, which develops above the geniohyoid muscle, presents a sublingual swelling in the midline of floor of the mouth.
- It often causes elevation of the tongue with difficulty in eating, talking, or sometimes even breathing.
- The cyst located below the geniohyoid muscle often produces a midline swelling in the submental region; which often produces a "double chin" appearance.
- The size of the cyst varies and the maximum size could be up to 2 cm or less in diameter.

Histopathology (Figs. 6.56A and B)
- A cystic cavity lined by orthokeratinized stratified squamous epithelium with prominent granular cell layer, which exhibits hair follicles, sebaceous glands, arrector pili muscles, etc.
- The cystic lumen is often filled with sebum, desquamated keratin, and hair shafts.
- The cyst capsule is composed of a narrow zone of compressed connective tissue that contains one or more skin appendages, such as sebaceous glands, hair follicles, or sweat glands.

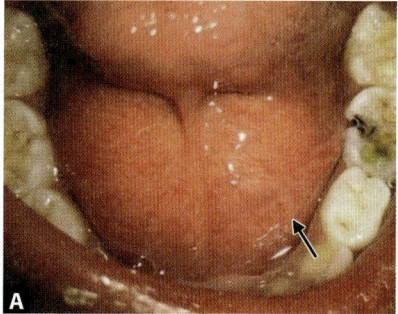 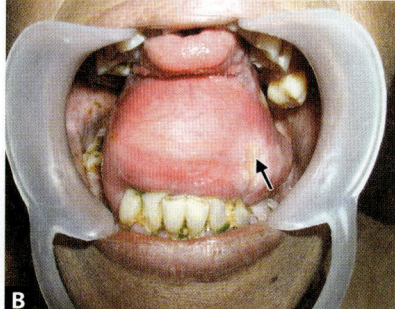

Figs. 6.55A and B: Dermoid cysts in the midline of floor of the mouth.

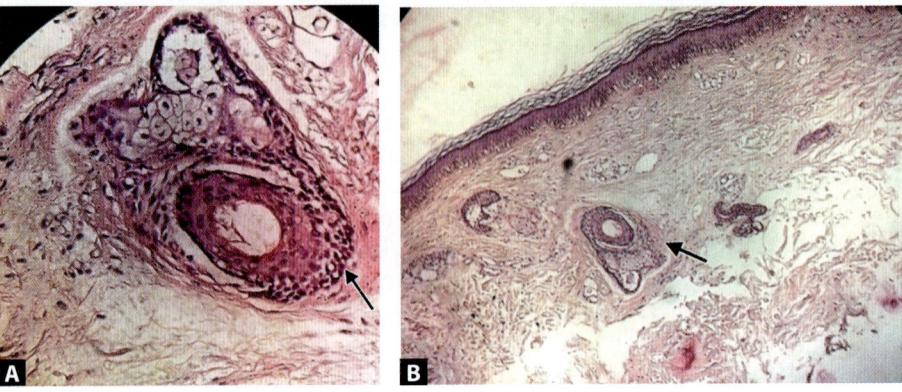

Figs. 6.56A and B: Photomicrograph of dermoid cyst showing sebaceous glands and hair follicle.

Treatment

Surgical enucleation.

SURGICAL CILIATED CYST OF MAXILLA

Definition

It is an iatrogenic cyst, which develops as result of surgery involving the maxillary sinus.

Clinical Features

- The cyst occurs in middle aged or older adults.
- It often causes pain and tenderness in the maxilla.
- All the patients have a previous history of surgery in the maxillary bone.

Radiographic Finding

X-ray reveals a well-circumscribed radiolucency in close proximity of the maxillary sinus.

Histopathology (Fig. 6.57)

- The cyst is lined by a pseudostratified ciliated columnar epithelium.
- The surrounding connective tissue is either normal or inflamed.

Treatment

Surgical enucleation.

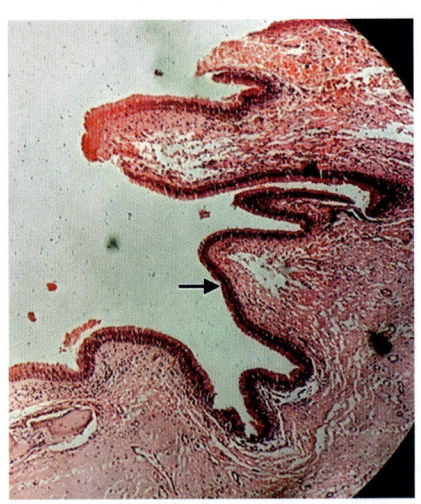

Fig. 6.57: Photomicrograph of surgical ciliated cyst of maxillary antrum.

BIBLIOGRAPHY

1. Abrams AM, Howell FV, Bullock WK. Nasopalatine cysts. Oral Surg Oral Med Oral Pathol. 1963;16:306-32.
2. Ackermann G, Cohen MA, Altini M. The paradental cyst: a clinicopathologic study of 50 cases. Oral Surg Oral Med Oral Pathol. 1987;64:308-12.
3. Adams A, Lovelock DJ. Nasolabial cyst. Oral Surg Oral Med Oral Pathol. 1985;60:118-9.
4. Aguilo L, Cibrian R, Bagan JV, et al. Eruption cysts: retrospective clinical study of 36 cases. ASDC J Dent Child. 1998;65(2):102-6.

5. Ahlfors E, Larsson A, Sjogren S. The odontogenic keratocyst: a benign cystic tumor? J Oral Maxillofac Surg. 1984;42:10-9.
6. Altini M, Cohen M. The follicular primordial cyst odontogenic keratocyst. Int J Oral Surg. 1982;11:175-82.
7. Anneroth G, Hall G, Stuge U. Nasopalatine duct cyst. Int T Oral Maxillofac Surg. 1986;15:572-80.
8. Bataineh AB, Rawashdeh MA, Al Qudah MA. The prevalence of inflammatory and developmental odontogenic cysts in a Jordanian population: a clinicopathologic study. Quintessence Int. 1984;5(10):815-9.
9. Brannon RB. The odontogenic keratocyst. A clinicopathologic study of 312 cases. II. Histopathologic features. Oral Surg Oral Med Oral Pathol. 1977;43:233-55.
10. Brannon RB. The odontogenic keratocyst. A clinocopathologic study of 312 cases. Part T. Clinical features. Oral Surg Oral Med Oral Pathol. 1976;42:54-72.
11. Brannon RB. The odontogenic keratocyst: a clinicopathologic study of 213 cases. Oral Surg Oral Med Oral Pathol. 1976;42:54.
12. Brawne RM, Gough NE. Malignant changes in the epithelium lining odontogenic cysts. Cancer. 1972;29:1199-207.
13. Brawne RM. Some observations on the fluids of odontogenic cysts. J Oral Pathol. 1976;5:74-87.
14. Brawne RM. The odontogenic keratocyst: clinical aspects. Br Dent J. 1970;128:225-31.
15. Brawne RM. The pathogenesis of odontogenic cysts: review. J Oral Pathol. 1975;4:31-46.
16. Brereton RJ, Symonds E. Thyroglossal cysts in children. Br T Surg. 1978;65:507.
17. Browne RM. The odontogenic keratocyst. Histological features and their correlation with clinical behavior. Br Dent J. 1971;131:249-59.
18. Buchner A, Hansen LS. Lymphoepithelial cysts of the oral mucosa. Oral Surg Oral Med Oral Pathol. 1980;50:441.
19. Buchner A, Hansen LS. The histomorphologic spectrum of the gingival cyst in the adult. Oral Surg Oral Med Oral Pathol. 1979;48:523-39.
20. Buchner A, Merrell PW, Hansen LS, et al. Peripheral (extraosseous) calcifying odontogenic cyst. Oral Surg Oral Med Oral Pathol. 1991;72:265-70.
21. Buchner A. The central (intraosseous) calcifying odontogenic cyst: an analysis of 215 cases. J Oral Maxillofac Surg. 1991;49:330-9.
22. Budnick SD. Compound and complex odontomas. Oral Surg Oral Med Oral Pathol. 1976;42:501-6.
23. Campbell RL, Burkes EJ. Nasolabial Cyst: report of case. T Am Dent Assoc. 1975;91:1210-3.
24. Cataldo E, Berkman MD. Cyst of the oral mucosa in newborns. Am T Dis Child 1968;116:44.
25. Chaudhry AP. A clinicopathologic study of intraoral lymphoepithelial cysts. T Oral Med. 1984;39:79.
26. Chehade A, Daley TD, Wysocki GP, et al. Peripheral odontogenic keratocyst. Oral Surg Oral Med Oral Pathol. 1994;77:494-7.
27. Cheng YSL, Wright JM, Walstad WR, et al. Calcifying epithelial odontogenic tumor showing microscopic features of potential malignant behavior. Oral Surg Oral Med Oral Pathol Oral Radiol Endod. 2002;93:287-95.
28. Christ TF. The globulomaxillary cyst: An embryologic misconception. Oral Surg Oral Med Oral Pathol. 1970;30:515-25.
29. Colgan CM, Henry J, Napier SS, et al. Paradental cysts: a role for food impaction in the pathogenesis? A review of cases from Northern Ireland. Br J Oral Maxillofac Surg. 2002;40(2);163-8.
30. Cohen MA, Shear M. Histological comparison of parakeratinized and orthokeratinized cysts (keratocysts). J Dent Assoc South Africa. 1980;35:161-5.
31. Dahlin DC, McLeod RA. Aneurysmal bone cyst and other non-neoplastic conditions. Skeletal Radiol. 1982;8:243-50.
32. Daley TD, Wysocki GP, Pringle GA. Relative incidence of odontogenic tumors and oral and jaw cysts in a Canadian population. Oral Surg Oral Med Oral Pathol. 1994;77:276-80.
33. Daley TD, Wysocki GP. The small dentigerous cyst. Oral Surg Oral Med Oral Pathol Oral Radiol Endod. 1995;79:77-81.
34. Deron PB, Nikolovski N, Hollander JC den, et al. Myxoma of the maxilla; a case with extremely aggressive biologic behavior. Head Neck. 1996;18:459-64.
35. Eversole LR, Sabes WR, Rovin S. Aggressive growth and neoplastic potential of odontogenic cysts. Cancer. 1975;35:270.
36. Foley WL, Terry BC, Jacoway JR. Malignant transformation of an odontogenic keratocyst: report of a case. T Oral Maxillofac Surg. 1991;49:768-71.

37. Forssell K. The primordial cyst: a clinical and radiographic study. Turku, Finland: Academic Dissertation; 1980.
38. Fowler CB, Brannon RB. The paradental cyst: a clinicopathologic study of six new cases and review of the literature. J Oral Maxillofac Surg. 1989;47:243-8.
39. Fowler CB, Branon RB. The paradental cyst: a clinicopathologic study of six new cases and review of the literature. T Oral Maxillofac Surg. 1989;47:243.
40. Fromm A. Epstein's pearls, Bohn's nodules and inclusion: cysts of the oral cavity. J Dent Child. 1967;34:275-87.
41. Gardner DG. Plexiform unicystic ameloblastoma: a diagnostic problem in dentigerous cysts. Cancer. 1984;47:1358.
42. Hansen J, Kobayasi T. Ultrastructural studies of odontogenic cysts. II Keratinizing cysts. Acta Morphol Neerl Scand. 1970;8:43-62.
43. Johnson L, Sapp JP, Melntire DN. Squamous cell carcinoma arising in a dentigerous cyst. T Oral Maxillofac Surg. 1994;52:987-90.
44. Kaugars GE, Cale AE. Traumatic bone cyst. Oral Surg Oral Med Oral Pathol. 1987;63:318-24.
45. Kaugars GE. Botryoid odontogenic cyst. Oral Surg Oral Med Oral Pathol. 1986;62:555-9.
46. Kramer IRH, Toller PA. The use of exfoliative cytology and protein estimations in preoperative diagnosis of odontogenic keratocysts. Int J Oral Surg. 1973;2:143-51.
47. Little JW, Jakobsen J. Origin of the globulomaxillary cyst. J Oral Surg. 1973;31:188-95.
48. Main DMG. Epithelial jaw cysts: 10-years of the WHO classification. J Oral Pathol. 1985;14:1-7.
49. Main DMG. Epithelial jaw cysts: a clinicopathological reappraisal. Br J Oral Surg. 1970; 8:114-25.
50. Mehregan DA, Al-sabah Hy, Mehregan AH. Basal cells epithelioma arising from epidermoid cyst. T Dermatol Surg Oncol.1994;20:405-6.
51. Nanavati SD, Gandhi PR. Median mandibular cyst. J Oral Surg. 1979;37:422-25.
52. Nethiananda S. Squamous cell carcinoma arising in the lining of an odontogenic cyst. Br J Oral Surg. 1983;21:56-62.
53. Ochlers FAC. Periapical lesions and residual dental cysts. Br T Oral Surg. 1970;8:103.
54. Pindborg JJ, Kramer IRH. Histological typing of odontogenic tumors, jaw cysts, and allied lesions. Geneva: World Health Organization; 1971.
55. Seward MH. Eruption cyst an analysis of the clinical features. T Oral Surg. 1973;31:31.
56. Shade NL, Carpenter WM, Delzer DD. Gingival Cyst of the adult: case report of a bacterial presentation. T Periodontol. 1987;58:796-9.
57. Shear M, Pindborg JJ. Macroscopic features of the lateral periodontal cyst. Scand J Dent Res. 1975;83:103-10.
58. Shear M. Cysts of the jaws: recent advances. J Oral Pathol. 1985;14:43-59.
59. Shear M. Cysts of the oral region, 2nd edition. Bristol: Wright; 1983.
60. Shear M. Primordial cysts. J Dent Assoc South Africa. 1960;15:211-7.
61. Sicher H. Anatomy and oral pathology. Oral Surg Oral Med Oral Pathol. 1962;15:1264-9.
62. Soskolne WA, Shear M. Observations on the pathogenesis of primordial cysts. Br Dent J. 1967;123:321-6.
63. Stoelinga PJW, Peters JH. A note on the origin of keratocysts. Int J Oral Surg. 1973;2:37-44.
64. Stoelinga PJW. Studies on the dental lamina as related to its role in the etiology of cysts and tumors. J Oral Pathol. 1976;5:65-73.
65. Strutthers PJ, Shear M. Root resorption produced by the enlargement of ameloblastomas and cysts of the jaws. Int J Oral Surg. 1976;5: 128-32.
66. Toller P. The origin and growth of the cysts of the jaws. Ann R Coll Surg Engl. 1967;40:306-36.
67. Toller PA. Newer concepts of odontogenic cysts. Int J Oral Surg. 1972;1:3-16.
68. Wang SZ, Chen XM, Li Y. Clinicopathologic analysis of glandular odontogenic cyst. Chung Hua Kou Chiang Hsueh Tsa Chih. 1994;29: 329-31.
69. Wright JM. Squamous odontogenic tumor like proliferations in odontogenic cysts. Oral Surg Oral Med Oral Pathol. 1979;47:354-8.

CHAPTER 7

Regressive Alterations of Teeth

◼ INTRODUCTION

Regressive alterations are the group of retrogressive changes in the teeth, which occur due to nonbacterial causes and results in wear and tear of the tooth structures with impairment of function.

Some of these regressive changes in teeth result from generalized aging process and others occur due to chronic persistent tissue injury (Box 7.1).

ATTRITION OF TEETH

◼ DEFINITION

Attrition is a constant form of retrogressive change in teeth, characterized by wear of tooth substance or restoration as a result of tooth-to-tooth contact during occlusion, mastication or parafunction.

It is mostly an age related physiologic process, which occurs over a long period of time and that is why older individuals often exhibit more attrition in their teeth as compared to the young.

The rate and severity of attrition depends upon several factors such as diet quality, dentition, force of the masticatory muscles and chewing habits, etc.

◼ TYPES OF ATTRITION

Although clinical distinction is difficult to make, attrition may be divided into two types:
1. Physiological attrition
2. Pathological attrition.

Physiological Attrition

- The tooth loss in physiological attrition is fairly constant and is proportionate to the age of the individual.
- Physiological attrition begins with wearing of the incisal edge of incisors; it is followed by the palatal cusp of maxillary molars and buccal cusp of mandibular molars.
- Attrition also occurs in the proximal surfaces of teeth in the contact point areas.

Pathological Attrition

Pathological attrition occurs due to certain abnormalities in occlusion, chewing pattern or due to some structural defects in the teeth. It often causes extensive loss of tooth structure, which results in disturbed function and loss of esthetics.

The tooth wear in this type of attrition does not maintain a consistent pattern and

Box 7.1	Causes of loss of enamel after tooth formation.

- Dental caries
- Trauma
- Attrition
- Abrasion
- Abfraction
- Erosion
- Bruxism
- Dentinogenesis imperfecta
- Amelogenesis imperfecta
- Radiation therapy

the amount of tooth loss is not proportionate to the age of the individual.

CAUSES OF PATHOLOGICAL ATTRITION

- *Abnormal occlusion:* May be developmental, e.g. crowding of teeth or malposed teeth. In these cases, abnormal occlusal positioning of teeth may lead to traumatic contact during chewing which may lead to more tooth wear.
- *Premature extraction of teeth:* Extraction of some teeth from the dental arch will increase occlusal load on the remaining teeth (overburdened teeth) as the chewing force for the individual remains constant.
- *Abnormal chewing habits:* Parafunctional chewing habits, e.g. bruxism (habitual grinding of teeth) and chronic persistent chewing of coarse and abrasive foods or other substance, e.g. tobacco and betel nut, etc.
- *Structural defects in teeth:* The structural defects, which make the tooth more vulnerable to attrition even under normal masticatory forces include—
  – Amelogenesis imperfecta
  – Dentinogenesis imperfecta

In these situations, the hardness of enamel or dentin is much more inferior as compared to the normal teeth and therefore, the rate of tooth wear is high even under normal chewing pressures.

CLINICAL FEATURES OF ATTRITION

- Attrition can occur in both deciduous as well as in the permanent teeth.
- Attrition of tooth is clinically manifested by the formation of flat, smooth, shiny, well-polished facets on those surfaces of teeth which come in contact with the opposing teeth (Fig. 7.1).
- Thus, attrition often occurs on the tip of the cusps, incisal edges, on the proximal contact areas, labial surface of lower anteriors and palatal surfaces of upper anteriors.
- In advanced cases, attrition may lead to severe reduction in the cuspal height with complete wearing of enamel and flattening of the entire occlusal surface (Fig. 7.2).
- When the enamel is lost on the occlusal surface, the dentin becomes attrited at a faster rate and the lesion may become cap shaped, surrounded by a rim of enamel at the periphery.
- When dentin becomes exposed it generally becomes discolored brown and sensitive.
- Attrition in the proximal surfaces of teeth occurs due to vertical movements of tooth within the socket during mastication.

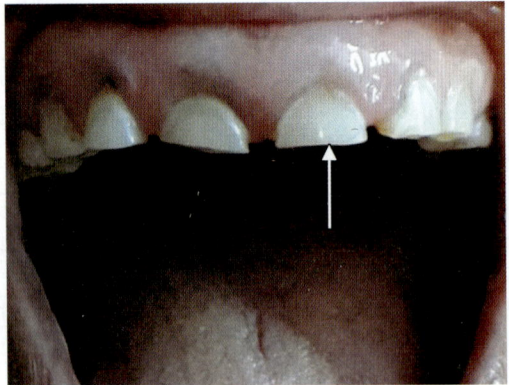

Fig. 7.1: Attrition of teeth.

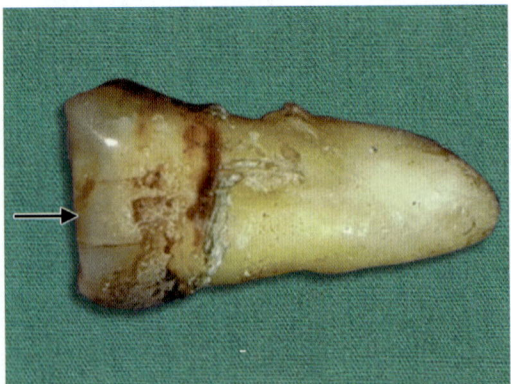

Fig. 7.2: Attrition of individual tooth with flattening of occlusal surface.

- Proximal surface attrition causes transformation of proximal "contact points" to relatively broad and flat "contact areas".
- This type of loss of tooth structure from the proximal surfaces may even lead to mesial migration of teeth in the dental arch.
- Normally, men often exhibit more severe attritions of teeth than women.
- Pulp exposure and subsequent pain are rare in case of attrition as the process is generally slow, and often allows sufficient time for formation of protective reparative dentin.
- Attrition may also occur on the restorations of teeth. A common example in this regard, is the development of shiny facets on the amalgam filled surfaces.
- Attrition may even possibly lead to fracture of the cusps of teeth or restorations.

TREATMENT

Treatment of attrition is difficult; however certain things can be done to reduce further tooth wear.
- Corrections of developmental abnormalities causing traumatic occlusion.
- Correction of parafunctional chewing habits.
- Protection of tooth by metal or metal ceramic crowns.
- Construction of occlusal guard, if the habit of bruxism is persisting.

ABRASION OF TEETH

DEFINITION

Abrasion is the pathological wearing of dental tissues or dental restorations by friction with foreign substances independent of occlusion (Fig. 7.3).

ETIOLOGY AND PATHOGENESIS

Different foreign substances produce different patterns of tooth abrasion. However, the process of tooth wear is similar in every case.

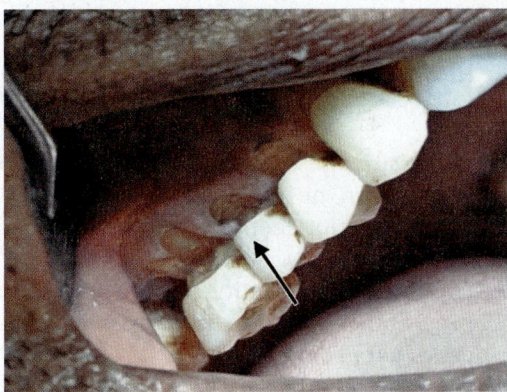

Fig. 7.3: Abrasion of teeth.

CAUSES OF ABRASION (BOX 7.2).

Toothbrush Abrasion
- It is the most common type of abrasion and is mostly associated with faulty tooth brushing technique.
- Abrasion mostly occurs when the brushing is done in horizontal brushing strokes rather than vertical strokes (Fig. 7.4).
- It also occurs if excessive force is applied on the teeth during brushing.
- The condition is made even worse when an abrasive dentifrice is used.

Box 7.2	Causes of abrasion.
- Toothbrush abrasion
- Habitual abrasion
- Occupational abrasions
- Abrasions by prosthetic appliances
- Ritual abrasions	

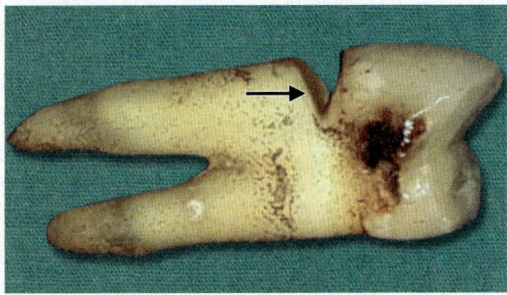

Fig. 7.4: Toothbrush abrasion making a "V"-shaped notch in the cervical area.

Habitual Abrasion

- Excessive habitual chewing of betel nut, tobacco and pan, etc. causes abrasion of teeth.
- Habitual pipe smokers may develop abrasion on the incisal edges of upper and lower anterior teeth due to continuous biting on the pipe stem.
- Chronic habitual biting of pencils, bobby pins (hair grips) and threads, etc. often cause abrasion.
- Improper and habitual use of tooth prick or dental floss, etc. can cause abrasions on the proximal surfaces of teeth.

Occupational Abrasion

Occupational abrasion develops when objects or instruments are habitually held between the teeth by professionals during work.

- Hairdressers often grip the hairpins between their teeth during work and this can cause tooth abrasions.
- Carpenters often keep small tools or nails between their teeth when they are at work and this practice cause abrasion of tooth resulting in notching on the tooth surface especially at the incisal edges of the anterior teeth.
- Similar occupational abrasions can also be seen among tailors and shoemakers.

Abrasion by Prosthetic Appliances

Faulty clasp design in removable partial denture prosthesis may also cause abrasion of tooth.

Ritual Abrasion

Ritual abrasions of tooth are uncommon nowadays and are mainly confined in Africa.

For example, ancient people used to believe in some pragmatic concepts and according to that they often used to mutilate their teeth with some instruments. These practices were aimed at making themselves immune from evil spirits.

Clinical Features of Abrasions

- In abrasion of tooth, the type and severity of surface wear will depend upon the duration and the type of faulty habit adopted by the person.
- Clinical manifestations differ in different types of habit, e.g. a defect in the tooth due to toothbrush abrasion will differ from that of the occupational abrasion or from the habitual abrasion.
- The abrasion produces a "V" shaped or wedge-shaped horizontal notch on the buccal surface of teeth. The notch will have sharp angles and highly polished dentin surface (Fig. 7.4).
- Toothbrush abrasions commonly occur on the cervical areas of the labial or buccal surfaces of teeth.
- Canines and premolars being the more prominent teeth are often more severely affected by abrasion.
- Teeth on the left side of the arch are more severely involved in right-handed persons and vice versa.
- Maxillary teeth are more commonly affected than mandibular teeth.
- In cervical abrasion, lesions are more often wide than deep.
- Toothbrush abrasion may also cause gingival recession.
- In pipe smokers, abrasions develop on the incisal surfaces of upper and lower anterior teeth. The lesion is characterized by a well-polished notch, whose shape typically matches with the shape of the pipe stem used by the smoker.
- Abrasion caused by habitual holding of nails or needles or other small tools by the tailors or shoe makers or carpenters, etc. often produces a small, deep, well-polished "ditch" on the incisal edge of teeth.
- Faulty use of tooth-prick or dental floss cause loss of dentin and cementum, especially of the root surfaces on the proximal walls of teeth.

- Severe abrasion (of any type) may cause opening up of the dentinal tubules and therefore, the patient may experience sensitivity in the affected teeth due to hot and cold substances.
- Secondary or reactionary dentin usually forms on the pulpal surfaces to protect the teeth from pulp exposures.
- In untreated cases, the lesion may deepen further and it may eventually expose the dental pulp with subsequent of pulpitis.

■ TREATMENT

Avoidance of abnormal brushing habits prevent abrasions, however in already developed cases, restorative treatment helps to keep the tooth surface intact and also it prevents further tooth wear.

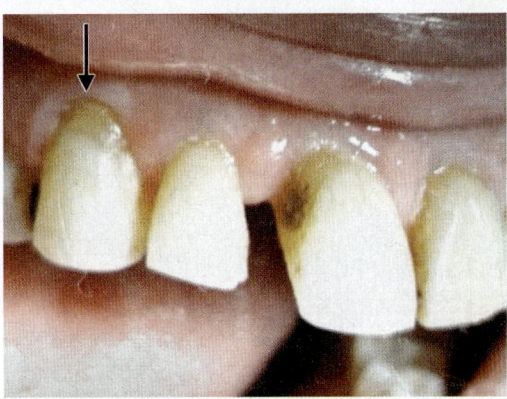

Fig. 7.5: Abfraction of tooth.

TOOTH ABFRACTION

■ DEFINITION

Abfraction is the pathologic loss of tooth enamel and dentin caused by biomechanical loading forces.

■ FORCES CAUSING ABFRACTION

- *Static forces:* Produced during swallowing, tongue thrusting and clenching.
- *Cyclic forces:* Forces produced during chewing.

These forces cause repeated flexure and ultimate material fatigue to the affected tooth at locations away from the point of loading.

■ CLINICAL FEATURES

- Abfraction causes breaking down of enamel on the buccal surface of tooth (Fig. 7.5).
- People with open bite or very deep class I cavity are more prone to develop abfraction of tooth.
- Sensitivity of tooth, sign of traumatic occlusion and wearing on the occlusal surface are often seen.
- Stress lines on the tooth surface and sometimes fracture of the tooth may occur.
- Repeated failure of restorations on the cervical area due to damaging lateral forces.

EROSION OF TEETH

■ DEFINITION

Erosion can be defined as progressive irreversible loss of hard dental tissues by some chemical process that does not involve bacterial action.

In erosion, dissolution of the mineralized tooth structure occurs upon contact with acids, which are introduced into the oral cavity either from intrinsic sources or from extrinsic sources. However, it is important to note that erosion may render the teeth more susceptible to other retrogressive changes like attrition and abrasion, etc.

■ ETIOLOGIC FACTORS FOR EROSION (BOX 7.3)

Extrinsic Factors

Acidic Foods and Beverages

Acids from extrinsic sources (source is outside the body), which can cause erosion

Box 7.3	Systemic diseases associated with erosion of teeth.

- Gastroesophageal reflux disease
- Chronic alcoholism
- Pregnancy
- Esophagitis
- Gastritis
- Peptic ulcer
- Hyperparathyroidism
- Bulimia
- Nervous system disorder

of tooth usually come from acidic beverages, foods, and medications, etc. or from the environment itself.

- Most of the fruits and fruits juices have a low pH and these can cause erosion of tooth if consumed regularly.
- Carbonated soft drinks and sports drinks are also very acidic in nature and frequent consumption of these drinks may result in erosion of tooth.
- Rate of erosion of tooth is proportional to the amount and frequency of consumption of acidic beverages/foods.

The erosive potential of acidic foods/beverages can be reduced if:

- They contain large amount of calcium, phosphate and fluoride, etc. which help in tooth remineralization.
- If tooth brushing is done after every intake of beverage.
- If drinks are taken by a straw rather than from a glass (it minimizes contact time with tooth).

Medications

Some medicines can be highly acidic in nature (e.g. vitamin C and hydrochloric acid preparations, etc.) and they can cause erosion of teeth when chewed or kept in the mouth for a long time prior to swallowing.

Occupational Erosions

- Occupational erosions are seen among workers who often come in contact with acids at their place of work. Commonly vapors of different acids, e.g. chromic acid, hydrochloric acid, sulfuric acid and nitric acids, etc. are released into the work environment during industrial electrolyte process. These vapors can cause erosion of teeth, on those surfaces, which are normally exposed to the atmosphere (incisal third of incisors).
- Commonly the workers involved in manufacturing of lead acid batteries or sanitary cleansers or soft drinks, etc. or those who are working in galvanizing or plating factories often develop occupational erosions of teeth.
- Occupational wine tasters often have erosion in their teeth.
- Swimmers who practice regularly in the pools can have erosion of their teeth if the pool water contains higher concentrations of acids.

Intrinsic Factors

The intrinsic pathway of erosion means the acids are produced within the body and cause erosion of tooth. This type of erosion occurs in cases of certain systemic diseases, which cause increased vomiting and regurgitations of bowel contents into the mouth.

CLINICAL FEATURES OF EROSION

- Acids from extrinsic source cause erosion on the labial or buccal surfaces of teeth and acids from intrinsic source cause erosion on the lingual or palatal surfaces of teeth (Fig. 7.6).
- The most common site of dental erosion is the gingival third of the labial surfaces of maxillary incisors.
- In chronic severe cases of erosion, the disease can involve even the proximal surfaces of teeth besides involving the labial and lingual surfaces.
- Clinically the condition is manifested by shallow, broad, "scooped-out" concavities on the enamel with highly polished surfaces.
- It usually involves multiple teeth.

Regressive Alterations of Teeth

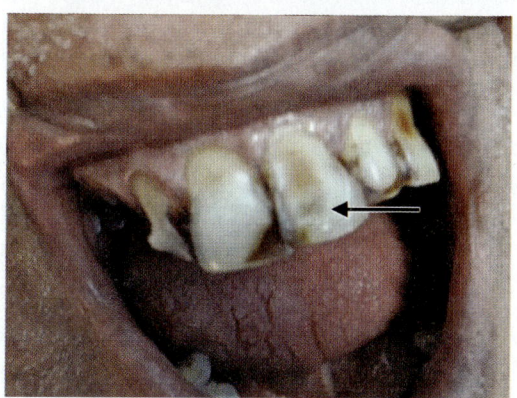

Fig. 7.6: Erosion of teeth.

- There will be cupping of occlusal surfaces of molar teeth or grooving of the incisal edges of anterior teeth with exposure of dentin.
- Increased incisal translucency of teeth also occurs.
- In severe erosion there may be loss of entire buccal cusp of the molar teeth which results in a "ski slope" like depression of the tooth that extends from lingual cusp up to the buccal cervical area.
- Amalgam restorations often have a clean, nontarnished appearance due to action of acids on the metal surface.
- Preservation of enamel "cuff" on the gingival crevice is common.
- Loss of enamel often causes hypersensitivity in the teeth; however the tooth sensitivity occurs only in cases of rapid erosions. Sensitivity of tooth does not occur in slowly progressing erosions; as there is enough time for formation of reactionary dentin in the tooth.
- Severe cases of erosion however can cause exposure of pulp in deciduous teeth.

TREATMENT

Preventive Treatment

Identification of etiology is important in the management of erosion. Avoidance of carbonated beverages.

Treatment of GERD if present.

Restorative Treatment

Proper restoration of the lost tooth structure.

Role of Salivary Function in the Prevention of Dental Erosion

Buffering action of saliva prevents erosion of teeth by neutralizing the acids in mouth.

Mineral ions in saliva cause re-mineralization of the damaged areas of teeth.

RESORPTION OF TEETH

■ DEFINITION

Resorption of teeth can be defined as a chronic progressive damage or loss of tooth structures (mostly roots of the teeth or sometimes crowns) due to the action of some specialized cells called odontoclasts.

Resorption is generally associated with some attempt at repair by the apposition of cementum or bone and the involved tooth may occasionally become ankylosed to the surrounding bone.

■ TYPES OF ROOT RESORPTION OF TEETH (TABLE 7.1)

- *Physiological resorption:* Resorption of root of deciduous teeth
- *Pathological resorption:* Abnormal damage to the permanent tooth structure due to resorption.
  - External resorption: Damage affecting the outer surface and progressing towards the inner areas of tooth.

Table 7.1: Resorption of teeth.

Physiological	Pathological	
Resorption of roots of the deciduous teeth	External resorption	Internal resorption
	• Secondary to periapical or other pathology • Idiopathic (burrowing)	• Secondary to pulpitis • Idiopathic

– Internal resorption: Damage beginning at the center of the tooth (dentin) and progressing outwardly.

Local Causes

- Trauma in the tooth
- Periapical or periodontal pathology, e.g. chronic abscess, granuloma or cyst
- Jaw cysts (odontogenic or nonodontogenic)
- Jaw tumors (odontogenic or nonodontogenic)
- Excessive mechanical forces (orthodontic treatment/faulty prosthesis or implants)
- Impacted teeth.

Systemic Causes

- Hypophosphatemia
- Hypophosphatasia
- Hyperparathyroidism
- Herpes-Zoster infection
- Hypothyroidism
- Hyperpituitarism.

Physiological Resorption

Physiological resorption occurs in the root of the deciduous teeth, which helps in their natural shedding before eruption of the permanent successors.

Physiological resorption occurs by the following mechanism:

- Reduced enamel epithelial cells present as a protective covering on the erupting permanent tooth crown release some chemical substances, which cause resorption of the roots of deciduous teeth.
- According to other investigators the pressure exerted by the permanent successor teeth on the deciduous teeth and alveolar bone during their eruption may cause resorption of the later.

External Resorption of Tooth

Definition

Pathological resorption that begins peripherally on the outer surface of the tooth root and moves towards the pulp is called the external resorption (Fig. 7.7A). Sometimes the process can affect the crowns of the unerupted teeth.

Role of Individual Factors (Box 7.4)

- *Periapical inflammation:* Often leads to the formation of granulation tissue around the root. The highly vascular granulation tissue triggers the process of bone or tooth resorption mainly by stimulating the osteoclast and odontoclast cells. The later cells, which can be either mononucleated or multinucleated, cause damage to the alveolar bone, cementum and dentin, etc. and leads to resorption of tooth surface.
- *Trauma in the tooth:* May initiate an inflammatory response in the periapical region of tooth, which triggers the odontoclast cells to resorb the roots.
- *Reimplanted teeth:* As the reimplanted or transplanted teeth are almost always nonvital and their roots have no surrounding viable periodontal ligaments, these are often resorbed externally and replaced by bone.
- *Cysts:* Cystic lesions may cause external resorption in the following mechanisms:
  - Cysts exert pressure on the roots of the adjacent teeth and cause their resorption.

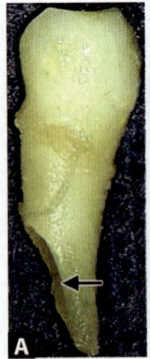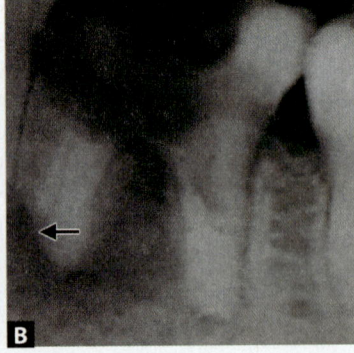

Figs. 7.7A and B: (A) Specimen of a permanent tooth showing external resorption of root; (B) X-ray showing the same.

Box 7.4   Causes of external resorption.

- Periapical or periradicular inflammation
- Trauma in the tooth
- Cysts in the jaw (especially dentigerous cyst)
- Excessive mechanical forces on teeth (orthodontic treatment)
- Excessive occlusal forces (faulty restoration/prosthesis)
- Tumors in the jaw (especially ameloblastoma)
- Reimplantation of tooth
- Periodontal surgery
- Pressure from impacted tooth
- Paget's disease of bone
- Alveolar bone grafting
- Hormonal imbalance
- Herpes zoster
- Intracoronal bleaching of pulpless teeth
- Idiopathic

– Epithelial cells of the lining epithelium of cyst can release some chemical mediators, which cause root resorption.
– The dentigenous cyst, which develops from the reduced enamel epithelial cells (these cells are responsible for deciduous root resorptions in normal conditions), often has a tendency for root resorption of the surrounding permanent teeth.
- *Tumors:* Benign and malignant tumors in the jawbone cause resorption of the roots of the adjacent teeth. Either due to pressure effect from the growing tumor or due to the action of the chemical mediators released by the tumor cells.
  Ameloblastoma is very much known for its ability to resorb the roots of the surrounding teeth.
- *Excessive mechanical or occlusal forces:* Trauma from malocclusion or excessive orthodontic forces can cause injury or necrosis of the periodontal ligaments, which may initiate resorption of the tooth roots.
- *Periodontal surgery:* As an after effect of periodontal surgery granulation tissue forms on the external surface of the root, which stimulates the odontoclast cells; as a result external resorption often occurs.

- *Impacted tooth:*
  – When an impacted tooth exerts pressure on the root of the adjoining erupted tooth, it can cause resorption.
  – An impacted tooth itself may undergo resorption in its crown portion and it probably happens due to partial loss of the protective covering of reduced enamel epithelium around the crown.
- *Idiopathic external resorption (Burrowing resorption):*
  – A burrowing type of external resorption is commonly seen in relation to a single or multiple erupted teeth.
  – Initially a localized area of the root surface near the cervical region (below the gingival epithelial attachment) is resorbed.
  – Following this, the resorption process borrows deeply into and ramifies throughout the dentin producing a "labyrinthine network" of lacunae and channels.
  – The resorbed tooth structures are replaced by granulation tissue and ankylosis sometimes develops.
  – The circumpulpal dentin and predentin are generally spared and they remain as narrow shell as the resorption encircles the pulp.
  – Radiographically burrowing type of resorption resembles the dental caries.
  – There is another pattern of external resorption of tooth, which starts at the root apex and progresses slowly in the occlusal direction.
  – Idiopathic external resorptions can affect almost all the teeth simultaneously.

Radiographic Appearances of External Resorption

- Loss of continuity in the peripheral or external outlines of teeth (Fig. 7.7B).
- External resorption sometimes appears as carious lesions.

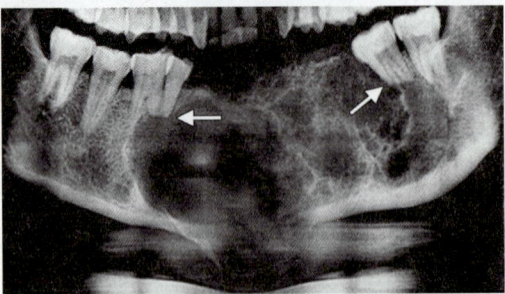

Fig. 7.8: External resorption of teeth due to a tumor (ameloblastoma).

- Lesions in the initial stages produce raggedness or blunting of the root apex (Fig. 7.8). Larger lesions may even produce a "moth-eaten" appearance due to irregular or uneven destruction patterns of tooth.
- Endodontically treated teeth radiographically exhibits as if the root canal filling materials are projecting beyond the apex.
- Often there is obliteration of the periodontal ligament space with development of ankylosis.
- When external resorption involves the crown of an impacted tooth, it may look like dental caries.

Consequences of External Resorption

External resorptions in severe cases may extend up to the pulp leading to loss of vitality of the affected tooth. However, there is always the danger of fracture of the tooth.

Internal Resorption of Tooth

Definition

Internal resorption of tooth refers to an uncommon condition in which the resorption process starts internally within the tooth itself and the dentin is gradually resorbed from the pulpal side towards the periphery.

Etiopathogenesis

- The disease can occur as part of an inflammatory response to pulpal injury, however, in many instances even no such initiating factors could be identified.
- The inflammatory reaction in the pulp causes activation of osteoclast or odontoclast cells in the internal surfaces of the root or crown, which result in the resorption of dentin.
- Gradually small resorption lacunae develop, which enlarge and coalesce together; and the entire dentin is eventually resorbed.
- Hyperplastic pulpal tissues gradually occupy the spaces created due to the dentinal resorption.

Clinical Features

- Internal resorption is often localized and affects a single anterior or posterior tooth in the jaw.
- The defect may involve either the crown portion of the tooth or the root portion
- As the disease initiates from the central portion of the tooth, there is no early symptom.
- In advanced stages when the coronal dentin is resorbed, the tooth often appears pink in color; because the hyperplastic and highly vascular pulp tissue fills up the resorbed spaces in dentin and is visible through the transparent enamel. This typical appearance is known as "'pink tooth of Mummery" (Fig. 7.9).
- The pink appearance of the tooth may also occur in cases of severe external resorptions (especially in burrowing type), when the gingival tissue projects into the resorbed spaces of dentin.

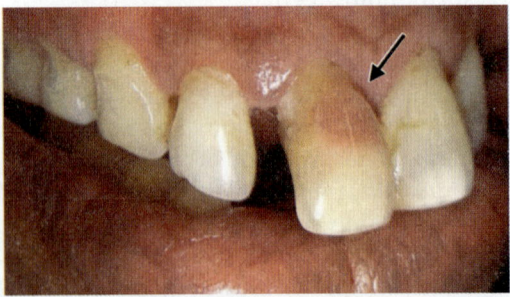

Fig. 7.9: Pink tooth in internal resorption.

- When internal resorption affects the root of the tooth no color change is usually evident.
- The affected tooth remains vital and asymptomatic, unless there is pulp necrosis due to fracture of the tooth or due to its perforation (which allows entry of infection causing agents).
- Untreated cases of internal resorption generally lead to perforations.

Radiological Features
- Radiographically, internal resorption presents a well-defined, spherical shaped, radiolucent area in the dentin, which is usually continuous with the pulp chamber or root canal.
- The radiographic image of the external outline of the tooth remains intact.
- When internal resorption leads to perforation of tooth, radiograph shows a communication between the pulp chamber or root canal and the periodontal ligament space.
- Sometimes there can be balloon type expansion of the root canal of the affected tooth.

Types of Internal Resorptions

Internal resorptions are of two types:
1. Internal inflammatory resorption
2. Internal replacement resorption.

Internal inflammatory resorption
- The condition occurs probably due to an intense inflammatory reaction within the pulp tissue.
- Microscopy reveals a chronically inflamed pulp tissue containing numerous inflammatory cells along with few multi-nucleated dentin resorbing cells (odontoclasts).
- Radiograph exhibits a uniform, spherical, and enlargement of the root canal.

Internal replacement resorption
- This resorption occurs in the absence of any inflammatory reaction within the pulp.
- Microscopy shows a fibrous granulation tissue in the pulp containing ectopic, bone-like calcified masses.
- Radiographically, an irregular "moth-eaten" type of radiolucency is formed in the dentin.

Treatment
- Extirpation of pulp tissue and conventional endodontic therapy.
- When the tooth is perforated, extraction is the only treatment possible.

The important differences between internal and external resorption of teeth are given in Table 7.2.

PULP CALCIFICATION

DEFINITION

Deposition of calcified mass(es) within the dental pulp for no apparent reason is called pulp calcification.

PATHOGENESIS OF PULP CALCIFICATION (FLOWCHART 7.1)

The etiology of pulp calcification (Box 7.5) is unknown and it appears to be not related to inflammation, trauma or any systemic disease.

Table 7.2: Differences between internal and external resorption of teeth.

	Internal resorption of teeth	External resorption of teeth
Incidence	Low	High
Direction	Inside-out	Outside-in
Pulp vitality	Vital	Nonvital
Outline of the defect	Smooth	Irregular
Root surface of affected tooth	Intact	Affected/resorbed
Root canal	Enlarged	Unchanged
Clinical symptoms	Asymptomatic	May be symptomatic

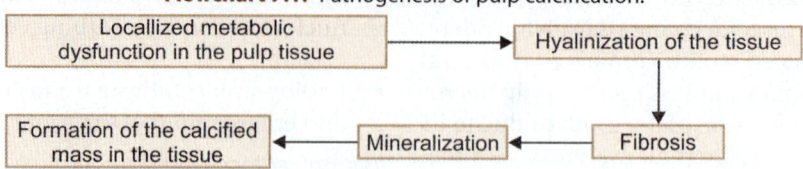

Flowchart 7.1: Pathogenesis of pulp calcification.

Box 7.5	Causes of pulp calcification.

- Idiopathic formation of pulp stones
- Formation of secondary dentin in response to caries
- Calcific metamorphosis—pulp obliteration due to aging or trauma
- Dentinogenesis imperfecta—excessive secondary dentin formation causing pulp obliteration
- Dentin dysplasia Type-I—chevron shaped pulp chambers
- Dentin dysplasia Type-II—pulp obliteration in deciduous teeth and pulp stone formation in permanent teeth
- Ehlers–Danlos syndrome
- Regional odontodysplasia

TYPES

Calcification in the pulp may be either diffuse (linear) or nodular (pulp stones) (Table 7.3).

- *Denticles:* These are small masses of tubular dentin formed within the pulp near the furcation area of tooth.
- *Pulp stones:* Pulp stones are nodular calcified bodies having an organic matrix and they occur frequently in relation to the coronal pulp. Pulp stones develop around a central nidus of pulp tissue (consisting of collagen fibrils, ground substance and necrotic cell debri).
- *Diffuse linear calcifications of pulp:* These are amorphous, unorganized, fine fibrillar strands of calcified masses and are typically formed within the radicular and coronal pulp.

TYPES OF PULP STONES

Pulp stones can be of two types—true and false.
1. True pulp stones are composed predominantly of dentin and have dentinal tubules.
2. False pulp stones are composed of concentric layers of calcified material with no tubular dentinal tubules.

According to their location in the dental pulp.
- Free pulp stones are surrounded on all sides by pulpal tissue and are not attached to the dentinal wall.
- Attached pulp stones are those, which are attached to the dentinal wall of the pulp chamber.
- Interstitial pulp stones are those where the pulp stones have become surrounded by reactionary or secondary dentin they are called interstitial pulp stones.

CLINICAL SYMPTOMS

Pulp stones do not cause any clinical symptoms and the affected tooth is vital, however mild, neurologic pain has sometimes been reported in the tooth because of their presence.

DIAGNOSIS

Pulp calcifications can be detected by the following methods:
- Large pulp stones are often detected by radiographs.

Table 7.3: Types of pulp calcification.

Nodular/discrete (pulp stone)			Diffuse calcification		
Pulp stones (Types)					
False			True		
Attached	Free	Interstitial	Attached	Free	Interstitial

- Ground section preparation of the affected tooth.
- Microscopic examination helps in differentiating between the true and false pulp stones (on the basis of presence or absence of dentinal tubules).
- Serial sectioning of tooth or multiple radiographs taken at different angles may help to detect whether the pulp stone is free or attached to the dentinal wall.

CLINICAL SIGNIFICANCE OF PULP CALCIFICATIONS

Both pulp stones and dystrophic pulp calcifications may cause difficulties during endodontic treatment of the affected tooth.

HYPERCEMENTOSIS

DEFINITION

Increase in the thickness of cementum (especially cellular cementum) on the root surfaces of tooth due to excessive cementogenesis is called hypercementosis.

ETIOLOGY OF HYPERCEMENTOSIS (TABLE 7.4)

Periapical inflammation: Low grade sustained periapical inflammation often causes stimulation of the apical cementoblasts cells. This produces thickening of cementum.
Mechanical stimulation: Mechanical stimulation (e.g. orthodontic force) into a tooth induce apposition of cementum, which results in hypercementosis.
Functionless or unerupted tooth: In such cases, cemental apposition overpowers cemental resorption due to the lack of adequate occlusal stress.
Paget's disease of bone: Hypercementosis of tooth is often associated with Paget's disease of bone.
Tooth repair: Excessive cementogenesis may occur during the repair process of a tooth root.

Table 7.4: Etiology of hypercementosis.

Local factors	Systemic factors
• Chronic periapical or periradicular inflammation • Occlusal trauma • Mechanical stress • Functionless tooth • Unerupted tooth • Tooth repair	• Aging • Paget's disease of bone • Cementoblastoma • Acromegaly • Pituitary gigantism • Arthritis • Calcinosis • Rheumatic fever • Thyroid goiter • Vitamin A deficiency • Idiopathic

Idiopathic: In most of the cases the exact cause of the disease is not known.

CLINICAL FEATURES

Clinically the involved teeth are completely asymptomatic and the condition is often discovered during routine radiographic examination. The condition is mostly seen in adults and either single or multiple teeth can be involved.

RADIOGRAPHIC FEATURES

Radiograph shows excessive cemental thickening with a typical bulbous appearance of the roots. The thickened or blunted root is separated from the surrounding alveolar bone by a well-defined periodontal ligament space.

MICROSCOPY

Microscopically hypercementosis reveals excessive disposition of normal cellular or acellular cementum on the root surfaces of tooth in concentric layers.

CLINICAL SIGNIFICANCE

- Hypercementosis sometimes causes obliteration of the periodontal ligament space resulting in ankylosis of tooth, especially when the cementum develops in continuity with the alveolar bone.

- It may result in concrescence of teeth.
- Because of ankylosis and bulbous nature of the root, the tooth is difficult to extract.

AGE CHANGES IN TEETH

Age changes in teeth include the changes in structure and composition of the dental tissues as well as the changes in morphology associated with tooth wear.

CHANGES IN ENAMEL

Following changes occur in advanced age:
- Increased brittleness
- Decreased permeability ionic exchange.
- Becomes darker in color
- More wear and tear
- Decreased water content
- Increased fluoride content
- Decreased caries incidence

CHANGES IN DENTIN

- Continuous formation of secondary dentin causing reduction in size and even obliteration of the pulp chamber.
- Dentinal sclerosis due to continued production of peritubular dentin.
- Sclerosis of dentin also causes increasing translucency of the roots.
- Root translucency of tooth starts at the apex and extends coronally with age.

CHANGES IN CEMENTUM

- Cementum continues to form in the apical third of the root throughout life.
- Increase in the thickness of cementum at the root-end helps to compensate for the occlusal and interproximal attrition of tooth.
- The amount of secondary cementum apposition increases with age.
- Besides cementum appositions, there can be areas of cemental resorptions with increasing age.

CHANGES IN PULP

Following changes always occur in the pulp tissue with age:
- Decreased cellularity.
- Reduced vascularity.
- Increased fibrosis due to continued formation of collagen fibers.
- Pulpal response to tissue injury can be impaired, which may cause reduced healing potential.
- Pulp volume gradually decreases with continued production of secondary dentin.
- Incidence of pulp calcification will be higher with age.

CEMENTICLES

Cementicles are small calcified bodies lying free in the periodontal ligament and are formed as a result of dystrophic calcifications.

PATHOGENESIS

Cementicles may develop in the following manner:
- Calcification of the epithelial cell rest of Malassez in the periodontal ligament tissue.
- Calcification of the soft tissue between the Sharpey's fiber bundles.
- Fragmentation and detachment of small piece of cementum from the root surface due to excessive force on the tooth.
- Calcification of thrombosed blood capillaries within the periodontal ligament.

Cementicles are not necessarily the mass of true cementum, any calcified tissue including alveolar bone are collectively referred to as cementicles. Their size can increase due to further disposition of calcium.

Cementicles are not usually visible in the radiograph and they do not have any clinical significance.

BIBLIOGRAPHY

1. Applebaum E. Internal resorption of teeth. Dental Cosmos. 1934;76:847.

2. Beaks H. Root resorption and their relation to pathologic bone formation. Int J Orthod Oral Surg. 1936;22:445.
3. Bergenholtz G. Inflammatory response of the dental pulp to bacterial irritation. J Endod. 1981;1:100-4.
4. Bernick S, Nedelman C. Effect of opening on the human pulp. J Endod. 1975;1:88-94.
5. Brown WG. Idiopathic tooth resorption in association with metaplasia. Oral Surg. 1954;7:1298.
6. Clark DC, Woo G, Silver JG, et al. The influence of frequent ingestion of acids in the diet on treatment for dentin sensitivity. J Can Dent Assoc. 1990;56:1101-3.
7. Eccles JD. Dental erosion and diet. J Dent. 1974;2:153-9.
8. Elvery MW, Savage NW, Wood WB. Radiographic study of the broadbeach aboriginal dentition. Am J Phys Anthropol. 1998;107:211-9.
9. Gandar BK, Truelove EL. Dangerous and management of dental erosion. J Contemp Dent Pract. 1996;1:1.
10. Giunta JL. Dental erosion resulting for chewable vitamin C tablets. JADA. 1983;107:253-6.
11. Grippo JO. Abfractions. A new classification of hard tissue lesions of teeth. J Esth Dent. 1991;3:14-8.
12. Hamasha A, Darwazeh A. Prevalence of pulp stones in Jordanian adults. Oral Surg Oral Med Oral Pathol Oral Radio Endod. 1998;86:730-2.
13. Heymann HO, Sturdevant JR, Bayne S, et al. Examining tooth flexure effects. J Am Dent Assoc. 1991;122:41-7.
14. Jarvinen V, Meurman JH, Hyvarinen H, et al. Dental erosion and upper gastrointestinal disorders. Oral Surg Oral Med Oral Pathol. 1988;65:298-303.
15. Jarvinen VK, Rytomaa II, Heinonen OP. Risk factors in dental erosion. J Dent Res. 1991;70:942-7.
16. Kitchen PC, Robinson HB. The abrasiveness of dentifrices as measured on the cortical areas of extracted teeth. J Dent Res. 1948;17:195.
17. Lussi A, Schaffner M, Hotz P, et al. Dental erosion in a population of Swiss adults community. Dent Oral Epidemiol. 1991;19:286-90.
18. Manly RS. The abrasion of cementum and dentin by modern dentifrices. J Dent Res 1941;20:583.
19. Mannerberg F. Salivary factors in cases of erosion odontol. Odontol Revy. 1963;14:156.
20. Maron FS. Enamel erosion resulting from hydrochloric acid tablets. JADA. 1996;127:781-4.
21. Mikola OJ, Baur WH. Cementicles and fragments of cementum in the periodontal membrane. Oral Surg. 1949;2:1063.
22. Milosevic A. Tooth wear: aetiology and presentation. Dent Update. 1998;25:6-11.
23. Mummery JH. The pathology of "Pink spots" on teeth. Br Dent J. 1920;41-300.
24. Neville BW, Damm DD, Allen CM, et al. Abnormalities of teeth. In: Neville BW, Damm DD, Allen CM, Bouquot JE (Eds). Oral and Maxillofacial Pathology. Philadelphia: WB Saunders; 2002. pp. 49-106.
25. Nunn JR. Prevalence of dental erosion and the implication for oral health. J Oral Sci. 1996;104:156-61.
26. Pindborg JJ. Pathology of Dental Hard Tissues. Copenhagen: Munksgaard; 1970. pp. 312-21.
27. Pindborg JJ. Pathology of the Dental Hard Tissues. Philadelphia: WB Saunders Company; 1970.
28. Rabinovitch BZ. Internal resorption. Oral Surg. 1957;10:193.
29. Robinson HB. Abrasion, attrition and erosion of the teeth. Health center J Ohio Univ. 1949;3:21.
30. Smith BG, Knight JK. An index for measuring the wear of teeth. Br Dent J. 1984;156:435-8.
31. Smith BG, Robb ND. The prevalence of tooth wear in 1007 dental patients. J Oral Rehab. 1996;23:232-9.
32. Tamse A, Kaffe I, Littner MM, et al. Statistical evaluation of radiologic survey of pulp stones. J Endod. 1982;8:455-8.
33. The chemical significance of hypercementosis. Oral Surg. 1954;7:79.
34. Vandenberghe JM, Panther B, Gound TG. Pulp stones throughout the dentition of monozygotic twins. Oral Surg Oral Med Oral Pathol Oral Radiol Endod. 1999;87:749-51.

CHAPTER 8

Bacterial, Viral and Fungal Infections

SPECIFIC BACTERIAL INFECTIONS

TUBERCULOSIS

Tuberculosis is a very contagious, chronic, granulomatous bacterial infection caused by *Mycobacterium tuberculosis* or rarely by *Mycobacterium bovis*.

Mycobacteria are acid fast bacilli, size about 2–3 μ × 0.4 μ, straight or slightly curved rods with rounded ends; nonmotile, nonsporing and non-capsulated. Their *acid fastness* is due to the presence of *"mycolic acid"* around the cell.

The incidence of tuberculosis has declined greatly all over the world due to the improvement in living standards, nutritional status and particularly due to the more and more availability of antitubercular drugs. However, the recent observations indicate that the disease is making an alarming and widespread comeback throughout the world, especially in the developed countries. This is partly due to human immunodeficiency virus (HIV) infections and emergence of many drug-resistant mycobacteria.

Pathogenesis (Flowchart 8.1)

Tuberculosis predominantly affects the lungs and the condition is called "pulmonary tuberculosis"; however sometimes the disease can also affect other organs, e.g. kidney, meninges, intestine and oral cavity, etc. and these lesions are called "extrapulmonary tuberculosis". Most of the people make the first contact with the bacteria in childhood through *airborne (droplet)* infections. Less frequently the disease can be caused by ingesting unpasteurized cow's milk infected

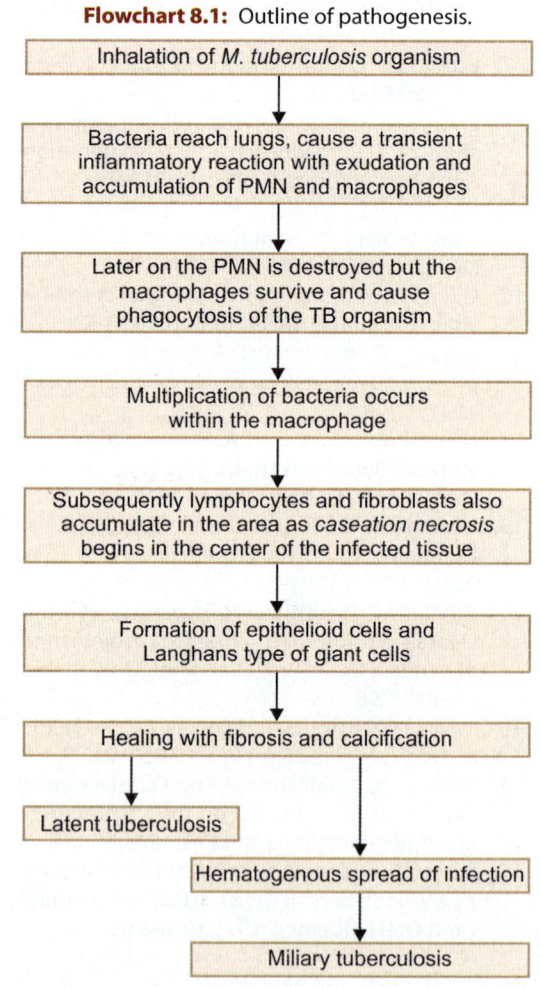

Flowchart 8.1: Outline of pathogenesis.

Inhalation of *M. tuberculosis* organism
↓
Bacteria reach lungs, cause a transient inflammatory reaction with exudation and accumulation of PMN and macrophages
↓
Later on the PMN is destroyed but the macrophages survive and cause phagocytosis of the TB organism
↓
Multiplication of bacteria occurs within the macrophage
↓
Subsequently lymphocytes and fibroblasts also accumulate in the area as *caseation necrosis* begins in the center of the infected tissue
↓
Formation of epithelioid cells and Langhans type of giant cells
↓
Healing with fibrosis and calcification
↓
Latent tuberculosis
↓
Hematogenous spread of infection
↓
Miliary tuberculosis

with *M. bovis* or other atypical mycobacterias. The initial exposure causes tissue hypersensitivity to the bacilli and it results in the development of host–response to the subsequent infections.

Types of Tuberculosis (Based on the Organ System Affected)

- Pulmonary tuberculosis (most common site)
- Extrapulmonary tuberculosis
  - Kidney: Renal tuberculosis
  - Lymph node: Scrofula
  - Bone: Osteomyelitis
  - Meninges: Tubercular meningitis
  - Multiorgan involvement: Miliary tuberculosis
  - Intestine: Intestinal tuberculosis
  - Skin tuberculosis: Lupus vulgaris
    - Mouth: Oral tuberculosis (ulcer, gingivitis, jaw osteomyelitis)
  - Vertebrae: Pott disease.

Clinical Features

- The disease commonly occurs in adult males although children are also often affected.
- *"Pulmonary tuberculosis"* is the most common form and patients often complain of the following:
  - Fever—evening rise of temperature
  - Persistent cough with expectoration
  - Hemoptysis (coughing of blood)
  - Gradual weight loss with anorexia
  - Chest pain, malaise, night sweats and easy fatigability
  - Signs of plural effusion/consolidation/cavitation in the lung.
- The untreated disease in people with low immunity spreads widely in the pulmonary and extra pulmonary organs of the body like bone, brain, kidney, intestine and liver, etc. and at this stage, the disease is known as *"miliary tuberculosis"*.
- *Tuberculous lymphadenopathy (Scrofula)*: Tuberculosis infection in the lymph node

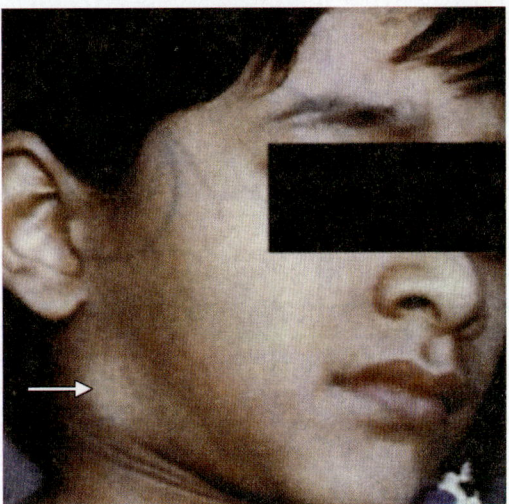

Fig. 8.1: Tuberculous lymphadenopathy (scrofula).

is called *"scrofula"* and usually a group of lymph nodes are involved (Fig. 8.1). The infected lymph nodes are often *enlarged*, with a *rubbery consistency* and are often *matted* in appearance.
- In untreated cases there may be *abscess formation* in these lymph nodes *(cold abscess)* with pain, swelling and development of pus discharging sinus, etc.
- Sometimes calcification occurs in these nodes, which indicates a past, healed disease rather than an active current infection.

Important Oral Lesions of Tuberculosis

- Tuberculous lesions of the oral cavity are rare and mostly occur as a complication of advanced pulmonary disease. Oral lesions mostly occur due to implantation of microorganisms in the oral mucosa during constant coughing. However, primary oral tuberculosis may occur in some cases. The overall incidence of oral tuberculosis is about 0.75–1.44%.
- The most common oral lesion of TB is tuberculous ulcer, besides this there can be some other lesions in the mouth like nonspecific erythema, chronic fissure,

> **Box 8.1 Oral manifestations of tuberculosis.**
> - Tuberculous ulcers
> - Tuberculous patches
> - Tuberculous gingivitis
> - Tuberculous nodules
> - Tuberculous osteomyelitis or simple bone radiolucency
> - Tuberculosis of the salivary glands
> - Tuberculosis of the lymph nodes
> - Tuberculous tonsillitis

granulomas or verrucal-papillary lesions (Box 8.1).

- *Tuberculous ulcer*: Tuberculous ulcers are most commonly seen on the mid-dorsum of the tongue, other sites include the gingiva, lips and palate, etc. The ulcers typically have undermined edges and are well-defined, superficial with irregular margins (Fig. 8.2). It is painless in the early stage but may become painful later. The base or floor of the ulcer is often granular with a yellowish-gray color. Tuberculous ulcers in the mouth are often not associated with cervical lymphadenopathy (Fig. 8.3A).
- *Tuberculous gingivitis*: Tuberculosis may produce erosive lesions with concomitant gingival hyperplasia along with nodular or papillary projections from the marginal gingiva.
- *Tuberculous lesions of salivary gland*: The infection may involve either the salivary gland tissue itself or it may affect the intra- or periglandular lymph nodes. There can be generalized glandular swelling or abscess formation along with pain, facial nerve palsy and fistulas tract formations, etc.
- *Tuberculous lesions of jaw bone*: Tuberculous infection may cause chronic osteomyelitis in the maxilla and mandible and in such cases the infection reaches the bone via the bloodstream or root canals of tooth or via the extraction sockets (Fig. 8.3B). Tuberculous osteomyelitis of the jaw bones clinically produce pain, swelling, sinus or

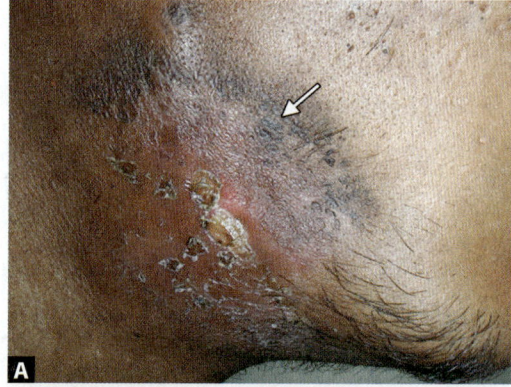

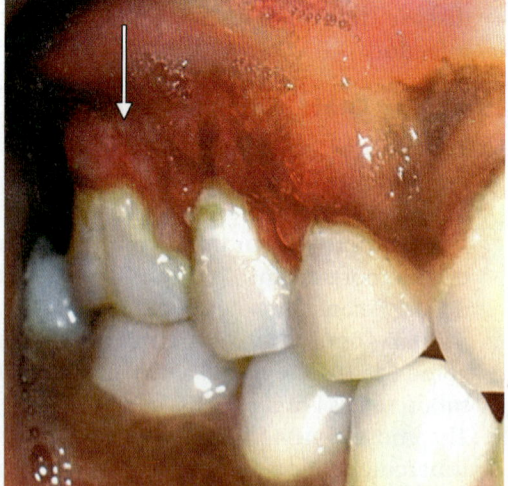

Fig. 8.2: Tubercular gingivitis with erosive lesion and areas of hyperplasia.

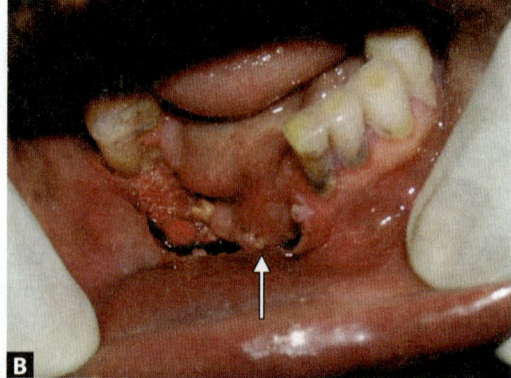

Figs. 8.3A and B: (A) Tuberculous lymph node (scrofula) with surface ulcer; (B) Tuberculous osteomyelitis.

fistula formation, trismus, paresthesia and lymphadenopathy.

Differential Diagnosis of Oral Tuberculous Lesions

- Squamous cell carcinoma
- Sarcoidosis
- Syphilis
- Aphthous ulcer
- Deep mycotic infections
- Traumatic ulcer
- Wegner's granulomatosis
- Tularemia
- Foreign body reaction.

Histopathology of Tuberculous Lesions

Microscopy reveals multiple tuberculous granulomas, which form in the connective tissue underlying an ulcer with undermined margins. Individual granuloma has the following character:
- Rounded outline
- Central caseous necrosis—appears eosinophilic with Hematoxylin and Eosin staining.
- Epithelioid cells—transformed macrophages looking like epithelial cells with ill-defined borders (occurs when macrophages cause phagocytosis of the tuberculous bacilli).
- Multinucleated "Langhans type" of giant cells: These giant cells form when multiple epithelioid cells fuse together; they have a typical horse-shoe shaped nuclear orientation.
- Chronic inflammatory cell infiltration: Mostly lymphocytes and plasma cells
- Peripheral fibrosis: The granuloma is usually surrounded by fibrous tissue, lymphocytes and plasma cells. They may undergo complete fibrosis and dystrophic calcification (Gohn complex).
- In some cases, tuberculous bacilli may be detected within the tissue in histologic sections (Figs. 8.4 to 8.6).

The important investigations in tuberculosis are given in Box 8.2.

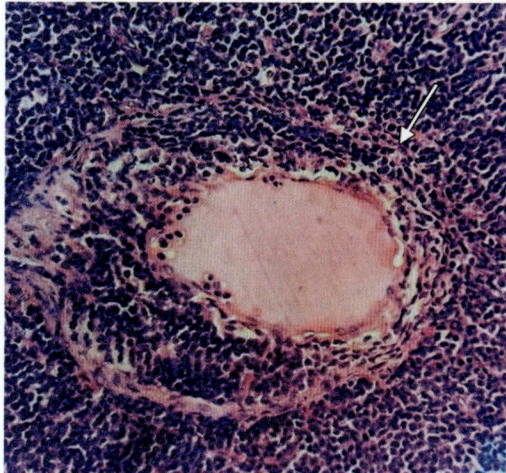

Fig. 8.4: Tuberculous lymph node with central caseous necrosis surrounded by epithelioid cells, Langhans type giant cells and lymphocytes.

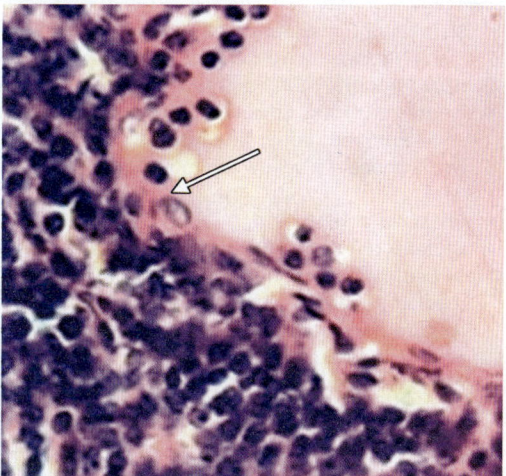

Fig. 8.5: Photomicrograph of TB showing "epithelioid cells".

Treatment

By antitubercular drugs, e.g. rifampicin, isoniazid, streptomycin, ethambutol, etc. in different standard regimens.

SYPHILIS (LUES)

Syphilis is a sexually transmitted disease (STD) caused by infection with a spirochete

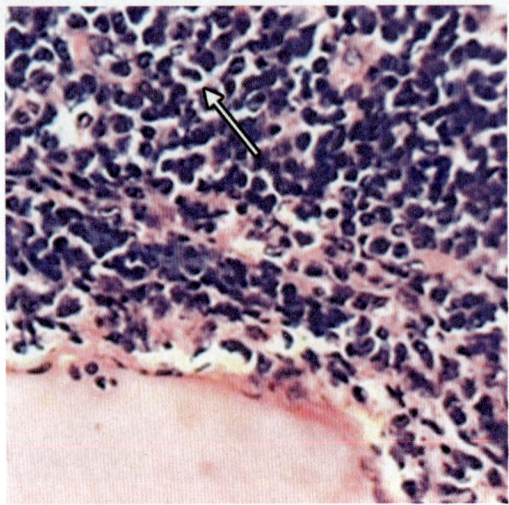

Fig. 8.6: Langhans type of giant cell.

Box 8.2	Investigations in tuberculosis.

- Staining of the smear prepared from sputum by Ziehl–Neelsen stain (bacilli appear red with blue background)
- Fluorescent stain: Smear stained with auramine and observed under fluorescent microscope. Bacilli appear as "yellow luminous rods" in a dark field
- Chest radiograph
- Bacterial culture in solid medium, e.g. Lowenstein-Jensen medium or in liquid medium, e.g. Dubos medium (materials used for culture may be sputum, laryngeal swab, gastric lavage, urine, cerebrospinal fluid and pus, etc.)
- Animal inoculation
- Histopathology
- Tuberculin test
- Enzyme-linked immunosorbent assay (ELISA) test
- PCR (polymerase chain reaction)

named *Treponema pallidum*. The disease is generally classified into two types:
1. Acquired syphilis
2. Congenital syphilis.

Acquired Syphilis

It is mostly contracted by venereal means, e.g. sexual intercourse with an infected partner, but in many cases, the disease may be acquired innocently by professionals like dental surgeons, nurses or other individuals while carelessly handling the infected patients.

The acquired syphilis manifests in three stages:
1. Primary syphilis
2. Secondary syphilis
3. Tertiary (late) syphilis.

Clinical Features of Syphilis

Primary Syphilis

General features (Box 8.3)
- There is an asymptomatic incubation period averaging about 21 days.
- The clinical symptoms appear at the site of inoculation, i.e. male and female genitalia and extragenital site like-fingers, perianal region and nipples, etc. (at these sites the spirochetes undergo rapid replication and enter into the lymphatics or blood stream).
- The characteristic primary lesion of syphilis is called "chancre" and it is a solitary, painless, indurated, non-tendered, non-hemorrhagic, ulcerated or eroded lesion.

Box 8.3	Oral manifestations of primary syphilis.

- Oral lesion of primary syphilis is called *"chancre"* which generally occurs 3 weeks after the contact with the organism.
- Most of the oral lesions occur on the lip (upper lip for males and lower lip for females); the other sites include tongue, palate, gingiva, uvula, tonsils, etc.
- The oral lesions of primary syphilis start as a painless nodule of about 1 centimeter in diameter, which gradually exhibits breakdown of the surface with development of an ulcer. The ulcers have indurated margins and are often covered by a grayish-white membrane. Tongue lesions often form on the dorsum of tongue and often there is enlargement of folate papilla.
- The chancres are often mistaken for oral squamous cell carcinomas.
- *STM—typical sites in the tongue: Syphilitic ulcer on "surface" (dorsum), tubercular ulcer at the "Tip" and malignant ulcer (carcinoma) at the "Margin" (lateral border).*

- The primary lesion appears between 3 and 90 days after the initial exposure.
- Initially the chancre starts as a dull red macule or papule, which later on becomes eroded or ulcerated.
- Regional lymph nodes are enlarged, painless and are rubbery in consistency.
- Both the chancre and the lymphadenopathy resolve within 6–8 weeks.

Secondary Syphilis

General features (Box 8.4)
- Secondary syphilis usually appears in about 6–8 weeks after the appearance of the primary chancre.
- This stage occurs due to the generalized hematogenous dissemination of the infection in the body.
- Secondary syphilis is generally characterized by skin lesions, mucosal lesions and few constitutional symptoms along with generalized lymphadenopathy.
- The skin lesions appear as diffuse painless macular, papular, follicular, lenticular or papulosquamous patches or rashes.

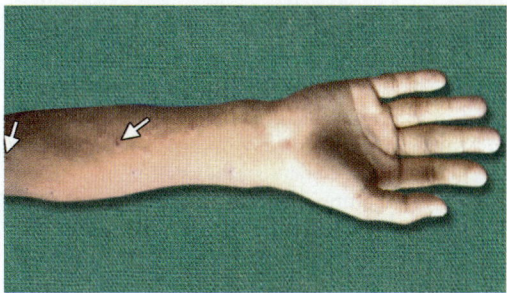

Fig. 8.7: "Coin-like" circular skin rashes of secondary syphilis.

- Skin lesions may also occur in the form of nodular, flat or papillary condition; which often resembles the viral papilloma, called condyloma lata.
- Circinate (coin-like) lesions on the face are characteristic of secondary syphilis (Fig. 8.7).
- Moreover there can be development of moist flat, papulonodular lesions at the mucocutaneous junctions and over the mucosal surfaces of genitalia.
- Areas of hyperpigmentations or hypopigmentations may be seen on the palms and soles.
- Constitutional symptoms associated with secondary syphilis include—malaise, headache, sore throat, anorexia, weight loss, fever, joint and muscle pain, laryngitis and pharyngitis, etc.
- Sometimes immunocompromised patients may exhibit a widespread and explosive form of secondary syphilis called "lues maligna"; characterized by large atypical necrotic ulcers of the face, scalp and oral mucosa, etc.

Tertiary (Late) Syphilis

General features (Box 8.5)
- Tertiary syphilis (third stage of the disease) usually occurs about 5–10 years after the primary infections; it affects nearly every organ of the body and this stage is associated with the most severe forms of systemic complications.

Box 8.4 Oral manifestations of secondary syphilis.

- The secondary lesions are mucocutaneous in nature and they usually occur 6–8 weeks after the primary infection.
- The oral lesions in this stage are called *"mucous patches"*, and these are commonly seen over the tongue, lips, buccal mucosa, gingiva, tonsils and palate, etc.
- These patches exhibit multiple, flat, irregular or circular, slightly raised, painless, white round erosions.
- Mucous patches are covered by a thin yellowish-gray (glistening) slough and are surrounded by a painful erythematous halo.
- Multiple "mucous patches" sometimes coalesce together to form irregularly linear "snail track" like ulcers. This stage is also contagious.
- Some moist papules are often seen at the angle of the mouth and they have a typical "split pea" like appearance.
- In secondary syphilis the tongue is often fissured.

> **Box 8.5** Oral manifestations of tertiary syphilis.
>
> - Intraoral lesions of tertiary syphilis are called "*gumma*" and are commonly seen on the hard and soft palate, tonsils, lips and tongue, etc.
> - These lesions begin as firm, small, pale, nodular masses in the midline of the palate.
> - They frequently ulcerate by central necrosis and produce painless, deep, rounded ulcers; which have punched-out edges and a wash-leathery floor.
> - Progressive necrosis and sloughing often leads to perforation of the palate and this is a very characteristic finding in tertiary syphilis.
> - Destruction of the soft palate and uvula may result in airway obstruction.
> - Tertiary syphilis causes *baldness* of tongue (*syphilitic glossitis*).
> - Many large, irregular leukoplakic patches develop on the dorsum of tongue (*syphilitic leukoplakia*). This stage of the disease is not contagious.
> - In tertiary syphilis, destruction of the nasal septum and collapse of the nasal cartilage results in "*saddle-nose*".

- It mainly affects skin, mucous membrane, CNS and cardiovascular systems. Besides this, muscles, bones and joints are also frequently affected.
- Typical lesion of tertiary syphilis is called "gumma", which is a localized, indurated, chronic granulomatous lesion; having either nodular or ulcerated surfaces. Moreover this lesion is also associated with extensive tissue destruction in the affected organs.
- Granulomatous ulcerative lesion often appears as a "punched-out" ulcer, having vertical walls and a dull red granulomatous base with an irregular outline.
- Skin lesions heal very slowly and often they leave "tissue paper" like scars.
- Tertiary syphilis occurring in pregnancy often results in congenital syphilis of the newborn.
- This disease also frequently occurs in association with AIDS.
- The most serious complication of tertiary syphilis is the destruction of the walls of large blood vessels, aneurysm of the arch of aorta, left ventricular hypertrophy and congestive cardiac failure, etc.
- Involvement of central nervous system (neurosyphilis) results in generalized paresis, dementia and strokes.
- Bone lesions cause osteomyelitis and destructions of the joints.

Congenital Syphilis

Definition

Congenital syphilis is a rare entity that occurs in children born of an infected mother. The condition occurs due to transplacental infection with *Treponema pallidum* during fetal development.

Pathogenesis of Congenital Syphilis

- In infected women, the organisms pass from mother to the fetus (before 5th month of gestation) and infection involve placenta and spread diffusely via blood inside the fetal body (Sometimes the infection may be contracted by the fetus during passage through the birth canal).
- Involvement of the developing tooth germs by *T. pallidum* is very common in congenital syphilis; the organisms cause inflammation in and around the tooth germs and results in hyperplasia of the epithelium of the enamel organ, particularly during the stage of morphodifferentiation. This is the reason why there are significant changes in the shape and size of teeth in congenital syphilis.

Clinical Features of Congenital Syphilis

The features of congenital syphilis may be divided into two groups—(1) early congenital syphilis and (2) late congenital syphilis.

Early congenital syphilis: Clinical manifestations occur within first 2 years of life and the features include the following:
- Hepatosplenomegaly
- Jaundice
- Generalized lymphadenopathy

- Maculopapular rashes
- Vesiculobullous eruptions on the palms and soles (pemphigus syphiliticus)
- Petechial spots
- Bony lesions like osteochondritis and periosteitis
- Desquamation.

Late congenital syphilis: Clinical manifestations after 2 years of life and the features include:

Hutchinson's triad (involving three structures—teeth, nerve and the eye): It is the pathognomonic feature of congenital syphilis, which involves three tissue:

1. Teeth: Hypoplasia of teeth, characterized by *screwdriver-shaped incisors*, also called Hutchinson's (notched) teeth and "peg laterals"; and *mulberry molars* (also known as Moon's molars). Deciduous teeth are more often affected than the permanent teeth.
2. Nerve: Eighth nerve deafness.
3. Eye: Interstitial keratitis of the eye characterized by corneal opacity and loss of vision.
   - The screwdriver-shaped incisors typically exhibit wide middle-third of the crown with tapered incisal edges and notched incisal edge. Peg-shaped lateral are also commonly seen.
   - The mulberry molars appear yellowish in color, the teeth have smaller occlusal table due to tapering of crowns; there is often presence of numerous globular projections from the occlusal surface, which resemble the surface of *"mulberries"*(hence the name mulberry molars is given).

Other features of congenital syphilis include:
- Clutton's joints (synovitis and restricted movements)
- Mental retardation
- Hydrocephalus
- Frontal bossing
- Saddle nose (bull-dog nose)—flat nose due to collapse of the nasal bridge
- Short maxilla with high arched palate
- Mandibular prognathism and increased interdental spaces
- Higoumenakis' sign—unilateral enlargement of clavicle due to neonatal periostitis
- Saber shins—sharp anterior bowing of tibia
- Rhagades—fissures, cracks or linear scars on the skin, mostly around the mouth and nose (due to Treponemal skin infection)
- Delayed eruptions of teeth
- Hypodontia and enamel hypoplasia.

Histopathology of Acquired Syphilitic Lesions

Primary syphilis

The chancre histologically presents the following features:
- A proliferative granulation tissue is present at the margin of the ulcer.
- Dense infiltrates of plasma cells, lymphocytes and macrophages.
- Obliterative endarteritis with perivascular infiltration of chronic inflammatory cells.
- *T. pallidum* may be seen when immunofluorescent studies or silver staining are done.

Secondary syphilis
- The macular lesion shows inflammatory cell infiltration and obliterating endarteritis.
- The papular lesion exhibits endothelial proliferation, swelling and perivascular chronic inflammatory cells infiltration.
- Condyloma lata reveals hyperplastic epithelium with hyperkeratosis and acanthosis.
- Obliterative endarteritis may also be seen and there may be occasional presence of epithelioid cells.

Tertiary syphilis
- The gumma microscopically presents a peripheral rim made up of fibroblasts, which surrounds a central zone of coagulative necrosis.
- Fibroblasts are plump and they often resemble epithelioid cells.

- Occasional presence of giant cells and regular presence of chronic inflammatory cells like plasma cells, lymphocytes and histiocytes, etc.

Diagnosis
- Detection of bacteria in smear by dark ground illumination microscopy.
- Bacterial culture in artificial media.
- Serological tests like Washerman reaction, Khan test, venereal disease research laboratory (VDRL) test, fluorescent treponemal antibody test (FTA), rapid plasma reagin (RPR) test, microhemagglutination assay-*T. pallidum* (MHA-TP) test
- ELISA
- Histopathology.

Treatment
High doses of penicillin.

GONORRHEA

Definition

Gonorrhea is a STD caused by *Neisseria gonorrhoeae* bacteria; the disease is often called "the clap". The microorganisms are often present in the moist part of the body, e.g. vagina, penis, eyes, throat and rectum, etc. The disease affects both males and females; and it can be spread through all forms of sexual activity including oral, vaginal and rectal sex.

Clinical Features

- Age: People of any age group can be affected; however, it is more prevalent in the age group of 15–30 years.
- Sex: Both sexes can be affected; however a man having sex with an infected woman has 30–50% chance of becoming infected, whereas a woman having sex with an infected partner has a higher (60–90) percentage of risk of getting infected.

  Moreover as the women do not develop many clinical symptoms of the disease like men, the disease often remains undetected and it can have a devastating effect on the reproductive system in these women. In gonorrhea, most of the lesions develop in the genital areas.

  The symptoms occur 2–10 days after the initial contact with the bacteria via the infected partner.

> **Box 8.6** Symptoms of gonorrhea in men.
> - Yellow, white or green pus-like discharge from tip of the penis
> - Fever and vomiting
> - Redness of the glans penis
> - Swelling of the testicles
> - Stinging during urination
> - Presence of blood in urine and frequent urination
> - Swelling of the lymph nodes in the groin region

> **Box 8.7** Symptoms of gonorrhea in women.
> - The initial infection occurs in the uterine cervix, however in severe cases it spreads to the deeper structures, e.g. uterus and ovarian tube
> - Bleeding during intercourse and pain
> - Fever and vomiting
> - Abnormal intermenstrual bleeding
> - Vaginal discharge
> - Pain in the abdomen
> - Burning or itching sensation during urination

Clinical Presentation of Gonorrhea

The important symptoms of gonorrhea in men and women are given in Boxes 8.6 and 8.7, respectively.

Oral Manifestations of Gonorrhea (Fig. 8.8)

- Oral lesions mostly occur due to fellatio and these mostly develop in the oropharynx, tonsils and uvula, etc.
- Diffuse erythema in the oropharynx with sore throat.
- Erythema, edema and discharge of pus from one or both tonsils.
- Cervical lymphadenopathy.
- Vomiting tendency due to irritation and soreness in the throat.
- Difficulty in swallowing.

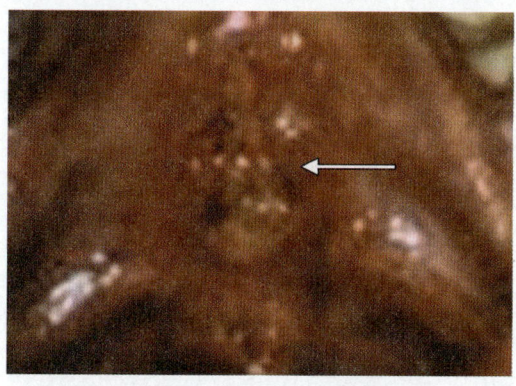

Fig. 8.8: Oral lesion of gonorrhea.

Diagnosis of Gonorrhea

- *Neisseria gonorrhoeae* can be demonstrated by gram staining and it appears as a gram negative diplococcus under microscope.
- Bacterial culture of the samples obtained from the purulent discharge. Thayer Martin agar medium is commonly used.
- Sugar fermentation test: *Neisseria gonorrhoeae* produces acid by fermentation of sugar, this is an important criteria for detection of the organism and for this a test called "Cystine Trypticase Agar (CTA) test is often done.
- Identification of bacterial DNA from the urine samples of the patient.

Treatment

High doses of antibiotics.

ACTINOMYCOSIS

Actinomycosis is a chronic granulomatous, suppurative and fibrosing infection; it was very common in the past but nowadays has become rare. The disease is caused by filamentous, gram positive, anaerobic actinomycotic group of organisms, namely *Actinomyces israelii, A naeslundii, A. bovis, A. odontolyticus* and *A. viscosus*, etc.

Types

Actinomycosis predominantly occurs in three forms:

1. Cervicofacial actinomycosis.
2. Abdominal actinomycosis.
3. Pulmonary actinomycosis.

The cervicofacial actinomycosis is the most common form (occurs almost in 50% cases) of the disease.

Pathogenesis

The disease is more common among cultivators. Normally *A. israelii* and other members of the family are present as normal inhabitants of the oral cavity and the tonsillar crypts; besides these areas they can be present within carious teeth, infected dental pulp and calculus deposits, etc. Infection often develops as the microorganisms take entry into the deeper tissues following tooth extraction, root canal treatment, trauma and jaw fracture, etc. The infection may also occur in presence of certain oral diseases like—periapical granuloma and pericoronitis, etc. Moreover, the actinomycotic group of organisms can also cause infection in combination with *Staphylococcus* and *Streptococcus*, etc.

Clinical Features

- Age: The disease occurs mostly in the 4th and 5th decade of life.
- Sex: More prevalent among males.
- Site: The disease commonly involves the jaw bones, upper neck and salivary glands, etc.

Presentation

- Initially, the disease starts as a soft tissue swelling over the upper part of the neck or below the ear, or near the angle of mandible with intense pain.
- The overlying skin appears dusky-red or bluish-red; which is firm and slightly tendered on palpation.
- The skin lesion is often classically described as "wooden indurated area of fibrosis".
- Later on, the swelling becomes fluctuant at the center and some areas of the skin gradually break down to produce multiple

pus discharging sinuses. Similar sinuses can also be seen intraorally.
- The pus contains clinically visible, small, yellowish-green granules which are known as "sulfur granules" and each of them represents a colony of organisms.
- The pus discharging sinuses heal-up with fibrosis but later on, some new sinuses appear in the region and the process continues for years. This leads to the formation of many disfiguring scars in the area with development of trismus.

Oral Manifestations

- The tonsillar tissue is most frequently affected along with buccal mucosa, submandibular and submental areas.
- Tonsillar lesions often cause tonsillar hyperplasia.
- There can be painful swelling of the salivary glands (mostly parotid and submandibular glands) followed by abscess formation.
- Trismus is a constant feature of this disease which develops before the pus formation begins.
- The abscess also can form in the submandibular and submasseteric spaces, which can further intensify the trismus.
- Involvement of the jaw bones by this disease often results in chronic osteomyelitis.
- Periapical abscess and granulomas frequently develop which cause pain, swelling in the jaw with formation of draining sinuses.
- The periapical lesions in actinomycosis frequently affect the maxillary anterior teeth and the mandibular molars.
- Actinomycosis infections do not spread to the lymph nodes; however the lymphadenopathy associated with the disease may be due to secondary infections caused by some other organisms.

Histopathology (Fig. 8.9)

- The cervicofacial actinomycosis microscopically exhibits chronic suppurative

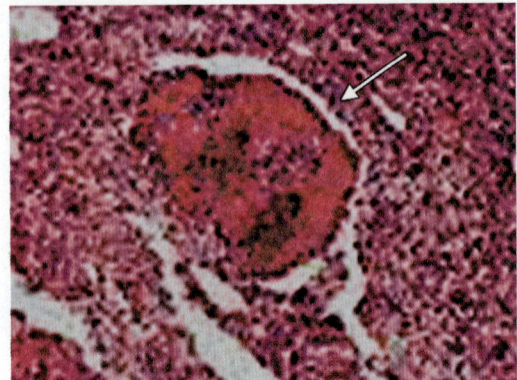

Fig. 8.9: Photomicrograph of actinomycosis.

inflammation in the affected tissue with formation of numerous abscesses; whose centers are typically occupied by the bacterial colonies.
- The abscess eventually drains through discharging sinuses over the skin and the pus often contains the so called "sulfur granules" which are nothing but colonies of actinomyces.
- The bacterial colonies in actinomycosis are characteristic and they often help in making the diagnosis; each colony is consisting of dense, eosinophilic mass of gram-positive filaments, as these club shaped filaments are arranged in a radiating rosette pattern, the colonies often produce a typical "ray fungus" like appearance.
- The colonies are gradually surrounded by polymorphonuclear neutrophils (PMN) followed by mononuclear cells (lymphocytes and plasma cells) and multinucleated giant cells. At the periphery the colonies are surrounded by a fibrous tissue wall.
- Bone tissue often exhibits extensive necrosis with multiple areas of granuloma formations.

Diagnosis

Actinomycosis is a rare disease and its diagnosis can be made in the following manner:

- Detection of sulfur granules from the pus.
- "Ray fungus" appearance of the bacterial colony
- Bacterial culture
- Immunofluorescence.

Treatment

By high doses of any of these drugs like penicillin, cephalosporin, clindamycin and lincomycin, etc.

STREPTOCOCCAL INFECTIONS

Impetigo

Impetigo is a superficial skin infection, often seen in children between 2 years and 6 years of age; it is mostly caused by *Streptococcus pyogenes* and sometimes by *Staphylococcus aureus*. Normally the Streptococcal organisms are often present on the skin surface and the infection begins when the microorganisms get inside the skin through some cuts, scratch, dermatitis or insect bite, etc. Infection can also spread by direct contact with wound or its secretions from an infected person. Outbreaks of this infection may be seen in unhygienic living conditions, and hot and humid climates.

Clinical Features

- Most common sites are skin over the face, arms and legs.
- The symptoms begin with erythematous macule over the skin followed by rapidly developing numerous small "pimple-like" pustules (Fig. 8.10).
- In other cases, longer lasting flaccid vesicles may also develop on the skin.
- As the pustules rupture, shallow erosions form covered with drying serum and this often produces a typical *yellow or honey colored crust*.
- If the crust is not removed, new lesions develop around the old pustules, thus causing extensive spread of the disease.
- Pruritus and regional lymphadenopathy may develop but fever is generally absent.

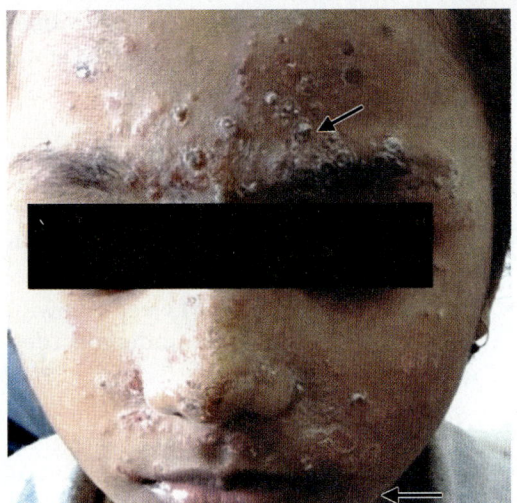

Fig. 8.10: Impetigo on the facial skin.

Treatment

Administration of antibiotics, especially *penicillin*.

Scarlet Fever

Scarlet fever is a rare specific bacterial disease caused by *Streptococcus B-haemolyticus* and it commonly occurs in children. The disease mostly begins in the throat with the development of tonsillitis and pharyngitis; but as the infection becomes systemically disseminated, the bacteria release erythrogenic toxins, which attack the blood vessels of the skin and produce the typical "skin rash".

Clinical Features

- The disease affects children between the ages of 3 years and 12 years.
- Fever, headache, vomiting, tonsillitis, pharyngitis and generalized lymphadenopathy, etc.
- The tonsils, soft palate and pharynx become erythematous and these areas often exhibit a yellowish exudation.
- A diffuse, bright red skin rash appears on the second or third day of the disease that starts on the chest and gradually spreads to the other body surfaces. The rash

occurs as a result of damage of the small superficial blood vessels by erythrogenic toxins liberated by the bacteria.
- Once the skin rash appears it becomes widespread within 24 hours and the rash is referred to as "sunburn with goose pimples".
- The lips, nose and chin, etc. are generally not involved.
- Skin rashes last for about 1 week following which the affected area undergoes desquamation.

Oral Manifestations

- The skin rash is particularly more noticeable over the face and the face is flushed, except for a zone of circumoral pallor.
- The oral cavity exhibits generalized edema, elongation of uvula and diffuse petechiae especially over the soft palate.
- The palate appears congested and inflamed, the hard palate exhibits punctiform redness, while the soft palate may have scattered petechial spots.
- During the first 2 days of the disease the tongue becomes covered with a white coat; through which only the enlarged and reddened fungiform papillae project like small, red knobs. This phenomenon is called "strawberry tongue".
- By the 4th or 5th day of the disease the white coating over the dorsum of the tongue is lost by desquamation; the tongue appears beefy red in color with many hyperplastic fungiform papillae and the condition is called "raspberry tongue".

Oral complications of scarlet fever: Several oral complications develop as the consequences of scarlet fever and these include cancrum oris, ulceration with perforation of the palate, osteomyelitis, peritonsillar abscess, mastoiditis and temporomandibular joint disturbances, etc.

Systemic Complications of Scarlet Fever

The disease usually subsides within a week or 10 days, but complications may occur in few cases due to the bacterial metastasis or hypersensitivity reactions.

These complications include pneumonia, meningitis, rheumatic fever, acute glomerulonephritis and septicemia, etc.

Rheumatic fever causes permanent damage to the heart valves and patients in future may become susceptible to subacute bacterial endocarditis.

Treatment

Administration of penicillin or erythromycin.

■ DIPHTHERIA

Diphtheria is a life-threatening acute bacterial infection caused by *Corynebacterium diphtheriae*, which commonly affects the children. The name *diphtheria* came from the word "diphtheros" (meaning—leather), as the disease produces "characteristic tough, leathery pseudomembrane". Humans are sole reservoir of these microorganisms and the infection can be acquired through contact with an infected person or a carrier.

Clinical Features

- The clinical manifestations begin to appear about 1–5 days after the initial contact with the infective organism.
- The disease starts with low-grade fever, malaise, vomiting, anorexia, headache, and lymphadenopathy, etc.
- There is extreme difficulty in taking food or drink due to severe sore-throat.
- The bacteria release strong exotoxin, which cause widespread damage to the various mucosal surfaces as well as the skin.
- The mucosal damage often causes exudation from the nasal, tonsillar, laryngeal, tracheal and pharyngeal areas.
- Initially exudation in the tonsillar area produces a thin, patchy yellowish-white film; which gradually thickens and later on forms a thick, fibrinous, grayish "pseudomembrane" or "diphtheric patch" (Fig. 8.11) that spreads over the tonsils, larynx, pharynx and uvula, etc.

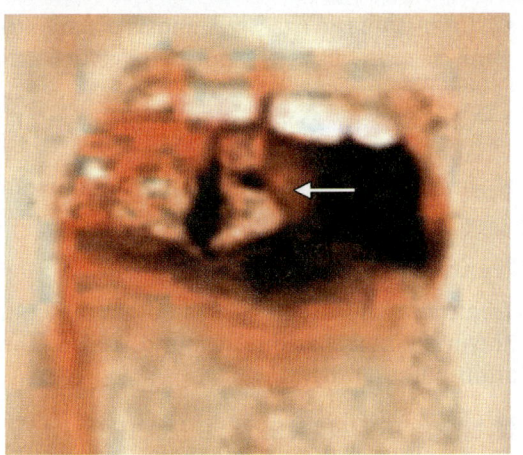

Fig. 8.11: Diphtheric patch in the throat.

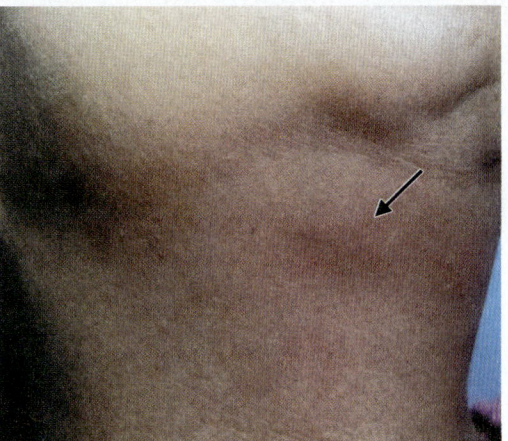

Fig. 8.12: Lymph node swelling in sarcoidosis.

- Development of this pseudomembrane (patch) is the most important clinical characteristic of diphtheria; the patch is very adherent and often difficult to remove. Whenever the patch is stripped off or is removed, it leaves a bleeding surface.
- In untreated cases the patch may cover the entire soft palate, uvula, larynx and trachea; which may cause respiratory obstruction and even death due to blockade of the airway.
- Paralysis of the soft palate may cause nasal regurgitations during swallowing; and there may be nasal intonation of voice.
- There may be severe cervical lymphadenopathy along with edematous swelling of the neck; and the later condition is often known as "bull neck".
- In diphtheria, complications may arise in the heart (myocarditis), nervous system and kidney, etc. during or after the disease.

Treatment

Diphtheria antitoxin injection, in combination with antibiotics.

SARCOIDOSIS

Sarcoidosis is a multisystem chronic granulomatous disease of unknown etiology; which resembles the tuberculosis in many respects.

Clinical Features

- The disease commonly affects the young adults between the ages of 20 years and 40 years; it affects females more than the males.
- The body organs which are often involved in sarcoidosis include the lymph nodes (Fig. 8.12), salivary glands, skin and bone, etc.
- Fever, malaise, dry cough, weight loss, chest pain and dyspnea, etc. are the usual symptoms of the disease.
- There may be multiple, slow growing, red patches occurring on the skin, which tend to ulcerate.
- In sarcoidosis, granulomatous lesions may also arise in relation to other organs such as kidney, GI tract, heart, liver, spleen and nervous system, etc.

Oral Manifestations (Fig. 8.13)

- Involvement of the lacrimal glands may produce a typical "keratoconjunctivitis" like symptoms.
- In the oral region, parotid gland is often (unilaterally or bilaterally) enlarged with concomitant facial nerve paralysis.
- There may be involvement of the minor salivary glands; which results in swelling and xerostomia.

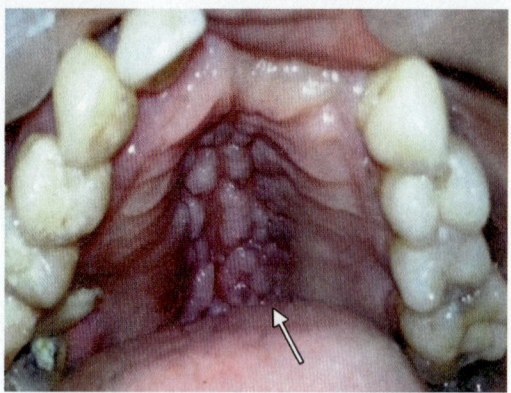

Fig 8.13: Sarcoidosis with nodular growths on palate.

- Occasionally small nodular submucosal growths over the soft palate, gingiva, floor of the mouth or cheek may be seen.
- Multiple erythematous nodules may develop over the cheek, labial mucosa and hard palate.
- In rare cases, central lesions in the maxilla, mandible or nasal bones may occur in sarcoidosis.

Histopathology

In the orofacial region, biopsy samples are usually obtained from the minor salivary glands.
- The microscopic picture of sarcoidosis reveals multiple, circumscribed, noncaseating granulomas within the affected organ.
- The granulomas are often consisting of clustered epithelioid cells, lymphocytes and multiple multinucleated giant cells.
- The giant cells are either Langhans type or foreign body type.
- The granulomas often contain star-shaped "asteroid bodies" or basophilic calcified "Schaumann bodies" (these are various inclusion bodies).

Diagnosis

- Elevated serum angiotensin-converting enzyme (ACE).
- In most of the cases, diagnosis of sarcoidosis is established by positive Kveim-Siltzbach skin test.
- Chest X-rays reveal bilateral hilar lymphadenopathy.
- Jaw X-rays reveal ill-defined radiolucent lesions with erosion of the cortical bone.

Treatment

Treatment of sarcoidosis is often difficult, however, many lesions respond well to the antitubercular drugs.

LEPROSY/HANSEN DISEASE

Leprosy is a chronic granulomatous infection caused by *Mycobacterium leprae* which primarily affects the skin and peripheral nerves.

This slightly contagious disease is broadly divided into four types—(1) tuberculoid leprosy, (2) lepromatous leprosy, (3) borderline leprosy and (4) intermediate leprosy. The disease progresses through the stages of invasion, proliferation, ulceration and resolution through fibrosis.

Clinical Features

- Multiple macules, papules or nodules develop over the facial skin (Fig. 8.14).

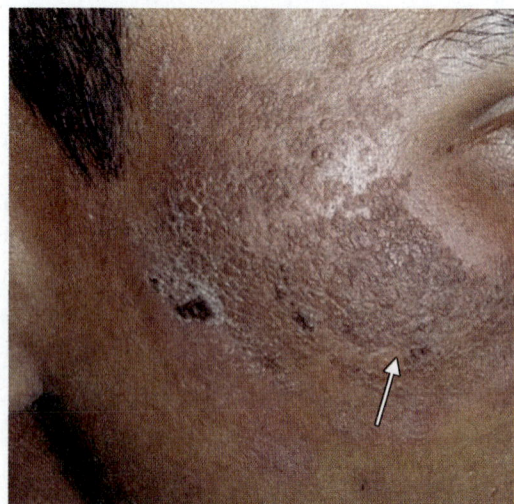

Fig. 8.14: Diffuse, dry macules and papules on facial skin in leprosy.

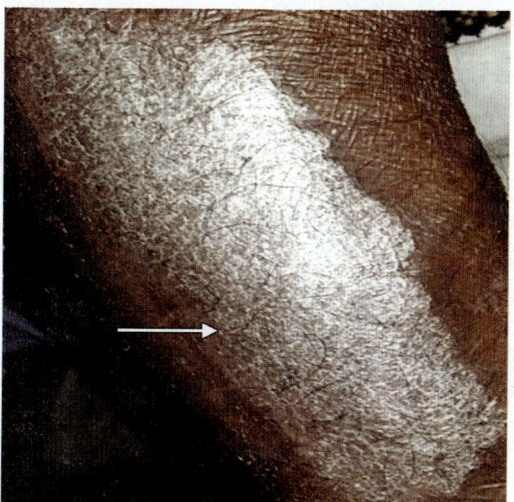

Fig. 8.15: Dry, wrinkled and burn-out shiny patches on skin in leprosy.

- Enlargement of these facial lesions causes considerable distortion in the facial appearance (leonine facies).
- Dry, wrinkled and burn-out shiny patches on skin of the body with absence of sweating (Fig. 8.15).
- Nose is very frequently damaged by the disease and it results in epistaxis, loss of nasal hard tissue with collapse of the nasal bridge and loss of sensation of smell.
- Loss of sensations in affected area as the nerves are destroyed.
- Facial and trigeminal paralysis are common, which results in loss of light touch, temperature and pressure sensations.
- Loss of hair including those of the eyebrows and eye lashes.
- Difficulty in closing the eyes resulting in corneal ulceration, keratitis and occasional blindness.

The oral manifestations of leprosy are given in Box 8.8.

Histopathology

- Microscopically the lesion shows granulomatous nodules consisting of epithelioid cells, lymphocytes, Langhans-type giant cells and vacuolated macrophages called "lepra cells".
- Nerves are infiltrated and destroyed.
- Acid fast bacilli may be seen within the nerves or within the macrophages.

Diagnosis

By determination of acid fast bacilli (*M. leprae*) in the smear or in the tissue.

Treatment

Treatment is done by long-term chemotherapy.

TETANUS

Tetanus is a serious type of bacterial disease caused by the bacteria named *Clostridium*

Box 8.8   Oral manifestations of leprosy.

- In the oral cavity, the disease produces tumor-like lesions called *"lepromas"*, which are found on the lips, gingiva, tongue, buccal mucosa, hard and soft palate, etc.
- Oral lesions appear as yellowish, soft or hard, sessile papules, which have a tendency to breakdown and ulcerate over time
- Repeated ulcerations in the mouth and attempted healing every time thereafter lead to ugly scarring and loss of tissue
- Ulcerations, necrosis and perforation of the palate are common
- Fixation of the soft palate with loss of uvula is also seen in some cases
- Difficulty in swallowing as regurgitation often occur
- Erosive lesions develop over the tongue followed by formation of large lobules; which gives a typical *"cobble-stone"* appearance of the tongue with loss of taste sensation
- Lip lesions cause severe disfigurement with development of macrocheilia
- Chronic gingivitis and periodontitis frequently seen
- Increased tendency for the development of candidiasis
- Enamel hypoplasia of teeth with pinkish-red discoloration and pulpitis
- Tapering of teeth, increased destruction of alveolar bone with premature loss of anterior teeth (especially upper teeth)

Essentials of Oral Pathology

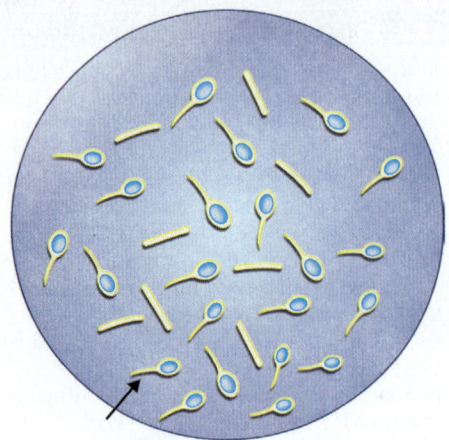

Fig. 8.16: *Clostridium tetani.*

tetani. The microorganism releases exotoxins that affect motor neurons and results in severe muscle spasms.

Pathogenesis

- *Clostridium tetani* is a gram-positive, non-encapsulated, motile organism having terminally located spore, with a typical drumstick like appearance (Fig. 8.16).
- Hot and damp climates with fertile soil rich in organic matter are favorable environment for the growth of these microorganisms.
- After introduction of the bacilli at the site of injury, tetanus can develop within few days to 2 months.
- In traumatized tissue the spores get converted into vegetative forms and during autolysis the vegetative form of the organism releases exotoxins, namely tetanospasmin and tetanolysin.
- The tetanospasmin affects brain, sympathetic nervous system, the skeletal muscle motor end plates and the spinal cord, etc.
- Initially tetanospasmin is bound to the peripheral nerves at the site of inoculation and then it is carried in a retrograde direction along the axons to the central nervous system.

Clinical Features

- Clinical manifestations usually appear 2 weeks after the infection and are characterized by severe pain and stiffness of the facial and neck muscles, resulting in trismus.
- Masseter muscle spasms can be so strong that it can cause severe tongue bite or even fracture of the anterior teeth or even jaw bones.
- Rigidity of the facial muscles may also produce a typical grinning expression called "risus sardonicus".
- In few cases, spasm of the entire body muscles produce "opisthotonus" and board-like rigidity of the abdomen.
- Laryngospasm occurs when the patient tries to swallow saliva.
- Body temperature is increased due to increased metabolic rate.
- Spasm of the muscles of deglutition results in dysphagia.
- Airway obstruction often occurs due to spasm of the pharyngeal, intercostal and diaphragmatic muscles.
- Patients often exhibit restlessness and irritability.
- Acute, paroxysmal, incoordinated spasm of the muscles is an indicator of the moderate to severe form of the disease.
- Patients with tetanus may die of anoxia or due to pulmonary complications like bronchopneumonia and pulmonary embolism, etc.

Key Points of Tetanus

- Tetanus is a serious bacterial disease caused by *Clostridium tetani*, which releases exotoxins *tetanospasmin* and *tetanolysin*.
- These enzymes attack the motor neurons and results in severe muscle spasms in various vital organs.
- Clinically the disease causes severe pain and stiffness of the facial and neck muscles, resulting in trismus.
- Rigidity of the facial muscles may also produce a typical grinning expression called *risus sardonicus*.
- Patients if left untreated often die of anoxia, bronchopneumonia and pulmonary embolism, etc.

Treatment

By injection of tetanus antitoxin, along with antibiotics, anticonvulsants and surgical wound care.

■ MIDLINE LETHAL GRANULOMA

Midline lethal granuloma is a serious disease that involves the nasal cavity, maxilla, palate and nasopharynx, etc.

Etiology

Etiology of the disease is unknown, according to different investigators, midline lethal granuloma can be of infective origin or it may develop as an immunopathologic collagen disorder.

Clinical Features

- Midline lethal granuloma begins with pain, stiffness in the nose and nonspecific ulceration over the palate or upper respiratory tract.
- The condition does not respond to any treatment.
- The disease progressively destroys the soft and hard palate and nose by causing extensive necrosis with concomitant purulent exudation.
- Perforation of the palate is a very common feature of this disease.
- Erythematous, granular, tumor-like lesions may be seen on the gingiva and other parts of the oral mucosa.
- With time the entire mid-face may be destroyed with involvement of the orbit.
- The patients often die due to exhaustion, hemorrhage, malnutrition and cachexia, etc.
- Clinically midline lethal granuloma often resembles a carcinoma but microscopically it appears as an innocuous, nonneoplastic lesion.

Histopathology

Destruction of the normal osseous and soft tissues of the face with replacement by an inflamed granulation tissue. Infiltration by mononuclear cells and scattered eosinophils are often evident.

Treatment

High dose of radiation therapy is the treatment of choice along with antibiotics and immunosuppressant drugs.

■ WEGENER'S GRANULOMATOSIS

Wegener's granulomatosis is a rare disease with poorly understood pathogenesis (probably having some immunological basis of origin). It is characterized by necrotizing vasculitis of the larynx, trachea, salivary glands, palate, etc. and is often associated with a fatal outcome.

Clinical Features

- This potentially lethal disease often starts with rhinitis, sinusitis and nasal crusting, etc. with gradual destruction of the nasal septum.
- It often results in a "saddle nose" deformity.
- Persistent cough with hemoptysis and uremia is common.
- The oral lesions include generalized severe proliferative or hyperplastic gingivitis and ulceration of the other mucosal surfaces.
- The gingival lesions produce swelling with a granular surface; the color of the gingiva is either dusky red or bright red (strawberry gingiva).
- These gingival lesions can be either localized or diffuse; and they often resemble the pregnancy gingivitis.
- Failure of healing of the extraction wounds is an important characteristic of this disease.
- Death usually results from renal failure.

Histopathology

Microscopically the disease shows necrosis and granulomatous inflammation of the tissue; with scattered giant cells, vasculitis and destruction of the small arteries.

Treatment

The disease is responsive to steroid and cytotoxic drug therapy.

NOMA (CANCRUM ORIS)

Noma is a rapidly spreading and extremely severe gangrenous infection of the orofacial tissues; which is characterized by perforation and destruction of large areas of the face. The disease is often fatal if not properly treated or left untreated.

Etiology

The disease probably develops as a result of infection caused by fusospirochetal organisms, in immunocompromised patients. The microorganisms include—*Fusobacterium necrophorum, F. nucleatum* and *Prevotella intermedia*, etc. However, other organisms which often complicate the disease process include *S. aureus* and *Borrelia vincentii*, etc.

Clinical Features

- The disease is more prevalent in children between the ages of 1 year and 10 years; it was very common among starving prisoners (particularly children) in the Nazi concentration camps during the Second World War.
- In the initial stage of the disease there is formation of a painful, red, indurated papule over the gingiva, at this stage it looks like typical acute necrotizing ulcerative gingivitis (ANUG) with extreme edema.
- It is soon followed by the formation of an ulcer over the gingiva, which spreads rapidly on both facial and lingual directions and exposes the underlying bone.
- The ulcer rapidly extends to the mucosal surfaces of the lips and cheek; and this condition is known as "necrotizing ulcerative mucositis".
- Within a few days a small, dark, reddish-purple area appears on the skin over the cheek, which rapidly undergoes gangrenous necrosis.
- As the tissue becomes ischemic, the overlying facial skin appears blue-black.
- Later on, a large hole of few inches size develops on the cheek due to sloughing of the tissue; which exposes the interior of the mouth (teeth and bone) with severe disfigurement.
- Severe sore mouth, increased salivation and diffuse edema of the face occur; along with extreme foul smell.
- Spread of infection into the jawbone results in osteomyelitis; which results in sequestration of bone with exfoliations of teeth.
- Noma eventually creates a large gaping facial defect in the mouth and death may occur due to aspiration pneumonia, severe diarrhea and dehydration, etc.

Treatment

Treatment is done by antibiotic therapy along with nutritional supplements.

PYOGENIC GRANULOMA

Pyogenic granuloma represents an overexuberant tissue reaction to some known stimuli or injuries. The term pyogenic granuloma is somewhat a misnomer since the condition is not associated with pus formation.

Clinical Features

- Age: The disease occurs at an early age.
- Sex: It is seen more frequently among females.
- Site: Pyogenic granuloma mostly occurs in relation to the gingiva, however on rare occasions other mucosal sites may be involved.

Presentation

- The lesion appears as a small, pedunculated or sessile, painless, soft, friable growth on the gingiva (Fig. 8.17).
- Labial surface of the gingiva is more frequently affected than the lingual surface.

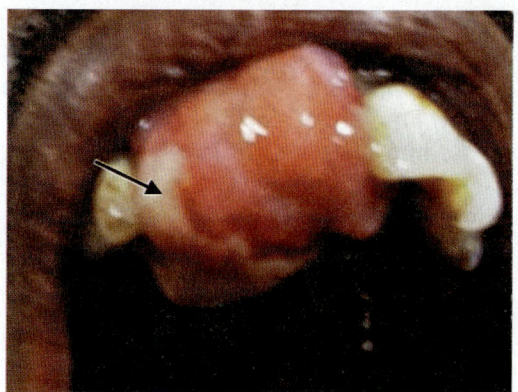

Fig. 8.17: Pyogenic granuloma developing from maxillary gingiva.

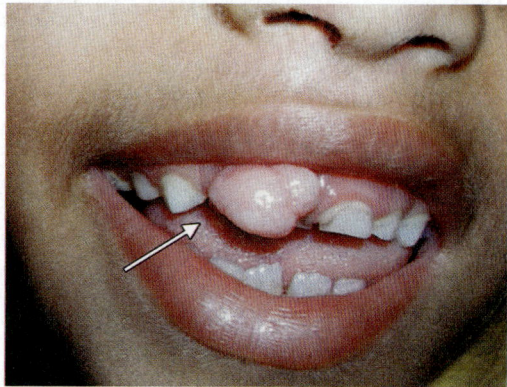

Fig. 8.18: Fibroepithelial polyp.

- The lesion often looks red and ulcerated; and it bleeds profusely, either upon provocation or spontaneously.
- The ulcerated area of the lesion is often covered by a yellow fibrinous slough.
- Sometimes a lesion similar to the pyogenic granuloma appears on the gingival tissue of pregnant women, which is known as "pregnancy tumor". This tumor is believed to develop due to hormonal alterations in the body during pregnancy, which causes as exuberant proliferative response in the gingiva against local irritants like plaque and calculus, etc.
- Older lesions of pyogenic granuloma undergo fibrosis due to decreased vascularity and reduction in the edema; in such cases they appear small, firm, painless, nodular growths with no surface ulceration and little tendency to bleed. Such lesions are called "fibroepithelial polyps" (Figs. 8.18 and 8.19).

Histopathology (Fig. 8.20)

- Histologically, pyogenic granuloma is composed of a lobular mass of hyperplastic granulation tissue; containing multiple proliferating fibroblasts, many thin walled and anastomosing blood capillaries and variable number of chronic inflammatory cells.

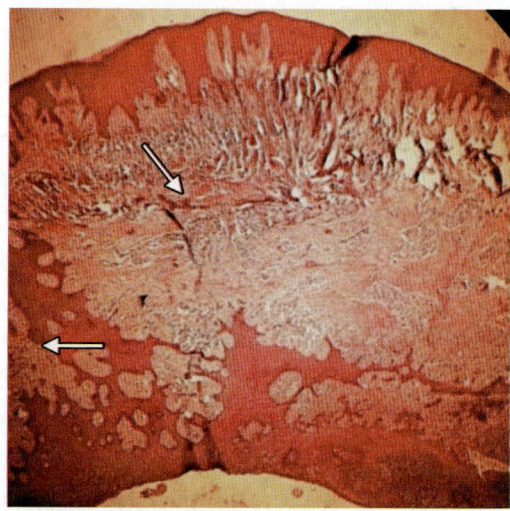

Fig. 8.19: Photomicrograph of fibroepithelial polyp.

- The overlying epithelium is thin and may be ulcerated, and in most of the cases the underlying connective tissue shows intercellular edema.
- Areas of hemorrhage and hemosiderin pigmentation are often seen within the connective tissue stroma.

Treatment

Pyogenic granuloma is treated by surgical excision.

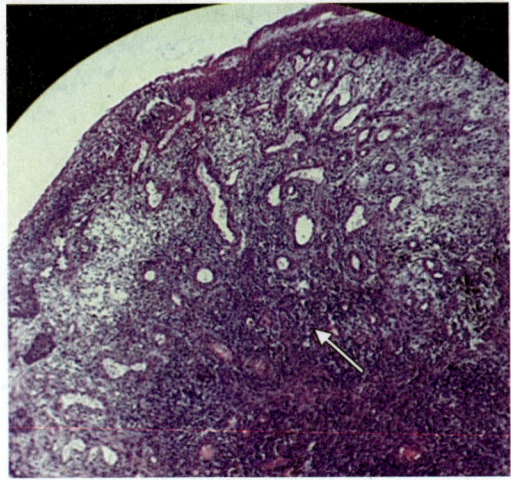

Fig. 8.20: Photomicrograph of pyogenic granulomas.

VIRAL INFECTIONS

A virus is an obligatory intracellular parasite, which codes the host cell by contributing its own nucleic acids to produce a new generation of virions.

The virus consists of a central core of either DNA or RNA, which is surrounded by a shell or capsid that is made up of protein. In some cases, there is another outer envelope composed of glycoproteins and lipids.

When a virus comes in contact with a susceptible cell, it adsorbs on to the cell surface at a "specific receptor site" which determines the susceptibility of the host cell to the particular virus. Subsequently, the virus penetrates the cell wall by a process of pinocytosis, during which the lipid envelope and the protein capsid is stripped off, to release the viral nucleic acid. The latter is then passed into the nucleus of the host cell and is coded for producing viral products.

Within the host cell, the virus may produce the following functions:
- It may influence the host cell to produce more and more virions, which come out of the cell by rupturing it and then they go on to attack the new cells.
- It can influence the host cell's own mitotic activity and cause increased host cell multiplication, eventually leading to the development of a neoplasm.
- In some instances, the viral infections may induce immunological changes either by causing direct infections to the cells of the immune system or by stimulating the production of antibodies, which may potentiate autoimmune reactions.

The methods of controlling the viral infection by killing these organisms is very difficult, because these organisms are always living intracellularly and one cannot kill them without killing the host cell itself. Another problem is difficulty in their identification inside the host cells, as the viruses are always changing their protein code, so that they can hide easily without being noticed by the body's own immunosurveillance network.

ACQUIRED IMMUNODEFICIENCY SYNDROME

Acquired immunodeficiency syndrome (AIDS) is a predominantly lethal type of viral infection, caused by HIV and is characterized by severe depletion of T4 lymphocytes in the body, with associated opportunistic infection of several varieties.

Etiology and Pathogenesis

The etiologic agent for AIDS is the HIV virus (type-I and type-II), which are nononcogenic "lentiviruses" of the human "retrovirus" family (Fig. 8.21, Table 8.1). Our body is protected by two types of immune systems-cell mediated immunity (by T lymphocytes) and humoral immunity (by B-lymphocytes through production of immunoglobulins). The CD4+ cells or the "helper -T4 lymphocytes" are the chief cellular elements for cell mediated immunity. These cells have CD4 receptor on the surface for recognition of foreign antigens.

The virus damages the immune system of the body by killing the CD4+T cells (helper -T lymphocytes), as a result body loses its

Bacterial, Viral and Fungal Infections

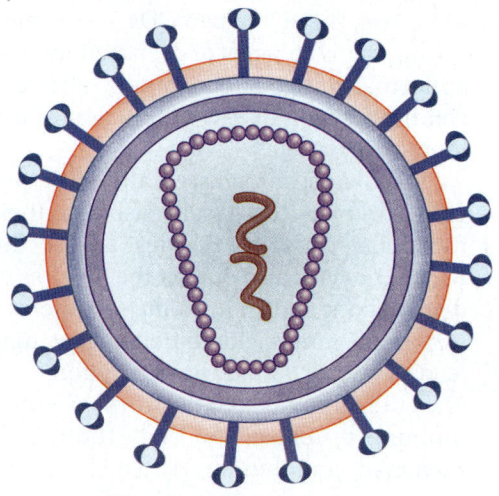

Fig. 8.21: Structure of HIV virus.

cell mediated immune capacity; and a large number of serious opportunistic infections and various malignancies develop that ultimately kill the patient.

Mode of Transmission of HIV

- *Sexual transmission*: It is the major mode of transmission of the virus and the infection can occur in both homosexuals and heterosexuals if one of the partners is infected.
- *Blood or blood products*: A person may be infected with HIV if he/she receives blood or blood products from an infected donor or if the transfusion kit used, is somehow contaminated by the virus.
- *Injection drug users*: Risk of HIV infection is more among the injection drug users because of sharing the contaminated needles by many people in the group.

- *Occupational transmission*: HIV transmission following skin puncture by needle or sharp instrument that was contaminated earlier by the virus, is a common risk for the doctors and other related professionals.
- *Maternal-fetal/infant transmission*: HIV can be transmitted from an infected mother to the fetus during pregnancy or to the infant during delivery.
- *Other body fluids*: The risk of transmission of the virus via the saliva, milk or tears, etc. from the infected person is reported, however, insects do not transmit the virus from one person to other.

Pathogenesis of HIV infection

The disease progresses in the following steps:
- *Entry of HIV virus into the body*: It occurs through various modes of transmission, e.g. sexual contact, through infected needles, from infected mother to child and via blood transfusions, etc.
- *Binding and fusion of HIV virus to the CD4+ cells*: HIV virus binds to this CD4 + receptor and fuses with the cell wall. After fusion the virus releases its RNA into the host cell.
- *Reverse Transcription*: The viral enzyme "reverse transcriptase" converts the single stranded HIV viral RNA into double stranded HIV viral DNA. The process is called "reverse transcription".
- *Integration*: The newly formed HIV-DNA enters into the host cell (T-4 cell) nucleus and hides within the host cells own DNA, the viral enzyme "integrase" helps in the hiding process. The integrated HIV DNA is called provirus, which may remain

Table 8.1: Major difference between HIV-1 and HIV-2 viruses.

HIV-1	HIV-2
• HIV-1 is more common virus causing AIDS • HIV-1 is more pathogenic • Duration of HIV-1 infection is much longer • Mother to child transmission (MTCT) is relatively common with HIV-1	• HIV-2 is mostly found in West Africa, Mozambique and Angola • HIV-2 is less pathogenic • Duration of HIV-2 infection is shorter • Mother to child transmission is rare with HIV-2

inactive for long time (latent stage) or may become active.
- *Transcription*: When the host cell receives signal to become active, the provirus uses a host enzyme "RNA polymerase" to create copies of the HIV genomic material as shorter strands of RNA, called messenger RNA (mRNA). The mRNA is used as a blueprint to make long chains of HIV proteins.
- *Assembly*: An HIV enzyme called "protease" cuts the long chain of HIV proteins into smaller individual proteins, the smaller proteins come together with copies of HIV's RNA material; this give rise to the formation of newly assembles virus particle.
- *Budding*: The new virus multiply through "budding" and increase in number, they subsequently rupture the cell and come out to infect other T4 cells. Killing of more and more T4 cells cause suppression of cell mediated immunity. The normal count of CD4+ T cells is 500–1,500/mm^3 of blood; if the count falls below 350/mm^3 then it should be assumed that the cell mediated immunity has been severely compromised.
- The normal ratio of CD4 helper lymphocytes and the CD8 suppressor lymphocytes is 2:1 but it is severely depleted in AIDS. Depletion of CD4 cells results in loss of production of noncellular components of the defense system of the body, e.g. interleukin-2, interferon, macrophage activating factor and factor that stimulates the production of natural killer cells, etc.
- Moreover, these infected CD4 T-cells also exhibit variable types of dysfunctions like abnormal antigen recognition, aberrant cell triggering and loss of function of the memory cells, etc.
- As the disease progresses, the HIV specific cytotoxic CD8 T-cells also lose their functional capacity. Besides T-cells, the B-lymphocytes also exhibit the features of dysfunctions and they produce compensatory hypergammaglobulinemia that may lead to several autoimmune reactions.
- Thus the HIV infection destroys the entire immune system of the body (both cell-mediated and humoral), which results in a variety of opportunistic infections as well as the development of many other pathologies, e.g. malignancies, etc. and the patient often fails to survive.
- *Viral load* (VL) is also an important parameter that indicates the disease progression; when the viral load is 550,000 copies/ml of blood, it is the time to start the treatment.

Clinical aspect of HIV

The stages of HIV and critical symptoms indicating progression of HIV to full blown AIDS are given in Table 8.2 and Box 8.9, respectively.

Clinical Spectrum of HIV/AIDS

Clinical manifestations of AIDS may be classified as follows (Table 8.3):

Group-I: Acute Infections
- Infectious mononucleosis
- Hepatitis

Table 8.2: Stages of human immunodeficiency virus (HIV).

Acute infection	Clinical latency	Full blown AIDS
Early stage of the disease characterized by large number of viral multiplication. Patients have mild symptoms of fever mimicking Flu or Influenza.	Rate of viral multiplication in the body is very slow during this period. Patients are relatively asymptomatic.	This is the most serious stage of HIV infection, the patient's immunity is severely compromised due very low Cd4+ cell count. Life threatening opportunistic infections and neoplasms develop that often kill the patient.

Bacterial, Viral and Fungal Infections

Box 8.9	Critical symptoms indicating progression of HIV into full-blown AIDS.

- Recurrent fever with profuse night sweats
- Rapid weight loss
- Extreme tiredness
- Persistent lymphadenopathy
- Prolonged diarrhea lasting for more than a week
- Oral, anal and genital ulcers
- Pneumonia
- Red, brown or pink spots on the skin and mucosa
- Memory loss and depression

- Meningitis
- Meningoencephalitis.

Group-II: Chronic Asymptomatic Infections

It is the potentially most dangerous group and seropositive individuals who are apparently healthy but capable of infecting others. Patient may have enlarged axillary glands as well as hematological and immunological abnormalities.

Table 8.3: AIDS defining opportunistic infections and neoplasms.

Protozoal and helminthic infections
- Cryptosporidiosis
- Pneumocystosis
- Toxoplasmosis

Fungal infections
- Candidiasis
- Cryptococcosis
- Histoplasmosis

Bacterial infections
- *Mycobacterium avium* intracellulare (atypical mycobacteria)
- Nocardiosis
- Salmonella

Viral infections
- Herpes simplex
- Cytomegalovirus

Neoplasms
- Kaposi sarcoma
- Non-Hodgkin's lymphoma
- Primary lymphoma of brain.

Main symptoms in Men	Main symptoms in Women
Neurological - Encephalitis - Meningitis - Dementia *Lymph node* - Persistent lymphadenopathy *Oral cavity and throat* - Candidiasis - Herpetic ulcers - Kaposi's sarcoma - Aphthous ulcers - Sore throat - Oropharyngeal ulcers *Systemic* - Fever, rapid weight loss, fatigue - Night sweats	*Neurological* - Cryptococcal meningitis - Dementia *Oral cavity and Throat* - Candidiasis - Herpetic ulcers - Aphthous ulcers - Sore throat - Oropharyngeal ulcers *Lungs* - Histoplasmosis - Tuberculosis - Pneumocystis pneumonia (PCP) *Heart* - Stroke *Eye* - Cytomegalovirus infection

Contd...

Contd...

Main symptoms in Men	Main symptoms in Women
Skin • Rashes/blotches • Kaposi's sarcoma *Respiratory* • Cough and shortness of breath • Pharyngitis • Pneumocystis pneumonia (PCP) *GI system* • Nausea, vomiting • Persistent diarrhea *Eye* • Blurred vision *Genitalia* • Ulcers • Warts *Liver* • Enlargement	*Blood* • Pancytopenia • Hyperglycemia *Liver* • Hepatitis C *Stomach* • Cytomegalovirus infection • Cryptosporidiosis • *Mycobacterium avium* complex *Reproductive system* • Genital ulcers • Menstrual irregularity • Human papilloma virus infection • Cervical cancer • Vaginal candidiasis • Pelvic inflammatory disease *Bone* • Osteoporosis

Group-III: Persistent Generalized Lymphadenopathy (PGL)

Unexplained lymphadenopathy in two or more extrainguinal sites persisting for more than 3 months in the absence of any concurrent illness or causative drugs.

Group-IV

- Constitutional diseases (AIDS-related complex): It is characterized by prolonged unexplained pyrexia, chronic persistent diarrhea, weight loss more than 10% of the previous normal body weight (Box 8.10).
- Neurologic diseases:
  - Progressive dementia.
  - Meningoencephalitis.
- Opportunistic infections:
  - Pneumonia or sinusitis:
    - *Pneumocystis carinii* pneumonia
    - Cryptococcosis
    - Mucormycosis
    - Toxoplasmosis
    - *Pseudomonas aeruginosa*
    - Tuberculosis (Box 8.11)
    - *Staphylococcus aureus*
    - *Streptococcus pneumoniae*
    - *Haemophilus influenzae*

Box 8.10 AIDS-related complex (ARC).

Definition: It is the stage of illness in a HIV infected person (who is HIV positive) and has developed some symptoms due to damage of the immune system, but without the opportunistic infections or the malignancies associated with AIDS.

Patients will have one or more of the following symptoms:
- Unexplained diarrhea for more than 1 month
- Malaise, fatigue, night sweats and fever continuing for over a month
- Weight loss of more than 10% of the body weight
- Lymphadenopathy
- Splenomegaly

Box 8.11 Tuberculosis in HIV patients.

- Tuberculosis (TB) is a common and serious opportunistic infection in HIV patients and is the cause of death for many of them
- In a normal patient, when the *Mycobacterium tuberculosis* organism enters the body the CD4 lymphocytes multiply to destroy them and thus tuberculosis is successfully prevented
- However, in HIV patients the same CD4+ lymphocytes are already reduced in number (as they are killed by the virus) and as a result the risk of active TB is much higher for them. That's why in many patients treatment of TB is started even before beginning the antiretroviral drug therapy against HIV virus

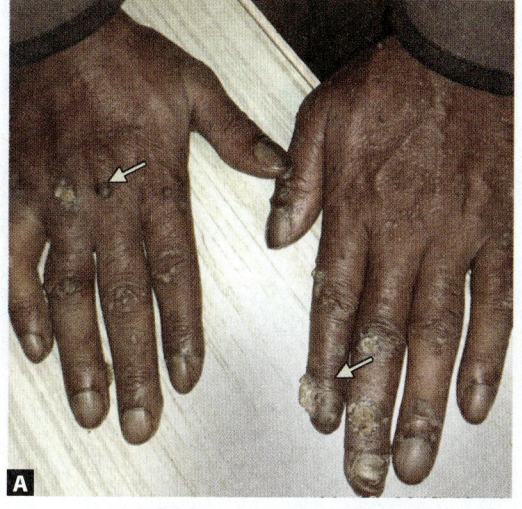 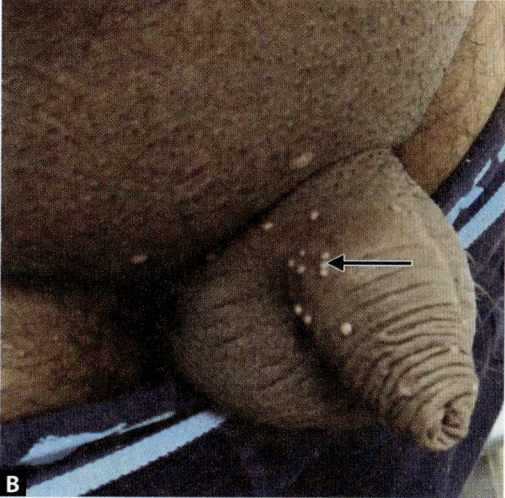

Figs. 8.22A and B: Verruca vulgaris on the (A) skin and (B) genitalia in a HIV-positive patient.

- Gastrointestinal infections (diarrhea):
  - Cryptosporidiosis
  - Isosporiasis
  - *Giardia*
- Mucocutaneous infections:
  - Herpes simplex
  - Herpes zoster
  - Candidiasis
  - *Staphylococcus aureus*
  - Histoplasmosis
  - Verruca (wart)
- Meningitis and encephalitis:
  - JC-virus (Jamestown Canyon virus)
  - Toxoplasmosis
- Disseminated infections:
  - Atypical mycobacteriosis
  - Cryptococcosis
  - Histoplasmosis
- Specified secondary neoplasms
  - Kaposi's sarcoma
  - Lymphoma (immunoblastic)
  - Burkitt's lymphoma
  - Squamous cell carcinoma of mouth, anus or rectum
  - Leukemia
- Others:
  - Encephalopathy
  - Purpura
  - Lupus erythematosus
  - Addison's disease
  - Seborrheic dermatitis
  - Thrombocytopenia.

The term "Wart" literally means "verruca" in Latin (a common wart is often known as "verruca vulgaris"). These are mainly caused by human papilloma virus (HPV), they are very common in HIV positive patients (Figs. 8.22 and 8.23; Table 8.4).

Key Points in Oral Manifestations of AIDS

Oral candidiasis (Fig. 8.29)	❖ Erythematous, hyperplastic and pseudomembranous (the last one is most common among children)
	❖ Esophageal candidiasis
	❖ Angular cheilitis
Viral infections of oral mucosa	❖ Herpes simplex and herpes zoster-causing atypical and chronic ulcers
	❖ Epstein-Barr virus—Causing hairy leukoplakia
	❖ Papilloma virus—causing proliferative lesions, e.g. verruca vulgaris, condyloma acuminatum and focal dermal hyperplasia
	❖ Cytomegalovirus infection

Bacterial infections	❖ Tuberculous ulcers ❖ Osteomyelitis of the jaw ❖ Submandibular cellulitis
Deep fungal infections (ulcers and proliferative lesions)	❖ Coccidioidomycosis ❖ Histoplasmosis ❖ Toxoplasmosis
Hairy leukoplakia, gingivitis and periodontitis (Figs. 8.24A and B)	❖ HIV-gingivitis ❖ HIV-rapidly progressive destructive periodontitis ❖ Necrotizing ulcerative gingivitis ❖ Exacerbation of atypical periodontitis ❖ Halitosis
Persistent generalized lymphadenopathy	
Tumors	❖ Kaposi's sarcoma—flat or nodular purplish lesion (mostly on the palate ❖ Non-Hodgkin's lymphoma ❖ Burkitt's lymphoma ❖ Squamous cell carcinoma
Stomatitis	❖ Progressive necrotizing ulcerations of the oral mucosa ❖ Recurrent major aphthous ulcers ❖ Atypical oropharyngeal ulcers ❖ Acute nonspecific ulcers of oral mucosa
Salivary gland disease	❖ Parotitis and enlarged parotids ❖ Sjogren's syndrome ❖ Xerostomia ❖ Unilateral or bilateral swelling of other salivary glands ❖ Cystic benign lymphoepithelial lesions
Neurological disorders	❖ Facial palsy ❖ Trigeminal neuropathy ❖ Paresthesia and hyperesthesia
Autoimmune disease	❖ Thrombocytopenic purpura ❖ Systemic lupus erythematosus
Miscellaneous diseases	❖ Sinusitis ❖ Vesiculobullous lesions ❖ Bacillary angiomatosis ❖ Addisonian pigmentations ❖ Delayed wound healing

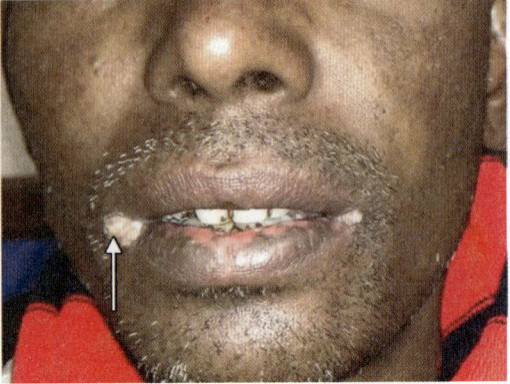

Fig. 8.23: Verruca of the mouth in a HIV-positive patient.

Table 8.4: Oral manifestations of AIDS*.

Group 1	Lesions strongly associated with HIV infection
	Candidiasis • Erythematous • Pseudomembranous
	Hairy leukoplakia
	Kaposi's sarcoma
	Non-Hodgkin's lymphoma
	Periodontal disease • Linear gingival erythema • Necrotizing ulcerative gingivitis • Necrotizing ulcerative periodontitis
Group 2	Lesions less commonly associated with HIV infections
	Bacterial lesions (*Mycobacterium avium, M. tuberculosis*)
	Melanotic hyperpigmentations
	Necrotizing ulcerative stomatitis Bacterial infections
Group 3	Lesions seen in HIV infection
	Bacterial infections • *Actinomyces israelii* • *Escherichia coli* • *Klebsiella pneumoniae* • Cat-scratch disease
	Drug reactions (ulcerative, erythema multiforme
	Lichenoid reaction, Toxic epidermolysis
	Epithelioid bacillary angiomatosis

Contd...

Contd...

| Fungal infections
• *Cryptococcus neoformans*
• *Histoplasma capsulatum*
• Mucormycosis
• *Aspergillus flavus* |
| Neurological disturbances (Facial palsy, Trigeminal neuralgia) |
| Viral infections
• Cytomegalovirus
• Molluscum contagiosum |

*Factors that predispose to oral lesions:
CD4 cell count < 200/μL of blood
Plasma HIV RNA levels > 3,000 copies/mL
Xerostomia, poor oral hygiene and smoking.
Source: European Commission Science and Knowledge Service. Clearinghouse classification of oral problems related to HIV infection. Luxembourg: European Commission; 1995.

Diagnosis of AIDS

- Clinical—according to WHO recommendations, existence of at least two major signs, e.g. chronic persistent diarrhea (more than one month), generalized pruritic dermatitis, recurrent herpes zoster, esophageal candidiasis, chronic progressive and disseminated HSV infection, Kaposi's sarcoma or cryptococcal meningitis suggests the diagnosis of AIDS.
- Western blot analysis
- Enzyme-linked immunosorbent assay (ELISA)
- Polymerase chain reaction (PCR)
- Detection of antibody to the virus in serum
- Detection of virus from the peripheral blood
- Lymphopenia
- Reversal of normal ratio of T helper to T suppressor lymphocytes
- Hypergammaglobulinemia
- Viral culture
- P24 antigen detection
- Immunological tests—CD4+ T cell count, CD4+ T cell% and CD4/CD8 ratio tests.
- Salivary tests to capture the HIV IgG antibody.

Treatment of AIDS

HIV anti-retroviral treatment (HAART) is the most standard and accepted mode of treatment in AIDS; in which 3-4 antiretroviral drugs are used at a time. The common antiretroviral drugs used in India are as follows:

- Nucleoside reverse transcriptase inhibitor (NRTI)—consisting of Zidovudine (AZT/ZDV), Stavudine (d4T), Lamivudine (3TC), Emtricitabine (FTC), Didanosine (DDI), Zalcitabine (ddC), Abacavir (ABC) and Tenofovir (TDF).
- Non-nucleoside reverse transcriptase inhibitor (NNRTI)—a group consisting of Nevirapine (NVP), Efavirenz (EFV).

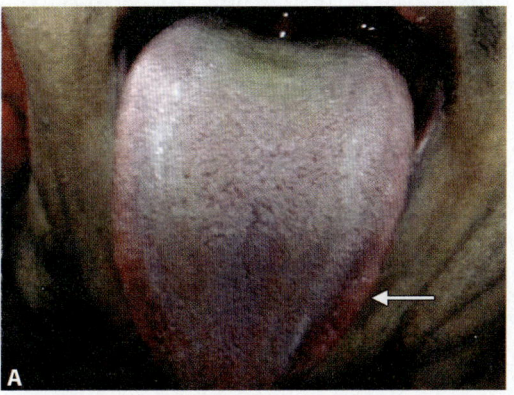 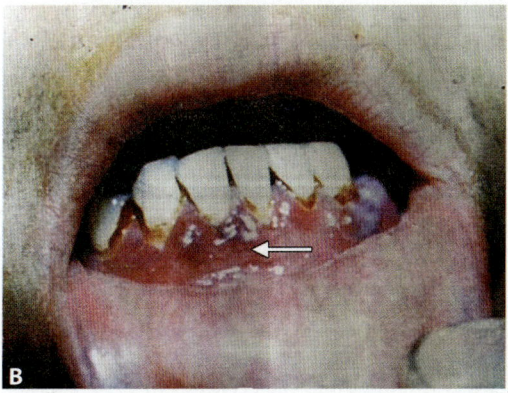

Figs. 8.24A and B: (A) Oral hairy leukoplakia in AIDS; (B) Kaposi's sarcoma of the gingiva.

- Protease inhibitor (PI)—consists of Saquinavir (SQV), Nelfinavir (NFV), Indinavir (IDV), Lopinavir (LPV), Ritonavir (RTV), Atazanavir.

Recommended Combination Regimens
- 2 NRTIs + 1 NNRTI or
- 2 NRTIs + 1 PI or
- 2 NRTIs + 2 PIs.

Administration of multiple drugs significantly prevents the development of resistant strains. Basically the disease is incurable so far and stress is given mostly to prevent or cure the secondary infections. Zidovudine may prolong and improve the quality of life in those with active AIDS. Cotrimoxazole is given for *Pneumocystis carinii* pneumonia and fluconazole is given for candidiasis.

HERPES VIRUS INFECTIONS

The term herpes is derived from the Greek word *herpein* which means to "creep or crawl" and it was used to describe the spreading nature of the skin lesions caused by this group of viruses.

Herpes virus family comprises of about 50 different DNA viruses and man is the host and exclusive reservoir of four important members of this group namely:
- Herpes simplex virus (HSV)—type I and type II (Fig. 8.25)
- Varicella-zoster virus
- Human cytomegalovirus
- Epstein-Barr virus.

Herpes Simplex Virus Type-I Diseases

It is responsible for a number of conditions such as:
- Acute herpetic gingivostomatitis
- Herpetic eczema
- Keratoconjunctivitis
- Meningoencephalitis
- Herpes labialis
- Genital herpes (occasional).

Herpes Simplex Virus Type-II Diseases

This virus is responsible for the following diseases:
- Genital herpes (very common)
- Neonatal herpes
- Uterocervical cancer
- Oral herpes (rare).

Varicella-Zoster Virus Diseases

This virus causes usually two diseases namely:
- Chickenpox
- Herpes zoster or shingles.

Human Cytomegalovirus Diseases

It produces the following diseases:
- Salivary gland disease
- Kaposi's sarcoma.

Epstein-Barr Virus Diseases

This virus is responsible for a variety of conditions like:
- Infectious mononucleosis
- Burkitt's lymphoma
- Nasopharyngeal carcinoma
- Hairy leukoplakia.

HERPES SIMPLEX VIRUS TYPE–I INFECTIONS

Primary Acute Herpetic Gingivostomatitis

This acute infection of the oral cavity is caused by the HSV type I and the disease usually

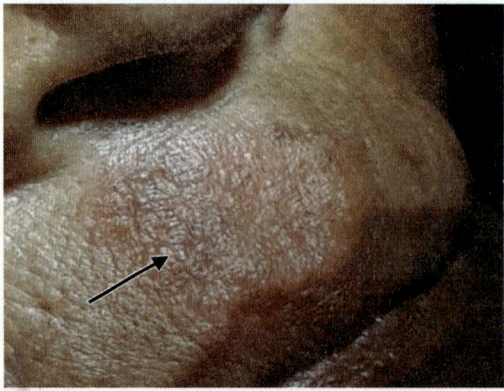

Fig. 8.25: Herpes simplex infection of facial skin.

occurs during childhood, between 3 years and 5 years of age. The disease is transmitted by close contact with an infected individual.

Clinical Features
- The disease is usually preceded by some other disease conditions, e.g. upper respiratory tract infection and fever, etc.
- The initial generalized signs and symptoms of the disease include: headache, nausea, anorexia, lack of tactile or sensory perceptions of the affected area, etc.
- These are followed by features like sore mouth, irritability, drooling, refusal of food, bilateral painful cervical lymphadenopathy and fever (103–105°F), etc.
- The oral lesion of primary herpes infection is called "primary herpetic gingivostomatitis" and it begins with reddening of the oral mucosa; followed by widespread vesicular lesions in the mouth.
- Both movable and attached mucosa can be affected and hard palate and dorsum of tongue are the most common sites. Other sites which may be involved are the gingiva,, lips, vermillion border, perioral skin and nasopharynx, etc. (Figs. 8.26 and 8.27).
- The vesicles are dome-shaped or pinhead type and measure about 2–3 mm in diameter and contain clear fluid; they rupture soon and leave shallow, painful,

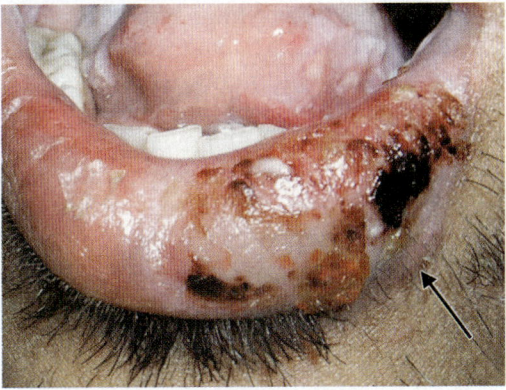

Fig. 8.27: Herpes labialis.

sharply demarcated ulcers with a red halo. These ulcers often have yellowish or grayish floor.
- Adjacent tiny ulcers coalesce to form diffuse, large, irregular lesions on the mucosa, which cause severe pain and difficulty in taking food.
- The gingiva strikingly red, swollen and painful; occasionally there may be presence of punched-out erosions on the free gingival margin (mostly on the facial aspect).
- Healing starts in about 3 days and the lesion is completely healed up within 7–14 days without any scar formation.
- In case of HIV infection, these herpetic ulcers will be larger, deeper, more painful and more persistent in nature.
- After the primary infection, the HSV can persist in latent form in the trigeminal ganglion and it may be reactivated later on to cause recurrent infections.

Histopathology
Acute herpetic gingivostomatitis histologically produces the following features:
- Formation of sharply defined vesicles in the superficial part of the keratinized epithelium.
- Infected tissue will have both intercellular and intracellular edema.
- Ballooning and vacuolization of the keratinocytes occur due to intracellular edema.

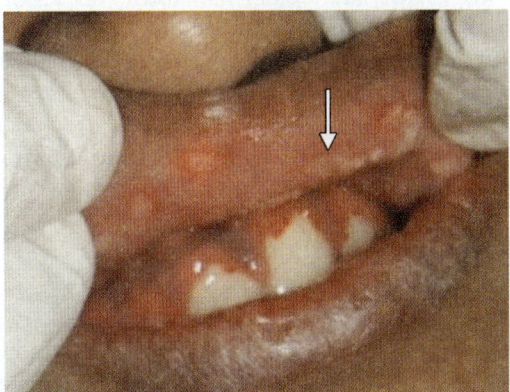

Fig. 8.26: Primary herpetic gingivostomatitis.

- The infected cells have enlarged nuclei with intranuclear inclusion body and marginated chromatin; (basophilic or eosinophilic nuclear inclusions with a clear halo are called *Lipschutz bodies*).
- Multiple multinucleated syncytial giant cells are occasionally present in the lesion (these are formed by fusion of adjacent degenerated prickle cells).

Differential Diagnosis

- Erythema multiforme
- Pemphigus
- Pemphigoid
- Chickenpox
- Allergic dermatitis.

Diagnosis

- Cytologic smear: Cytologic examination of vesicular fluid reveals the presence of inclusion bodies and ballooning degeneration of infected cells.
- Biopsy: See the histopathological features.
- Culture: Aspiration of vesicle contents and subsequent tissue culture produces change in the culture cells in 24 hours.
- Fluorescent antibody test: HSV specific antibodies are labeled with fluorescent dye and seen microscopically.
- Serology: Examination of blood (serum) for detection of HSV specific antibodies.

Treatment

In acute herpetic gingivostomatitis, only the palliative treatment is done (e.g. antibiotics are given to prevent secondary infections and antipyretics are given to control fever). Acyclovir shortens the recovery period of primary herpetic gingivostomatitis.

Recurrent Herpetic Infections

After the primary infection is over, the herpes virus retreats to the trigeminal ganglion where it lies dormant in a latent form. Later on, under some appropriate stimulation the virus becomes reactivated once again and it proceeds from the ganglion and moves centrifugally down the axon of the sensory nerve to the epithelium. The virus then produces secondary herpetic lesions over the lips, palate, nasal cavity and gingiva, etc.

Factors causing stimulation or reactivation of the virus:
- Common cold (fever blister)
- Exposure to sun light
- Emotional stress
- Trauma
- Fever
- Menstrual cycle
- Immunosuppressant therapy
- Radiations.

Clinical Features

- Recurrent infection by HSV 1 most frequently affects the vermillion border of the lips or skin adjacent to the lips; these lesions are commonly known as "herpes labialis" or "cold sores".
- The lesion starts with pain, paresthesia and burning or itching sensation over the lips; with reddening of the mucosa.
- Within 24–40 hours, clusters of fluid filled vesicles appear in these areas, which rupture soon and form multiple ulcers.

Herpetic Eczema

Herpetic eczema is an uncommon infection caused by HSV type-I virus and the disease consists of an epidermal form of lesion superimposed upon a preexisting disease like eczema, seborrheic dermatitis, impetigo or scabies, etc. The lesion is characterized by diffuse, vesicular eruptions in a typical umbilicated pattern and it commonly involves the children.

Keratoconjunctivitis

This eye lesion caused by HSV type-I virus presents severe swelling and congestion of the palpebral conjunctiva with or without corneal ulceration and keratitis. The initial lesion heals up rapidly, but recurrent attacks may cause serious corneal scarring which may ultimately lead to blindness.

Meningoencephalitis

Meningoencephalitis is a serious form of HSV type-I infection of the brain and it is characterized by fever, headache, convulsions, paralysis of different muscle groups and even death.

■ HERPES SIMPLEX VIRUS TYPE-II INFECTIONS

Genital Herpes

The HSV type-II viruses are commonly found in the genitalia, and they often produce vesicular lesions in the genital mucosa of both sexes along with fever, and inguinal lymphadenopathy. Genital herpes is a somewhat more virulent infection than the oral herpes and is more significantly associated with the development of uterocervical cancer in females. However due to the altered sexual practices, the HSV-II virus may sometimes be transported to the oral cavity where these viruses may produce oral herpes as well.

Neonatal Herpes

The neonatal herpes is an uncommon disease in which, the newborn infant acquires the HSV type-II infection during the passage through the birth canal of the mother suffering from herpetic vulvovaginitis. The disease usually manifests in the 4th to 7th day of life, and it exhibits widespread signs and symptoms, which eventually cause death of the infant in most cases or cause severe neurologic abnormalities in those who survive.

■ HERPES ZOSTER (VARICELLA-ZOSTER VIRUS INFECTIONS)

Chickenpox

Chickenpox is a highly contagious infection caused by the herpes virus *Varicella-zoster*, it is a minor self-limiting disease, which usually affects children and on rare occasions, non-immune adults. The virus is usually transmitted by direct contact and has an incubation period of 2–3 weeks.

Clinical Features (Figs. 8.28 and 8.29)
- The disease begins with slight fever, headache, anorexia, nausea, vomiting, myalgia, sore throat, etc.
- The skin lesions start with as itchy macular rash, first appearing over the trunk and then rapidly spreading over the face and limbs.

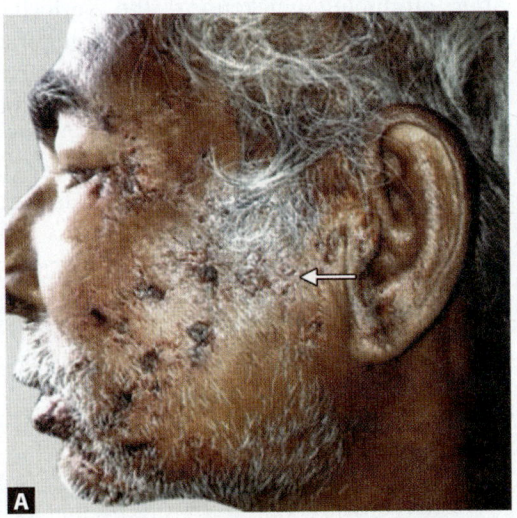
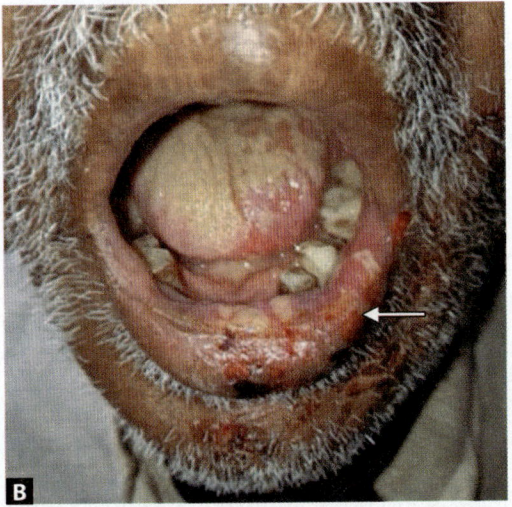

Figs. 8.28A and B: Herpes zoster showing vesicle formation unilaterally.

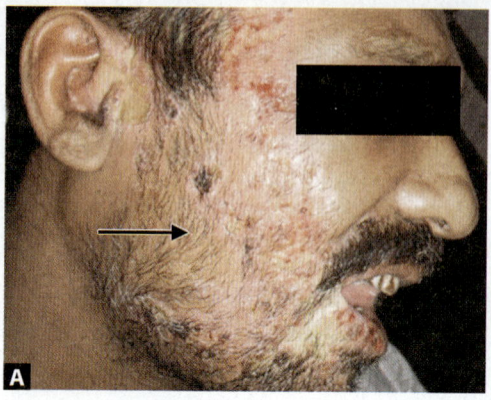 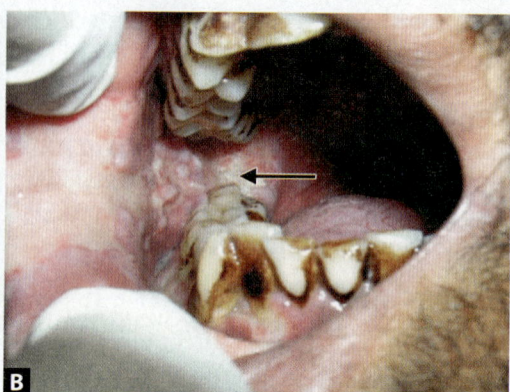

Figs. 8.29A and B: Herpes zoster—(A) Extraoral view, and (B) numerous crateriform ulcers on buccal mucosa.

- After 3-4 days, crops of pruritic vesicles appear on the skin and similar vesicles also develop on the oral mucosa, conjunctiva and genital mucosa as well.
- The individual vesicle appears as "dew drop" on rose petals and is often surrounded by a zone of erythema at the periphery.
- The oral lesions often precede the skin lesions and they develop mostly on the palate, buccal mucosa and gingiva; moreover, oral lesions often look similar to those of the skin lesions.
- The vesicles of the skin become pustular before breaking down to form focal crusting lesions.
- Following rupture of the oral vesicles painless, aphthous-like ulcers form in the mouth.
- Occasionally, skin lesions become secondarily infected and these lesions heal with formation of a depressed scar (pock).

Diagnosis

The diagnosis is made on the basis of clinical findings and by the detection of virus specific antibodies in the serum.

Treatment

Only palliative treatment is given, which includes antibiotics, antipyretics and vitamins, etc.

Herpes-Zoster (Shingles)

Definition

Herpes zoster is a recurrent regional infection caused by the Herpes Zoster virus, which occurs due to reactivation of the virus after the primary infection (Chickenpox). The disease is characterized by unilateral extreme pain along with vesicular eruptions and stomatitis in the related dermatome. Unlike the primary herpes simplex infection, herpes zoster occurs in a distinctively unilateral pattern and it does not recur often (Box 8.12).

Pathogenesis

After producing chickenpox, the Varicella-zoster virus remains dormant in the trigeminal ganglion for decades; later on it may be reactivated again. The virus may become reactivated following stress, trauma, malnutrition and immunosuppression, etc. Moreover these lesions also frequently develop among patients with

Box 8.12	Factors causing reactivation of Varicella zoster virus.
• Advanced age • Stress • Trauma • Malnutrition • HIV infection • Hodgkin's lymphoma • Organ transplant • Radiotherapy and chemotherapy	

organ transplant, HIV infection and Hodgkin's, etc. Following their reactivation the virus travel along the first, second and third branch of the trigeminal nerve and produce the disease called herpes-zoster or shingles in the sensory dermatome.

Clinical Features (Fig. 8.30)

- The herpes zoster occurs in the 5th, 6th and 7th decade of life; rarely the disease affects the children.
- The disease is often preceded by mild fever, malaise, headache and painful lymphadenopathy, etc.
- The first signs of the disease are pain, irritation or tenderness in one or more divisions of the trigeminal nerve.
- Gradually the pain becomes extremely severe with development of clusters of vesicles over the skin and oral mucosa; which characteristically develop on one side of the face up to the midline (other side of the face remains completely free of symptoms).
- The first branch of the trigeminal nerve is most commonly affected and the disease beside affecting the first branch, may also involve the following other branches like:
  - Nasociliary nerve—causing herpetic keratitis
  - Ciliary nerve—causing Argyll Robertson pupil
  - Facial nerve—causing Ramsay Hunt syndrome.
- Within the oral cavity the numerous, white opaque vesicles also develop unilaterally over the buccal mucosa, soft palate and tongue, etc. and cause stinging pain, paresthesia and severe stomatitis.
- In due course of time the fragile vesicular lesions of the skin and the oral mucosa rupture and they leave painful and often extensive "crateriform" ulcers. The ulcers eventually heal up in a few days time without scar formation.
- In herpes zoster, the neuralgic pain in the oral cavity often simulates "toothache"
- Paralysis of the facial nerve is also sometimes reported.
- The acute phase of the disease often lasts for about 7–10 days.
- A large number of patients develop severe pain in the same parts of the body long after the herpes zoster lesions have healed up and this unpleasant condition is often known as "post-herpetic neuralgia".

Key Points of Herpes-Zoster

- Herpes-zoster is a recurrent viral infection caused by the Herpes-zoster virus.
- It causes severe pain and burning sensations in the dermatome along the course of sensory nerve (fifth cranial nerve is more frequently affected).
- The disease begins with fever, malaise, headache and painful lymphadenopathy, etc.
- These are followed by intense pain with development of clusters of vesicles over the skin and oral mucosa.
- The painful vesicles characteristically develop unilaterally on one side of the face up to the midline; the other side of the face remains completely free of symptoms.
- The vesicles also develop unilaterally inside the oral cavity, which cause stinging pain, paresthesia and severe stomatitis, etc.
- Herpes-zoster histologically presents swelling of the infected epithelial cell due to intracellular edema (ballooning degeneration) and margination of the nuclear chromatin.
- Treatment is done by antiviral drugs and antibiotics to prevent secondary infections.

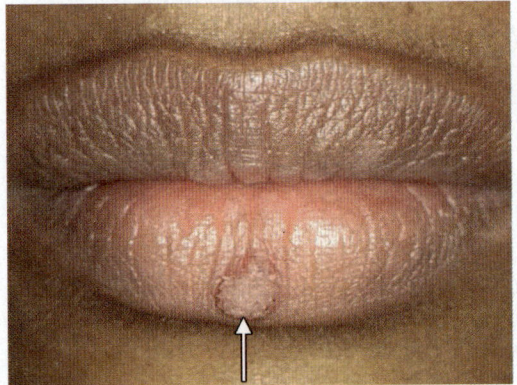

Fig. 8.30: Verruca vulgaris (wart) on the lower lip.

Histopathology
- Herpes-zoster is histologically characterized by swelling of the infected epithelial cell cytoplasms due to intracellular edema (ballooning degeneration).
- Margination of the nuclear chromatin and formation of intranuclear inclusion bodies.
- Reticular degeneration of the epithelial cells along with presence of multiple multinucleated giant cells and polymorphonuclear neutrophilic infiltration in the connective tissue.

Diagnosis of Herpes-Zoster
Clinical: The disease is nearly always diagnosed on the basis of its very characteristic clinical findings, e.g.
- Unilateral distribution of the lesion
- Early severe pain and paresthesia
- Facial rash accompanying the stomatitis.

Histopathology: See histopathological features.

Serology: The disease is diagnosed by the detection of virus-specific antibodies in the serum.

Cytologic smear: Cytologic smears prepared from the vesicular fluid reveal inclusion bodies and ballooning degeneration of the infected cell.

Culture: Tissue culture using vesicular contents produces change in the culture cells which could be correlated with the clinical findings found in the primary infection.

Immunofluorescence: H-Z virus specific antibodies are labeled with fluorescent dye and seen microscopically.

Molecular techniques: Dot blot hybridization and PCR.

Treatment
Antiviral drugs such as acyclovir is given along with antibiotics to prevent secondary infections.

CYTOMEGALOVIRUS INFECTION

In cytomegalovirus infection, the infected cells often contain large intranuclear or paranuclear inclusion bodies, which make the cells dramatically swollen (cytomegaly).

The disease primarily affects the salivary gland tissue during early childhood. It is mostly transmitted via the saliva, blood, milk, semen and urine, etc.

Clinical Features
- Cytomegalovirus infections are mostly subclinical in nature and during the initial period it produces fever, malaise, pharyngitis, myalgia and lymphadenopathy, etc.
- Painful swelling of the parotid and submandibular glands often occurs.
- Aphthous-like ulcers may develop in the mouth, in which cytomegalovirus can be demonstrated.
- In severe cases the disease may produce hepatosplenomegaly, jaundice, pneumonia, purpura, microcephaly, cerebral calcification and dental or neurological abnormalities, etc.
- On rare occasions this virus may produce Kaposi's sarcoma in AIDS patients.

Histopathology
- Vascular endothelial cells, salivary ductal epithelial cells and odontogenic epithelial cells are frequently affected.
- Infected cells contain large intracytoplasmic and intranuclear inclusion bodies and as a result the affected cells are dramatically swollen (cytomegaly) with presence of large nuclei and prominent nucleoli. These cells are often termed as "owl-eye" cells.

Treatment
Only palliative treatment with analgesics, antipyretics and antibiotics are given. No standard antiviral agent is available against this virus.

EPSTEIN–BARR VIRUS INFECTIONS

Epstein–Barr virus is a member of the herpes virus group and it exhibits tropism for the human B-lymphocytes. The virus produces several diseases, namely
- Infectious mononucleosis,
- Burkitt's lymphoma and
- Nasopharyngeal carcinoma, etc.

Epstein–Barr virus can also cause B-cell lymphomas and in hairy leukoplakias of the tongue.

Infectious Mononucleosis/Glandular Fever/Kissing Disease

Infectious mononucleosis or glandular fever is a self-limiting disease which commonly involves the children and young adults. The virus is mainly transmitted via saliva and the common mode of transmission is via intimate kissing with an infected person. The incubation period for the disease is about 7 weeks.

Clinical features
- Initially the disease manifests only in the oral cavity by producing features like gingivostomatitis, gingival bleeding and multiple pinpoint petechiae at the junction of the hard and soft palate.
- About 3–5 days after the appearance of the oral symptoms, other features appear like fever, malaise, fatigue, pharyngitis and severe sore throat, etc.
- The fully developed disease exhibits pharyngitis, severe cough, pharyngeal edema, generalized as well as cervical lymphadenopathy, hyperplastic tonsillar glands with tonsillar exudation, thrombocytopenia and hepatosplenomegaly, etc.
- Acute necrotizing ulcerative gingivitis (ANUG) type of lesion commonly develops in mouth.
- The disease terminates spontaneously within about 1 month time.

Diagnosis
Infectious mononucleosis is diagnosed by a heterophile antibody test called "Paul-Bunnell test".

Treatment
Only palliative treatment is done, complete bed rest is essential.

HUMAN PAPILLOMAVIRUS INFECTION

Human papillomavirus (HPV) belongs to the family of papovavirus; these are DNA viruses, which enter the body by direct or indirect contact and finally reach the basal or suprabasal parts of the skin and epithelium.

The virus replicates in the stratum spinosum, and produces diseases like squamous papilloma, verruca vulgaris and occasionally condyloma acuminatum, etc.

Verruca vulgaris (Common Wart)
It is a type of benign, focal hyperplasia of the oral mucosa and skin, caused by the HPV. The skin lesions more frequently develop in the hands and they appear as painless, white, pink or yellow nodules with papillary projections on the surface (Fig. 8.30). Mucosal lesions also appear as pedunculated or sessile, white colored nodules or papules, which are often seen on lips and tongue. The lesions are more commonly seen in patients with HIV infection.

Condyloma Acuminatum (Venereal Wart)
It is a STD characterized by localized proliferation of the genital, oral and anal epithelium. The HPV is believed to be responsible for the development of this lesion and HPV types 2, 11, 6, 53 have more prominent roles. Condyloma acuminatum is also commonly seen in patients with HIV infection.

Clinically condyloma acuminatum presents clusters of well-defined, exophytic, sessile growths with blunt projections on the surface. Although both have a warty look, condyloma acuminatum differs from papilloma by the fact that the former is larger in size and always occurs in multiple clusters.

PARAMYXOVIRUS INFECTION

Measles (Rubeola)

Measles is a catarrhal inflammation of the dermal, respiratory and oral epithelium which is characterized by focal degeneration and exfoliation of the affected cells.

Etiology and Pathogenesis

The disease is caused by paramyxovirus, these are a group of large RNA viruses responsible for causing measles and mumps. Both viruses are transmitted through saliva and easily contracts young individuals. Measles is one of the most common viral diseases affecting humans.

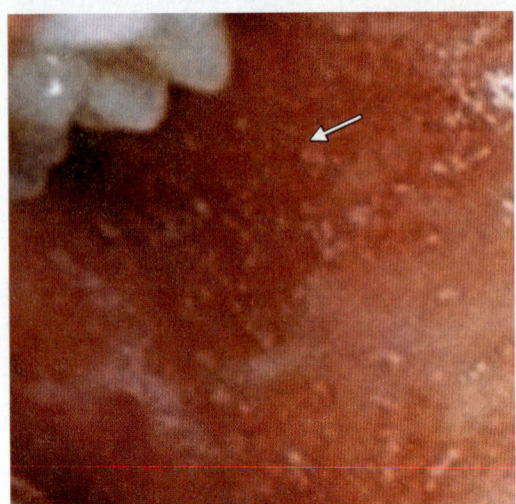

Fig. 8.31: Koplik's spots on the buccal mucosa.

Clinical Features

- Measles is a highly contagious disease which often occurs among children and sometimes, in immunocompromised adults.
- Initially the disease produces severe headache, skin rash, high fever, malaise, photophobia and cough, etc.
- One of the most important features of the disease is the presence of "Koplik's spots" in the mouth, which consist of a cluster of white or white-yellow pinpoint papules on an inflamed, red background (Fig. 8.31).
- Koplik's spots often make a typical "grain of salt" appearance on the buccal mucosa, labial mucosa and soft palate, etc.
- About 2–4 days after the development of Koplik's spots in the oral cavity, diffuse erythematous maculopapular skin rashes begin to appear over the facial skin followed by skin of the trunk and extremities.
- Severe measles during early childhood can produce "pitted enamel hypoplasia" in the permanent dentition (Fig. 8.32).

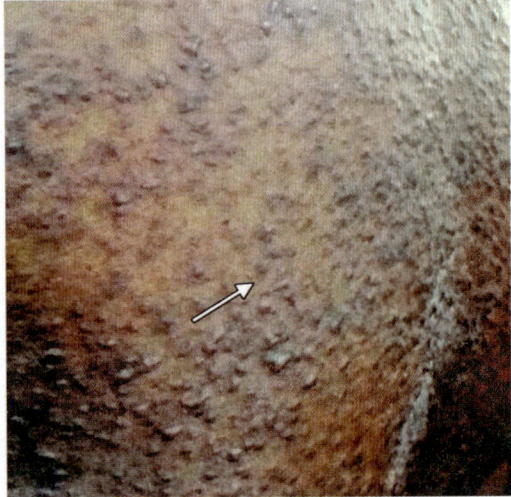

Fig. 8.32: Measles showing erythematous maculopapular skin rash.

Treatment

Only palliative treatment is done and antibiotic therapy is necessary to combat secondary infections.

Mumps

Mumps is an acute contagious, localized viral infection, caused by the paramyxovirus;

Bacterial, Viral and Fungal Infections

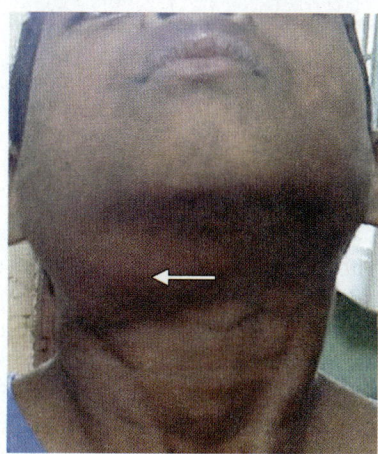

Fig. 8.33: Mumps causing swelling of the Rt. sided parotid gland

which primarily affects the salivary glands. The disease is characterized by unilateral or bilateral, nonsuppurative enlargement of the parotid glands and sometimes other major salivary glands.

Clinical Features

- The disease occurs more commonly among children and young adults and the incubation period is about 2–3 weeks.
- The initial features of the disease include low-grade fever, myalgia, headache, malaise, loss of taste sensation and loss of appetite, etc.
- Pain in the parotid region with subsequent unilateral or bilateral parotid swelling is the most common clinical manifestations of the disease. However in some cases submandibular and sublingual salivary glands are also involved (Fig. 8.33).
- In case of parotid enlargement, elevation of the ear-lobe on one or both sides can be seen when it is clinically viewed from behind the patient. The swelling can extend below up to the posterior inferior border of the mandible.
- The enlarged glands are very painful during meals.

- Intraorally the parotid papilla over the opening of the Stensen's duct is enlarged.
- Painful swelling of the testicles occurs frequently.
- Involvement of pancreas, breast and other salivary glands are also seen in adult patients.

Complications

Pancreatitis, meningitis, oophoritis, etc. occur commonly but the most important complication is the occurrence of "orchitis" in adult males which may sometimes lead to sterility.

Treatment

Only symptomatic treatment is done.

COXSACKIE VIRUS INFECTIONS

Herpangina

Herpangina is a viral disease caused by coxsackie viruses type A1 to 6,8,10 and 22; it is a highly contagious disease and often affects young children during the summer and early autumn seasons.

The virus is transmitted via saliva or by inhalation of air-borne droplets; often the disease spreads rapidly through close-knit groups such as children of the same school.

Clinical Features

- The disease usually occurs in localized fashion and typically involves the soft palate, uvula, anterior pillars of fauces and palatine tonsils.
- Initially it produces acute pharyngitis with anorexia and dysphagia with or without lymphadenopathy.
- The other related symptoms could be headache, nausea, vomiting, fever, malaise and myalgia.
- Oral lesions start as erythematous macules on the soft palate near uvula and anterior pharynx (oropharyngeal

erythema); lesions are never seen anterior to these locations.
- Later on there is formation of multiple, small, fragile vesicles in the locations mentioned earlier.
- Soon the fragile vesicles rupture and leave shallow, pinpoint ulcers.
- The ulcers often resemble herpetic infections and each ulcer is surrounded by a zone of intense erythema (halo).
- The ulcers heal spontaneously within 1–2 weeks.

Treatment

Only palliative treatment is done.

Hand, Foot and Mouth Disease

Hand, foot and mouth disease is caused by coxsackie virus (A-16 and A-9) type and it can spread as minor epidemic among the school children and teachers; Moreover, parents are also sometimes affected by the disease. Incubation period is between 3–10 days.

Clinical Features

- It is a highly contagious systemic infection characterized by simultaneous occurrence of oral ulcerations and vesicular eruptions (rash) on the extremities (rashes are often seen on the palm of the hand, sole of the foot).
- The disease starts with mild symptoms like fever, sore throat, dysphagia and malaise, etc.
- The skin lesions consist of small vesicles or occasionally large blisters that form mainly around the base of the fingers or toes.
- In the oral cavity there is often formation of vesicles and ulcerations on the hard palate, tongue, labial mucosa and buccal mucosa. The ulcers occur more anteriorly and unlike herpangina, these are uncommon in the oropharyngeal area.
- The ulcers often resemble herpetic ulcers but the significant difference is that gingiva is rarely affected.

Treatment

Only symptomatic treatment is advised in this disease.

Aphthous Ulcers

Definition of Ulcer

Loss of surface tissue due to a sloughing of necrotic inflammatory tissue; the defect extends into the underlying lamina propria.

Aphthous ulcer is the most common type of nontraumatic, ulcerative condition of the oral mucosa, which may affect up to 15–20% of the population at some time in their lives. It is characterized by persistently recurrent, painful ulcers of the mouth (Box 8.13).

There are two distinct age groups for the disease:
- More common group comprises of young people between early childhood to late teenage.
- Second group of people are adults, many of whom have anemia and history of smoking cessation (highly placed professionals and people of higher socioeconomic status tend to suffer from this disease more often than others).

Etiology

The exact etiology is not known and only few probable factors have been identified which are as follows:
- *Genetic predisposition*: The disease often affects several members of the same family

Box 8.13	List of etiological factors in aphthous ulcer
<ul><li>Genetic predisposition</li><li>Exaggerated response to trauma</li><li>Immunological factors</li><li>Microbiologic factors</li><li>Nutritional factors</li><li>Systemic conditions</li><li>Hormonal imbalance</li><li>Non-smoking</li><li>Allergy and chronic asthma</li><li>Miscellaneous factors</li></ul>	

and moreover identical twins are more frequently affected.
- *Exaggerated response to trauma*: The ulcer develops in those mucosal sites which are subjected to trauma in the past (e.g. tooth prick injury).
- *Immunological factors*: The disease may occur due to some autoimmune reactions, or in patients with immunosuppression (e.g. AIDS).
- *Microbiologic factors*: The disease may be caused by herpes simplex virus type-I or *Streptococcus sanguis* or L forms organisms.
- *Nutritional factors*: Deficiency of vitamin B12, folate and iron, etc. often reported in patients with aphthous ulcer.
- *Systemic conditions*: Behcet's syndrome, Crohn's disease and celiac disease are often associated with aphthous ulcer (Box 8.14).
- *Hormonal imbalance*: Hormonal change during menstrual cycle may increase the incidence of aphthous ulcer.
- *Nonsmoking*: The disease almost exclusively occurs in nonsmokers or the people those who have given up smoking recently.
- *Miscellaneous factors*: Stress and anxiety.

Clinical Features

- Aphthous ulcers usually develop over the movable, nonkeratinized oral mucosa like the tongue (lateral borders), vestibule, lips, buccal mucosa, soft palate and floor of the mouth, etc.
- Highest incidence of the disease is reported during early adult life.

- Before the appearance of the ulcer, the involved area produces a burning or tingling sensation, but the ulcers are never preceded by vesiculations.
- These ulcers recur in an interval of about 3–4 weeks.

Types

There are three clinically recognizable forms aphthous ulcer:
1. Minor aphthous ulcer
2. Major aphthous ulcer
3. Herpetiform ulcer.

Minor Aphthous Ulcer (Fig. 8.34)

- It is the most common type of aphthous ulcer (85%) and appears episodically either as single ulcer or in clusters of 1–5 ulcers.
- These are very painful, shallow, round or elliptical ulcers, measuring about 2–8 mm in diameter with a crateriform margin.
- The lesions are often surrounded by an erythematous "halo" and have yellowish-gray, fibrinous floor.
- Minor aphthous ulcer mostly develops over the nonkeratinized mucosa, e.g. inner surface of lips, soft palate, anterior fauces, floor of the mouth and ventral surface of the tongue (gland bearing mucosa), etc.
- The ulcer lasts for about 7–10 days and then heals up without scarring by regeneration of epithelium across the floor of the ulcer.

Box 8.14	Systemic conditions associated with aphthous ulcer.
<ul><li>HIV infection</li><li>Behcet's syndrome</li><li>Cyclic neutropenia</li><li>Celiac disease</li><li>Nutritional deficiency</li><li>MAGIC syndrome (mouth and genital ulcers with inflamed cartilage</li><li>Reiter's disease</li></ul>	

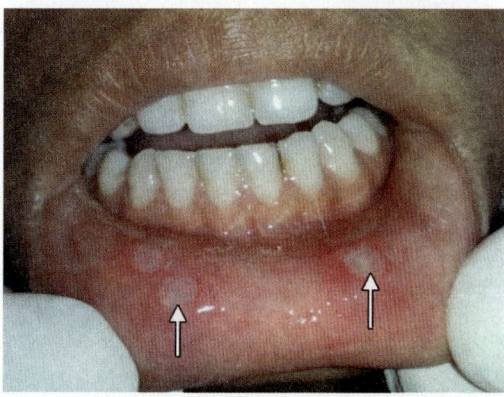

Fig. 8.34: Minor aphthous ulcer of the lower lip.

- Recurrence is common and often occurs at an interval of 2–3 weeks.
- The disease mostly causes difficulty in taking food, mastication and speech, etc.

Major Aphthous Ulcer (Fig. 8.35)

- Major aphthous ulcers are less common (10%) and are considered to be the most severe among all types.
- Ulcers are generally single and are much larger in size (0.5 cm to several centimeters in diameter) and can involve both keratinized as well as nonkeratinized mucosae.
- Mostly seen over the lips, soft palate and fauces (nonkeratinized mucosa) but can also involve dorsum of tongue and gingiva (keratinized mucosa).
- Major aphthous ulcers are more painful and much deeper lesions and appear crateriform (owing to its increased depth) and it heals with scar formation in about 6 weeks time.
- They often make the patients ill (due to the psychologic stress and difficulty in food intake).
- Few lesions may look like malignant ulcers, moreover sometimes these lesions occur in association with HIV infections.
- Severe scarring following healing of major aphthous ulcer may cause trismus and microstomia.

Herpetiform Ulcer

- Herpetiform type of aphthous ulcers are much uncommon lesions (seen in less than 5% cases) and these ulcers are named so because they resemble herpetic ulcers (Fig. 8.36).
- Herpetiform ulcers are characterized by formation of several (sometimes hundreds) extremely painful, small (less than 2 mm), superficial ulcers in the oral mucosa.
- These ulcers develop on a background of generalized mucosal erythema and they frequently coalesce.
- The ulcers last for several weeks or months (duration is much longer than the other two types).
- Children in their late teens often suffer from this disease and the lesions occur in both gland-bearing mucosa as well as over the keratinized mucosa.

Histopathology of Aphthous Ulcer

The histopathologic findings are nonspecific and are not pathognomonic:
- Aphthous ulcer microscopically shows the presence of an overlying degenerated and ulcerated epithelium being covered by a fibrinopurulent exudate.
- Vacuolization and necrosis of the individual epithelial cells occur.

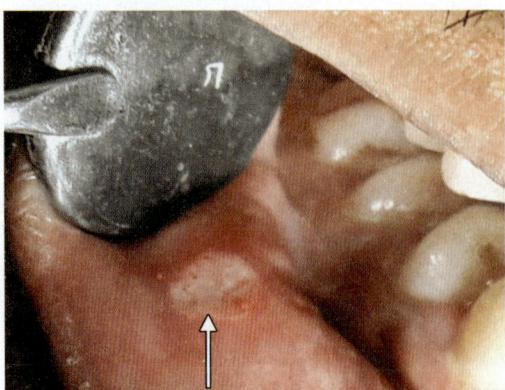

Fig. 8.35: Major aphthous ulcer of the lip.

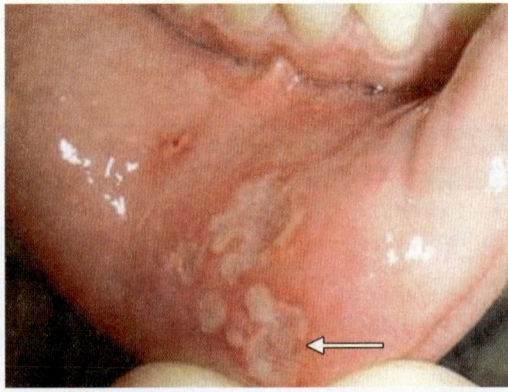

Fig. 8.36: Herpetiform type of aphthous ulcer.

- In the underlying connective tissue, dense infiltration of neutrophils is found in the superficial layer.
- In the deeper layers of connective tissue lymphocytes, macrophages, plasma cells and mast cells, etc. often predominate.
- Mononuclear cells are often seen to surround the small blood vessels (perivascular cuffing).

Cytology
Cytologic smears prepared from the materials obtained from around the recurrent aphthous ulcer reveals the presence of "Anitschkow's cells". These cells are characterized by the presence of elongated nuclei containing a linear bar of chromatin, with few radiating processes extending towards the nuclear membrane.

Differential Diagnosis
- Herpetic ulcers
- Traumatic ulcers
- Pemphigus vulgaris
- Cicatricial pemphigoid
- Ulcers due to neutropenia
- Crohn's disease.

Treatment
Treatment of aphthous ulcers is unsatisfactory and empirical. Topical and systemic administration of steroids is useful for the containment of the disease and in few cases immunomodulator drugs produce some beneficial effects. Recurrence is very common.

Behçet's Syndrome
Behçet's syndrome is a multisystem disease that predominantly affects young males and is characterized by multiple superficial, painful "aphthous-like ulcers" in the oral cavity. However to fulfill the criteria of being Behçet's syndrome, clinically there should be presence of aphthous-like ulcer in the oral cavity along with at least two of the following lesions, e.g. skin lesion, eye lesion or genital lesion, etc.

Etiology
Etiology is unknown; may be caused by some immunologic abnormality.

Clinical Features
- *Oral lesions*: Aphthous-like ulceration in the oral cavity.
- *Skin lesions*: Erythematous macular, papular, vesicular or pustular lesions in the skin; thrombophlebitis may also sometimes develop.
- *Eye lesions*: Ocular lesions in Behçet's syndrome include uveitis, conjunctivitis, photophobia and retinitis, etc.
- *Genital lesions*: Ulceration in the genitalia, which looks similar to those of the oral cavity.
- *Other lesions*: Behçet's syndrome sometimes presents some additional features like neural, vascular, articular, renal or gastrointestinal lesions of various kinds.

Histopathology
Microscopically the lesions produce similar feature to what is found in minor aphthous ulcer. However there can be some additional features like severe vasculitis and vascular damage, etc.

Treatment
Behçet's syndrome is treated by systemic steroid therapy.

Reiter's Syndrome
Reiter's syndrome is a disease commonly found among white adult males, which produces the classic triad comprising of nongonococcal urethritis, arthritis and conjunctivitis.

Etiology
Mostly unknown, however it is believed to be an immunologically mediated disorder; which is often triggered by some infections.

Clinical Features

- Age: The disease commonly occurs between the ages of 20 years and 35 years.
- Genital lesions: Genital lesions produce a characteristic "balanitis circinata" over the glans penis; moreover genital ulcers are also commonly seen.
- Oral lesions: Oral lesions are mostly seen over the buccal mucosa, palate and gingiva, etc. and these lesions present painless, aphthous-like ulcers. In addition to this a tongue lesion is often seen that resembles the typical 'geographic tongue'. Pruritic spots are also seen on the palate.
- Skin lesions: Well circumscribed erythematous erosions with irregular white linear boundary.

Histopathology

The oral epithelium exhibits hyperkeratosis with elongation of rete-pegs; formation of few microabscesses occur in the superficial part of the epithelium. Histologically, the lesion often resembles "psoriasis".

Treatment

Systemic steroid therapy and administration of antibiotics.

Rabies

Rabies as an acute fatal viral disease of CNS caused by rabies virus that affects all animals and the virus is transmitted by the infected secretions (usually saliva).

Mostly the diseases are caused due to the bite of infected animals like dogs, cats, foxes, wolves and bats, etc.

Pathogenesis

After the introduction of the live virus through the skin following animal bite, the virus replicates within the striated muscle cells at the site of inoculation. Then the virus reaches the peripheral nerve and moves centripetally up the nerve to the CNS via the nerve axoplasm. In brain it replicates exclusively within the gray matter and then again it passes centrifugally along the autonomic nerves to reach different body tissues like salivary glands, adrenal medulla, liver, kidney, lungs, heart and skin, etc.

The incubation period of rabies is about 10 days to 1 year (mean being 1–2 months).

Clinical Manifestations

The clinical manifestation of rabies can be divided into four stages:
1. Prodromal stage
2. Encephalitic stage
3. Stage of brainstem centers dysfunction
4. Recovery stage (very rare).

The prodromal stage persists for about 1–4 days and is marked by fever, headache, malaise, nausea, vomiting, anorexia, sore throat and paresthesia at the site of inoculation.

The encephalitic stage is characterized by excitation, anger, confusion, hallucination, paralysis of the vocal cord, high fever (105°F), excessive salivation and lacrimation.

There can be excessive sensitivity to bright, loud noise, touch or even gentle breeze, etc.

The stage of brainstem dysfunction presents the features like facial palsies, difficulty in deglutition, foaming from the mouth. One of the most important features of this stage is "hydrophobia"—(the violent, painful, involuntary contraction of diaphragm with accessory respiratory, pharyngeal and laryngeal muscles which is initiated by drinking water or even while thinking of any drink).

Most of the patients die following coma and respiratory arrest, and the median survival rate is only about 4–20 days.

Laboratory Findings

- WBC count is elevated up to 17,000–30,000 per cm of blood
- Isolation of virus from saliva

- Mouse inoculation study for viral antigens
- Detection of Negri bodies in the brain tissue
- Fluorescent antibody (FA) staining for viral antigen.

Treatment
- The animal should be captured, confined and observed for 10 days and if any illness or abnormality in its behavior is noticed during that period, it should be killed for fluorescent antibody examination and detection of "Negri body" in the brain.
- Local wound should be cleaned by generous scrubbing with soap water and 1–4% benzalkonium chloride.
- Passive immunization with antirabies antiserum.
- Active immunization with antirabies vaccine.

Box 8.15	Local and systemic conditions predisposing to the development of candidiasis.

- Immunologic immaturity in infants or in old aged persons
- Suppression of oral microflora by broad spectrum antibiotics
- Hormonal disturbances like diabetes mellitus, hypoparathyroidism, oral pills and pregnancy, etc.
- Long-term local or systemic steroid therapy
- Xerostomia with Sjogren's syndrome
- Chronic denture wearing
- Heavy smoking
- Advanced malignancy, acute leukemia and squamous cell carcinoma, etc.
- Malabsorption and malnutrition—iron, folic acid and other vitamin deficiencies
- Prolonged broad spectrum antibiotic therapy causing suppression of oral flora
- Immunosuppression (e.g. AIDS)
- Chemotherapy and radiotherapy
- Tricyclic antidepressant therapy
- Blood group "O" individuals (Tend to suffer more)

FUNGAL INFECTION

CANDIDIASIS

Candidiasis is the most common type of mycotic or fungal infection that occurs in the oral cavity and is predominantly caused by *Candida albicans*. The disease can also be produced by *C. tropicalis, C. glabrata, C. krusei* and *C. pseudotropicalis*, etc. but far less commonly. Candida is also called "monila" and hence the disease is known as "moniliasis".

Candida albicans is the most prominent member in the candida family; it is a yeast-like fungus, which multiplies primarily by the production of buds from ovoid yeast cells. This fungus may be present in two forms (the character called dimorphism)—(1) "yeast form" (mostly inactive) and (2) "hyphal/filament form" (it is the infective form).

The candidal "yeasts" can multiply only inside the body (outside the host they cannot multiply), these organisms are present as commensal organisms in the oral cavity, digestive tract and vaginal tract, etc. in many healthy persons; however they become pathogenic due to some local or systemic changes in the body (mostly in debilitating diseases and immunosuppression). The infective phase of the organism is characterized by the presence of "hyphae" that can directly invade oral keratinocytes (Box 8.15).

Pathogenesis

Candidal organisms produce the disease by tissue invasion or by inducing a hypersensitivity reaction or by releasing some potent toxins. They produce large number of opportunistic infections in immunocompromised patients.

Clinical Features

Candida albicans can cause acute or chronic white lesions and also atrophic, red lesions in the mouth. Candidiasis occurs mostly as superficial infection and besides oral cavity it can involve skin and occasionally the deeper structures, e.g. esophagus, lungs or endocardium, etc. in severely debilitated or immunosuppressed persons.

Table 8.5: Classification of oral candidiasis.

Acute candidiasis	Chronic candidiasis	Systemic candidiasis	Mucocutaneous candidiasis
• Pseudomembranous type	• Atrophic type • Hypertrophic type	• Candidal endocarditis	• Localized type (oral cavity, face, nails, and scalp, etc.)
• Atrophic type	• Candida-associated angular cheilitis	• Candidal meningitis • Candidal septicemia	• Familial type • Syndrome-associated candidiasis

The oral candidiasis can be classified into the following types (Table 8.5):

Acute Pseudomembranous Candidiasis

- It is commonly known as "oral thrush" and it appears as a smooth, thick, creamy-white or yellow, soft and friable plaque (pseudomembrane) on the oral mucosa (Fig. 8.37).
- The plaque can be easily wiped off by gentle scraping, which leaves an erythematous, raw, bleeding surface in the underlying area.
- The lesions may occur at any mucosal site.
- The plaque consists of fungal organisms, keratotic debris, inflammatory cells, desquamated epithelial cells and fibrin, etc.
- Oral thrush commonly occurs among children, debilitated elderly persons, AIDS patients and patients with xerostomia due to Sjogren's syndrome or irradiation.
- In neonates, the disease is contracted from birth canal of an infected mother.

Acute Atrophic Candidiasis

- It occurs when the pseudomembranous covering of the oral thrush is lost.
- The lesion presents generalized red, painful, "peeling patches" over the mucosa, which often causes tenderness, dysphagia and burning sensation, etc.
- The condition is commonly seen on the dorsum of the tongue and palate in patients receiving long-term antibiotic or steroid therapy (Fig. 8.38).

Chronic Atrophic Candidiasis

- This form of candidiasis is also known as "denture-induced stomatitis" and seen

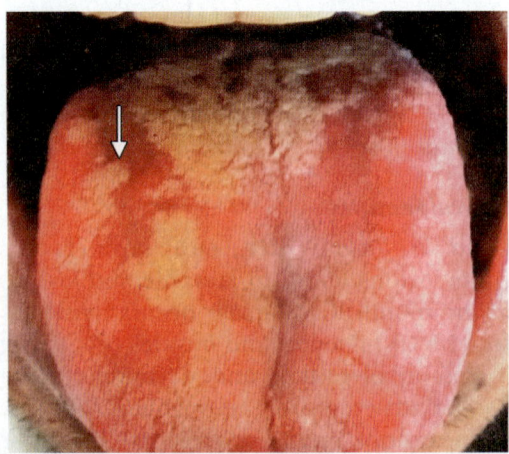

Fig. 8.37: Acute pseudomembranous candidiasis of the tongue.

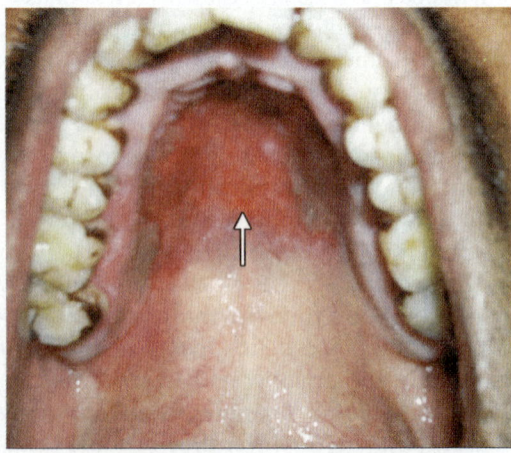

Fig. 8.38: Atrophic candidiasis of palate.

typically on the hard palate beneath the prosthesis among the denture wearing elderly persons.
- The lesion clinically appears as a bright red, edematous, velvety area limited by the extent of the prosthesis; at some points there may be flecks of thrush.

Candida-associated Angular Cheilitis
- An important form of chronic atrophic candidiasis is "angular cheilitis". It occurs at the angle of the mouth among persons having deep commissural folds secondary to overclosure of mouth (Fig. 8.39).
- It can also occur among persons with lip-licking habits, denture wearing, or deficiency of riboflavin, vitamin B12 and folic acid deficiency, etc.
- The infection starts due to the colonization of fungi in the skin folds following deposition of saliva due to repeated lip-licking.
- Clinically the patients often have soreness, erythema and fissuring (red cracks) at the corner of the mouth. In some cases the defect can extend over the adjoining skin surfaces. The cracks are often covered with pseudomembrane.

Chronic Hyperplastic Candidiasis
- It is form of chronic candidiasis, which produces persistent, adherent, firm, white

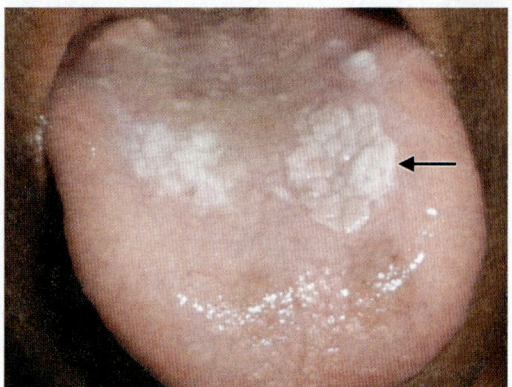

Fig. 8.40: Chronic hyperplastic candidiasis.

plaques or patches on the oral mucosa that often resembles oral leukoplakia. The patchy areas are of irregular thickness and density and they have a rough, nodular surface (Fig. 8.40).
- The lesions are mostly seen in middle aged male smokers, which develop on the dorsum of tongue, buccal mucosa near the commissure (often bilaterally) and the palate.
- These lesions cannot be removed by scraping and in some cases there may be presence of erythematous areas within the patch.

Localized Mucocutaneous Candidiasis
- This is characterized by long standing and persistent candidal infections in the oral cavity, skin, nails and vaginal mucosa, etc.

Familial Mucocutaneous Candidiasis
- It is believed to be transmitted genetically as autosomal recessive trait and most of the patients are mildly affected.
- A triad of mucocutaneous candidiasis, thymoma and myositis has been reported in 1968.

Syndrome-associated Candidiasis
Severe candidiasis (both acute and chronic variety) are well recognized opportunistic infections in immunosuppressed patients,

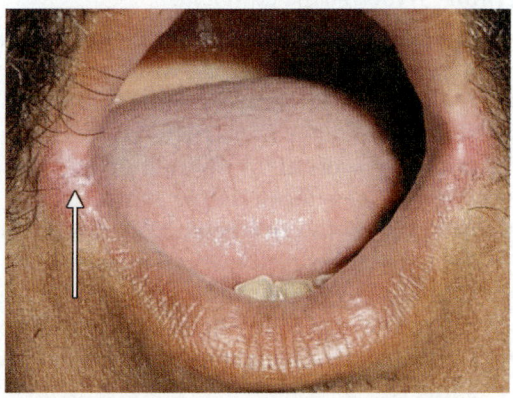

Fig. 8.39: Candida associated angular cheilitis.

particularly those suffering from AIDS. Depressed cell-mediated immunity is believed to be the cause.

Candidiasis Endocrinopathy Syndrome

- Transmitted as autosomal recessive trait.
- Chronic oral candidiasis occurring mostly in the second decade of life.
- Hypoparathyroidism, Addison's disease, diabetes mellitus and hypothyroidism.

Systemic Candidiasis

Candidal Endocarditis

- Patients who have undergone prosthetic heart valve replacements and those who are using for a long time venous catheters are at risk for developing candidal endocarditis.
- Candidal growth in the valve may result in the development of major venous embolism.
- Clinically, the patient often develops fever, dyspnea, edema and congestive cardiac failure, etc.

Candidal Meningitis

- Spread of candidal organisms into the brain results in meningitis, which could be a consequence of oral candidiasis and in such cases, the organisms can be detected from the CSF.
- Patients often develop fever, headache, stiffness in the body and hemiplegia.
- The condition is often fatal.

Candidal Septicemia

- It occurs due to disseminated spread of candidal organisms throughout the body and it can be secondary to severe oral or oropharyngeal candidiasis.
- Clinically the patient often develops fever, chill, nausea, vomiting, shock and coma, etc.
- The condition can be fatal if not treated in time.

Histopathology of Candidiasis

Acute Pseudomembranous Candidiasis

- The layer of thrush develops due to invasion of the candidal hyphae into the superficial layers of the epithelium with subsequent proliferation.
- Hyperplastic epithelium exhibits superficial necrotic and desquamating parakeratinized layer along with candidal hyphae, yeast cells and PMN.
- Often there is separation between the superficial pseudomembrane and the deeper layers of epithelium.
- The candidal hyphae penetrate the epithelium vertically and extend downwards up to the glycogen rich zone; lamina propria is infiltrated by chronic inflammatory cells.
- In H&E stained sections the hyphae often appear as a weakly basophilic thread-like structure.
- These are readily visualized by periodic acid Schiff (PAS) or Grocott's silver stain (Figs. 8.41A and B).

Acute Atrophic Candidiasis

- Thin, atrophic, nonkeratinized epithelium with occasional presence of candidal hyphae.
- Chronic inflammatory cell infiltration is seen in the epithelium as well as in the lamina propria.

Chronic Hyperplastic Candidiasis

- Hyperplastic, acanthotic epithelium with parakeratosis in clinically white areas.
- Intercellular edema and PMN infiltration sometimes causing separation between different layers of the epithelium.
- Microabscess formation in some cases.
- Atrophy of the epithelium with loss of keratin in the clinically erythematous areas.
- Candidal hyphae invading the parakeratinized layer at right angles to the surface.
- Epithelial dysplasia may be present in some cases.

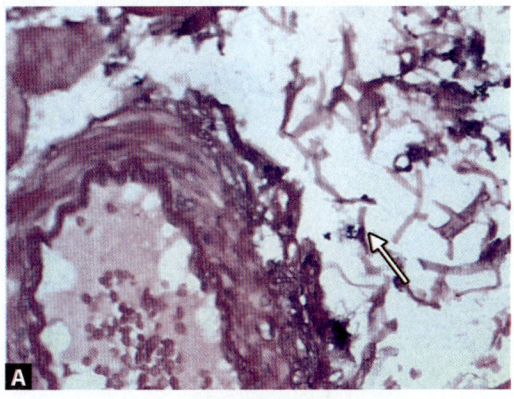
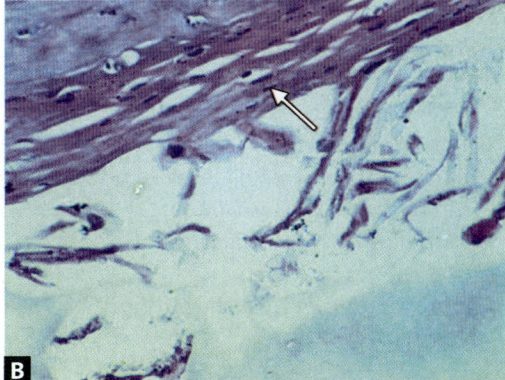

Figs. 8.41A and B: Photomicrographs of candidal hyphae (PAS stain).

Differential Diagnosis

- Chemical burn
- Mucous patch of syphilis
- Traumatic ulcer
- Leukoplakia
- Lichen planus
- Discoid lupus erythematosus (DLE).

Treatment

Topical and systemic administration of nystatin is done in conventional cases. In immunosuppressed patients, systemic administration of amphotericin-B and fluconazole may be necessary. Removal of primary etiological factors and improvement of oral hygiene is essential

DEEP FUNGAL INFECTIONS

Coccidioidomycosis

It is deep fungal infection of the lung and caused by *Coccidioides immitis* (Fig. 8.42). The disease is commonly seen in North and South America, where it occurs in endemic form. Since the disease occurs predominantly in the central valley of California, it is often known as "valley fever".

Clinical Features

- The disease starts with a flu-like illness characterized by fever, malaise, fatigue, headache, myalgia, cough and dyspnea, etc.

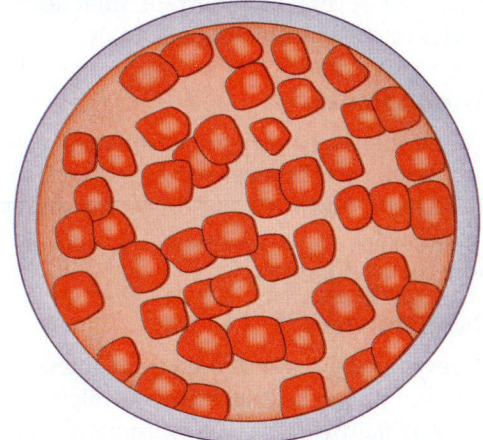

Fig. 8.42: *Coccidioides immitis* (spherule enclosing endospores).

- Lymphadenopathy, chest congestion and joint pain, etc. develop after that.
- Pulmonary lesions produce tuberculosis like features, e.g. chest pain, weight loss, persistent cough and low-grade fever, etc.
- Granulomatous, verrucous or necrotic ulcers of the skin (more often on the facial skin).

Oral Manifestation

- Granulomatous proliferation of oral mucosa with ulceration and induration.
- Regional lymphadenopathy and occasional jaw swelling.
- Oral lesions heal with scarring.

Histopathology

- Multiple focal granulomas containing large number of macrophages, lymphocytes, plasma cells and multiple multinucleated giant cells.
- Liquefaction necrosis and exudation at the margin of the lesion.
- Epithelial hyperplasia with microabscess formation.
- Large double contoured "spherules" are seen with silver stain.

Treatment

Ketoconazole is effective in mild infections. In case of severe or recurrent infections—amphotericin-B is the drug of choice.

Histoplasmosis

Histoplasmosis is a deep fungal infection of the lung tissue, which is caused by *Histoplasma capsulatum* (Figs. 8.43 and 8.44). The disease is contracted by inhalation of the airborne spores of the organism.

Clinical Features

- Fever, malaise, nonproductive cough, dyspnea, anorexia, headache, myalgia and chest pain (in case of pulmonary infections).

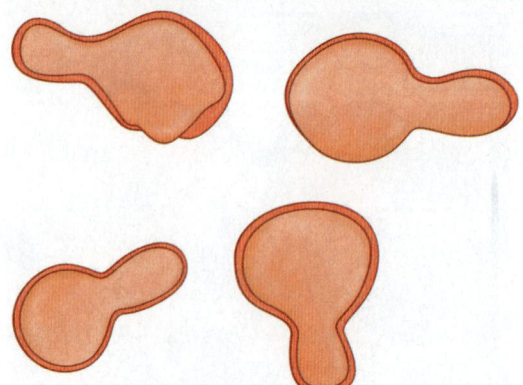

Fig. 8.44: *Histoplasma capsulatum* (yeast form).

- In disseminated cases the disease manifests with hepatosplenomegaly and lymphadenopathy.
- Involvement of kidney and bone marrow.
- Granulomatous lesions may also be seen over the skin.
- Calcification of the hilar lymph nodes.

Oral Manifestations

- Oral lesions occur in the forms of nodules over the mucosa, which frequently undergoes ulceration with raised, rolled borders and induration of the surrounding tissue.
- The ulcers are painful and are often clinically confused with squamous cell carcinoma.
- Most of the oral lesions develop in the gingiva, tongue, palate and buccal mucosa, etc.
- Some lesions may be papular, verrucous or plaque-like.
- Sore throat, pain during chewing, hoarseness of voice and dysphagia are common.
- Granulomatous lesions often cause destruction of the alveolar bone with loosening or exfoliation of teeth.
- Oral lesions of histoplasmosis may occur secondary to HIV infections and uncontrolled diabetes and in many cases they resemble carcinoma or tuberculous ulcers (Fig. 8.45).

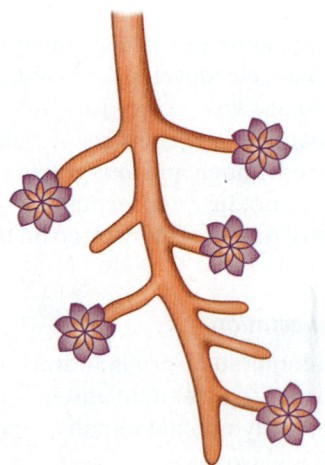

8.43: *Histoplasma capsulatum* (mycelial form).

Bacterial, Viral and Fungal Infections

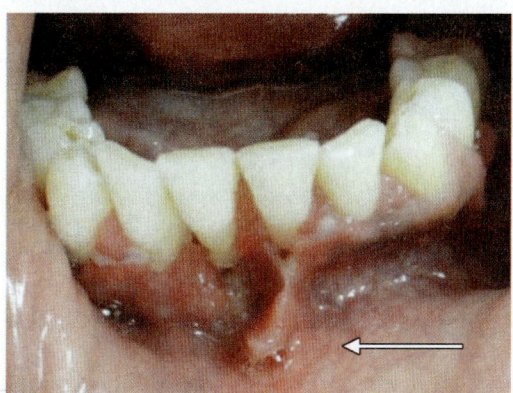

Fig. 8.45: Histoplasmosis of mouth in a diabetic patient.

Differential Diagnosis
- Squamous cell carcinoma
- Tuberculosis
- Actinomycosis
- Leishmaniasis.

Histopathology (Fig. 8.46)
- Histologically the disease reveals a granulomatous lesion characterized by the formation of multiple, small, granulomas containing histiocytes and the fungi.
- The granulomas are often surrounded by histiocytes, lymphocytes, plasma cells and few scattered multinucleated giant cells.

- Pseudoepitheliomatous hyperplasia can be seen in nonulcerated lesions.

Treatment
Administration of amphotericin-B.

Cryptococcosis

Cryptococcosis is a chronic fungal infection caused by *Cryptococcus neoformans*. The disease commonly affects the lung, kidney, skin and the mucous membrane (Fig. 8.47). It has a particular tendency to spread to the CNS.

Clinical Features
- Cough with mucoid expectoration, pleuritic pain and hemoptysis, etc.
- Pustular lesions which may also discharge pus-like material.
- Papular, nodular or ulcerative lesions over the skin.
- Brain infection results in meningoencephalitis with associated neurogenic symptoms.
- Cryptococcosis may occur as an opportunistic infection in patients suffering from lymphoma, leukemia, diabetes and sarcoidosis, etc.

Oral Manifestation
- Oral lesions often appear as nodular or granulomatous areas which undergo ulceration within a few days.

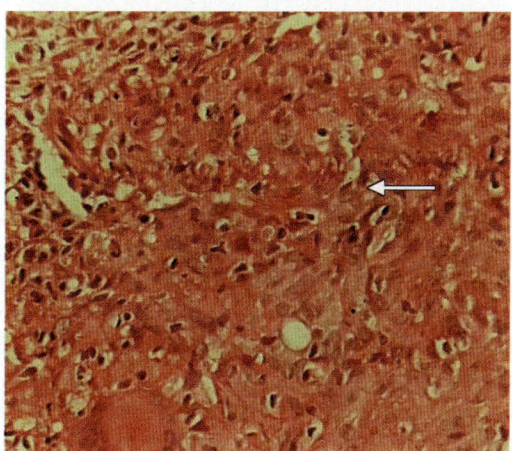

Fig. 8.46: Photomicrograph of histoplasmosis.

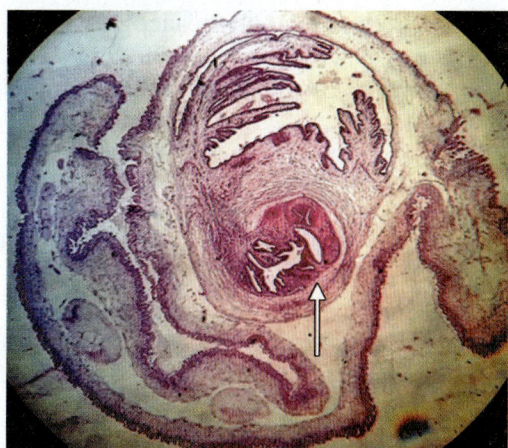

Fig. 8.47: Photomicrograph of cryptococcosis.

- The ulcers are nonhealing crater-like, which are often painful.
- These lesions are commonly seen over the hard and soft palate, gingiva, tongue, tonsillar pillars and extraction sockets, etc.
- Some lesions may cause perforation of the palate.

Histopathology
- Multiple focal granulomas exhibiting epithelioid cells, macrophages, lymphocytes, plasma cells and multinucleated giant cells.
- Encysted cryptococcal organisms can be seen in PAS stained sections.
- The infective form of the fungus is a budding yeast that exhibits a thick, mucicarmine-positive capsule, which resembles a halo.

Treatment
Administration of amphotericin-B.

North American Blastomycosis

It is a chronic fungal infection caused by *Blastomyces dermatitidis*.

Clinical Features
- Low-grade fever, weight loss, cough and purulent sputum.
- Elevated, verrucous crusted lesion (either single or multiple) on the face and hands.
- Lesions heal by scarring at the center.
- Bone involvement is seen in large number of cases.

Oral Manifestations
- Proliferative, ulcerated lesions developing over the palate, lips, tongue, gingiva and maxilla or mandible.
- Loosening of teeth and draining sinuses.
- Oropharyngeal pain and cervical lymphadenopathy.

Treatment
Administration of amphotericin-B.

Mucormycosis

Mucormycosis or *phycomycosis* is a fungal disease caused by a fungus belonging to the order Mucorales.

Clinical Features
- Cervicofacial mucormycosis is characterized by the occurrence of a triad comprising of—uncontrolled diabetes mellitus, periorbital infection and meningoencephalitis.
- Nasal infection with dark blood-stained discharge.
- Facial pain and swelling is common with occasional facial nerve paralysis.
- Necrosis of nasal septum and turbinates.

Oral Manifestations
- Maxillary sinusitis with swelling alveolar ridge and palate are the most common manifestations of this disease.
- Paresthesia of the branches of trigeminal nerve is also common.
- Ulcerative lesions on the palate are the common oral manifestation of this disease.
- The area looks black or gray and often there is perforation of the bone.

Treatment
Administration of amphotericin-B.

ORAL MYASIS (MAGGOT INFECTION)

It is a rare disease caused by larvae of certain dipteran flies; the disease begins if the flies lay eggs on an open wound from where the eggs can hatch into the larva which are known as "maggots" (Fig. 8.48). The maggots feed on live or necrotic tissues and keep on multiplying inside the wound and if proper care is not taken these organisms burrow into deeper tissues causing extensive damage to the tissues or organs.

Maggots can be removed by applying turpentine oil on the wound or they can be mechanically removed one by one.

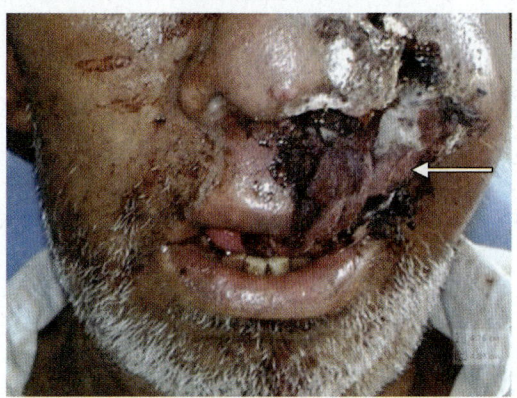

Fig. 8.48: Oral maggot infection.

BIBLIOGRAPHY

1. Aaby P, Bukh J, Lisse IM, et al. Measles mortality, state of nutrition, and family structure: a commonly study from Guinea-Bissau. J Infect Dis. 1983;147:693-701.
2. Abbot JN, Briney AT, Denaro SA. Recovery of tubercle bacilli from mouth washings of tuberculous dental patients. J Am Dent Assoc. 1955;50:49-52.
3. Agnew RG. Cancrum oris. J Periodontol. 1947;18:22-3.
4. Akinosi JO. African histoplasmosis presenting as a dental problem. Br J Oral Surg. 1970;8:58-63.
5. Andris JS, Capra JD. The molecular structure of human antibodies specific for the human immunodeficiency virus. T Clin Immunol. 1995;15:17-26.
6. Babajews A, Nicholls MW. Tetanus associated with dental sepsis. Br J Oral Maxillofac Surg. 1985;23:36-40.
7. Barton RP. Lesions of the mouth, pharynx and larynx in lepromatous leprosy. Lepr India. 1974;46:130-4.
8. Bauer WH. Tooth buds and jaws in patients with congenital syphilis. Correlation between distribution of Treponema pallidum and tissue reaction. Am J Pathol. 1944;20:297.
9. Bell WA, Gamble GE, Garrington GE. North American blastomycosis with oral lesions. Oral Surg Oral Med Oral Pathol. 1969;28:914-23.
10. Benoliel EH, Asquith J. Actinomycosis of the jaws. Int Jo Oral Surg. 1985;14:195-9.
11. Bhatti SA. Cervicofacial actinomycosis in pregnancy. Br Dent T. 1989;166:83-5.
12. Bjorlin G. Oral tuberculosis. Odontologisk Revy. 1967;18:395-9.
13. Blankson JM. Measles and its problems as seen in Ghana. Environ Child Health. 1975;21:51-4.
14. Bleck TP. *Clostridium tetani* (tetanus). In: G Mandell (Ed). Principles and Practice of Infectious Diseases, 5th edition. New York: Churchill Livingstone; 2000.
15. Bogliolo L. South American blastomycosis (Lutz's disease): a contribution of knowledge of its pathogenesis. Arch Dermatol Syphilol. 1950;61:470-5.
16. Bradnum P. Tuberculous sinus of the face association with an abscessed lower third molar. Dent Pract Dent Rec. 1961;12:127-8.
17. Brennan TF, Vrabec DP. Tuberculosis of the oral mucosa. Report of a case. Ann Otol Rhinol Laryngol. 1970;80:601-5.
18. Brodsky RH, Klattel JS. The tuberculous dental periapical granuloma. Am J Orthodont Oral Surg. 1943;29:498-502.
19. Brodsky RH. Oral tuberculous lesion. Am J Orthodont Oral Surg. 1942;28:132-9.
20. Brown OE, Finn R. Mucormycosis of the mandible. J Oral Maxillofoc Surg. 1986;44:132-6.
21. Bruce KW. Tuberculosis of the alveolar gingiva. Oral Surg Oral Med Oral Pathol. 1954;7:894-900.
22. Brunell PA. Mumps. In: Feigin RD, Cherry JD (Eds). Textbook of pediatric infectious diseases. Philadelphia: WB Saunders; 1981. pp. 1231-5.
23. Brunell PA. Varicella-zoster infections. In: Feigin RD, Cherry JD (Eds). Textbook of pediatric infectious diseases. Philadelphia: WB Saunders; 1981. pp. 1206-10.
24. Brunet LB, Ancelle RA. The international occurrence of the acquired immunodeficiency syndrome. Ann Int Med. 1985;103:670-4.
25. Burkitt DP. Aetiology of Burkitt's lymphoma—an alternative hypothesis to a vectored virus. J Nat Can Inst. 1969;42:19-28.
26. Cassingham RJ, Cassingham ML. Palatal petechiae in infectious mononucleosis. J Oral Med. 1970;25:133-6.
27. Cawson RA, Odell EW. Essentials of oral pathology and oral medicine, 6th edition, Edinburgh: Churchill Livingstone; 1998.
28. Cawson RA. Chronic oral candidiasis and leukoplakia. Oral Surg Oral Med Oral Pathol. 1966;22:582-91.

29. Centres for Disease control and Prevention. Measles, mumps and rubella vaccine use and strategies for elimination of measles, rubella and congenital rubella syndrome and control of mumps. MMWR. 1998;47:1.
30. Chue PW. Gonococcal arthritis of the temporomandibular joint. Oral Surg Oral Med Oral Pathol. 1975;39:572-7.
31. Cobb HB, Courts F. Chronic mucocutaneous candidiasis: report of case. J Dent Child. 1980;47:352.
32. Cole ST. Deciphering the biology of *Mycobacterium tuberculosis* from the complete genome sequence. Nature. 1998;392:537.
33. Cowen L. Gonococcal dermatitis syndrome. Br J Ven Dis. 1969;45:228-31.
34. Crawford JT. New technologies in the diagnosis of tuberculosis. Semin Respir Infect. 1994;9:62-70.
35. Cruickshank R. Tetanus and diphtheria. In: Cruickshank R, Standard KL, Russel HB (Eds). Epidemiology and community health in warm climate countries. Edinburg:Churchill Livingstone; 1976. pp. 77-82.
36. Curran JW. The epidemiology and prevention of the acquired immunodeficiency syndrome. Ann Int Med. 1985;103:657-62.
37. Dalgleish AG, Beverley PC, Clapham PR. The CDA (T4) antigen is an essential component of the receptor for the AIDS retrovirus. Nature. 1985;312:763.
38. Dismukes WE, Delgado DG, Mallernee SV, et al. Destructive bone disease in early syphilis. JAMA. 1976;236:2646-8.
39. Dohvoma CN. Primary herpetic gingivostomatitis with multiple herpetic whitlows. Br Dent T. 1994;177:251-2.
40. Donohue WB, Bolden TE. Tuberculosis of the salivary glands. A collective review. Oral Surg Oral Med Oral Pathol. 1961;14:576-88.
41. Dorph-peterson L, Pindborg JJ. Actinomycosis of the tongue. Oral Surg Oral Med Oral Pathol. 1954;7:1178-80.
42. Dorrucci M, Rezza G, Vlahow D, et al. Clinical characteristics and prognostic value of acute retroviral syndrome among injecting drug users. AIDS. 1995;9:597.
43. Dyment PG, Klink LB, Jackson DW.Hoarseness and palatal petechiae as clues in identifying streptococcal throat infections. Pediatrics. 1968;41:821-3.
44. Eddleston M, Peacock S, Juniper M, et al. Severe cytomegalovirus infection in immunocompetent patients. Clin Infect Dis. 1997;24:52.
45. Epstein JB, Sherlock CH, Wolber RA. Oral manifestations of cytomegalovirus infections. Oral Surg Oral Med Oral Pathol. 1993;75: 443-51.
46. Epstein MA. Burkitt's lymphoma.Clues to the role of malaria. Nature. 1984;312:398.
47. Eversole LR, Laipis PJ. Oral squamous papillomas: detection of HPV DNA by in situ hybridization. Oral Surg Oral Med Oral Pathol. 1988;65:545-50.
48. Farmanm AG. Clinical and cytological features of the oral lesions caused by chickenpox (varicella). J Oral Med. 1976;31:94-8.
49. Farmer ED, Lawton FE. In: Stone's oral and dental disease, 5th edition. Edinburgh: Livingstone, Edinburgh; 1966. pp. 768.
50. Fish DG, Ampel NM, Galgiani JN, et al. Coccidioidomycosis during human immunodeficiency virus infection. A review of 77 patients. Medicine. 1990;69:384.
51. Fiumara NJ, Wise HM, Many M. Gonorrheal pharyngitis. N Engl J Med. 1967;276:1248-50.
52. Fiumara NJ. The diagnosis and treatment of gonorrhoea. Symposium on venereal disease. Med Clin North Am. 1972;56:1105-13.
53. Flumara NJ, Berg M. Primary syphilis in the oral cavity. Br J Vene Dis. 1974;50:463-4.
54. Frauenfelder D, Schwartz AW. Coccidioidomycosis involving head and neck. Plast Reconst Surg. 1967;39:549-53.
55. Gershon AA. Varicella-zoster virus:immunity and latent infection. In: JJ Hooks, GW Jordan (Eds). Viral Infections of Oral Medicine. Elsevier: Amsterdam; 1982. pp. 123-32.
56. Giles HV. Local histoplasmosis. Buccolingual form. Oral Surg Oral Med Oral Pathol. 1968; 25:167-70.
57. Gold RS, Sager E. Oral sarcoidosis: a review of the literature. J Oral Surg. 1976;34:237-44.
58. Goldsand G. Actinomycosis. In: Heoprich PD. Infections Disease, 2nd edition. Hagerstown Maryland: Harper and Rowe; 1977. pp. 365-71.
59. Goodwin RA Jr, Shapiro JL, Thurman GH, et al. Disseminated histoplasmosis: clinical and pathologic correlations. Medicine. 1980;59:1.
60. Goodwin RA, Loyd JE, Des Prez RM. Histoplasmosis in normal hosts. Medicine. 1981;60:231.

61. Gordon Smith EC. Virus diseases. In: Woodruff AW, Wright SG (Eds). Medicine in the Tropics. Churchill Livingstone: Edinburgh; 1984. pp. 305-48.
62. Gottlieb GJ Ackerman AB. Kaposi's sarcoma: an extensively disseminated form in young homosexual men. Hum Pathol. 1982;13,882-92.
63. Greenberg MS. Herpesvirus infections. Dent Clin North Am. 1996;40:359-68.
64. Hadfield TL. The pathology of diphtheria. J Infect Dis. 2000;181(Suppl 1):S116.
65. Harnisch J. Diphtheria. In: Isselbacher KL, Adams RD, Braunwald E, Petersdrf R, Wilson RD (Eds). Harrison's principles of internal medicine, 9th edition). New York: McGraw Hill; 1980. pp. 671-5.
66. Henrard DR, Phillips JE, Muenz LR, et al. Natural history of HIV-1 cell free viremia. JAMA. 1995;274;554.
67. Hillerup S. Diagnosis of sarcoidosis from oral manifestations. Int J Oral Surg. 1976;5:95-9.
68. Holbrook WP, Rodgers GD. Candidal infections: experience in a British dental hospital. Oral Surg. 1980;49:122.
69. Holland J. Emerging zygomycoses of human: *Saksenaea vasiformis* and *Apophysomyces elegans*. Curr Top Med Mycol. 1997;8:27.
70. Hornstein OP, Gorlin RJ. Infectious oral disease. In: Gorlin RJ, Anf HM (Eds). Goldman Thomas Oral Pathology, 6th edition.St. Louis: CV Mosby; 1970. pp. 708-74.
71. Hyypia T, Stanway G. Biology of coxsackie A viruses. Adv Virus Res. 1993;42:343-73.
72. Igo RM, Taylor CG, Scott AS, et al. Coccidioidomycosis involving the mandible: report of a case. J Oral Surg. 1978; 36:72-5.
73. Jakush J. AIDS. The disease and its implications for dentistry. J Am Dent Assoc. 1987;115:395-55.
74. Jamsky RJ, Christen AG. Oral gonococcal infections. Oral Surg Oral Med Oral Pathol. 1982;53:358-62.
75. Barlett JG. Medical management of HIV infection. Baltimore (MD): Johns Hopkins University, Department of Infectious Diseases; 2000.
76. Kadirova T, Kartoglu HU, Strebel PM. Clinical characteristics and management of 676 hospitalised diphtheria cases, Kyrgyz Republic, 1995. J Infect Dis. 2000;181(Suppl 1):S 110.
77. Keen GA. Human cytomegalovirus infection. South African Med J. 1985;68:159-61.
78. Kessel LJ, Taylor WD. Chronic mucocutaneous candidiasis-treatment of the oral lesions with miconazole: two case reports. Br J Oral Surg. 1980;18:51.
79. Kirkland TN, Fierer J. Coccidioidomycosis: a reemerging infectious disease. Emerg Infect Dis. 1996;2:192.
80. Kornet H, Scheffer RF, McHoney PL. Bilateral tuberculous granulomas of the tongue. Arch Otolaryngol. 1965;82:649-61.
81. Lahner T. Oral thrush or pseudomembranous candidiasis. Oral Surg Oral Med Oral Pathol. 1964;18:27-37.
82. Larsen SA, Steiner BM, Rudolph AH. Laboratory diagnosis and interpretation of tests for syphilis. Clin Microbiol Rev. 1995;8:1-21.
83. Laskaris G, Sklavounou A. Molluscum contagiosum of the oral mucosa. Oral Surg Oral Med Oral Pathol. 1984;58:688-91.
84. Levitt GW. The surgical treatment of deep neck infections. Laryngoscope. 1971;81: 403-11.
85. Lger M, Larson J. Coccidioidal osteomyelitis. In: Ajello L (Ed). Coccidioidomycosis.Tucson:The University of Arizona Press; 1967. pp. 89.
86. Lifson AR. Oral lesions and the epidemiology of HIV. In: Greenspan JS, Greenspan D (Eds). Oral manifestations of HIV infection: proceedings of the 2nd International Workshop on the Oral Manifestations of HIV infection. San Francisco, California: Quintessence Publishing Co.; 1995. pp. 38.
87. Lynch MA, Brightman VJ, Greenberg MS. Burket's Oral Medicine: Diagnosis and Treatment, 9th edition. Philadelphia: JP Lippincott Company; 1994.
88. Lynch PJ. Condylomata acuminate (anogential warts). Clin Obstet Gynecol. 1985;28:142-51.
89. Mace MC. Oral African histoplasmosis resembling Burkitt's lymphoma. Oral Surg Oral Medi Oral Pathol. 1978;46:407-12.
90. Mackewicz CE, Yang LC, Lifson JD, et al. Non-cytolytic CD8 T-cell anti-HIV responses in primary HIV-1 infection. Lancet. 1994;344:1671.
91. Marsh P. Oral microbiology. Walton-on-Thames: Thomas Nelson & Sons; 1980.
92. McCracken AW, Cawson RA. Clinical and oral microbiology. New York: McGraw-Hill; 1983.
93. Miller CS. Herpes simplex virus and human papillomavirus infections of the oral cavity. Semin Dermatol. 1994;13:108-17.

94. Morse HE, Kent JN, Rothschild H. Tetanus. Review of literature and report of a case. J Oral Surg. 1978;36:462-6.
95. Musher DM. *Streptococcus pneumoniae.* In:Mandell GL (Ed). Principles and practice of Infections of cases, 5th edition. New York: Churchill Livingstone; 1999.
96. Nalesnik MA, Starzl TE, Epstein-Barr virus, infectious mononucleosis, and post-transplant lymphoproliferative disorders. Transplant Sci. 1994;4:61-79.
97. Nawman CW, Rosenbaun D. Oral cryptococcosis. J Periodontol. 1962;33:266-9.
98. Neville BW, Damm DD, Allen CA, et al. Oral and Maxillofacial Pathology, 2nd edition, Philadelphia: Saunders, an imprint of Elsevier; 2002.
99. Oxman MN. Herpes stomatitis. In: Braude AI (Ed). Medical microbiology and infectious disease.Philadelphia: WB Saunders; 1981; 1:860.
100. Phelan JA, Saltzman BR, Friedland GH, et al. Oral findings in patients with acquired immunodeficiency syndrome. Oral Surg Oral Med Oral Pathol. 1987;64:50-6.
101. Pindborg JJ. Atlas of disease of the oral mucosa, 4th edition. Copenhagen: Munksgaard; 1985.
102. Pindborg JJ. Atlas of the disease of the oral Mucosa. Copenhagen Munksgaard; 1980.
103. Pindborg JJ. Classification of oral lesions associated with HIV infection. Oral Surg Oral Med Oral Pathol. 1989; 67:292-5.
104. Prabhu SR, Daftary DK. Clinical evaluation of orofacial lesions in leprosy. Odontostomatologic Tropicale. 1981;IV:83-95.
105. Prabhu SR, Wilson DF, Johnson NW. Oral diseases in the tropics, 1st edition. Delhi: Oxford University Press; 1993.
106. Raab-Traub N. Epstein-Barr virus infection in nasopharyngeal carcinoma. Infect Agents Dis. 1992;1:173-84.
107. Richards JM. Notes on AIDS. Br Dent J. 1985; 158:199-201.
108. Rosenberg ES, Billingsley JM, Caliendo AM, et al. Vigorous HIV-1 specific CD4+T cell responses associated with control of viremia. Science. 1997;278:1447.
109. Rowe NH, Drach JC, Brooks SL. Management of recurrent herpes labialis. In: McDonald RE (Ed). Current therapy in dentistry. St. Louis: CV Mosby; 1980. pp. 55-9.
110. Ruso TA. Actinomycosis.In:Mandell GL (Ed). Principles and Practice of infectious Diseases. New York: Churchill Livingstone; 1999.
111. Samaranayake L. Oral mycoses in HIV infection. Oral Surg Oral Med Oral Pathol. 1992;73:171-80.
112. Samaranayake LP. Nutritional factors and oral candidiasis. J Oral Pathol. 1986;15:61-5.
113. Schmid GP. Treatment of chancroid, 1997. Clin Infect Dis. 1999;28 (Suppl 1):S14.
114. Sciubba JJ. Oral aspects of sexually transmitted disease. Ann Dent. 1978;37:17.
115. Scully C. Orofacial herpes simplex virus infections: current concepts in the epidemiology, pathogenesis, and treatment, and disorders in which the virus may be implicated. Oral Surg Oral Med Oral Pathol. 1989;68:701-10.
116. Shafer WG, Hine MK, Levy BM. A textbook of oral pathology, 4th edition. Philadelphia: WB Saunders; 1983.
117. Shafer WG, Hine MK, Levy BM. Bacterial viral and mycotic infections. In: A text book of oral pathology. Philadelphia: CV Mosby; 1983. pp. 340-450.
118. Shillitoe EJ, Greenspan JS. Adeno, coxsackie, measles and mumps viruses. In: Hooks JJ, Jorden GW (Eds). Viral infections in oral medicine. Amsterdam: Elsevier; 1982. pp. 142-52.
119. Silverman S, Beumer J. Primary herpetic gingivo stomatitis of adult onset. Clinical, laboratory and ultrastructural correlations identifying viral etiology. Oral Surg Oral Med Oral Pathol. 1973;36:496-503.
120. Soames JV, Southam JC. Oral pathology, 3rd edition.London: Oxford University Press; 1999.
121. Spector WG. Epithelioid cells, giant cells and sarcoidosis. Ann NY Acad Sci. 1976;278:3-6.
122. Stoll BJ. Congenital syphilis: evaluation and management of neonates born to mothers with reactive serologic tests for syphilis. Pediatr Infect Dis T. 1994;13:845-52.
123. Straus SE. Overview of the biology of varicella-zoster virus infection. Ann Neurol. 1994;35 (Suppl):S4-8.
124. Van Brakel WH1, de Soldenhoff R, McDougall AC. The allocation of leprosy patients into paucibacillary and multibacillary groups for multidrug therapy, taking into account the

number of body areas affected by skin or skin and nerve lesions. Lep Rev. 1992;63:231.
125. Wood TA Jr, DeWitt SH, Chu EW, et al. Anitschkow nuclear changes observed in oral smears. Acta Cytol. 1975;19:434.
126. Wyngaarden JB, Smith LH Jr. Cecil Textbook of Medicine 16th ed. Philadelphia. WB Saunders Company; 1982.
127. Young RC, Carbone PP, DeVita VT, et al. Aspergillosis: the spectrum of the disease in 98 patients. Medicine. 1970;49:147-73.
128. Young SK, Rowe NH, Buchanan RA. A clinical study of the control of facial mucocutaneous herpes virus infections I Characterization of natural history in a professional school population. Oral Surg. 1976;41:498.

CHAPTER 9

Dental Caries

DEFINITION OF DENTAL CARIES

Dental caries can be defined as *"a microbial disease of the calcified tissues of tooth, characterized by demineralization of the inorganic portions and destruction of its organic structures".*

Dental caries is a complex, continuous, and dynamic biological process of tooth decay, and comprising periods of progression alternating with periods of arrest or even partial repair.

It has neither any dramatic or recognizable starting point nor any endpoint, unless that is regarded as an acute pulpitis resulting in excruciating pain (Figs. 9.1A and B).

The periods of the disease activity in dental caries vary widely in their duration and intensity between different populations groups, between different individuals, and within a single patient at different ages or even throughout the day. Even within a single mouth, individual sites of each tooth vary greatly in their susceptibility.

Like any other infectious disease, the progress of dental caries depends upon a constantly changing balance between the nature and intensity of the injurious stimulus on one hand, and the nature and quality of the host's biological responses on the other; many factors influence this balance.

The initiation of a carious lesion at a given tooth surface, be it enamel of the crown or cementum of the exposed root surface, is customarily explained as a series of physicochemical phenomena.

Acids produced by fermentation of carbohydrates by the plaque bacteria cause subsurface demineralization of tooth enamel; and this is considered as the earliest defining manifestation of caries progression.

EPIDEMIOLOGY OF DENTAL CARIES

Dental caries has been recognized throughout history and exists around the world with variable frequency.

The epidemiological studies on dental caries have been very useful in the determination of the need for, and effectiveness of, the dental treatments.

The most common epidemiological measure of dental caries is the DMF index (decayed, missing, or filled teeth); this is a measure of the number of teeth that are diseased, missing, or filled at the time of examination.

The DMF may be reported as the number of teeth (DMFT) or surface affected (DMFS). These measures are cumulative because they

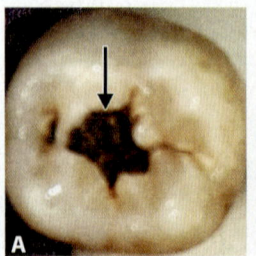
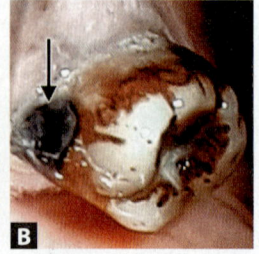

Figs. 9.1A and B: Dental caries.

not only indicate the number of missing or filled teeth, but also reveal the total number of teeth removed in the past as well as the total number of restorations done in the mouth. In addition to this, the index also states number of teeth having active caries and the number of their surfaces involved.

According to the target of WHO, no country should have a DMFT of 3 at the age of 12 by the year 2000 AD.

In the earlier days, it was a trend that the people from the developed countries, e.g. USA, UK, Australia, New Zealand, Western Europe, Scandinavia, and North America use to have more dental caries in comparison to the people of the underdeveloped or developing countries from Africa and Asia.

The basic reason behind this fact was that the people from the developed countries used to take more refined foods that contained large amounts of easily fermentable sugars, especially the sucrose.

Moreover, people of these countries could also afford to take frequent in-between meals that contained large amounts of sugar.

Both these factors contributed greatly to their higher incidences of caries, whereas at the same time, the people from Africa, Asia, etc. did continue to take their traditional foods, which were usually more fibrous and unrefined in nature and were not readily fermentable, thereby, contributed very little to the causation of dental caries.

In the western world, there has been a sharp increase in the disease activity in the first half of the century. However, since early 1970s, there has been a steady decrease in the prevalence of caries among the population of these countries because people have undertaken a wide range of caries preventive measures.

However, the recent reports indicate that the people from the underdeveloped countries are also showing higher incidences of dental caries. The basic reason behind this fact is that the people from the underdeveloped countries nowadays have also adopted more of urbanized lifestyle and westernized pattern of food habits.

The people of the Asian and African continents have diverted from the so-called traditional food habits and have widely adopted the so-called easily fermentable and highly sugar-containing diets, which highly increase the risk of caries in them.

Moreover, the people of Asian and African continents, though, have access to the high sugar-containing foods, and they don't have much access to the caries prevention measures available either individually or socially.

PATHOPHYSIOLOGY OF DENTAL CARIES

The pathophysiology of dental caries is a very complex reaction and it cannot be explained in terms of a single event or observation.

For this purpose, the process of dental caries is often explained with the help of many theories (Box 9.1).

Acidogenic Theory

This theory is also known as Miller's chemicoparasitic theory, as it was first postulated by WD Miller in the year 1889 and it proposes that "Acids formed due to the fermentation of dietary carbohydrates by oral bacteria lead to progressive decalcification of the tooth structures with subsequent disintegration of the organic matrix".

Therefore, acidogenic theory states that the process of dental caries involves two stages:
1. *Initial stage*: Production of organic acids occurs as a result of fermentation of carbohydrates by the plaque bacteria.

Box 9.1	Major theories of dental caries.
• Acidogenic theory • Proteolytic theory • Proteolytic chelation theory • Sucrose chelation theory • Autoimmune theory	

2. *Late stage*: The acids cause decalcification of enamel followed by dentin and thereby cause total destruction of these two structures along with dissolution of their softened residues.

The final result is the loss of integrity of the tooth structures at a particular point on the surface with formation of a cavity.

According to Miller, there are four important factors, which can influence the process of tooth destruction in the process of dental caries and these factors are as follows:
1. Dietary carbohydrates
2. Microorganisms
3. Acids
4. Dental plaque.

Role of Carbohydrates in Dental Caries

Numerous epidemiological studies have shown that the fermentable dietary carbohydrates play an important role in the causation of caries, especially the readily fermentable types of carbohydrates, e.g. glucose, sucrose, fructose, etc. Among them, sucrose is implicated to be the most potent one. These sugars are easily and rapidly fermented by cariogenic bacteria in the oral cavity to produce acids at or near the tooth surface and cause dissolution of the hydroxyapatite crystals of the enamel followed by the dentin. Once a small defect forms in the enamel, it facilitates more and more plaque accumulation and thereby cause more acid formation leading to more decay in the tooth, which becomes unstopable.

The evidences that support the role of carbohydrates in the causation of caries include the following:
- Increased prevalence of caries in developing countries due to westernization or urbanization of the society and an increase in the availability of refined carbohydrates (sucrose) in the diet.
- Decrease in the prevalence of caries during World War-II because of sugar restrictions followed by rise of caries incidence to previous levels, when sucrose became available once again.
- "The Hopewood House Study"—in children's home in Australia, where sucrose and white breads were eliminated from diet, the children had low caries rate. However, the caries index was increased dramatically when these children moved out of the said house and started taking conventional carbohydrate-rich diet.
- Patient with hereditary fructose intolerance, who cannot tolerate fructose or sucrose develop little or virtually no caries.

Types of carbohydrates and Their Caries Risk

Dietary carbohydrates undoubtedly cause caries; however, the rate of caries attack always depends upon the forms of carbohydrate consumed by a person and the frequency of intake of such carbohydrates.
- The risk of caries attack increases greatly, if sugar is taken repeatedly in-between two major meals. It provides an almost constant supply of carbohydrate to the plaque bacteria for fermentation and subsequent production of acids to cause caries.
- Normal pH of saliva is 6.2–7.6 (average is 6.7); this pH falls rapidly after consumption of sugar with subsequent acid production in mouth by carbohydrate fermentation by cariogenic bacteria slowly the pH gets back to the normal level again as the acids are neutralized by the salivary bicarbonates (Buffering action).
- This pH alteration can be recorded with the help of a graph called Stephan's curve, it demonstrates the pH curves of plaque in response to consumption of sugar. It is observed that following consumption of sugar, the pH of the plaque falls to 4.5–5 within 1–3 minutes and it takes another 10–30 minutes to return to neutrality. The critical pH of plaque is 5.5 and tooth demineralization starts, if the pH drops below this level.

Table 9.1: Different types of carbohydrate and their cariogenic potential.

Compound	Nature	Cariogenicity
Sucrose	Disaccharide (glucose and fructose)	Highest cariogenicity
Galactose (milk sugar)	Disaccharide	Less cariogenic than sucrose
Glucose, fructose	Monosaccharide	Less cariogenic than sucrose
Lactose	Monosaccharide	Less cariogenic than sucrose
Xylitol, sorbitol, mannitol and lactitol	Sugar alcohols	Noncariogenic
Saccharin, aspartame, thaumatin, and cyclamate	Non-sugar sweeteners	Noncariogenic

- Risk of caries incidence increases greatly, if the dietary sugar is sticky in nature, which can remain adhered to the tooth surfaces for a longtime after taking the meal.
- The glucose, sucrose, fructose, etc. are rapidly diffused into the plaque due to their low-molecular weight and, therefore, make themselves easily available for fermentation by the plaque bacteria.
- However, the principal carbohydrates available in human diet are sucrose and starches.
- Interestingly, if there are repeated intakes of sugar during this period in the form of in-between meals, the pH will fall further and it will take an even longer time to return back to neutrality. The continuous and prolonged fall in the plaque pH results in more tooth demineralization (Table 9.1 and Box 9.2).
- **Extracellular polysaccharide (Dextran):** It is a sticky, insoluble substance produced by cariogenic bacteria with the help of sucrose and it helps in strongly adhering the bacteria on to the tooth surface. The enzyme glucosyl transferase plays an important role in the synthesis of dextran. Dextran thus increases the risk of caries, although besides dextran, other extracellular polysaccharides are also synthesized by the cariogenic bacteria, for example, the glucan—(synthesized from glucose), and levan—(from fructose) but, both are soluble and weakly adhering substances, play a less significant role in caries formation as compared to dextran.
- **Intracellular polysaccharides:** Few cariogenic bacteria, especially *S.mutans* has the unique property of storing sugars

> **Box 9.2** Sucrose—the most potent cariogenic carbohydrate.
>
> - Sucrose is the most important cariogenic carbohydrate. It is disaccharide and forms about one-third of our carbohydrate diet
> - It has the maximum capacity to produce acids and promote tooth decay
> - The caries producing microorganisms, especially the *Streptococcus mutans*, readily use up sucrose to synthesize an *extracellular insoluble polysaccharide* with the help of their enzyme glucosyl transferase
> - The disaccharide bond of sucrose contains enough energy to react with the bacterial enzymes to synthesize extracellular polysaccharide
> - This sticky polysaccharide is called *dextran* and *it helps in adhering or binding the plaque firmly onto the tooth surface to enable a direct contact between the acids and the tooth and thus cause more tooth decay*
> - Sucrose promotes colonization of tooth by *S. mutans*
> - Its small molecules help it to diffuse readily into the plaque
> - Bacterial metabolism of sucrose is very rapid as compared to any other carbohydrate
> - When sucrose is fermented by cariogenic bacteria and there are production acids, they quickly start to demineralize the tooth
> - Sucrose is also readily converted into *intracellular "glucan-like" polymers*, which can also be metabolized into acids in future at the time of dietary restrictions of sucrose.

inside its cell body as future reserve and this stored sugar can be utilized to continue caries at the time of dietary sugar restrictions by the patient (when sugar is not available to cause caries).
- The role of dietary carbohydrates in the formation of caries can further be established by the fact that, when the dietary sucrose is replaced by sorbitol, xylitol, mannitol, or lactitol, etc., the nonfermentable carbohydrates, the possibility of caries formation is greatly reduced.
- Starches produce little or no caries because they are very slowly diffused into the plaque and they also require extracellular amylase to become hydrolyzed before they can be assimilated and metabolized by plaque bacteria.
- Moreover, nonsugar sweeteners, e.g. saccharin, aspartame and thaumatin, etc. are noncariogenic.

Role of Microorganisms in Dental Caries

Goadby, in 1903, stated that caries occurs due to combined action of many common bacteria, some of which are acid producers and some are dentin liquefiers. Since the time of Miller (1889), most investigators acknowledged that microorganisms cause decalcification of tooth by means of carbohydrate fermentation with subsequent acid production (Box 9.3).

Box 9.3	The common cariogenic microorganisms.

- *Streptococcus mutans*
- *Streptococcus sanguis*
- *Streptococcus mitior*
- *Streptococcus salivarius*
- *Streptococcus milleri*
- *Peptostreptococcus*
- *Lactobacillus acidophilus*
- *Actinomyces israelii*
- *Actinomyces viscosus*
- *Actinomyces naeslundii*

Box 9.4	Essential qualities of cariogenic bacteria.

- Should be able to produce acids
- Should be able to produce a low pH in the mouth (usually <5) to demineralize the tooth
- Should be able to survive and continue to produce acid at low levels of pH
- Should be able to attach strongly onto the tooth surface (even the smooth surface)
- Should be able to synthesize insoluble, sticky polysaccharides, e.g. dextran, glucan, etc.

The evidence for the role of bacteria in the genesis of dental caries can further be established by the following facts:
- If the mouth becomes free of bacteria, as in germfree animals, the dental caries will never develop.
- Use of antibiotics effectively reduces the caries incidence in humans as well as in animals.
- Oral bacteria can demineralize tooth enamel in vitro and produce lesions similar to the naturally occurring dental caries.
- Specific bacterial groups (known for their cariogenic potential) can be isolated and identified from the carious lesions (Box 9.4).

A large number of microorganisms play their individual roles in the development of dental caries and among them, the most important one is the *Streptococcus mutans* (Box 9.5).

This organism is mostly responsible for the initiation of enamel caries and moreover, it plays at least three very important roles to facilitate caries formation, which are as follows (Boxes 9.6 and 9.7):

Box 9.5	Laboratory culture of *S. mutans*.

S. mutans produces a grayish-white colony in glucose agar medium; the colony is about 1 mm in diameter, firm and it typically slides along the surface of the medium. The bacterial colony is distinctive in its appearance of being sunk into the agar, as if it had eaten its way into the medium

Dental Caries

Box 9.6	Colonization mechanism of *Streptococcus mutans*.

- Initial adherence
- Interbacterial adherence
- Glucan mediated binding to pellicle
- Sucrose dependent accumulation

Box 9.7	Characteristics that makes *Streptococcus mutans* the most potent cariogenic bacteria.

- There are some very important characteristics of *S. mutans* that give the organism more edge over others in terms of caries production
- *S. mutans* produces acids from fermentation of sucrose, glucose, lactose, mannitol and mucin, etc.
- It is present in large numbers in normal saliva, always ready to attack the tooth as soon as the suitable carbohydrates are available
- *S. mutans* can be isolated in pure culture from the dentin of carious tooth
- It can survive at a pH as low as 4.2
- *S. mutans* synthesizes extracellular insoluble polysaccharide "dextran"; which helps in adhering plaque bacteria to the tooth surface to enable more tooth decay
- *S. mutans* can produce 'intracellular polysaccharide' (they store sugars inside their cell body as future reserve), which are used to continue caries even if the patient is no longer taking sugar
- *S. mutans* can produce caries in a tooth in laboratory environment
- It can adhere to acquired pellicle and thus facilitates in plaque formation
- *Streptococcus mutans* also has the ability to adhere and grow even on hard and smooth surfaces of tooth
- A special type of adhesive known as protein B contributes in colonization of mutans on tooth
- It can cause pit and fissure, smooth surface and root caries.

- Besides *S. mutans*, other streptococci which are cariogenic include *Streptococcus sanguis, Streptococcus mitior, Streptococcus salivarius, Streptococcus milleri* and *Peptostreptococcus*, etc.
- The actinomycotic group of organisms namely the *Actinomyces israelii, Actinomyces viscosus* and *Actinomyces naeslundii,* etc. are the important organisms that produce root caries in teeth. Among all organisms in the group, *A. viscosus* is considered to be the most active agent to cause root caries.
- *Actinomyces viscosus* is acidogenic bacteria which, in addition to having intracellular polysaccharide stores, also forms extracellular levans and heteropolysaccharides consisting of hexosamine and hexose.
- The *Lactobacillus acidophilus* organisms were considered to be important cariogenic organisms in the past due to their presence within the carious cavities in large numbers. They are both acidogenic as well as aciduric and could therefore multiply in the low pH of plaque and inside the carious lesions. However, higher *Lactobacillus* counts in saliva also indicate the presence of more active carious lesions in the oral cavity. Since these organisms cannot adhere onto the smooth surfaces of teeth, they are not capable of producing smooth surface caries. However, these organisms are important for the progression of "dentinal" caries.

Role of Acids in Dental Caries

During the process of caries formation, *S. mutans* and *L. acidophilus produce* a large variety of organic acids in the oral cavity due to fermentation of dietary carbohydrates. (Box 9.8). These acids can cause demineralization of enamel followed by dentin and eventually cause the tooth decay. The decay begins due to sharp drop in the pH at the "plaque-tooth interface" (Box 9.9).

Box 9.8	Important acids produced in caries to cause tooth decay.

- Lactic acid
- Aspartic acid
- Butyric acid
- Acetic acid
- Propionic acid
- Glutamic acid

Box 9.9	Plaque pH and tooth demineralization.
pH 5.5 or above—No demineralization of tooth
pH 5 to 4.5—Subsurface demineralization of enamel
pH 4 to 3—Surface demineralization of enamel

Stephan's Curve

- Stephan curve graphically demonstrates the pH curves of plaque in response to sugars; it is carried out by measuring the pH levels of dental plaque after rinsing the mouth with a 10% glucose or sucrose solution.
- Following the ingestion of sugar, the pH of the plaque in mouth falls from 6.5 (normal pH of saliva) to about 4.5–5 within 1–3 minutes.
- It takes another 10–30 minutes to return to normal pH.
- Repeated intakes of sugar cause pH to fall further and each time, it takes even longer time to return back to normal (Box 9.10 and Fig. 9.2). Stephan studied the pH in dental plaques after rinsing of the mouth with a 10% glucose or sucrose solution. Within 2–5 minutes after the rinse, the pH in the plaque dropped to between pH 4.5 and 5.0 and gradually returned to the initial pH level within 1–2 hours. Further studies indicated differences in reductions in pH between caries free and caries active subjects. The plaque pH in the caries free group did not fall below 5.0 after the glucose rinse, while the pH in the caries active group dropped below 5.0 units after the glucose rinse in over half the cases (Box 9.11).

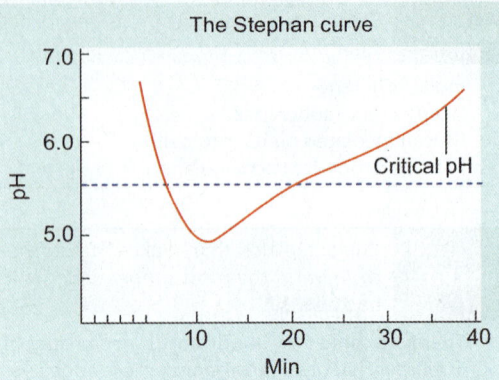

Fig. 9.2: "Stephan curve" showing alteration of pH graph with intake of sugar.

Role of Bacterial Plaque in Dental Caries

Plaque is a thin, transparent film produced on the tooth surface and it consists

Box 9.10	Significant observations through Stephan curve.

- It establishes the basic principles of acidogenic theory
- It demonstrates the ill effects of consumption of repeated "in-between meals"
- It shows the variable degrees of pH changes in caries-immune and caries-susceptible individuals following intake of same amount of sugar
- The curve can show the variable levels of pH changes with intake of food containing lower or higher levels of sugar

Box 9.11	Factors determining the "rate of acid demineralization" of tooth in caries.

- Rate of acid production—faster the rate more is the decay
- Volume of production of acid—more volume of acid more decay
- Type of acid—some acids produced by carbohydrate fermentation is strong and some are weak in their tooth demineralizing capacity
- Degree of fall of pH—lower the fall of pH, greater the decay
- Persistence of acid attack on tooth—longer the acids remain on tooth, greater the decay
- Localization of acids on the tooth surface—dextran helps to keep the plaque and acids firmly held onto the tooth surface and this cause more decay
- Repetition of acid production (through in between meals)—means more decay
- Protection of acid if acid on the tooth surface remains under the cover of plaque and does not get neutralized by the buffering action of saliva, it causes more tooth decay
- Surface quality of tooth enamel—weaker the enamel, faster the decay.

Dental Caries

> **Box 9.12** Stages of plaque formation on teeth.
> - Deposition of cell-free, structureless, acquired pellicle
> - Thickening of acquired pellicle due to further deposition salivary glycoproteins following bacterial stimulation
> - Colonization of *S. mutans* and *S. sanguis* within 24 hours
> - Progressive build-up of plaque substance by bacterial polysaccharides
> - Colonization of filamentous and other organisms as the plaque matures.

> **Box 9.13** How dental plaque helps in the initiation of dental caries
> - It harbors the cariogenic bacteria on the tooth surface
> - Rapid production of high amounts of acids within the plaque occurs through fermentation of carbohydrates by cariogenic bacteria
> - Plaque helps to hold these acids onto the tooth surface for a long duration
> - Increased thickness of plaque does not allow the salivary buffers to enter into it to neutralize the acids produced by the cariogenic bacteria
> - Plaque protects the acids produced by the cariogenic bacteria from getting neutralized in two ways—(a) It has diffusion limiting property that does not allow acids to escape, and (b) the same property of plaque does not allow the buffering agents from saliva to enter into it and cause neutralization of acids
> - Continued sugar production from bacterial intracellular polysaccharides helps to maintain a low pH and facilitates more tooth decay. All these purposes served by the dental plaque enhance the tooth decay.

predominantly of microorganisms suspended in salivary mucins and extracellular bacterial polysaccharides (glucans). There is also presence of desquamated epithelial cells, leukocytes, food debris, etc. in it (Box 9.12).

Acquired pellicle is a component of the dental plaque, which is made by the salivary glycoprotein and is formed just prior to the bacterial colonization.

- One hour after the formation of acquired pellicle, some organisms such as *S. sanguis, A. viscous, A. naeslundii* and *Peptostreptococcus*, etc. become attached to it. These organisms are called "pioneering organisms" in dental caries.
- These initial organisms lack in caries producing potential since they are mostly aerobic in nature and produce very little amount of acid by the fermentation of the carbohydrates.
- As the plaque matures with time, *S. mutans* group becomes more predominant within the plaque (Box 9.13).

Limitations of Acidogenic Theory

Although the acidogenic theory of dental caries has got a wide acceptance, it has the following limitations:
- It cannot explain subsurface demineralization.
- It fails to justify the rampant caries.
- It cannot explain the caries in impacted tooth.

Proteolytic Theory

- *"The proteolytic enzymes liberated by cariogenic bacteria cause destruction of the organic matrix of enamel; as a result the inorganic crystals of enamel get disintegrated, which leads to the formation of a cavity on the tooth"* –this is theory is called the proteolytic theory of dental caries. It was first proposed by Gottlieb in 1944.
- The concept of proteolytic theory was further extended by Pincus in 1949 and he proposed that the "sulfatase enzyme" liberated by gram-negative bacilli, hydrolyze the sulfated mucosubstances of enamel matrix and thereby liberate sulfuric acid, glutamic acid and aspartic acid, etc. which subsequently dissolve the mineral portion of the enamel.
- The scope of the proteolytic mechanism in initiating the enamel caries is very limited because two reasons:
    a. The organic (protein) content of enamel matrix is very scanty.

b. Proteolytic microorganisms are also very less in mouth.

However, this mechanism can be a more appropriate one in cases of dentinal and cemental caries.

Limitations of Proteolytic Theory
- The carious lesion cannot be reproduced in vitro by the proteolytic mechanism.
- Proteolytic bacteria are very uncommon in the oral cavity.
- This theory cannot explain the role of sucrose, pH, fluoride, etc. in dental caries.

Proteolytic Chelation Theory

The proteolytic chelation theory explains the process of dental caries in the following way, during caries, initially there is proteolytic breakdown of the organic matrix of enamel. Following this, a 'chelation process' begins with the interaction of proteolytic breakdown products, acquired pellicle and food debris, etc. that forms a 'chelating agent'.

The chelating agent, which is formed, is always negatively charged (mostly due to its protein content) and it releases the positively charged calcium ions (Ca^{++}) from the enamel or dentin. This process is called chelation, and it eventually results in tooth decay.

Chelation: It is the process that involves in the complexing of a metallic ion to a complex substance by a coordinate covalent bond, which results in a highly stable, poorly dissociated and weakly ionized compound called chelate.

The proteolytic-chelation theory explains that the destruction of the organic matrix of the enamel as well as its mineral parts both occur simultaneously and interdependently.

Sucrose Chelation Theory

Sucrose chelation theory proposes that "very high concentration of sucrose in the mouth of a caries-active individual may result in the formation of complex substances like calcium saccharates and calcium complexing intermediaries, etc. by the action of phosphorylating enzymes". These complexes cause release of the calcium and phosphorus ions from the enamel and thereby result in tooth decay.

This theory is unlikely to be significant because once the sucrose is in the oral cavity, it readily gets metabolized to form acids, and there is hardly any scope for formation of calcium saccharates, etc. Moreover, for the formation of calcium saccharate, a very high level of pH is required, the range which is never achieved in the oral cavity.

Autoimmune Theory

The autoimmune theory of dental caries suggests that a few odontoblast cells at some specific sites, within the pulp of a few specific teeth, are damaged by the autoimmune mechanisms. For this reason, the defense capacity and integrity of the overlying enamel or dentin in those specific areas are compromised, and they can be the potential sites for caries development in future.

■ CONTRIBUTING FACTORS IN DENTAL CARIES

A large number of factors influence the caries process directly or indirectly and they are as follows:

Intrinsic factors: Tooth factor

Extrinsic factors: These include the following:
- Saliva factor
- Diet factor
- Systemic factors
- Immunity.

Tooth Factor

Few teeth in mouth are more susceptible to than others and also some surface of an individual tooth can have more caries; therefore the rate of progression of caries is not always equal in every tooth. Factors influencing the site of attack and the rate of caries progression in a tooth depend upon several factors which are as follows:

Composition of Tooth

- There is an inverse relationship between enamel solubility and the mineral ion concentration of the enamel surface of a tooth. If the enamel surface is highly mineralized (due to the presence of Ca^{++}, F^-, Zn^{++} and Fe^{+++}, etc. in higher concentrations), it is obviously less soluble and such teeth are less prone to caries.
- On the other hand, if the solubility of the surface enamel is higher (hypomineralized tooth), the chance of caries formation is more in it.
- Increased permeability of the enamel (in hypoplastic tooth) also increases the possibility of caries.
- A graded increase in the mineral content of enamel with age may account for an increased resistance to caries in older individuals.

Effective Pulp-dentin Complex

If the functional status of the pulp-dentin complex within the tooth remains very sound, the rate of tooth destruction is less. The complex actually resists the progress of caries and subsequent invasion of pulp by forming reparative dentin.

Morphology of Tooth

Presence of deep, narrow and retentive pits and fissures on the tooth surface may contribute to a higher caries incidence, because these developmental surface defects favor the colonization of plaque microorganisms.

Position of Tooth

The malaligned, rotated or out-of-position teeth in the dental arch are attacked by caries more frequently as there is more possibility of plaque accumulation and also these teeth are difficult to keep clean.

Saliva Factor

The saliva factors play a very important role in the prevention of dental caries.

Flow rate: When the salivary flow rate is adequate in the oral cavity, it causes cleaning of the bacteria from the tooth surface by its flushing action and thus the chances of caries formation remain less. Xerostomia/Desalivation—When there is decrease in the amount of salivary secretion, an increased caries incidence is obvious; as the salivary cleaning action is missing.

Viscosity: When viscosity of saliva is increased, there will be more deposition of plaque on the tooth surfaces causing more caries. Moreover, saliva with lower viscosity also causes more caries as the normal minerals (causing remineralization) and bicarbonates (causing buffering action), etc. will be less in it.

[*Buffering capacity*: High concentrations of salivary bicarbonate ions cause neutralization of acids produced by the cariogenic bacteria by their buffering action and this results in a decrease in the rate of tooth decay]. Whenever the buffering action of saliva is suppressed, the risk of caries becomes high.

Moreover, saliva also contains urea, which gets hydrolyzed to produce ammonia and the later agent can cause rise in the salivary pH. This rise in pH can counter the acid attacks on the tooth surface and thus prevent caries. Moreover, the buffering capacity of saliva is often enhanced with increased salivary flow rate.

Salivary enzymes: Salivary "amylase" causes breakdown of starch (residual carbohydrates) from the tooth surface and make them more soluble. As a result, these are easily washed away from the mouth.

Fluoride action: Saliva acts as a vehicle for fluoride ions, which enter into the plaque and prevent tooth decay.

Salivary immunoglobulins: Salivary immunoglobulins (IgA and IgG) inhibit the cariogenic bacteria especially the *S. mutans*, by facilitating their destruction process through phagocytosis and thus eventually reduce the possibility of caries.

Remineralization of tooth: Calcium and phosphate ions present in the saliva help in the partial repair of tooth damaged by caries and this process called remineralization of tooth. Remineralization can control the rate of tooth destruction in caries and this process starts when the salivary pH is above 5.5.

Direct antibacterial action: Several antibacterial agents are found in saliva like lysozyme, thiocyanate, lactoferrin and lactoperoxidase, etc. These agents cause destruction of the cariogenic bacteria by their direct antibacterial action and thereby reduce the caries incidence in the mouth.

Key salivary factors in dental caries in Table 9.2.

Role of Fluorides in the Prevention of Dental Caries

The fluoride reduces the caries incidence in the following mechanisms:
- During the development of tooth, systemic fluorides cause conversion of the hydroxyapatite crystals of enamel into fluoroapatite crystals, since these crystals are highly resistant to acids, the risk of caries becomes less.
- Fluorides also help in the remineralization of tooth after caries by redepositing or by reprecipitating the mineral ions lost from the tooth. Fluorides prevent the activity of the enzyme "glucosyl transferase" which is essential for the formation of extracellular polysaccharides (dextran, levan, etc.) and thereby reduce the bacterial (cariogenic) adhesion onto the tooth surface.
- The fluoride ions can limit the rate of carbohydrate metabolism by the cariogenic bacteria and thereby reduce the acid attacks on the tooth.
- Fluorides inhibit the enzyme "enolase" which is essential for carbohydrate metabolism, and thus prevent the carbohydrate degradation and acid production.
- In high concentrations, the fluoride ions can be directly toxic to the *S. mutans*.

Diet Factor

Physical Nature of Diet

If the diet contains sufficient amount of fibrous foods that help to keep the teeth clean as well as stimulates the salivary flow, the chances of caries becomes less.

Composition of the Diet

Presence of vegetables, fat, phosphates, vitamins (A, D, K and B Complex) and minerals significantly reduce the risk of caries.

Systemic Factor

Some people hereditarily have an increased tendency to develop caries while other people show just the reverse tendency.

Table 9.2: Key salivary factors in dental caries.

Factors associated with low caries	Factors associated with high caries
High flow rate	Low salivary flow rate
Proper salivation	Desalivation (xerostomia)
Normal viscosity	Too high or too low viscosity
Buffering capacity	Lack of salivary buffering action
Salivary enzymes	Salivary glycoproteins may contribute to plaque formation
Fluoride action	
Salivary immunoglobulins	Sucrose in saliva may be used up by the plaque bacteria to produce caries
Remineralization	
Direct antibacterial action	

Immunity

Immune mechanism plays an important role in the prevention of caries in humans. It is facilitated by serum and salivary immunoglobulines as well as cell mediated immune systems.

The immune-mediated prevention of caries is mostly associated with the reduction in the number of *S. mutans* organisms in plaque.

In gingival crevicular fluid there is presence of immunoglobulins (IgG, IgM and IgA), complements, neutrophil leukocytes, sensitized lymphocytes and macrophages, etc. which cam prevent dental caries.

CLINICAL ASPECTS OF DENTAL CARIES

Clinical Types

Pit and Fissure Caries (Fig. 9.3)

- This type of lesion occurs in the developmental pits and fissures of the teeth (especially if these areas are deep, narrow and retentive in nature and thereby facilitate plaque accumulation).
- The pit and fissure caries often occurs on the occlusal surfaces of molars and premolars, buccal and lingual surfaces of molars and lingual surfaces of maxillary incisors.
- The lesions usually appear brown or black, with little softening and opaqueness of the surface. Enamel directly bordering the pit or fissure may appear opaque and bluish-white as it becomes undermined.
- When the lesion is examined by a fine explorer tip, a "catch point" is often felt.
- The lesions are smaller in the beginning but become wider as they spread towards the dentin due to the typical orientation of the enamel rods.
- When the lesions reach the dentinoenamel junction (DEJ), they spread laterally to cause undermining of the enamel.

Incipient Caries

Definition: When initial caries occurs in a tooth with no cavity formation, it is called 'incipient caries'; it develops due to subsurface demineralization of enamel (but surface remains intact).

- With further progression of caries in untreated cases, the surface enamel becomes undermined and breaks down to form cavity.
- Clinically, incipient caries presents a "chalky-white" appearance of the tooth surface and it is only found when the surface of the tooth is dry and the typical chalky-white condition disappears, if the surface of the tooth becomes wet.
- The incipient caries is a reversible process and the lesion can be cured due to remineralization by salivary mineral ions.
- Incipient caries can be prevented by topical fluorides, which help to maintain the integrity of enamel undermined by dentinal caries.

Smooth Surface Caries (Fig. 9.4)

- This type of carious lesion occurs on the smooth surfaces of teeth, e.g. proximal surfaces or gingival areas of the buccal and lingual aspect of tooth.

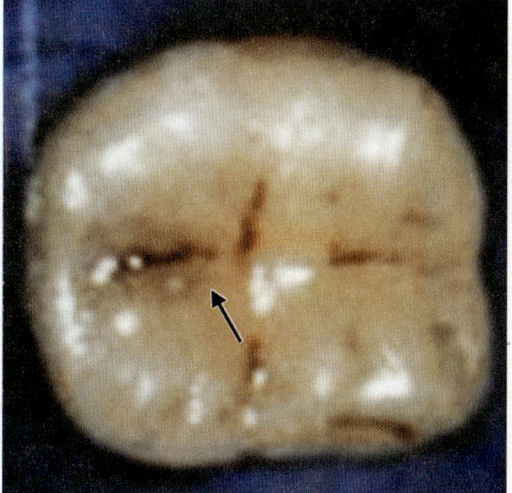

Fig. 9.3: Pit and fissure caries in early stage.

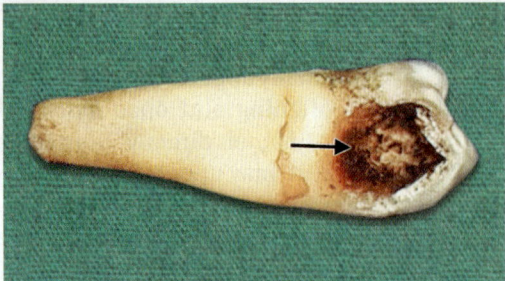

Fig. 9.4: Smooth surface caries on the proximal surface.

- Smooth surface caries most commonly occurs in the proximal surface of the teeth just below the contact point.
- The initial lesion appears as a well-demarcated, chalky-white opacity of enamel with no loss of continuity of the surface.
- The white spot lesion becomes pigmented yellow or brown and it often extends buccally and lingually.
- The surrounding enamel becomes bluish white as the lesion continues to progress.
- The surface of the affected enamel becomes rough and later on, there is formation of a cavity.

Rampant Caries (Fig. 9.5)

The word 'rampant' means unrestrained or something unstoppable; rampant caries is an acute fulminating type of carious process, which is characterized by simultaneous involvement of multiple number of teeth (may be all teeth) in multiple surfaces.
- Rapid coronal destruction occurs within a short span of time, causing early involvement of the pulp.
- The common age of occurrence of rampant caries is about 4–8 years for the deciduous teeth and 11–19 years for the permanent teeth.
- Interestingly, the rampant caries can occur in persons with no previous history of dental caries and in those persons who maintain a good level of oral hygiene regularly.

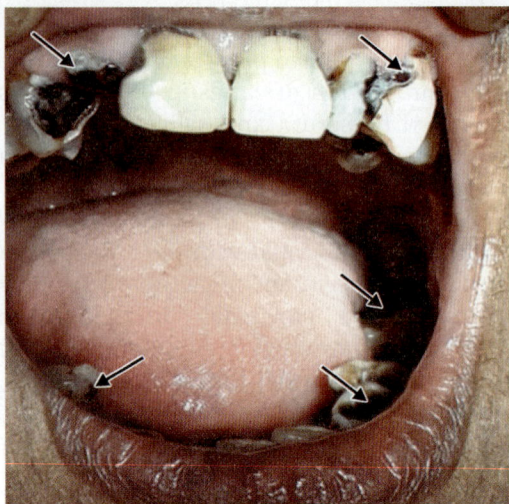

Fig. 9.5: Rampant caries.

- Moreover, rampant caries attacks those surfaces of teeth, which are otherwise considered immune to the disease.

Nursing Bottle Caries (Fig. 9.6)

- This is also another type of acute carious lesion, which occurs among children who take sweetened milk or fruit juices by the nursing bottle, for long hours, preferably during sleep.
- Large amount of sugar in the milk, that is also kept inside the mouth for long durations, these two are the key factors

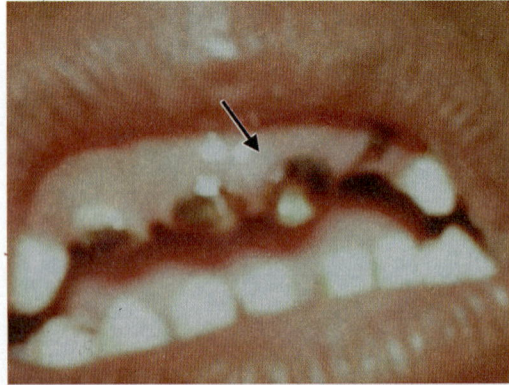

Fig. 9.6: Nursing bottle caries affecting the upper deciduous incisor teeth.

Table 9.3: Comparison of rampant caries and nursing bottle caries.

Rampant caries	Nursing bottle caries
• Acute, widespread caries with early pulpal involvement of teeth, which are usually immune to decay • Seen at all ages, including adolescence • Affects the primary and permanent dentition • Any tooth of any arch in the mouth can be involved • Surfaces considered immune to decay are involved. Thus, mandibular incisors are affected • No specific etiology	• Specific form of rampant caries • Seen in infants and toddlers • Affects the primary dentition • The maxillary incisors most frequently involved • Mandibular incisors are not involved • Bottle-feeding before sleep is the main cause

in nursing bottle caries. Because the sugar facilitates the cariogenic bacteria to produce caries at a rapid pace by fermenting those sugars.
- Nursing bottle caries commonly occurs in the upper anterior teeth (as these are constantly coming in contact with the sweetened milk); while the lower teeth are not usually affected as they remain under the cover of the tongue (sweetened milk does not the lower teeth) .
- Both the nursing bottle caries and rampant caries cause early pulp involvement because they spread at a very rapid pace and as a result, the pulp hardly gets any time to protect itself by forming reparative dentin (Table 9.3).

Chronic Caries

This type of caries progresses at a slower pace and it rarely causes pulp involvement (unless the tooth is left untreated for many years) because the pulp gets sufficient time to produce secondary dentin or reactionary dentin to protect itself.

Arrested Caries (Fig. 9.7)

Arrested caries is a lesion whose progression is ceased after the initial development. It can occur both in enamel and in dentin.

Arrested caries of enamel

Arrested caries in enamel may occur when the carious process stops before cavity formation. It occurs when the adjacent carious tooth (from which the disease has actually spread to this new tooth) is lost or is extracted, so that the carious lesion in the new tooth becomes easily accessible for cleaning and plaque control measures. It is commonly seen in smooth surfaces of tooth.

Arrested caries of dentin

The arrested caries of dentin usually occurs when a carious cavity becomes wide open, so that it gets exposed to the cleaning measures like tooth brushing, salivary secretions and mastication, etc. The arrested caries presents a hard, black or brown-colored dentinal surface at its base (eburnated dentin). Its surface is highly mineralized due to remineralization from oral fluids and has increased fluoride content.

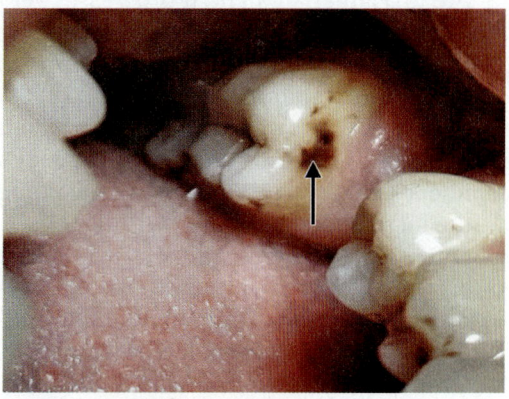

Fig. 9.7: Arrested caries.

Recurrent Caries

Recurrent caries refers to a carious lesion that begins around the margins or at the base of a preexisting defective restoration.

Forward Caries

When a carious lesion progresses unidirectionally from enamel to dentin and then towards the pulp, it is called a forward caries.

Backward Caries

After reaching the DEJ caries often spreads laterally and involve a wide area of dentin. From here sometimes, caries proceeds in a backwardly direction again towards the surface (i.e. from dentin back to enamel).

Root Caries

These are carious lesions, which involve the (cemental wall) of the exposed root surfaces of teeth.

Important features of root caries are as follows:
- Before development of root caries, the root of the tooth must be exposed due to gingival recession (more often seen in elderly people).
- Because of the roughness of the cemental wall, plaque accumulates readily and cause caries. Root caries often cause damage to a larger area and it progresses very fast and cause early pulp involvement due to the relative softness of cementum as compared to enamel.
- In root caries, the cementum is often invaded along the direction of "Sharpey's fibers" and microorganisms spread along the incremental lines.
- Once the cementum is destroyed, root caries reaches dentin and the later is progressively destroyed by a combination of both demineralization and proteolysis.
- Clinically, these lesions are extensive, shallow and saucer-shaped, with ill-defined margins. The lesions often have soft surfaces with brownish discoloration of the affected area.
- There may be formation of sclerotic dentin as the caries progresses into the dentin from cementum.
- Sometimes, the carious lesion may encircle the entire root of the affected tooth
- The actinomycotic groups of organisms are mostly responsible for the causation of root caries. However, *S. mutans* and *L. acidophilus*, etc. may also be associated with this disease.
- Microradiograph reveals subsurface demineralization of the root, which extend to the dentin. Surface remineralization is also seen in some areas.

Radiation Caries

Patients receiving large doses of radiation mostly for the treatment of cancer in the head and neck region, often develop a specific type of large "caries-like lesions" in the cervical areas of the teeth. These lesions begin a few weeks to few months after radiotherapy. They often surround the entire crowns of the affected teeth, gradually weaken them and even sometimes can cause amputations of tooth.

The exact cause of radiation caries is not known, but it may be due to the reduced salivary secretions, secondary to the radiotherapy (Fig. 9.8).

Radiological Features of Dental Caries (Figs. 9.9 and 9.10)

Radiographs are often helpful in the detection of dental caries since the damage caused by caries is shown in radiographs as distinct radiolucent areas on the surfaces teeth. The common X-rays used for detection of caries include the intraoral periapical (IOPA), orthopantomogram (OPG) and bitewing radiographs are advised for this purpose.

Dental Caries

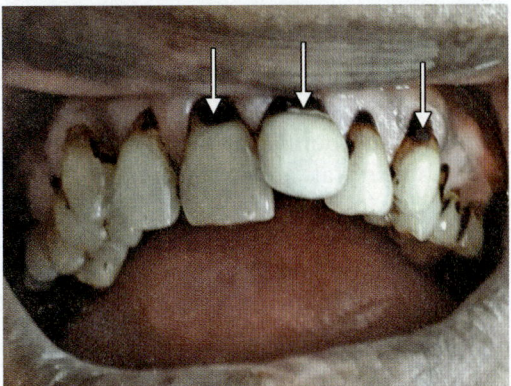

Fig. 9.8: Radiation of caries.

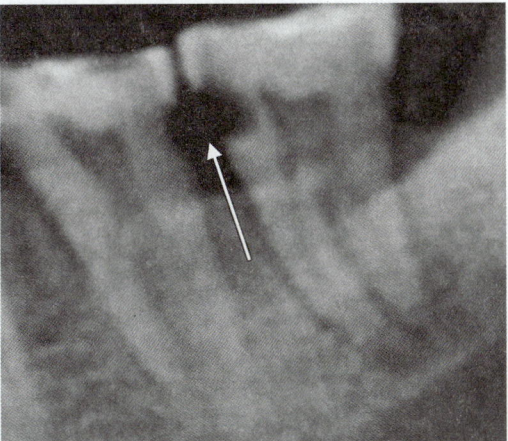

Fig. 9.9: Proximal caries.

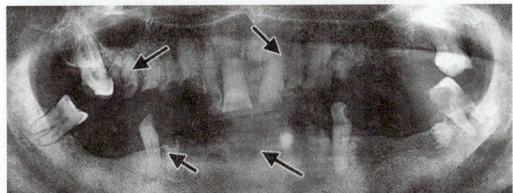

Fig. 9.10: Orthopantomogram (OPG) showing rampant caries.

The bitewing radiographs are especially indicated for the detection of proximal caries. IOPA radiograph produces very distinct images of few teeth in small section of jaw, it is less costly. OPG (Orthopantomogram) produces image of the entire dentition and both the jawbones.

Interpretation: The shape of the lesion varies in pit and fissure from smooth surface caries because carious lesions follow the direction of enamel rods.

Smooth surface caries particularly of proximal surface, has a distinctive shape. It forms a triangular or cone-shaped lesion with the apex toward the junction and the base toward the surface of tooth.

Pit and fissure caries: Characteristically forms a triangular or cone-shaped lesion with the apex at the outer surface and base toward the DEJ. It produces greater cavitations than smooth surface caries.

The root caries on the radiograph usually produces a U-shaped radiolucent area with irregular margin.

In dental X-rays if the enamel radiolucency is extending up to the DEJ, it is considered that the tooth will have a cavity and there is definite involvement of the underlying dentin. Whereas if the enamel radiolucency does not extend to the DEJ, there should be no clinically detectable cavity in the tooth, although there is caries in the tooth.

■ HISTOPATHOLOGICAL ASPECT OF DENTAL CARIES

Enamel Caries

For the microscopic examination of enamel caries, ground section preparations are used because the decalcified sections of enamel become useless owing to the very high concentration minerals in this tissue. The ground section preparation is examined by transmitted or polarized lights.

Enamel caries is discussed as:

Histologic Features of Early Enamel Caries

- There will be loss of interprismatic or inter-rod substances with increase in the prominence of the enamel rods.
- Appearance of transverse striations of the enamel rods due to segmental demineralization.

- Dark lines often appear at right angles to the enamel rods, suggesting segments.
- Accentuation of the incremental striae of Retzius often occurs.

Histologic Features of Advanced Enamel Caries

Advanced enamel caries microscopically presents several zones in the tissue, which are as follows:

Zone I: Translucent zone

- It is the deepest zone in the carious enamel and is the first recognizable histological change at the advancing front of the lesion.
- This zone is slightly more porous than the normal sound enamel and contains 1% by volume of spaces (the pore volume), which is 0.1% in sound normal enamel.
- The pores are larger than the usual smaller pores seen in normal enamel. Dissolution of mineral occurs mainly at the junction of prismatic and interprismatic enamel.

Zone II: Dark zone

The dark zone is located just superficial to the translucent zone and its dark appearance is due to the excessive demineralization of the enamel due to caries.

- This zone is narrower in rapidly advancing caries and it is wider in slowly advancing lesions.
- This zone contains 2–4% pore volume.
- Some pores are larger but other pores are smaller than those of the translucent zone.
- This zone also reveals some degrees of remineralization of the carious enamel.

Zone III: Body of the lesion

This zone is situated between the dark zone and the surface layer of enamel, and it represents the area of greatest demineralization.

- It has a pore volume of between 5% and 25%.
- This zone contains apatite crystals larger than those of the normal enamel.

- Large crystals result from reprecipitation of minerals dissolved from deeper zones.
- With continuing acid attacks on the enamel, there may be further dissolution of minerals both from the periphery of the apatite crystals and their cores.
- The lost minerals in the enamel are often replaced by unbound H_2O and organic matters.
- This zone shows increased prominence of the striae of Retzius.

Zone IV: Surface zone

Initially, the surface zone of a carious enamel remains comparatively unaffected despite subsurface demineralization and also to the surface remineralization.

- It is about 40 μm thick.
- However, in untreated cases, the surface enamel often gets destroyed and a cavity is formed.
- Surface remineralization results from active precipitation of mineral ions derived from both plaque and the saliva.

Ultrastructural studies (of enamel caries): Ultrastructural studies suggest that the initial dissolution of enamel begins along prism boundaries and later on there is demineralization occurring both within and between the prisms, which results in an increase in the intercrystalline gap.

Along with dissolution, there is also remineralization of enamel and change in enamel crystal structures due to the combined effects of demineralization and remineralization of enamel.

Histology of Dentinal Caries (Caries in Dentin)

The dentinal caries, histologically, presents five zones in the tissue, which are as follows:

Zone I (Normal Dentin)

- This zone represents the innermost layer of the carious dentin and here the dentinal tubules appear normal.

- There is evidence of fatty degeneration of the Tomes' processes.
- No crystals in the lumen of the tubules.
- No bacteria in the tubules.
- Intertubular dentin has normal cross-banded collagen and normal dense apatite crystals.

Zone II (Subtransparent Dentin)
- This is the zone of dentinal sclerosis and it is characterized by the deposition of very fine crystal structures within the dentinal tubules at the advancing front.
- Superficial layer shows areas of demineralization and damage of the odontoblastic processes.
- No bacteria in the tubules.
- This dentin is capable of remineralization.

Zone III (Transparent Dentin)
- This zone appears transparent and this is because of the demineralization of dentin due to caries.
- It is softer than normal dentin.
- Further loss of mineral ions from intertubular dentin.
- Large crystals within the lumen of the dentinal tubules.
- No bacteria in tubules.
- Cross-banded intertubular collagen still intact.
- This zone is capable of self-repair and remineralization.

Zone IV (Turbid Dentin)
- This zone is called the "turbid dentin" and is marked by the widening and distortion of the dentinal tubules, which are packed with microorganisms. There is very little amount of mineral present in the dentin and, moreover, denaturation of collagen fibers also takes place.
- This zone cannot undergo self-repair or remineralization.
- Must be removed before restorative treatment.

Zone V (Infected Dentin)
- This is the outermost zone of the carious dentin and is characterized by complete destruction of the dentinal tubules (it happens due to severe expansion of dentinal tubules due to accumulation of a large number of microorganisms and their by-products) (Fig. 9.11).
- The expanded tubules also cause compression and bending of the adjacent tubules and eventually destroy them.
- In this zone, the areas of decomposition of dentin, which occur along the direction of the dentinal tubules, are called the "liquefaction foci of Miller" (Fig. 9.12).
- In some areas, the cariogenic microorganisms spread laterally and

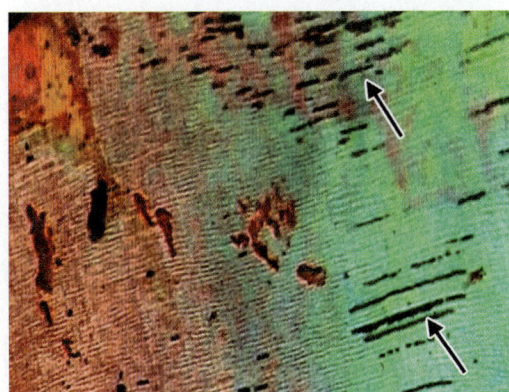

Fig. 9.11: Photomicrograph of infected dentin with presence of microorganisms within dentinal tubules.

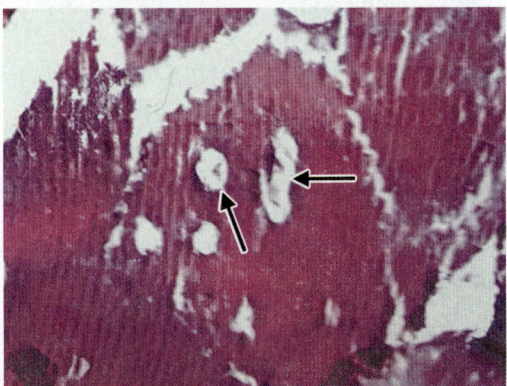

Fig. 9.12: Photomicrograph of infected dentin showing "liquefaction foci of Miller" (arrows).

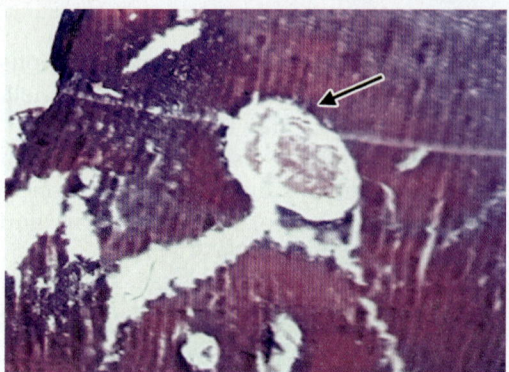

Fig. 9.13: Photomicrograph of infected dentin showing "transversec left" (arrow).

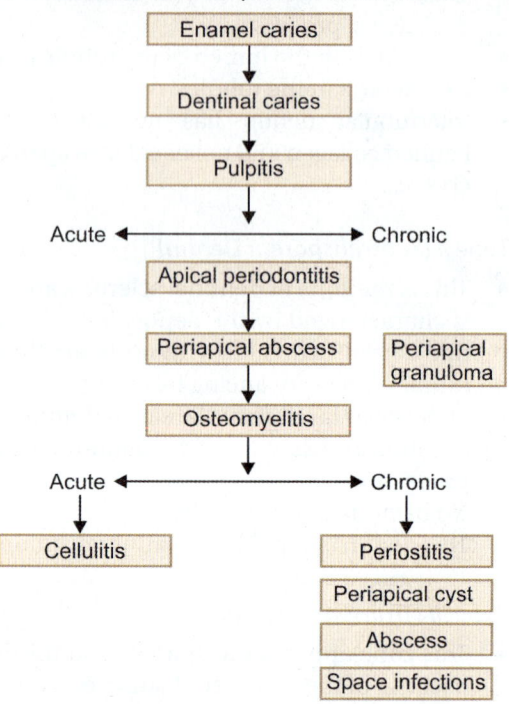

Flowchart 9.1: Sequelae of dental caries.

large bacteria-filled clefts develop at right angles to the direction of the tubules due to decomposition of dentin. These clefts are called the "transverse clefts".
- The mechanism of formation of transverse clefts is not clearly known; they may follow the course of incremental lines, or result from the coalescence of liquefaction of adjacent tubules.
- Transverse clefts may also arise by extensive proteolytic activity along the interconnecting lateral branches of odontoblastic processes (Fig. 9.13).
- In Zone V, bacteria may no longer remain confined within the dentinal tubules and they invade and destroy the peri- and intertubular dentin. In the process, the entire dentinal structure becomes destroyed (Flowchart 9.1).

■ PROTECTIVE RESPONSES OF DENTIN AND PULP AGAINST CARIES

Hectic odontoblastic activity takes place in the dentin-pulp complex in order to protect the tooth from the invasion of caries.

Following are the protective responses from the pulp-dentin complex:

Tubular Sclerosis

Peritubular dentin reduces the size of the individual dentinal tubules and thus prevents the bacterial penetration.

Regular Reactionary Dentin

Reactionary dentin develops on regular basis as a result of localized, nonspecific mild irritation to the odontoblast cells. However, this dentin seems to develop mostly during caries attack in a tooth.

In regular reactionary dentin, a layer of dentin forms at the surface of the pulp chamber deep to the progressive front of dentin caries and it contains normal tubular structures.

It is often hypermineralized as compared to the primary dentin and it delays the pulp exposure by caries by increasing the depth of the tissue between carious dentin and the pulp.

Irregular Reactionary Dentin

This type of dentin forms under moderate to severe insult by caries and this irregular reactionary dentin contains only few irregularly shaped and tortuous tubules. Sometimes, the dentinal tubules can be even absent.

Dead Tracts

The dead tracts form when the odontoblast cells die and their tubules become sealed off. They often prevent the further progression of caries in dentin towards the pulp.

CARIES ACTIVITY TESTS

A number of caries activity tests have been evolved to help detect the presence of oral conditions associated with increased risk of caries. However, no single test can be relied upon to predict the caries susceptibility of a person with a high degree of confidence. Caries activity tests are more useful than clinical examinations since these can predict the need for preventive treatment before the caries has actually started.

Snyder Test

Snyder test is the qualitative determination of acidogenic organisms in the mouth; it measures the ability of salivary microorganisms to produce organic acids from a carbohydrate medium. Glucose-agar media containing an indicator dye (bromocresol green) is used for this test. The indicator dye changes from green to yellow in the range of pH from 5.4 to 3.8.

Paraffin-stimulated saliva (0.2 mL) is added into the medium, change of the medium from green to yellow is indicative of the degrees of caries activity.

Results

If the color of the medium changes from green to yellow within 24 hours, caries susceptibility of the patient should be considered very high.

If the similar color change occurs within 48 hours, the patient is considered to have a definite caries susceptibility.

If the color change occurs in 72 hours, a limited caries susceptibility is indicated.

Finally, if the color change does not occur in 72 hours, the patient should be considered caries immune.

Table 9.4: Change of color and its relation to caries conduciveness.

Change of color	Caries conduciveness
No change in color in 15 minutes	Nonconducive
Color changes from blue to orchid in 15 minutes	Slightly conducive
Color changes from blue to red in 15 minutes	Moderately conducive
Color changes from blue to red immediately on mixing	Highly conducive
Color changes from blue to color less in 15 minutes	Extremely conducive

Salivary Reductase Test

Salivary reductase test measures the activity of reductase enzyme present in salivary bacteria. Paraffin-stimulated saliva is collected in a plastic container and an indicator dye "diazoresorcinol" is added to it, which colors the saliva blue.

The reductase enzyme liberated by the cariogenic bacteria causes color changes in the medium from blue to other colors, which indicates the caries "conduciveness" of the patient.

Results

Table 9.4 depicts the results of the test.

Salivary Buffering Capacity Test

Salivary buffering capacity test is a chair side test to measure the buffering capacity of the saliva. A special kit called "Dentobuff" is used for this test, which contains a small vial of weak HCl and a color indicator chart.

If one milliliter saliva is put into the acid solution, its pH will rise gradually depending upon the buffering capacity of the saliva, and this change of pH is measured by the accompanying color chart.

Results

If the buffering capacity of saliva is normal, the final pH of the solution will rise up to 5–7, and if the buffering capacity is low, the pH will rise up to 4 only.

However, it is understood that more is the buffering capacity of saliva, less will be the acid demineralization of the tooth due to caries.

Microbiological Test

Microbiological test helps to measure the number of *S. mutans* and *L. acidophilus* per microliter of saliva.

Two samples of paraffin-stimulated saliva (1 mL each) are collected from the patient; these are diluted 10 times and each is cultivated in two different special media—(1) Rogosa's SL agar medium for *Lactobacillus;* and (2) Mitis salivarius agar medium for *S. mutans*.

After incubation, the number of colonies that developed into two separate media are counted and then are multiplied by 10 (dilution factor) to estimate the number of bacteria in 1 mL of saliva.

Result

If the count is more than 1,000,000 *S. mutans* and more than 100,000 *L. acidophilus*, the caries susceptibility of the individual should be considered very high.

If the count is less than 100,000 *S. mutans* and less than 1,000 *L. acidophilus*, the individual is considered less susceptible to caries.

Streptococcus mutans Dip-slide Method

This test measures the number of *S. mutans* colonies in modified mitis-salivarius agar; the saliva is collected for 5 minutes and is poured over the agar-coated slide. Slides are then dried and bacitracin disks are placed in the middle of the inoculated agar about 1 cm from each other. The slide is then incubated in a tube containing CO_2 for 48 hours. A zone of inhibition 10–20 mm in diameter is formed around each bacitracin disk. *S. mutans* presents small blue colonies with the zone of inhibition.

Result

The colony density is compared with a model chart and classified as 0 (negligible), 1 (less than 100,000), 2 (100,000–1,000,000) and 3 (more than 1,000,000) *S. mutans* colony forming units per milliliter of saliva.

Enamel Solubility Test

Popularly known as "Fosdick calcium dissolution test", in this test, the patient's saliva is mixed with glucose and, thereafter, measured amount (in milligram) of powdered enamel is mixed with it and kept for 4 hours.

Acid which is produced due to fermentation of glucose by the cariogenic bacteria present in the saliva causes dissolution of powdered enamel. The test measures the amount of enamel powder dissolved during the 4-hour period.

METHODS OF CARIES PREVENTION

The dental caries can be prevented by the following methods:

Limit Substrate

- Eliminate sucrose from the diet or reduce its amount.
- Eliminate sucrose from the "in-between" meals and snacks.

Modify Oral Microflora

- Bactericidal mouth-rinse by chlorhexidine
- Topical fluoride treatments
- Antibiotic treatment by vancomycin and tetracyclines

Plaque Disruption

Plaque disruption by brushing and flossing, etc.

Modify Tooth

- Systemic fluorides
- Topical fluorides
- Maintain a smooth surface of the tooth

Stimulate Salivary Flow

- Eat noncariogenic fibrous foods that require lots of chewing.
- Use sugarless chewing gums
- Administer sialogogues.

Restore Tooth Surface

- Restore all cavitated lesions
- Seal pits and fissures at caries risk
- Correct all defects, e.g. marginal crevice, proximal overhangs.

■ CARIES VACCINE

Dental caries fulfills the criteria of an infectious disease and the possibility of preventing it by vaccination has been persuaded over a long period of time. The rationale is that immunization with *S. mutans* should induce an immune response, which might prevent the dental caries in the following ways:

- It will prevent the ability of the microorganisms to colonize onto the tooth surface.
- It can alter the pattern of polysaccharide metabolism by the bacteria and thereby reduce their adhering capacity onto the tooth surface.
- It can reduce ability of microorganisms to produce acids also.
- It can reduce caries by helping in the process of killing the cariogenic microorganisms.

The caries vaccines are usually given at the age of about 6 months, before the eruption of the deciduous teeth. Oral administration or subcutaneous injection of killed *S. mutans* can induce the formation of specific IgA, IgG and IgM in the blood.

Passive immunization against caries can also be done by injecting specific IgG class of antibody against the *S. mutans*.

Caries vaccination can be given by oral, intranasal, tonsillar route, minor salivary gland and rectal routes.

Poor Success of Caries Vaccine

The concept of caries vaccine may be theoretically very convincing but there is a very high risk of other problems due to its administration in humans. Since the vaccine is prepared against the "M-protein", which is a surface antigen of *Streptococcus* but it shares similar antigenic characteristics with human heart muscles. As a result, the caries vaccine given against streptococcal surface antigen (M protein) may also act as "cross-reacting foreign antigen" and therefore induce autoimmune reaction against heart muscles once given to the humans. That is why caries vaccine produced from *S. mutans* surface antigen could not be successfully implemented. *Other vaccine*—the enzyme glucosyltransferase converts sucrose into glucans, which are important for accumulation of *S. mutans* on the tooth surfaces. Antibodies against glucosyltransferase enzyme have been tested in experimental animals and it has been observed that these antibodies can reduce the accumulation of plaque and the incidences of caries. However, this mechanism is more effective in rodents and it has got little effect on primates.

Experimental Caries in Animals

Dogs have been used as experimental animals for producing experimental caries; however, no caries could be produced in this way probably because dogs are naturally immune to caries.

■ BIBLIOGRAPHY

1. Alaluusua S, Kleemola-Kujala E, Grönroos L, et al. Salivary caries related tests as predictors of future caries increments in teenagers; a three-year longitudinal study. Oral Microl Immunol. 1990;5:77-81.
2. Amamo J. The decline of caries in European Countries. In: RM Frank, S O'Hickey (Eds). Strategy for dental caries prevention in European countries according to their laws and regulations. Oxford: IRL Press; 1987. pp. 21-36.
3. Arends J, Jongebloed WL. Mechanism of enamel dissolution and its prevention. Journale de Biologic Buccale. 1977;5:219-37.
4. Arnold RR, Russell JE, Devine SM, et al. Antimicrobial activity of the secretory innate defense factors lactoferrin, lactoperoxidase, and lysozyme. In: Guggenheim B (Ed.). Cariology Today. Basel: Karger; 1984.

5. Baum LJ. Dentinal pulp conditions in relation to caries lesions. Int Dent J. 1970;20:309-37.
6. Beighton D. *Streptococcus mutans* and other streptococci from the oral cavity. Society of Applied Bacteriology Technical Series. 1985;21:177-90.
7. Bowden GH, Hardie JM, Slack GL. Microbial variations in approximal dental plaque. Caries Res. 1975;9:253-77.
8. Bowen WH, Genco RN, O'Brien TC. Immunologic aspects of dental caries special supplement to immunology abstracts. Washington DC: Information Retrieval Inc.; 1976.
9. Bowen WH. Nature of plaque. Oral Sci Rev. 1976;9:3.
10. Brannston M, Lind PO. Pulpal response to early dentinal caries. J Dent Res. 1965;44:1045-50.
11. Brooks JD, Mertz-Fairhurst EJ, Della-Giustiana VE, et al. A comparative study of two pit and fissure sealants: three-year results in Augusta, Georgia. J Am Dent Assoc. 1979;99:42.
12. Brunelle JA, Carlos JP. Changes in the prevalence of dental caries in US schoolchildren, 1961-1980. J Dent Res. 1982;61:1346.
13. Carlesson J, Grahnen H, Jonsson G. Lactobacilli and streptococci in the mouths of children. Caries Res. 1975;9:333-9.
14. Chen WC, Noncillis GH. The kinetics of dissolution of tooth enamel-a constant composition study. J Dent Res. 1986;65:663-8.
15. Cohen S, Burns RC. Pathways of the pulp. St Louis: CV Mosby; 1984.
16. Darling AI. The pathology and prevention of caries. Br Dent J. 1959;107:287-302.
17. Dawes C. The nature of dental plaque, films and calcarious deposits. Ann NY Acad Sci. 1968;153:102-19.
18. DePaola PF, Soparkar PM, Tavares M, et al. A dental survey of Massachusetts school children. J Dent Res. 1982;61:1356.
19. Douglass CW, Gammon MD. The epidemiology of dental caries and its impact on the operative dentistry curriculum. J Dent Ed. 1984;48:547-55.
20. Easpelid I. Radiographic diagnosis and treatment decision on approximal caries. Community Dent Oral Epidemol. 1986;14:265-70.
21. Fejerskov O, Thylstrup A, Larsen MJ. Rational use of fluorides in caries prevention: a concept based on possible cariostatic mechanisms. Acta Odontol Scand. 1981;39:241.
22. Fitzgerald DB, Stevens R, Fitzgerald RJ, et al. Comparative cariogenicity of *Streptococcus mutansstrains* isolated from caries-active and caries-resistant adults. J Dent Res. 1977;56:894.
23. Fusayama T, Okusa K, Hosoda H. Relationship between hardness, discoloration and microbial invasion in carious dentin. J Dent Res. 1966;45:1033.
24. Fusayama T. Two layers of carious dentin: diagnosis and treatment. Oper Dent. 1969;42:63.
25. Garn SM, Rowe NH, Clark DC. Parent child similarities in dental caries rates. J Dent Res. 1976;55:1129.
26. Glass RL. Secular changes in caries prevalence in two Massachusetts towns. J Dent Res. 1982;61:1352.
27. Hadden WC. Basic data on health care needs of adults ages 25-74 years, United States, 1971-75 Vital and Health statistics: Series 11, Data from the National Health Survey; no 218 DHHS publication no. (PHS) 81-1668. Washington, DC: Government Printing Office; 1980.
28. Harper DS, Loesche WJ. Growth and acid tolerance of human dental plaque bacteria. Arch Oral Biol. 1984;29:843-8.
29. Harvey CR, Kelly JE. Decayed, missing and filled teeth among persons 1-74 years, United States, 1971-74. Vital and health statistics: Series 11, Data from the National Health Survey; no 223 DHHS publication no (PHS) 81-1673. Washington, DC: Government Printing Office; 1981.
30. Hillman JD, Yaphe BI, Johnson KP. Colonization of the human oral cavity by a *Streptococcus mutans*. J Dent Res. 1985;64(11):1272-4.
31. Hodge HC. The concentration of fluorides in drinking water to give the point of minimum caries with maximum safety. J Am Dent Assoc. 1950;40:436.
32. Jenkins GN. Salivary effects on plaque pH. In: Kleinberg I, Ellison SA, Mandel ID (Eds). Saliva and Dental Caries (supplement to Microbiology Abstracts). Washington, DC: Information Retrieval, Inc.; 1979.
33. Johnson RH, Rozanis J. A review of chemotherapeutic plaque control. Oral Surg. 1979;47:136.
34. Kammerman AM, Starkey PE. Nursing caries: a case history. J Ind Dent Assoc. 1981;60:7.
35. Katz RV. Root caries: clinical implications of the current epidemiologic data. Northwest Dent. 1981;60:306.

36. Loesche WJ. Dental caries: a treatable infection. Springfield, Illinois: Charles C Thomas Publisher; 1982.
37. Loesche WJ. Role of *Streptococcus mutans* in human dental decay. Microbial Rev. 1986;50: 353-80.
38. Loeschw WJ. Clinical and microbiological aspects of the therapeutic agents used according to the specific plaque hypothesis. J Dent Res. 1979;58:2404.
39. Mandel ID, Ellison SA. Naturally occurring defense mechanisms in saliva. In: Tanzer JM (Ed.). Animal models in cariology (supplement to Microbiology abstracts). Washington, DC: Information Retrieval, Inc.; 1981.
40. Marthaler TM. Explanations for changing patterns of disease in the western world. In: Guggenheim B (Ed). Cariology Today. Basel: Karger; 1984.
41. Massler M. Pulpal reactions to dental caries. Int Dent J. 1967;17:441-60.
42. Milnes AR, Bowden GHW. The microflora associated with developing lesions of nursing caries. Caries Res. 1985;19:289-97.
43. Minah GE, Loesche WJ. Sucrose metabolism in resting-cell suspensions of caries-associated and non-caries-associated dental plaque. InfectImmun. 1977;17:43-61.
44. Miyauchi H, Lwaku M, Fusayama T. Physiological recalcification of carious dentin. Bull Tokyo Med Dent Univ. 1978;25:169-79.
45. Nikiforuk G. Understanding dental caries: Prevention—Basic and Clinical Aspects. Basel, New York: Karger; 1985.
46. Nolte WA. Oral microbiology with basic microbiology and immunology, 4th Edition. St Louis: CV Mosby Company; 1982.
47. O'Brien TC. Microbial aspects of dental caries. Microbial Abstr Spec Suppl. 1976;1:263.
48. Ripa LW, Leske GS, Sposato A, et al. NaF solution: results of a demonstration program after four school years. J Am Dent Assoc. 1981; 102:482.
49. Ripa LW. Fluoride rinsing: what dentists should know. J Am Dent Assoc. 1981;102:477.
50. Schupbach P, Guggenheim B, Latz F. Human root caries: histopathology of initial lesions in cementum and dentin. J Oral Pathol Med. 1989;18:146-56.
51. Sheiham A. Dental caries in underdeveloped countries. In: Guggenheim B (Ed.). Cariology Today. Basel: Karger; 1984.
52. Silverstone LM. In vitro studies with special reference to the enamel surface and the enamel-resin interface. In: Silverstone LM, Dogon IC (Eds). Proceedings of an international symposium on the acid etch technique. St. Paul, Minn: North Central Publishing;1975.
53. Silverstone LM. Remineralization and enamel caries: New concepts. Dent Update. 1983;10: 261-73.
54. Svanberg M, Loesche WJ. Salivary concentration of *Streptococcus mutans* and *Streptococcus sanguis* and the colonization of artificial fissures in humans by these organisms. Arch Oral Biol. 1977;22:441-7.
55. Taubman MA, Smith DS. Effects of local immunization with glucosyltransferase fraction from *Streptococcus mutans* on dental caries in rats and hamsters. J Immunol. 1977;118:710.
56. Thylstrup A, Fejerskov O. Textbook of Clinical Cariology, 2nd edition. Copenhagen: Munksgaard; 1996.
57. Weddell JA, Klein Al. Socioeconomic correlation of oral disease in six to thirty six months children. Pediatr Dent. 1981;3:306-11.

CHAPTER 10

Disease of Dentin-pulp Complex and Periapical Tissues

PULPAL DISEASES

■ INTRODUCTION

Dental pain is probably one of the most common sufferings experienced by most patients due to various dental diseases but the commonest disease that causes pain in teeth is dental caries. Large numbers of patients take refuse to the dentist only when they are cornered by the misery of pain in the tooth as a result of caries.

Dental pulp is the main component part of tooth, where the pain actually begins in caries. Pulp is the soft delicate connective tissue that occupies the central portion of the tooth and it has got two parts namely—(1) the pulp chamber (the coronal portion) and (2) the root canals (the radicular portion).

Pulp is richly innervated by numerous nerve fibers, which enter the pulp through the apical foramina. The nerve bundle entering the pulp consists mainly of sensory fibers of the trigeminal (5th cranial) nerve and sympathetic branches from the superior cervical ganglion. Each bundle contains both myelinated and unmyelinated axons.

The myelinated fibers are of two types namely the Aα fibers and Aβ fibers, whereas the unmyelinated fibers are designated as C-fibers. Physiologically the Aα fibers are responsible for transmitting the sharp localized pain in the pulp and the Aβ fibers are responsible for transmitting the mechanical, thermal and tactile sensations. The C-fibers are associated with the transmission of dull, diffuse pain in the dental pulp.

■ DENTIN-PULP COMPLEX

Dentin is the vital and cellular hard tissue, ultimately and inseparably related to the ground substance to the dental pulp. It is important to note that the dentin and the pulp together act as a unit called the "dentin-pulp complex", while responding to the injurious stimuli of various nature in the tooth. The complex forms reactionary dentin to protect the pulp from being damaged due to injury, especially in caries.

■ ETIOLOGY OF PULPAL DISEASES

A large number of factors causing injury to dentin-pulp complex have been identified, which may cause either acute or chronic injury. As a general rule, the response to the injurious stimuli, which can cause damage or necrosis to cells, varies with the stimulus intensity and with the defense capacity of the body.

As the pulpal tissue is lying within the solid confinement of dentinal walls and because its entire blood supply depends upon the smaller blood vessels passing through the tiny apical foramina, (often it makes the pulpal tissue a little more extra vulnerable) moderate degree of injury to pulp often elicits an exaggerated amount of damage (Fig. 10.1).

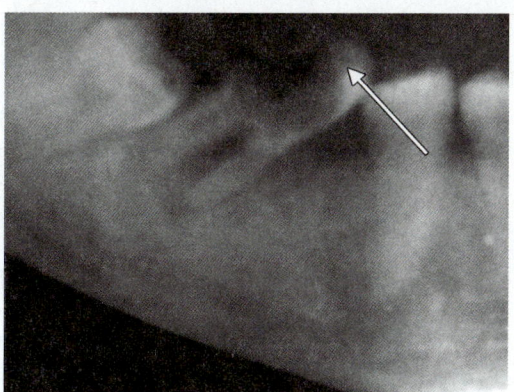

Fig. 10.1: X-ray of large carious tooth with pulp exposure.

CLASSIFICATION OF THE PULPAL DISEASES

The classification of the pulpal diseases has been described in Table 10.1.

Miscellaneous Diseases of the Pulp

- Aerodontalgia
- Necrosis
- Reticular atrophy
- Calcifications
- Pulpal metaplasia.

Focal Reversible Pulpitis

Focal reversible pulpitis or pulp hyperemia is a mild, transient, localized inflammatory reaction in the pulp, which can be treated by conservative means, without involving any form of direct pulp therapy (Box 10.1).

Clinical Features

- The tooth with focal reversible pulpitis is sensitive to thermal changes, especially to cold.
- Pain often results while drinking cold fluids or when ice or cold air is applied to the tooth.

Box 10.1	Etiology of focal reversible pulpitis.
• Slowly progressing chronic carious lesion • Stimuli of short duration, e.g. cutting dentin while cavity preparation • Metallic restoration without proper thermal insulation • Chemical irritation to the pulp (e.g. acid etching in cervical margin of tooth) • Excessive pressure by orthodontic appliances • Severe attrition or abrasion of tooth with minimal dentin thickness	

Table 10.1: Classification of pulpitis.

According to severity of inflammation			

1. Reversible pulpitis
• Asymptomatic
• Symptomatic
• Focal/subtotal
• Generalized/total
	2. Irreversible pulpitis
	• Acute irreversible pulpitis
	  – Abnormally responsive to cold
	  – Abnormally responsive heat
	• Chronic irreversible pulpitis
	  – Chronic asymptomatic pulpitis with pulp exposure
	  – Chronic hyperplastic pulpitis
	  – Chronic pulpitis with internal resorption of tooth
		3. Pulp degeneration with/without calcification	4. Pulp necrosis

According to extent of involvement			
Focal/subtotal pulpitis • Open pulpitis • Closed pulpitis		Total/generalized pulpitis • Open pulpitis • Closed pulpitis	

- The pain is of very short duration and it disappears as soon as the thermal irritant is withdrawn.
- Pain also results when the tooth is exposed to extremely high temperatures.
- Young people develop focal reversible pulpitis more often than the older individuals because of the more reparative capacity of the pulp tissue among the former group.
- Pulpal stimuli, which cause reversible pulpitis in young people often causes irreversible pulpitis to the older individuals because of the less pulpal tissue viability.
- The affected tooth responds to stimulation by electric pulp tester at a lower level of current (including a lower pain threshold) when compared with an adjacent normal tooth.
- The involved tooth often shows large carious lesions or improper restoration.

Histopathology

Histologically, focal reversible pulpitis presents the following features (Fig. 10.2):
- Acute inflammatory reaction in the pulp limited to the odontoblastic or subodontoblastic regions, adjacent to the irritated dentinal tubules.
- Dilatation of pulpal blood vessels with increased vascular permeability.

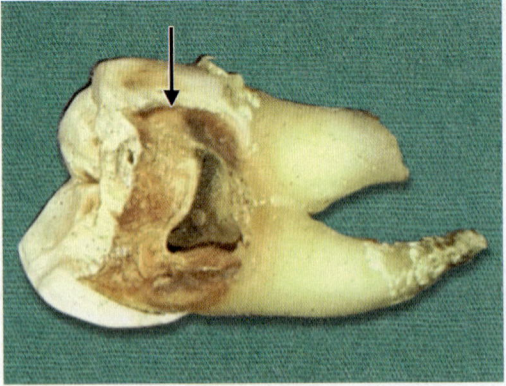

Fig. 10.2: A grossly carious tooth specimen with involvement of pulp.

- Edema in the pulp with infiltration by the polymorphonuclear leukocytes in the area.
- Odontoblast cell nuclei may be displaced into the dentinal tubules due to either increased local tissue pressure or due to abnormal dentinal fluid movements during injury.
- Few odontoblast cells could be damaged in the localized area of injury.
- Thrombosis of pulpal blood vessels may occur in some cases.

Treatment

Treatment of focal reversible pulpitis is mostly directed toward elimination of the primary irritating factors and restoration of tooth wherever necessary.

Acute Pulpitis

Acute pulpitis is an irreversible condition characterized by acute, intense inflammatory reaction in the pulpal tissue.

Mode of Development

Acute pulpitis can occur in the following pathways:
- As an extension of the focal reversible pulpitis.
- As a *de novo* condition, where the inflammation is acute from the beginning.
- As an acute exacerbation of the chronic pulpitis.

The etiology of acute pulpitis is given in Box 10.2.

Clinical Features

Acute pulpitis is often considered as one of the most dreaded diseases of tooth because of the horrific nature of pain involved in it. The disease usually presents the following features:
- The tooth is extremely sensitive to hot and cold stimuli; however the pain in acute pulpitis can start spontaneously in the absence of any stimulus.

Disease of Dentin-pulp Complex and Periapical Tissues

> **Box 10.2** Etiology of acute pulpitis.
> - Caries progressing beyond the dentinal barrier and reaching the pulp
> - Pulp exposure due to faulty cavity preparation
> - Blow to tooth with subsequent damage to pulp
> - Excessive heating of tooth during cavity preparation without water spray
> - Chemical irritation to the pulp
> - Cracked tooth syndrome
> - Tooth or teeth coming in the line of fracture when the jaw is traumatized
> - Anachoretic infection to the pulp
> - Recurrent caries around a preexisting restoration
> - Metallic restoration in a tooth without proper thermal insulation

> **Box 10.3** Characteristics of pain in acute pulpitis.
> - **Radiating pain** (*means extension of pain to another site whilst the original pain persists at its original site*): Pain in acute pulpitis often radiates to other parts of the orofacial region; for example pain in lower molar teeth may radiate to the ear and to the tongue. Similarly pain from the upper molars may spread to the forehead and zygomatic region. Pain in the posterior teeth may radiate to the anterior teeth up to the midline of the jaw.
> - **Referred pain** (*when pain is felt at a distance from its source and there is no pain at the site of the disease*): In acute pulpitis, patient may experience pain in upper teeth while the actual pain may be from the lower teeth. Pain from lower molars may be so really and truly felt in the ear that patients often go to consult an ENT specialist before consulting a dental surgeon. Referred pain in teeth may sometimes lead to unnecessary removal of a healthy tooth by the doctor by mistake while the undiagnosed diseased tooth remains in the mouth, this might lead to unpleasant professional situations.

- A short and severe "lancinating" type of pain is often elicited from the affected tooth (Box 10.3).
- Application of hot or cold stimuli causes an increase in the intensity of pain and such type of pain persists for a longer duration even after the stimuli are removed.
- As the dental pulp is located within the solid confinement of dentinal walls, intrapulpal pressure builds up quickly and so is the pain, since there is lack of escape route of inflammatory exudates during pulpal inflammations.
- In the initial stages the pain can be localized and patient can identify the offending tooth, however in the more severe later stages the pain becomes regional and the patient is unable to identify the offending tooth.
- *Special times of occurrence of pain*: The intensity of pain increases during sleep because there is a rise in local blood pressure in head and neck region in supine position, which results in increased venous return leading to higher blood flow into the pulp chamber. More flow of blood in the pulp chamber causes more compression of the nerves resulting in higher intensity of pain. As soon as the patient gets up from bed, the pulpal pressure becomes less and pain intensity becomes significantly less.
- Application of cold (e.g. patients often keep water in mouth) often relieves the pain temporarily as it prevents expansion of the pulpal exudates causing less pressure on the nerves. Moreover, in low temperature peripheral nerve endings in pulp becomes slightly numb.
- If the entrance to the pulp opening is not wide, acute pulpitis not only causes an excruciating pain but also helps in quickly spreading the inflammation throughout the pulp with subsequent necrosis.
- Acute pulpitis is often associated with microabscess formation in the pulp along with liquefaction degeneration.
- When drainage is established, small amount of pus exudes from the opening, which has a noxious odor.
- The affected tooth responds to a lower level of current, if electric pulp tester is used.
- Pain subsides when the drainage is established or when the pulp undergoes complete necrosis.

- The tooth is neither mobile and nor tendered to percussion; unless the pulpal inflammation has spread beyond the root apex into the periapical region.
- Patients with acute pulpitis are often apprehensive and moderately ill.
- When intrapulpal pressure becomes very high during acute inflammation, it can cause collapse of the apical blood vessel. This phenomenon is known as "pulp-strangulation".

Histopathology

Acute pulpitis presents the following histopathological features (Fig. 10.3):
- Severe edema in the pulp with vasodilatation.
- Moderate to dense infiltration of polymorphonuclear leukocytes.
- Focal or complete destruction of the odontoblast cells at the pulp dentin border.
- Many microabscess formations, characterized by areas of liquefaction degeneration in the pulp being surrounded by dense band of neutrophils and microorganisms.
- In severe cases, there may be complete liquefaction and necrosis of the pulp with total destruction of the odontoblastic cell layer. This phenomenon is known as acute suppurative pulpitis.
- Death of the pulp may also be accompanied by tissue dehydration and the condition is known as "dry gangrene of the pulp".

Treatment

- Drainage of exudate or pus from the pulp chamber.
- Root canal treatment (RCT) or extraction of tooth.

Chronic Pulpitis

Chronic pulpitis is a condition characterized by a low grade, often persistent inflammatory reaction in the pulpal tissue with little or no constitutional symptoms.

Etiology

Etiology for chronic pulpitis is same as that of the acute pulpitis but here the irritants are of low virulence.

Mode of Development

- Chronic pulpitis mostly occurs as a chronic inflammatory reaction in the pulp from the very beginning.
- Occasionally, it may be present as a quiescent phase of the preexisting acute pulpitis.

Clinical Features

Generally in chronic pulpitis the signs and symptoms are much milder in comparison to the acute pulpitis.
- The tooth with chronic pulpitis may be asymptomatic for quite some time.
- In other cases there may be an intermittent dull and throbbing pain in the tooth.
- The tooth is less sensitive to hot and cold stimuli and it responds to a higher level of current when electric pulp tester is used. It happens due to degeneration of most of the nerve fibers in the chronically inflamed pulp.
- Even if the pulp is exposed to the oral environment through a large open cavity in the tooth, still a very little pain is felt.
- Touching or manipulation of the exposed, chronically inflamed pulp by small

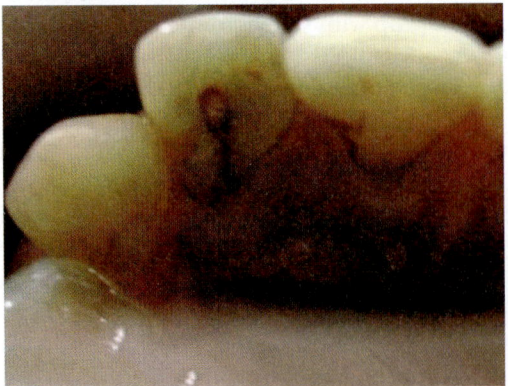

Fig. 10.3: Dens-invaginatus causing pulp exposure.

instruments often elicits bleeding but causes little pain.

Histopathology

- The chronic inflammatory response in the pulp is characterized by cellular infiltration by lymphocytes, plasma cell and macrophages, etc.
- The chronic nature of the inflammation may continue for a long-time with occasional periods of acute exacerbations.
- Blood capillaries are prominent and few microorganisms are also found in the pulpal tissue.
- Prolonged chronic inflammation may encourage fibroblastic activity in the pulp with formation of collagen bundles.
- Persisting chronic pulpitis may cause diffuse or solitary areas of calcification in the pulp.
- Chronic inflammation of the pulp in some cases may result in internal resorption of the tooth.

Treatment

- RCT or
- Extraction of tooth.

Pulp Polyp (Chronic Hyperplastic Pulpitis)

Pulp polyp is an unusual type of hyperplastic granulation tissue response in the pulp, which is characterized by an overgrowth of the tissue outside the boundary of the pulp chamber as a protruding mass.

Pathogenesis

Pulp polyp exhibits an intense proliferation of the pulpal connective tissue and this type of hyperplastic tissue growth depends on several factors, which are given in Box 10.4.

Clinical Features

- Pulp polyp clinically appears as a small, pinkish-red, lobulated mass, which

Box 10.4 Contributing factors for pulp polyp.
- Persistence of balance between injurious agents and tissue resistance
- Presence of a low-grade sustained inflammation
- Pulp tissue should be well-vascularized with excellent tissue reactivity
- The carious cavity should be wide open
- The patients must be young with good body resistance
- The apical foramen of the affected tooth must be wide so that pulpal strangulation and complete necrosis due to inflammation does not occur

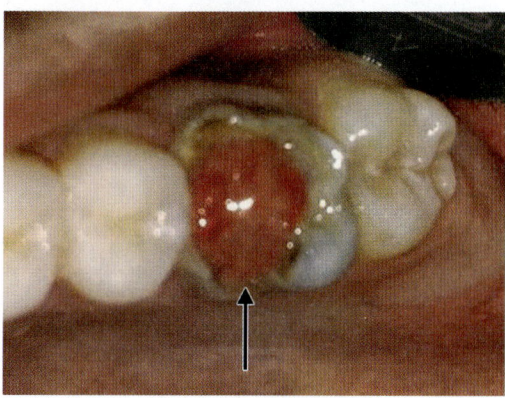

Fig. 10.4: Pulp polyp.

protrudes from the pulp chamber and often fills up the carious cavity (Fig. 10.4).
- The teeth in which pulp polyp commonly develops are often the deciduous molars and first permanent molars.
- The condition is obviously seen in either children or young adults.
- The affected tooth always has a large open carious cavity, which is present for a long duration.
- The lesion bleeds profusely upon provocation.
- If traumatized, the pulp polyp becomes ulcerated and appears as a dark red, fleshy mass with fibrinous exudate on the surface.
- The involved tooth is usually painless but it may be sensitive to thermal stimuli.

- Although pulp polyp is a purely connective tissue growth, it may be sometimes superficially epithelized.

Histopathology

Pulp polyp histologically presents the following features:
- The hyperplastic pulpal tissue lesion presents the features of a granulation tissue mass, consisting of numerous proliferating fibroblasts and young blood capillaries.
- There may be edema and hyperemia with focal areas of pulp necrosis, which are surrounded by areas of fibrosis.
- Inflammatory cell infiltration chiefly by the lymphocytes, plasma cells and sometimes polymorphonuclear neutrophils in the tissue are common.
- Reparative secondary dentin may be formed occasionally adjacent to the dentinal wall of the affected tooth.
- Stratified squamous type epithelial lining is sometimes found on the surface of the pulp polyp, which resembles oral epithelium.
- The epithelial cells on the surface of the polyp are believed to be the desquamated epithelial cells, which came either from the buccal mucosa, gingiva or from the salivary gland ducts.
- These cells are carried via saliva and are transplanted on to the surface of the pulp polyp.
- When the pulp polyp is present for a longtime, persistent rubbing of the buccal mucosa against the lesion may help in the grafting of epithelial cells on its surface.
- The epithelized surface of the pulp polyp may sometimes show even well-formed retes peg-formation.

Treatment

Treatment is done either by RCT or by extraction of the affected tooth.

Aerodontalgia

Aerodontalgia is an unusual type of dental pain, which occurs as an effect of change in the altitude.

Clinical Features

- Aerodontalgia affects some persons who, experience pain in the tooth during high altitude flight or during deep sea diving.
- At ground levels the tooth is completely asymptomatic.
- In some cases the pain may not start immediately during the flight or during diving, instead it may occur few hours or days later.
- The condition may be related to subclinical pulpitis.
- Sometimes, similar problem may happen in an endodontically treated tooth with improper obturation of the root canals (with some voids present).
- The entrapped air in the voids may expand during flight or during diving (due to alteration in the atmospheric pressure), which creates pressure in the periapical nerve bundles at the root apex and produce pain.

Pulp Necrosis

Pulp necrosis may occur either due to pulpitis or due to injury and subsequent occlusion of the apical blood vessels.
- A coagulative type of necrosis of the pulp occurs due to ischemia.
- When the necrosis follows pulpitis, the breakdown of inflammatory cells may lead to liquefactive degeneration in the pulp.
- The necrosed pulp may become secondarily infected by putrefactive bacteria from caries.
- The gangrenous necrosis of pulp is usually associated with a foul odor, when the pulp chamber is opened for endodontic therapy.

- In sickle cell anemia, blockage of the pulpal vessel by sickled or defective RBCs may result in pulp necrosis.

DIAGNOSIS OF PULPAL DISEASES

Several clinical tests are performed for the evaluation of pulpal disease, which are discussed here.

History

- In pulpitis, history often reveals the state of the disease:
- Intense pain in the tooth, which increases at night indicates an irreversible pulpal damage.
- Pain or sensitivity with thermal change indicates focal reversible pulpitis.
- A tooth having dull pain of late but has passed through previous bouts of sharp acute pain, indicates either chronic pulpitis or pulp necrosis.

Clinical Examination

Clinical examination of tooth either visually or with hand instruments may help in establishing the diagnosis of the pulpal diseases. A tooth having large caries with pulp exposure or a fractured tooth or a discolored tooth, all should be suspected for possible pulp pathology.

Radiographic Examination

Intraoral periapical radiographs or bitewing radiographs, etc. can help in establishing a diagnosis in pulpal disease. Radiographs often indicate if the caries has reached the pulp or if the pulpal inflammation has already progressed beyond the apical foramen into the periapical tissue.

Clinical Test for Evaluation of Pulp Response (Pulp Vitality Tests)

If the dental pulp is not in a healthy state it will generate abnormal responses to different stimuli and this can help in making a diagnosis of the pulpal disease (Box 10.5).

Box 10.5 Pulp vitality tests.

- *Heat test*: Sensitivity to heat may be tested by application of hot water or heated gutta-percha stick on the suspected tooth. A tooth having pulpitis will respond to a lower level of heat as compared to a normal tooth
- *Cold test*: Selective application of cold water or water ice or dry ice can help in assessing the pulpal health. This is by far the most reliable method of pulp testing
- *Percussion*: Sensitivity to percussion indicates periapical inflammation as sequlae of pulpitis
- *Palpation*: Palpation of the apical tissues may elicit tenderness or swelling in periapical inflammations
- *Pressure*: Gentle pressure on the tooth often helps to diagnose fracture or cracked tooth syndrome
- *Electrical pulp test*: The electric pulp testing reveals varying degrees of sensory reply in the pulp electric current is passed through the pulp
  In reversible pulpitis the pulp gets stimulated at a lower level of current as compared to that of a normal pulp (because of lower pain threshold). In irreversible pulpitis the pulp responds to an even lower level of current. In chronic pulpitis the pulp responds to a higher level of current due to the decreased number of sensory nerve fibers in the pulp as a result of necrosis
- *Laser Doppler flowmetry*: It can be used as an advanced diagnostic aid for accurate diagnosis of pulpal pathology

Bacteriology of Pulpal Infections

The commonly encountered microorganisms in the dental pulp during acute or chronic pulpitis are as follows:

Anaerobic organisms:	
Gram-negative rods	Gram-positive rods
• Bacteroides buccae	• Actinomyces israelii
• Bacteroides denticola	• Actinomyces odontolyticus
• Bacteroides endodontalis	• Eubacterium alactolyticum
• Bacteroides gingivalis	• Eubacterium brachy
• Fusobacterium nucleatum	• Eubacterium lentum
• Wolinella recta	• Eubacterium nodatum
• Selenomonas sputigena	• Lactobacillus catenaforme
	• Lactobailus minutus

Contd...

Contd...

Gram-negative cocci	Gram-positive cocci
Veillonella parvula	• *Streptococcus constellatus* • *Streptococcus intermedius* • *Streptococcus morbillorum* • *Peptostreptococcus anaerobius* • *Peptostreptococcus magnus* • *Peptostreptococcus prevotii*
Aerobic and facultative anaerobic organisms:	
Gram-negative rods • *Capnocytophaga ochracea* • *Eikenella corrodens* • *Campylobacter sputorum*	Gram-positive rods • *Actinomyces naeslundii* • *Actinomyces viscosus* Gram-positive cocci • *Streptococcus mutans* • *Streptococcus milleri* • *Streptococcus mitior* • *Streptococcus sanguis*

DISEASES OF THE PERIAPICAL TISSUES

■ PRIMARY ACUTE APICAL PERIODONTITIS

Primary acute apical periodontitis mostly occurs as a result of extension of the pulpal inflammation into the periapical tissues. The lesion may also occur as a result of occlusal trauma and in such cases the pulp is vital.

Clinical Features
- Moderate pain and sensitivity in the tooth.
- Slight extrusion of the tooth due to escape of inflammatory exudates into the apical periodontal ligament.
- The most important and determining feature is the severe pain on slight pressure during mastication. Thooth is tendered to purcussion
- Thermal changes (hot and cold) do not aggravate the pain.
- Pain is intense and throbbing later when apical abscess develops.
- The gingiva overlying the affected root may be red and tendered.
- The regional lymph nodes are often enlarged and tendered.

Possible Complications
- Periapical abscess formation
- Regional lymphadenopathy
- Cellulitis
- Development of periapical granuloma.

Treatment
Extraction or endodontic treatment of the diseased tooth.

■ PERIAPICAL GRANULOMA (CHRONIC APICAL PERIODONTITIS)

Definition
Granuloma: It is the focal collection of inflammatory cells at the site of tissue infection, surrounded by fibrous tissue wall; the cells present in a granuloma include lymphocytes, macrophages and giant cells.

Periapical granuloma is a localized mass of granulation tissue around the root apex of a nonvital tooth, which develops in response to a low-grade infection or inflammation.

Pathogenesis
Most of the periapical granulomas develop due to the spread of pulpal infections beyond the root apex. The root canal of a nonvital tooth is an ideal environment for bacterial growth because it protects the organisms from normal body defenses, as well as it provides them with good nutrition. In case of periapical granuloma a balance between the pathogenicity of bacteria within the canal and the defense capacity of the periapical tissue is established.

Inflammation in the periapical region causes destruction of the apical periodontal ligaments, adjoining alveolar bone and cementum, etc. Later on, these tissues are replaced by a mass of "granulation tissue". The granuloma increases in size due to the gradual resorption of the surrounding bone by chemical mediators like osteoclast activating factor (OAF) and collagenase, etc. which are released by the chronic inflammatory cells.

Clinical Features

- The offending tooth produces sensitivity to percussion, which occurs due to edema, hyperemia and inflammation of the apical periodontal ligaments (Fig. 10.5).
- There can be mild pain and discomfort in the tooth during chewing solid foods.
- Patient may give a previous history of pain in the tooth (earlier when pulpitis was present), which had subsided thereafter.
- The involved tooth is always nonvital and it does not responds to thermal or electric pulp testers.
- The tooth may be slightly elongated from its socket and is tendered to the chewing pressure.
- In many cases, periapical granuloma may be asymptomatic throughout its course.
- There may be severe pain and sensitivity in the tooth during acute exacerbations of the disease.

Radiological Features

- Most of the lesions are detected incidentally during routine radiographic examinations.
- In the initial stages, periapical granuloma radiographically shows widening of the periodontal ligament space at the root apex (Fig. 10.6).
- Fully developed lesions usually produce a well-defined, radiolucent area of varying size, which appears to be in continuity with the root apex.
- Sometimes, the radiolucent lesion is well-demarcated from the surrounding normal bone by a thin sclerotic margin.
- In other cases, the radiolucency blends gradually with the surrounding tissue.
- Long-standing periapical granuloma may show varying degrees of root resorption and loss of apical lamina dura.

Histopathology

Histologically, periapical granuloma presents the following features:

- There will be a granulation tissue mass consisting of proliferating fibroblasts, endothelial cells and numerous immature blood capillaries.

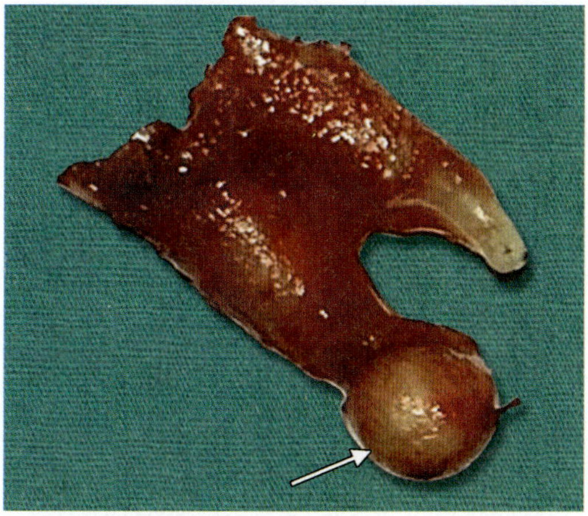

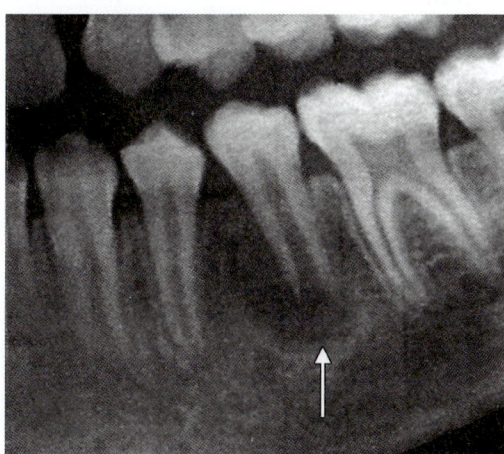

Fig. 10.5: Periapical granuloma.

Fig. 10.6: Radiograph of periapical granuloma.

- Chronic inflammatory cells, e.g. macrophages, lymphocytes and plasma cells, etc. are often present in the lesion.
- Some lesions show the presence of epithelial islands, cholesterol clefts and foam cells.
- Giant cells are also found on rare occasions.
- Although periapical granuloma is a "sterile" lesion, few bacteria (e.g. *Actinomyces israelii*, *Actinomyces naeslundii* and *Arachnia propionica*) are almost always present in the lesion.
- The epithelial cell rests of Malassez, a natural component of the periodontal ligament, sometimes proliferate in response to chronic inflammation and these proliferating cells later on may undergo cystification to produce radicular cyst.
- The bony tissue at the periphery of the lesion is usually lined by osteoclast cells with areas of bone resorptions.
- Resorption of cementum and dentin may also occur as a result of the chronic inflammation.

Treatment
The lesion is treated either by extracting the tooth or by performing RCT in the tooth with apicoectomy or apical curettage.

Sequelae
Sequelae of periapical granuloma:
- Resorptions of root apex or apical bone.
- Acute exacerbation with severe pain.
- Development of acute periapical abscess.
- Formation of radicular cyst
- Hypercementosis of tooth

ACUTE EXACERBATION OF CHRONIC PERIAPICAL GRANULOMA/ABSCESS (PHOENIX ABSCESS)

- Most of the periapical granulomas clinically remain quite as long as the balance between the bacteria contained within the root canal and body's defense in the granuloma is maintained.
- If this balance is lost somehow, an explosive type of acute exacerbation occurs in the preexisting chronic lesion, which is known as "phoenix abscess".
- Clinically phoenix abscess presents severe pain, local swelling, extreme tenderness in the tooth upon pressure and sometimes facial cellulitis, etc.

PERIAPICAL ABSCESS (DENTOALVEOLAR ABSCESS)

Definition
Periapical abscess can be defined as a localized, acute or chronic suppurative infection in the periapical region of a nonvital tooth.

Pathogenesis
Periapical abscess often results from a mixed bacterial infection caused by strict anaerobes, e.g. *Prevotella* and *Porphyromonas*, etc. Anaerobic streptococci and staphylococci also play major roles in causing the disease.

The etiological factors of periapical abscess are given in Box 10.6.

Clinical Features (Figs. 10.7 and 10.8)
- Periapical abscess is a common odontogenic infection and constitutes about 2% of all apical radiolucencies.

Box 10.6	Etiological factors of periapical abscess.
	• Extension of pulpal infection into the periapical tissue
	• Fracture of tooth with pulp exposure
	• Accidental perforation of the apical foramen during root canal treatment, which results in entry of pulpal microorganisms into the periapical area
	• Extension of periodontal infection into the periapical tissues
	• Secondary bacterial invasion into the preexisting periapical granuloma or cyst or scar
	• Anachoretic infection of the periapical tissues

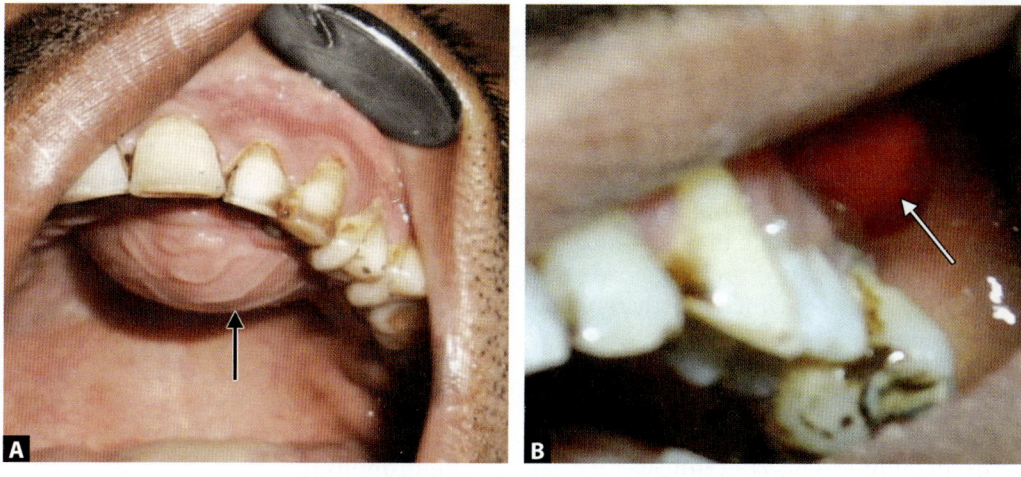

Figs. 10.7A and B: Acute periapical abscess.

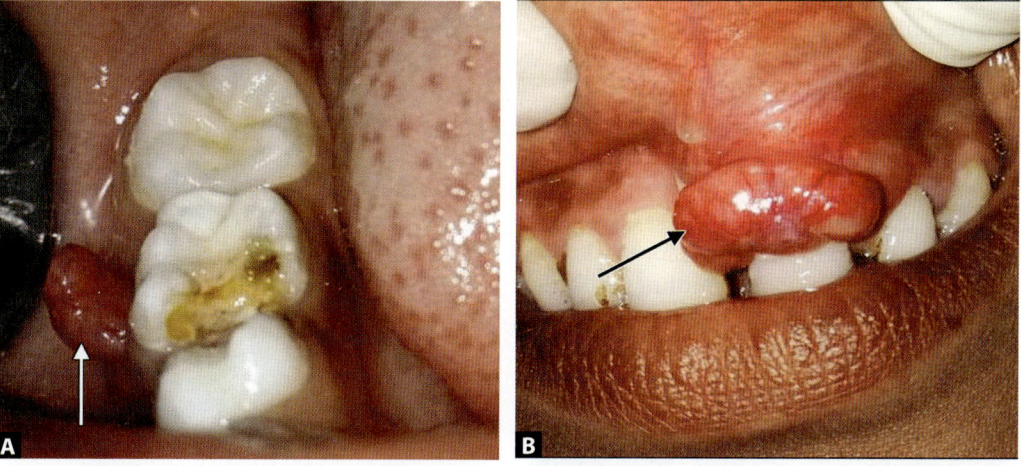

Figs. 10.8A and B: (A) Chronic periapical abscess with pus discharging sinus; (B) Acute exacerbation of chronic periapical abscess.

- Acute abscess produces severe pain in the affected tooth with localized swelling and erythema.
- The pain aggravates when pressure is applied with the opposing tooth.
- The affected tooth may be extruded from the socket due to pressure from purulent exudates and inflammatory infiltrates in the periapical area.
- The associated tooth is nonvital and sometimes it can be mobile also.
- The affected area of the jaw may be tender on palpation.
- Elevated body temperature and localized lymphadenitis are common.
- Application of heat on the tooth intensifies pain, whereas application of cold relieves the pain temporarily.

- Spread of infection into the adjacent soft tissues may cause cellulitis.
- Pus discharging sinus often develops on the alveolar mucosa over the affected root apex and sometimes on the skin overlying the jawbone.
- If the host resistance is high or the virulence of the organisms involved in periapical abscess is low, a chronic stage of the abscess sets in, which mostly remains asymptomatic.
- Unlike the acute lesions, chronic periapical abscess usually produces mild, dull pain and it also produces intraoral or extraoral pus discharging sinuses.

Complications of acute periapical abscess:
- Development of cellulitis
- Osteomyelitis
- Space infections
- Septicemia
- Ludwig's angina
- Cavernous sinus thrombosis

Radiological Features

As the acute periapical abscess develops quite rapidly, there is little time for the lesion to cause any significant amount of bone resorption (Fig. 10.9). Therefore, radiographic changes in acute abscess are minimum and are limited to only slight thickening of the periodontal ligament space in apex region of the involved tooth.

However, in chronic periapical abscess, radiographs often reveal small radiolucent areas at the root apex with poorly defined margins.

Histopathology

Histologically, periapical abscess presents the following features (Fig. 10.10):
- The lesion appears as a zone of liquefaction necrosis, which is made up of proteinaceous exudates, necrotic tissue and a large number of viable or dead neutrophils (pus).
- The adjacent tissues surrounding the abscess have many dilated blood capillaries and infiltration with neutrophils.
- Inflammatory change is also observed in the periodontal ligament and adjoining bone marrow.
- Bony trabeculae in the periapical region may show empty lacunae, which results from the death of the osteocytes.
- In chronic periapical abscess the inflammatory cell pattern is different and in these lesions often exhibit infiltration by lymphocytes, plasma cells and macrophages, etc.

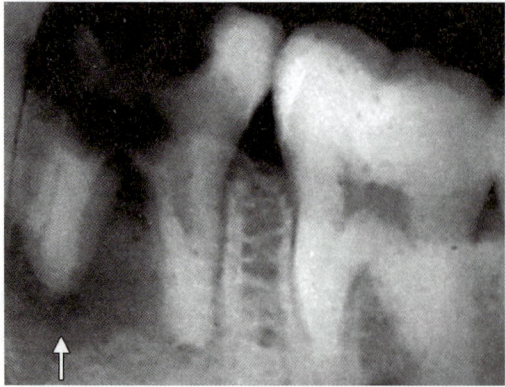

Fig. 10.9: X-ray showing periapical abscess with irregular bone loss.

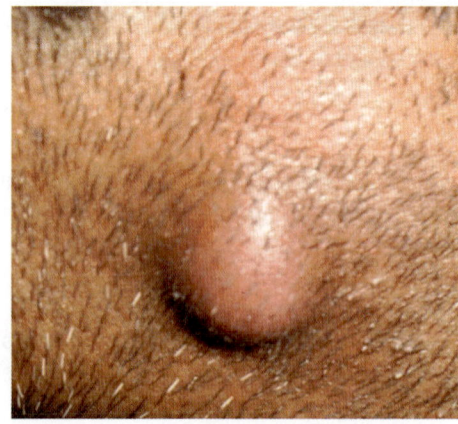

Fig. 10.10: Extraoral spread of periapical infection.

- Areas of bone destruction are also accompanied by areas of fibrosis as well as bone regeneration in chronic lesions.
- Pus discharging sinus in chronic abscess is often lined either by a granulation tissue or by a squamous epithelial lining.

Treatment

- Drainage through an opening in the tooth or by an incision over the soft tissue swelling.
- Antibiotics.
- Root canal treatment or extraction of tooth after the acute phase is over.

The radiographic comparison in periapical abscess, periapical granuloma and periapical cyst is described in Figure 10.11.

■ OSTEOMYELITIS

Definition

Osteomyelitis can be defined as the inflammation of bone and bone marrow along with the surrounding periosteum.

The inflammatory condition involves all the structures of bone, e.g. the bone marrow, bone cells, Haversian systems, periosteum, blood vessels, nerves and epiphyses, etc.

It should be noted that bone reactions in osteomyelitis often vary depending upon the severity of the inflammatory process involved; hence bone necrosis often occurs in severe acute osteomyelitis, while bone formation occurs in chronic osteomyelitis.

The classification of osteomyelitis is given in Box 10.7.

Box 10.7 Classification of osteomyelitis.

There are various types of osteomyelitic lesions occurring in the jawbones, which can be broadly divided into *two groups—(1) acute osteomyelitis* and *(2) chronic osteomyelitis*. According to the specificity of the causative microorganisms, osteomyelitis may be of two types—specific osteomyelitis and nonspecific osteomyelitis.
Acute osteomyelitis
Most commonly encountered (nonspecific) lesions in this category include:
- Acute suppurative osteomyelitis
- Acute subperiosteal osteomyelitis
- Acute periostitis

Chronic osteomyelitis (nonspecific type)
- Chronic intramedullary osteomyelitis
- Chronic focal sclerosing osteomyelitis
- Chronic diffuse sclerosing osteomyelitis
- Chronic osteomyelitis with proliferative periostitis
- Chronic subperiosteal osteomyelitis
- Chronic periostitis

Specific type
- Tuberculous osteomyelitis.
- Syphilitic osteomyelitis.
- Actinomycotic osteomyelitis.

Radiation induced osteomyelitis
Idiopathic osteomyelitis

Periapical abscess	Periapical granuloma	Periapical cyst
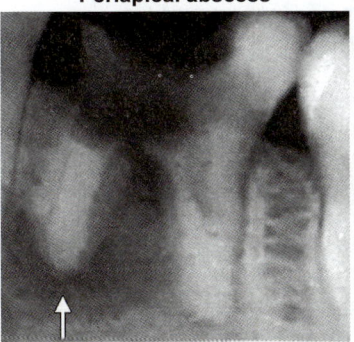	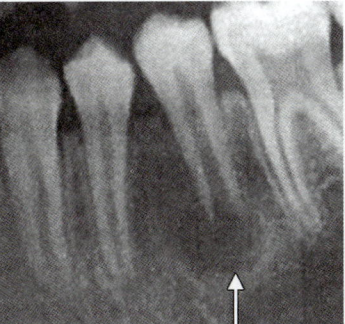	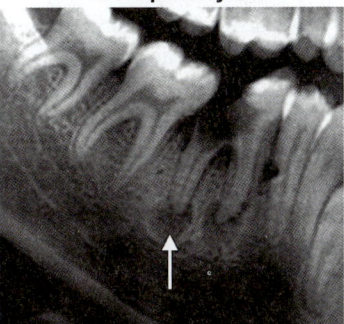
Apical radiolucency with ill-defined and irregular margin	Apical radiolucency with well-defined and smooth margin	Apical radiolucency with well-defined and well-corticated margin

Fig. 10.11: Radiograph of various periapical lesions.

Etiology of Osteomyelitis

- Direct spread of infection from dental pulp into the jawbone.
- Spread of infection into the bone from the preexisting suppurative odontogenic infections, e.g.
  - Periapical abscess
  - Periodontal pocket involved in a fractured jaw bone
  - Infected periapical granuloma
  - Infected periapical cyst
  - Acute necrotizing ulcerative gingivitis
  - Periodontal abscess
  - Pericoronitis
  - Infected and fractured tooth/retained root tip
- Spread of infection following removal of tooth without proper asepsis and antibiotic coverage.
- Compound fracture of the jawbone with exposure of bone outside the skin or mucosa.
- Gunshot injuries in the jaw with soft tissue laceration and exposure of bone.
- Spread of microorganisms from overlying soft tissue (skin or mucosa) infections.
- Post-radiation secondary infection.
- Infection to the preexisting bony diseases, e.g. Paget's disease of bone, fibrous dysplasia and osteopetrosis, etc.
- Phosphorus poisoning
- Anachoretic infections
- Idiopathic factors.

Being an inflammatory disease, development of osteomyelitis depends mainly upon the balance between the virulence and number of microorganisms present in the bone and the local or systemic defense capacity of the patient's body to infection.

However, besides these two main factors there are several other predisposing factors which play determining role in the pathogenesis of osteomyelitis (Box 10.8).

> **Box 10.8** Predisposing factors of osteomyelitis.
> - Malnutrition and chronic alcoholism
> - Drug addiction
> - Radiotherapy
> - Anemia, especially sickle cell anemia
> - Diabetes (poorly controlled)
> - Acute leukemia
> - Agranulocytosis
> - Syphilis
> - Measles and typhoid fever
> - HIV infection and AIDS
> - Extremes of age
> - Urinary tract infection

Microorganisms Involved in Osteomyelitis

Osteomyelitis due to specific bacterial infections like tuberculous, syphilitic and actinomycotic group of organisms occurs in the jawbones quite often. Osteomyelitis of the jaws due to nonspecific bacterial infections is far more common as compared to the specific types and microorganisms responsible for this type of infections are as follows:
- Aerobic organisms
  - *Staphylococcus aureus*
  - Hemolytic *Streptococcus*
- Anaerobic organisms
  - *Bacteroides*
  - Anaerobic *Streptococcus*

Pathogenesis of Osteomyelitis (Flowchart 10.1)

In osteomyelitis, inflammation and destruction of bone take place by the following mechanisms:
- Infection first reaches the bone marrow first and from there it extends into the cancellous bony spaces.
- The nutrient vessels in the infected area of bone become thrombosed and are occluded with dead or viable neutrophils, microorganisms and necrotic tissue debri, etc.)

Flowchart 10.1: Outline of pathogenesis of osteomyelitis.

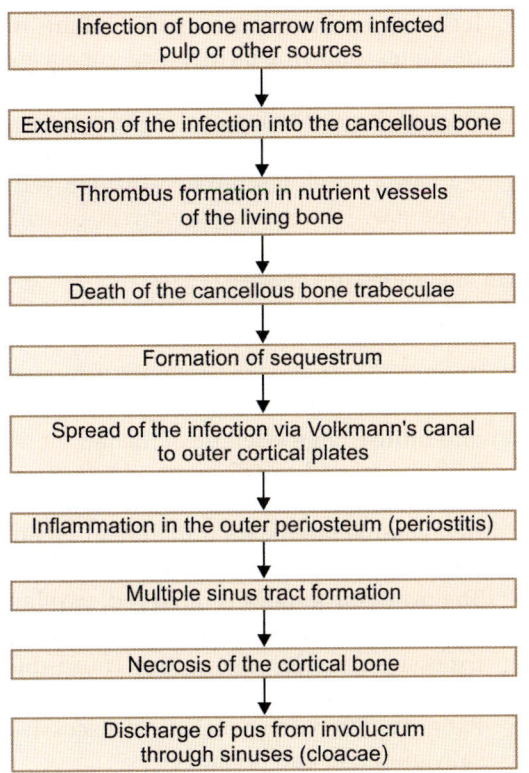

- Due to thrombosis of the nutrient vessels and excessive pressure from the inflammatory exudates against the rigid and confined space in the bone, the *nutrition supply to the bone cells is completely disturbed and it results in the necrosis of cancellous bone.*
- The infection then spreads via the Volkmann's canals in the cortical plates and reaches to the external surface of bone below the periosteum, inflammation at this area results in periostitis.
- As inflammation intensifies on the outer surface of bone, periosteum gets separated from bone due to accumulation of more and more exudates and pus; *the separation of periosteum results in necrosis of the cortical bone (as nutrient supply to the cortical bone mostly comes from the periosteum).*
- Therefore in osteomyelitis, damage of bone takes place from both periosteal as well as endosteal (bone marrow) sides, which cause complete necrosis of bone in the area and results in formation of *"sequestrum"* (dead piece of bone).
- Further extension of the inflammation may lead to single or multiple sinus tracts formation on the overlying skin or mucosa.
- Once the acute phase of the disease is over, repair work begins in the area with formation of new bones by the osteoblast cells still surviving in the damaged periosteum.
- As the repair continues, the dead bone (sequestrum) gets either resolved or is pushed out of the bone.
  However sometimes few small pieces of sequestra may still remain in the area and they get completely covered by newly formed bone; thus the enclosed sequestrum within the new bone is called the *"involucrum".*
- *Cloaca*: it is an opening or hole in the bony cortex connecting with the involucrum and it allows drainage of pus out of the dead bone.
- *Brodie's abscess* is a small localized intraosseous abscess involving the bony cortex, which is surrounded (walled off) by newly formed reactive bone. This abscess may remain as a sterile lesion within the confinement of healthy bone or it may act as future source of infection. In case of chronic non-suppurative osteomyelitis, bone destruction and bone formation take place simultaneously.

Acute Suppurative Osteomyelitis

Acute suppurative osteomyelitis is a serious type of diffusely spreading acute inflammation of the bone, characterized by extensive tissue necrosis.

Clinical Features (Figs. 10.12A and B)

- *Age*: Acute osteomyelitis usually occurs after 30 years of age as there is more probability of systemic diseases from this age and onwards and moreover there is also decreased bony resistance to infection (due to reduced bone vascularity).
- *Sex*: Incidence is more among males than females.
- *Site*: The mandible is involved more often than the maxilla as it has a limited blood supply and it is a dense bone with thicker cortical plates. The mandibular lesions are usually diffuse in nature, while the maxillary lesions are mostly well-localized. Moreover the maxillary lesions are rare and are seen in infants or neonates following birth injuries or severe otitis media, etc.

Bacteriology: *Staphylococci* and *Streptococci* are the organisms, which predominantly cause acute suppurative osteomyelitis of the jaw. However, *Actinomyces israelii*, *Prevotella*, *Porphyromonas* and *Bacteroides* can also cause the disease.

Clinical Presentation

- Acute suppurative osteomyelitis often causes severe throbbing, deep seated pain and diffuse large swelling of the jaw along with the related soft tissues.
- Often there is loosening and soreness of the regional teeth with difficulty in taking food.
- The overlying gingiva is often red, swollen and tendered to palpation.
- Excessive muscle edema may cause difficulty in mouth opening and swallowing.
- Patients often complain of excessive salivation and bad breath, etc.
- Multiple intraoral or extraoral pus discharging sinuses often develop (Fig. 10.13).
- Regional lymph nodes are enlarged and tendered in most cases.

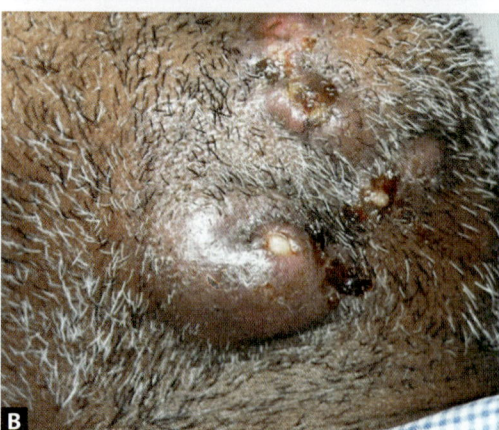

Figs. 10.12A and B: (A) Acute osteomyelitis of the jaws; (B) Acute osteomyelitis of the jaw causing severe infection of overlying soft tissue.

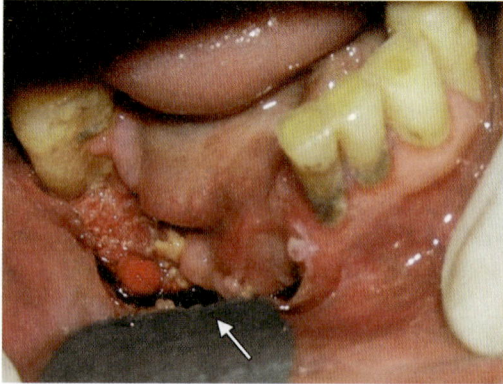

Fig. 10.13: Osteomyelitis mandible with necrosis of bone and overlying soft tissue of mouth

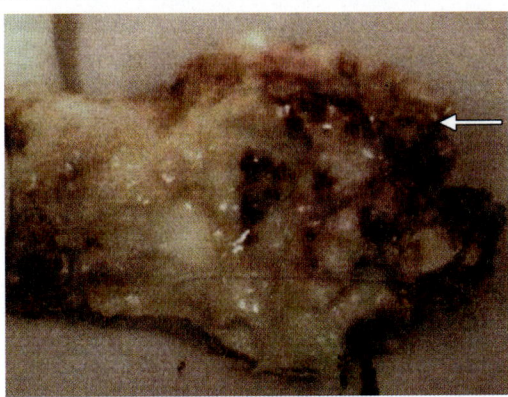

Fig. 10.14: A piece of dead bone (sequestrum).

- Paresthesia or anesthesia of the lip (either on the affected side or the entire lip) is a common and characteristic phenomenon.
- Necrotic bone fragment or sequestrum may exfoliate spontaneously from the bony wound (Fig. 10.14).
- Pathologic fracture may occur sometimes due to weakening of bone as a result of progressive destruction.

Radiological Features (Fig. 10.15)

- In the initial stage of the disease, when bone destruction is yet to occur, no noticeable radiographic change is observed in the jaw.
- At this stage of the disease, a radionucleotide scan may be helpful in documenting the subtle bony changes occurring in the jaw.
- Radiographic changes become more apparent in about 10 days' time since the onset of the disease and these radiographic changes are characterized by large areas of radiolucencies in the jaw bone, with ill-defined, moth-eaten margins.
- Sequestra are frequently seen as multiple radiopaque foci of diminished radiodensity within the lesion.
- The sequestra become more sharply defined as they are gradually separated from the normal bone.
- In the chronic stages of the disease, subperiosteal new bone formation may be seen in the jaw (especially in young patients); and the new bone often appears as thin, curved strip of radiopacity on the outer surface of the bony cortex.
- The involucrum radiographically appears as a gray shadow on the outer surface of the cortical plate.
- "Cloacae" may be seen as dark shadow traversing the bony opacity.

Brodie's abscess appears a localized radiolucent cavity within the cortical bone.

Histopathology

- In acute suppurative osteomyelitis, the bone marrow undergoes liquefaction necrosis and purulent exudates occupy the marrow space.
- Thrombosis of the blood vessels also occurs in the medullary spaces.
- A large number of acute inflammatory cell infiltrations occur in the Haversian canal and the periphery of the bone, which predominantly contains polymorphonuclear neutrophils with occasional presence of lymphocytes and plasma cells.
- Increased osteoclastic resorptions of bone often produces scalloping at the bony margins.

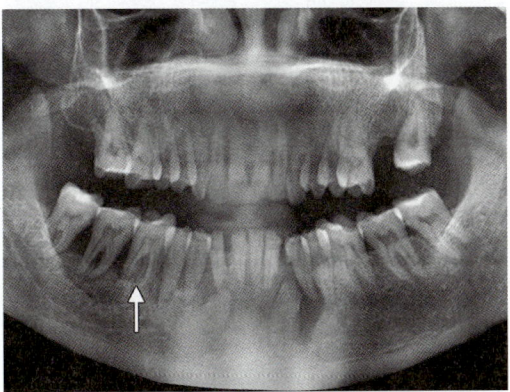

Fig. 10.15: Radiograph of osteomyelitis of right mandible.

- Bacterial colonies are often seen within the marrow tissue of the inflamed bone and sinus tracts may also form in the oral cavity.
- Some areas of the affected bone undergo complete necrosis with degeneration of both osteoblast cells (bordering the bony trabeculae) and osteocyte cells (inside the lacunae) and therefore results in the development of sequestrum (dead piece of bone).
- Sequestrum is separated from the remaining viable bone but is often surrounded by granulation tissue.

Differential Diagnosis
- Metastatic tumor in the bone with secondary infection.
- Primary intra-alveolar carcinoma.
- Primary mesenchymal malignant neoplasm.
- Primary lymphoma of bone.
- Intraosseous salivary gland neoplasm.

Treatment
- Incision and drainage of the inflammatory exudates and pus
- Antibiotic therapy
- Removal of the sequestrum is important without which healing will not occur
- Elimination of the primary source of infection, e.g. offending tooth, etc.

Chronic Suppurative Osteomyelitis

Depending on the severity of symptoms and the course of the disease over the time, suppurative osteomyelitis is divided into two varieties—(1) acute and (2) chronic. The disease, which is persisting for more than a month, is called *chronic suppurative osteomyelitis*.
- Chronic suppurative osteomyelitis may be the sequelae of acute suppurative osteomyelitis, in which proper treatment is either not done or inadequately done.
- The disease may also arise primarily as a chronic, low-grade inflammatory reaction in the bone, without any preexisting acute phase.

Etiology
Nonspecific microorganisms like staphylococci, streptococci, Bacteroides and Actinomyces, etc. mostly cause the disease.

Clinical Features (Figs. 10.16A and B)
- The molar area of mandible is more frequently affected.
- In case of chronic suppurative osteomyelitis, the pain is usually mild and dull vague in nature even if the disease is very extensive.
- Patients often give history of dull vague pain in the jaw for several weeks, which had started following an acute tooth abscess, tooth fracture or extraction, etc.

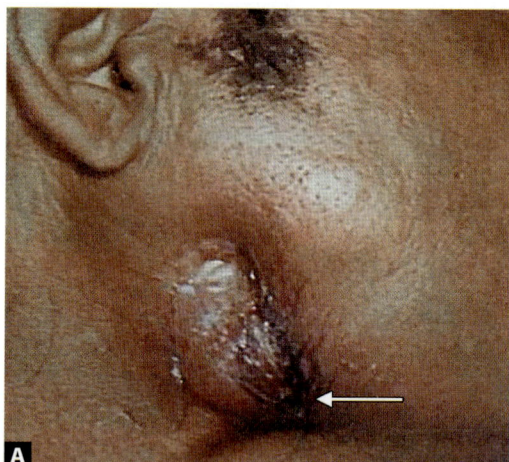

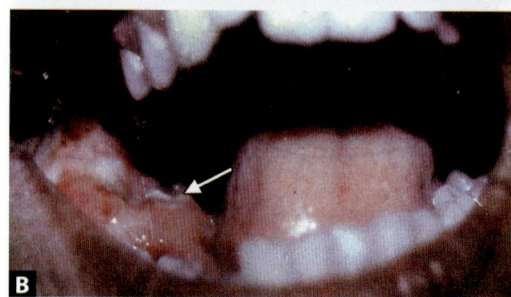

Figs. 10.16A and B: Chronic suppurative osteomyelitis causing formation of extraoral sinus.

- Jaw swelling is a common feature but mobility of teeth and sinus tract formations, etc. are rare.
- On rare occasions sinus tracts may develop both intraorally and extraorally with intermittent discharge of purulent materials.
- Anesthesia and paresthesia of the lip are very uncommon.
- Acute exacerbations of the chronic disease may occur from time to time.
- Sequestrum is often found, which protrudes from the ulcerated skin or mucosal surfaces.

Radiology
- Radiographically chronic suppurative osteomyelitis mostly presents a "moth-eaten" radiolucent area in the bone with poorly defined margins.
- Within the radiolucent area multiple radiopaque foci are evident, which represent areas of "sequestrum" formations.

Chronic osteomyelitis may exhibit at least four different radiographic images, which are as follows:
1. An ill-defined radiolucency in the bone with ragged borders.
2. A radiolucency with multiple radiopaque foci within it, the later structures represent sequestra.
3. A dense zone of radiopacity with faint radiolucency at the margin.
4. A "salt and pepper" radiographic effect in the bone.

Histopathology
Chronic suppurative osteomyelitis often presents the following features:
- Chronic inflammatory reaction in the bone with accumulation of exudates and pus within the medullary spaces.
- The lymphocytes, plasma cells and macrophages, etc. predominate among the inflammatory cells.
- Osteoblastic and osteoclastic activity occur parallel with formation of irregular bony trabeculae having reversal lines.

Treatment
- Administration of antibiotics after bacterial culture and sensitivity testing
- Surgical intervention in order to remove the sequestrum (saucerization of the bone).

Chronic Focal Sclerosing Osteomyelitis (Condensing Osteitis)

Definition
Chronic focal sclerosing osteomyelitis or condensing osteitis is a rare nonsuppurative inflammatory condition of bone characterized by sclerotic bone formation around the root apex of a nonvital tooth.

Pathogenesis
The condition develops as a result of chronic persistent inflammation in the bone, where resistance of the tissue against infection is very high or where the virulence of the infective organisms is low.

A low-grade inflammation in the jaw bone causes stimulation of the osteoblast cells, which results in the formation of dense trabecular bone in the area and this process is known as *osteosclerosis*.

Osteosclerosis with additional bone formation may sometimes results in decreased marrow spaces.

Etiology
The common conditions, which can precipitate chronic focal sclerosing osteomyelitis, include the following:
- Chronic pulpitis
- Traumatic malocclusion.

Clinical Features
- The disease frequently develops in children or young adults before the age of 20 years.

- Mandibular first molars are mostly involved with this condition. However, mandibular second molars or premolars can also be involved on rare occasions.
- The condition is mostly asymptomatic and there is no bony expansion seen.
- Majority of the lesions are discovered incidentally during routine radiographic examination of the jawbone.
- The associated tooth is nonvital and usually presents a large carious lesion, it is mostly asymptomatic or is associated with occasional mild pain.
- The disease can also occur in relation to a noncarious tooth and in such cases, traumatic malocclusion is the most likely factor.
- When the associated tooth is removed, the lesion may remain within the jaw for an indefinite to period of time without symptoms.

Radiological Features

The lesion radiographically presents the following features (Fig. 10.17):
- Well-circumscribed radiopaque mass with uniform radiodensity; seen around the root apex of a nonvital tooth.
- There is no radiolucent border around the lesion as may be seen in cemento-osseous dysplasia.
- The affected tooth exhibits an apical inflammatory process with widening of periodontal ligament space.
- The radiopacity is not separated from the root apex and the root tips are usually identified within the radiopaque lesion.
- A residual area of condensing osteitis that is seen after resolution of the inflammatory focus is known as "bone scar".
- The radiodensity of the lesion is much higher as compared to the surrounding normal bone.

Histological Features
- There is usually presence of a dense mass of sclerotic bone in the lesion with little or no interstitial marrow tissue.
- Wherever the bone marrow is present it is usually fibrotic and is often infiltrated by chronic inflammatory cells.

Differential Diagnosis
- Mature cementoma
- Osteoma
- Complex odontoma
- Cementoblastoma
- Osteoblastoma
- Metastatic tumor.

Treatment
- The affected tooth should be treated endodontically or it should be removed.
- No treatment required for the bony lesion.

Diffuse Sclerosing Osteomyelitis

Definition

Diffuse sclerosing osteomyelitis is a different entity which is mainly confined to the mandible and it typically involves a large section of the bone.

Etiology

Diffuse sclerosing osteomyelitis is a proliferative reaction in response to a low-grade inflammation or infection in the jaw bone.

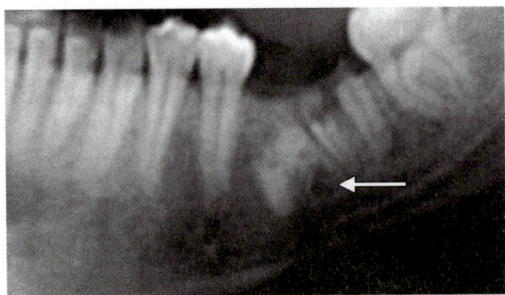

Fig. 10.17: Chronic focal sclerosing osteomyelitis.

The infections in such cases are usually wide spread or diffuse in nature and are derived either from the periodontal tissue or from the periapical tissue.

Low grade, sustained and subclinical infection caused by *Propionibacterium acnes* and *Peptostreptococcus intermedium* may cause this disease.

Clinical Features

- Diffuse sclerosing osteomyelitis is usually seen among elderly people.
- It is mostly seen among blacks and racial groups.
- More common among females.
- Mandible is mostly affected in diffuse sclerosing osteomyelitis especially in edentulous areas (Fig. 10.18). The disease can affect the maxilla as well and even sometimes all four quadrants of both jaw could be affected at a time.
- It is usually asymptomatic but sometimes the patients may complain of a vague pain in the jaw with foul taste in the mouth.
- *SAPHO syndrome*: It is a special entity characterized by chronic multifocal osteomyelitis with hyperostosis and osteitis of the bone. The condition is associated with negative bacterial culture and is nonresponsive to antibiotic therapy.

Radiographic Features

- Radiograph in diffuse sclerosing osteomyelitis shows areas of diffuse or nodular sclerosis of the bone (Fig. 10.19).
- The appearance may be similar to the "cotton-wool" radiopacities seen in Paget's disease of bone.
- The border between the sclerotic bone and the normal bone is not well-demarcated.

Histopathology

- Diffuse sclerosing osteomyelitis shows formation of dense irregular bone within a hypocellular fibrous stroma (Fig. 10.12)
- Bony trabeculae often reveal multiple reversal and resting lines.
- Patchy distribution of chronic inflammatory cells is often found in the marrow tissue.

Differential Diagnosis

- Paget's disease of bone
- Osteopetrosis
- Cementomas
- Gardner's syndrome
- Late stage of fibrous dysplasia.

Treatment

No treatment is required as the disease is often asymptomatic and is too extensive for surgical removal. In case of acute exacerbations, surgical debridement and

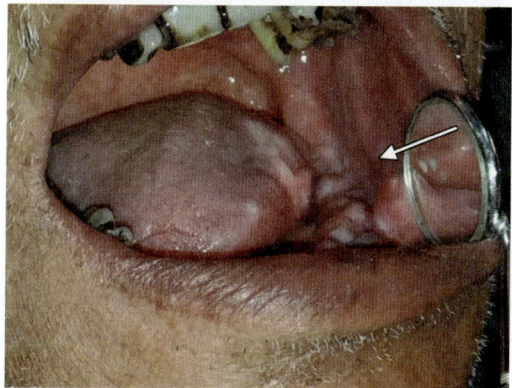

Fig. 10.18: Diffuse sclerosing osteomyelitis involving left mandible.

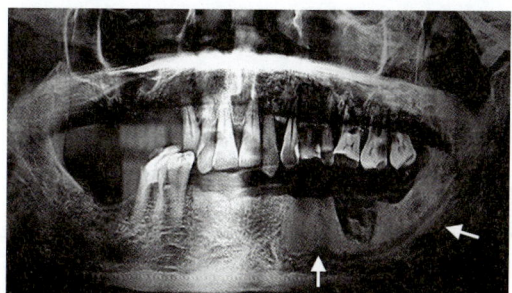

Fig. 10.19: Diffuse sclerosing osteomyelitis showing large area of sclerotic bone and a sequestrum on the left side of mandible.

removal of the sequestrum is done along with antibiotic therapy.

Chronic Osteomyelitis with Proliferative Periostitis (Garre's Osteomyelitis)

Definition
Garre's osteomyelitis mainly involves the periosteum and exhibits reactive periosteal osteogenesis in response to low-grade infection or trauma. The condition was first authentically reported in 1893 by German physician C Garre and it is characterized by focal gross thickening of the involved bone due to subperiosteal new bone deposition (duplication of the cortex). The predisposing factors for the development of Garre's osteomyelitis are given.

Pathogenesis
It is usually believed that a low-grade, sustained infection of the jaw bone, occurring in a young person with high degree of body resistance and excellent tissue reactivity, may often precipitate Garre's osteomyelitis.

All the above mentioned factors contribute to a strong osteogenic potential of the periosteal osteoblast cells in the affected jaw bone.

Generally in Garre's osteomyelitis, a low-grade chronic inflammation spreads through the cortical bone of the jaw and it initiates a proliferative reaction in the periosteum, leading to subperiosteal new bone formations.

It is important to note that an acute and intense type of inflammation or infection in the jaw bone usually does not produce Garre's osteomyelitis, since this type of infection does not permit sufficient time for the bone to undergo any subperiosteal osteogenesis.

Clinical Features
- *Age*: Children and young adults (mean age is 13 years).
- *Sex*: There is no sex predilection.
- *Site*: Mandible is commonly involved in Garre's osteomyelitis in its posterior part. Maxilla can be affected on rare occasion.

Clinical Presentations (Fig. 10.20)
- The involved jaw bone often presents a grossly carious, nonvital tooth (mostly lower first permanent molar tooth).
- The tooth is always associated with periapical or sometimes other inflammatory foci.
- There is thickening and swelling of the affected bone with little or no pain.
- The size of the swelling may be ranging from centimeters to a lesion spanning the entire length of the mandible (Box 10.9).
- The thickness of the bone may be up to 1 cm.
- Occasionally slight tenderness or a vague pain may be felt in the affected area of bone.
- The overlying skin and oral mucosa appears normal.
- Garre's osteomyelitis is generally a solitary lesion, however multifocal lesions are also sometimes reported.
- Slight pyrexia and moderate leukocytosis may be present but the erythrocyte sedimentation rate (ESR) is normal.

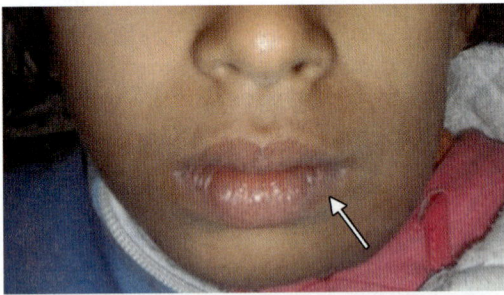

Fig. 10.20: Garre's osteomyelitis of mandible.

Box 10.9	Common diseases associated with periosteal new bone formation in the jaw.

- Osteomyelitis
- Trauma
- Cyst
- Malignancy, e.g. osteosarcoma and chondrosarcoma
- Fracture of bone

Radiographic Appearance
- Garre's osteomyelitis radiographically presents a central jaw lesion with a mottled, predominantly radiolucent appearance, the lesion often has few radiopaque foci (Fig. 10.21).
- The affected periosteum forms several layers of reactive vital bone and as a result the expanded cortex of bone radiographically exhibits many concentric or parallel opaque layers, which often produce a typical "onion skin" appearance.
- The standard occlusal radiograph reveals a smooth, convex, bony overgrowth on the outer cortex of the jaw. This is often called *"duplication" of the cortex*.
- Few newly formed bony trabeculae are often oriented perpendicular to the "onion skin" layers.

Histopathology
- The lesion histologically presents areas of newly formed bone, consisting of multiple osteoids and primitive bony tissues in the subperiosteal region.
- The bony trabeculae are arranged in linear parallel rows with presence of highly cellular intervening connective tissue.
- Osteoblastic activity dominates the outer surface of bone while both osteoblastic as well as osteoclastic activities can be observed in the central part of bone.

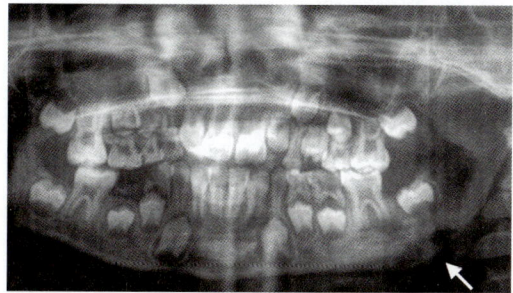

Fig. 10.21: Radiograph showing Garre's osteomyelitis of mandible (left 1st molar area) with "duplication of cortex".

- The marrow spaces contain fibrous tissue showing patchy areas of chronic inflammatory cell infiltration.
- On rare occasions there may be presence of small sequestra.

Differential Diagnosis
- Ossifying fibroma
- Immature fibrous dysplasia
- Ewing's sarcoma
- Osteoblastic osteosarcoma
- Metastatic tumor of the jaw bone
- Pulse granuloma.

Treatment
- Elimination of the causative agent.
- Extraction of the offending tooth and antibiotic therapy.
- The cortical swelling undergoes spontaneous physiologic remodeling and does not required any additional surgical intervention.

Giant Cell Periostitis with Hyaline Change (Pulse Granuloma)

Definition
A large variety of foreign materials can be implanted into the oral tissues, some of which can initiate a granulomatous reaction. Such reactions are characterized by chronic inflammation and subsequent formation of a ring-shaped hyaline eosinophilic structure in the tissue and few giant cells.

The term "pulse granuloma" has been coined since vegetable materials especially pulses are believed to cause this disease more often than others. The disease occurs when the vegetable material is introduced into the oral tissue via extraction socket or surgical flaps or open root canals, or through ulceration in the oral mucosa.

Clinical Features
- Clinically the lesion is either dome-shaped or multinodular and it is usually soft or firm in consistency.

- Mucobuccal fold is the most common site for the development of pulse granuloma and often there is thickening of the periosteum due to proliferative periostitis.
- Pain is not a prominent feature

Histopathology

- Fibrosis in the submucosa with presence of granulation tissue showing few inflammatory cells.
- Multiple ring-like hyaline structures are found, which are enclosing connective tissue including blood vessels.
- Pulse granuloma produces multiple compartmentalized spaces containing giant cells.
- Oil-granuloma produces many empty vacuoles.

Treatment

Local excision is the treatment of choice.

ENDODONTIC-PERIODONTIC LESIONS

Sometimes infections of the pulpal origin may spread into the periodontal tissue and likewise the periodontal infections may also sometimes spread to involve the dental pulp secondarily. Therefore, a possibility is always there for the development of a combined endodontic-periodontic lesion, which is facilitated by two important factors.

1. Dynamic nature of both pulpal and periodontal diseases.
2. Communication between pulp and periodontium via accessory canals or the apical foramen.

BIBLIOGRAPHY

1. Ackerman F, Klein JP, Franx RM. Ultrastructural localization of *Streptococcus mutans* and *Streptococcus mutans*, sanguis antigens in carious (Buccale) human dentine. J Biol Buccale. 1981;9:203-17.
2. Adarms D. The granulomatous inflammatory response. Am J Pathol. 1976;84:164.
3. Aison EL. Osteomyelitis of the jaw. J Am Dent Assoc. 1938;25:1261.
4. Allison TR. Electron microscopic study of "Rushton" hyaline bodies in cyst linings. Brit Dent J.1974;137:102.
5. Andreasen JO. Traumatic injuries of the teeth, 2nd edition. Copenhagen: Munksgaard; 1983.
6. Barker BC, Ehrmann EH. Human pulp reactions to glucocorticosteroid-antibiotic compound. Aust Dent J. 1969;14:104-19.
7. Baumgartener JC, Falker WA Jr. Bacteria in the apical 5 mm of infected root canals. Endodont. 1991;17:380.
8. Bell WH. Sclerosing osteomyelitis of the mandible and maxilla. Oral Surg. 1959;12: 391.
9. Blair VP, Brown JB, Moore S. Osteomyelitis of the jaws. Int J Orthod. 1931;17:168.
10. Boalger EA. Histologic study of a hypertrophied pulp. J Dent Res. 1931;11:256.
11. Boling LR, Robinson HB. Vascular changes in inflamed dental pulp. J Dent Res. 1938; 17:310.
12. Bourgoyne JR, Quinn JH. The periapical abscess. J Oral Surg. 1949;7:320.
13. Brunnstrom M, Astrom A. The hydrodynamics of the dentin, its possible relationship to dental pain. IntDent J. 1972;2:219-27.
14. Brunnstrom M, Lind PO. Pulpal response to early dental caries. J Dent Res. 1965;44: 1045-50.
15. Brook I, Frazier E, Gtter M. Aerobic and anaerobic microbiology of periapical abscess. Oral MicrobiolImmunol. 1991;6:123-5.
16. Cameron CE. Cracked tooth syndrome. J Am Dent Assoc. 1964;68:405-11.
17. Cawson RA, Odell EW. Essentials of oral pathology and oral medicine, 6th edition. Edinburgh: Churchill Livingstone; 1998.
18. Cawson RA. Essentials of dental surgery and pathology, 4th edition. Edinburgh: Churchill Livingstone; 1984.
19. Cecic P, Hartwell G, Belli R. Cold as diagnostic aid in cases of irreversible pulpitis. Oral Surg Oral Med Oral Pathol. 1983;56:647-50.
20. Cohen S, Burns RC. Pathways of the pulp, 4th edition. St. Louis: CV Mosby; 1987.
21. Cvek M. A clinical report on partial pulpotomy and capping with calcium hydroxide in permanent incisors with complicated gawn fracture. J Endodont. 1978;4:232-7.

22. Dachi SF. The relationship of pulpitis and hyperemia to thermal sensitivity. Oral Surg. 1965;19:776.
23. Daramola J, Ajagbe H. Chronic osteomyelitis of the mandible in adults a clinical study of 34 cases. Br J Oral Surg. 1982;20:58-62.
24. Dunlap CL, Barker BF. Giant cell hyaline angiopathy. Oral Surg. 1977;44:587.
25. Ehrmann EH. Pulp testers and pulp testing with particular represented to the use of dry ice. Aust Dent J. 1977;22:272-9.
26. Eisenbud L, Miler J, Roberts J. Garre's proliferative periostitis occurring simultaneously in four quadrants of the jaws. Oral Surg. 1981;51:172-8.
27. El-Labban NG, Kramer RH. The nature of the hyaline rings in chronic periostitis and other conditions-an ultrastructural study. Oral Surg. 1981;51:509.
28. Eversole L, Stone C, Strub D. Focal sclerosing osteomyelitis/focal periapical osteomyelitis. Radiographic patterns. Oral Surg. 1984;58: 456-60.
29. Eversole LR, Leider AC, Crowin JO, et al. Proliferative periostitis of Garre: its differentiation for other neoperiostoses. J Oral Surg. 1979;3:725.
30. Fabe SS. Acute hematogenous osteomyelitis of the mandible. Oral Surg Oral Med Oral Pathol. 1950;3(1):22-6.
31. Guo X, Niu Z, Xiao M, et al. Detection of interleukin-8 in exudates from normal and inflamed human dental pulp tissues Int Endod J. 2000;33(2):132.
32. Hahn C, Falkler W, Minah G. Microbiological studies of carious dentin for human teeth with irreversible pulpitis. Arch Oral Biol. 1991;36:147-53.
33. Harsis R, Griffin CJ. Histogenesis of the fibroblasts in the human dental pulp. Arch Oral Biol. 1967;12:459.
34. Hymn J, Cohen M. The predictive value of the endodontic diagnostic tests. Oral Surg. 1984;58:343-6.
35. Iwu C, MacFarlane TW, MacKenzie D, et al. The microbiology of periapical granulomas. Oral Surg Oral Med Oral Pathol. 1990;69:502-5.
36. Jack Obsen I, Kerekes K. Long-term prognosis of traumatized permanent anterior teeth showing calcifying process in the pulp cavity. Scand J Dent Res. 1977;85:588-98.
37. Jack Obsen S, Hollender L. Treatment and prognosis of diffuse sclerosing osteomyelitis (DSO) of the mandible. Oral Surg. 1980;49:7-14.
38. Kim S. Neurovascular interactions in the dental pulp in health and inflammation. J Endo. 1990;16:48-58.
39. Lichty G, Langlais RP, Aufdemorte T. Garre's osteomyelitis. Oral Surg. 1980;50:309.
40. Mathiesen A. Prevention and demonstration of mast cells in human apical granuloma and radicular cysts. Scand J Dent Res. 1973;81: 218.
41. McMillan MD, Kardos TB, Edwards JL, et al. Giant cell hyaline angiopathy or pulse granuloma. Oral Surg. 1981;52:178.
42. Mincer HH, McCoy JM, Turner JE. Pulse granuloma of the alveolar ridge. Oral Surg. 1979;48:126.
43. Neville BW, Damm DD, Allen CA, et al. Oral and Maxillofacial Pathology, 2nd edition, Saunders (an imprint of Elsevier): Philadelphia; 2002.
44. Ohnishi T, Suwa M, Oyama T, et al. Prostaglandin E2 predominantly induces production of hepatocyte growth factor/scatter factor in human dental pulp in acute inflammation. J Dent Res. 2000;79(2):748.
45. Orban B, Ritehery BT. Toothache under conditions simulating high altitude flight. J Am Dent Assoc. 1945;32:145.
46. Robertson PB, Luscher B, Spangberg LS, et al. Pulpal and periodontal effects of electrosurgery involving cervical metallic restoration. Oral Surg. 1978;46:702.
47. Robinson HB, Boling LR. Diagnosis and pathology of anachoretic pulpitis I. Bacteriologic Studies. J Am Dent Assoc. 1941;28:268.
48. Russell W. An address on a characteristic organism of cancer. Brit Med J. 1980;2:1356.
49. Shafer WG. Chronic sclerosing osteomyelitis. J Oral Surg. 1957;15:138.
50. Shear M. Cysts of the oral regions, 3rd edition. Oxford, London: Wright (an imprint of Butterworth-Heinemann Ltd.); 1996.
51. Soames JV, Southam JC. Oral pathology,3rd edition. London: Oxford University Press; 1999.
52. Stanley HR. The cells of the dental pulp. Oral Surg. 1962;15:849.

53. Stanley HR. The effect of systemic diseases on the human pulp. Oral Surg Oral Med Oral Pathol. 1972;33(4):606-48.
54. Stern MH, Dreizen S, Mackler BF, et al. Antibody-producing cells in human periapical granulomas and cysts. J Endod. 1981;7:447.
55. Stern MH, Dreizen S, Mackler BF, et al. Quantitative analysis of cellular composition of human periapical granuloma. J Endod. 1981;7:117.
56. Torabinejad M, Bakland LK. Immunopathogenesis of chronic periapical lesions. Oral Surg. 1978;46:685.
57. Trowbridge HO, Kim S. Pulp structure and function. In: Cohen S, Burns R (Eds). Pathways of the pulp, 4th edition. St Louis: CV Mosby; 1987.
58. Waldron CA, Giansanti JS, Browand BC. Sclerotic cemental masses of the jaws (so-called chronic sclerosing osteomyelitis, sclerosingosteitis, multiple enostosis, and gigantiformcementoma). Oral Surg. 1975;39:590.
59. Weber DF. Human dentin sclerosis: a microradiographic survey. Arch Oral Biol. 1974;19:163.
60. Weine FS. Endodontic therapy, 2nd edition. St Louis: CV Mosby Company; 1976.

CHAPTER 11

Spread of the Oral Infection

INTRODUCTION

An infective process involving the tooth and its supporting structures is known as odontogenic infections.

In the oral cavity, a large number of such odontogenic infective lesions are often encountered, which originate either from the gingival tissue or from the periapical sites.

Infections from the gingival tissue often involve the deeper periodontal ligaments and the supporting alveolar bone and they may even progress to the periapical region of tooth.

In most instances of periapical infections, the microorganisms are derived from the necrosed dental pulp as a sequel of dental caries.

Common odontogenic infections in the oral cavity:

- Pericoronitis
- Periodontal abscess
- Periapical abscess
- Subperiosteal abscess
- Osteomyelitis.

Once the odontogenic infections reach the bone or muscle or mucosa or lymph nodes, etc. they may either resolve spontaneously or spread to the local or the distant sites.

IMPORTANT FACTORS FOR ODONTOGENIC INFECTIONS (BOX 11.1)

Factors Relating to Organisms

Some organisms producing odontogenic infections are more virulent than others, moreover, a few organisms, e.g. Group A streptococci can produce enzymes like hyaluronidase and fibrinolysins, etc. which help in the diffuse spread of infection into distant areas by breaking down tissue barriers.

Box 11.1	Factors determining spread of oral infections to distant sites.

- Virulence of the microorganisms
- Immunity of the host
- Anatomical site of the initial infection

Factors Relating to the Host

If the host or the patient has a high degree of body immunity or resistance power, the distant spread of infection from the oral cavity is less likely to occur and vice versa.

Factors Relating to the Site of Infection

The site of initial infection also determines whether it will remain localized or will make a distant spread.

The thinner cortical plates of bone or loose tissue spaces around the wound may offer little resistance to the spread of infection, therefore, infections from such areas may often spread diffusely.

However, thicker cortical plates of bone and tough tissue sites (e.g. areas of muscle attachments) may actually prevent the distant spread of infection.

SPACE INFECTIONS

Odontogenic infections often spread through natural pathways into potential tissue spaces situated between different planes of fascia.

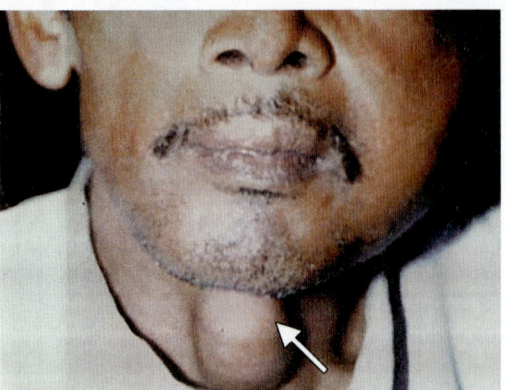

Fig. 11.1: Space infection spreading into the neck.

Infections into the various tissue spaces are known as the "space infections". Such infections in the vicinity of the jaw bones can be divided into two broad groups, namely, those related to the maxilla and those related to the mandible (Fig. 11.1)

SPACE INFECTIONS RELATED TO MAXILLA

Canine Fossa Infection

Source of Infection

Maxillary canine tooth.

Clinical Features

- Pain and tenderness over infraorbital region, fever.
- Submandibular lymphadenopathy.

Treatment

Treatment of offending tooth and antibiotics.

Palatal Space Infection

Source of Infection

Maxillary lateral incisors and infection via palatal roots of maxillary molars.

Clinical Features

Pain and an extremely tendered swelling over the palate.

Treatment

Antibiotic therapy and treatment of the involved tooth.

Infratemporal Space Infection

Boundary: Infratemporal space is bordered by the following structures:
- *Anteriorly*: Maxillary tuberosity
- *Posteriorly*: Lateral pterygoid muscle, condyle of the mandible, temporalis muscle
- *Laterally*: Tendon of the temporalis muscle, coronoid process of mandible
- *Medially*: Lateral pterygoid plate, inferior belly of the lateral pterygoid muscle.

Contents of Infratemporal Space
- Pterygoid plexus, internal maxillary artery
- Mandibular, myelohyoid, lingual, buccinator and chorda tympani nerves
- External pterygoid muscle

Source of Infection
- Infected maxillary molar teeth
- Infected needles or solution used for injection of the maxillary tuberosity.

Clinical Features
- Trismus and pain
- Swelling of the eyelids when postzygomatic fossa is involved
- Dysphagia due to involvement of pharynx
- Swelling in the preauricular region, which may extend up to the cheek.

Treatment

Surgical drainage, antibiotics and treatment of the involved tooth.

Pterygomandibular Space Infection

Pterygomandibular space is the inferior portion of the infratemporal space.

Boundary: The space lies between the internal pterygoid muscle and the ramus of the mandible.

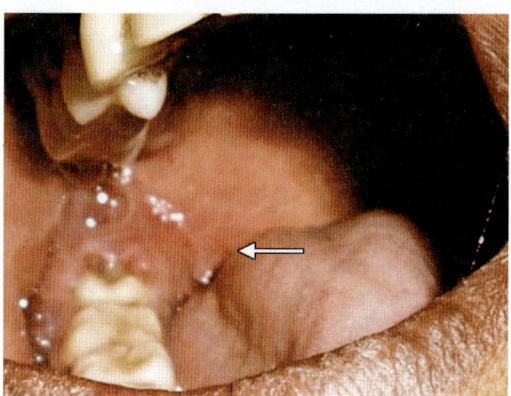

Fig. 11.2: Pericoronitis, a common cause of space infections.

Sources of Infection
- Pericoronitis of mandibular third molar tooth
- Infected needles or injection into the space.

Clinical Features
- Severe trismus
- Radiating pain
- Swelling of the lateral-posterior region of soft palate may be seen (Fig. 11.2).

Treatment
Surgical drainage, antibiotics and treatment of the infected 3rd molar.

Temporal Pouch Infection

Source of Infection
Secondary infections from the submasseteric, pterygopalatine and infratemporal spaces. Maxillary molars are the common offending teeth.

Clinical Features
- Pain and trismus
- Swelling may be an occasional feature.

Treatment
Surgical drainage, antibiotics and treatment of the involved tooth.

Parotid Space Infection

Parotid space is a compartment formed by splitting of the investing layer of deep cervical fascia.

Contents
- Parotid glands and extra- and intraglandular lymph nodes
- Facial nerve, auriculotemporal nerve and posterior facial vein
- External carotid, internal maxillary and superficial temporal arteries.

Source of Infection
Secondary infections from lateral pharyngeal and submasseteric spaces.

Clinical Features
- A smooth, painful swelling in front and below the external ear.
- Fever, chills, etc.
- Sometimes, the entire side of the face may be swollen.

Treatment
Surgical drainage, antibiotics and treatment of the offending tooth.

SPACE INFECTIONS RELATED TO MANDIBLE

Mental Space Infections

Source of Infection
Mandibular anterior teeth.

Clinical Features
- A tense painful swelling in the chin region.
- This kind of swelling can also occur in the localized nonodontogenic infections.

Treatment
Surgical drainage, antibiotics and treatment of the offending tooth.

Submental Space Infection

Boundary: Anteriorly the midline of mandible, posteriorly the anterior border of the submaxillary space and inferiorly by the myelohyoid muscle.

Source of Infection
Mandibular anterior teeth.

Clinical Features
- Painful swelling in the submental area.
- Occasionally dyspnea and dysphagia.

Treatment
- Antibiotic therapy and treatment of the offending tooth.

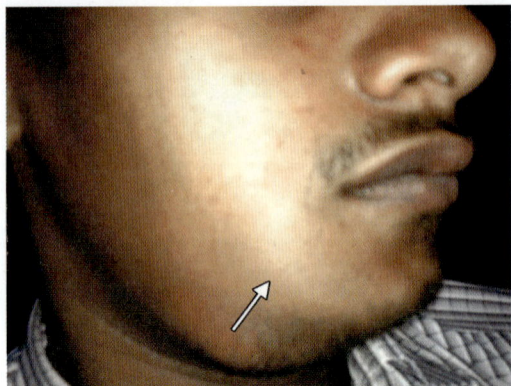

Fig. 11.3: Acute submandibular space infection.

Submandibular Space Infection

Boundary: Submandibular or submaxillary space is bordered by the following structures:
- *Medially*: Hyoglossus and digastric muscles
- *Laterally*: Superficial fascia and skin
- *Superiorly*: Posterior portion of hyoglossus muscle.

Contents
Submandibular salivary gland and lymph nodes.

Source of Infection
Infected mandibular molars.

Clinical Features
- Submandibular space infection is the most common of all space infections in the orofacial region (Figs. 11.3 and 11.4).
- Fever, chill and anorexia.
- Pain with swelling near the angle of the mandible.
- Submandibular lymphadenitis and submandibular sialadenitis.
- Infections from the submandibular space may extend to the sublingual and submental spaces, and rarely to the lateral pharyngeal spaces.
- Involvement of the pharynx and the larynx may cause dyspnea and dysphagia.

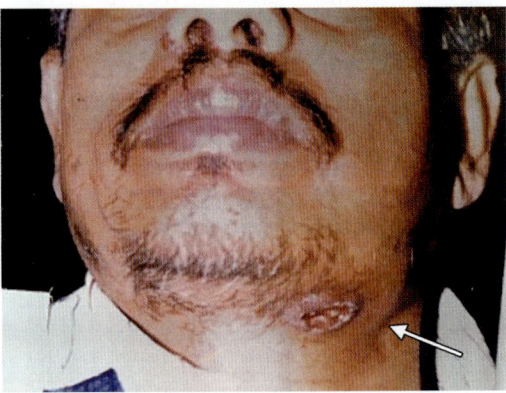

Fig. 11.4: Submandibular space infection with extraoral sinus.

- Distant spread of infection into the cranial fossa or of the mediastinum.

Treatment
- Surgical drainage, antibiotics, treatment of the offending tooth
- Tracheotomy may be required in cases of airway obstruction.

Sublingual Space Infection

Boundary: Sublingual space is situated above the submandibular space and it is bordered by the following structures:
- *Superiorly*: Mucosa of the floor of the mouth.
- *Inferiorly*: Mylohyoid muscle.
- *Anterolaterally*: Body of the mandible.

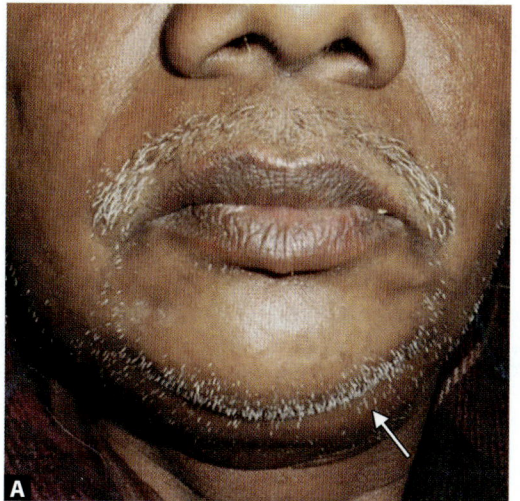 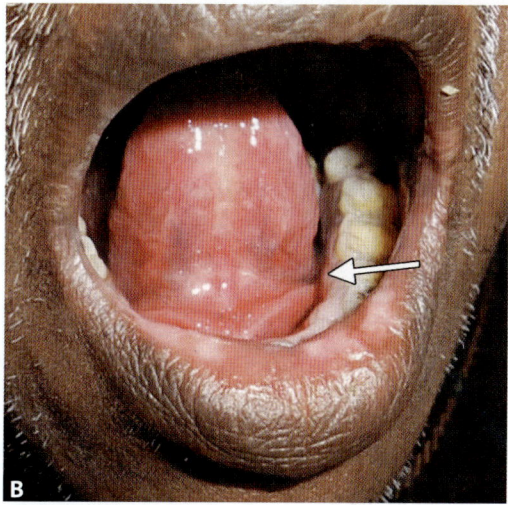

Figs. 11.5A and B: Sublingual space infection.

- *Posteriorly*: Hyoid bone.
- *Medially*: Median raphae of the tongue.

Source of Infection
- Mandibular teeth except second and third molars.
- Sublingual infections may be transported from the submandibular space.

Clinical Features
- Swelling of the floor of the mouth
- Airway obstructions in severe cases
- Dysphagia
- Infections can spread to involve the tongue (Figs. 11.5A and B).

Treatment
Surgical drainage, antibiotics and treatment of the involved tooth.

Lateral Pharyngeal Space Infection

Lateral pharyngeal or parapharyngeal space is situated deep in the neck and infection of this space often terminates fatally.

Boundary: It is bordered by the following structures:
- *Anteriorly*: Buccopharyngeal aponeurosis, parotid gland and pterygoid muscles
- *Posteriorly*: Prevertebral fascia
- *Laterally*: Carotid sheath
- *Medially*: Lateral wall of the pharynx.

Source of Infection
- Mandibular third molar.
- Infection of the palatine tonsils, mastoid air cells and parotid glands.
- Infection may also come from the retromandibular space.

Clinical Features
- Pain, trismus with fever and chill
- Dysphagia and dyspnea due to involvement of the pharynx and larynx
- Infection from lateral pharyngeal space may spread to the mediastinum via the prevertebral fascia.

Complications
- Septicemia
- Respiratory paralysis
- Thrombosis of the internal jugular vein
- Erosions of the internal carotid artery.

Treatment
- Surgical drainage, antibiotics and treatment of the involved tooth.
- Maintenance of airway patency.

Retropharyngeal Space Infection

Boundary: It is bordered by the following structures:
- *Anteriorly*: Wall of the pharynx.
- *Posteriorly*: Prevertebral fascia.
- *Laterally*: Lateral pharyngeal space and carotid sheath.

Source of Infection
Lateral pharyngeal space.

Clinical Features
- Pain, swelling and dysphagia, etc.
- Retropharyngeal space infection may spread to the mediastinum as the prevertebral fascia extends to the posterior mediastinum.

Infection of the Space of Body of Mandible

Boundary: A natural tissue space exists around the body of the mandible as it is enclosed by a layer of fascia derived from the outer layer of deep cervical fascia.
- *Inferiorly*: The fascia attaches on the inferior border of mandible and then covers its body from both buccal and lingual side.
- *Superiorly*: It becomes continuous with the alveolar periosteum and muscles of the facial expression having attachment to the mandible.

Contents
- Body of mandible excluding the ramus, along with the covering periosteum
- Fascia and muscle attachments
- Teeth and periodontium.

Source of Infection
- Mandibular teeth, periodontal pocket, fractured mandible
- Blood-borne infections
- Extension of infection from neighboring tissue spaces.

Clinical Features
- The odontogenic infections perforate either buccal or the lingual cortical plates of mandible and spread to the mandibular body space.
- The clinical manifestation varies and it depends upon factors like the source of infection, which cortical plate (buccal or lingual) has been perforated and at what level of the bone.
- If infections from incisors, cuspids and bicuspids are spreading into the space by perforating the buccal cortical plate, an induration, swelling and fluctuation of the labial sulcus will be observed.
- When infections from the same sources are perforating the lingual cortical plate, swelling of the floor of the mouth will occur.
- Infections from mandibular molar teeth when perforate the buccal cortical plate above the attachment of buccinator muscle, a swelling of the oral vestibule is seen.
- If buccal perforation takes place below the level of attachment of buccinator muscle, a swelling of the covering skin over mandible is noticed.
- When infections of mandibular molars and premolars perforate the lingual cortical plate of bone above the level of attachment of the mylohyoid muscle, swelling of the floor of the mouth occurs.
- If lingual perforation occurs below the myelohyoid attachment, the infection spreads either into the submandibular space or into the lateral pharyngeal space.

Treatment
Surgical drainage, antibiotics and treatment of the involved tooth.

Submasseteric Space Infection

Boundary: Submasseteric space is bordered by the following structures:
- *Medially*: Lateral surface of the mandibular ramus.

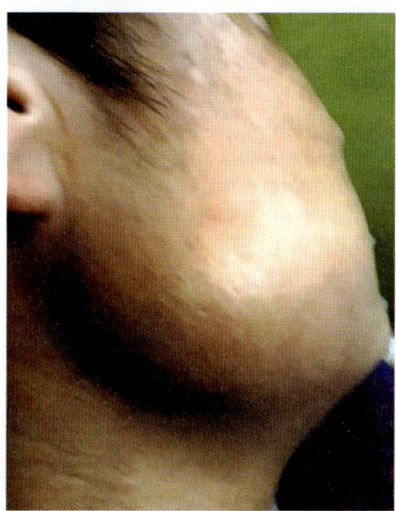

Fig. 11.6: Submasseteric space infection.

- *Laterally*: Masseter muscle.
- *Anteriorly*: Retromolar fossa.
- *Posteriorly*: Parotid gland.

Source of Infection
- Mandibular 3rd molars
- Infection from this tooth passes through the retromolar fossa and moves into the submasseteric space.

Clinical Features
- Pain and swelling due to subperiosteal abscess formation (Fig. 11.6)
- Trismus.

Treatment

Surgical drainage, antibiotics and treatment of the involved tooth.

The sequelae of odontogenic infections are given in Box 11.2.

Box 11.2	Sequelae of odontogenic infections.
• Localized abscess formation • Acute cellulitis • Space infections • Ludwig's angina • Cavernous sinus thrombosis • Bacteremia, septicemia, toxemia and pyemia	

CELLULITIS

DEFINITION

Cellulitis is an acute edematous, purulent inflammatory process, which spreads diffusely through different tissue spaces or fascial planes.

PATHOGENESIS

- Acute cellulitis is mostly caused by some unusually virulent bacteria, which often produce hyaluronidase and fibrinolysins, etc, (mostly released by Group A streptococci).
- Hyaluronidase and fibrinolysins cause help the infective process to spread diffusely into tissue spaces.
- Diminished body immunity, bacterial resistance to antibiotics, favorable anatomic locations, etc. also help in the process development of cellulitis.
- Microorganisms such as *Streptococcus pyogenes* and anaerobes, particularly bacteroides most commonly produce facial cellulitis.
- In acute cellulitis, infection from the lower anterior teeth perforates the lingual cortical plate of bone and moves into the superficial sublingual space, and from there tracks backward.
- Infection from lower molar teeth, after penetrating the lingual cortical plate spread either to the sublingual and submandibular space or into the parapharyngeal spaces.

CLINICAL FEATURES

Cellulitis clinically presents the following features (Table 11.1):
- Development of a large, diffuse, painful swelling over the face or neck with facial asymmetry.
- The soft tissue swelling is usually firm and brawny.
- When cellulitis involves the superficial tissue spaces, the overlying skin becomes warm and purplish-red.

Table 11.1: Primary sources of infections and risk factors for orofacial cellulitis.

Primary sources of infections for orofacial cellulitis	Risk factors in orofacial cellulitis
• Periapical abscess • Pericoronitis or pericoronal abscess • Periodontal abscess • Osteomyelitis • Infected postextraction wound • Gunshot injuries • Oral soft tissue infections • Oral infection in HIV • Blood-borne infections	• Poor oral hygiene • Suppressed immunity, e.g. HIV, diabetes, chronic leukemia, liver and kidney diseases, and circulatory disorder • Long-term steroid therapy • Previous history of cellulitis • Drug addicts • Obesity

- In untreated cases, the redness spreads over a large area of skin and small deep red spots appear over the reddened area. Even small vesicles may form on the affected area of skin, which rupture later.
- However, when the infection spreads along the deeper tissue spaces, the skin appears normal.
- Fever, chill, leukocytosis, etc. are often present, which make the patient slightly ill.
- Regional lymphadenopathy frequently develops and in untreated cases cellulitis may spread over a wide area and sometimes involve the entire face (Fig. 11.7).

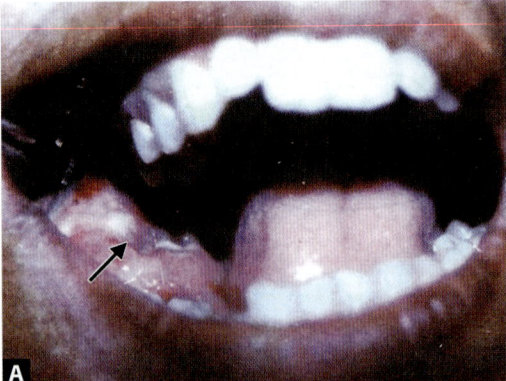

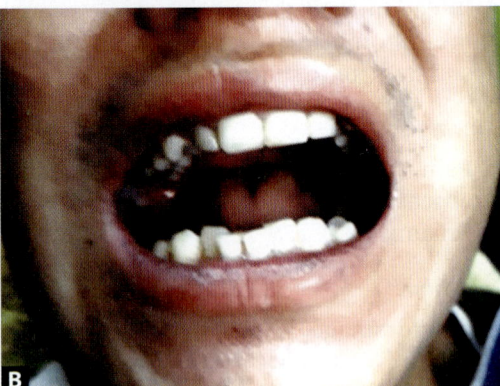

Figs. 11.8A and B: (A) Extensive 3rd molar infection causing cellulitis; (B) Trismus developed from 3rd molar infection.

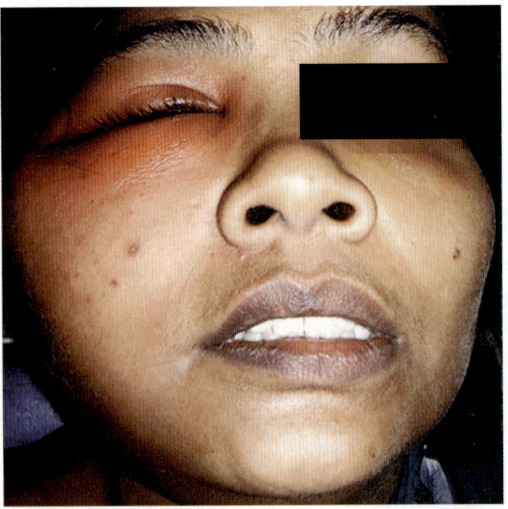

Fig. 11.7: Cellulitis causing massive facial swelling spreading up to the orbital area.

- Trismus, dyspnea, and dysphagia are the common complications (Figs. 11.8A and B).
- Some lesions resolve completely, however, in other cases pus discharging intraoral or extraoral sinuses may develop.

HISTOPATHOLOGIC FEATURES

- Collection of a large amount of fibrin and serum fluid in the tissue.
- Separation of periosteum and muscles from the bony surface due to accumulation of fluid.
- Acute inflammatory cell infiltration by PMN and occasionally lymphocytes.
- Pus may develop in the later stages of the disease.
- Formation of sinus tracts over skin or mucosal surfaces.

TREATMENT

- Bacteriological examination of the exudate or pus, etc.
- Surgical drainage, antibiotics and elimination of the primary source of infection.

LUDWIG'S ANGINA

DEFINITION

Ludwig's angina is an overwhelming diffuse, suppurative cellulitis, which simultaneously involves the submaxillary, sublingual, and submental spaces.

The sublingual space lies below the tongue above the mylohyoid muscle, while the submaxillary and submental spaces lie below the mylohyoid; the compartments are continuous around the posterior border of mylohyoid muscle and therefore can be involved by the space infections simultaneously resulting in Ludwig's angina (Box 11.3).

CAUSATIVE MICROORGANISMS

Mixed infections involving both aerobes and anaerobes are responsible; alpha-hemolytic streptococci are the most frequently encountered organisms to cause Ludwig's angina, followed by staphylococci and bacteroides. Rarely *Haemophilus influenzae, E. coli* and Pseudomonas may also be involved (Box 11.4).

Box 11.3	Predisposing factors for Ludwig's angina.

- Diabetes mellitus
- HIV infection
- Oral transplants
- Aplastic anemia
- Long-term steroid therapy
- Liver and kidney diseases

Box 11.4	Primary sources of infections in Ludwig's angina.

- Periapical, pericoronal or periodontal infections from mandibular molar teeth (80% cases).
- Submandibular sialadenitis
- Infection of the other orofacial soft tissues
- Gunshot injury or stab wounds in the floor of the mouth with secondary infection
- Infection following fracture of mandible
- Osteomyelitis of the jawbones
- Spread of infection from peritonsillar or parapharyngeal abscesses

PATHOGENESIS OF LUDWIG'S ANGINA

- In Ludwig's angina, all the three important spaces in the submandibular region—(1) the submandibular space, (2) sublingual space and (3) the submental space, are involved simultaneously.
- Infection from multiple decayed lower teeth (both premolars and molars) can be crucial for the development of this condition; since lower premolar roots lie above the attachment of mylohyoid muscle and cause sublingual space infection. While the lower molar roots extend up to or below the mylohyoid line and cause submaxillary space infection; as this space is also continuous with the submental space around the posterior border of mylohyoid, both can be infected together.
- Although involvement of these spaces occurs one after the another, the spread of infection is so rapid as if it is involving all the spaces together.

CLINICAL FEATURES

- Ludwig's angina produces a rapidly spreading, large, diffuse and "woody-

hard" type aggressive swelling; which involves the upper part of neck and floor of the mouth bilaterally with brawny induration.
- The swelling in the floor of mouth region causes elevation of the tongue; which may be pushed up against the palate and the patient often has a typical open mouthed appearance.
- As the tongue is pushed upward and backward it may threaten airway obstruction.
- The enlarged tongue may protrude outside the mouth and the condition is called woody tongue.
- The swollen area of the neck is firm, painful, nonfluctuant and does not pit upon pressure.
- The condition is always bilateral and the patient is often unable to open the mouth, speak or swallow properly.
- Usually, the patient is very toxic with high fever, chill, rapid pulse, dysphagia, sore throat, drooling and fast respiration, etc.
- In untreated cases, cellulitis may spread further and cause a massive swelling in the neck above the hyoid bone; this condition is often known as "bull neck" (Fig. 11.9).

- As the condition deteriorates further there may be development of edema glottis; which is a serious condition and can result in death due to asphyxia.
- Other serious consequences of Ludwig's angina include the development of cavernous sinus thrombosis, meningitis, brain abscess and suppurative encephalitis, etc.

■ DIAGNOSIS

Diagnosis is usually established by the following methods:
- Clinical features of the disease are often very specific.
- Leukocytosis
- Bacterial culture with identification of specific microorganisms.

Treatment
- High dose of antibiotics
- Drainage by incision at the anterior part of the neck
- Emergency tracheostomy may be required in cases of airway obstructions.

CAVERNOUS SINUS THROMBOSIS (THROMBOPHLEBITIS)

■ DEFINITION

Cavernous sinus thrombosis is a serious life-threatening condition characterized by formation of septic thrombi within the cavernous sinus and its numerous communicating branches.

■ ROUTES OF SPREAD OF INFECTIONS

External Route
- The veins of the maxillary regions of face anatomically drain into the cavernous sinus and because of this, infections from upper lip, face, eye and nares, etc. often reach cavernous sinus directly through facial and angular veins.
- Since facial and angular veins are quite longer vessels and, moreover, they have no value systems in them, infections

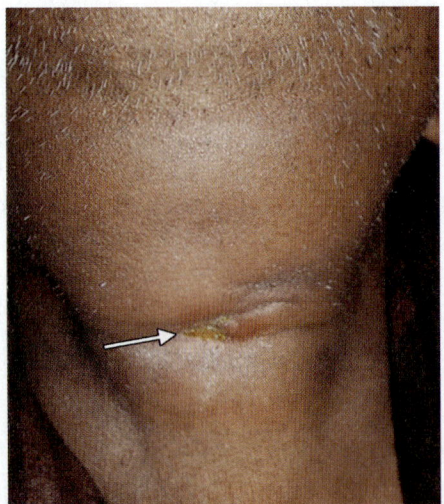

Fig. 11.9: Ludwig's angina causing "bull neck".

from the outer face spread rapidly to the cavernous sinus via this route.

Internal Route

- Infections from internal structures (especially upper and lower third molar teeth) reach cavernous sinus via the pterygoid plexus.
- Spread of infection via the internal route usually occurs at a much slower pace, since the infection has to pass through many small and twisted venous passages of the pterygoid plexus.

■ CLINICAL FEATURES

- Patients with cavernous sinus thrombosis are often gravely ill and if timely intervention is not done the disease can terminate fatally.
- Headache, fever, vomiting, nausea and chill, etc. are present in the initial stages.
- Patients may also develop tachycardia, tachypnea, stiffness of the neck and irregular breathing, etc. with alarming severity.
- Occlusion of the ophthalmic veins causes photophobia, increased lacrimation, proptosis, chemosis, dilatation of pupil and edema of the eyelids, etc.
- Paralysis of the external ocular muscles, exophthalmos, fixation of the eyeball, intraocular hemorrhage, and even blindness can occur.
- Massive swelling of the nose and forehead areas.
- Complete paralysis of the third, fourth and sixth cranial nerves common.
- Pain above the eye and diminished sensation over the forehead.
- The condition is initially unilateral but, it often becomes bilateral within 2–3 days.
- Death may occur due to brain abscess, meningitis, septicemia, toxemia or pyemia, etc.

■ TREATMENT

- Maintenance of airway in cases of respiratory distress

- High doses of antibiotic therapy
- Drainage
- Anticoagulant therapy.

MAXILLARY SINUSITIS

■ DEFINITION

Maxillary sinusitis can be defined as the acute or chronic inflammations of the maxillary sinus.

■ ETIOLOGY

- Maxillary sinusitis often occurs due to direct extension of odontogenic infections from upper premolars and molars.
- Displacement of root fragments of these teeth into the sinus.
- However, there are a few other causes of maxillary sinusitis, which are as follows:
  – Common cold
  – Influenza
  – Exanthematous diseases
  – Spread of infections from the neighboring frontal or parietal sinuses
  – Phycomycosis infection
  – Traumatic injury to the maxillary tuberosity followed by secondary infection.

■ CLINICAL FEATURES

- Acute maxillary sinusitis produces moderate to severe pain in the sinus region with swelling.
- The pain usually increases when digital pressure is applied over the maxilla.
- Patient feels pain in the teeth or in the ear because the sinusitis pain is often referred to these structures.
- Fever, malaise, discharge of pus into the nose with fetid breath, etc.
- Chronic maxillary sinusitis presents vague pain or no pain, stuffy sensation in the face, nasal discharge and foul breath.

■ RADIOLOGICAL FEATURES

- For detailed visualization of the maxillary sinus, Water's view radiographs are specifically needed.

- Acute maxillary sinusitis radiographically does not produce any significant diagnostic findings.
- However, chronic maxillary sinusitis often produces clouding of the maxillary sinus due to the presence of fluid and hyperplastic epithelial tissues which fill up the sinus.

HISTOLOGICAL FEATURES

- In acute maxillary sinusitis, the lining epithelium of the maxillary sinus shows edema, occasional hemorrhage and infiltration by acute inflammatory cells.
- Chronic maxillary sinusitis often produces marked thickening of the lining epithelium with formation of numerous epithelial polyps. Squamous metaplasia of the ciliated columnar epithelium may be seen.
- The polyps are made up of hyperplastic, granulation tissue with lymphocytic and sometimes plasma cell infiltrations.

TREATMENT

- Removal of primary sources of infection by currettage, drainage and antibiotics.

FOCAL INFECTION

It has been observed since long time that infections from oral cavity can spread to distant parts of the body and produce fresh lesions over there.

Orofacial tissues especially the teeth and the periodontium normally harbor numerous microorganisms, which are otherwise nonpathogenic as long as they are within the oral cavity. However, once these organisms spread to the distant organs of the body, they behave as strictly pathogenic organisms and produce diseases.

DEFINITION

Focal Infection

Metastases of microorganisms or their toxins from a localized site of infection to any distant part of the body with subsequent injury are called "focal infections".

Focus of Infection

Circumscribed area of tissue, which is infected by exogenous pathogenic organisms and is usually located near the skin or mucosal surface is called a "focus of infection".

MECHANISM OF FOCAL INFECTION

Focal infections mostly occur by the following mechanisms:
- Spread of "microorganisms" via the blood vessels or lymphatics.
- Spread of "bacterial toxins" through blood vessels or lymphatics (erythrogenic toxins liberated by beta-hemolytic streptococci produce diffuse, bright skin rashes in scarlet fever) (Box 11.5).

COMMON CONSEQUENCES OF "FOCAL INFECTIONS" FROM THE OROFACIAL REGION

- Bacteremia, septicemia, toxemia and pyemia
- Subacute bacterial endocarditis
- Cavernous sinus thrombosis
- Meningitis and brain abscess
- Subdural empyema
- Suppurative encephalitis
- Ocular diseases
- Renal diseases
- Gastrointestinal diseases

Box 11.5	Examples of various oral "foci" of infections.
• Periapical abscess (acute or chronic) • Pericoronitis • Infected periapical granuloma or cyst • Periodontal abscess • Infected dental pulp or root canals • Infected root fragments of teeth • Osteomyelitis • Syphilitic chancre • Infections in the maxillary sinus, nasal sinus, throat and tonsils, etc.	

- Upper respiratory tract disease
- Dermatological lesions
- Bacteremia, septicemia, toxemia and pyemia
- Rheumatoid arthritis and rheumatic fever.

Bacteremia and Septicemia

Bacteremia

Bacteremia is the condition in which there is "transient presence of bacteria in blood stream" without their multiplication.

Toxemia

Toxemia is the condition characterized by the formation of toxins or toxic products in blood by the bacteria.

Pyemia

Pyemia is septicemia caused by pyogenic bacteria with formation of multiple abscesses in internal organs like liver, lung, kidney, brain and heart, etc.

Septicemia

Septicemia literally means "sepsis of blood" and the condition is characterized by presence of actively multiplying bacteria in the blood stream with formation of their toxic products in blood.

Common infective organisms to cause septicemia
- Bacterial agents
  - *Staphylococcus aureus*
  - *Streptococcus pneumoniae*
  - *E. coli*
  - *Streptococcus viridans*
  - *Streptococcus pyogenes*
  - *Haemophilus influenzae*
  - *Klebsiella spp.*
- Fungal agents
  - *Candida albicans* and other species
  - *Cryptococcus neoformans*
  - *Histoplasma capsulatum*
  - *Mucor spp.*
  - *Aspergillus spp.*

Clinical features of septicemia
- Hyperthermia (fever) or hypothermia
- Rigors, tachycardia and tachypnea
- Hypoxia, dyspnea and cyanosis
- Hypotension
- Agitation in elderly
- Mental confusion.

Complications in septicemia
- Septic or toxic shock
- Disseminated intravascular coagulation (DIC)
- Multiorgan failure (e.g. heart, lung, liver and kidneys).

BIBLIOGRAPHY

1. Allan BP, Egbert MA, Myall RW. Orbital abscess of odontogenic origin: case report and review of the literature. Int T Oral Maxillofac Surg. 1991;20:268-70.
2. Bullock JD Fleischman JA. The spread of odontogenic infections to the orbit: diagnosis and management. T Oral Maxillofac Surg. 1985;43:749-55.
3. Cogan MIC. Necrotizing mediastinitis secondary to descending cervical cellulitis. Oral Surg. 1973;36:307.
4. Dajani AS, Taubert KA, Wilson W, et al. Prevention of bacterial endocarditis: Recommendations by the American Heart Association. J Am Med Assoc. 1997;277(22):1794-801.
5. De Leo AA, Schoenknecht FD, Anderson MW, et al. The incidence of bacteremia following oral prophylaxis on pediatric patients. Oral Surg. 1974;37:36.
6. Giunta JL. Comparison of erysipelas and odontogenic cellulitis. T Endod. 1987;13:291-4.
7. Gonty AA, Costich ER. Service facial and cervical infections associated with gas-producing bacteria report of two cases. T Oral Surg. 1981; 39:702-7.
8. Heilelman JF, Dirlam JH. Severe cellulitis of dental origin with gas-producing bacteria. T Indiana Dent Assoc. 1982;61:11-3.
9. Kaban LB, McGill T. Orbital cellulitis of dental origin: differential diagnosis and the use of the computed tomography as a diagnostic aid. T Oral Surg. 1980;38:682-5.
10. Lacassin F, Hoen B, Leport C, et al. Procedures associated with infective endocarditis in

adults: a case-control study. Eur Heart J. 1995; 16(12):1968-74.
11. Madden GJ, Smith OP. Lingual cellulitis causing upper airway obstruction. Br T Oral Maxillofac Surg.1990;28:309-10.
12. Matusow RJ. Acute pulpal-alveolar cellulitis syndrome: V: apical closure of immature teeth by infection control: the importance of an endodontic seal with therapeutic factors: part 2. Oral Surg Oral Med Oral Pathol. 1991;72:96-100.
13. Matusow RJ. The acute primary endodontic cellulitis syndrome: etiologic, pathogenic, and therapeutic factors. Compendium. 1988;9: 682-90.
14. Ochs MW, Dolwick MF. Facial erysipelas: report of a case and review of the literature. T Oral Maxillofac Surg. 1991;49:1116-20.
15. Ogundiya DA, Keith DA, Mirowski J. Cavernous sinus thrombosis and blindness as complications of an odontogenic infection: report of a case and review of literature. T Oral Maxillofac Surg. 1989;47:1317-21.
16. Soames JV, Southam JC. Oral pathology, 3rd edition, London: Oxford University Press; 1999.
17. Soffin CB, Morse DR, Seltzer S, et al. Thermography and oral inflammatory conditions. Oral Surg Oral Med Oral Pathol. 1983;56:256-62.
18. Srinivasan B. Textbook of oral and maxillofacial surgery, 1st edition. New Delhi: Churchill Livingstone; 1994.
19. Strauss HR, Tilghman DM, Hankins J. Ludwig. Angina, empyema, pulmonary infiltration, and pericarditis secondary to extraction of a tooth. T Oral Surg. 1980;38:223-9.
20. Strom BL, Abrutyn E, Berlin JA, et al. Dental and cardiac risk factors for infective endocarditis: a population-based, case-control study. Ann Int Med. 1998;129(10):761-9.
21. Suei Y, Tanimoto K, Taguchi A, et al. Chronic recurrent multifocal osteomyelitis involving the mandible. Oral Surg Oral Med Oral Pathol. 1994;78:156-62.
22. Tomaselli DL, Feldman RS, Krochtengel AL, et al. Osteomyelitis associated with chronic periodontitis in a patient with end-stage renal disease; a case report. Periodontal Clin Invest. 1993;15:8-12.
23. Travis RT, Steinle CJ. The effects of odontogenic infection on the complete blood count in children and adolescents. Pediatr Dent. 1984; 6:214-9.
24. Van der Meer JT, Thompson J, Michel MF, et al. Epidemiology of bacterial endocarditis in the Netherlands. II. Antecedent procedures and use of prophylaxis. Arch Int Med. 1992; 152(9):1869-73.
25. Van Merkesteyn JP, Bakker DJ der Waal I, Kusen GJ, et al. Hyperbaric oxygen treatment of chronic osteomyelitis of the jaws. Int J Oral Surg. 1984;13:386-95.
26. Wannfors K, Hammarstrom L. Periapical lesions of mandibular bone: difficulties in early diagnostics. Oral Surg Oral Med Oral Pathol. 1990;70:483-9.

CHAPTER 12

Physical and Chemical Injuries of the Oral Cavity

PHYSICAL INJURIES

FRACTURES OF TEETH

Tooth fracture is a common type of injury and it occurs in a variety of situations, e.g. sudden severe trauma, tooth weakened by a large restoration, nonvital tooth and internal resorptions, etc.

It is important to note that the boys usually have more tooth fractures in comparison to the girls, and class II malocclusion is associated with more cases of anterior tooth fractures (Figs. 12.1A and B).

ROOT FRACTURE

Root fracture represents a small percentage of total number of tooth fractures. Most cases occur due to trauma between the ages of 10 years and 20 years (Fig. 12.2).

CEMENTAL TEAR

Cemental tears cause detachment of part of cementum often due to sudden rotational forces, which remains within the periodontal ligament. The condition is usually asymptomatic.

BRUXISM

Definition

Bruxism can be defined as the habitual, unintentional grinding or clenching of teeth, it occurs periodically either during sleep in the night or during day-time. The person, who has the habit of bruxism does grinding or clinching of teeth at inappropriate moments along with repeated tapping. The act causes considerable amount of damage to the teeth and the related structures (Table 12.1).

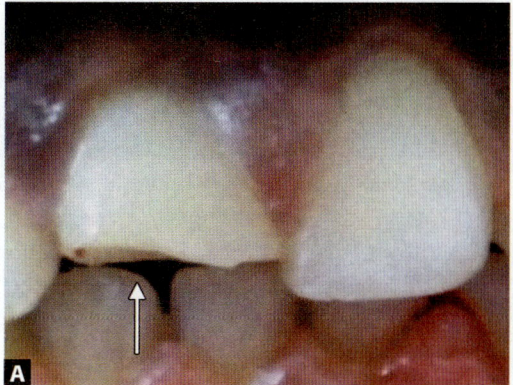 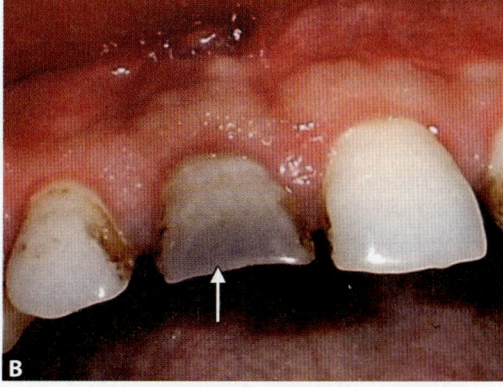

Figs.12.1A and B: (A) Anterior tooth fractures due to injury; (B) Injury with loss of vitality of tooth.

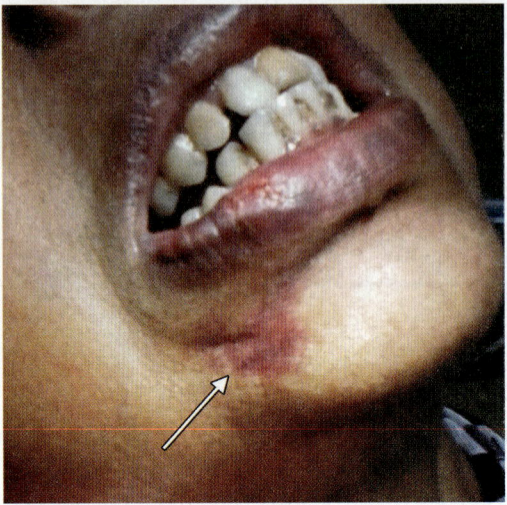

Fig.12.2: Hematoma on the face due to injury.

Causes
- Local factor: Occlusal disturbances
- Systematic causes: Unrecognized mental tension due to the following reasons:
  - Chronic GI upset
  - Sleep disorder
  - Heredity
  - Physical disability
  - Endocrine disorder
- Psychological factor
  - Emotional upsets due to fear, pain, anger, rejection, nervousness or frustrations, etc.
  - Persons with aggressive, hurried or overly competitive tendencies.

Types of Bruxism
There are two types of bruxism:
1. Nocturnal
2. Day-time habit.

Clinical Features (Fig. 12.3)
- Severe attrition of teeth with loss of enamel and exposure of dentin (both occlusally and interproximally)
- Noise during grinding of teeth

Table 12.1: Causes of premature loss of teeth.

Trauma	• Due to accidents • Psychotic patients • Radiation
Periodontal diseases	• Aggressive juvenile periodontitis • AIDS related periodontal diseases
Hereditary conditions	• Acatalasia • Chediak-Higashi disease • Cyclic neutropenia • Dentin dysplasia-type I (rootless tooth) • Hypophosphatasia • Hypophosphatemia • Lesch-Nyhan syndrome • Papillon-lefevre syndrome • Down's syndrome
Immunocompromised states	• HIV/AIDS • Leukemia • Chemotherapy
Neoplasms	• Benign and malignant neoplasm of the jaws • Lymphomas • Tumor-like conditions
Miscellaneous factors	• Diabetes mellitus • Histiocytosis–X • Acrodynia • Regional odontodysplasia (ghost teeth) • Osteomyelitis • Vitamin-C deficiency • Langerhans cell disease

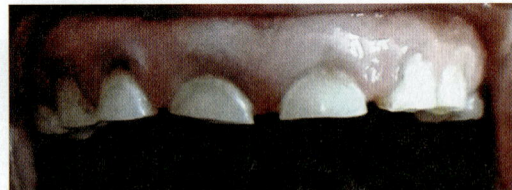

Fig. 12.3: Bruxism causing severe attrition of teeth.

- Multiple wear facets on the occlusal surface with occasional fracture of cusps or restorations
- Loosening and drifting of teeth
- Gingival recession

- Hypertrophy of the masticatory muscles (predominantly masseter and anterior temporalis)
- Facial pain, myalgia and headache
- Tenderness on palpation of muscles of mastication
- Sensitivity of teeth
- A popping or clicking sound in the TM joint.

Treatment
- Removal of the irritating factors (local and systemic)
- Use of occlusal splints
- Behavior modification.

ANKYLOSIS OF TEETH

Tooth ankylosis is a pathological condition in which the root of the tooth becomes completely united with the bony socket.

Pathogenesis
Ankylosis of tooth occurs due to partial resorption of root with subsequent deposition of cementum or alveolar bone causing obliteration of periodontal ligament space.

Clinical Features
- Ankylosis can occur in both deciduous as well as in permanent dentitions and it can develop during any stage of tooth development or tooth eruption.
- The ankylosed teeth are asymptomatic and often produce a dull, high pitched, muffled sound on percussion, instead of a sharp normal sound.
- Ankylosed deciduous tooth often blocks the path of eruption of permanent tooth.

Common Symptoms Associated with Ankylosed Tooth
- Congenital absence of single or multiple tooth
- Malocclusion of teeth especially infraocclusion
- Abnormal tooth eruption pattern in the jaw.

Radiographic Features
Radiographically, these teeth often show obliteration of the periodontal ligament spaces around their roots.

Treatment
- Orthodontic treatment to help the tooth to erupt
- Surgical repositioning of the affected tooth may be required
- Wherever required, these teeth should be extracted by surgical method only.

SUBMERGED TEETH

Definition
A tooth which has not erupted to the point of making contact with the opposing maxillary or mandibular tooth, during mastication. In other words a submerged tooth is the one, whose relative occlusal movement in the dental arch has stopped during or after the period of active eruption.

Clinical Features
- Submerged teeth are ankylosed deciduous teeth, usually located in the mandibular posterior region.
- They can be single or multiple in numbers.
- The submerged appearance occurs as the occlusal plane of the retained smaller sized tooth is located below the occlusal plane of the rest of the teeth in the arch.
- Submerged tooth often gets ankylosed in the jaw and blocks the path of eruption of permanent successor.

Radiographic Features
Radiograph reveals obliteration of the periodontal ligament space around the root of the submerged tooth with variable degree of root resorptions. It also reveals missing or

impacted permanent successor tooth below the submerged tooth.

Treatment
Extract and orthodontically move the permanent successor.

TOOTHBRUSH INJURY

Toothbrush injuries are caused by chronic physical irritation from the toothbrush bristles to the marginal and the attached gingiva (Fig. 12.4).

Clinical Features
- The lesions commonly appear as superficial linear erosions in an erythematous background.
- Some lesions may appear as white, red or ulcerated areas.
- Most lesions produce pain, especially during taking food and some of these lesions can be infected secondarily.
- When the injury is very severe, it can produce deep clefts on the gingival margin with severe gingival recession.

TOOTHPICK INJURY

Toothpick injury is almost similar to that of toothbrush injury as discussed earlier. It usually results from habitual, overzealous use of common utensils for maintaining oral hygiene.

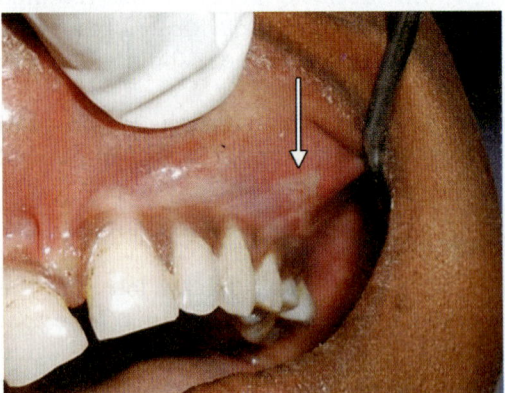

Fig. 12.4: Toothbrush injury causing traumatic ulcer.

Clinical Features
- It is usually a localized problem and having involvement of only one or two areas of the dental arch.
- Since toothpicks are often inserted into the interproximal areas, the interdental papillae are often damaged or lost.
- Typically, there is a depression involving both buccal and lingual aspects of the gingiva.
- Besides the gingival tissue, toothpick injury also causes injury and subsequent loss of the cementum, dentin, and cervical enamel on the mesial and distal aspect of the tooth.
- Patients may have pain and sensitivity in the teeth.

LINEA ALBA

Linea alba is a Latin name which means "white line" and it is more popularly used to describe a white fibrous structure that runs down the midline of our abdomen. However in the oral cavity a similar white line is often seen on the buccal mucosa (mostly bilaterally) at the level where the occlusal surfaces of upper and lower teeth meet and it is called the "linea alba" of the cheek.

This line runs from the angle of the mouth to the posterior teeth region and is often believed to be caused by friction or trauma from the teeth.

TRAUMATIC ATROPHIC GLOSSITIS

Definition
These are focal sensitive erythematous areas of the tongue due to physical (traumatic) injury or irritation.

Causes
- Recent restorations or other changes in oral environment
- Broken fillings or prosthesis
- Chipped cusps or sharp incisal edges
- Extensive calculus in lower anterior teeth
- Malaligned or crowded teeth

- As a symptom of familial dysautonomia or Riley-Day syndrome.

Clinical Features
- Site: Tip of the tongue and occasionally the lateral margin.
- The affected area shows thinning and reddening of the mucosa.
- The filiform papilla is lost and the fungi form papilla appears enlarged and reddened.
- Patients usually move their tongue repeatedly over the restorations or broken edges in a compulsive manner to explore these areas and thereby injure the tongue.

Treatment
Elimination of the irritating factor.

TRAUMATIC ULCER

An ulcer can be defined as the breach in continuity of the skin or the epithelium, extending below the basement membrane due to molecular cell death.

If an ulcer develops as a result of trauma, it is known as the traumatic ulcer.

Causes of Traumatic Ulcer
Traumatic ulcers in the oral cavity may occur due to the following reasons:
- Accidental biting of the mucosa while eating or chewing.
- Injury from the orthodontic or prosthetic appliances.
- Injury from a sharp broken tooth, carious or malposed tooth.
- Toothbrush injury.
- Injury due to iatrogenic causes (e.g. violent rubbing of mucosa with the cotton roll during dental procedures).
- Injury from ill-fitting or misaligned prosthesis.
- Thermal, chemical or electrical injury to the oral mucosa.
- Nocturnal parafunctional habits, e.g. bruxism, cheek biting, thumb sucking.
- Improper feeding of children.
- Factitious injury.
- Xerostomia.

Clinical Features (Fig. 12.5)
- Traumatic ulcers frequently develop on the tongue, vestibule, alveolar ridge or palate, etc.
- The lesion often exhibits a solitary, painful ulcer of short duration.
- The ulcers are often covered with a yellow, fibrinopurulent exudate.
- Most of the time, the cause of the ulcer is easily detected from the patient's history.
- There is considerable difficulty in taking foods.
- Secondary infections often make the situation complicated.
- Long standing ulcers may be associated with premalignant or malignant changes.

Treatment
Removal of the primary cause and symptomatic treatment will easily cure the condition. Systemic conditions should be duly treated wherever required.

FACTITIOUS INJURIES (SELF-INFLICTED ORAL WOUNDS)

Factitious injuries are self-inflicted injuries caused by the patient himself or herself and

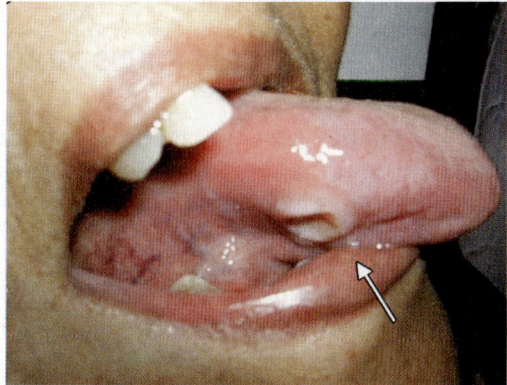

Fig. 12.5: Traumatic ulcers on the tongue from sharp teeth.

Box 12.1	Characteristics of wound in factitious injuries.

- Presence of a wound in absence of any recognizable disease or any apparent cause
- Bizarre shape or outline of the wound is often inconsistent with the history given by the patient.
- Wounds found in the mouth of an otherwise healthy individual
- Wounds are found only in accessible parts of the body (where the patient can cause self-injury with nails, teeth or hands, etc.)

these are either habitual or inadvertent. These injuries are commonly seen in persons with disturbed mental state and injuries are purposefully created for "seeking attention and sympathy from family members" (Box 12.1). In some cases, the emotionally disturbed patients may even carefully try to maintain or continue with the factitious wounds in their mouth, either by interfering with its healing process or by causing repeated injuries in the same area.

Following are the examples of few factitious injuries:
- Cheek and lip biting
- Self extraction of tooth
- Fingernail injuries
- Nasal ulcerations and facial emphysema
- Periorbital ecchymosis
- Persistent oral mucosal and gingival ulcerations
- Mandibular subluxation.

■ DENTURE RELATED INJURIES OR LESIONS

Denture injuries may be either acute or chronic in nature and there are several types of such injuries, which are as follows:
- Traumatic ulcer
- Denture hyperplasia
- Denture stomatitis or sore mouth
- Angular stomatitis (due to improper vertical height in dentures)
- Papillary palatal hyperplasia
- Frictional keratosis

- Pain due to pressure on a buried tooth in the gums.

Acute Injuries

Acute denture injuries commonly occur due to wearing of a new prosthesis, which is yet to be adjusted. New dentures may cause injury to the oral mucosa resulting in pain and ulceration.

Denture Sore Mouth

This is an uncommon condition of oral mucosa, which occurs due to irritation from denture coupled with superadded candidal infections.

Clinically, the lesion presents a fiery red, smooth, swollen and painful oral mucosa, which was in direct contact with the denture base. A burning sensation due to hot and spicy food is also common.

Epulis Fissuratum

It is a common denture injury produced by chronically ill-fitting dentures.

In these patients, ridge support becomes gradually diminished due to pressure from the artificial prosthesis, which causes resorption of the alveolar ridge.

Due to increased resorption of the ridge, the denture flanges extend deep into the sulcus and cause impingement of the soft tissue.

Clinical Features

- Clinically, epulis fissuratum appears as elongated rolls of tissue or large nodular masses in the mucoabial or mucobuccal fold area into which the denture flanges easily and perfectly fit (Fig. 12.6).
- The lesions are painless, firm and there may be occasional ulceration.

Papillary Hyperplasia of the Palate

It is an unusual condition characterized by numerous, small, "wart-like" outgrowths on the mucosal surface of palate.

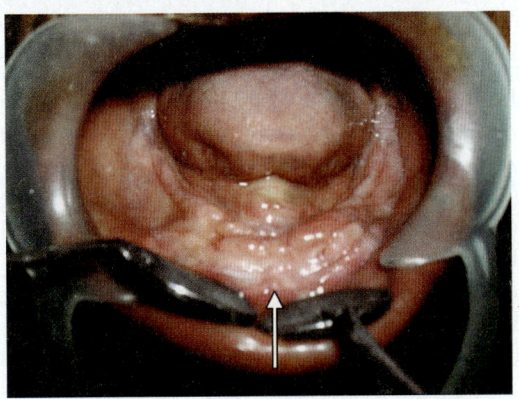

Fig. 12.6: Epulis fissuratum.

Poor oral hygiene and ill-fitting dentures, etc. are frequently associated with the development of this condition.

ELECTRICAL BURNS IN THE MOUTH

Electrical burns of the oral and paraoral tissues are commonly seen in children usually between the ages of 2-4 years.

The injury occurs in the following situations:
- Due to biting on the plugged cord of an electrical appliance by the child
- Sucking on the receptacle (female) end of an extension cord.

Pathogenesis
- Electrical burns are produced by an arc, which results from the electric current passing through the electrolyte rich saliva.
- The arc reaches temperatures as high as 3000°C and causes deep thermal burns and local tissue destruction within moments.

Clinical Features
- Electrical burns mostly occur in the lower lips and angle of mouth. It can also occur in the gingiva and the tongue.
- Electrical burns differ from thermal burns and produce one or more deep craters in the tissue, measuring about 1-3 cm in diameter with a light yellow base.

Table 12.2: Complications of electrical burns of the mouth.

Anodontia	Electrical burns cause damage to the developing tooth buds and results in anodontia
Microstomia	Due to damage to the growth centers of the developing jawbone
Lip deformities	Due to abnormal post burn healing
Malocclusion	Due to poor growth and development of the damaged jawbones
Facial deformity	Due to severe damage and necrosis of facial soft tissue and jawbones

- These lesions are mostly painless and bloodless.
- Often the normal appearing tissue surrounding the crater becomes ischemic and these areas produce a peculiar "cold" sensation.
- Within next 3-4 weeks the base of the crater and the surrounding tissue slough out, leaving a large disfiguring defect (Table 12.2).

Treatment
Cosmetic reconstruction of face and mouth.

THERMAL BURNS IN MOUTH

Thermal burns of the oral tissues occur mostly due to contact with hot foods and beverages. It can also occur rarely during dental procedures when hot instruments accidentally come in contact with oral soft tissues.

Mild Burns

Hot foods and beverages generally cause this and the areas commonly affected are the tip of the tongue and anterior part of the palate, (since these anatomical structures come in contact with foods first).

In cases of mild thermal burn, the area shows slight erythema which resolves spontaneously in few hours' time.

Moderate Burns

This type of burn often occurs when hot sticky foods become adhered to the palate (especially hot cheese).

Injured area becomes erythematous with sloughing of the epithelium, and it causes pain and burning sensation for many days.

Severe Burn

Severe burns occur mostly during dental procedures, when an overheated instrument or material comes in direct contact with the oral soft tissues. It can occur during taking impression with an overheated hydrocolloid impression material. The gingival tissue is often damaged and it shows mucosal erythema and sloughing with intense pain.

Lip and commissural tissue may often get burnt if touched with a hot instrument (e.g. tip of the hot ball burnisher or root canal plugger, etc.). There is often severe pain in the area and it heals with scar formation.

■ RADIATION INJURIES

Radiation injuries occur due to the ionizing effects of electromagnetic waves or energized particles on living cells.

Radiation injuries may occur from sun, X-ray machines and radioactive elements, etc. As radiations (which are tremendously powerful rays of energy) pass through any living cell, they destroy the cells by damaging the cell organelles.

This effect of radiation is used therapeutically in the management of cancers. Radiotherapy is the process of controlled elimination of the diseased cells by radiation, the cancer cells often die or even if they survive they lose their capacity to multiply. During this process some normal cells in and around the field of radiation are also damaged.

Types of Therapeutic Radiations

Therapeutic electromagnetic waves may be of *low energy (less than 1,000 KeV or orthovoltage)* or it may be of *high energy (4 million to 25 million KeV or super voltage)*.

The low-energy waves are used for the treatment of superficial skin or mucosal lesions, especially cancers, because the energy absorption in such cases mostly occur at the point of initial contact with the tissue.

When high-energy electromagnetic waves are used, the energy absorption mostly takes place in the deeper tissues and as a result the surface tissue like skin or epithelium, etc. is spared. High-energy electromagnetic waves are useful in the treatment of deep tissue neoplasms or metastatic lesions.

Dose Selection

During radiotherapy treatment, the amount of cell damage depends upon the amount of energy the tissue absorbs. Generally, the amount of energy is measured as "rad" (radiation absorbed dose) or as gray (Gy). Normally, 1 rad is equivalent to the absorption of 100 ergs/g and 1 Gy equals to 100 rads.

Therapeutic Effects of Radiation

Therapeutic radiation causes injury and subsequent necrosis of the neoplastic cells either by virtue of its *direct effect* or by its *indirect effect*.

Direct Effect

Electromagnetic energy destroys the chemicals inside the cell and as a result the cell looses its ability to function, multiply or it may die.

Indirect Effect

In this case the cell necrosis occurs indirectly by means of the toxic compounds produced by the ionizing radiation, when the energy is absorbed.

The indirect process occurs through the production of free radicals that combine to form toxic substances such as H2O2, which damages the cell. Radiation can interrupt with cell division process.

Factors Determining the Effectiveness of Radiation (Box 12.2)

- *Stage of the cell cycle*: Cells in the initial stages of maturation or cells which are growing rapidly, e.g. bone marrow cells or cells of the fetus, etc. are very sensitive to radiation as compared to those of the more mature stages.
- *Mitotic index*: Lesions with high index of mitotic activity are more responsive to radiotherapy than the lesions with little or no mitotic activity.
- *Nature of tissue*: Besides the cancer cells certain normal cell, e.g. lymphoblasts, bone marrow cells, germ cells of ovaries and testes, and lining epithelial cells of the intestine are highly sensitive to radiation. Whereas the tissues like nerve, brain, endocrine glands muscles, bone and mature cartilage, etc. are relatively insensitive or resistant to radiotherapy.

X-ray Radiation and its Effects on Various Normal Tissues

Persons, who work with radioactive materials or those who are working at nuclear fission reactors, or those who are receiving therapeutic radiations are most susceptible to cellular injury from radiation.

Various effects of radiation in different parts of the body, with special emphasis to the orofacial structures are discussed in the following section.

Box 12.2	Factors determining the degrees of radiation injury.

- Type of radiation
- Amount of radiation
- Part of the body treated
- Amount of normal tissue included in the zone of irradiation

The amount of radiation different tissues can tolerate without being damaged [Measurement is done by the unit Gray (Gy) which is the SI unit of absorbed radiation dose of ionizing radiation]:

- Fetus: 2 Gy
- Bone marrow: 2 Gy
- Ovaries: 2–3 Gy
- Lens of the eye: 5 Gy
- A child's bone: 20 Gy
- Adult's bone: 60 Gy
- A child's muscle: 20–30 Gy
- Adult's muscle: 100 Gy or more.

Various Damaging Effects of Radiation on Individual Organs or Tissues

The list of major radiation-induced complications is provided in Box 12.3.

Effects of Radiation on Cells

- Cells may be undamaged
- Cells may be damaged but remain functionally viable

Box 12.3	List of major radiation-induced complications.

- *Acute complications* (appear 1–2 weeks after the radiotherapy and they occur due to acute injury to the oral tissues):
  - Oropharyngeal mucositis
  - Change in salivary composition
  - Altered taste sensations (Dysgeusia)
  - Secondary bacterial, fungal and viral infections in mouth
  - Periodontal pain
- *Chronic complications* (occur due to change in vascularity and cellularity of soft tissue, bone and the salivary glands):
  - Trismus and fibrosis
  - Oral ulcers
  - Candidiasis
  - Malnutrition
  - Osteoradionecrosis
  - Dental caries
  - Tooth demineralization
  - Xerostomia
  - Pain in temporomandibular joint
  - Psychological impact

- Cells may be damaged and function abnormally
- Cells are completely necrosed.

Effects of Radiation on Skin
- 2–3 weeks after radiation erythema appears on the skin, the initial erythema fades away quickly, but it reappears within 2–4 weeks.
- Very high doses of radiation cause edema, swelling and desquamation of the skin with ulcerations.
- The ectodermal components of the body, e.g. sweat glands, sebaceous glands and hair follicles, etc. are destroyed initially and the loss of *hair follicles* results in alopecia within the radiation field.
- Scarring occurs eventually with atrophy, dryness, and pigmentations of skin.
- Telangiectasia may develop on the skin. The skin becomes rigid and less resistant to injury.
- Most of the skin reactions heal up within 4–6 weeks' time.

Effects of Radiation on Oral Mucosa
- Initially oral mucosa becomes dry, erythematous and atrophic.
- Mucositis develops later on with necrosis, denudation, ulcerations, and sloughing of the epithelium.
- The ulcer is often covered by a plaque-like yellow or pale fibrinous exudates.
- Pain, discomfort in the mouth especially during meals and moreover secondary infections also commonly occur.
- Dental procedures are often difficult to perform due to dry mouth, increased risk of secondary infections and delayed healing, etc.
- Dysphasia, cough and hoarseness of voice are also common.
- Very often, there is loss or alteration of taste sensations due to degeneration of the taste buds (dysgeusia or hypogeusia).
- Pain and discomfort remain for about 2 weeks, and complete regeneration of the epithelium occurs in 1 month time.
- Mucosa becomes coarse and atrophic after healing, and in many cases, dysplastic changes also develop.

Effects of Radiation on Salivary Glands
- Salivary glands are extremely sensitive to the effect of radiation, which cause damage to parenchyma and the glands exhibit inflammatory change with painful swelling.
- Xerostomia or dryness of mouth is the earliest and most common manifestation. If gland is partially damaged xerostomia is temporary but when the glands are completely destroyed, xerostomia will be permanent.
- The saliva becomes thick and its flow is stagnant, and there is difficulty in food intake due to sore mouth.
- Increased chances of development of candidiasis along with pain and discomfort.
- Altered pH and electrolyte content of saliva along with decreased secretions of immunoglobulin.
- Often there is reduction in the buffering capacity of saliva along with fall in pH, which leads to an increased caries susceptibility of teeth.

Effects of Radiation on TM Joint and Muscles
- Degenerative changes in the joint with subsequent fibrous ankylosis and trismus
- Muscle fibers are often damaged and replaced by fibrous tissue
- Osteoradionecrosis of the bony component of the TMJ may sometimes occur.

Effects of Radiation on Blood Vessels
- Small vessels become thickened and distorted, which results in diminished blood supply.

- Vascular insufficiency due to radiation may result in some serious complications like increased susceptibility to infection, delayed wound healing and bone necrosis.

Effects of Radiation on Teeth

- If radiation is given during the formative stage of teeth, there can be complete degeneration of the tooth buds with development of anodontia.
- In other cases, there may be incomplete root formation and delayed eruption of teeth.
- The tooth may exhibit white, chalky or opaque areas on the enamel.
- After several months, the enamel becomes soft with loss of its translucency and it may chip off.
- The erupted teeth often become nonvital and brittle with increased risk of fracture.
- A peculiar form of tooth destruction occurs in the cervical areas of teeth following radiation, which resembles dental caries and is often known as "radiation caries".
- Serious destruction of the periodontal tissue resulting in weakness of the teeth.
- Xerostomia and osteoradionecrosis may contribute greatly to the premature loss of teeth.

Effects of Radiation on Bone

- Radiation causes injury or damage to both the bone tissue as well as the metaphyseal growth cartilage.
- Effects of radiation on bone is often secondary to the damages occurred in its nutrient vessels.
- Normal balance of bone formation and bone resorption is disturbed, also there is increased risk of fracture of bone with slight trauma.
- In cases of high dose of radiation there can be complete degeneration of the osteoblast and osteocyte cells with loss of vitality of bone.
- Trauma to the affected bone (e.g. during tooth extraction) may lead to the development of "osteoradionecrosis". It is characterized by a chronic, painful infection and necrosis of the bone, accompanied by late sequestration and permanent deformity.
- Osteomyelitis sometimes occurs due to infection to the bone that is already devitalized by the direct effects of radiation.
- The weakened bone may undergo pathological fracture.

Effects of Radiation in the Blood

- There will be decrease in certain components of blood either due to direct damaging action of radiation or due to depression of bone marrow.
- The RBC count remains normal while the platelet count falls considerably.
- There is increased incidence of bleeding.

Effects of Whole Body Radiation (Table 12.3)

Initially after receiving the radiotherapy, the patients often develop nausea, vomiting, fatigue, malaise, anorexia and diarrhea, etc.

Table 12.3: Effects of extremely high doses of ionizing radiation in the body Sievert (Sv).*

Dose	Effect in the body
1–2 Sv	Vomiting, loss of appetite and generalized discomfort, etc. symptoms disappear within a short period
2–6 Sv	Good chance of survival, provided the patient is given immediate blood transfusions and antibiotics
6–10 Sv	Massive destruction of bone marrow with lack of formation of blood cells. Patients often die of infections and uncontrolled hemorrhage
10–20 Sv	Patient dies of vomiting, diarrhea, infection and starvation, etc.
Above 20 Sv	Massive destruction of central nervous system, cardiovascular system; patients die within a few days

*Sievert (Sv) is the SI unit of absorbed radiation dose.

- Abnormal mutations and genetic diseases; failure of conceptions and abnormal child birth.
- Elevation of serum and urinary amylase.
- Increased risk of cancer like leukemia, carcinoma of the thyroid, breast, lung, brain, skin and stomach, etc.

Effects of Radiation in Embryo and Fetus
- Growth retardation with small head and brain.
- Poorly developed immune system and mental retardation.
- Increased incidences of developmental anomalies.
- Increased risk of childhood cancers, e.g. leukemia and solid tumors, etc.
- Genetic diseases due to the mutational change.

OSTEORADIONECROSIS

Definition
Osteoradionecrosis is an acute form of osteomyelitis that occurs after the bone has been exposed to therapeutic doses of radiation, usually given for any malignancy in the head and neck area. The condition occurs secondary to radiation-induced damage of the intraosseous microvasculature and the osteocytes and leads to formations of sequestrum (Box 12.4).

Pathogenesis
Osteoradionecrosis generally occurs if the radiation dose in the body exceeds 60 Gy; radiation therapy at this dose kills the osteocytes and also severely damages the intraosseous microvessels, which results in reduced healing capacity of the bone. The compromised bone tissue easily becomes necrosed with formation of sequestrum following trauma due to lack of inflammatory defense mechanism. Mandible is more often affected by osteoradionecrosis, since normally this bone has minimum vascularity. Dental extractions, periodontal diseases, bone trauma, etc. following radiotherapy often trigger the process of osteoradionecrosis.

Bacterial infections initially enter the nonvital bone via the portals created by extractions of teeth, periodontal pockets, periapical lesions, traumatic injuries in the tissue due to surgery or wearing of prosthesis, etc. The inflammation results in acute osteomyelitis in the bone with sequestrum formation.

The risk of development of osteoradionecrosis is less during the first 4 months after radiation (called the golden period) and risk is highest during the next 8 months (5th to 12th month).

Clinical Features
- *Age*: Elderly adults.
- *Sex*: More frequent among males.
- *Site*: More often in mandible than maxilla.

Presentation
- Ulceration, severe pain, swelling and formation of draining sinuses or fistulas on the alveolar ridge.
- Exudation of pus from the area and presence of severe foul smell.
- Malocclusion is common with development of trismus.
- Sequestration of large fragments of necrotic bone from the affected area.
- Possibilities of pathological fracture and permanent deformity in the bone.

Radiological Features
Large areas of "moth-eaten" radiolucency are seen in the affected area of bone with presence of opaque sequestra. There is often

---

Box 12.4   Grades of osteoradionecrosis.
- **Grade I:** Represents osteoradionecrosis of the jaw with exposure of the alveolar bone
- **Grade II:** Osteoradionecrosis not responding to hyperbaric oxygen therapy and requires sequestrectomy or saucerization
- **Grade III:** Osteoradionecrosis with full thickness involvement of bone and/or pathological fracture

enlargement of the marrow space in the affected part of the bone.

Histopathology
- The overlying soft tissue exhibits necrosis with acute inflammatory cell infiltrations.
- Absence of osteoblasts and lacunar osteocytes in the bone.
- The marrow tissue contains necrotic cells, microorganisms and inflammatory cells.

Treatment
Debridement of necrotic tissues should be done along with removal of the sequestrum. Administration of intravenous antibiotics and hyperbaric oxygen therapy are essential. Maintenance of strict oral hygiene is necessary.

LASER RADIATION

Light amplification by stimulated emission of radiation or simply LASER is frequently used in different surgical procedures including those of the oral cavity.

The Laser induced hazards to the tissues occur mostly due to the intense heat that is generated at the tip of the instrument during surgery.

Following are the common Laser-induced injuries, which affect the oral tissues:
- A chalky spot or a crater or a hole formation on the enamel surface.
- Charring of the dentin.
- Hemorrhagic necrosis of the pulp tissue, with acute or chronic inflammatory cell infiltrations.
- Coagulation necrosis of the odontoblast cells.
- Nonspecific ulceration on the oral epithelium with purulent inflammation.

CHEMICAL INJURIES

CONGENITAL PORPHYRIA

Definition
Congenital porphyria is inherited as an autosomal recessive trait, which is responsible for the development of a defective pathway for the metabolism of hematoporphyrin and resulting in the accumulation of excessive porphyrins in the blood or urine. The circulatory porphyrins get deposited in the teeth at the time of their mineralization and cause discoloration; Similar types of porphyria depositions also take place in the bone and the skin.

Clinical Features
- Clinically, the teeth exhibit a "pinkish-brown" discoloration and bright-red fluorescence under ultraviolet light (erythrodontia).
- The skin appears light brown and is extremely sensitive to sunlight.
- Hemolytic anemia develops frequently with splenomegaly.
- Bones are fragile with increased incidence of pathological fractures.
- Vesiculobullous lesions often develop on the exposed skin surfaces of face and extremities, which heal with scarring.
- Ocular damage can lead to development of blindness.

BILIARY ATRESIA

Biliary atresia is an uncommon congenital disease of newborn infants characterized by narrowing or absence of the common bile duct, which results in elevated bilirubin levels in blood and discoloration of teeth.

Clinical Features
- Patients with biliary atresia often develop severe jaundice, clay colored stool and dark yellow-brown urine, etc.
- The liver is often enlarged and tendered, and the affected child shows poor weight gain.
- Discoloration of teeth, mainly the teeth of deciduous series is a common feature of the disease.
- The affected teeth appear dark or greenish in color, with roots of the teeth more intensely stained than the crowns.

ERYTHROBLASTOSIS FETALIS

Erythroblastosis fetalis is a hemolytic anemia of newborn, which develops during intrauterine life and results from incompatible factors in the blood of the mother and the fetus.

An Rh-negative mother normally develops antibodies against the erythrocytes of an Rh-positive fetus. These antibodies when cross the placental barrier, attack and destroy the fetal erythrocytes resulting in severe hemolysis.

Because of this hemolysis, large amounts of biliverdin and bilirubin (blood pigments) are produced in the blood, which later on become deposited into the skin and teeth.

The discolorations affect only the primary teeth and their color varies from green or bluish-green or yellowish gray.

The pigments are largely confined to the dentine and in some cases enamel hypoplasia may also be present.

FLUOROSIS

See enamel hypoplasia in Chapter 1.

ORAL MANIFESTATIONS OF VARIOUS METAL POISONING

Heavy metals are those, whose specific gravity is at least five times more than that of water. Generally they have no function nor they can be metabolized in our body but these elements can gradually accumulate in the body from environment and cause toxicity or poisoning. Systemic poisoning is often caused by a large number of metal salts, e.g. arsenic, lead, bismuth, mercury, silver and phosphorus, etc. Moreover some metals are essential for our health in small amounts, e.g. iron, zinc, etc. but these are often toxic in higher concentrations (Table 12.4).

ORAL MANIFESTATIONS OF CYTOTOXIC DRUG THERAPY

Cytotoxic drugs are often administered to children suffering from leukemia or other malignant conditions (Figs. 12.7A and B). If such therapy is given at the time of development of tooth, the following dental abnormalities can

Table 12.4: The clinical manifestations of different metal poisoning.

Name of the metal	Features of poisoning
Arsenic	• Gingivitis and stomatitis • Painful mucosal ulcerations, hyperpigmentations and hyperkeratosis • Excessive salivation • Vomiting, diarrhea and neurological disturbances
Lead	• Excessive salivary secretions • Metallic taste in the oral cavity • Swelling of the salivary glands • Development of a dark "lead-line" along the gingival margin (due to the perivascular depositions of lead-sulfide in the submucosa and basement membrane zone)
Bismuth	• Burning sensations in the oral mucosa • Metallic taste • A blue-black "bismuth line" on the marginal gingiva • Blue-black pigmentation of the lips, buccal mucosa, vestibule and undersurface of the tongue, etc.
Mercury	• Extreme exhaustion, fever and weight loss, etc. • Excessive salivation with salivary gland swelling • Stomatitis and glossitis • A dark black line on the free gingival margin
Silver	• An *"Ashen-Gray"* discoloration of the skin and oral mucosa • Microscopy reveals a fine black, granular, deposition of silver salts in the submucosa

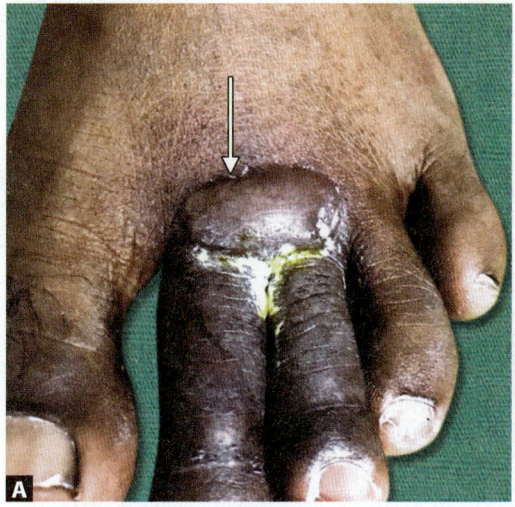
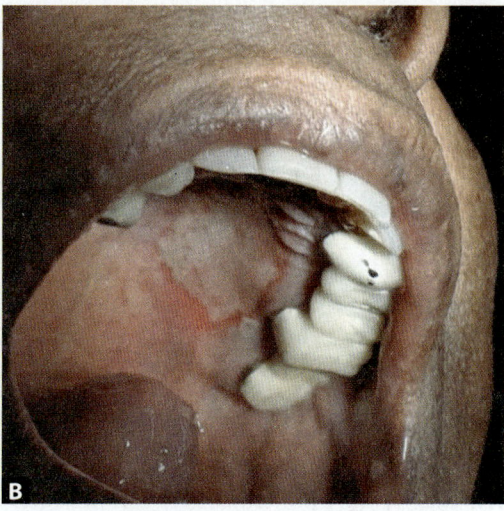

Figs. 12.7A and B: (A) Skin eruption; (B) Oral mucosal ulcer following cytotoxic drug therapy.

be seen, e.g. anodontia, hypoplastic crowns, short roots of teeth and enamel defects, etc.

The important drug reactions in the mouth are given in Table 12.5.

ORAL MANIFESTATIONS OF TETRACYCLINE STAINING

Tetracycline drug has got selective affinity for the calcium ions of the teeth and bone; it causes abnormal staining of these structures.

Tetracycline staining occurs frequently due to the prophylactic or therapeutic use of the drug to the pregnant mothers (in the second and third trimester) or the infants (up to the age of 7 years). During the development of teeth and bone, the tetracycline chemically reacts with their calcium and make a complex substance, which causes discoloration of teeth and bone.

Clinical Findings

- Both deciduous and the permanent teeth are affected by this staining.
- The intensity and distribution of the color vary depending upon the specific form of tetracycline used and their duration of administration (Fig. 12.8).

Table 12.5: Important drug reactions in the mouth.

Local reactions	• Chemical irritation • Disturbance of oral microflora
Systemic reactions	• Bone marrow depression • Depressed cell mediated immunity • Lichenoid reactions • Stevens–Johnson syndrome • Fixed drug rash • Toxic epidermal necrolysis
Miscellaneous reactions	• Gingival hyperplasia • Dry mouth • Mucosal pigmentation

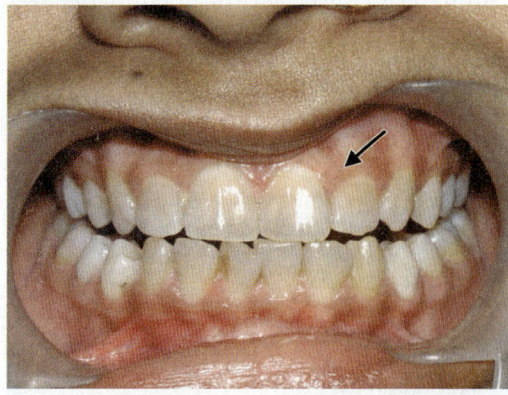

Fig. 12.8: Tetracycline staining.

- Chlortetracycline produces brownish-gray color while oxytetracycline tends to produce a yellowish discoloration of teeth.
- The discoloration is intense at the time of eruption of teeth and gradually the teeth become only "brownish" following exposure to light.
- The discoloration is always internal.
- The section of the tooth often produces bright yellow fluorescence under ultraviolet light.

ANGIONEUROTIC EDEMA

Angioneurotic edema is a type of allergy that is often triggered by pollen, drugs, venom, food or medications. It frequently produces a rapidly developing, painless, smooth, diffuse, edematous swelling, which often involves the face, lips, eyes, tongue, and extremities (Fig. 12.9).

- The edema develops very rapidly and it also subsides rapidly, after lasting for about 24–36 hours.
- On rare occasions, angioneurotic edema may cause edema glottis that result in suffocation or even death.

CHEMICAL BURNS

Acetylsalicylic Acid (Aspirin)

Acetylsalicylic acid tablets are often kept over the gingiva near the root of a painful tooth or within the carious cavity of a painful decayed tooth in order to get relief from pain. The drug has no local effect and the pain if relieved is because of the systemic effect due to its slow absorption through the oral mucosa.

If acetylsalicylic acid is put in direct contact with the oral mucosa it slowly gets dissolved in the saliva and liberates a strong acidic solution, which often causes necrosis of the mucosa.

Clinical Features

- This type of chemical burn is often known as "aspirin burn" (Fig. 12.10).
- It produces a localized, white, friable area on the mucosa with burning pain.
- In severe cases, removal of the superficial white layer of the epithelium reveals a raw, erosive surface with bleeding tendency.
- Upon stoppage of the practice, the lesion heals within 1–2 weeks.

CHEMICAL BURNS DUE TO OTHER MEDICAMENTS

Many other chemicals used in dentistry may also produce chemical burns of the facial skin and oral mucosa. In the following section effect of some of these agents are discussed.

- *Phenol*: Used as disinfectant.
- *Silver nitrate*: Used as cauterizing agent.
- *Trichloroacetic acid (TCA)*: Used as chemical cauterizing and gingival retracting agent.

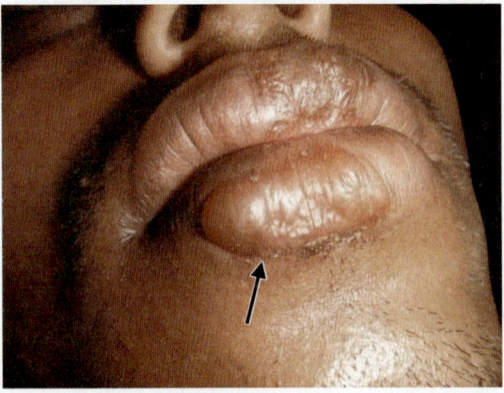

Fig. 12.9: Angioneurotic edema.

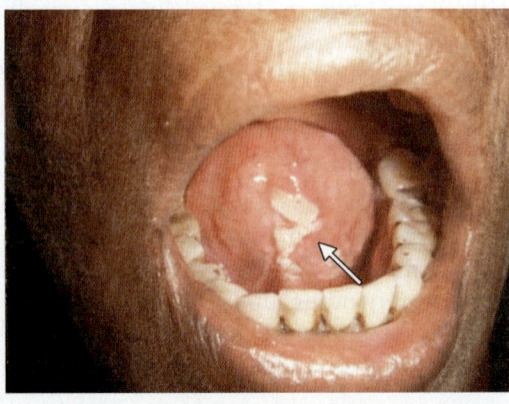

Fig. 12.10: Aspirin burn.

- H_2O_2: Used as root canal medicaments and bleaching agent.

All these agents cause sloughing of the mucosa in the area of contact and produce pain, irritation and discomfort, etc.

BIBLIOGRAPHY

1. Abrams RG, Josell SD. Common oral and dental emergencies and problems. Pediatr Clin North Am. 1982;29: 681-715.
2. Adrian RM, Hood AF, Skarin AT. Mucocutaneous reactions to antineoplastic agents. CA Cancer J Clin. 1980;30(3): 143-57.
3. Aeinehchi M, Eslami B, Ghanbariha M, et al. Mineral trioxide aggregate (MTA) and calcium hydroxide as pulp-capping agents in human teeth a preliminary report. Int Endod J. 2003;36(3): 225-31.
4. Arendorf TM, Walker DM. Denture stomatitis: a review. T Oral Rehab. 1987;14: 217-27.
5. Attanasio R. Nocturnal bruxism and its clinical management. Dent Clin North Am. 1991;35: 235-52.
6. Balogh JM, Sutherland SE. Osteoradionecrosis of the mandible: a review. T Otolaryngol. 1989;18: 245-50.
7. Bishop K, Briggs P, Kelleher M. The aetiology and management of localized anterior tooth wear in the young adult. Dent Update. 1995;22: 28-32.
8. Blackhe DD, Brady FA. The maxillary antrolith. Oral Surg. 1979;48:187.
9. Brown LR, Dreizen S, Handler S, et al. Effect of radiation-induced xerostomia on human oral microflora. J Dent Res. 1975;54: 740.
10. Bruchner A, Hansen LS. Amalgam pigmentation (amalgam tattoo) of the oral mucosa. Oral Surg. 1980;49: 139.
11. Budtz-Jorgensen E. Oral mucosal lesions associated with the wearing of removable dentures. T Oral Pathol. 1981;10: 65-80.
12. Carl W, Wood R. Effects of radiation on the developing dentition and supporting bone. J Am Dent Assoc. 1980;101: 646.
13. Carlson ER. The radiobiology, treatment and prevention of osteoradionecrosis of the mandible. Recent Results Cancer Res. 1994;134: 191-9.
14. Casamassimo PS, Lilly GE. Mucosal cysts of the maxillary sinus: a clinical and radiographic study. Oral Surg. 1980;50: 282.
15. Cawson RA. Essentials of dental surgery and pathology, 4th edition. Edinburgh: Churchill Livingstone; 1984.
16. Cohen S, Burns RC. Pathways of the pulp, 7th edition. St. Louis: Mosby Inc.; 1998.
17. Edlich RF, Nichter LS, Morgan RF, et al. Burns of the head and neck. Otolaryngol Clin North Am. 1984;17: 361-88.
18. Friedman RB. Osteoradionecrosis: causes and prevention. NCI Monogr. 1990;(9): 145-9.
19. Glaros AG, Rao SM. Effects of bruxism: a review of the literature. J Prosthet Dent. 1977;38: 149.
20. Gordon NC, Brown S, Khosla VM, et al. Lead poisoning. Oral Surg. 1979;47: 500.
21. Harrison JD, Rowley PS, Peters PD. Amalgam tattoos: light and electron microscopy and electron-probe microanalysis. J Pathol. 1977; 121:83.
22. Jacob RF. Management of xerostomia in the irradiated patient. Clin Plast Surg. 1993;20: 507-16.
23. Jacobs SG. Ankylosis of permanent teeth: a case report and literature review. Aust Orthod T. 1989;11: 38-44.
24. Jeganathan S, Lin CC. Denture stomatitis—a review of the aetiology, diagnosis and management. Aust Dent T. 1992;87: 107-14.
25. Jensen JD, Resnick SD. Porphyria in childhood. Semin Dermatol. 1995;14: 33-9.
26. Jensen JL, Howell FV, Rick GM, et al. Minor salivary gland calculi. Oral Surg. 1979;47: 44.
27. Johnson R. Traumatic dental injuries in children: part 2—treatment of injuries to Permanent teeth. Update Pediatr Dent. 1989: 2: 1-8.
28. Johnson R. Traumatic dental injuries in children: part—evaluation of traumatic dental injuries and treatment of injuries to primary teeth. Update Pediatr Dent. 1989;2: 1-7.
29. Kaneshiro S, Nakajima T, Yoshikawa Y, et al. The postoperative maxillary cyst: report of 71 cases. J Oral Surg. 1981;39: 194.
30. Levitch LC, Bader JD, Shugars DA, et al. Non-carious cervical lesions. T Dent. 1994;22: 195-207.
31. Lynch MA, Brightman VJ, Greenberg MS. Burker's Oral Medicine: Diagnosis and Treatment, 9th edition. Philadelphia: JB Lippincott Company; 1994.
32. Mello HS. The mechanism of tetracycline staining in primary and permanent teeth. T Dent Child. 1967;34: 478-87.
33. Miller G. Fat embolism: a comprehensive review. J Oral Surg. 1975;33: 91.

34. Milosevic A. Tooth wear: an aetiological and diagnostic problem. Eur T Prosthodont Restor Dent. 1993;1: 173-8.
35. Miserendino LJ, Pirk RM. Lasers in dentistry. New York: Quintessence Publishing Co Inc.; 1995.
36. Morrish RB Jr, Chan E, Silverman S Jr, et al. Osteonecrosis in patients irradiated for head and neck carcinoma cancer. Cancer. 1981; 47(8):1980-3.
37. Neville BW, Damm DD, Allen CA, et al. Oral and Maxillofacial Pathology, 2nd edition. Philadelphia: Saunders (an imprint of Elsevier); 2002.
38. Ohba T, Yang RC, Chen CY, et al. Postoperative maxillary cyst. Int J Oral Surg. 1980;9: 480.
39. Parirokh M, Asgary S, Eghbal MJ, et al. A comparative study of white and gray mineral trioxide aggregate as pulp capping agents in dog's teeth. Dent Traumatol. 2005;21(3): 150-4.
40. Paterson JR. Tetracycline stained vital teeth—review of literature. T Indiana Dent Assoc. 1979: 58: 18-22.
41. Phillips RW. Skinner's Science of Dental Materials. 8th edition. Philadelphia: WB Saunders Company; 1982.
42. Quincke H. UberakutesumschirebenesHaautodemMonatschrPrakDemat. 1882;1: 129.
43. Regezi JA, Scuibba J. Oral pathology: clinical-pathologic correlations, 2nd edition. Philadelphia: WB Saunders Company; 1993.
44. Seals RR Cain JR. Prosthetic treatment for chemical burns of the oral cavity. T Prosthet Dent. 1985;53: 688-91.
45. Smith RG, Burtner AP. Oral side-effects of the most frequently prescribed drugs. Spec Care Dentist. 1994;14: 96-102.
46. Soames JV, Southam JC. Oral pathology, 3rd edition. London: Oxford University Press; 1999.
47. Spieler EL. Toothbrush abrasion: prevention and the alert toothbrush. Compend Contin Educ Dent. 1994;15: 306-12.
48. Thompson JC, Ashwal S. Electrical injuries in children. Am T Dis Child. 1983;137: 231: 5.
49. Westernman GH, Hicks MJ, Flaitz CM, et al. Argon laser irradiation in root surface caries: In vitro study examines laser's effects. J Am Dent Assoc. 1994;125: 401-7.
50. White JM, Swift EJ Jr. Lasers for use in dentistry. J Esthet Restor Dentist. 2005;17(1): 60-5.
51. With TK. Porphyrias in animals. Clin Hematol. 1980;9: 345-70.
52. Wood JF. Mucosal reaction to cobalt-chromium alloy. Brit Dent J. 1974;136: 423.
53. Wright JM, Barton FE, Ryrd DL, et al. Complications of the treatment of oral cancer. In: Oral cancer: clinical and pathological considerations. Boca Raton, FL: CRC Press, 1988.
54. Yamamoto H, Okabe H, Ooya K, et al. Laser effect on vital oral tissues: a preliminary investigation. J Oral Path. 1973;1: 256.

CHAPTER 13

Biopsy and Healing of Oral Wounds

BIOPSY

DEFINITION

Biopsy is the removal of tissue from the living organism for the purpose of microscopic examination and diagnosis.

Biopsy is generally advised for confirmation of diagnosis in patients with suspected oral lesions, where clinical and radiographic or other methods have failed to make a satisfactory diagnosis.

The main objective of biopsy is to obtain sufficient amount of viable tissue from the most representative site a suspected lesion for histopathological interpretation and diagnosis.

It should be remembered that during performing biopsy of any oral epithelial tissue lesion, the biopsy sample should include full thickness of the epithelium as well as sufficient connective tissue. Inclusion of the connective tissue helps to determine if the epithelial lesion has created any change in the underlying tissue (e.g. invasion, inflammatory change, fibrosis, necrosis, giant cell formation or calcification, etc.) and also it (connective tissue) provides physical support to the specimen, so that tissue will not curl or lose its shape after biopsy. Moreover, during biopsy of an oral lesion of mesenchymal tissue origin, tissue sample must be obtained from a greater depth since the lesion is present below the mucosa as well as the lamina propria (Table 13.1).

INDICATIONS OF BIOPSY

The common oral lesions where biopsy should be indicated are as follows:
- Any clinically suspected case of malignancy, unhealed ulcer of long duration, induration,

Table 13.1: Important stromal changes caused by oral epithelial lesions.

Stromal changes	Name of the lesion
• Invasion	• Squamous cell carcinoma
• Pushing margins	• Verrucous carcinoma
• Subepithelial bullae	• Pemphigoid
• Band-like infiltration of lymphocytes	• Lichen planus
• Excessive fibrosis and hyalinization of collagen	• OSF
• Giant cells	• Peripheral giant cell granuloma
• Ossification	• Peripheral ossifying fibroma
• Melanin pigmentation	• Malignant melanoma
• Caseous necrosis	• Tuberculosis
• Hyphae formation: Candidiasis	• Candidiasis
• Edema and hypervascularity	• Pyogenic granuloma
• Islands of healthy epithelium within stroma	• Tangential sectioning

hemorrhage, sudden onset of anesthesia or paresthesia, red or red-white lesions with irregular border and sudden growth in a nevus with color change, etc.
- All suspected benign and malignant tumors of the jawbone
- All precancerous lesions and conditions, e.g. leukoplakia, erythroplakia, OSF and lichen planus, etc. to see dysplastic changes and suspected malignant transformation.
- Confirmation of clinical diagnosis of lesions like pemphigus, pemphigoid and erythema multiforme, etc.
- Sudden acceleration of growth in preexisting bony diseases like Paget's disease of bone, fibrous dysplasia and osteogenesis imperfecta, etc.
- Second biopsy from the margin of a cancerous lesion after surgery, to confirm if the lesion has been completely removed or not.
- Follow-up biopsy in suspected cases of recurrence in already treated cases of cancer and precancer.

■ CONTRAINDICATIONS OF BIOPSY

- Medically compromised patients like-coronary artery disease, renal failure, hepatic impairment and immunocompromised patients, etc.
- Lesions having life-threatening risk of hemorrhage during biopsy, e.g. large hemangioma
- Lesions in close proximity to vital structures like external carotid artery, facial artery and nerve, parotid or submandibular duct, etc.
- Although not fully contraindicated but precautions must be taken before performing biopsy in the following cases—pregnancy (especially in 1st and 3rd trimesters), uncontrolled diabetes, steroid therapy, HIV or hepatitis B infections, hemophilia, purpura, severe anemia and in malignant melanoma (in which disseminated spread of the tumor can occur even with slight trauma during biopsy),

Box 13.1 Different types of biopsy.
- Surgical biopsy—incisional biopsy, excisional biopsy and punch biopsy
- Fine needle aspiration cytology and CT guided FNAC
- Exfoliative cytology
- Brush biopsy
- Frozen section biopsy
- Endoscopic biopsy
- Cone biopsy
- Core needle biopsy
- Suction assisted core needle biopsy
- Laser biopsy

lesion in esthetic areas like vermilion border of lips, etc.

■ TYPES OF BIOPSY

The types of biopsy are given in Box 13.1.

Excisional Biopsy

If a lesion is totally excised for histological evaluation, it is called "excisional biopsy", and this type of biopsy is usually done in case of small lesions (Fig. 13.1).

Generally small, pedunculated, and exophytic lesions in accessible sites of the mouth are often considered for this type of biopsy.

An elliptical deep incision is given around the pedunculated base of the lesion and a wedge-shaped tissue is removed along with the entire lesion.

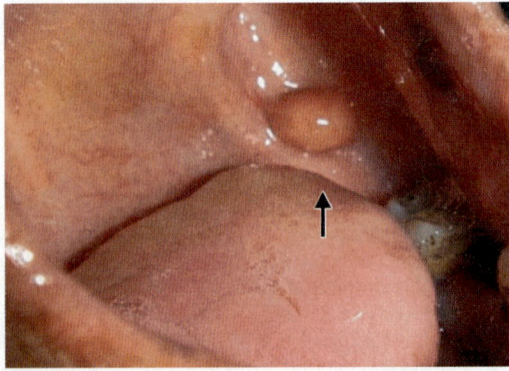

Fig. 13.1: A case for excisional biopsy

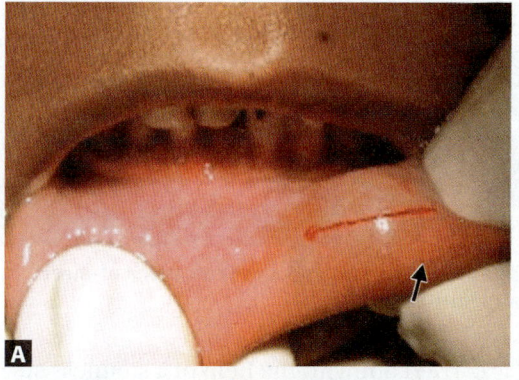 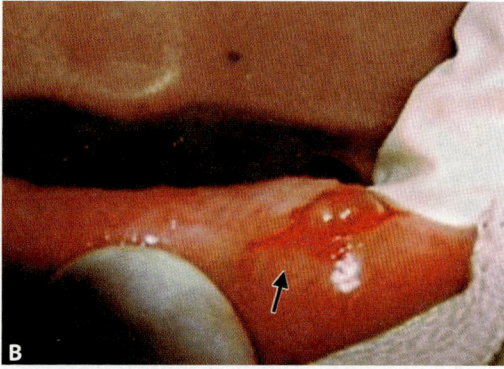

Figs. 13.2A and B: Lower incision given first followed by the upper incision (semilunar type).

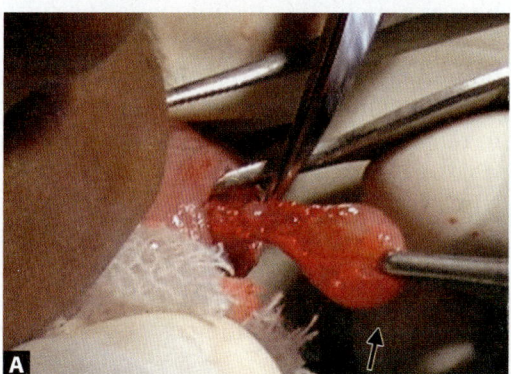 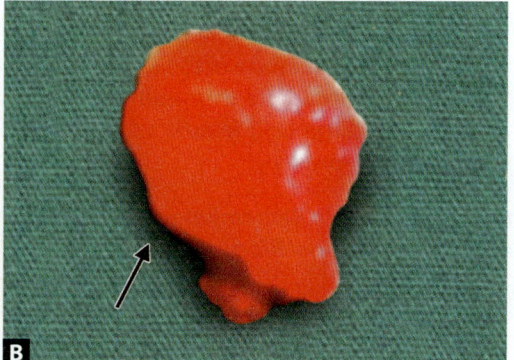

Figs. 13.3A and B: (A) Procedure of excisional biopsy; (B) Tissue sample obtained after excisional biopsy.

Advantage of Excisional Biopsy

Excisional biopsy ensures complete removal of the lesion and no extra surgery is required (Figs. 13.2A and B).

Limitations of Excisional Biopsy

- Can be done only in small lesions, which are expected to be benign.
- Cannot be done is very large lesions with unconfirmed diagnosis.
- It should not be attempted in suspected malignant lesions.

Incisional Biopsy

When only a small section of tissue is removed from a lesion for the purpose of histological evaluation, it is called "incisional biopsy". This type of biopsy is indicated in the case where the lesion is too large to excise initially without knowing the exact diagnosis, or if the lesion is of such nature that the total excision would be irrational (Figs. 13.3A and B).

It is the ideal biopsy technique for suspected malignancies, precancerous lesions spread over a wide area, dermal lesions (e.g. pemphigus and pemphigoid), etc.

Multiple biopsies must be taken in surface lesions, which are spreading over a wide area and exhibiting varying surface characters at different parts of the lesion; for example a single lesion may have areas of redness, pain, ulceration, keratosis, necrosis, and border irregularities, etc. (Figs. 13.4A to C).

Advantage of Incisional Biopsy

Much easier procedure, less chance of postoperative complications, quicker healing, facilitates accurate surgical planning for a

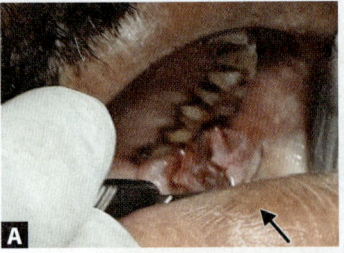 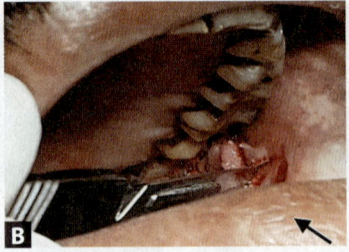 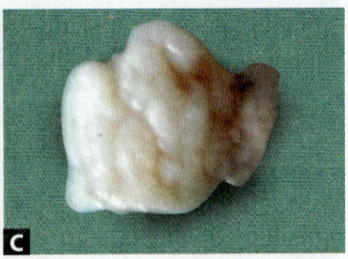

Figs. 13.4A to C: (A and B) Incisional biopsy being done in a case of squamous cell carcinoma of cheek; (C) Tissue sample after the biopsy.

lesion since the diagnosis is confirmed before surgery.

Limitation of Incisional Biopsy

- It does not allow study of the entire lesion.
- Procedure often fails if proper site selection is not done or if insufficient amount of tissue is removed.

Important Points to Remember while Performing Incisional Biopsy

- Selection of most representative site of the lesion
- Anesthetic solution should not be injected directly inside the lesion
- Necrotic tissue from the surface or other debris should be removed before biopsy
- Number 15 scalpel blade should be used
- Elliptical incision should be given as it facilitates quicker healing (by primary intension)
- Length and width ratio of the incision should be 3:1
- Lower incision should be given first so that bleeding does not obscure the field
- A suture may be passed through the lesion for holding it easily while removing the tissue.
- Anterior tip of the ellipse to be lifted first with tissue forceps and the base is cut with blade.

Punch Biopsy

Punch biopsy, the name came from the word 'punch' that means dissection or removal; it is carried out with the help of a stainless steel round ended cutting instrument called 'tissue biopsy punch'. This technique is useful for both incisional or excisional purposes and it particularly useful in obtaining tissue samples from the skin and mucous membrane. It helps in removing tissue samples from a variety of lesions, e.g. oral cancers and precancers, red-white lesions, moles and small lumps, etc.

In the mouth, tongue and buccal mucosa are the ideal areas for punch biopsy; since the instrument can be placed perpendicularly over these areas for cutting.

Procedure of Punch Biopsy

Punch is placed on the lesion and a downward, twisting motion is applied to ensure a circular incision; the tissue is cut from the base with a curved scissor.

Advantages of Punch Biopsy

Easier technique and unnecessary tissue cutting can be avoided.

Limitations of Punch Biopsy

- Only applicable in certain accessible parts of mouth, e.g. tongue, lip and buccal mucosa, etc.
- Cannot be performed in areas like floor of mouth, soft palate and gingiva, etc.
- Twisting action in punch biopsy often cause detachment between different layers of epithelium or between the epithelium and the connective tissue; hence this technique is not applicable in vesiculobu-

lous lesions, where intraepithelial or subepithelial bullae are important diagnostic clues.
- The wound in punch biopsy is circular and not elliptical in shape and is difficult for suturing.

Cone Biopsy

It is a surgical biopsy and it removes the tissue which is cylindrical or cone shaped. The advantage of this technique is that it provides a large sample of tissue.

Fine Needle Aspiration Cytology

Fine needle aspiration cytology (FNAC) is done by aspirating tissue materials from inside a lesion and is commonly performed in cases of glandular or cystic lesions. This biopsy is done with a fine needle attached to a syringe; during biopsy the needle is inserted into the lesion and then vacuum is created so that tissue samples are sucked into the syringe. The sample is used to prepare a smear and seen under microscope after staining (Figs. 13.5 and 13.6).

CT-guided FNAC

Here, the technique is same as conventional FNAC but the imaging facility attached with the instrument helps in locating the wound to be biopsied.

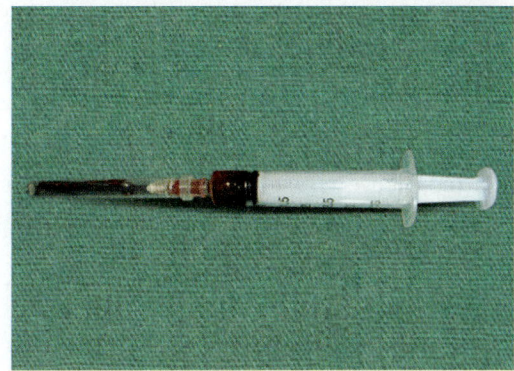

Fig. 13.6: Aspirated sample after fine needle aspiration cytology.

Core Needle Biopsy (Core Biopsy)

The technique is partly same as FNAC but here after the needle (2 mm in diameter) has been inserted into the target lesion, the needle is advanced further within the deeper cell layer to remove the core tissue. The needle has a cutting tip that helps in removing tissue. The advantage of this technique is that it is more definitive procedure than FNAC and can be used in inaccessible lesions.

Vacuum-assisted Core Biopsy

Here, the core biopsy syringe is attached to a suction associated with a vacuum device. Advantage of this technique is that it helps in removing multiple samples in one needle insertion.

Frozen Section Biopsy

Frozen section biopsy is performed in order to get an immediate histological report of a lesion (e.g. often performed during surgery to determine whether a lesion is malignant or not, or to evaluate the margin of an excised cancer to ascertain that the entire lesion is removed). The tissue is obtained from a lesion and the fresh tissue is quickly frozen at about –70°C in liquid nitrogen or dry ice. The frozen tissue is then sectioned in a refrigerated microtome and then stained to get a prompt diagnosis. In this type of biopsy the slides

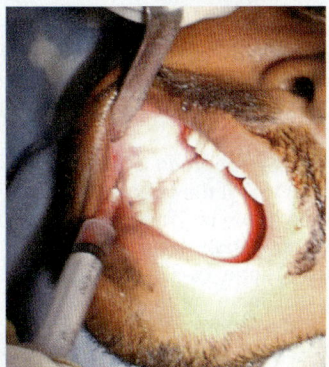

Fig. 13.5: Procedure of fine needle aspiration cytology.

Brush Biopsy

This technique is used to collect cells from the surface as well as subsurface layers of a suspected lesion for microscopic examination. A round stiff bristle brush is rotated vigorously at a particular site of the lesion until bleeding starts, which ensures a sufficiently deep sample. Smear is prepared from the sample, which is scanned under microscope to detect any abnormal cells.

Advantage: Removes deeper cells than what is obtained in simple scrapping of surface during conventional FNAC.

Liquid Biopsy

It is the diagnostic test to detect the cancer biomarkers in the body fluids, especially the blood; the procedure is also called "fluid biopsy" or "fluid phase" biopsy. It is a noninvasive, much painless, more simple and less expensive procedure than the traditional "tissue biopsy"; moreover this biopsy can be repeated several time in different stages of the disease, especially for monitoring purposes.

Materials examined in liquid biopsy: These can be circulating tumor cells (CTCs), circulating cell-free tumor DNA (ctDNA) and circulating tumor RNA (among these, ctDNAs are mostly looked for).

Principle of liquid biopsy: Like normal cells, cancer cells may sometimes be present in blood, moreover these cells may shed or release fragmented DNA (circulating tumor DNA or ctDNA) and RNA into the blood through apoptosis. In liquid biopsy, especially these fragmented DNA (ctDNA) particles are collected from intravenous blood samples and immunohistochemically tested for detection of cancer mutations in them.

cannot be preserved for future references; hence photomicrographs of the slides are important.

PROCEDURE OF TISSUE BIOPSY (BOXES 13.2 AND 13.3)

Box 13.2 Important points to remember while performing biopsy.

- Most suspected or representative site of the lesion should be chosen for biopsy
- The wound should not be painted by any coloring agent before biopsy
- The anesthetic solution should not be injected directly inside the lesion to avoid distortion of the tissue
- Slough or necrotic areas to be avoided for sampling
- Sharp instruments are to be used to avoid tissue tearing
- A suture can be placed through the lesion for holding the tissue, which helps in controlling its movements while cutting and protects it from being swallowed by the patient or absorbed by the suction
- Repeated cutting of the tissue during incision should be avoided
- During biopsy, the tissue is obtained in such a way that it includes both the diseased as well as some normal tissue at the border of the wound
- If the lesion is multifocal or large, it is ideal to obtain more than one sample from different sites for making more accurate diagnosis
- The biopsy specimen should be of sufficient thickness and depth (size of the sample should be at least 1 cm × 0.6 cm and the depth should be 2 mm)
- Edge of the specimen should be vertical and not beveled
- After obtaining the tissue, it should be immediately placed on a glazed paper to avoid tissue curling
- The sample should be labeled properly with patient's name and the clinical details of the lesion
- The wound should be sutured and bleeding must be controlled
- If the biopsy specimen is a calcified tissue (e.g. bone and tooth) then decalcification of the said specimen is to be done before the standard processing and sectioning. Decalcification is usually done by keeping the specimen in ethylenediamine tetra-acetic acid (EDTA) or other acid solutions
- Biopsy should be repeated, if the diagnosis is not consistent with the clinical findings or the provisional diagnosis

> **Box 13.3** Fixation of biopsy specimen.
> - Fixation of the tissue specimen is necessary immediately after biopsy to avoid autolysis; which may cause loss of microscopic details
> - 10% formal saline (formaldehyde solution in normal saline or a neutral pH buffer) is the routinely used fixative in biopsy
> - Small specimens are generally fixed overnight and large specimens are fixed for 24 hours; so that the fixative can penetrate and diffuse into the tissue specimen
> - Tissue specimens must be fixed before it is processed
> - The volume of the fixative should be at least 10 times to that of the tissue
> - For large specimens, proper incisions to be given to allow penetration of the fixative up to the center of the specimen

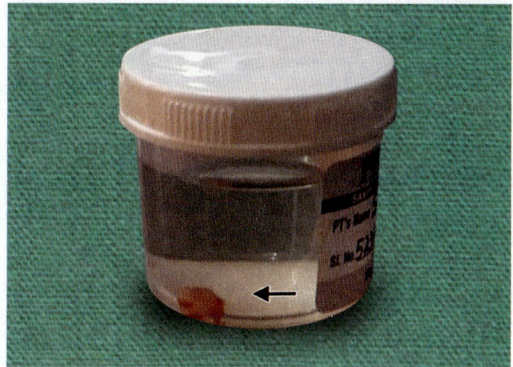

Fig. 13.7: Biopsy sample in formalin fixative.

- The area of the wound from where the biopsy will be taken is cleaned first.
- The area is anesthetized.
- The most representative site of the wound is identified.
- Elliptical incision given, lower incision given first then upper; so that bleeding does not hamper visibility.
- A section of tissue from the identified site of wound (or sometimes the entire wound) is removed.
- The tissue is cleaned and put into 10% formalin solution for fixation (Fig. 13.7).
- The biopsy site is sutured after achieving hemostasis.
- The biopsy specimen is sent for processing, sectioning, staining and microscopic diagnosis.

LABELLING OF SPECIMEN

After the biopsy, the specimen should be properly labeled in the following manners.
- Mention the name, age and sex of the patient.
- Mention the date and time of biopsy.
- Mention the type of biopsy, the site from where it is obtained and the nature of the tissue (e.g. bone tissue or soft tissue, etc.).
- Mention the brief clinical, radiological and other relevant features of the lesion (if any).
- Mention the provisional diagnosis.

Tissue Processing

- After fixation of the tissue, it is dehydrated in a series of solvents.
- It is then impregnated with paraffin wax and a wax block is prepared.
- The wax block is mounted on a microtome and ultrathin sections (4 μm) are made.
- The section is mounted on a glass microscope slide for staining.
- Hematoxylin and eosin stain is often routinely used for staining of the tissue (Table 13.2).

BIOPSY REPORT

- A negative report should not be considered final, especially if it is totally unexpected than what was thought earlier.
- Biopsy should be repeated, if there is any doubt regarding the diagnosis (Box 13.4).
- If further investigations are required, e.g. histochemistry, immunohistochemistry, tissue culture or animal inoculation, etc. should be done.

Exfoliative Cytology

Exfoliative cytology is the microscopic study of cells obtained from the surface of an organ or lesion after suitable staining.

Table 13.2: Staining characteristics of various tissues with hematoxylin and eosin (H/E).

Hematoxylin (basic dye) stains the tissue blue-black	Eosin (acidic dye) stains the tissue red
• Nucleus (DNA, RNA)	• Cell cytoplasm
• Ground substance of connective tissue	• Keratin • Muscle cytoplasm
• Reversal lines of bone	• Decalcified bone • Collagen

The neoplastic cells are less cohesive than the other normal cells and usually they shed on the surface of the lesion or into the secretion (e.g. the saliva). The shed neoplastic cells are obtained from the lesion by scrapping its surface and are then evaluated for possible changes like dysplasia (indicative of their cancerous origin) or malignancy, etc.

Technique of Exfoliative Cytology
- First of all the surface of the lesion is cleaned by removing all the debris and mucins, etc.
- After that, gentle scrapping is done on the surface of the lesion with a metal cement spatula or a moistened tongue blade for several times.
- Thus, materials present on the surface of the lesion are adhered or collected at the border of the instrument.
- The collected material is then evenly spread over a microscopic slide and is fixed immediately with either 95% alcohol or equal parts of alcohol and ether (Fig. 13.8).

Box 13.4	Causes of failure of biopsy.

- Specimen obtained from unrepresentative site of the lesion
- Damaged or improperly fixed specimen
- Specimen of insufficient depth
- Incorrect processing, sectioning or staining
- Inflammation or secondary infection may mask the exact diagnosis
- Microscopic features are too difficult to interpret as in poorly differentiated lesions
- Lesion with nonspecific histological findings, e.g. aphthous ulcer

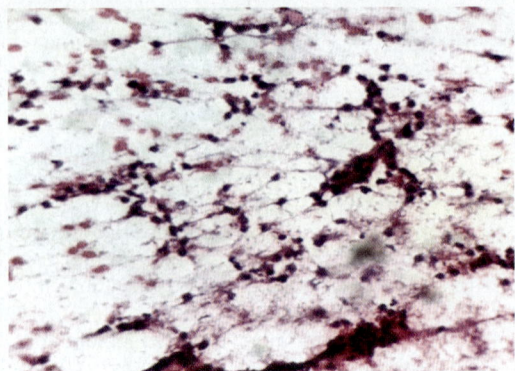

Fig. 13.8: Photomicrograph of exfoliative cytology.

- The slide is then air-dried and is stained by a special stain called PAP stain (Papanicolaou stain).

Important Points in Exfoliative Cytology
- It is not a substitute for, but an adjunct to the conventional surgical biopsy.
- Anesthesia is not required in this technique and it is most useful for screening of cancer, detection of virally infected cells, acantholytic cells and candidal hyphae, etc.
- It is a quick, simple, painless, and bloodless procedure.
- It helps to check the false-negative biopsy cases.
- Special procedures like immunohistochemistry can be performed in exfoliative cytology samples.
- The procedure is especially helpful in follow-up detection of recurrent cancer cases.
- It helps in screening a large number of lesions, which do not look like cancers clinically.
- However, it is unreliable for confirmatory diagnosis of cancers (Box 13.5 and Table 13.3).

HEALING OF ORAL WOUNDS

Individual factors affecting the healing of oral wounds are as follows:
- *Age*: The rate of wound healing in younger individuals is faster in comparison to that of the older individuals.

> **Box 13.5** Indications of exfoliative cytology.
>
> The exfoliative cytology can be helpful for the diagnosis of the following oral lesions:
> - Herpes simplex
> - Herpes zoster
> - Pemphigus vulgaris
> - Pemphigoid
> - Squamous cell carcinoma
> - Aphthous ulcer
> - Candidiasis

- *Type of tissue*: Different types of tissue in our body exhibit variation in their healing potential. For example, the epithelial tissue heals up at a much faster rate in comparison to the neural tissue.
- *Location of the wound*: Wounds in an area where there is a good vascular supply heal more rapidly than those located in the relatively avascular areas.
- *Mobility of the wound*: If the wound site is subjected to constant movements, the rate of wound healing is delayed and it may be due to repeated disruptions of the newly formed connective tissue. The immobilized soft tissue or bony wounds usually heal at a faster pace.
- *Trauma*: Mild trauma to the tissue may hasten its healing process, but severe trauma definitely retards the healing.
- *Local temperature*: If the local temperature in the area is high and is well maintained, the healing process occurs at a faster rate. But, if the local temperature in the area is low, the healing process can be delayed.
- *Radiation*: Low dose of radiation in the tissue stimulates its healing process, whereas a high dose of radiation disturbs the same.
- *Nutritional factors*: Nutritionally deficient persons (especially with deficiency of vitamin C, proteins and minerals, etc.) usually exhibit a slower rate of wound healing.
- *Circulatory factors*: Tissue with a very good blood supply heals at a faster rate in comparison to the tissue whose blood supply is diminished due to certain reasons, e.g. anemia, tissue dehydration or aging, etc.
- *Infections*: A low-grade infection in the tissue may stimulate its healing process. A sterile wound on the other hand heals at a slower pace, however, severe infections in the tissue always disturb the healing process.
- *Hormonal factors*: The trephones (wound hormones) released by proteolytic breakdown of cellular debris, accelerate the healing process. Administration of other hormones, e.g. ACTH, cortisone, etc. causes an inhibition in the growth of granulation tissue and thereby results in a delayed wound healing.

Table 13.3: Interpretation of findings in exfoliative cytology.

Class I (normal)	The findings indicate that only normal cells are present in the smear
Class II (atypical)	The findings indicate the presence of minor cellular atypia, but no evidence of malignancy
Class III (intermediate)	This is an in between cytology that separates cancer from noncancer diagnosis. The cells display wider atypia that may be suggestive of cancer, but the features are not clear-cut. Biopsy is recommended for further confirmation of the diagnosis
Class IV (suggestive of cancer)	The findings indicate that in the lesion, there is presence of few cells with malignant characteristics or many cells with borderline characteristics. Biopsy is mandatory
Class V (positive of cancer)	The cells exhibit definite features of malignancy. Biopsy is mandatory

HEALING OF BIOPSY WOUND

Healing by First Intention (Primary Healing)

When the cut surfaces of the biopsy wound can be approximated or closely sutured, the wound heals up by primary intention. The process occurs in the following manners:
- In the initial phase, there will be formation of blood clot, which helps to hold the parts of the wound together.
- The tissue becomes edematous and an inflammatory process starts, with the infiltration of polymorphonuclear neutrophils (PMN) and lymphocytes into the area.
- The tissue debris collected in the wound are cleared either by the process of phagocytosis or by their lysis with the help of proteolytic enzymes, liberated by the inflammatory cells.
- Once the tissue debris are cleared, granulation tissue forms that replaces the blood clot in the wound, and it usually consists of young blood capillaries, proliferating fibroblasts, PMN and other leukocytes.
- The epithelium at the edge of the wound starts to proliferate and gradually it covers the entire wound surface.
- Finally, the healing process is complete with progressive increase in the amount of dense collagen bundles and decrease in the number of inflammatory cells in the area (Figs. 13.9A and B).

Healing by Secondary Intention

When the opposing margins of the wound cannot be approximated together by suturing, the wound fills in from the base with the formation of a larger amount of granulation tissue, such type of healing of the open wound is known as "healing by secondary intention" or "secondary healing". It takes place in the following way (Fig. 13.9C):
- The secondary healing occurs essentially by the same process as seen in the primary healing, the only difference is that a more severe inflammatory reaction and an exuberant fibroblastic and endothelial cell proliferation occur in the later.
- In secondary healing, once the blood clot is removed, the granulation tissue fills up the entire area and the epithelium begins to grow over it, until the wound surface is completely epithelized.
- Later on, the inflammatory exudates disappear slowly and the fibroblasts produce large amounts of collagen.
- Most of the healing processes occurring due to secondary intention, result in scar formation at the healing site. However, in the oral cavity these are rare (Figs. 13.10 and 13.11).

HEALING OF GINGIVECTOMY WOUND

Early Healing Phase

Almost immediately after the procedure there is formation of blood clot, which actually

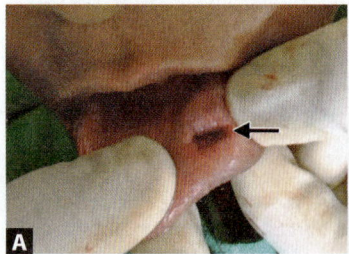 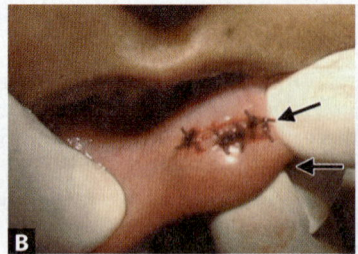 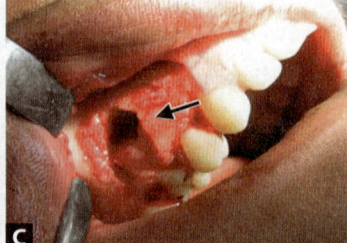

Figs. 13.9A to C: (A) A fresh biopsy wound; (B) A biopsy wound to be healed by primary intention; (C) A wound to be healed by secondary intention.

of the wound, the epithelial cells also start proliferating and approximately 72 hours after the surgery the deeper part of the blood clot is converted into a layer of young, granulation tissue. The superficial portion of the tissue is filled with PMN. The epithelium progresses to cover up the wound below the surface layer of the clot.

Late Healing Phase

Organization of the clot is completed with formation of a dense connective tissue mass. The epithelium is thin but if it covers up the entire wound surface it matures gradually and there is formation of rete-pegs. There is gradual decrease in the number of inflammatory cells. Formation of the labial and lingual surface occurs first and finally, within few days, there will be development of the interproximal gingiva. The later occurs by union of the labial and lingual gingiva.

HEALING OF THE EXTRACTION WOUND

Healing in an *extraction socket* occurs in the following steps (Figs. 13.12A and B):
- Soon after a tooth is extracted, bleeding occurs in the socket and the clot is formed.
- Within a day, the periphery of the clot shows edema and neutrophilic cell infiltrations.

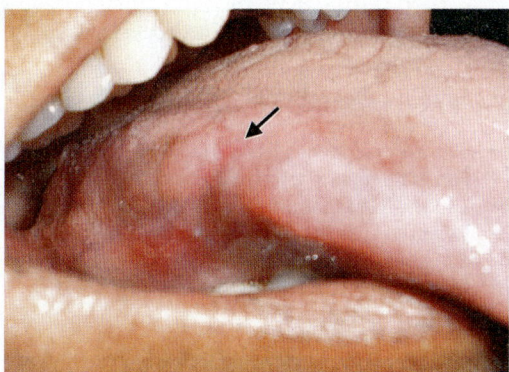

Fig. 13.10: Healing of biopsy wound after 5 days.

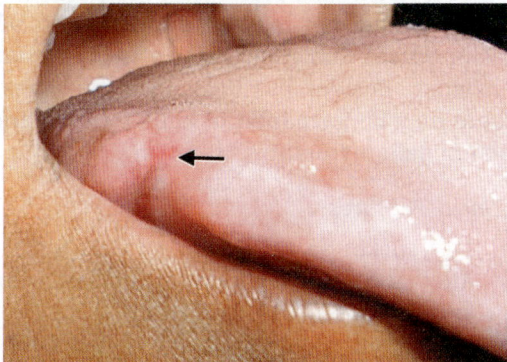

Fig. 13.11: Healing of wound in tongue after 7 days.

keeps the area covered. Approximately, 48 hours after gingivectomy, proliferation of fibroblast and young blood capillaries begin just beneath the blood clot. At the margin

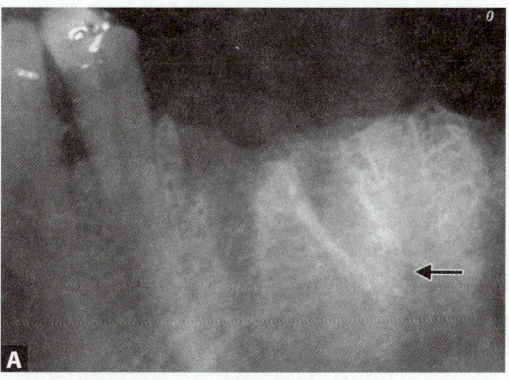
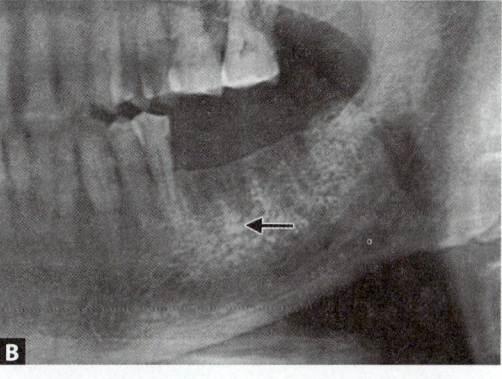

Figs. 13.12A and B: (A) Wound of extraction socket before healing; (B) Healing of same wound after 1 month.

- In the next 2–4 days, fibroblasts and endothelial cells proliferate into the surrounding bone marrow spaces and they gradually enter into the clot. This process is called "organization of the clot".
- At the same time, removal of the debris (e.g. necrotic tissue, dead cells and dead pieces of bone, etc.) from the wound also takes place, and it is done by the neutrophils, macrophages and the osteoclast cells, etc. (they cause either phagocytosis or proteolysis of the said debris).
- The clot organization process is completed usually by a week and following this, the epithelium at the periphery of the wound starts growing and it gradually covers of the entire socket area.
- Later on, the inflammatory cells decrease in number and the collagen fibers increase in the area.
- In about 10–15 days, immature bone or osteoids start forming at the margin of the socket. They move into the socket and gradually fill up the entire socket by replacing the granulation tissue.
- Finally, in about 3 weeks to 6 months' time, the entire socket is filled with mature bone that replaces the osteoids.

Dry Socket (Alveolar Osteitis)

Definition

Dry socket can be defined as the failure of appropriate healing after tooth extraction due to disruption of initial clot with eventual lack of organization by granulation tissue.

Dry socket is the most common complication of an extraction and it develops in about 5% cases in all extractions. However, the incidence rate is much higher in relation to impacted 3rd molars (Box 13.6).

Pathogenesis

After a tooth is extracted blood clot forms, which stops further bleeding, protects the wound and promotes healing. Dry socket develops if the blood clot is lost from the wound and the bony wall of the socket is exposed to the air, food and fluids, etc. The loss of blood clot may be due to excessive localized fibrinolytic action or bacterial enzymes. Besides the fibrinolytic enzymes, there may be formation of kinins, which are potent pain mediators.

Box 13.6 Possible causes of dry socket.
- Traumatic extraction
- Smoking after extraction
- Excessive rinsing after tooth extraction
- Oral contraceptives use during extraction
- Foods being impacted in the socket
- Limited local blood supply
- Excessive use of vasoconstrictors in the local anesthesia
- Osteosclerotic bone disease
- Previous radiotherapy
- Preexisting pericoronitis

Clinical Features

- Dry socket generally develops 2–4 days after tooth extraction and it lasts for several days.
- Maximum numbers of dry socket cases are seen in relation to the mandibular 3rd molar teeth.
- Women suffer from the condition more often than men.
- The dry socket is usually a very painful condition; the nature of pain is intense, deep seated and throbbing type and the patient often has a foul breath.
- The pain may be continuous for weeks or months and the dead bones from the socket wall may shed as "crumb-like" fragments.
- Clinical examination reveals a socket devoid of clot and the bony walls of the socket are bare, whitish, and visible.
- Mucosa around the dry socket is red, inflamed looking and tendered.
- Sometimes the socket may be filled with decomposing food debris and the dead bone; the bony walls of the socket may be felt as a rough area with probe.

- Local swelling and lymphadenopathy, etc. are less frequently seen.
- Sometimes the gingival tissue from the adjacent area may overgrow and fills up the socket.

Radiological Finding

Radiologically, dry socket presents unhealed bony socket long time after the extraction, and sometimes there may be formation of sequestrum.

Histopathology
- Histologic sections of the socket wall reveal the formation of necrotic bone, containing empty lacunae.
- There is intense inflammatory reaction in the surrounding bone.
- Dry socket is a localized osteitis and not an osteomyelitis and the condition heals very slowly.

Treatment

Zinc oxide eugenol pack is often given in the socket for palliative reaction.

HEALING OF THE FRACTURED JAWBONE

Once a jawbone is fractured, bleeding occurs immediately at the site and a hematoma forms, which is converted into a mass of blood clot. From this clot formation onwards, the healing is completed in three stages (Fig. 13.13).

Stage I: Formation of Fibrous Callus

- At this stage, inflammatory reactions take place in the bone at the periphery of the fracture site and there is proliferation of fibroblasts and endothelial cells in the bone marrow as well as in the periosteum. These cellular elements enter into the fracture site and organize the clot.
- Along with the clot organization, edema develops and inflammatory cell (e.g.

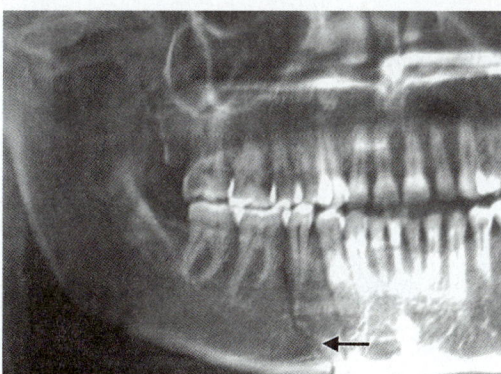

Fig. 13.13: Fracture wound in body of mandible.

neutrophils, plasma cells and lymphocytes, etc.) infiltration also gradually occurs in the area.
- The necrotic cells, connective tissue and bone fragments are removed from the fracture site by phagocytosis, proteolysis and osteolysis, etc.
- Within few days, the clot is replaced by granulation tissue, which later on forms a fibrous tissue mass (fibrous callus) at the fracture site.

Stage II: Formation of Primary Bone Callus

During this stage, the fibrous callus is gradually replaced by immature bone or osteoids at the fracture site. Generally, the primary bone callus forms in an amount which is far in excess to its requirement, and it usually extends to cover up areas beyond the fracture line in all directions.

Both the fibrous and primary bone callus binds the fractured fragments of bone together, and they appear radiolucent when a radiograph is taken (Fig. 13.14).

Stage III: Formation of Secondary Bone Callus

During this stage, the mature bone replaces the primary bone callus gradually. This mature bone callus is not exuberant in amount and it usually appears radiopaque.

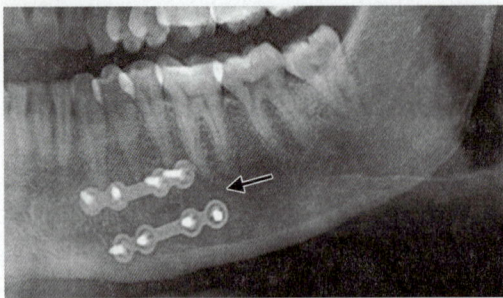

Fig. 13.14: Healing of wound after jaw fracture.

Later on, the secondary callus is remodeled by resorption of its excess bony tissue and finally a normal jaw outline is restored.

Replantation of Tooth

Definition

Replantation can be defined as the purposeful removal of a tooth and its almost immediate replacement with the object of obturating the canals apically while the tooth is out of its socket.

Replantation is planned to save a tooth where conventional endodontic therapy or endodontic surgery has failed. It is a system of organization, sterility, and quickness.

Indications

- Difficult access in the tooth (it is true in case of lower 2nd molar).
- *Anatomic limitation*: Tooth apex in close proximity to the important nerves and vessels.
- Perforations in areas not accessible surgically.
- *Medically compromised patients*: Handicapped, geriatric and non-cooperating.
- Failed previous apical surgery.
- When apical surgery can possibly create defects in other teeth.
- Deciduous teeth needed as space maintainers.
- To preserve postextraction alveolar bone for a prosthesis.
- Persistent chronic pain.
- Accidental avulsion of tooth.

Contraindications

- Preexisting moderate to severe periodontitis
- Curved or flared roots
- Nonrestorable tooth
- Missing interseptal bone.

Procedure of Replantation

Case selection
The ideal tooth for replantation is one that has relatively straight roots and some furcation area, because they can be more stable when replanted. A tooth with fused roots and no furcation area is not a good case for replacement, since it is difficult to stabilize such tooth in the socket. If the tooth breaks or fractures during extraction, replantation will be impossible.

Process of extraction
- Exaction should be done under block anesthesia and there should be least amount of trauma or compression to the periodontal ligament. Severe luxation should be avoided to protect the integrity of the cortical and inter-radicular bone.
- No elevators to be used during extraction to avoid damage to the periodontal ligament and the cementum.
- Beaks of the forceps should not go beyond the cementoenamel junction while holding the tooth for extraction, otherwise there will be damage of the cemental tissue.
- Extraction is done with a slow rocking movement and for the said purpose extraction of one tooth might take time as long as 20–30 minutes.

Postextraction Tooth Care

- Once the intact tooth is removed from the socket, it should be immediately placed into a solution, which can maintain the viability of the periodontal ligament.
- A solution called Hank's balanced salt solution (HBSS), whose composition and pH is similar to that of normal saliva can be used for this purpose.

- The socket should not be curetted and no granulation tissue should be removed from the apical region.
- If the socket is touched, there will be postoperative resorption of bone.

External RCT and Apicectomy

Once the tooth is removed, apicectomy is done and root canals are filled; and the root ends are polished.

Replantation

- Once the tooth is endodontically treated (extraorally), it is placed back into the socket and the buccal and lingual cortical plates are compressed manually.
- Patient is advised to bite for few minutes on the tooth with the help of a wooden stick to stabilize it. Once the tooth is properly placed and gentle pressure is given, it often pops back into the socket with little mobility remaining. Splinting may be used in some cases.

Causes of failure of replantation:

- *Resorption*: Mild resorption may result in ankylosis of the tooth and in such cases the replantation may not fail, however, in severe cases of inflammatory root resorption, the procedure may fail.
- *Infections*: Severe chronic infection may prevent proper healing and may result in failure of the procedure.
- *Pain*: In case of chronic uncontrolled pain the tooth should be removed.
- *Fracture*: Fracture of the tooth or the cortical bone during replantation results in automatic failure of the procedure.

Transplantation of Teeth

Definition

Transplantation refers to the replacement of one damaged tooth by another tooth.

Most common example of transplantation is replacement of mandibular first molar tooth by a developing mandibular 3rd molar.

Types of Transplantation

Transplantations may be of two types:
1. *Autogenous transplantation*: When the replacing tooth is obtained from the same person.
2. *Homologous transplantation*: When the replacing tooth is collected from another person.

Once the tooth is transplanted it remains stable in the new location because it develops fresh periodontal ligament, cementum, gingiva, epithelial attachment and alveolar bone, etc. The pulp remains vital and becomes revascularized. Therefore, the transplanted tooth behaves clinically and physiologically like a normal viable tooth.

Criteria of a Successful Transplantation

- The transplanted tooth must develop attachment in the new socket.
- There should be development of new periodontal ligament, alveolar bone, gingiva and epithelial attachment, etc.
- The tooth should be physiologically, clinically, and radiographically normal and vital.
- The transplanted tooth should perform masticatory functions as good as any other tooth in the jaw.
- It must be cosmetically acceptable.
- There should not be any periodontal or peri-apical lesion or any abnormal resorption.

Causes of Failure of Transplantation

- Lack of generation of fresh attachment tissues in the new socket
- Infections
- Resorption.

HEALING AROUND OSTEOINTEGRATED IMPLANTS

Definition

Osteointegrated implants are those in which a direct, functional, and structural union develops between the living bone and the surface of the implant (Fig. 13.15).

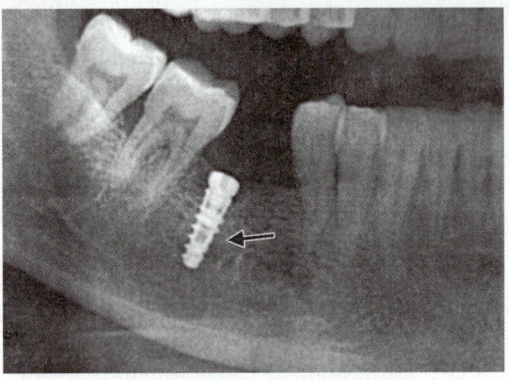

Fig. 13.15: Healing around osteo-integrated implant.

Criteria for a Successful Implant

- The material should be biocompatible.
- The surface of the implant should be rough so that it can provide a greater surface area for bone contact.
- Strict aseptic techniques should be employed to prevent any postsurgical infection.
- While drilling the bone to prepare holes for inserting the implant post, overheating must be avoided.
- Temperature above 47°C causes damage of the bone and interferes with healing.
- Plaque accumulation should be avoided around the implant margins.
- Sufficient healing period should be permitted (about 3 months) for proper osteointegration and during that period no load should be applied on the implant.

Healing: Once the implant is placed in the bone, first of all there is formation of a thin layer of blood clot along the surface of the implant.

The clot organizes, as there is proliferation of fibroblasts and blood capillaries from the adjacent normal connective tissue. A layer of granulation tissue forms in the process and with time, it is replaced by cancellous and compact bone and fibrous marrow.

The alveolar connective tissue comes in close contact with the implant surface and dense bundles of collagen run parallel to the long axis of the implant.

The gingival epithelium encircles around the implant as a collar and it attaches with the implant surface by a basal lamina and hemidesmosomal junction similar to that of the junctional epithelium. Although, light microscopically the implant appears to be in direct contact with the bone, electron microscopy reveals the presence of an electron dense, nonmineralized layer of tissue, which separates the two tissues.

BIBLIOGRAPHY

1. Prabhu SR, Daftury DK, Johnson NW. Oral diseases in the tropic. Oxford: Oxford University Press; 1992.
2. Andreason JO, Andreason FM. Avulsions. In: Andreason JO, AndreasonFM(Eds). Text book and color atlas of traumatic injuries to the teeth, 3rd edition. St. Louis: Mosby; 1994.
3. Birn J. Etiology and pathogenesis of fibrinolyticalveolitis ("dry socker"). Int J Oral Surg. 1973;2:211.
4. Borea G. Tooth germ transplantation. Int Dent J. 1972;22:301.
5. Brånemark PI, Albektsson T. An introduction to osseointegration. Tissue-integrated Prostheses: Osseointegration in Clinical Dentistry. Chicago: Quintessence; 1985. pp. 11-53.
6. Cawson JW, Eveson RA. Oral pathology and diagnosis-color atlas with integrated text, 1st edition. Portsmouth, New Hampshire: William Heinemann Medical Books Limited; 1987.
7. Cook RM. The current status of autogenous transplantation as applied to the maxillary canine. Int Dent J. 1972;22:286.
8. Dunlap CL, Barker BF. Myospherulosis of the jaws. Oral Surg. 1980;50:238,1.
9. Eveson JW, Shear M. Cysts of the Oral region, 3rd edition. Oxford: Butterworth-Heinemann Ltd.; 1992.
10. White SC, Goaz PW. Oral radiology: principles and interpretations. Philadelphia: Elsevier Health; 2014.
11. Hansen J, Fiboek B. Clinical experience of auto-and allotransplantation of teeth. Int Dent J. 1972;22:270.
12. Philip SJ, Eversole LR, Wysocki JP. Contemporary oral and maxillofacial pathology. St. Louis: Mosby; 2003.

13. Macleod J. Davidson's Principles and Practice of medicine, 14th edition. Philadelphia: Churchill Livingstone; 1977.
14. Lang NP, Karring T. Proceedings of the First European workshop on periodontology. Chicago: Quintessence Publishing; 1994.
15. Eversole LR. Clinical outline of oral pathology: diagnosis and treatment. New York: People's Medical Publishing House; 2001.
16. Lilly GE, Osbon DB, Rael EM, et al. Alveolar osteitis associated with mandibular third molar extractions. J Am Dent Assoc. 1974; 88:802.
17. Lynch MA, Brightman VJ, Greenberg MS. Burket's oral medicine–diagnosis and treatment, 9th edition. Philadelphia: Lippincott Williams and Wilkins; 1994.
18. Regezi J, Sciubba J, Jordan R. Oral Pathology, 6th edition. New York: Elsevier; 2011.
19. Natiella JR, Armitage JE, Greene GW. The replantation and transplantation of teeth. A Review. Oral Surg.1970;29:397.
20. Newman MG, Takei J, Carranza FA. Carranza's clinical periodontology, 9th edition. Philadelphia: Saunders, 2002.
21. Ahmed R. Special issue on 102nd birth anniversary celebration. WB State Dent J. 2013.
22. Regezi J, Sciubba J, Jordan R. Oral Pathology, 6th edition. New York: Elsevier; 2011.
23. Shafer WG. A textbook of oral pathology, 4th edition. Philadelphia: WB Saunders Co.; 1983.
24. Soames JV, Southam JC. Oral Pathology, 3rd edition. Oxford: Oxford University Press; 1998.
25. Tencate AR. Oral Histology: development, structure, and function, 3rd edition. St. Louis: Mosby; 1989.
26. The Lippincott Manual of Nursing Practice, 2nd edition. Philadelphia: JB Lippincott Company; 1978.
27. Van Winkle W Jr, Hastngs JC, Hinbes D, et al. Effect of suture materials on healing skin wounds. Surg Gynecol Obstet. 1975;140:1.
28. Wood NK, Goaz PW. Differential Diagnosis of Oral Lesions, 4th edition. St. Louis: Mosby; 1997.

CHAPTER 14

Oral Aspects of Metabolic Disorders

DISTURBANCES IN MINERAL METABOLISM

Many essential body functions require the participation and interaction of various mineral ions. These minerals could be involved in bone formation or activation of endocrine functions or maintenance of cardiovascular functions, etc. Moreover, they can also act as co-factors in various enzymatic functions. In the following section metabolic aspect of certain essential minerals will be discussed.

■ CALCIUM

Calcium is primarily required for making the structural form of skeleton, where it is present in large quantity (about 1–2 Kg), which is much more than any other minerals found in our body. Besides the skeleton (where about 98% of all body calcium is present in the form of calcium phosphate salts), some amount of calcium is present in blood serum and very little portion is present in ionic form. The normal serum calcium concentration in adult humans is about 9–10 mg/dL. Parathyroid hormone (PTH) controls the plasma calcium levels; when blood calcium level drops it releases calcium ions into the serum by resorbing the bone minerals. On the other hand, it can withdraw calcium from blood if its level becomes high (Boxes 14.1 and 14.2). Thus nearly 0.5 mg of calcium is entering and leaving the skeleton daily.

> **Box 14.1** Effects of low calcium levels in plasma.
> - Increased neuromuscular irritability
> - Tetany—characterized by perioral muscular spasm and carpopedal spasm
> - Convulsions and laryngospasms
> - Defective blood coagulation
> - Disturbance in normal heart rhythm
> - Irregularity in normal membrane permeability
> - Defective formation of bones and teeth
> - Bone resorptions and increased osteoporosis

> **Box 14.2** Effects of increased calcium levels in plasma.
> - Anorexia, nausea, vomiting, constipation, depression and lethargy, etc.
> - Depressed nerve conductivity and muscle rigor
> - Coma
> - Deposition of solid calcium and phosphorus stones within the blood vessels, mucous membrane, skin and kidney, etc.

Calcitonin is the hormone that helps to reduce the serum calcium level by incorporation of calcium into the bone and thus oppose the action of parathyroid. Calmodulin is a small calcium binding messenger protein that modifies the activity of many enzymes and other proteins in response to changes in serum concentration of calcium.

Dietary Source

Dietary source of calcium mostly comes from milk; the other sources include dairy products, fruits, calcium rich water and green leafy vegetables, etc.

The calcium enters the plasma either via its absorption from the intestinal tract or through resorption of calcium ions from the bone mineral. The bone serves as the important storage.

Calcium leaves the plasma via secretion into the gastrointestinal tract, urinary excretion, and sweating and further redeposition into bone mineral.

Factors affecting the absorption of calcium into the body from diet:
- Vitamin D is an important cofactor, which increases the absorption of calcium from the intestine.
- Reduction in the level of parathyroid hormone in blood causes increased calcium absorption.
- Chemicals like, citrates or oxalates and pathological conditions, e.g. sprue, etc. cause decreased calcium absorption.

Pathologic Calcifications

Pathologic calcification is the abnormal deposition of calcium salts in any tissues except the teeth and bones.

Types
- Dystrophic
- Metastatic
- Calcinosis.

Dystrophic Calcification

It is a type of pathologic calcification characterized by deposition of calcium salts in dead or degenerated tissues; with normal calcium metabolism and normal serum calcium levels. It is not associated with increased levels of serum calcium but related to the change in the local environment, e.g. increased local tissue alkalinity, etc.

Pathogenesis of dystrophic calcification: As calcium salts enter into the dead tissue, they bind to the phosphate and produce apatite crystals of calcium phosphate.

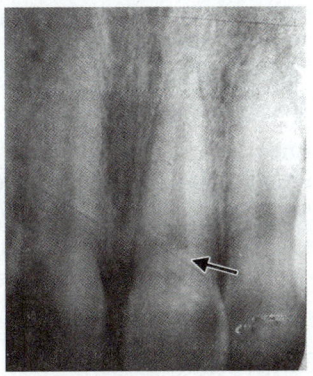

Fig. 14.1: Radiograph showing pulp stone.

Examples of dystrophic calcification
- Tuberculosis (calcification in the areas of caseous necrosis) and lymph node.
- Pulp stones (Fig. 14.1)
- Calcification of the gingival tissue, tongue and buccal mucosa
- Calcification in CEOT, ossifying fibroma, cementifying fibroma and cysts like COC
- Blood vessel arteriosclerosis.

Metastatic Calcification

Abnormal deposition of calcium in apparently normal tissues due to increased serum calcium (hyperkalemia) and abnormal calcium metabolism in the body. This type of calcification usually involves tissues, e.g. lung, kidney, gastrointestinal tract (GIT), blood vessels and oral mucosa and jawbones.

Examples of metastatic calcifications
- Primary hyperparathyroidism
- Multiple myeloma
- Hypervitaminosis-D
- Sarcoidosis
- Paget's disease of bone
- Metastatic tumor of bone
- Renal failure
- Parathyroid adenomas.

Calcinosis

Abnormal deposition of calcium under or within the skin or epithelium. It is often seen in cases of scleroderma and dermatomyositis, etc.

PHOSPHORUS

Phosphorous is an essential mineral element in bone metabolism and plays crucial roles in the formation of bones and teeth. Besides this, phosphorus plays some other important roles in body functions, which are as given in Box 14.3.

Hyperphosphatemia

Increased phosphorus levels (above 4.5 mg/dL results in hyperphosphatemia; which may cause abnormal calcification in different parts of the body. The possible causes of the condition include—renal failure with decreased excretion, hypoparathyroidism and excess phosphorus given in IV injections, etc.

Hypophosphatemia

Decreased phosphorus levels or hypophosphatemia occurs when the serum phosphorus level goes below 2.5 mg/dL.

Causes
- Renal failure with increased excretion
- Heavy metal poisoning
- Starvation
- Respiratory alkalosis
- Sepsis.

Clinical Features

Hypophosphatemia may result in anorexia, bone pain, muscular weakness, waddling gait, defective growth in children, thrombocytopenia, decreased WBC formation, and hemolytic anemia, etc.

Hypophosphatasia

Hypophosphatasia is a hereditary disorder characterized by the deficiency of alkaline phosphatase in the blood and in the tissues. The condition causes defective bone mineralization and there is also defective cementogenesis.

Clinical Features
- Premature loss of primary teeth
- Enlarged pulp chambers of the primary teeth
- Lack of cementum formation on the root surface
- Hypoplasia of enamel
- Inadequate mineralization of the long bones with rickets-like change
- Premature exfoliation of permanent teeth (sometimes it is the only manifestation of the disease).

IRON

Iron deficiency is a common finding in protein energy malnutrition and it occurs due to the following causes:
- Chronic blood loss due to worm infestations
- Decreased absorption of iron
- Increased hepatic sequestration of iron.

Absorption

Iron is absorbed as ferrous or ferric salts from the upper part of duodenum.

Clinical Features

- Esophageal web in Plummer-Vinson's syndrome
- Spooning of nails
- Oral ulceration and sore tongue
- loss of color of the facial skin
- Fissuring in the angle of the mouth
  Myeloperoxidase is an iron-containing enzyme involved in antibacterial activation of

---

Box 14.3 Functions of phosphorus in the body.

- It helps in the metabolism of carbohydrates and fat by the process of phosphorylation
- It forms phosphoproteins, nucleoproteins and nerve phosphatides, etc.
- Adenosine triphosphate (ATP) is the energy resource for various biologic functions of the body and phosphorus plays an important role in the formation of ATP
- Normal plasma concentration of phosphorus is about 2–4 mg/dL

neutrophilis (PMN) and it is frequently seen that iron deficiency anemia causes a decrease in the myeloperoxidase activity, which results in decreased antibacterial activity of PMN.

Hemochromatosis is a condition resulting from increased iron absorption in the body and it causes pigmentation of skin and mucosa due to excessive iron deposition. The other features of the disease include red, raw fissured tongue or the tongue may be pale in color with smooth, atrophic, depapillated surface.

ZINC

Zinc helps in proper functioning of our immune system and it also has role in cell division, cell growth, wound healing, bone growth and carbohydrate metabolism. Zinc is a powerful antioxidant acts as an anticancer agent as well. Deficiency of zinc occurs due to chronic intake of poor quality protein especially the vegetable proteins.

Effects of Zinc Deficiency

- Delayed wound healing
- Retarded bone growth and defective epithelial keratinization
- Infertility in men and women
- Premature ageing
- Increased risk of cancer due to free radical injury
- The most common oral manifestation of zinc deficiency is altered taste sensations; patients has increased liking for saltier and sweeter foods.

DISTURBANCE IN VITAMIN METABOLISM

VITAMIN D

Although vitamin D belongs to the category of vitamins, it chemically behaves like a hormone or prohormone in many instances. Vitamin D is fat soluble and it can be produced in the sun-exposed skin or it can be absorbed in the intestine as dietary vitamin D (Box 14.4). The active form of vitamin D is known as 1-25 dihydroxycholecalciferol and it is metabolized by the pathways and it is shown in Flowchart 14.1.

Osteoporosis

Osteoporosis is a common disease of bone characterized severe weakness in the bone

Box 14.4	Functions of vitamin D.

- Vitamin D helps in the absorption of calcium and phosphorus from the foods in intestine by stimulating the calcium binding proteins in the GI tract
- It helps in calcium and phosphorus metabolism
- It promotes the calcification or mineralization of bone, cartilage and teeth; however very high levels of vitamin D can cause bone resorptions
- Vitamin D acts on immune system by promoting phagocytosis and by inducing immunomodulatory functions
- It antagonistically acts against the action of parathyroid hormone
- It increases the renal reabsorption of calcium

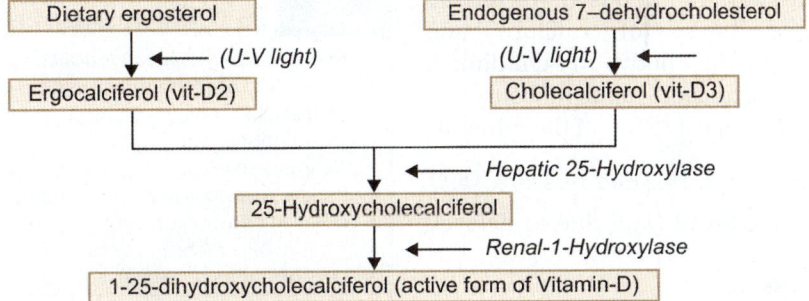

Flowchart 14.1: Metabolic pathway of vitamin D.

with increased susceptibility to fracture. It occurs when bone resorption in the body becomes far more than bone formation; causing gradual loss of mineral content in the bone. This disease is more prevalent among older individuals.

Etiology

- Low intake of calcium and the minerals
- Lack of intestinal absorption of minerals
- Decreased estrogen levels in blood leading to demineralization of bone
- Increased urinary loss of calcium
- Hyperparathyroidism
- Stress
- Long-term steroid therapy
- Tetracycline and anticonvulsant therapy.

Clinical Features

- It is frequently seen in postmenopausal women and older males.
- Chronic bone pain, bending in the bone and difficulty in performing normal activities.
- Increased incidences of spontaneous fracture of bone especially femoral neck fracture.
- Loss of lamina dura of alveolar bone with increased tooth mobility and tooth exfoliation.
- Increased incidences of jawbone fracture. In osteoporosis, X-ray reveals bone rarefaction and thinning of the cortex.

Rickets

It is a hereditary disorder transmitted as X-linked dominant trait and is characterized by decreased levels of calcium and phosphorus in the body in childhood; coupled with decreased renal reabsorption and increased renal excretion of the mineral.

Clinical Features (Figs. 14.2 and 14.3, Box 14.5)

- Wide fontanelles of skull due to delayed closure
- Frontal bossing

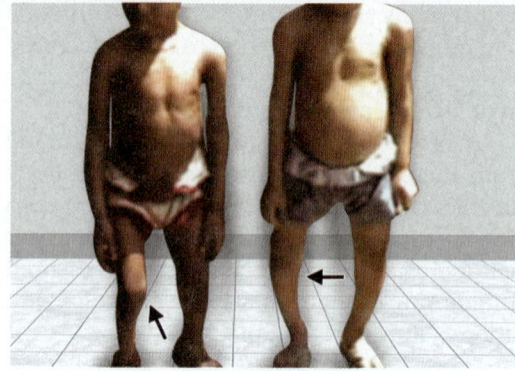

Fig. 14.2: Familial rickets.

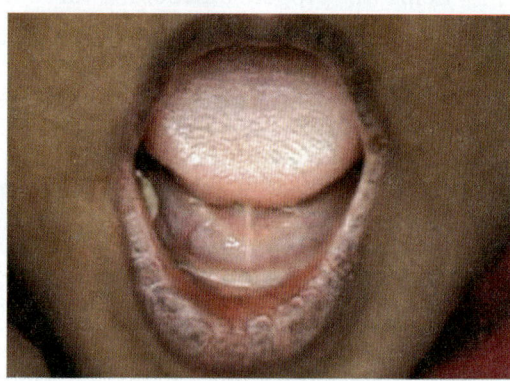

Fig. 14.3: Lack of tooth development in rickets.

- Decrease in the body length
- Swelling of the wrist and ankle joints
- Bowing of legs as the bones are soft and weak
- Wide knee joints
- Increased incidence of bone fracture
- Muscular weakness

Box 14.5	Oral manifestations of rickets.
<ul><li>Formation of globular hypocalcified dentin</li><li>Wide band of predentin formation</li><li>Large pulp horns, which may be extending up to the dentinoenamel junction</li><li>No increase in the caries susceptibility</li><li>Periapical lesions in multiple teeth</li><li>Delayed eruption of teeth</li><li>Abnormal cementum formation</li><li>Loss of lamina dura of alveolar bone</li></ul>	

- Pigeon chest (protrusion of the sternum and ribs).

VITAMIN A

Vitamin A is a fat-soluble vitamin, which is derived from the carotenes (plant pigments). It is commonly found in the fish oils, butter and eggs, etc. The transformation of carotenes into vitamin A and its absorption takes place in the small intestine.

Functions

- Vitamin A helps in the maintenance of the structure and function of specialized epithelium.
- It produces photosensitive pigments in the eye.
- It prevents the growth of epithelial malignant tumors.
- It maintains the normal skeletal growth.
- Maintenance of lysosomal stability and synthesis of glycoprotein (Box 14.6).

Effects of Hypervitaminosis A (Excess Vitamin A in the Body)

- *Among children*: Cortical thickening of bone, retarded bone growth, hemorrhage and bulging of the fontanelles.
- *Among adults*: Fatigue, anorexia, bone pain, skin pigmentations and alopecia, etc.

VITAMIN E

Vitamin E is an antioxidant and it protects the body from free radical injury, increases body immunity, regulates platelet aggregation and prevents premature aging.

Features of Vitamin E Deficiency

- Cell membrane damage
- Increased risk of thromboembolic diseases
- Hemolytic anemia
- Posterior column abnormalities
- Cerebellar ataxia.

VITAMIN B COMPLEX

Thiamine (B_1)

Thiamine plays an important role in carbohydrate metabolism and its deficiency produces "beriberi". The oral manifestations of beriberi include edema of the tongue, loss of its papillae, and glossodynia.

Riboflavin (B_2)

The riboflavin deficiency mostly occurs due to malabsorption syndrome and it has profound impact in the oral tissues.

Clinical Features of Riboflavin Deficiency

- The disease causes reddening, inflammation and depapillation of the tongue.
- Tongue is often sore and it also sometimes becomes ulcerated.
- Magenta glossitis is a peculiar form of glossitis, which occurs due to riboflavin deficiency. In this disease the tongue is magenta in color and its surface appears granular or "pebbly" due to flattening and mushrooming of the papillae.
- *Angular cheilitis*: The lips show reddening with fissures, painful cracks, dry scaling and maceration at the corner of the mouth (Fig. 14.4).
- Lip lesions may extend into the oral mucosa and give rise to white patchy lesions.
- Oral mucosa in general looks red and shiny; the gingiva is not affected in riboflavin deficiency.

Box 14.6 Effects of vitamin A deficiency.

- Night blindness and impaired vision
- Bitot's spot—a gray, triangular, elevated spot in the conjunctiva
- Xerophthalmia (dry conjunctiva)
- Corneal ulceration
- Follicular keratosis of the skin
- Squamous metaplasia of the columnar epithelium and gingivitis
- Decreased salivary secretions due to metaplasia of the secretory epithelium of salivary glands
- Hyperkeratosis of the oral mucosa, etc.

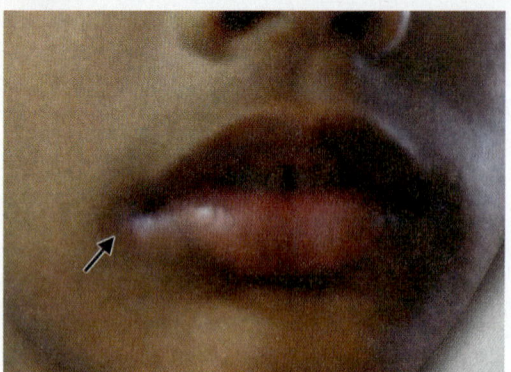

Fig. 14.4: Angular cheilitis in riboflavin deficiency.

Niacin (Vitamin B3)

Niacin plays an important role in the intracellular oxidation process and its deficiency causes pellagra.

Clinical Features of Niacin Deficiency

- The disease pellagra is summarized by four Ds—dementia, dermatitis, diarrhea, and death.
- Nasolabial seborrhea and malar pigmentations.
- The oral mucous membrane in pellagra presents generalized stomatitis with burning sensation, swelling, redness, pain and ulceration, etc.
- The tongue becomes red, enlarged and depapillated, with a "bald" surface. The tongue can also be thickly coated with a grayish pigmentation of the surface.
- Deep ulcers on the tongue may be seen in severe cases.
- Gingival margins are often red, swollen and ulcerated.
- Painful lips and angular cheilitis often develop.
- Dermatitis involving the exposed parts of the body, especially around the neck above the cloths margin (Casal necklace).

Folic Acid (Vitamin B9)

If folic acid is given during pregnancy, it can reduce the risk of neurological defects in the child and moreover, it can also reduce the risk development of orofacial clefts.

Causes of Folic Acid Deficiency

- Malnutrition
- Pregnancy
- Malabsorption
- Drug treatment with phenytoin.

Deficiency of folic acid causes the following:
- Loss of filiform and fungiform papilla of tongue; which results in a smooth, shiny appearance.
- Defective keratinization and increased susceptibility to infection in the oral mucosa.
- Gingivitis and oral ulceration.
- Atrophy of the tongue papillae with glossitis.

VITAMIN C (ASCORBIC ACID)

Vitamin C or ascorbic acid is a water soluble vitamin and it plays very important role in the synthesis of collagen fibers. The collagen fibers form the ground substance of all the connective tissues, i.e. connective tissue proper, bone, cartilage and blood vessels, etc.

Humans do not have the ability to synthesize their own vitamin C and must obtain through diet. Vitamin C is available in fresh foods, however, heating or drying of fruits cause loss of considerable amount of this vitamin (Box 14.7).

Box 14.7	Functions of vitamin C.

- Synthesis of collagen
- Helps in the synthesis of neurotransmitter norepinephrine
- Synthesis of carnitine, a molecule that helps in transport of fat to mitochondria to produce energy
- Metabolism of cholesterol
- Highly effective antioxidant
- Decreases the risk of cardiac diseases, strokes and cancer, etc.
- Decreases the oxidative stress and thereby reduce the risk of diabetes mellitus

Deficiency of Vitamin C

Deficiency of vitamin C leads to many disorders but scurvy is the most serious and important among them; the symptoms of scurvy generally develop after at least three months of severe or total deficiency of vitamin C. The hallmark feature of the disease is poor collagen synthesis, which seriously weakens the blood vessels, connective tissue, and bone.

Following are the manifestations of scurvy:
- Petechiae and ecchymosis in the oral mucous membrane (Fig. 14.5).
- Fatigue, weakness due to defective fat metabolism in the body.
- Hyperemia, edema and enlargement of the gingiva, with an increased bleeding tendency.
- Gingivitis is followed by detachment of periosteum from bone, resulting in severe pain, bleeding and swelling, etc. This often leads to marked loosening of teeth and sometimes premature exfoliations of teeth.
- Pain, swelling, and bleeding in the mouth with bad breath and difficulty in taking food.
- Retardation of wound healing due to lack of formation of connective tissue and bone.
- Defective function of odontoblast and osteoblast cells.
- Disturbed bone growth in children due to defective collagen synthesis and osteoid matrix formations.
- Premature loss of hair and small bleeding around the hair follicles (corkscrew hair)
- Follicular hyperkeratosis—a skin condition characterized by excessive synthesis of keratin in the hair follicles; which results in rough, cone-shaped, elevated papules in the skin.
- Joint pain and swelling due to weakness in the ligaments, muscles, and bones.

VITAMIN K

Vitamin K is essential for synthesis of prothrombin (clotting factor-II) and it also helps in synthesis of other clotting factors, e.g. factor VIII, IX, and X. Most of vitamin K is synthesized by intestinal microflora in humans and some amount of it can be available from natural fruits.

Deficiency of vitamin K causes decreased prothrombin levels in blood with increased tendency for hemorrhage and bruising. There can also be increased bleeding after tooth extraction and following minor surgical procedures, etc.

DISTURBANCES IN PROTEIN METABOLISM

AMYLOIDOSIS

Amyloids are abnormal fibrillar proteins, which have a peculiar homogenous, translucent appearance and a characteristic staining property.

Amyloidosis is a pathological condition characterized by the extracellular deposition of amyloids within the tissue.

Types

Amyloidosis is of two types:
1. *Primary (idiopathic) type*: Arising as a result of derangement of immunoglobulin synthesis and consists of fragments of IgG molecules in the tissues.

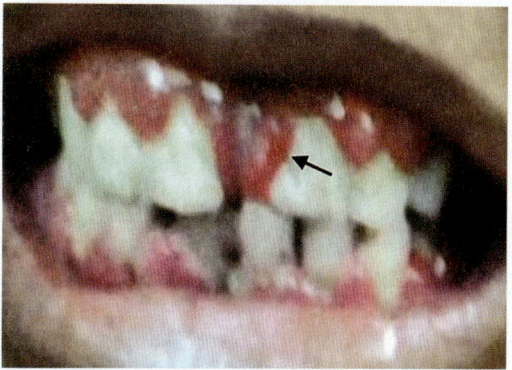

Fig. 14.5: Oral lesions of scurvy.

2. *Secondary (reactive) type*: Occurs as a complication of many diseases, especially the chronic destructive inflammatory lesions like rheumatoid arthritis and few malignant conditions.

Clinical Features

- Oral amyloidosis is commonly seen among patients suffering from multiple myeloma or monoclonal gammopathy, etc. and the disease occurs due to overproduction of immunoglobulin light chains.
- Smooth surfaced, waxy papules or plaques may be found on the lips, eyelids and neck, etc.
- Localized amyloidosis in the oral cavity commonly produces macroglossia and gingival swelling, etc. and the swelling is usually firm and indurated.
- There can be presence of hemorrhagic bullae on the surface of the lesion, which ruptures to produce shallow ulcer.
- The tongue lesion may present a lobulated growth, which sometimes may be so massive that it will prevent the closure of mouth.
- The surface of the lesion appears pale or purplish and the lateral border of the tongue often shows indentations of teeth.
- Petechiae and ecchymosis can be present in other parts of the oral mucous membrane in amyloidosis.
- Systemic amyloidosis may cause claudication (severe cramp-like pain, mostly occurs in legs) of jaw muscles due to infiltration of amyloids into blood vessels.
- Reactive amyloidosis occurs secondary to chronic infections like tuberculosis, sarcoidosis or osteomyelitis, etc.
- Amyloids can also be found in large amounts in Pindborg's tumor.
- Amyloidosis of the salivary glands may produce xerostomia with dryness of mouth and hoarseness of voice.

Histopathology

- Microscopically amyloids appear as weakly eosinophilic, homogenous, amorphous hyaline materials, which often show a perivascular distribution.
- Amyloids are generally deposited extracellularly within the submucosal connective tissue.
- Congo red is the special stain used for the detection of amyloids in the tissue and it produces a typical "apple-green" birefringence, when viewed with polarized light.
- Crystal violet stain exhibits red colored amyloid materials in the tissue.

Treatment

By surgical excision. Prognosis can be poor in some cases due to cardiac, hepatic or renal failures.

PORPHYRIA

Porphyria refers to an in born error of porphyrin metabolism and it is characterized by the overproduction of uroporphyrin and other related substances. The condition may also results from certain infections.

Porphyria is commonly of two types:
1. Erythropoietic porphyria
2. Hepatic porphyria.

Clinical Features

- The erythropoietic porphyria is characterized by red urine, photophobia, hairy face and reddish or brownish colored teeth.
- The tooth discoloration is due to deposition of porphyrins in enamel, dentin and cementum, etc.
- The discoloration is more intense in deciduous teeth with both enamel and dentin is affected; discoloration is less severe in permanent teeth.
- The discolored areas or zones of teeth exhibit a red fluorescence when exposed to Wood's UV light.
- The disease sometimes produces vesiculobullous skin lesions.
- Porphyria does not require any treatment, only veneering of discolored teeth is done to improve esthetics.

DISTURBANCES IN CARBOHYDRATE METABOLISM

■ HURLER'S SYNDROME

Hurler's syndrome is a disturbance of carbohydrate metabolism and is characterized by elevated mucopolysaccharide levels in urine. The disease is sometimes fatal in nature and it commonly affects children.

Clinical Manifestations
- Mental retardation
- Dwarfism with large head and prominent foreheads
- Hypertelorism
- Puffy eyelids and corneal clouding
- Hepatosplenomegaly.

Oral Manifestations
- Deformed face with broad saddle-nose
- Short and broad mandible
- Coarse and thick lips
- Lack of tooth eruption or delayed eruption
- Large tongue and open mouth
- Microdontia and diastema formation
- Gingival hyperplasia.

Radiographic Features
Radiolucencies around the crowns of unerupted teeth in the jaw due to mucopolysaccharide deposition are common findings in this disease. Localized bone destruction in the jaw.

Histopathology
- Abnormal deposition of intracellular mucopolysaccharides in different vital organs, e.g. liver, spleen, heart and nervous system, etc.
- Presence of "hunter's cells" in the tissue, these cells are large with crescent shaped nuclei and metachromatically staining cytoplasms.

Treatment
No treatment is possible, death often occurs from cardiac or lung involvement.

DISTURBANCES IN LIPID METABOLISM

The diseases, which occur due to the disturbance in lipid metabolism, are classified into two broad groups:
1. *Histiocytosis "X"*: The histiocytosis X group includes three diseases, namely:
   i. Hand-Schuller-Christian disease
   ii. Eosinophilic granuloma.
   iii. Letterer-Siwe disease.
2. *Lipid reticuloendotheliosis*: It also includes two diseases and these are:
   i. Gaucher's disease
   ii. Niemann-Pick disease.

■ HAND-SCHULLER-CHRISTIAN DISEASE

Hand-Schuller-Christian disease occurs among young children and it primarily causes replacement of the normal bone marrow cells by proliferating macrophages.

Clinical Features
- Hepatosplenomegaly, skin rash, diabetes insipidus, and exophthalmos.
- Ulceration and necrosis of oral mucous membrane with halitosis
- Loosening and premature exfoliation of teeth, delayed wound healing.

Radiographic Features
Presence of multiple, punched-out radiolucent areas in the skull bone. Diffuse radiolucency of the jaw, with destruction of alveolar bone and displacement of teeth.

Histopathology
- Microscopically the lesion reveals, multiple, large, vacuolated foam cells and small non-vacuolated cells. Both types of cells are histiocytic in nature.
- Treatment is done by surgery, chemotherapy, and occasionally by radiotherapy.
- Some patients may undergo spontaneous remission.

EOSINOPHILIC GRANULOMA

Eosinophilic granuloma is a chronic, localized form of bone disorder, which commonly occurs in the second and third decade of life.

Clinical Features (Figs. 14.6 and 14.7)
- Fever, malaise, headache, and anorexia
- Localized pain, swelling, and tenderness in the jawbones
- Gingival soft tissue swelling (sometimes), halitosis, and mobility of teeth.

Radiographic Findings
Radiographs present single or multiple areas of bone destruction and the teeth in the X-rays appear as "hanging-in-the air" like condition.

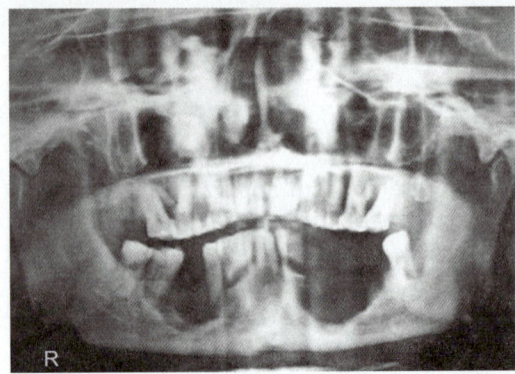

Fig. 14.8: Radiograph of eosinophilic granuloma.

Often there is increased possibility of pathological fractures of the bone (Fig. 14.8).

Histopathology
Microscopically, eosinophilic granuloma shows numerous proliferating histiocytes in diffuse sheets, within which many eosinophils are dispersed. Individual cells club together to form multinucleated giant cells (Fig. 14.9).

Treatment
Surgical curettage and radiotherapy. Prognosis is good.

LETTERER-SIWE DISEASE

Letterer-Siwe disease is the most fatal form of histiocytosis X and it usually occurs before the age of 2 years.

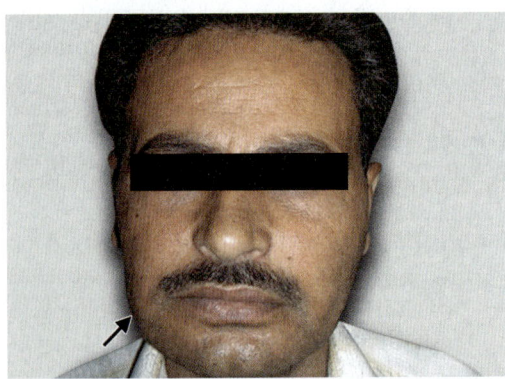

Fig. 14.6: Eosinophilic granuloma (extraoral).

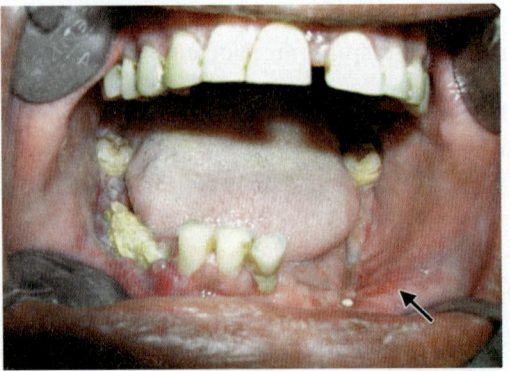

Fig. 14.7: Eosinophilic granuloma (intraoral).

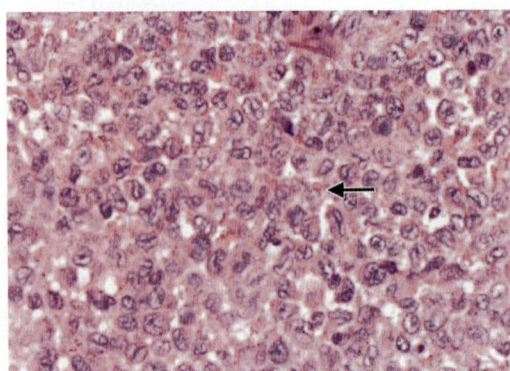

Fig. 14.9: Photomicrograph of eosinophilic granuloma.

Clinical Features
- The disease primarily affects the viscera, like spleen, liver, lung, lymph nodes, bone marrow and skin, etc.
- Hepatosplenomegaly, anemia, and lymphadenopathy.
- Fever, malaise, and irritability.
- Petechiae or ecchymosis of skin and mucous membrane.
- Mucosal ulcerations and gingival hyperplasia.
- Loosening and premature exfoliation of teeth.
- Radiographs reveal diffuse areas of bone destruction in the jaws.

Histopathology
The lesion microscopically shows marked proliferations of non-lipidized histiocytes.

Treatment
No specific treatment is possible. Prognosis is grave.

GAUCHER'S DISEASE
Gaucher's disease is characterized by the deposition of kerasin (a lipid) in the reticular cells of liver, spleen, bone marrow and lymph nodes.

It can occur at any age and females are affected more often than males. Skin pigmentation, gingival bleeding, hepatosplenomegaly and ecchymosis, etc. are the common clinical manifestations.

Microscopically, large foam cells with "crumpled silk" cytoplasm (Gaucher's cells) are found in the lesion.

NIEMANN-PICK DISEASE
Niemann-Pick disease is characterized by the accumulation of sphingomyelins (a lipid) in the cells of the reticuloendothelial system. It is a fatal disease and occurs most commonly among infants. Destructive jaw lesions, mental retardation and blindness, etc. are the usual manifestations of this disease.

DISTURBANCES IN HORMONE METABOLISM

HYPOPITUITARISM
Dwarfism
Hypopituitarism in infancy leads to dwarfism, in which the patients usually have a much shorter but well-proportioned body.

Causes
The disease occurs due to reduced synthesis of growth hormone in childhood.

Clinical Features (Box 14.8)
- Short stature of the body
- Sparse hair on the head and other hairy regions
- Atrophy of all organs of the body
- Wrinkled atrophic skin and childish face
- Hypogonadism, impotence, and amenorrhea
- Extreme weight loss.
- Coma and death in several cases.

Diagnosis
- Hypoglycemia
- Decreased serum growth hormone levels
- Skull X-rays reveal tumor in sellar region
- CT scans and MRI to detect tumors in the brain.

PITUITARY INSUFFICIENCY IN ADULTS
Clinical Features
- Easy fatigability and weakness, hypotension and cold intolerance

Box 14.8	Oral manifestations of hypopituitarism.
<ul><li>Small face in comparison to the skull</li><li>Delayed exfoliation of deciduous teeth</li><li>Delayed completion of tooth roots</li><li>Delayed eruption of permanent teeth</li><li>Crowding of teeth</li><li>Underdevelopment of maxilla and mandible</li><li>Smaller crown size of the teeth and smaller root length</li><li>Lack of development of third molars</li></ul>	

- Irregular menstrual cycle in females
- Lack of development of secondary sexual characteristics
- Failure of lactation, dry, and wrinkled skin.

Treatment

Administration of corticosteroids, estrogens, androgens and thyroxin, etc.

DIABETES INSIPIDUS

Definition

Diabetes insipidus is a disorder of water metabolism characterized by polyuria; it is caused by the deficiency of vasopressin, the antidiuretic hormone (ADH) secreted by the posterior pituitary.

Etiology

- *Neurogenic cause*: Central, hypothalamic, pituitary and neurohypophyseal disturbances cause deficiency of ADH, vasopressin.
- *Nephrogenic cause*: Vasopressin resistance caused by the insensitivity of the kidneys to the effect of vasopressin.
- *Gestagenic (gestational) cause*: Caused by the deficiency of vasopressin that occurs during pregnancy.
- *Dipsogenic*: Caused by abnormal thirst with excessive consumption of water resulting in polyuria.

Clinical Features

- *Marked polyuria*: Daily output of 5–25 liters of urine.
- *Polydipsia (increased thirst)*: 4–40 liters of fluid required daily.
- Patients have a craving for cold water.
- Dehydration, headache, fatigue, and irritability.
- Xerostomia (dry mouth) is the most significant oral manifestation.
- There can be noninflammatory swelling of the salivary glands (sialosis), which particularly involves the parotids.

Diagnosis

- Increase in plasma osmolarity
- Low specific gravity of urine (1.001–1.005)
- *Fluid deprivation test*: Fluid intake is restricted for 8–12 hours and even after that if there is no increase in the specific gravity or osmolality of urine, the case should be diagnosed as diabetes insipidus.

Treatment

- Administration of vasopressin
- Administration of chlorpropamide to reduce urine volume and to potentiate the action of vasopressin
- Detection and treatment of cranial lesion, if any.

HYPERPITUITARISM

Hyperpituitarism or increased production of growth hormone from the anterior pituitary, it leads to two diseases:
1. *Gigantism*: Due to hypersecretion of growth hormone in infants (before the fusion of bone epiphyses)
2. *Acromegaly*: Due to hypersecretion of growth hormone in adults (after the fusion of bone epiphyses).

Causes

- Hypersecretion of growth hormone due to functional pituitary adenoma
- Increased function of anterior pituitary, which regulates the secretion of growth hormone.

PITUITARY GIGANTISM (BOX 14.9)

The following features characterize gigantism clinically:
- Generalized symmetric overgrowth of the body.
- Extreme body height (above 7 feet) with long extremities.
- Genital underdevelopment and excessive perspiration.
- Headache, lassitude, joint, and muscle pain.
- Defective vision.

Oral Aspects of Metabolic Disorders

> **Box 14.9** Oral manifestations of gigantism.
> - Enlarged maxilla and mandible with severe growth of the facial soft tissues
> - Marked increase in the vertical dimension of face
> - Large size of teeth (true generalized macrodontia) and early eruption of teeth
> - Root length is generally greater than normal
> - Macroglossia and hypercementosis of teeth, etc.

- A large number of cases occur as part of Albright's syndrome.

ACROMEGALY

The disease occurs in adults due to hypersecretion of growth hormone in adults after the closure of epiphyseal end plates.

Clinical Features

The patients with acromegaly do not have a gigantic body but they often develop the following general features:
- Thick bones with larger hands and feet; which often have a "spade-like" appearance.
- Hypertrophy of sweat and sebaceous glands with excessive sweating.
- Abnormal glucose tolerance and sexual dysfunction.
- Enlarged skull with increased intracranial pressure causing headache, photophobia, and visual disturbances.
- Hypertension, cardiomegaly, hepatomegaly and peripheral neuropathy, etc.
- Osteoporosis, arthralgia, and myalgia.
- Bowing of the legs and barrel-shaped chest (Box 14.10).

Diagnosis

- Increased serum inorganic phosphorus level.
- Glycosuria and hypercalciuria.
- T_4 level is normal or low.
- X-ray of skull reveals large sella.
- Serum growth hormone level is increased.

Treatment

Surgery or radiotherapy to the pituitary tumor.

> **Box 14.10** Oral manifestations of acromegaly.
> Some interesting changes take place in the orofacial region of the patient suffering from acromegaly and these changes are as follows:
> - Overproduction of growth hormone in adults causes activation of condylar growth center in mandible with abnormal increase in the size of the bone.
> - Loss of oval facial feature, frontal bossing and thickening of nasolabial sulcus.
> - Large mandible often leads to gross skeletal deformity with development of class III malocclusion, diastema and anterior open bite.
> - Macroglossia with indentations of teeth on the lateral border of tongue.
> - Thick lips, which often produce a Negroid appearance to the patient.
> - Hypercementosis in tooth.
> - Increase in the thickness of the jaw bones (like other bones) due to subperiosteal new bone deposition.
> - Hypertrophy of tissues of soft palate, which often causes disturbance in sleep.
> - Large nose, ears and prominent eyebrows with brow furrow.
> - Increased incidence of periodontitis.
> - Poor fitting of old prosthesis due to large size of the jaw (especially lower).
> - Enlargement of maxillary air sinuses.
> - A typical coarse facial features due to abnormal soft tissue growth.

HYPOTHYROIDISM

Hypothyroidism is the acquired disease of decreased levels of thyroid hormone in the body, usually causes decreased metabolic rate, which often results in the retardation of *growth, differentiation,* and *function* of the entire body systems.
- During childhood, hypothyroidism produces a disease called *cretinism*
- It produces another disease *myxedema* among adults.

Causes

- Decreased secretion of TSH (thyroid stimulating hormone) by pituitary gland (necessary for secretion of thyroid hormone)

- Atrophy or damage to the thyroid gland, especially due to radiation therapy and medications
- Congenital absence of thyroid gland
- Iodine deficiency
- Autoimmune disease causing damage to the thyroid gland (Hashimoto's disease)
- Metabolic disturbances
- Surgical removal of thyroid gland (either due to unavoidable surgery or by any mistake); sometimes removal of lingual thyroid nodule may lead to this problem, if that is the only thyroid tissue patient had.

General Features of Hypothyroidism
- Depression, poor memory, and slow heart beats.
- Dry coarse hair, dry skin, and puffy face.
- Enlarged thyroid, weight gain, and menstrual irregularity.
- Constipation, brittle nails, and infertility.

CRETINISM (BOX 14.11)

It is the congenital disease due to absence or deficiency of normal thyroid secretion in children; it is clinically manifested by the following features:
- Neonatal jaundice, horse-cry, constipation, and low body temperature.
- A short, poorly developed (dwarfed) body due to delayed ossification of bone.
- Mentally retarded, often dull and apathetic child.
- Delayed development of speech and walking capability.
- Larger size of the skull and generalized non-pitting edema.
- Coarse dry skin and sparse brittle hair
- Brittleness of the fingernails.
- Hypotension, protuberant abdomen with umbilical hernia.
- Flat nose due to retraction of nasal bridge.
- Poor development of teeth with delayed eruption.
- Broad and puffy face with enlarged tongue and thick lips.
- Atrophy of the sweat glands.

MYXEDEMA

Myxedema is the disease caused by deficiency of thyroid hormone (hypothyroidism) in adults.

General Symptoms (Box 14.12)
- It frequently develops among the middle-aged males.
- Patients often suffer from weakness, weight gain, fatigue, lethargy, low blood pressure and mental retardation, etc.
- Dry cold skin with loss of hair, swelling of the face (puffy face) and extremities.
- Cold intolerance, husky voice, decreased sweating, and anorexia.
- Loss of memory, hearing impairment, arthralgia, muscle cramps, and paresthesia.
- The lethargic stage may progress to coma in severe cases.

Diagnosis
- Reduction in serum T_3 and T_4 levels
- Elevation of serum TSH level
- Increased BMR.

Box 14.11 Oral manifestations of cretinism.
- Delayed eruption and exfoliation of deciduous teeth
- Broad flat face due to defective growth of the skull and facial bones
- Macroglossia with protruding tongue and thick lips
- Dull expressionless face with dry coarse skin
- Constant drooling of saliva from the mouth
- Malocclusion and under development of mandible

Box 14.12 Oral manifestations of myxedema.
- Dull expressionless face with periorbital puffiness and loss of hair
- The tongue, lips and eyelids, etc. are edematous (nonpitting) and swollen
- The large tongue often interferes with speech
- Underdevelopment of maxilla and mandible

Treatment
Administration of thyroid preparations.

■ HYPERTHYROIDISM (BOX 14.13)
Hyperthyroidism is the disease, caused by excessive production of thyroid hormone in the body.

Causes
- Hyperplasia of thyroid gland with increased function (goiter)
- Increased secretion of thyroid hormone due to benign tumor in the gland
- Increased TSH secretion due to pituitary overfunction.

Clinical Features
Clinically, the disease produces the following features:
- The disease mostly occurs in third and fourth decade of life, more common in females
- Osteoporosis, excessive sweating, and hair loss and menstrual problems.
- Hypertension and exhaustion.
- Excitability, nervousness, anxiety, irritability.
- Weight loss (despite increased appetite), palpitations (tachycardia) and anorexia.
- Widened pulse pressure (increased systolic and decreased diastolic pressure)
- Increased risk of cardiovascular disease.
- Emotional instability with easy tearing, photophobia, and warm smooth skin.
- Nervousness, muscle weakness, and tremors.
- Exophthalmos (swollen eyes) and hyper-defecation.

Diagnosis
- Increased BMR
- Elevated serum protein bound iodine concentration
- Decreased urinary excretion of iodine.

Treatment
- Administration of antithyroid drugs
- Surgery or radiotherapy to the thyroid gland tumor, if any.

■ HYPERPARATHYROIDISM
In the human body, there are four parathyroid glands present, and these glands release the hormone called the parathormone. The primary function of parathormone is to maintain the normal calcium and phosphorus levels in blood.

Whenever there is a decrease in the calcium or phosphorus levels in blood, the parathormone cause erosion of bone from the skeleton in order to liberate free calcium or phosphorus ions to make up the deficit. Parathormone also increases the blood phosphorus levels by inhibiting its urinary excretion.

Excessive concentration of parathormone in the blood is known as hyperparathyroidism (Fig 14.10), and it is of two types: (1) primary hyperparathyroidism, and (2) secondary hyperparathyroidism.
- The primary hyperparathyroidism occurs due to excessive parathormone production as a result of adenoma, hyperplasia or functional carcinoma of the parathyroid glands.
- Secondary hyperparathyroidism occurs as a result of hyperplasia of the gland secondary to some diseases, like end-stage of renal disease, osteomalacia and multiple myeloma, etc. The clinicopathological manifestations of both types of hyperparathyroidism are almost same.

Box 14.13   Oral manifestations of hyperthyroidism.
- Early exfoliation of deciduous teeth
- Premature eruption of permanent teeth
- Alveolar bone atrophy
- Increased susceptibility to oral infections
- Difficulty in undergoing dental extractions or other dental surgical procedures because of the cardiac abnormality

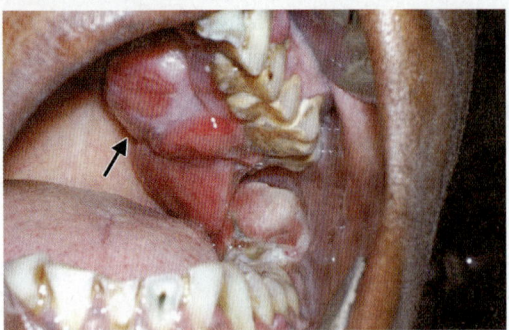

Fig. 14.10: Hyperparathyroidism.

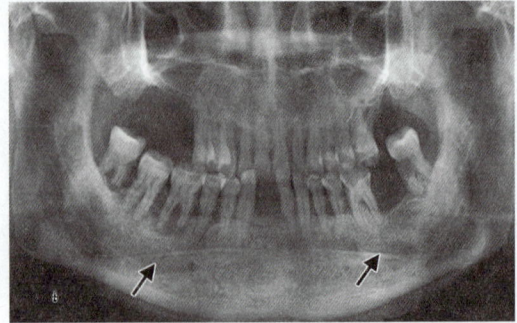

Fig. 14.11: Radiograph of hyperparathyroidism with severe bone loss in the jaw.

Clinical Manifestations

- The disease occurs more commonly among the middle-aged females (post-menopausal).
- The early symptoms include fatigue, weakness, anorexia, polyurea, thirst, and constipation, etc.
- Depression, insomnia, vomiting, headache, and loss of memory of recent events.
- Peptic ulcers and itching sensations in the skin.
- Hypertension and CVS due to renal damage.
- Kidney stones (due to increased excretion of calcium) and joint stiffness.
- Bone pain, pathological fractures and coma, etc. may occur
- The common oral manifestations are loosening and mobility of teeth, and fracture of the jawbones, etc.
- Swelling of the jaw with development of brown tumor.

Radiological Features (Fig. 14.11)

- Generalized osteoporosis with thinning of the bony trabeculae.
- Loss of lamina dura around the roots of teeth is an early manifestation of the disease.
- In severe cases multiple, well-defined, unilocular or multilocular radiolucent areas in the jawbones, which often resemble cysts or tumors (osteitis fibrosa cystica).
- Similar osteoclastic lesions can also be seen in other bones, e.g. pelvic bones, ribs and clavicles, etc.
- Thinning and expansion of the cortical plates and increased resorptions of medullary bone.
- Decrease in the trabecular density and blurring of normal trabecular pattern often produce a typical "ground-glass" appearance in the jawbone.
- Lateral skull radiograph reveals a "salt and pepper" effect.
- Subperiosteal resorption of bone in fingers and resorption of the terminal phalanges.

Histopathology (Fig. 14.12, Box 14.14)

- Microscopy reveals increased osteoclastic activity with resorptions of bony trabeculae, as well as formation of some new bones by the osteoblast cells.
- "Dissecting osteitis" is a peculiar pattern of bone resorption seen in hyperparathyroidism; in which the osteoclast cells create elongated tunnel or hole in the bony trabaculum by boring through its center along the length and thus cause complete dissection of it. The dissecting osteitis often results a "railroad-tract" like defects in the bone.
- The marrow spaces around the areas of resorption are replaced by fibrovascular

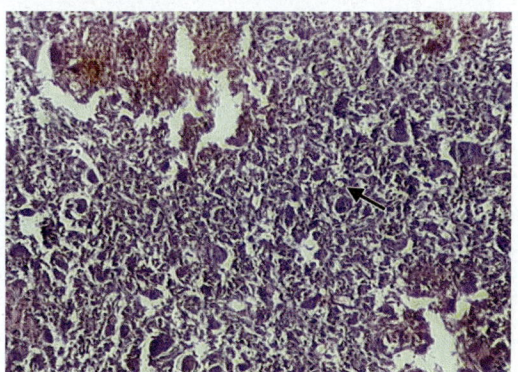

Fig. 14.12: Photomicrograph of hyperparathyroidism multiple giant cells and areas of hemorrhage.

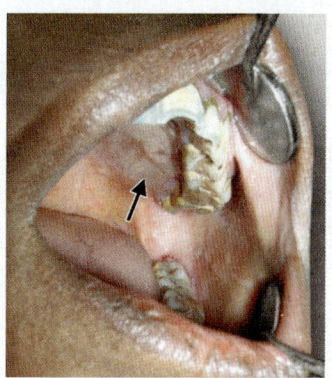

Fig. 14.13: Hyperparathyroidism after treatment.

tissue characterized by large number of blood capillaries and endothelium-lined spaces; along with multiple multinucleated osteoclast type of giant cells, areas of excessive hemorrhage and hemosiderin pigmentations.
- The gross tissue specimen often has a reddish-brown appearance due to so many large vessels and hemorrhage with presence of blood pigments and hence the lesion is often referred to as the "brown tumor or brown nodules".
- Sometimes there can be fibrosis around the resorbed bony trabeculae.
- The combination of increased bone resorption, peritrabecular fibrosis and the cystic brown tumors are the hallmark of severe hyperparathyroidism and it is also called generalized osteitis fibrosa cystica (von Recklinghausen disease of bone).
- Histologically, the tissue looks very similar to giant cell granuloma.

However, multiple bone involvement, which is commonly seen in hyperparathyroidism, is not seen in giant cell granulomas. Moreover, parathormone assay helps in differentiating these two lesions accurately.

Treatment

Excision of the parathyroid tumor, administration of vitamin D and dietary phosphate supplements (Fig. 14.13).

■ HYPOPARATHYROIDISM

Hypoparathyroidism refers to the deficiency of parathyroid hormone levels in the body and it is a much more rare entity as compared to hyperparathyroidism.

Causes

- If parathyroid gland is mistakenly removed during surgical intervention of the thyroid.
- Autoimmune damage of the parathyroid gland.
- Rare diseases like DiGeorge syndrome or endocrine candidiasis syndrome.

Box 14.14	Laboratory investigations of hyperparathyroidism.

- Serum calcium level may be as high as 15–17 mg/dL (normal is 9–12 mg/dL)
- Serum alkaline phosphatase and urinary hydroxyproline levels are not elevated unless the condition is extremely severe
- Serum phosphate level may be as low as 2.5 mg/dL
- USG, CT scan, etc. are done to detect the tumor in the gland
- Urinary calcium and phosphate levels are elevated
- Serum parathormone level is elevated (could be detected by immunoassay)

Clinical Features

- Hypocalcemia follows the loss of parathyroid hormone.
- Increased neuromuscular excitability if the calcium level falls below 7–8 mg/dL.
- Tetany with carpopedal spasm occurs if serum calcium level falls below 5–6 mg/dL (Box 14.15).

Laboratory Diagnosis

- Decreased level of parathormone in blood as seen in radioimmunoassay.
- Decreased serum calcium concentration.
- Decreased serum phosphate level.
- Normal renal functions initially.

Treatment

Administration of vitamin D precursor (ergocalciferol).

ADRENAL HORMONES

Adrenal glands are located above the kidney (hence are also called suprarenal glands); each gland has two parts—(1) an outer cortex and (2) an inner medulla and both parts liberate several hormones (called adrenal hormones).

Adrenal cortex liberates three hormones:
1. Mineralocorticoids, e.g. aldosterone.
2. Glucocorticoids, e.g. cortisol (steroid).
3. Sex hormones, e.g. adrenal androgens.

Adrenal medulla liberates two hormones:
1. Epinephrine (adrenaline)
2. Norepinephrine.

Function of Mineralocorticoids

These hormones are concerned with sodium and water retentions and potassium excretions in the body.

Function of Glucocorticoids (Steroids) (Table 14.1, Box 14.16)

- To antagonize the action of insulin (promotes gluconeogenesis, which provides glucose).
- Increases breakdown of protein.
- Increases breakdown of fatty acids.
- Suppresses inflammation, inhibits scar formation.
- Blocks allergic reactions and produces strong anti-inflammatory action.

Table 14.1: Indications of steroid therapy.

Hormone disorder	Addison's disease
Rheumatic condition	Rheumatoid arthritis
	Acute rheumatic fever
Blood disorders	ITP (idiopathic thrombocytopenic purpura) Leukemia Hemolytic anemia
Allergic conditions	Bronchial asthma, allergic rhinitis
Dermatologic conditions	Drug rashes, giant hives, lichen planus, atopic dermatitis
Ocular diseases	Conjunctivitis, uveitis.
Collagen diseases	Lupus erythematosus, polyarteritis nodosa
GI problems	Ulcerative colitis
Organ transplant recipients	As an immunosuppressive drug
Neurological problems	Cerebral edema
Miscellaneous conditions	Gout, multiple sclerosis, etc.

Box 14.15 Oral manifestations of hypoparathyroidism.

- *Chvostek's sign* is an important finding associated with hypocalcemia, which is characterized by twitching of the upper lip when the facial nerve is tapped just below the zygomatic process
- Aplasia or hypoplasia of teeth with failure of eruption
- Short roots of teeth but thick lamina dura
- Incompletely mineralized dentin
- Enamel hypoplasia (pitting type) and short roots of teeth
- Chronic persistent candidiasis in young people

Oral Aspects of Metabolic Disorders

Box 14.16	Common side effects of long-term steroid therapy.

- Suppression of adrenocortical function with risk of circulatory failure
- Suppressed inflammatory response
- Immunosuppression
- Increased susceptibility to opportunistic infections
- Depressed protein metabolism
- Impaired wound healing
- Moon face
- Raised blood sugar
- Sodium and water retention
- Mood change

- Decreases the number of circulating eosinophils and leukocytes.

Indications of Glucocorticoids

- Status asthmaticus
- Acute adrenal insufficiency
- Anaphylactic reaction (only after adrenaline has been given).

Steroid Crisis

The steroid hormone plays an essential role in maintaining life because it performs important metabolic activity of the body. It provides the capacity to resist all types of noxious stimuli and stressful environmental changes. The secretion of steroid hormone is controlled by the pituitary hormone called the adrenocorticotropic hormone (ACTH).

If a patient takes steroid (cortisol) from outside sources for a longer duration of time, the function of the adrenal cortex becomes diminished in the body. Such exogenous steroid-dependent person if stops taking the drug abruptly, he or she may go into severe shock when exposed to some kind of stress or strain.

Such type of condition is known as "steroid crisis" and it occurs due to the lack of steroid production by the adrenal cortex during emergency. For such reason, in steroid-dependent persons, the therapy should not be stopped abruptly; rather the therapy should be ended by gradually tapering the dose of steroid.

Mineralocorticoids

Aldosterone

It is a steroid hormone of mineralocorticoid group, produced by the outer section (zona glomerulosa) of the adrenal cortex in the adrenal gland. It acts on the kidney nephrons to conserve sodium (Na) ion and secrete potassium (K) ions in order to increase blood pressure. Aldosterone is decreased in Addison's disease and it is increased in Conn syndrome.

Aldosteronism

It is an abnormality of electrolyte balance in the body caused by excessive secretion of aldosterone.

Features

Hypokalemia, alkalosis, polyurea, hypertension, and increased risk of heart failure.

■ WATERHOUSE–FRIDERICHSEN SYNDROME

Waterhouse–Friderichsen syndrome occurs as a result of acute adrenocortical insufficiency, in association with infection by *Meningococci, Streptococci, Pneumococci*, etc.

The disease is often characterized by rapidly fulminating septicemia, purpura and death within 48–72 hours.

■ CHRONIC ADRENOCORTICAL INSUFFICIENCY (ADDISON'S DISEASE)

Addison's disease is a debilitating and potentially fatal condition, which occurs due to chronic insufficiency of the adrenocortical hormone; as a result of destruction of adrenal cortex (Fig. 14.14).

The clinical manifestations include:
- Postural hypotension, weakness, anorexia, etc.
- Fatigue, irritability, weight loss, nausea, vomiting and diarrhea, etc.

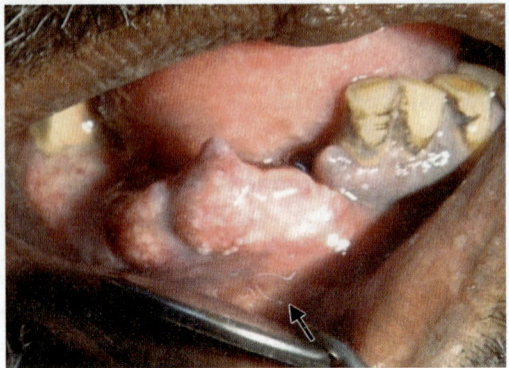

Fig. 14.14: Extensive oral infection in patient receiving steroid therapy.

- Brown hyperpigmentations of skin including orofacial region (this is called bronzing hyperpigmentations and it occurs due to increased level of beta-lipoprotein or increased ACTH, both cause stimulations to the melanocytes to produce more melanin in the skin or mucosa).
- Chronic mucocutaneous candidiasis.

Hyperfunction of Adrenocortical Hormone (Cushing's Syndrome)

Cushing's syndrome results from over activity of the adrenal glands with consequent hypersecretion of glucocorticoids (Boxes 14.17 and 14.18).

Causes

- Administration of high dose of ACTH or increased ACTH production in a pituitary tumor.
- Administration of high dose of corticosteroids.
- Adrenocortical hyperplasia with over production of glucocorticoids.
- Adenoma or carcinoma of the adrenal cortex.
- Ectopic ACTH syndrome.

Diagnosis

- Increased levels of urinary 17-hydroxycorticosteroids.

Box 14.17 Clinical features of Cushing's syndrome.

- Generalized obesity and lowered resistance to stress
- Facial plethora (markedly edematous face with reddish complexion)
- Decreased libido, menstrual irregularity
- Decreased linear growth of children
- Mental changes include memory loss, poor concentration and depression (steroid psychosis)
- Persistent hyperglycemia (steroid diabetes)
- Weakness due to muscle wasting
- Thin skin with increased capillary fragility resulting in ecchymosis and easy bruising
- *Severe osteoporosis* leads to pathological bone fracture under low impact trauma
- Potassium depletion leading to hypokalemia, arrhythmias, muscle weakness, and renal disorder
- Sodium and water retention which causes hypertension and edema
- Abnormal fat deposition in the orofacial region produces a puffy and bilateral edematous swelling of the face *(moon facies)*
- Development of abnormal fat pad on the neck *(buffalo-hump)*
- *Decreased immunity* with increased susceptibility to infection and poor wound healing
- Increased production of androgens causes virilism (development of secondary male characters in females) and hirsutism (abnormal growth of facial and body hair in women)
- Occasional chloasma like pigmentations of face and pressure points

Box 14.18 Oral manifestations of Cushing's syndrome.

- Facial plethora (rounded face with flushing or redness) or puffy "moon" facies
- Hirsutism (abnormal growth of facial and body hair in women)
- "Buffalo-hump" development of abnormal fat pad on the neck
- Increased susceptibility to oral infections due to depressed immunity
- Delayed healing of oral wounds including postextraction wounds
- Increased susceptibility to jaw fracture due to osteoporosis
- Easy bruising on the facial skin during dental procedures
- Occasional chloasma (melasma) like pigmentations on the facial skin

- Increased plasma cortisol levels.
- Glycosuria not controlled by insulin.
- Albuminuria.
- Adrenal tumor can be detected by MRI.

Treatment
Surgical removal of the gland tumor or radiotherapy.

PANCREATIC HORMONE (INSULIN)

Diabetes Mellitus
Diabetes mellitus is the metabolic disorder characterized by glucose intolerance, and it is caused by an imbalance between insulin supply and insulin demand in the body.

Insulin is a natural hormone secreted by the "beta cells of the islets of Langerhans" of pancreas.

Importance of Insulin
It helps in transporting or carrying the glucose (sugar) molecules from bloodstream to the cells and thus controls the level of glucose in blood. Glucose is the main fuel or source of energy for most of our body functions; once the glucose reaches the cell, it is burnt in the cell to produce energy. If there is any excess glucose, it is sent to the liver for preservation in the form of glycogen.

In absence of insulin excess glucose accumulates or builds up in the bloodstream (hyperglycemia) leading to diabetes mellitus. Diabetes not only occurs due to the lack of insulin, it can also occur due to reduced effectiveness of insulin. The disease affects the metabolism of carbohydrates, proteins, fat, water, and electrolytes.

Other important functions of insulin, besides maintaining blood glucose are as follows:
- Stimulates lipogenesis
- Diminishes lipolysis
- Increases amino acid transport into cells
- Modulates transcription
- Altering the cell content of numerous mRNAs
- Stimulates growth
- DNA synthesis
- Cell replication.

Types of Diabetes Mellitus
There are two main types of diabetes mellitus:
1. Insulin-dependent diabetes mellitus (IDDM), which is also called "Type I diabetes" or "Juvenile diabetes" (occurs in 3–5% cases only).
2. Noninsulin-dependent diabetes mellitus (NIDDM), which is also called "Type II diabetes" or "Adult onset diabetes" (occurs in 95% cases).

- The type I diabetes mellitus (IDDM) occurs if the beta cells produce little or no insulin (occurs in children, peak age is 20 years).
- The type II diabetes mellitus (NIDDM) occurs when the beta cells produce insulin but our body cells do not respond to that insulin (hence called *insulin resistance*) (it occurs mostly between ages of 35 years and 40 years).

Clinical Manifestations (Box 14.19)
There are four cardinal signs of diabetes mellitus:
1. Polyuria (frequent urination)
2. Polydipsia (extreme thirst)
3. Polyphagia (increased hunger)
4. Sudden weight loss occurs due to breakdown of body proteins to provide energy in absence of insulin.

Other important features of diabetes mellitus (Fig. 14.15, Box 14.20):
- Unexplained fatigue, irritability, and tiredness
- Nocturia (nocturnal polyuria)—frequent urination at night.
- Drowsiness or lethargy
- Breathing difficulty (hyperventilation)
- Increased susceptibility to infection
- Delayed wound healing
- Myopia with sudden blurred vision
- Numbness of the extremities
- Nausea, vomiting and abdominal pain.

| Box 14.19 | Oral manifestations of diabetes mellitus. |

- Pronounced hyperplasia of the attached gingiva
- Severe rapidly destructive, periodontitis and periodontal abscess formations (diabetes increases the progression of periodontal disease by altering the tissue response to local irritants)
- Pain and inflammation of gingiva, with frequent bleeding
- Dry mouth due to polyuria and dehydration
- Delayed wound healing is one of the most common and important manifestations of the disease
- Diabetic sialosis (symmetrical, painless, recurrent swelling of the salivary glands, particularly parotids) and sialorrhea (excessive secretion of saliva) may also occur
- Increased caries susceptibility in poorly controlled diabetes with higher DMFT caries index
- Increased tendency for oral infections by hemolytic *Streptococci* and *Staphylococci*
- Unusually prolonged oral candidiasis, especially erythematous candidiasis with central papillary atrophy of tongue
- Burning mouth syndrome due to dry and damaged mucosa
- Occasional presence of erosive lichen planus-like lesions in the mouth
- Increased prevalence of "dry socket" after tooth extraction
- Loss of taste sensation or altered taste sensations (dysgeusia)
- Increased incidence of enamel hypoplasia
- Atypical dental pain
- Benign migratory glossitis and mucormycosis may occur in IDDM cases

| Box 14.20 | Complications of diabetes mellitus. |

- Diabetic ketoacidosis
- Diabetic neuropathy
- Diabetic nephropathy
- Diabetic retinopathy
- Vascular disorders
- Ischemic heart disease
- Increased susceptibility to infection
- Hypoglycemic coma and death
- Increased risk of hypoglycemic shock following dental extractions especially in case of delay in taking normal diet.
- Oral lichenoid reactions
- Sialadenosis

Diagnosis

Blood examinations for:

- Fasting blood glucose level—diabetes is diagnosed if it is higher than 126 mg/dL two times.
- Hemoglobin A1c test (HbA1C)—reveals long-term status of blood sugar
  - *Normal*: Less than 5.7%
  - *Prediabetes*: 5.7–6.4%
  - *Diabetes*: 6.5% or higher.
- Random blood sugar level—you may have diabetes if it is higher than 200 mg/dL.
- Glucose tolerance test (GTT)—if sugar concentration in venous blood is above 130 mg/dL, diabetes is confirmed.
- Urinary glucose estimations—if the level is above 10–20 mg/dL, diabetes should be suspected.
- Detection of ketone bodies in urine.

Diabetic Ketoacidosis

Diabetic ketoacidosis (DKA) is a serious complication that occurs mostly in people with uncontrolled type 1 diabetes; the condition develops when the insulin level is very low or absent; hence there is no possibility of energy production by glucose metabolism. In this situation body tries to produce energy through alternate metabolic pathway and it breaks down stored fat and muscles of the body.

Break down of fat produces ketone bodies, which mix up with blood causing

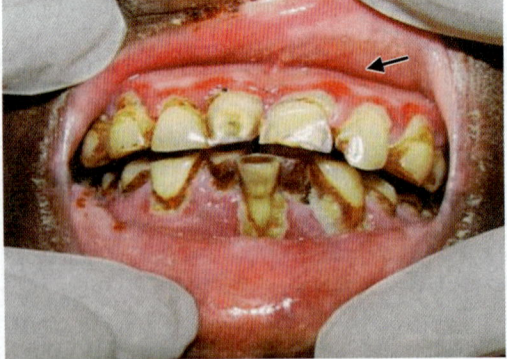

Fig. 14.15: Severe gingivitis in a diabetic patient.

fall of blood pH and metabolic acidosis (the blood becomes acidic and toxic), this often leads to coma.

Features of diabetic ketoacidosis:
- Deep and rapid breathing
- Dry skin and mouth with flushed face
- Acetone smell in mouth (nail polish like smell) or sometimes "sweet and fruity" odor in breath
- Nausea or vomiting, inability to keep down fluids
- Stomach pain
- Patients often have ketone in blood and urine and the sugar level is above 400–800 mg/dL
- Children often die with brain edema.

Gestational (Pregnancy) Diabetes

Gestational diabetes is hyperglycemia (high-blood sugar level) that occurs during pregnancy in otherwise nondiabetic women. It occurs due to hormonal changes during the period of pregnancy and blood sugar level automatically comes back to normal after delivery.

Cause of gestational diabetes: It occurs due to hypersecretion of some hormones particularly the *estrogens, cortisol, and the human placental lactogen,* which suppress the action of insulin and result in hyperglycemia (such type of hormonal actions are called contra-insulin effect). Gestational diabetes usually begins about 20–24 weeks into the pregnancy.

Steroid Diabetes

Steroid diabetes or "steroid-induced diabetes" refers to the prolonged hyperglycemia due to *glucocorticoid therapy* for another medical condition. Prednisolone and dexamethasone are the common hormonal drugs which can cause steroid diabetes.

Cause of steroid diabetes: Steroid diabetes occurs because glucocorticoid hormones oppose the action of insulin and cause increase in blood sugar level either by decreasing the peripheral uptake of sugar or by increasing the process of gluconeogenesis in liver.

Treatment of Diabetes Mellitus
- Diet control
- Administration of oral hypoglycemic drugs
- Insulin therapy whenever necessary.

HYPOGLYCEMIA

When the blood sugar level falls below 70 mg/dL the condition can be called hypoglycemia, it may develop rapidly in people with diabetes who are receive insulin therapy.

Features of Hypoglycemia
- Headache, hunger, and nervousness
- Rapid heartbeat (palpitations), shaking, and sweating
- Severe weakness.

PROGERIA

Progeria is a disease of unknown etiology and it is characterized by dwarfism and premature senility. The affected infants exhibit alopecia, skin pigmentation, atrophic skin, high-pitched voice, smaller mandible, muscular atrophy and joint deformity, etc. The patients usually have an above normal IQ and they resemble a "wizened little old person". Delayed eruption of teeth and excessive secondary dentin formation are the common oral findings.

IMBALANCE OF SEX HORMONES

Imbalance of sex hormones in the body and their related changes in the oral tissue take place during puberty, menstruation, pregnancy, and menopause.

The following oral manifestations are seen due to imbalance in sex hormones:
- *Puberty*: Hyperplastic gingivitis and gingival bleeding
- *Pregnancy*: Gingivitis, gingival bleeding and pregnancy tumor

- *Menstruation*: Transitory gingivitis and cyclical oral ulcerations
- *Menopause*: Desquamative gingivitis, dry mouth, and glossodynia.

BIBLIOGRAPHY

1. Alorecht M, Banoczy J, Tamas G Jr. Dental and oral symptoms of diabetes mellitus. Community Dent Oral Epidemiol. 1988;16:378-80.
2. Aponte-Merced L, Navia JM. Pre-eruptive protein energy malnutrition and acid solubility of rat molar enamel surfaces. Arch Oral Biol. 1980;25:701.
3. Arnaud CD. The parathyroid glands. In: Wyngaarden JB, Smith LHJ (Eds). Cecil Text Book of Medicine, 16th edition. Philadelphia: WB Saunders; 1982. pp. 1286-302.
4. Avioli LV, Krane SM. Metabolic bone disease and clinically related disorders. Philadelphia: WB Saunders Co.; 1990.
5. Baird JD, Strong JA. Endocrine and metabolic diseases. In: Macleod J (Ed). Davidson's Principles and Practice of Medicine. London: Churchill Livingstone; 1979. pp. 506-89.
6. Baxter JD. Endocrine and reproductive disease. In: Wyngarrden JB, Smith LHJ (Eds). Cecil Text Book of Medicine, 16th edition. Philadelphia: WB Saunders; 1982. pp. 1142-56.
7. Bilezikian JP, Levine MA, Marcus R, et al. The parathyroid: Basic and clinical concepts. New York: Raven Press; 1994.
8. Bohme M, Wahlgren CF. Lipoid proteinosis in three children. Acta Paediatr. 1996;85:1003-5.
9. Camargo CA, Kolb EA. Endocrine disorders. In: Krupp MA (Ed). Current Medical Diagnosis and Treatment. Los Altos, California: Appleton and Lange; 1987. pp. 677-748.
10. Campbell MJA. Epidemiology of periodontal disease in the diabetic and the non-diabetic. Aus Dent J. 1972;17:274-83.
11. Chan I, EL-Zurgany A, Zendah B, et al. Molecular basis of lipoid proteinosis in a Libyan family. Clin Exp Dermatol. 2003;28:545.
12. Chatterjee MN, Shinde R. Text book of medical biochemistry, 6th edition. New Delhi: Jaypee Publisher; 2005.
13. Cohen RD. The metabolic and molecular basis of acquired disease. Philadelphia: WB Saunders Co.; 1990.
14. Cotter FE, Pritchard J. Clonality in Langerhans' cell histiocytosis. Br Med J. 1995;310:74.
15. Di Orio LP, Miller SA, Navia JM. The separate effects of protein and calorie malnutrition on the development and growth of rat bones and teeth. J Nutr. 1973;103:856.
16. Edington GM, Gilles HM. The Endocrine Glands in Pathology in the Tropics. London: Edward Arnold; 1969.pp. 551-62.
17. Egeler RM, Favara BE, van Meurs M, et al. Differential in situ cytokine profiles of Langerhans-like cells and T cells in Langerhans cell histiocytosis: Abundant expression cytokines relevant to disease and treatment. Blood. 1999;94:4195.
18. Farrell PM, Bieri JG, Megavitamin E supplementation in man. Am J Clin Nutr. 1975;28:1381.
19. Finestone AJ, Boorujy SR. Diabetes mellitus and periodontal disease. Diabetes. 1967;16:336-43.
20. Franklin EC. Amyloidosis. Bull Rheum Dis. 1975;26:832.
21. Goodman DS. Vitamin A and retinoids: recent advances. Fed Proc. 1969;38:2501.
22. Hamada T, Wessagowit V, South AP, et al. Extracellular matrix protein 1 gene (ECM1) mutations in lipoid proteinosis and genotype-phenotype correlation. J Invest Dermatol. 2003;120:345.
23. Hinrichs EH. Dental changes in juvenile hypothyroidism. J Dent Child. 1966;23:167.
24. Jolly M. Vitamin A deficiency: a review I. J Oral Therapeut Pharmacol. 1971;3:364.
25. Karam JH. Diabetes mellitus, hypoglycaemia and lipoprotein disorders. In: Krupp MA (Ed). Current Medical Diagnosis and Treatment 1987. Los Altos, California: Appleton & Lange; 1987. pp. 749-81.
26. Kyle RA, Bayrd ED. Amyloidosis: review of 236 cases. Medicine. 1975;54:271.
27. Leahy MA, Krejci SM, Friednash M, et al. Human Herpes virus 6 is present in lesions of Langerhans cell histiocytosis. J Invest Dermatol. 1993;101:642.
28. McClain K, Jin H, Gresik V, et al. Langerhans cell histiocytosis: lack of a viral etiology. Am J Hematol. 1994;47:16.
29. Miller MF. Diseases of the endocrine organs. In: Lynch MA (Ed). Burkitt's Oral Medicine. Diagnosis and treatment, 7th edition. Philadelphia: Lippincott; 1977.pp. 443-69.
30. Moy LS, Moy RL, Matsuka LY, et al. Lipoid proteinosis: ultrastructural and biochemical studies. J Am Acad Dermatol. 1987;16:1193.

31. Newton JA, Rasbridge S, Temple A, et al. Lipoid proteinosis—new immunopathological observations. Clin Exp Dermatol. 1991;16:350.
32. Nizel A. Nutrition in clinical dentistry, 3rd edition. Philadelphia: WB Saunders Co.; 1989.
33. Ramsay I, Bayliss R. A Synopsis of Endocrinology and Metabolism. Bristol, England: Wright; 1986.
34. Rao GS. Dietary intake and bioavailability of fluoride. Annu Rev Nutr. 1984;4:115.
35. Rotruck JT, Pope AL, Ganther HE, et al. Selenium: biochemical role as a component of glutathione peroxidase. Science. 1973;179:588.
36. Scully C, Cawson RA. Endocrine and metabolic disease including pregnancy and menopause. In: C Scully, RA Cawson (Eds). Medical Problems in Dentistry. Philadelphia: Elsevier; 1982. pp. 195-241.
37. Sethuraman G, Tejasvi T, Khaitan BK, et al. Lipoid proteinosis in two siblings: a report from India. J Dermatol. 2003;30:562.
38. Shafer WG, Hine MK, levy BM. Oral aspects of metabolic disease. In: Shafer WG, Hine MK, Levy BM (Eds). A Textbook of Oral Pathology, 4th edition. Philadelphia: WB Saunders; 1983. pp. 616-67.
39. Sonis ST, Fazio RC, Fang L. Principles and practice of Oral Medicine. Philadelphia: W.B. Saunders; 1984.
40. Spolnik KJ, Patterson SS, Maxwell DR, et al. Dental radiographic manifestations of end-stage rental disease. Dent Radiogr Photogr. 1981;54:21.
41. Van Dis ML, Allen CM, Neville BW. Erythematous gingival enlargement in diabetic patients: a report of four cases. J Oral Maxillofac Surg. 1988;46:794.
42. Vasilakis GJ, Nygard VK, Dipalma DM. Vitamin D resistant rickets—a review and case report of an adolescent boy with a history of dental problems. J Oral Med. 1980;35:19.
43. Willman CL, McClain KL. An update on clonality, cytokines, and viral etiology in Langerhans cell histiocytosis. Hematol Oncol Clin North Am. 1998;12:408.
44. Witkop CJ, Roa S. Inherited defects in tooth structure. Birth Defects. 1971;7:153.

CHAPTER 15

Diseases of Bone

BASIC STRUCTURE AND FUNCTION OF BONE

Bone tissue is made up of two main components—bone matrix and cellular components (Flowchart 15.1).

Bone matrix is made up of an organic component called "osteoid", constituting 35% of the bone structure and rest are minerals (65%).

Osteoid

It is the organic part of bone matrix, which constitutes about 35% of the extracellular components of bone. It is made up predominantly of type I collagen, some amount of glycosaminoglycans (GAG), and bone proteins derived from osteoblast cells, e.g. osteonectin, osteopontin, fibronectin, and osteocalcin. Among these bone proteins, osteocalcin is the most crucial one because it helps in bone formation, bone mineralization, and calcium homeostasis.

Minerals

Minerals in the bone are present in the form of hydroxyapatite crystals of calcium and phosphorus $[Ca_{10}(PO_4)_6(OH)_2]$ which provide strength and hardness to the organic matrix and also act as the premium reservoir of body's 99% calcium and 85% phosphorus.

Osteoblasts

They are the chief bone-forming cells which synthesize, transport and assemble bone matrix and control its mineralization.

Osteocytes

These are inactive osteoblasts (not dead) which become embedded within the mature bone matrix; osteocyte cells and their cytoplasmic processes reside within the spaces called "lacunae" and "canaliculi", respectively. These cells are interconnected within the bone by their cytoplasmic processes. They help in regulating the bone calcium and phosphate

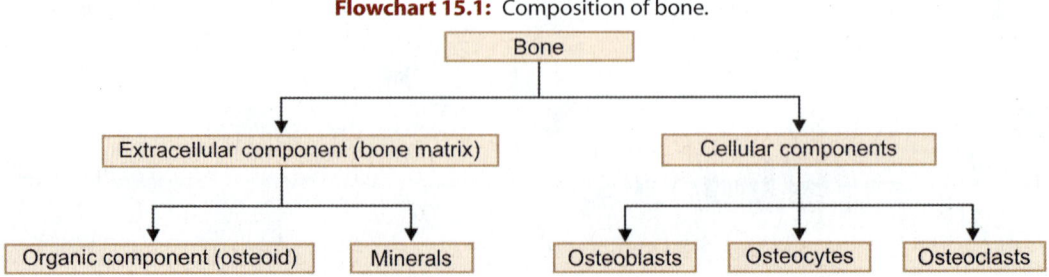

Flowchart 15.1: Composition of bone.

levels; moreover osteocytes also detect the mechanical forces in bone and translate them into biologic activity.

Osteoclast

These are specialized multinucleated macrophages derived from circulating monocytes and are responsible for bone resorption. Osteoclasts have a chemical substance "integrin" on their cell surface, which helps them to attach with bone matrix; after attachment these cells create a trench or "resorption pit" on the bony wall. The osteoclast cells then release acids and enzyme matrix metalloprotease (MMP) into the pit, which cause dissolution of the organic and inorganic components of bone and result in resorption.

Facial profiles in some important diseases are described in Table 15.1.

▰ PAGET'S DISEASE OF BONE (OSTEITIS DEFORMANS)

Definition

Paget's disease is a relatively uncommon bony disorder characterized by repeated phases of extensive bone resorption followed by phases of excessive and uncoordinated new bone formation in the same area. It finally results in formation of large masses of structurally unsound bone in different parts of the skeleton, which often cause severe distortion and weakening of the affected bones.

The disease is named after Sir James Paget who first reported it in the year 1877. It is more prevalent among white populations in England, France, Austria, Germany, and New Zealand, etc.

Etiology

The exact etiology of the diseases is not known, although several factors have been implicated, which probably trigger the disease, these factors include the following:
- Genetic abnormality
- Inflammatory reaction to the bone
- Circulatory disturbances
- Defective connective tissue metabolism
- Slow viral infections (measles and paramyxovirus)
- Autoimmune disorders
- Endocrine abnormality.

Table 15.1: Typical facial profiles in some important diseases.

Mona Lisa facies	Scleroderma
Lion-like (leonine) face	Paget's disease and Lepromatous leprosy
Wolf-like face	Lupus erythematosus
Chubby face	Cherubism
Mask-like face	Facial paralysis
Moon-like face	Cushing's syndrome
Mongoloid facies	Down syndrome
Coarse facies	Acromegaly
"Wizened old man" like face in a child	Progeria
Fish-like face	Crouzon syndrome
Man-like face in women	Androgenital syndrome
Bird facies	Pierre Robin syndrome
Bovine facies (cattle-like)	Craniofacial dysostosis
Chipmunk facies (squirrel -like)	Thalassemia major
Frog-like face	Intranasal disease
Gargoyle facies (ugly animal-like face)	Hurler syndrome
Hippocratic/Cachectic facies	Close to death after severe and prolonged illness, e.g. cancer
Monkey-like face	Marasmus (severely malnourished child)
Snarling (dog-like) facies	Myasthenia gravis
Torpid (dull) facies	Myxedema
Plethoric facies	Polycythemia vera and Cushing's syndrome
Ricketic facies	Rickets
Potter facies	Oligohydramnios (deficiency of amniotic fluid in pregnancy)

Clinical Features

- *Incidence*: The incidence rate is about 2.5% of all persons over 40 years of age.
- *Age*: The disease can occur at any age but usually most of the patients are in their fifth, sixth, and seventh decade of life.
- *Sex*: Males are slightly more commonly affected than females (3:2).
- *Sites*: Paget's disease has a predilection for the weight-bearing areas of the body, especially the vertebral column and femur, etc. The skull, pelvis, and sternum, etc. are also commonly involved. Among the jaw bones, maxilla is affected twice as often as mandible.

Natural History of the Disease

In Paget's disease, the affected bones are abnormal in nature (often referred to as *Pagetic bones*) and the various changes, which take place in these bones during the disease, are divided into three progressive and overlapping phases:

1. *Initially*: Predominantly *osteolytic phase.*
2. *A mixed osteolytic and osteoblastic phase* in the middle.
3. *Finally*: Osteosclerotic phase.

Presentation (Figs. 15.1 and 15.2)

- In many cases, Paget's disease can be asymptomatic, which are detected only during radiographic examinations and the disease is mostly polyostotic but few cases can be monostotic.
- Most of the patients complain initially of a localized deep and aching pain in the affected bone along with bilaterally symmetrical swelling.
- The pain may either be due to microfracture in the affected bone or due to nerve compression by the abnormally growing bone and it is sometimes so severe that the patient is unable to move the affected organ.
- More deformity in the bone is usually observed in the stress-bearing areas, e.g. spine, femur, sacrum, and pelvis, etc.

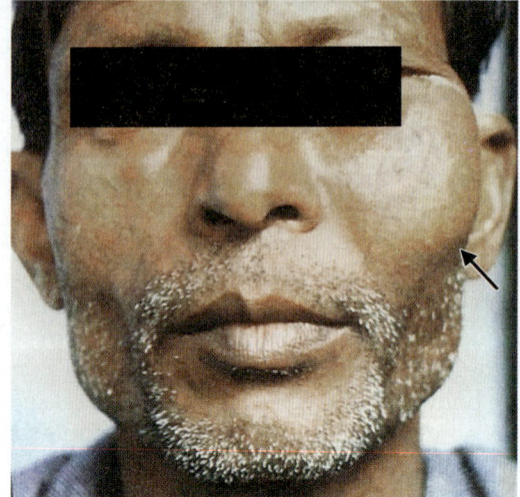

Fig. 15.1: Paget's disease of bone causing swelling of the maxilla.

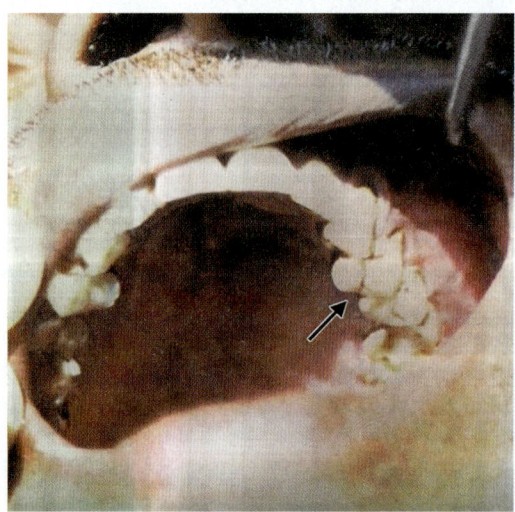

Fig. 15.2: Intraoral view of the same patient showing expansion of the maxillary bone.

- The disease in the weight-bearing areas of the body may cause severe bowing deformity and thereby result in a typical *"monkey-like stance"*. Moreover, these patients often have a characteristic waddling gait.
- Involvement of the craniofacial skeleton often produce *"leontiasis ossea"* (lion-face)

and such patients often have a *grotesque* (ugly and distorted) face due to severe bony deformity.
- Progressive enlargement of the cranium makes it so heavy that *patient is often unable to hold the head erect*; such patients often feel *difficulty in wearing their old hats* (which is an important diagnostic clue for the disease).
- Weakening of the cranial bone may sometimes cause invagination of skull base (platybasia).
- The patients may develop headache, deafness, blindness, and facial paralysis, etc. which occur due to the narrowing of the skull foramina and subsequent compression of the cranial nerves passing through them (both sensory and motor disturbances are seen).
- The defect in long bones (femurs and tibiae) often causes bowing of the legs with localized thickening of the bone in the affected area. The defective long bones in Paget's disease may be further weakened by secondary osteoarthritis and these bones easily get fractured (*"chalk stick-type fracture"*).
- Involvement of spine may cause kyphosis (curvature of the spine); moreover compression fracture of spine in severe cases may result in spinal cord injury.
- *Increased localized temperature of the skin* in the affected areas of bone is often noticed, which is due to hypervascularity in the underlying Pagetic bones.
- Many tumors or tumor-like conditions may develop from the affected bones in Paget's disease, e.g. giant cell tumor of bone, central giant cell granuloma, etc.
- The most serious complication of Paget's disease is the malignant transformation in the affected bone that leads to osteosarcoma and fibrosarcoma.

Radiological Features

The radiographic findings of Paget's disease of bone are highly variable depending upon the stage of the disease.
- Initially, there is presence of only radiolucent areas in the affected bone due to decreased density.
- In the next stage, radiographs of the involved bone reveal haphazard arrangement of newly formed bony trabeculae within the radiolucent area, which often produces a patchy radiopaque pattern called "cotton-wool" appearance (Figs. 15.3A and B).

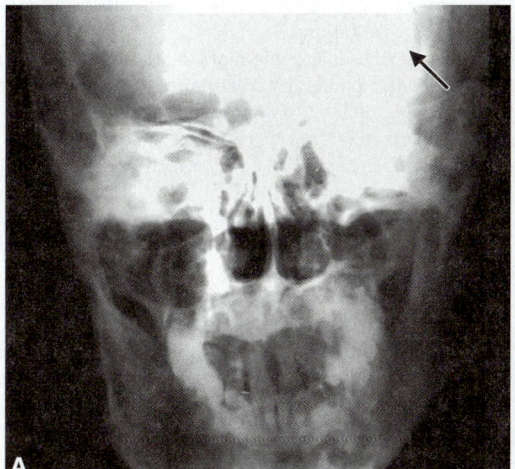
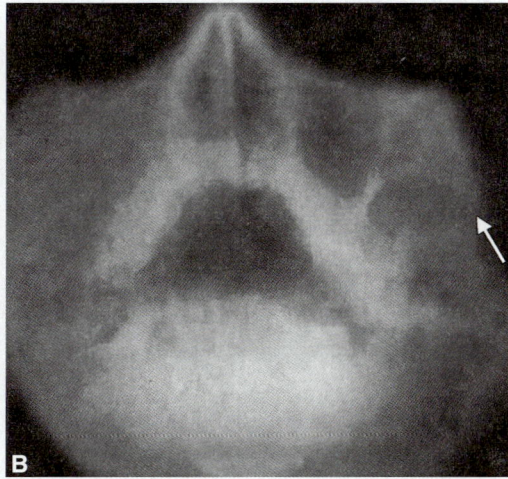

Figs. 15.3A and B: Paget's disease: Increased radiodensity of the skull and jaw bone with a typical "cotton-wool" appearance.

- The lesions become more and more radiopaque due to increased osteosclerosis with loss of normal trabeculations in the later phases of the disease.
- Lateral skull projection reveals a large, prognathic, and pagetoid mandible. The maxillary lesions often extend to the sinuses and cause decreased air-space or obliteration.
- Hypercementosis of the tooth which involves the entire dentition.
- Loss of lamina dura and ankylosis with obliteration of the periodontal ligament space.
- Root resorptions are also commonly observed.
- Monostotic form (involving only a single bone) of Paget's disease of mandible presents a typical "black beard" image on bone scan.

Diseases with "cotton-wool" radiographic appearance:
- Paget's disease of bone
- Chronic diffuse sclerosing osteomyelitis.

Oral Manifestations of Paget's Disease

- Denture-wearing people often complain of tightness of their old dentures with poor fit due to progressive enlargement of maxilla, especially the alveolar ridge.
- Facial paralysis due to compression of the nerve as a result of obliteration of the cranial foramina.
- Diastema, loosening of teeth with malocclusion and difficulty in lip closure are common and all the teeth in the jaw are vital.
- Flattening of palate, retroclination of incisors, and palatoversion of posterior teeth often occurs.
- Moreover, the disease may cause necrosis of the gingiva and the underlying alveolar bone; due to excessive internal pressure in the jaw.
- Gross hypercementosis of teeth is a characteristic finding of Paget's disease and the teeth are often fused with the jaw bone.
- Extraction can be difficult in these patients because of fusion of tooth with the jaws, post-extraction hemorrhage and chances of development of osteomyelitis, etc.
- Maxillary lesions often cross the midline and involve both quadrants of the jaw.
- Pathological fractures in the affected bones may occur, since these bones are very weak despite their gross thickening.

Histopathology

- Rapid, irregular bone resorption, and subsequent exaggerated bone deposition in the same affected area are the hallmark features of Paget's disease.
- The disease begins with random osteoclastic bone resorption and the affected area of bone is replaced by a highly vascularized cellular connective tissue. This stage shows only osteoclastic activity in the bone and there is no osteoblastic activity. The active osteoclasts are often larger in size and their cytoplasm contains several nuclei; few cells can have as many as hundred nuclei or more.

Key Points of Paget's Disease

- Paget's disease is a bony disorder characterized by repeated resorption and deposition with severe weakening and deformity of the affected bone.
- The disease mostly affects older individuals who complain of deep and aching pain, with swelling of the involved bone.
- Progressive enlargement of skull causes difficulty in wearing old hats and enlargement of alveolar ridge makes it difficult to wear dentures.
- Patients may have headache, deafness, blindness, and facial paralysis, etc. due to the narrowing of the skull foramina.
- Flattening of palate, retroclination of incisors, and palatoversion of posterior teeth, diastema, and malocclusion often occurs.
- Radiograph reveals a typical *"cotton-wool"* appearance in the bone and hypercementosis of the teeth.
- Histologically, the bone exhibits rapid resorption and subsequent bone deposition with the presence of multiple reversal and resting lines.
- Laboratory investigation shows markedly raised serum alkaline phosphatase level.
- Paget's disease increases the tendency for pathological fracture of the affected bone as well as increases the risk of development of osteosarcoma.

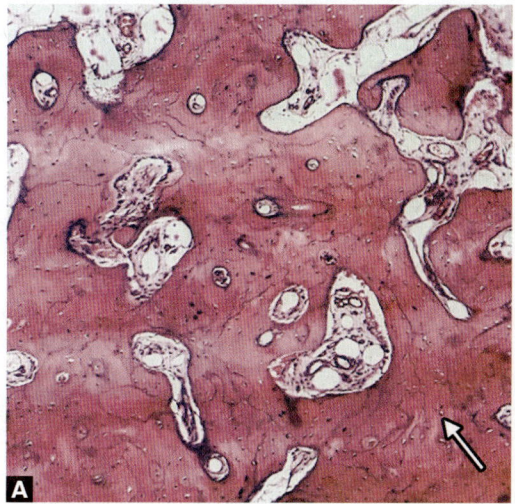 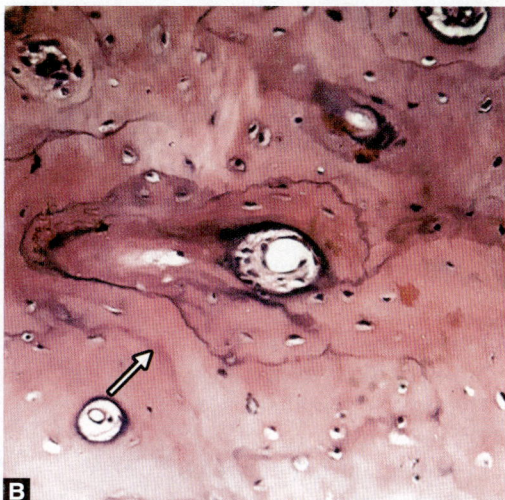

Figs. 15.4A and B: Photomicrographs of Paget's disease showing hypermineralized bone with multiple "reversal" and "resting" lines.

- The second stage of the disease, both osteoclastic and osteoblastic activities occur simultaneously; the lesion shows formation of new lamellar or woven bones within the same connective tissue that has formed due to bone resorption in the earlier stage. The affected area of bone also shows fibrosis of bone marrow tissue.
- The newly formed bone may again be resorbed by the osteoclast cells and this type of repeated bone formation and resorption often cause loss of normal architecture of the bone.
- The final stage of the disease shows increased bone thickening with abnormally increased density of bone (osteosclerosis). The alternate phases of bone resorption and bone deposition are often marked by prominent basophilic "reversal and resting lines" (these lines indicate the junction between alternating areas of bone resorptions and bone formations) (Figs. 15.4A and B).

Reversal Line

A line between two segment bones that have formed at different times (it demarcates the end of osteoclastic activity and the beginning of osteoblastic activity). In Paget's disease, reversal lines are scalloped or wavy and not smooth (scalloped margin indicates that there was bone resorption earlier in the same area).

Resting Line

These are parallel vertical lines representing the periods of rest (or relative quiescence) in between the rhythmic phases of bone deposition.

- The irregular pattern of such lines often characteristically produces a "jigsaw-puzzle" or "mosaic pattern" in the bone.
- The affected bone becomes thick, sclerosed, and the medullary cavity becomes obliterated.
- Chronic inflammatory cells and many dilated blood capillaries are present within the bone.

Laboratory Findings

- During the osteoblastic phase of the disease, the serum alkaline phosphatase level may be markedly elevated up to 250 Bodansky units (normal 1.5–5 units).
- There may be an increased urinary calcium hydroxyproline level during the osteolytic phase of the disease.

- Bone scan may be helpful in determining the exact extent of the disease.
- Although considerable amount of loss of bone minerals occurs due to resorption, the serum calcium and phosphorus levels, however, are always normal or near normal.

Differential Diagnosis
- Acromegaly
- Fibrous dysplasia of bone
- Florid osseous dysplasia
- Hyperparathyroidism
- Osteopetrosis
- Cementifying or ossifying fibromas
- Osteosarcoma
- Metastatic carcinoma
- Sclerosing osteomyelitis.

Treatment
It is not a fatal disease unless there is malignant transformation; symptomatic treatments can be done with analgesics to relieve bone pain. Administration of calcitonin and bisphosphonates may help by suppressing the bone resorption.

Surgery may be required in cases of severe bony deformities and in cases of pathological fractures of the affected bone.

Common lesions exhibiting ossification or calcification within them have been described in Table 15.2.

FIBROUS DYSPLASIA OF BONE

Definition
Fibrous dysplasia is a nonhereditary, idiopathic skeletal developmental disorder of bone-forming mesenchyme that manifests as a defect in osteoblastic differentiation and maturation.

The disease begins with osteolysis, in which an area of normal bone is gradually replaced by fibrous connective tissue, later on the same fibrous tissue undergoes osseous metaplasia and there is again formation of new bone in the area. Although the new bones which form as part of the disease process are entirely different from those present in the normal bone before. Histologically the diseased bone shows all of the components of normal bone but

Table 15.2: Common lesions which exhibit ossification or calcification within them.

A. Inflammatory lesions	• Chronic sclerosing osteomyelitis (focal and diffuse) • Garrey's osteomyelitis • Condensing osteitis • Tuberculosis • Chronic sinusitis • Tonsillolithiasis (stone in tonsil)
B. Neoplastic conditions	• Ossifying fibroma (central and peripheral) • Osteoma or osteoid osteoma • Osteoblastoma • Osteosarcoma • Chondrosarcoma • Cementoma • Cementifying fibroma • Cementoblastoma • Pindborg tumor (CEOT) • Calcifying epithelial odontogenic cyst COC • Adenomatoid odontogenic tumor (AOT) • Odontoma • Ameloblastic fibro-odontoma • Desmoplastic ameloblastoma • Metastatic carcinoma • Mucoepidermoid tumor • Pleomorphic adenoma
C. Fibro-osseous lesions	• Fibrous dysplasia of bone • Paget's disease • Cherubism • Osteogenesis imperfecta • Osteopetrosis
D. Miscellaneous conditions	• Sialolithiasis (stone in salivary gland) • Pulp stone • Calcinosis cutis: CREST syndrome • Traumatic bone cyst • Aneurysmal bone cyst • Exostoses

they fail to differentiate into a fully mature bone probably due to some localized developmental arrest.

Types
Fibrous dysplasia is broadly divided into two types:
1. *Monostotic fibrous dysplasia*: When a single bone is involved by the disease in a localized area. This type accounts for about 80–85% of all cases. Jaw bones are frequently affected in this type.
2. *Polyostotic fibrous dysplasia*: When multiple bones (more than two) of the skeleton are involved by the disease.

The polyostotic fibrous dysplasia of bone has two subtypes:
1. Polyostotic fibrous dysplasia of *Jaffey's type*: In which several bones of the skeleton are affected in association with café-au-lait skin pigmentations (it is often known as Jaffe–Lichtenstein syndrome).
2. Polyostotic fibrous dysplasia in association with *McCune-Albright syndrome*: The condition is characterized by fibrous dysplasia of multiple bones, café-au-lait skin pigmentation, and endocrine abnormalities, especially precocious puberty.

Mazabraud Syndrome
It is a clinical type in which fibrous dysplasia (usually polyostotic) occurs in association with soft tissue myxomas.

Etiology
The exact etiology of the disease is not known, however it is believed to be a nonneoplastic self-limiting condition caused by some genetic abnormality (mutation in *GNAS1* gene). It is believed that the clinical manifestations and severity of fibrous dysplasia varies according to time of mutation in the *GNAS1* gene, for example:
- Albright syndrome develops if mutation occurs during embryogenesis.
- Polyostotic fibrous dysplasia develops if mutation takes place during very early stage of skeleton formation.
- Monostotic fibrous dysplasia develops if mutation occurs during the late stage or after completion of skeleton formation.

Predisposing Factors
- Liver damage
- Infections
- Glandular dysfunctions
- Neurofibromatosis
- Lipoid granulomatosis
- Trauma
- Abnormal osteoclastic maturation of bone forming mesenchyme.

Clinical Features
Age: Fibrous dysplasia usually occurs in the first and second decade of life. Abnormal bony growth continues upto late teens or early twenties.

Sex: The polyostotic type of the disease occurs 2–3 times more often among females, however in monostotic type, males and females are almost equally affected.

Sites: The polyostotic fibrous dysplasia commonly involves the skull, facial bones, clavicles, pelvic bones, and long bones, etc.

The monostotic fibrous dysplasia frequently involves the femur, tibia, ribs, and jaw bones; maxilla is usually more commonly affected than mandible.

The mandibular lesions are often truly monostotic in most cases, whereas the maxillary lesions are frequently associated with involvement in other bones, e.g. frontal, zygomatic, and sphenoid, etc.

Clinical Presentation
(Figs. 15.5 and 15.6)
- The monostotic type of fibrous dysplasia is more common (80-85%) than the polyostotic type.

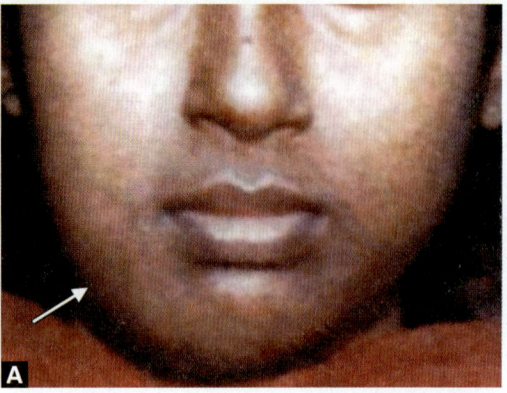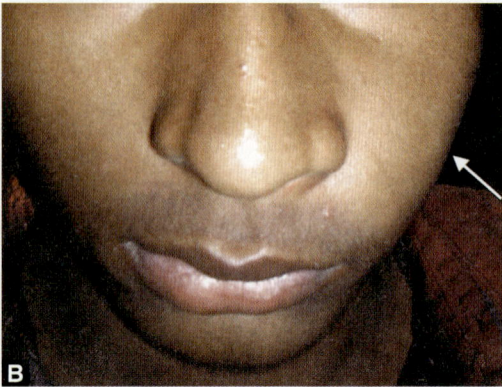

Figs. 15.5A and B: (A) Fibrous dysplasia of right side of mandible; (B) Left side of maxilla.

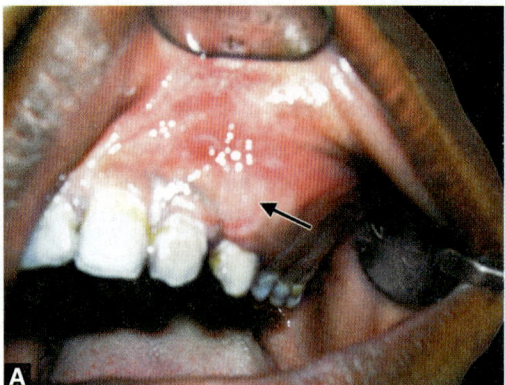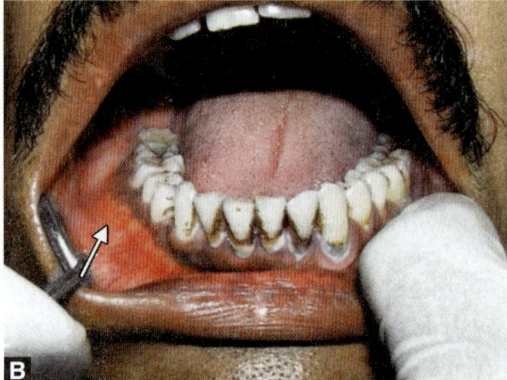

Figs. 15.6A and B: Fibrous dysplasia (intraoral view) of maxillary and mandibular lesions.

- It begins during early adolescent period and often stops spontaneously at the time of skeletal maturation.
- Monostotic type of the disease is mostly asymptomatic and only few patients complain of slow enlarging swelling in the bone with occasional pain. Sometimes severe involvement of the bone may cause fracture and discrepancy in the length of long bone. The monostotic form of the disease never transforms into polyostotic form with time.
- Maxillary or mandibular lesions cause mostly painless, localized unilateral smooth swelling in the jaw.
- Polyostotic fibrous dysplasia occurs at an early age than the monostotic variant and it often shows gradual enlargement of multiple bones at a time.
- Involvement of the jaw bones may cause severe facial asymmetry with marked swelling of the cheek (this may be the first sign of fibrous dysplasia in many children); the disease eventually causes huge deformity of the orofacial region.
- Expansion and gradual distortion of the cortical plates, displacement of teeth, disturbances in tooth eruption (many teeth may even fail to erupt), etc. are commonly observed.
- The teeth may be drifted, rotated or misaligned in the jaw due to the growing bony mass, and in many patients severe malocclusion often develops.

- Although the process is slow enlarging, some lesions may be very aggressive however, palpation in the affected area does not elicit pain. There may be gross deformity in the bones with pathological fractures.
- The maxillary lesions may sometime extend into the maxillary air-sinus and occasionally into the orbital floor; the latter often results in exophthalmos, proptosis, and nasal obstructions, etc. Moreover, maxillary lesions may also exhibit obliteration of the canine fossa.
- Mandibular lesions mostly concentrate near the molar–premolar area and if lower border of the mandible is involved, there is often presence of a bulging and an increase in the depth of the jaw.
- Larger lesions may sometimes become traumatized and ulcerated due to impingement by the teeth during chewing.
- The polyostotic fibrous dysplasia with multiple bone involvement and skin "café-au-lait" pigmentation but without any endocrine disturbances is known as "Jaffe–Lichtenstein syndrome".
- The "café-au-lait" skin pigmentations are characterized by light-brown pigmented areas on the skin overlying the affected bone. The pigmentation is mostly seen in the neck, buttock, back, trunk, thigh, and sacral areas; it shows a typically irregular serpiginous border (jagged periphery). The café-au-lait pigmentations are rarely seen in the oral mucosa.
- This pigmentation can also be seen in Von-Recklinghausen's disease, where they have a characteristic "smooth border" rather than a "jagged border".
- Polyostotic fibrous dysplasia of bone with "café-au-lait" skin pigmentations and multiple endocrinopathies like precocious puberty in females, pituitary adenoma, acromegaly, goiter, Cushing syndrome, hyperparathyroidism, and hyperthyroidism, etc. constitute the syndrome called "McCune–Albright syndrome".
- The precocious puberty in Albright syndrome occurs in young women and it consists of premature vaginal bleeding in the first few months of life, breast development, and axillary and pubic hair growth, etc. at the age of about 2–3 years.
- On rare occasions, fibrous dysplasia lesions may undergo malignant transformation and develop fibrosarcomas.

Radiological Features
- In the initial stages, both monostotic and polyostotic forms of the disease produce unilocular or multilocular radiolucent areas in the bone containing faint bony trabeculae (Figs. 15.7A and B).
- The disease often produces expansion and distortion of cortical plates of bone with displacement of teeth.

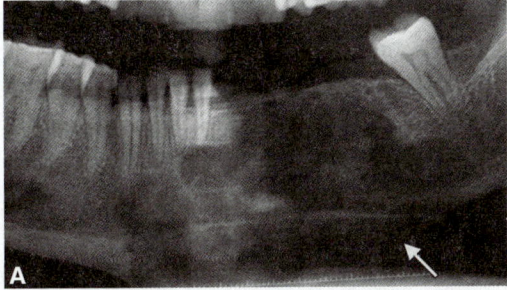 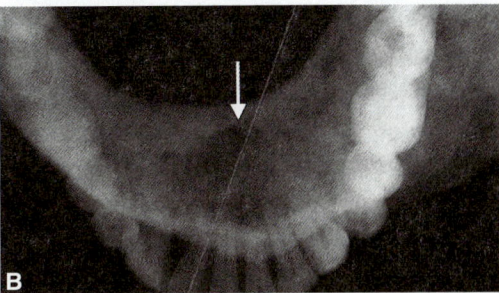

Figs. 15.7A and B: (A) X-ray showing a typical "ground glass" appearance in mandible; (B) X-ray showing severe expansion with a typical "orange peel" appearance of mandible.

- Sometimes "egg-shell" crackling of the expanded cortex of the affected bone may be seen.
- Later on, as the lesion matures, a classical "ground-glass" or "orange peel" or "pebbled" appearance of bone is observed in radiographs and ground-glass type is the most common radiographic appearance of fibrous dysplasia.
- The margin of the lesion is not well-demarcated and it gradually blends imperceptibly with the adjacent normal bone.
- Mandibular lesions exhibit expansion of both buccal and lingual cortical plates with bulging distortion of the lower borders.
- The inferior alveolar canal is often displaced superiorly from its normal position due to the expanding bony lesion.
- Both erupted and unerupted teeth are randomly distributed within the lesion.
- Fibrous dysplasia often radiographically exhibits narrowing of the periodontal ligament space and an ill-defined lamina dura.
- Maxillary lesions present obliteration of the maxillary sinus with superior displacement of the sinus floor.
- Involvement of multiple skull bones, e.g. occipital, frontal, and sphenoid, etc. by the disease along with the maxillary bone often characteristically produces increased density of the base of the skull.

Lesions with ground-glass radiographic appearance:
- Fibrous dysplasia of bone
- Cherubism
- Hyperparathyroidism.

Key Points of Fibrous Dysplasia of Bones

- ❖ Fibrous dysplasia is a fibro-osseous disorder, in which an area of normal bone is gradually replaced by abnormal fibrous connective tissue.
- ❖ The disease occurs in two main forms—monostotic (when a single bone is affected) and polyostotic (when multiple bones are affected).
- ❖ The disease causes progressive, painless, and smooth swelling of the jaw with facial asymmetry.
- ❖ Polyostotic fibrous dysplasia may be associated with McCune–Albright syndrome, which presents multiple bone swelling, "café-au-lait" skin pigmentations, and precocious puberty, etc.
- ❖ On radiographs, the disease produces a classical, "ground-glass" appearance of bone.
- ❖ Histologically, fibrous dysplasia exhibits a highly cellular and well-vascularized fibrillar connective tissue that replaces the normal bone.
- ❖ Multiple irregular trabeculae of immature bone are found within the fibrous tissue, typically producing a "*Chinese letter*" pattern.

Differential Diagnosis

- Ossifying fibroma enchondroma
- Giant cell tumor of bone
- Paget's disease of bone
- Garre's osteomyelitis
- Brown tumor of hyperparathyroidism
- Low grade osteosarcoma
- Eosinophilic granuloma.

Laboratory Findings

- The serum calcium, phosphorus, and alkaline phosphatase levels are within normal limits.
- Occasionally, there may be elevated serum alkaline phosphatase levels in polyostotic form of the disease.
- Basal metabolic rate may be moderately high.
- Premature secretion of pituitary follicle-stimulating hormone may occur in some cases.

Macroscopic Findings

Macroscopically the lesion is well-circumscribed and present within the medullary cavity, causing variable degrees of bone expansion and distortion. The lesional tissue looks glossy, tan-white in color, and it gives a gritty feeling while cutting (the gritty feeling may be due to the presence of many thin bony trabeculae within the tissue).

Few lesions may be bluish-white in color, which is due to chondroid metaplasia of the lesional bone.

Histopathology (Fig. 15.8)

- Histologically, fibrous dysplasia reveals the presence of a highly cellular and relatively avascular fibrillar connective tissue that replaces the normal bone.
- The diseased tissue contains multiple, bland spindle-shaped fibroblast cells of uniform size which are arranged in a "whorled pattern" and moreover, the collagen fiber bundles completely lack their orientation.
- Multiple thin, irregular, curvilinear trabeculae of woven bone are distributed within the fibrous tissue and their abnormal arrangement or distribution within the lesion often produces a "Chinese letter" pattern. These bony trabeculae often lack prominent osteoblastic rimming and these are formed due to osseous metaplasia of the connective tissue stroma.
- These bony trabeculae are evenly spaced, uniformly distributed, and are separated from one another, the trabeculae are not bordered by osteoblast cells as seen in the normal bone, instead there may be few osteoblast cells scattered throughout the bone trabeculae.
- Spheroidal areas of calcification resembling cementum may be present within the lesion and occasionally there may be presence of foci of giant cells in the lesion.
- In jaw lesions, the bony trabeculae may be thicker and blunter than that of the long bone lesions.
- At the margin, the lesion gradually blends with the surrounding normal bone (this feature particularly distinguishes fibrous dysplasia from ossifying fibroma of bone, since the latter lesion is well-demarcated from the surrounding bone by a capsule).
- With increase in the age of the lesion, the amount of cellularity within the fibrous tissue decreases, and the amount of bone tissue increases. This feature is more commonly evident in the jaw lesions rather than the long bone lesions.
- Occasionally, fibrous dysplasia of bone may be associated with the development of aneurysmal bone cyst.

Treatment

Fibrous dysplasia is a self-limiting disease and the growth usually ceases after puberty, with spontaneous bone remodeling. However, surgical recontouring of bone may be needed in larger lesions for cosmetic or functional reasons. Fibrosarcoma may develop from these lesions, especially, following radiotherapy.

■ CHERUBISM/FAMILIAL FIBROUS DYSPLASIA OR DISSEMINATED JUVENILE FIBROUS DYSPLASIA

Definition

Cherubism is a rare benign hereditary (autosomal dominant type) familial fibrous dysplasia of the jaws, involving more than one quadrant and it often causes "bilaterally symmetrical enlargement" of mandible or sometimes the maxilla that stabilizes after puberty. Cherubism was first reported by Jones in the year 1933.

Pathogenesis

Cherubism is a hereditary disease (autosomal dominant disorder) however, according to

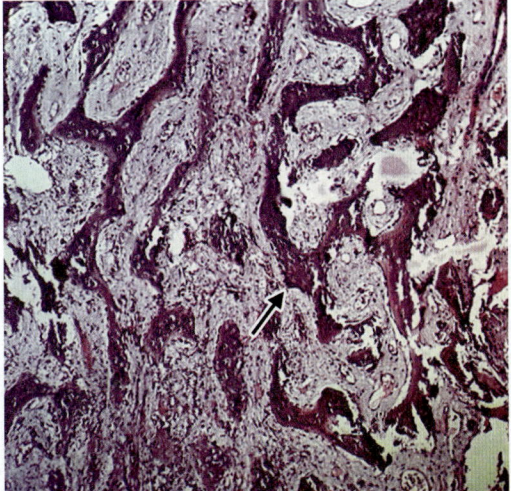

Fig. 15.8: Photomicrograph of fibrous dysplasia of bone.

many investigators, it can occur as a result of the following reasons:
- Anomalous development of bone
- Latent hyperparathyroidism
- Hormone-dependent neoplasm
- Trauma
- Disturbance in the development of bone forming mesenchyme.

Clinical Features

Age: The disease commonly affects the young individuals, usually at the age between 1 year and 5 years.

Sex: More common among males than females; it is also more severe in boys than girls.

Presentation

- The disease follows a familial pattern and several members of the same family may be affected. Some nonfamilial cases are also reported, which occur due to new mutations.
- At birth, the appearance of the patient is absolutely normal. However, between the age of 1 year and 5 years, painless, bilateral, and symmetric swelling develops in mandible or sometimes in maxilla in severe cases (Figs. 15.9A and B).
- In cherubism, symmetrical, broad, and protruding mandibular swelling (which starts at the angle region on both sides) causes excessive cheek fullness. This often gives rise to the typical appearance of "chubby face" to the child. Since most little children naturally have a somewhat chubby face, the parents may not appreciate the abnormality unless the mandibular swelling becomes substantial.
- When the maxillary swelling is very extensive, pressure on the floor of the orbit may result in an upward turn of pupils of the patient's eyes and thus revealing a rim of white sclera below the iris; this phenomenon is often referred to as the "heavenward look (eye toward heaven)". This so called heavenward look often gives patient an "angelic appearance".
- Moreover, the severe maxillary swelling in cherubism may cause stretching of the facial skin and retraction of the lower eyelids.
- Patients with cherubism also exhibit expansion, and widening of the alveolar ridge, premature exfoliation of deciduous teeth; extensive diastema formation, delayed eruption of permanent teeth and flattening of the palatal vault, which may be "V"-shaped.
- Noninflammatory submandibular lymph-adenopathy also develops in cherubism, which occurs due to reactive hyperplasia, etc.

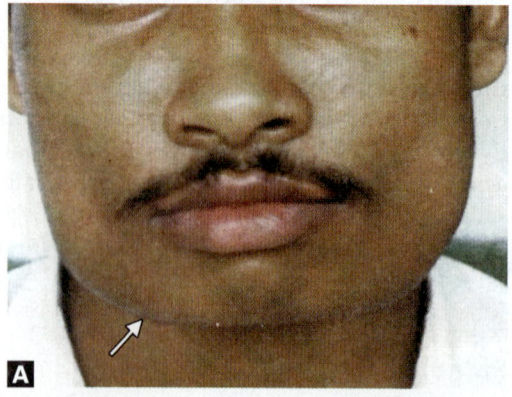 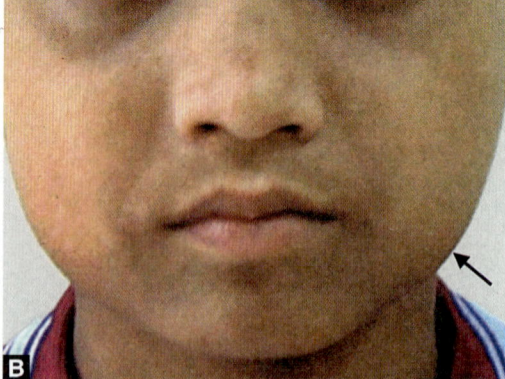

Figs. 15.9A and B: (A) Cherubism producing typical bilateral mandibular swelling; (B) Bilateral mandibular swelling with 'chubby face' in cherubism.

- Cherubism can also exhibit partial anodontia, rotation or transposition teeth and occasional resorption of roots of teeth.
- In severe cases of cherubism, the jaw swelling can be so massive that the patients may have masticatory, swallowing, speech, and even breathing difficulties.
- Compression of the cranial nerves may cause visual and auditory disturbances in cherubism. On rare occasions, there can be destruction of the infraorbital ridge.
- Pathological fracture of the affected bone may occur in some cases.
- The bony swelling continues till puberty and then it starts to regress; face becomes normal by 25–40 years of age. Moreover, there may be development of central giant cell granuloma from a preexisting lesion of cherubism.
- Cherubism has been reported to occur in conjunction with Noonan syndrome, which is characterized by congenital heart disease, chest deformity, mental retardation, facial bone anomalies, webbed neck, gingival fibromatosis, blood coagulation disorder, and obstructive sleep apnea, etc.

Radiological Features

- In cherubism, the involved jaw bone radiographically shows well-defined, multilocular, and "cyst-like" or "soap bubble" type radiolucent areas or cavities on both sides of mandible (Figs. 15.10 and 15.11).

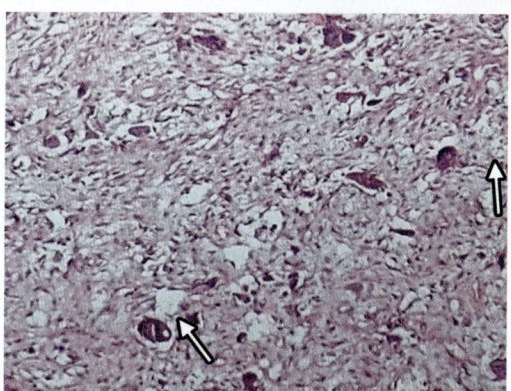

Fig. 15.11: Photomicrograph of cherubism.

- The small radiolucent areas often coalesce together to from larger defects in the bone.
- The initial destruction of bone starts at the angle of the mandible, which can be detected by X-rays even before the clinical symptoms appear.
- Cherubism in later stages causes severe bilateral expansion of the jaw with thinning of the cortical plates. However, the radiographic changes in cherubism are often more overwhelming and extensive than the actual clinical swelling produced by the disease.
- In few cases, there may be presence of the classic "ground-glass" appearance in cherubism.

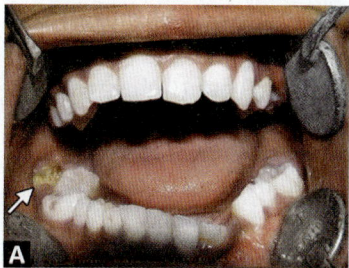
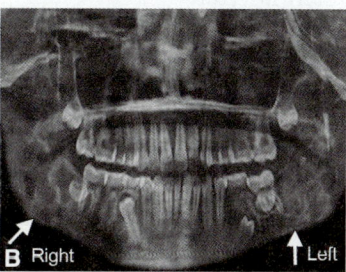
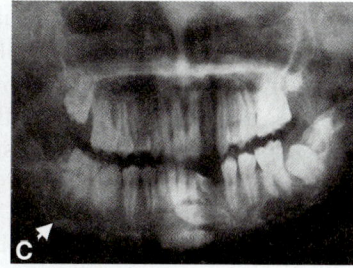

Figs. 15.10A to C: (A) Severe mandibular bony expansion in cherubism; (B) Cherubism: OPG showing bilateral, multicystic lesions in the mandible; (C) Failure of eruption of many teeth in cherubism.

- Radiographs also reveal displacement of the inferior alveolar canal or obliteration of the maxillary antrum in few cases.
- Sometimes, multiple unerupted and displaced teeth appear to be floating within the cyst-like spaces and the condition is often referred to as "floating tooth syndrome".
- Cortical perforations rarely occur and maxillary lesions often extend to the sinus.
- Moreover, the radiographic defects in the bone may persist even after the disease had clinically subsided.

Grading System in Cherubism

According to Ramon and Engelberg, cherubism lesions can be divided into the following grades depending upon the extent and severity of the disease process:
- *Grade I*: Cherubism involving ascending ramus of mandible on both sides.
- *Grade II*: Cherubism involving ascending ramus bilaterally along with both maxillary tuberosities.
- *Grade III*: Massive involvement of whole maxilla and mandible except the condylar processes.
- *Grade IV*: Same as grade III with involvement of floor of orbits causing orbital compression.

Histopathology

- Microscopic section from the lesion presents a highly cellular and vascular connective tissue stroma, which is often arranged in a "whorled pattern".
- Numerous proliferating fibroblasts and variable numbers of multinucleated giant cells are also found within the stroma.
- Giant cells are relatively smaller in size and they often aggregate around the thin-walled blood capillaries.
- The number of giant cells gets fewer and fewer as there is more and more spontaneous repair of the bony defect.
- A distinctive feature of the disease is the presence of an "*eosinophilic perivascular cuffing*" of collagen fibers around the blood capillaries.
- Varying amounts of metaplastic bony tissues are found within the stroma.
- Within the connective tissue, extravasated blood and deposits of hemosiderin pigments are sometimes seen.
- Lymph nodes exhibit reactive hyperplasia, fibrosis, and chronic inflammatory cell infiltration.

Laboratory Investigations

Serum alkaline phosphate levels are raised during the late osteoblastic phase (phase of repair) of the disease. CT scans can be used to determine the extent to which the disease has involved the jaw.

Differential Diagnosis

- Enchondroma
- Fibrous dysplasia of bone
- Hyperparathyroidism
- Eosinophilic granuloma
- Caffey's disease
- Central giant cell granuloma
- Aneurysmal bone cyst.

Treatment

No treatment is required since cherubism is a self-limiting disease and with skeletal maturation the disease regresses spontaneously after puberty.

OSTEOGENESIS IMPERFECTA (BRITTLE BONE DISEASE)

Osteogenesis imperfecta is a genetically transmitted disease of bone characterized by lack of synthesis of type I collagen in bone, which results in defective matrix formation and lack of mineralization with increased bone fragility. Although the disease predominantly affects the bone, it can also disturb other tissues rich in type I collagen, e.g. joints, eyes, teeth, ear, and skin, etc.

Pathogenesis

Osteogenesis imperfecta is a hereditary disease, in which mutations occur in the genes that encode the α1 and α2 chains of type I collagen and as a result there is defective assembly of higher order of collagen polypeptides. This hampers the synthesis of type I collagen and results in defective bone tissue formation and bone mineralization (since type I collagen is the most important component of organic matrix of bone). In osteogenesis imperfecta, there is too little compact bone that results in extreme skeletal fragility (the bones may grow to their normal length but are often thin with lack of usual cortex formation).

Clinical Features (Fig. 15.12)

There are at least four types of osteogenesis imperfecta; two of them are inherited as autosomal recessive traits, while the other two are inherited as autosomal dominant traits.

Interestingly, the recessive variants of the disease are more severe in nature.
General clinical manifestations of osteogenesis imperfecta include the following:
- Bowing deformity of the bone with multiple fractures due to increased skeletal fragility.

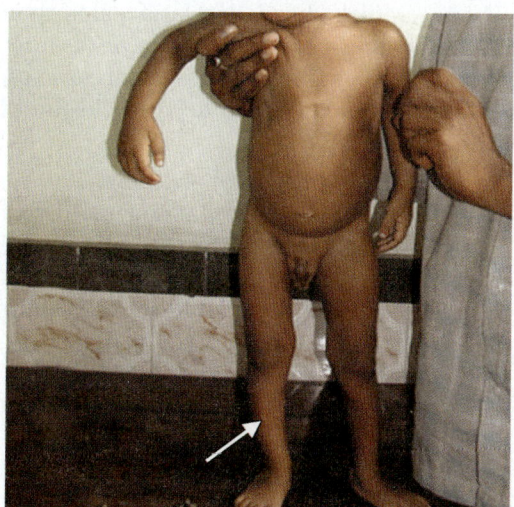

Fig. 15.12: Osteogenesis imperfecta.

- Blue sclera—lack of collagen makes the sclera thin and translucent, as a result the bluish venous plexus of the underlying choroid becomes partially visible.
- Defective teeth—in the form of small teeth with bulbous crowns, dentinogenesis imperfecta with increased secondary dentin formation and development of blue or brown translucency (opalescent teeth).
- Loss of hearing due to defective formation of the bones of middle and inner ear as well as disturbance in sensorineural mechanism.
- Hypermobility of the joints.
- Increased incidence of class III malocclusion due to maxillary hypoplasia.
- Excessive bruising tendency due to defective skin.

Types of Osteogenesis Imperfecta
- Neonatal lethal type
- Severe nonlethal type
- Moderate and deforming type
- Mild and nondeforming type.

Neonatal Lethal Type

This type of osteogenesis imperfecta is the most severe form of the disease (10%) and it is characterized by multiple fractures of bone *in utero* or during parturition and the child seldom survives.

Severe Nonlethal Type

In this form of osteogenesis imperfecta, the disease is not evident until the late childhood and the patient shows fractures of bone with minimum trauma. Sometimes the fractures may occur at birth and the patients often have generalized bony deformity. Although the fractured bone heals up rapidly, considerable skeletal deformity and a dwarfed stature often develop.

Moderate and Deforming Type

Patients in this type are less severely affected than the other two types already mentioned.

This type of osteogenesis imperfecta may be associated with dentinogenesis imperfecta (more in relation to deciduous teeth) and blue sclera in about 25–50% cases.

Mild and Nondeforming Type

This type of the disease occurs in nearly 60% cases and the patients are clinically normal, although they have an increased tendency for bone fracture due to trauma. These patients also have blue sclera and the associated dentinogenesis imperfecta in about 25% cases.

Oral Manifestations of Osteogenesis Imperfecta

- Large head size, frontal bossing, and maxillary hypoplasia.
- Bulbous crowns of teeth with dentinogenesis imperfecta and blue or brown translucence (opalescent teeth).
- Class III malocclusion with anterior and posterior cross bite.
- Severe attrition of deciduous as well as permanent teeth due to poor bonding strength between enamel and dentin at the DEJ (which appears straight instead of being scalloped as seen in normal teeth).
- Multiple impacted permanent teeth.
- Excessive bruising tendency.
- Increased incidences of development of osteitis and osteomyelitis following extraction of teeth.

Radiological Features

Radiographically, osteogenesis imperfecta reveals the following features:
- Shortened and deformed extremities with large areas of cyst-like radiolucencies.
- Multiple fractures or healed areas of previous fractures are often present in the bone.
- The teeth exhibit features of dentinogenesis imperfecta with bulbous crowns, obliteration of pulp chamber and short roots.
- Radiolucent or mixed "radiolucent-radiopaque" lesions are found in the mandible with extreme thinning of the cortex.
- "Wormin bones" in the skull characterized by multiple small sutural bones in the skull arranged in a mosaic pattern.

Histopathology

- Severe form of osteogenesis imperfecta histologically reveals thinning of the cortex, which is composed of immature woven bone.
- Bony trabeculae are short, thin, and fragile and they are widely spaced and disorganized.
- Bony tissue displays increased number of osteoblasts with severely reduced bone matrix.
- The immature woven bones do not transform into mature lamellar bones.

Treatment

No treatment is possible to alter the course of the disease. Some improvements in the condition occur automatically after puberty. Care should be taken during extraction of tooth, so that alveolar bone is not fractured.

CLEIDOCRANIAL DYSPLASIA

Definition

Cleidocranial dysplasia (CCD) [cleido = collarbone, cranial = head, dysplasia = abnormal formation], a rare genetic skeletal disorder characterized by abnormal growth of clavicles, dental abnormalities, and delayed closure of the fontaneles.

There are two important phenomena:
1. *Cleidocranial dysostosis*—skeletal defect involving a single bone or only a small group of closely related bones (in this disease only clavicle is defective with or without defect in the cranial bones).
2. *Cleidocranial dysplasia*—is a widespread, diffuse skeletal defect with absence or hypoplasia of clavicles, defective craniofacial bones, growth retardation, and dental abnormality, especially delayed or failure of eruption of teeth.

Origin
The disease may be hereditary in nature with autosomal dominant trait or it may occur as a result of spontaneous mutations.

Clinical Features
- There may be complete absence or hypoplasia of one or both clavicles with hypermobility of the shoulder joints and it is the most important feature of cleidocranial dysplasia.
- The disease affects both sexes equally.
- Interestingly, the patients can bring their opposing shoulders medially up to the midline due to partial or complete absence of the clavicles and weakness of the muscles attached to them.
- Frontal and parietal skull plates are elongated (bossing), although the other bones of the skull are normal.

> **Key Points of Cleidocranial Dysplasia**
> - Cleidocranial dysplasia is a rare genetic disorder characterized by abnormal growth of clavicles, skull, and the face with a tendency for failure of tooth eruption.
> - Due to abnormal development of clavicles, patients can often move their opposing shoulders medially up to the midline.
> - Patients also have short stature, big head, frontal bossing, delayed closure of fontanels, etc.
> - Oral manifestations of the disease include hypoplasia of the jaws and multiple impacted or unerupted supernumerary teeth.
> - Radiograph reveals partial or complete loss of clavicles, warmin bone in the skull with open fontanels, and multiple impacted teeth in the jaw.

- Patients often have short stature, big head, long neck, and narrow shoulders, etc.
- Delayed closures of the fontaneles, underdeveloped paranasal sinuses, ocular hypertelorism, and photophobia, etc. are the other important features of the disease.

Oral Manifestations
- Entire mid-face is underdeveloped with retrusion maxilla and decreased lower facial height.
- Nose is flat, broad-based, and lacks the bridge.
- Although, the mandible is of normal size, it appears elongated because of the hypoplastic maxilla.
- High and narrow arched palate is almost always seen with increased incidences of cleft palate.
- In the oral cavity, multiple impacted permanent teeth and several retained deciduous teeth are often present.
- Large numbers impacted supernumerary teeth are also found in the jaws, which exhibit defective crowns and abnormal root patterns.
- Roots of the permanent teeth are often thin and short, moreover there may be absence of cellular cementum on the roots.
- Development of partial or complete anodontia may be seen in few cases.
- Cystic lesions (especially dentigerous cysts) may develop in the jaws, mostly in association with the impacted teeth.

Radiographic Features
- Tortuous suture lines in the skull bones (wormin bones) with open fontaneles and open sutures.
- Partial or complete loss of clavicles.
- Multiple unerupted and impacted teeth in the jaws, some of which are deciduous and some are supernumerary teeth.
- Roots of the teeth are thin and short.
- Maxillary sinus is small and rudimentary.
- Ascending ramus of the mandible is narrow.
- There may be hypoplasia of the alveolar process.

Histopathology
The permanent teeth have no cellular cementum.

Differential Diagnosis
- Craniofacial dysostosis
- Cleidocranial dysostosis.

Treatment

No treatment is possible.

OSTEOPETROSIS/MARBLE BONE DISEASE/ALBERS-SCHÖNBERG DISEASE

Definition

Osteopetrosis is an uncommon hereditary bone disorder characterized by reduced physiologic bone resorption and an abnormal increase in the bone density (skeletal sclerosis), which occurs due to impaired function of osteoclast cells. In the disease, the density of bones is extremely high ("stone-like" or "chalk-stick" like bones) and such bones are more brittle and susceptible to fracture.

Types

- Autosomal dominant—benign type (adult osteopetrosis).
- Autosomal recessive—malignant type (infantile osteopetrosis).

Pathogenesis

The defect is a genetic one, characterized by lack of balance between bone deposition and bone resorption in the skeleton. In this disease, bone deposition by the osteoblast cells is normal but the normal physiologic bone resorption by osteoclast cells is hampered due to impairment in the process of acidification in the osteoclast resorption pit that is essential for the dissolution of the calcium hydroxyapatite of bone.

The disease eventually results in the development of hypermineralized, inelastic, "chalk-stick" like bones with extreme brittleness.

Clinical Features

- In osteopetrosis, the abnormalities in the bone often result in altered sutures, compression of cranial nerves, and frequent fractures, etc.
- Decreased bone marrow hematopoietic functions (as the medullary space is often completely obliterated by abnormal bone deposition) result in anemia, thrombocytopenia, and leucopenia, etc.
- Lack of bone marrow activity results in compensatory extramedullary hemopoiesis within the liver and spleen, which often results in hepatosplenomegaly.
- The infants suffering from malignant version of this disease generally have osteopetrosis at birth or in the early childhood and they rarely survive longer.
- Patients often have broad face, hypertelorism, and snub nose, etc.
- Patients often suffer from deafness, blindness, pain, and facial paralysis, etc. due to narrowing of the cranial foramina and the resultant compression of nerves.
- Enlarged cranium, frequent bone pain, and prominent frontal bossing, etc. are also frequently seen.
- Long bones are often shortened and are extremely fragile.
- Severe cases of osteopetrosis result in breathing and hearing difficulties due to oversized facial bones and mastoid process.
- The teeth often have defective enamel and short roots. Their eruption process can be delayed.
- There can be increased incidence of dental caries and many of the teeth in the dental arch can be ankylosed.
- Increased bone density and fragility may cause frequent fractures of jawbone and osteomyelitis following tooth extractions; these occur due to decreased blood supply to the bone with poor healing capacity along with increased susceptibility to infections.

Radiology

In osteopetrosis, radiographs often show the classical feature of *"bone within the bone appearance"*. It results from increased thickening of the cortex and obliteration of the medullary spaces of bone. Radiographs of the jaw bone exhibit increased *radiodensity of the bone, which is almost equal to that of the tooth.*

The cartilaginous portions of the rib also exhibit an uncharacteristic increase in the opacity. Cranial bones appear thickened and sinus cavities are reduced in size.

Differential Diagnosis
- Endosteal hyperostosis
- Van Buchem disease
- Sclerosteosis.

Histopathology
- Microscopy shows a very dense and sclerotic bone with little compensatory remodeling.
- The medullary cavities are small and they contain very little amount of marrow tissue and large amounts of amorphous bone.
- In the bone marrow, osteoblasts are present in normal numbers, but the osteoclasts are almost absent.
- In some cases, normal number of osteoclast cells may be present in the bone, but these cells are not functionally viable.

Treatment
No treatment except bone marrow transplantations. Supportive therapies like repeated blood transfusions and antibiotics are essential for the survival of the patient.

■ MARFAN SYNDROME

Definition
Marfan syndrome is a hereditary disease transmitted or inherited as autosomal dominant trait and is characterized by defective organization of collagen.

Clinical Features (Fig. 15.13)
- The classic clinical finding in this disease is the presence of abnormally long, thin extremities, and spidery fingers (Fig. 15.14).

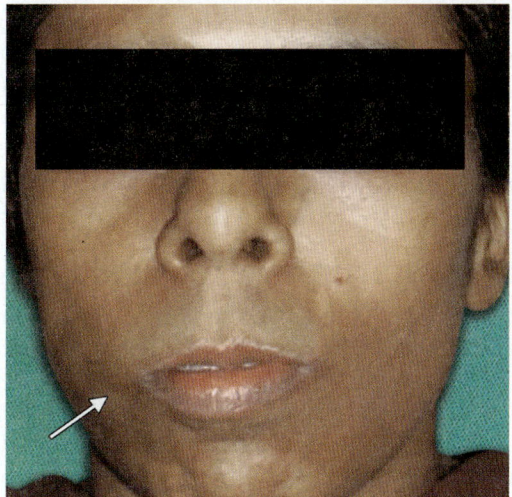

Fig. 15.13: Marfan's syndrome-I.

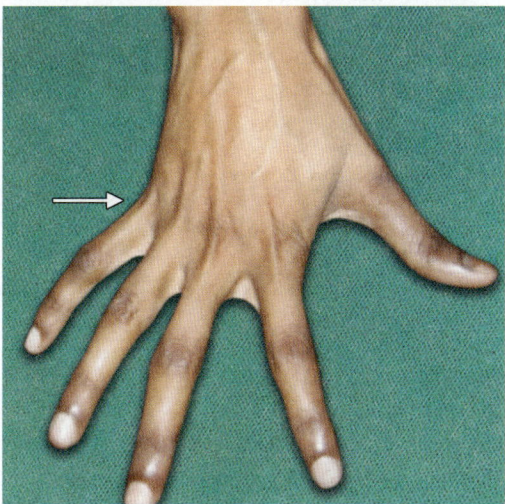

Fig. 15.14: Marfan's syndrome "spidery fingers".

- Patients are usually very tall and slim, and they often have muscle hypotonia.
- The patients often show hyperextensibility of joints, with recurrent habitual dislocations, frontal bossing, large external ears, and shrunken eyes, etc.
- Cardiac abnormalities like aortic aneurysm, aortic regurgitation, and valvular defects, etc. are also commonly associated with this disease.

Oral Manifestations (Fig. 15.15)

- Patients often have a long and narrow face, bifid uvula, cleft palate, and high palatal vault.
- Malocclusion of teeth, TMJ dysarthrosis.
- Increased chances of development of multicystic lesions in the jaw bone.

DOWN SYNDROME (TRISOMY 21)

Down syndrome is the most common chromosomal abnormality to occur in man. There are many forms of the disease but the most common one is trisomy 21 (about 94%), which is caused by the chromosomal nondisjunction, thereby resulting in an extra chromosome with the chromosome pair of 21.

The Down syndrome of trisomy 21 type involves almost all organs of the body and it affects the child more often, if the maternal age is above 45 years.

Clinical Features (Figs. 15.16 and 15.17)

- Patients with Down syndrome present a variety of defects like—short stature, flat face, depressed nasal bridge, and small slanting eyes with epicanthal folds (features of typical mongoloid facies).
- Mental retardation, large anterior fontaneles, open cranial sutures, small ears and sexual underdevelopment, etc. are often present.
- Patients often have broad and short hands with small feet and digits, protuberant abdomen, and delayed puberty, etc.
- These patients often have heart anomalies (40% cases); moreover they come in the higher risk category for development of leukemia and Alzheimer-like dementia in later life.
- The iris shows Brushfield spots.

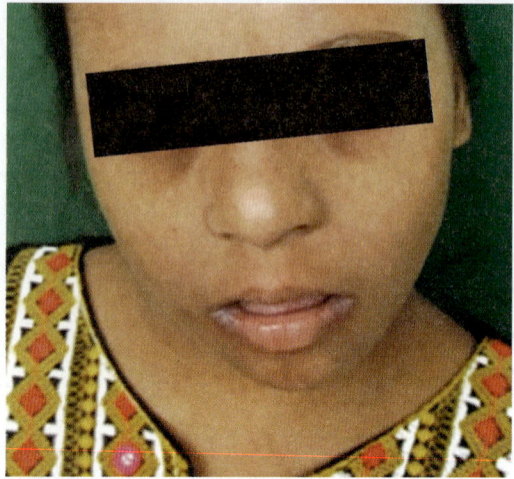

Fig. 15.16: Down syndrome with typical "mongoloid facies "Showing frontal bossing, depressed nasal bridge, and open mouth.

Oral Manifestations of Down Syndrome

- Short head, small and open mouth with protrusion of tongue due to macroglossia.
- High-arched palate, hypoplastic maxilla.
- Mandibular prognathism with class III malocclusion, delayed eruption of teeth.
- There may be presence of cleft lip or palate with difficulty in speech.
- Tongue is generally large (macroglossia), it is pebbly and fissured (scrotal tongue).
- Lips are often thick, everted, dry and fissured with presence of angular cheilitis

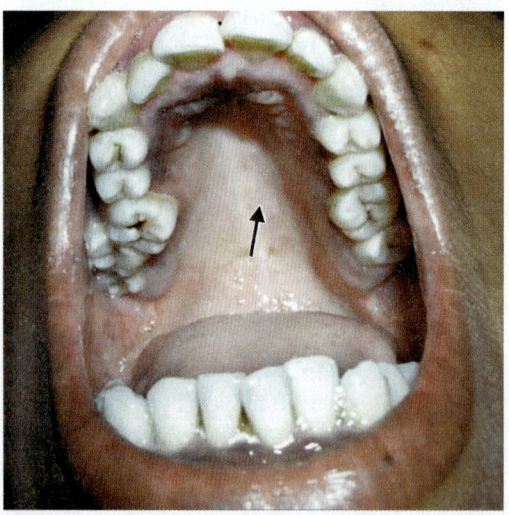

Fig. 15.15: Marfan's syndrome showing "high arched" palate.

Diseases of Bone

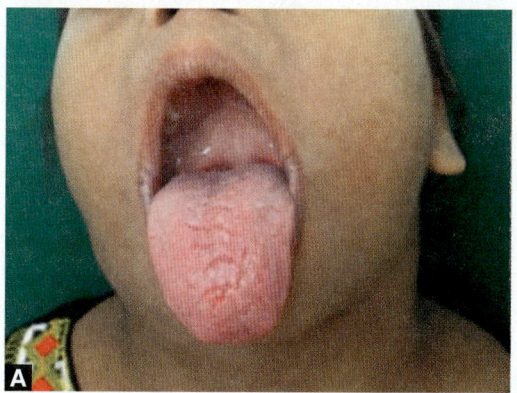 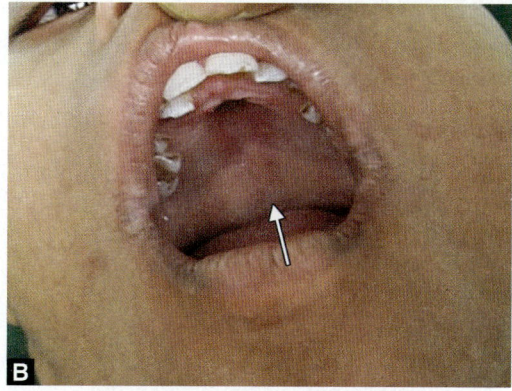

Figs. 15.17A and B: Down syndrome with macroglossia: (A) Scrotal tongue; (B) High-arched palate.

- Malocclusion, partial anodontia and microdontia with short roots of teeth.
- Malformed teeth, taurodontism, supernumerary teeth and enamel hypoplasia, etc. are frequently seen.
- Low caries activity.
- These patients may have an increased tendency to develop acute necrotizing ulcerative gingivitis (ANUG) and juvenile periodontitis.

Treatment
No treatment is required.

INFANTILE CORTICAL HYPEROSTOSIS (CAFFEY'S DISEASE)

Definition
Caffey's disease is a perplexing anomaly of unknown etiology and it is characterized by an abnormal enlargement of bone in children, along with other systemic complications.

Types
Two types—familial and sporadic, the familial type arises usually earlier than the sporadic type and some lesions can be present even at birth.

Clinical Features
- Most of the patients are below 6 months of age and in few cases it may even develop in the intrauterine life.
- Patients often exhibit rapidly developing, bilaterally symmetrical mandibular swelling, which disappears in 3–12 months. However, the disease should not be confused with cherubism, which also presents bilateral mandibular swelling.
- There may be presence of few deep-seated, tendered, and soft tissue swellings.
- The patients are often highly irritable and are unable to take food, and they may also have fever, leukocytosis, raised ESR, and elevated serum alkaline phosphatase levels, etc.
- Dysphagia, pseudoparalysis, anemia, and leukocytosis often occur.
- Soft tissue swellings usually develop in those areas of the body from where hyperostosis of the bone occurs in future.

Oral Manifestations
- Frequent mandibular bone involvement with deformity and facial swelling.
- Soft tissue or muscle swelling of the face.
- Difficulty in swallowing.
- Refusal of food by the child.
- Malocclusion of teeth.

Radiographic Features
Radiographically, the disease exhibits abnormal thickening of mandibular cortical bone and bulging of its lower border due to subperiosteal

new bone formation. The subperiosteal new bone formation with cortical thickening is often known as periosteal cloaking.

Histopathology
Microscopy reveals edema and thickening of the periosteum, with apposition of many thin bony trabeculae parallel to one another.

Differential Diagnosis
- Osteomyelitis
- Osteoma
- Abnormally healed fractured bone
- Cherubism
- Osteopetrosis.

Treatment
No surgical intervention is required and prognosis is good. Steroids may be given to eliminate the symptoms.

MANDIBULOFACIAL DYSOSTOSIS (TREACHER–COLLINS SYNDROME)

Mandibulofacial dysostosis is rare hereditary or familial disease characterized by defects in the structures derived from first and second branchial arches. The disease often shows multiple closely related defects of the head and face area.

Clinical Features
- Malformation of the external ear (distorted pinna) with absence of external auditory canal; there is occasional deformity in the middle and internal ear.
- Antimongoloid palpebral fissures with coloboma of the outer portion of the lower eyelids.
- Marked hypoplasia of the mandibular body and zygoma with narrow face and depressed cheek.
- All these facial changes give the patient a typical "bird-face" or "fish-face" like appearance.
- Patients often have a down turned mouth with presence of lateral facial clefts.
- Important oral manifestations of this disease include crowding and malocclusion of teeth, high arched palate, and occasional clefts, etc.
- Atypical hair growth in the form of 'tongue shaped" hairline.
- Parotid hypoplasia.
- Narrowing of larynx and trachea combined with mandibular hypoplasia often causes respiratory and speech difficulties in children.

Radiographic Changes
Radiographs reveal partial or complete agenesis of mandible and malar bones with small paranasal sinuses.

Treatment
No treatment is required.

ACHONDROPLASIA

Definition
Achondroplasia is the most common skeletal dysplasia, which occurs due to hereditary defect in endochondral ossification. The disease is caused by retarded cartilage growth due to failure of normal cartilage proliferation at the epiphysis and it results in failure of longitudinal growth of the long bones.

Clinical Features
- Achondroplasia is the major cause of dwarfism and patients with the disease often exhibit short and muscular extremities, bowed legs, and large head with prominent forehead, etc.
- The limbs are extremely short in relation to the trunk and head and these short-limbed dwarfs of achondroplasia traditionally become circus clowns.
- Except the skeletal abnormality, these patients usually have normal intelligence, reproductive status, and lifespan.
- Oral manifestations of this disease include short maxilla, depressed nasal bridge,

relative mandibular prognathism, and malocclusion, etc.

MASSIVE OSTEOLYSIS (VANISHING BONE DISEASE)

Definition

It is an uncommon and unusual disease characterized by sudden, spontaneous, and massive resorption of bones leading to their complete disappearance and subsequent replacement by fibrous tissue.

Clinical Features

Age: Teen age and young adults.
Sex: Commonly affected bones by the disease are clavicle, scapula, humerus, ribs and sacrum, etc.
- Among the jaw bones, mandible is more frequently affected than maxilla.
- The disease is spontaneous and asymptomatic, and it progresses rapidly; sometimes the entire jaw can be destroyed.
- Some patients have past history of trauma in the bone of the affected area.
- Sometimes, there may be pain in the jaw bone with displacement and mobility of teeth, in the absence of any underlying cause.
- Pathological fractures occur following minor trauma, as the bone.

Radiographic Features

Initially the disease produces small, localized, and ill-defined osteoporotic foci in the bone, which coalesce to form massive zones of osteolysis. The borders of the lesion are ill-defined and non-corticated. Moreover, there are no signs of reossification in the osteolytic areas of bone.

Histopathology

- In the earlier stages of the disease, normal bony trabeculae exhibit foci of resorption.
- Bone is completely resorbed within a short span of time and is replaced by a fibrovascular connective tissue with some evidence of chronic inflammatory cell infiltration.

Differential Diagnosis

- Hyperparathyroidism
- Cherubism
- Histiocytosis–X
- Malignancy (predominantly metastatic)
- Osteolytic phase of osteosarcoma.

Treatment

Radiation therapy may prevent the progression of the disease otherwise, there is no successful treatment.

BIBLIOGRAPHY

1. Ablin DS. Osteogenesis imperfecta: a review. Can Assoc Radiol J. 1998;9(2):110-23.
2. Adekeye EO, Edwards MB, Goubran GF. Fibro osseous lesions of the skull, face and jaws in Kaduna, Nigeria. Br J Oral Surg. 1980;18:57-72.
3. Afzal AR, Rajab A, Fenske C, et al. Linkage of recessive Robinow syndrome to a 4 cm interval on chromosome 9q22. Hum Genet. 2000;106:351-4.
4. Agus ZS. Etiology of hypocalcemia. Up To Date CD-ROM. Wellesley, MA: Up To Date, Inc; 2000.
5. Bahadur S, Shenoy AM, Singh MK. Fibro-osseous lesions of the maxilla. J Laryngol Otol. 1986;100:653-7.
6. Barker BF, Jensen JL, Howell FV. Focal osteoporotic bone marrow defects of the jaws. Oral Surg Oral Med Oral Pathol. 1974;38:404-13.
7. Barker D, Welbury RR. Dental findings, in Morquio syndrome (mucopolysaccharidoses type IVa). ASDC J Dent Child. 2000;67(6):431-3.
8. Barnet F, Elfenbein L. Paget's disease of the mandible-a review and report of a case. Endod Dent Traumatol. 1985;1:39-42.
9. Bays RA. The influence of systemic bone disease in bone resorption following mandibular augmentation. Oral Surg Oral Med Oral Pathol. 1983;55:223-30.

10. Bellus GA, Bamshad MJ, Przylepa KA, et al. Severe achondroplasia with developmental delay and acanthosis nigricans (SADDAN): phenotypic analysis of a new skeletal dysplasia caused by a Lys650Mer mutation in fibroblast growth factor receptor 3. Am J Med Genet. 1999;2;85(1):53-65.
11. Bodo M, Baronni T, Carinci F. Interleukin secretion, proteoglycan and procollagen alpha (1)(1) gene expression in Crouzon fibroblasts growth factor. Cytokine. 2000;12(8):1280-3.
12. Brannon RB, Fowler CB. Benign fibro-osseous lesions: a review of current concepts. Adv Anat Pathol. 2001;8:126-43.
13. Cabral CE, Guedes P, Fonseca T. Polyostotic fibrous dysplasia associated with intramuscular myxomas: Mazabraud's syndrome. Skeletal Radiol. 1998;27:278-82.
14. Caillaud C, Poenaru L. Gene therapy in lysosomal diseases. Biomed Pharmacother. 2000;54(10):505-12.
15. Chen CP, Chern SR, Wang W, et al. Second-trimester molecular diagnosis of a heterozygous 742 - > T (R248C) mutation in the FGFR3 gene in a thanatophoric dysplasia variant following suspicious ultrasound findings. Ultrasound Obstet Gynecol. 2001;17(3):272-3.
16. Cuerda E, delPozo J, Rodriguez-Lozano J, et al. Acne in Apert's syndrome: treatment with isotretinoin. J Dermatolog Treat. 2003;14(1):43-5.
17. De Smet A, Travers H, Neff JR. Chondrosarcoma occurring in a patient with polyostotic fibrous dysplasia. Skeletal Radiol. 1981;7:197.
18. DelBalso AM, Werning JT. The role of computed tomography in the evaluation of cement-osseous lesions. Oral Surg Oral Med Oral Pathol. 1986;62:354-7.
19. Demitsu T, Kakurai M, Okubo Y, et al. Skin eruption as the presenting sign of Hunter syndrome HB. Clin Exp Dermatol. 1999;24(3):179-82.
20. Dickinson CJ. The possible role of osteoclastogenic oral bacterial products in etiology of Paget's disease. Bone. 2000; 26(2):101-2.
21. Dourmishev A, Miteva L, Mitev V, et al. Cutaneous aspects of Down syndrome. Cutis. 2000;66(6):420-4.
22. Ebata K, Takeshi U, Tohnai I, et al. Chondrosarcoma and osteosarcoma arising in polyostotic fibrous dysplasia. J Oral Maxillofac Surg. 1992;50:761-4.
23. Edelson JG, Obad S, Geiger R, et al. Pyknodysostosis: orthopaedic aspects with a description of 14 new cases. Clin Orthop. 1992;280:273-6.
24. Edwards PA. Benign fibro-osseous lesions of the jaws. Ear Nose Throat J. 1984;63:383-92.
25. Engelbert RH, Pruijs HE, Beemer FA, et al. Osteogenesis imperfecta in childhood: treatment strategies. Arch Phys Med Rehabil. 1998;79(12):1590-4.
26. Eversole LR, Leider AS, Nelson K. Ossifying fibroma: a clinicopathologic study of sixty-four cases. Oral Surg Oral Med Oral Pathol. 1985;60:505-11.
27. Eversole LR, Sabes WR, Rovin S. Fibrous dysplasia: a nosologic problem in the diagnosis of fibro-osseous lesions of the jaws. J Oral Pathol. 1972;1:180-220.
28. Eversole LR. Clinical Outline of Oral Pathology, 2nd edition. Philadelphia: Lea & Febiger; 1984.
29. Eyre DR, Upton MP, Shapiro FD, et al. Non expression of cartilage type II collagen in a case of Langer-Saldinoachondrogenesis. Am J Hum Genet. 1986;39(1):52-67.
30. Feingold M, Schneller S. Down syndrome and systemic lupus erythematosus. Clin Genet. 1995;48(5):277.
31. Felix R, Hofstetter W, Cecchini MG. Recent developments in the understanding of the pathophysiology of osteopetrosis. Eur J Endocrinol. 1996;134(2):143-56.
32. Fernbach SK. Craniosynostosis 1998: concepts and controversies. Pediatr Radiol. 1998; 28(9):722-8.
33. Gallegos-Arreola MP, Machorno-Lazo MV, Flores-Martinez SE, et al.
34. Garjian KV, Pretorius DH, Budorick NE, et al. Fetal skeletal dysplasia: three-dimensional US-initial experience. Radiology. 2000;214(3): 717-23.
35. Girschick HJ, Schneider P, Kruse K, et al. Bone metabolism and bone mineral density in childhood hypophosphatasia. Bone. 1999; 25(3):361-7.
36. Golan I, Baumert U, Held P, et al. Radiological findings and molecular genetic confirmation of cleidocranial dysplasia. Clin Radiol. 2001; 56:525-9.
37. Hall EH, Naylor GD, Mohr RW, et al. Early aggressive cemento-ossifying fibroma: a diagnosis and treatment dilemma. Oral Surg Oral Med Oral Pathol. 1987;63:132-6.

38. Hammner JE, Scofield HH, Cornyn J. Benign fibro osseous jaw lesions of periodontal membrane origin: An Analysis of 249 Cases. Cancer. 1968;22:861-78.
39. Hart TC, Bowden DW, Bolyard J, et al. Genetic linkage of the tricho-dento-osseous syndrome to chromosome 17q21. Hum Mol Genet. 1997;6:2279-84.
40. Jesen BL. Cleidocranial dysplasia: craniofacial morphology in adult patients. J Craniofac Genet Dev Biol. 1994;14:163-76.
41. Kabukcuoglu F, Kabukcuoglu Y, Yilmaz B, et al. Mazabraud's syndrome: intramuscular myxoma associated with fibrous dysplasia. Pathol Oncol Res. 2004;10(2):121-3.
42. Khosla S, Melton III LJ, Wermers RA. Primary hyperparathyroidism and the risk of fractures: a population-based study. J Bone Miner Res. 1999;14:1700-7.
43. Kolble N, Sobetzko D, Ersch J. Diagnosis of skeletal dysplasia by multidisciplinary assessment: a report of two cases of thanatophoric dysplasia. Ultrasound Obstet Gynecol. 2002;19(1):92-8.
44. Kress W, Collmann H, Busse M. Clustering of FGFR2 gene mutations impatients with Pfeiffer and Crouzon syndromes (FGFR2-associated craniosynostoses). Cytogenet Cell Genet. 2000;91(1-4):134-7.
45. Lindsay R, Dempster DW. Osteoporosis: current concepts, Bull N Y Acad Med. 1985;61:307-22.
46. Lomri A, Lemonnier J, Hott M, et al. Increased calvaria cell differentiation and bone matrix formation induced by fibroblast growth factor receptor 2 mutations in Apert syndrome. J Clin Invest. 1998;101(6):1310-7.
47. Lucus RB. Pathology of Tumors of the Oral Tissues, 4th edition. Edinburgh: Churchill Livingstone; 1984.
48. Marques IL, Barbieri MA, Bettiol H. Etiopathogenesis of isolated Robin sequence. Cleft Palate Craniofac J. 1998;35(6):517-25.
49. Marx SJ. Causes of Hypocalcemia or Osteomalaci. A Review of Endocrinology Diagnosis and Treatment. NH Syllabus. 1999;506-12.
50. Mock D, Rosen IB. Osteosarcoma in irradiated fibrous dysplasia. J Oral Pathol. 1986;15:1-4.
51. National Institutes of Health. (2001). NIH Osteoporosis and Related Bone Disorders-National Resource Center. Fast Facts on Fibrous Dysplasia. Washington DC: NIH.
52. Obisesan AA, Lagundoye SB, Daramola JO, et al. The radiologic features of fibrous dysplasia of the craniofacial bones. Oral Surg Oral Med Oral Pathol. 1977;44:949-59.
53. Odeku EL, Martinson FD, Akinosi JO. Craniofacial fibrous dysplasia in Nigerian Africans. Int Surg. 1969;51:170-82.
54. Oldridge M, Zackai EH, McDonald-McGinn DM, et al. Denovo alu-element insertions in FGFR2 identify a distinct pathological basis for Apert syndrome. Am J Hum Genet. 1999;64(2):446-61.
55. Pal BR, Shaw NJ. Rickets resurgence in the United Kingdom: improving antenatal management in Asians. J Pediatr. 2001;139(2):337-8.
56. Posnick JC, Ruiz RL. The craniofacial dysostosis syndromes: current surgical thinking and future directions. Cleft Palate Craniofac J. 2000;37(5):433.
57. Roughley PJ, Rauch F, Glorieux FH. Osteogenesis imperfecta-clinical and molecular diversity. Eu Cell Mater. 2003;30;5:41-7.
58. Schlumberger HG. Fibrous dysplasia of single bones (monostotc fibrous dysplasia). Milit Surgeon. 1946;99:504-27.
59. Singer FR, Mills BG. The etiology of Paget's disease of bone. Clin Orthop Relat Res. 1977;127:37-42.
60. Thomas DW, Shepherd JP. Paget's disease of bone: current concepts in pathogenesis and treatment. J Oral Pathol Med. 1994;23:12-6.
61. Whinery JG. Progressive bone cavities of the mandible. Oral Surg Oral Med Oral Pathol. 1955;8:903-16.
62. Whitaker SB, Waldron A. Central giant cell lesions of the laws. Oral Surg Oral Med Oral Pathol. 1993;75:199-208.
63. Wilson DF, D'Rozario R, Bosanqut A. Focal osteoporotic bone marrow defect. Aust Dent J. 1985;33:77-80.

CHAPTER 16

Diseases of Temporomandibular Joint

DEVELOPMENTAL DISORDERS

Hypoplasia of the Mandibular Condyle

Condylar hypoplasia is characterized by reduction in the size of condylar process.

Etiology

- Heredity
- Birth injury
- Infections to the adjoining structures
- Developmental anomalies, e.g. Treacher Collins syndrome, hemifacial microsomia, etc.

Clinical Features

- Underdevelopment of ramus
- Deviation of mandible to the affected side during mouth opening
- Antegonial notch is deeper on the involved side
- Midline shift of dentition toward the affected side
- Masticatory insufficiency
- Cosmetically poor appearance of the face.

Treatment

Genioplasty or osteotomy.

Hyperplasia of the Mandibular Condyle

Condylar hyperplasia is a rare defect, which is often characterized by a unilateral enlargement of the mandibular condyle with facial asymmetry.

Etiology

The condition develops probably due to some localized proliferative reactions in the jawbone.

Clinical Features

The clinical features of condylar hyperplasia include deviation of chin to the opposite side during mouth opening, cross-bite, excessive vertical lengthening of the ramus, and occasional pain in the temporomandibular joint (TMJ), etc.

Treatment

The condition is treated by surgical recontouring of the condyle.

TRAUMATIC DISORDERS

Luxation and Subluxation

Both conditions occur due to partial or complete dislocations of the head of condyle out of the glenoid fossa. Luxation or dislocation of TMJ occurs when the head of the condyle excessively moves anteriorly over the articular eminence into such a position, from where it cannot return back to its original position inside glenoid fossa by itself.

When the condyle is completely dislocated out of the glenoid fossa, it is called luxation, while the partial dislocation of the same is called subluxation.

Diseases of Temporomandibular Joint

Etiology
Luxation or subluxation occurs mostly due to:
- Trauma to the TMJ
- Wide mouth opening for an extended period of time (e.g. dental procedures, etc.).

Clinical Features
The patients usually complain of "sudden locking" of the jaw with inability to close the mouth. In the initial phases, the problem happens rarely, but later on, patients may have such situation quite frequently, thereby, making eating and talking very difficult.

Treatment
In case of luxation or subluxation, the dislocated condyle is to be guided into its normal position by giving inferior and posterior pressure by holding the mandible firmly in the molar region.

Patients should be advised not to open the mouth too widely. In recurrent cases, flattening of the articular eminence is done.

Ankylosis of Temporomandibular Joint

Ankylosis of the TMJ is characterized by lack of movement of the condylar head within the glenoid fossa, due to fusion of the opposing components of the joint with obliteration of the joint space. It results in the limitation of mouth opening.

Etiology
A large number of factors can cause the development of TMJ ankylosis and important among them are described in Table 16.1.

Clinical Features
Age: Ankylosis usually occurs in children below the age of 10 years.
Sex: Both sexes are almost equally affected.

Types of Ankylosis
False ankylosis: False ankylosis is extra-articular and it occurs due to pathological conditions outside the joint resulting in fibrous or bony union between the coronoid process and maxilla or zygoma. Here the joint itself is not deformed or damaged. False ankylosis often develops due to muscle trismus in odontogenic infections and also jaw fractures.

True ankylosis: True ankylosis is intra-articular and it is again of two types—true bony ankylosis and true fibrous ankylosis.
- *True bony ankylosis*: When there is complete loss of mouth opening due to

Table 16.1: Etiology of ankylosis of temporomandibular joint (TMJ).

Trauma	- Birth injury due to forceps delivery
	- Intracapsular fracture with bleeding
	- Accidental trauma to the mandible that pushes the head of the condyle into the glenoid fossa
	- Lack of early mobilization after TMJ fracture
	- Malunion of the condylar fractures
	- Radiotherapy to the TMJ
Infections	- Otitis media
	- Mastoiditis
	- Congenital syphilis
	- Osteomyelitis
	- Pyogenic arthritis of TMJ from hematogenous infections
Systemic juvenile arthritis	- Psoriatic arthritis
	- Osteoarthritis
	- Rheumatoid arthritis
Neoplasms	- Chondroma
	- Osteochondroma
	- Osteoma
	- Metastatic tumors
Miscellaneous	- Congenital developmental defect in the joint
	- Synovial chondromatosis

complete bony fusion between the head of the condyle and the glenoid fossa. True bony ankylosis shows the following features:
- Complete obliteration of the joint space
- Deposition of bone with destruction and subsequent fusion of temporal fossa, meniscus, and head of the condyle
- Antegonial notching anterior to the angle of mandible
- Elongation of the coronoid process.

- *True fibrous ankylosis*: Intra-articular fibrous ankylosis occurs, if the TMJ space is obliterated by the deposition of a fibrous tissue mass (e.g. scar). Fibrous ankylosis mostly occurs due to hemorrhage in the joint space due to trauma with subsequent fibrosis (hemarthrosis). The TMJ shows haziness and narrowing of the joint space. In such cases, limited degree of mouth opening is possible.

Presentation

- Mostly seen in young people and both sexes are equally affected.
- Difficulty in mouth opening is the chief complain in TMJ ankylosis, patients can open the mouth partly in case of fibrous ankylosis, but in case of bony ankylosis complete lack of mouth opening is seen (Fig. 16.1).
- Facial asymmetry with deviation of the chin to the affected side.
- TMJ ankylosis in young age hampers the growth of jawbones, often causes micrognathia, retrusion of mandible, increased over-jet with severe malocclusion, etc.
- Difficulty in taking food and difficulty in speech.
- Maximum numbers of ankylosis cases are of unilateral type, patients exhibit displacement of chin (backward and laterally) toward the involved side on attempted mouth opening.

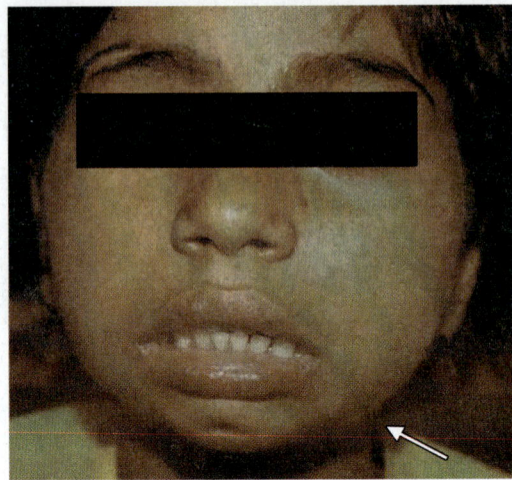

Fig. 16.1: Ankylosis of temporomandibular joint with complete lack of mouth opening.

- Bilateral ankylosis in the younger age causes microstomia and receding chin (Fig. 16.2).
- Occasionally, during the early stage of development, patient may complain of pain and tenderness in the TMJ area.

Radiological Features

In case of bony ankylosis, radiograph shows the loss of normal architecture of TMJ and obliteration of the joint space due to

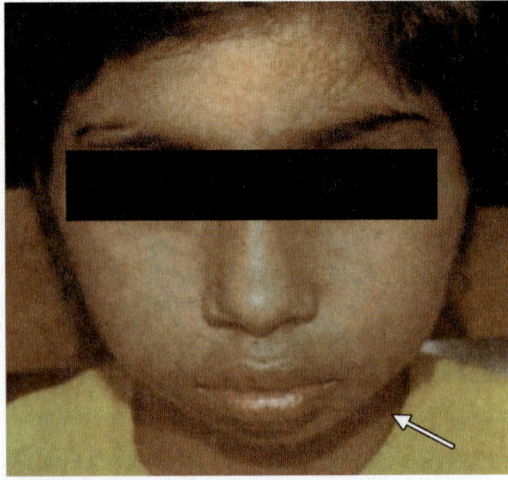

Fig. 16.2: Ankylosis of the TM Joint causing microstomia.

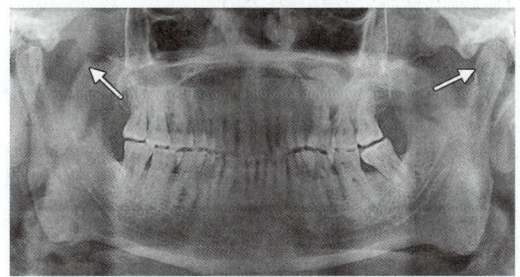

Fig. 16.3: Ankylosis of TM Joint showing obliteration of the joint space.

deposition of bone. In case of false ankylosis, the TMJ appears normal (Fig. 16.3).

Histopathology

Microscopically the ankylosed joint shows destruction of the component parts of TMJ, e.g. head of the condyle, meniscus and the fossa, etc. The joint space is completely filled up with either fibrous tissue or by bone.

Treatment

Temporomandibular joint ankylosis is treated by surgical correction of the joint (arthroplasty). Moreover to eliminate further possibility of ankylosis or recurrence, a gap is constantly maintained between the head of the condyle and the glenoid fossa, by placing some non-absorbing material, e.g. tendon sheath, in the joint space. This procedure is known as "gap arthroplasty".

Costochondral grafting is done sometimes in young patients to facilitate the growth of mandible.

■ INFLAMMATORY DISORDERS

Ankylosing Spondylitis

Ankylosing spondylitis is a chronic inflammatory disease of the connective tissue, which primarily affects the axial skeleton and the central joints including the TMJ.

Etiology
- Exactly not known
- Trauma and rheumatoid arthritis could cause this disease.

Clinical Features
- Stiffness resulting from immobility of the joint during sleep.
- Stiffness is relieved by heat and exercise. It is more common in men and there may be some facial asymmetry.

Radiographic Features

Flattening of the condyle with presence of osteophytes, bony erosion, and sclerosis.

Treatment

Intra-articular injections of corticosteroids.

Osteoarthritis

Osteoarthritis is a degenerative and destructive disease of the weight-bearing joints, although TMJ is not a weight-bearing joint, osteoarthritis can still occur in it due to the aging process or trauma.

Clinical Features

Clinically, osteoarthritis presents the following features:
- Clicking sounds in the joint while opening and closing movements of the jaw.
- Limitation of movements of the joint.
- Sometimes there may be deep ache or pain in the joint.
- Muscles of mastication are often tendered due to strain caused by non-use or restricted use of the painful joint.

Radiographic Features (Fig. 16.4)

Radiograph shows "osteophytic lipping" or protuberance on the articular disc with flattening of the articular surfaces of the joint.
- In few cases, subarticular radiolucent areas (Ely's cysts) can be seen.
- Narrowing of the joint space due to abnormal ossifications.

Other Investigations
- CT scanning
- Arthroscopy
- MRI.

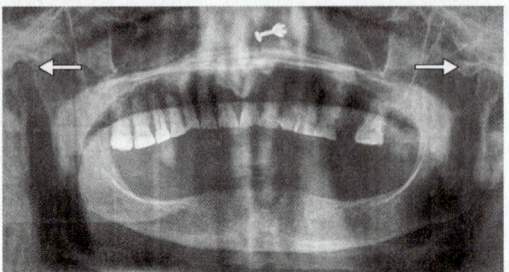

Fig. 16.4: Erosion of the head of condyles in osteoarthritis.

Histopathology

- Osteoarthritis histologically shows vertical and horizontal cracks on the articular cartilage. In more chronic cases, these cracks may even extend up to the underlying bone.
- The cartilage also becomes less elastic with decrease in the number of chondrocytes.
- Degeneration of chondrocytes, localized destruction of cartilage, and eburnation of bone, etc. are also seen.
- Large degenerating spaces or subchondral cysts may develop beneath the articular cartilage.
- In few cases, localized areas of repair produce multiple elevations on the disk surface and the condition is known as "lipping".

Treatment

There is no satisfactory treatment for osteoarthritis, however condylectomy should be considered in very severe cases.

Rheumatoid Arthritis

Rheumatoid arthritis is a systemic disease that usually affects many joints including the TMJ and the disease is characterized by progressive autoimmune destruction of the joint structures.

Etiology

Detection of increased serum IgG, rheumatoid factor, and antinuclear antibodies, etc. indicates that an "autoimmune mechanism" probably initiates the disease. The autoimmune reaction brings about inflammatory change in the synovial membrane of the joint with subsequent fibroblastic proliferations. The inflammatory process also generates collagenase and other enzymes, which cause destruction of the joint cartilage and the underlying bone.

Clinical Features

- The disease usually occurs in the third and fourth decade of life and females are more commonly affected.
- During the acute phase of the disease, patient may suffer from fever, malaise, fatigability, weight loss, anemia, and raised ESR, etc.
- The TMJ is involved mostly bilaterally along with other joints.
- It becomes swollen, tendered, and stiff.
- The maximum feeling of stiffness is experienced in the early mornings and it diminishes gradually as the day progresses.
- There may be occasional presence of pain, crepitations, and tenderness in the joint, resulting in restricted jaw movements.
- Clicking sounds in the joint may develop in chronic cases, where structural alterations have taken place in the meniscus and the articular cartilage.
- There may be presence of salivary gland swelling and dryness of mouth.
- On rare occasions, rheumatoid arthritis patients may develop secondary Sjögren's syndrome.
- In cases of rheumatoid arthritis in children (Still's disease), restricted jaw movements may cause mandibular underdevelopment with concomitant occurrence of class II division I malocclusion.
- Ankylosis of the TMJ may develop on rare occasions due to rheumatoid arthritis.

Radiology

Radiograph shows irregularity of the condylar as well as the articular surfaces, with flattening of condyle and widening of TMJ space.

Histopathology

- Microscopy reveals edema, exudation, and other inflammatory changes within the synovial membrane of the joint.
- The articular surface is ultimately destroyed and is replaced by the granulation tissue.
- Chronic inflammatory cell infiltration by lymphocytes, macrophages, and neutrophils is often seen in the damaged tissue of the joint.
- There can be development of fibrous or even bony ankylosis of the joint in some cases.

Treatment

Systemic steroid therapy and antibiotics.

Acute Traumatic Arthritis

Acute traumatic arthritis occurs due to trauma to the mandible which results in inflammatory changes within the TM joint space. It may also occur due to hemarthrosis, in case blood vessel is torn inside the joint.

Clinical Features

- Pain and tenderness in the joint
- Inability to close the mouth completely
- Pain increases while opening and closing the mouth.

Treatment

Giving adequate rest to the joint and application of heat. Mobilization of the joint after 10 days.

Myofascial Pain Dysfunction Syndrome

Myofascial pain dysfunction (MPD) syndrome is a disease complex that disturbs the entire masticatory apparatus and is characterized by pain and limitation of movement of the TMJ.

Etiology

- The disease occurs due to defective neuromuscular coordination coupled with emotional stress, which eventually results in masticatory muscle spasm and fatigue.
- The condition is further aggravated by occlusal disharmonies like defective restoration, lack of posterior occlusion due to loss of molar teeth and faulty dentures, etc.
- Habitual grinding of teeth (bruxism) can also initiate the disease.
- Anxiety, stress, and personality disorders can play a major role in the initiation of the disease.
- Minor injury to the TMJ caused by violent yawning, laughing, and strenuous dental treatment of long durations.

Clinical Features (Table 16.2)

- More than 80% of the patients are females and they are usually aged between 20 years and 30 years.
- The pain in this disease is dull in nature and it is usually present unilaterally in the preauricular area or in the ear.
- In many cases, the pain radiates to the angle of mandible or temporal region.
- The intensity of pain varies at different times of the day.

The associated symptoms of MPD:
- Neurologic—tingling, numbness, blurred vision, and twitches.
- Musculoskeletal—fatigue, tension, tiredness, and joint pain.
- Otologic—tingling, ear pain, dizziness, vertigo, and diminished hearing.
- Gastrointestinal tract—nausea, vomiting, diarrhea, xerostomia, and constipation.

Laboratory Investigations

- Complete blood count (CBC) to rule out any systemic infection.
- ESR, rheumatoid factor (RF), and antinuclear antibody (ANA) are done to rule out possible diagnosis of rheumatoid arthritis.
- Serum uric acid should be checked to rule out the underlying disease "gout".

Table 16.2: Clinically four positive features and two negative features of myofascial pain dysfunction (MPD).

Positive features (Laskin's cardinal symptoms of MPD)	Negative features
• Pain and discomfort in the temporomandibular joint and anywhere about the head and neck	• Absence of any clinical, radiological, and biochemical evidence of organic change in the joint
• Tenderness in the muscles of mastication on palpation	
• Limitation of movements and deviation of the jaw	• Absence of tenderness in the joint when palpated via external auditory meatus
• Joint noise-clicking, grating or snapping sounds in the temporomandibular joint during opening and closing of the mouth	

Differential Diagnosis

- Referred pain from the nearby teeth.
- Organic disease in the TMJ, e.g. inflammation with fluid accumulation in the joint space.
- Trigeminal or glossopharyngeal neuralgia.
- Migraine.

Treatment

The disease is self-limiting and does not progress to any permanent disability or damage. Conservative treatment is often done by administering analgesics, muscle relaxants, and tranquilizers, etc. Besides this, correction of occlusal disharmonies, psychological counseling, and warm compress, etc. are also done.

Neoplasia of Temporomandibular Joint

Both benign and malignant neoplasms can develop from the TMJ, but their incidence is usually rare (Table 16.3).

Site of Origin

Neoplasms of TMJ can occur from any structural components of the joint like head of condyle, articular fossa, disc or the capsule, etc.

Clinical Features

Neoplasms of TMJ can cause the following problems:
- Temporomandibular joint dysfunctions
- Facial asymmetry
- Malocclusion
- Prognathic deviation of mandible to the opposite side
- Pain and swelling.

Tomography

Malignant neoplasms can cause destruction of the joint structures which could be easily detected by tomography.

Treatment

It depends upon the specific nature of the lesion.

BIBLIOGRAPHY

1. Abdel-Hakim AM. Stomatognathic dysfunction in the western desert of Egypt: an epidemiological survey. J Oral Rehab. 1983;10:461-8.
2. De Bont LGM. Temporomandibular joint, articular structure and function. Rijksuniversiteit Groningen. 1985.pp.1-83.
3. Gazit E, Lieberman M, Ein R, et al. Prevalence of mandibular function in 10-18 years old Israeli school children. J Oral Rehab. 1984;11:307-17.
4. Ginhrass RO. Chondrosarcoma of the mandibular joint. J Oral Surg. 1954;12:614.
5. Goss AN, Burns RJ. Facial pain. Aust Dent J. 1975; 20:287-9.
6. Kummoona R. Functional rehabilitation of ankylosed temporomandibular joints. Oral Surg Oral Med Oral Pathol. 1978;46:495-505.
7. Muir CM, Goss AN. The radiographic morphology of painful temporomandibular joints. Oral Surg Oral Med Oral Pathol. 1990;70:355-9.

8. Norman JE, De B, Painter DM. Hyperplasia of the mandibular condyle. J Maxillofac Surg.1980;8:161-75.
9. Nwoku AL. Rehabilitating children with temporo-mandibular joint ankylosis. Int J Oral Surg. 1979;8:271-5.
10. Pereira FJ Jr, Lundh H, Westesson PL. Age related changes in retrodiscal tissue in the temporomandibular joint. J Oral Maxillofac Surg. 1996;54:55-61.
11. Toller PA, Glynn LE. Degenerative disease of the mandibular joint. In: B Cohen, IRH Kramer (Eds). Scientific Foundations of Dentistry. London: Heinemann; 1976. pp. 605-19.
12. Widmaml SE, Westesson PL, Kim LK, et al. Temporomandibular joint pathosis related to sex, age, and dentition in autopsy material. Oral Surg Oral Med Oral Pathol. 1994;78: 416-25.
13. Yagi K, Abbas K. A study of ankylosis of the temporomandibular joint in the Sudan. Report Submitted to the Faculty of Medicine, University of Khartoum; 1981.

CHAPTER 17

Oral Aspects of Hematological Disorders

INTRODUCTION

Types of human blood cells and the common blood disorders are described in Flowchart 17.1 and Table 17.1, respectively.

PERNICIOUS ANEMIA

Definition

Pernicious anemia is a type of chronic, progressive, megaloblastic anemia of adults and is characterized by impaired maturation of RBC secondary to insufficient vitamin B_{12}. It occurs due to deficiency of an intrinsic factor (transport protein) in the stomach, which is essential for the absorption of vitamin B_{12}.

Vitamin B_{12} and folic acid act as essential co-factors for the maturation of RBC within the bone marrow. Although folic acid deficiency can be ameliorated by dietary supplements, the vitamin B_{12} deficiency cannot be rectified in pernicious anemia by dietary supplements, as there is lack of a transport protein (intrinsic factor) in the intestine which is essential for its absorption.

Clinical Features

There are four major cardinal features of pernicious anemia:
1. Abnormally large red blood cells
2. Hypochlorhydria of stomach

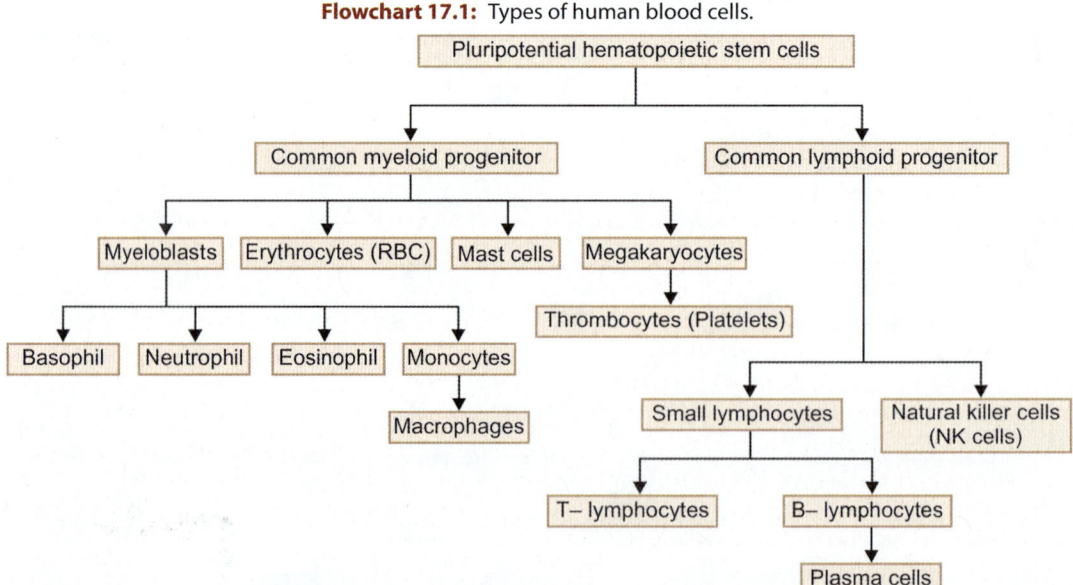

Flowchart 17.1: Types of human blood cells.

Oral Aspects of Hematological Disorders

Table 17.1: Common blood disorders.

Disorders affecting RBCs	Disorders affecting WBCs	Disorders affecting platelets	Disorders affecting plasma
• Pernicious anemia • Iron deficiency anemia • Aplastic anemia • Hemolytic anemia • Thalassemia • Sickle cell anemia • Polycythemia • Erythroblastosis fetalis	• Leukemia • Lymphoma • Multiple myeloma • Agranulocytosis • Cyclic neutropenia	Purpura	• Hemophilia • Von Willebrand disease • Deep venous thrombosis • Disseminated intravascular coagulation (DIC)

3. Neurologic and gastrointestinal symptoms
4. A fatal outcome, unless the patient receives lifelong injections of vitamin B_{12}.

Clinical Presentation
- Generalized weakness, fatigue, palpitations, dyspnea, headache and feeling of faint, etc. due to reduced oxygen-carrying capacity of blood.
- Patients often have a smooth, dry and yellow skin, nausea, vomiting, anorexia, diarrhea and weight loss, etc.
- Neurological manifestations include tingling sensations in the hands and feet, paresthesia and numbness of the extremities due to peripheral nerve degeneration.

Oral Manifestation
- Glossitis, glossodynia (painful tongue), loss of taste sensation, and glossopyrosis (burning tongue), etc. are the hallmark features of pernicious anemia.
- Tongue lesions may develop even before the fall of blood hemoglobin (Hb) level.
- The tongue often appears "beefy red" in color with areas of patchy ulcerations on the dorsum and lateral borders.
- Sometimes, atrophy and inflammation of the filiform papillae produces a "bald" appearance of the tongue and the condition is often known as "Hunter's glossitis".
- Generalized inflammation of oral mucosa causes burning sensation, dysphagia, and difficulty in denture wearing.
- There may be pallor in the oral mucosa with purpuric spots and occasional aphthous-like ulcerations.

Diagnostic Assessment
- Total RBC count is reduced to less than 3 million per mm^3 of blood, elevated mean cell volume (MCV), mean cell hemoglobin (MCH) and mean cell hemoglobin concentration (MCHC).
- Decreased WBC count
- If MCV is less than 96 fL (RBC is large), it frequently indicates pernicious anemia.
- Peripheral blood smear shows oval, macrocytic, and hyperchromic red blood cells.
- Bone marrow contains large number of megaloblasts.
- Unconjugated bilirubin is elevated due to increased hemolysis.
- Serum lactate dehydrogenase (an enzyme liberated from damaged tissue) level is extremely high.
- Schilling's test detects the absence of intrinsic factor in the stomach.
- Gastric secretion analysis reveals the presence of higher level of free hydrochloric acid.

Treatment

Intramuscular injections of vitamin B_{12}.

IRON DEFICIENCY ANEMIA

Iron deficiency anemia is a chronic, microcytic, hypochromic type of anemia, which occurs either due to inadequate absorption or excessive loss of iron from the body.

It is the most common form of anemia and the erythrocytes, besides being hypochromic and microcytic, are also severely decreased in number.

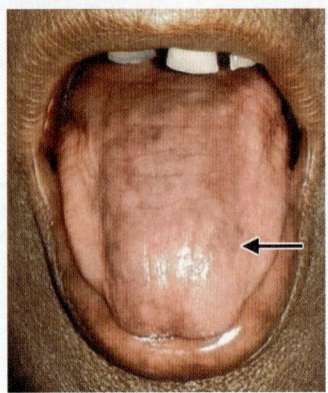

Fig. 17.1: Bald tongue in iron deficiency anemia.

Causes
- Inadequate absorption of iron in the body
- Excessive loss of blood
- Increased demand for RBC
- Decreased intake of iron in the body.

Clinical Manifestation
- Fatigue, easy tiring, lightheadedness, and lack of energy
- Palpitations, dizziness, and sensitivity to cold
- Lemon-tinted pallor of the skin and generalized weakness
- Koilonychia (spoon-shaped brittle finger nails) is an important feature in iron deficiency anemia.

Oral Manifestation
- Mucosal pallor with loss of keratinization (atrophic mucositis) (Fig. 17.1).
- In some patients, atrophic mucositis in the aerodigestive tract or oropharynx may predispose to the occurrence of squamous cell carcinoma.
- Depapillations and mucosal atrophy produces smooth, bald, red, and glazed appearance of the tongue.
- Often there is burning sensations in the tongue (glossopyrosis) and glossodynia (painful tongue).
- Angular cheilitis, dysphagia (difficulty in swallowing), recurrent aphthous ulcer and candidiasis of the oral mucosa.
- Plummer-Vinson syndrome—which presents a triad of symptoms comprising of dysphagia, stomatitis (inflammation of the oral mucosa), and atrophic glossitis.

Diagnostic Assessment
- Peripheral blood smear shows small (microcytic) and pale (hypochromic) RBCs.
- Hemoglobin level is decreased to as low as 3.6 g/100 mL.
- Total RBC count is dropped moderately but rarely it goes to below 3 million per mm^3.
- Mean cell volume, MCH, and MCHC—all are reduced.
- Serum iron level is decreased to 10 mg (normal 50–150 mg).
- Hemosiderin is completely absent from the bone marrow.
- If gastrointestinal tract bleeding is the suspected cause of iron deficiency anemia, then the following additional investigations are to be done:
  – X-rays (GI tract series)
  – Stool examination for occult blood
  – Esophagoscopy, gastroscopy, and sigmoidoscopy, etc.

Histopathology
- Tongue shows atrophy of the covering epithelium with loss of papillae.
- Leukocytic infiltrations in the spinous cell layer as well as in the underlying connective tissue.

Treatment
300 mg ferrous sulfate tablet; 3-4 tablets per day for 6 months.

■ APLASTIC ANEMIA

Aplastic anemia is a rare life-threatening hemorrhagic disease characterized by general lack of bone marrow activity that results in decreased formation of RBC, WBC, and platelet cells.

Decreased production of RBC causes anemia, decreased production of WBC causes leukopenia, and decreased production of platelets results in thrombocytopenia (severe depletion of all cell types of blood is often known as pancytopenia).

Etiology
- Hereditary factor—e.g. Fanconi's syndrome
- Drugs and chemicals such as chloramphenicol, phenylbutazone, sulphonamides, DDT and benzene etc.
- Radiation
- Infections—tuberculosis and viral hepatitis
- Idiopathic.

Clinical Manifestations
The systemic and oral manifestations of aplastic anemia are almost similar to leukemia (in terms of anemic severity, bleeding tendency, and susceptibility to infections). It is more common in young adults and elderly individuals.

Common Symptoms
- Weakness, lightheadedness with dyspnea, tachycardia, and fatigue due to slight physical exertion.
- Marked pallor, edema, cold and yellow skin, and petechiae.
- Yellowish discoloration of the eyes.
- Frequent episodes of epistaxis, fatal hemorrhage, and bruises.
- Numbness and tingling of the extremities.
- Fever and severe infections often occur due to neutropenia.

Oral Manifestations
- Petechiae, ecchymoses, purpuric spots, and frank hematoma formations in the oral cavity.
- Spontaneous gingival bleeding, mucosal pallor, and ulcerations.
- Persistent oral infections including candidiasis.
- Fulminating conditions like bacteremia and septicemia, etc. may develop from simple oral infections.

Histopathology
Histologically oral mucosa exhibits accumulation of numerous microorganisms with extreme lack of inflammatory cell infiltration in the connective tissue.

Diagnostic Assessment
- RBC count is usually below 1 million/mm^3.
- WBC count may be as low as 2,000/mm^3.
- Platelet count may fall below 20,000/mm^3.
- Bone marrow is fatty and contains only few developing blood cells.
- Bleeding time prolonged but clotting time is normal.

Treatment
Blood transfusion, antibiotics, splenectomy, and bone marrow transplant, etc. Approximately, 50% patients die within 6 months after detection of the disease due to severe infections and hemorrhage.

■ HEMOLYTIC ANEMIA

Definition
Anemia occurring due to increased hemolysis in the body, which the bone marrow cannot compensate even by increasing the production of RBCs.

Causes

- Hereditary causes:
  - Hereditary spherocytosis
  - Glucose-6-phosphate dehydrogenase deficiency (G6PD)
  - Sickle cell anemia
  - Thalassemia.
- Acquired causes:
  - Antibody-mediated hemolytic disorders:
    - Acquired autoimmune hemolysis
    - Paroxysmal cold hemoglobinuria
    - Erythroblastosis fetalis.
  - Hemolysis due to physical, chemical or biological agents:
    - Physical agents: Hemolysis due to prolonged physical exercise
    - Chemical agents: Chemical agents and drugs can cause damage to RBC cells to produce anemia.
      » Important chemical agents, which can cause hemolysis are—arsenic, lead, sulfonamides, potassium chlorate, methyldopa, naphthalene, mefenamic acid, etc.
    - *Biological agents*: Several microorganisms can cause hemolysis which include:
      » *Plasmodium falciparum*
      » *Clostridia*
      » *Streptococcus pyogenes.*

Clinical Features

- Pallor, weakness, lightheadedness, and fatigability.
- Jaundice, recurrent infections, leg ulcers, etc.
- Dyspnea or other cardiovascular symptoms.
- Dark colored stool (due to hemolysis).

Oral Manifestations

- Pallor or yellow tinge of the oral mucosa.
- Discoloration of teeth in erythroblastosis fetalis.
- Gingival hemorrhage.

Diagnostic Assessment

- Blood Hb percentage is often below to 10 g/dL.
- Erythrocyte survival rate about 12 days (normal 120 days).
- Reticulocyte count, unconjugated serum bilirubin, fecal urobilinogen, and serum iron level all are—raised.
- Coombs' test—negative.

Treatment

Treatment of anemia and effective management of the underlying diseases.

- Blood transfusion in severe cases.
- Steroids may be used in case of immune-mediated disorders.
- Splenectomy should be done in case of spherocytosis.
- Administration of folic acid.

THALASSEMIAS

Thalassemias are a group of inherited, chronic, hemolytic disorder characterized by defective synthesis of hemoglobin in the RBC that results in the production of extremely thin, fragile, and functionally compromised erythrocytes called "target cells". In thalassemia patients, the defective RBCs survive only few days in the peripheral circulation as they are readily recognized by the spleen and are destroyed leading to anemia.

There is bone marrow hyperplasia in order to compensate the anemia and patients also require frequent blood transfusions.

Pathogenesis: Blood Hb is made up of two types of proteins—α-chain protein and β-chain protein; in thalassemia patients, there is genetically induced deficiency of either of these proteins in the Hb, which causes formation of defective RBCs.

- *α-thalassemia*: If α-chain synthesis of Hb is disturbed (also called thalassemia minor)

- *β-thalassemia*: If β-chain synthesis of Hb is disturbed (also called thalassemia major)
- *Thalassemia intermedia*: A rare type with features of intermediate severity.

Since the β-thalassemia is more common among the two types, it is called "classic or major thalassemia" and its other name is "*Cooley's anemia*."

Thalassemia is an autosomal recessive disease, it can be transmitted by either mother or father or both of them (both parents can be carriers) (Table 17.2); moreover both male and female children can be affected in this disease (*contrary to hemophilia, which is transmitted by the mother only and the male child is exclusively affected and not the female child*).

In thalassemia, the heterozygous form (*transmitted by a single parent*) of the disease is often mild which is known as *thalassemia minor* and the homozygous form (*transmitted by both the parents*) of the disease is very severe and is known as *thalassemia major*.

Thalassemia minor patients are *carriers* of the disease as they carry the defective genes, but they do not have much symptoms of the disease throughout their life, this is also called *"thalassemia trait"*.

Clinical Manifestation

The disease is commonly detected in the first 2 years of life and siblings are commonly affected.

- Persistent anemia, jaundice, and hepatosplenomegaly.
- Fever, chills, malaise, generalized weakness, and lethargy.
- Bone marrow hyperplasia often produces painless enlargement of mandible and maxilla; which often results in a typical "chipmunk facies"
- Cholelithiasis and leg ulcers also develop frequently.
- Most of the patients have a mongoloid facies with prominent forehead, depressed nasal bridge, prominent cheek bones, protrusion of the maxillary anterior teeth and slanting eyes, etc.
- Severe form of the disease arising during infancy may terminate in death as early in the adolescence. High output cardiac failure is often the cause of death in such patients.

Radiographic Appearance

- The skull bones radiographically exhibit thin and poorly-defined inner and outer cortex and the trabeculae between them are coarse, elongated, and bristle-like, which produce a typical "hair-on-end" or a "crew-cut" appearance.
- Radiograph of the ribs exhibit a typical "rib within a rib" appearance due to increased radiodensity within or overlapping the medullary space of the ribs.
- Sometimes, the jaw bones show coarsening of some bony trabeculae and blurring or disappearance of others; it often produces a typical radiographic appearance called "salt-and-pepper effect".
- Delayed pneumatization of the paranasal sinuses, especially the maxillary sinuses.

Table 17.2: Parental genetic status and possible risk of thalassemia in children.

Parental status	Risk in children
If one parent is a carrier and other is normal	50% children normal and maximum 50% carrier
If both parents are carriers	25% children will have thalassemia and 50% carrier
If one parent has thalassemia and the other is a carrier	50% children will have thalassemia and rest 50% carrier (none is normal)
If both parents have thalassemia	All children will have thalassemia
If one parent has thalassemia and the other is normal	No children will be normal; each one will be either a carrier or diseased

Oral Manifestations of Thalassemia
- Bimaxillary protrusion with painless enlargement of the jawbones and retracted lips.
- Spacing or flaring of anterior maxillary teeth, marked open bite, and malocclusion.
- Pallor of the oral mucosa.
- Xerostomia due to salivary gland dysfunctions as a result of iron overload.
- Prominent malar bones, depressed nasal bridge with mongoloid facies.
- Delayed pneumatization of maxillary sinuses.
- Discoloration of teeth due to iron deposition.

Diagnostic Assessment
Laboratory findings in thalassemia include the following:
- Presence of "target cells" and "safety pin" cells in peripheral blood.
- Presence of abnormal nucleated RBCs in blood
- WBC count can rise up to 10,000 to 25,000/cu mm of blood.
- The serum bilirubin and fetal hemoglobin levels
- Elevated fecal and urinary urobilinogen due to severe hemolysis.
- Bone marrow is hyperplastic and produces large numbers of immature, primitive looking, stem forms of RBCs.
- Excessive accumulations of alpha chains within the RBCs are called inclusion bodies (Fessas bodies).

Treatment
Multiple blood transfusions and splenectomy, etc. Desferrioxamine and chelating agent may reduce the effect of iron overload in tissues.

■ SICKLE CELL ANEMIA
Definition
Sickle cell anemia is an inherited defect in the synthesis of Hb molecule, in which the erythrocytes assume a sickle or crescent shape. These defective erythrocytes are easily destroyed causing severe anemia.

Pathogenesis
Sickle cell anemia is an autosomal recessive type of inherited disease, which is characterized by a point mutation in the Hb gene, which results in an abnormal Hb molecule (HbS).

Each person inherits one gene from each parent, which governs the synthesis of Hb. HbS is less soluble than HbA (normal adult hemoglobin) and the former forms long fibers, which deform the RBC into sickle shape. These crescent-shaped or sickle-shaped RBCs in sickle cell anemia are more prone to agglutination. More agglutinations (hemolysis) of RBCs lead to more anemia and increased viscosity of blood, moreover increased risk of blocking of capillaries may result in ischemic damage in various organs and the situation is known as "sickle cell crisis".

Clinical Features
- Symptoms develop about the age of one year with delayed physical growth and development.
- Malaise, weakness, and pallor and jaundice with a yellow sclera due to hemolysis.
- Loss of consciousness is a common feature in severe cases (sickle cell crisis).
- Extreme susceptibility to infections, renal failure, and CNS disturbances are common.
- There can be death due to widespread ischemia, hypoxia, and hypothermia.
- Extreme pain in abdomen, lung, long bones, and joints due to ischemia and infarction.

Oral Manifestations
- Oral mucosal polar with occasional yellowish color due to hemolytic jaundice.

- Asymptomatic pulpal necrosis, anesthesia, and paresthesia of the mandibular nerve.
- Extraction of tooth may lead to the development of osteomyelitis especially in mandible.
- Thrombosis of blood vessels and infraction in the jawbone often produce "painful cries".

Radiographic Features

- Skull radiographs reveal multiple, small icicle like spicules across the calvarium, which produces a "hair-on-end" appearance.
- Occasionally infracts develop in the jawbones, which radiographically mimic osteomyelitis.
- Intraoral periapical radiographs reveal "step–ladder" like trabeculae between roots of contagious posterior teeth.

Diagnostic Assessment

Sickle cells are viewed on a stained smear of blood under microscope.
- Total RBC count—decreased
- Hb%—lowered
- Hematocrit value—decreased
- Serum unconjugated bilirubin—raised
- Hemoglobin electrophoresis reveals the presence of Hb-S in blood.

Treatment

No specific treatment. Oxygen and blood transfusions in serious emergencies.

ERYTHROBLASTOSIS FETALIS

Erythroblastosis fetalis is a congenital hemolytic anemia of newborn, which occurs due to the Rh incompatibility. The disease results from the destruction of fetal RBC due to the reaction between maternal and fetal blood factors.

Pathogenesis

If the mother is Rh-negative, but the fetus is Rh-positive, then the mother's blood can develop antibodies (anti-Rh agglutinins) against the Rh-factor of the fetus.

These antibodies may pass onto the fetus by crossing the placenta and destroy its RBCs; this often results in hemolysis, jaundice, and anemia, etc.

Oral Manifestation

- Black, brown or bluish discoloration of the deciduous teeth in the child due to deposition of blood pigments.
- Enamel hypoplasia, which may produce a "ring-like" defect on the tooth crowns and is often termed as "Rh-hump".

POLYCYTHEMIA VERA

Polycythemia vera is chronic disease characterized by excessive proliferation of RBCs, usually with an increased Hb level and total blood volume.

Secondary polycythemia: It is commonly associated with hypoxia (cardiac or pulmonary disease), excessive production of erythropoietin, steroid therapy or chronic exposure to chemicals, etc.

Clinical Features

- Dyspnea, fullness of head and face, pruritus, fatigue, and visual disturbances.
- Plethoric appearance of face, slurring of speech, splenomegaly, coronary thrombosis and paresthesia of the cranial nerves, etc.
- Peptic ulcers, epigastric pain along with intestinal, nasal or cerebral hemorrhages.
- A characteristic finding of the disease is the "ruddy cyanosis" or a reddish-purple hue of the face, extremities and lips due to the presence of deoxygenated blood in the cutaneous vessels.

Oral manifestations of polycythemia vera:
- Deep purplish-red discoloration of the oral mucosa; especially in the tongue, gingiva, cheek, and lip.
- Engorged and swollen gingiva with extreme bleeding tendency.

- Submucosal petechiae, hematoma, and ecchymoses.

Laboratory findings in of polycythemia vera:
- RBC count as high as 8–12 million/mm^3 of blood.
- Increase in the total blood volume and blood viscosity.
- Hemoglobin level may be high (18–20 g/100 mL)
- Greater hematocrit level with thrombocytosis and leukocytosis.

Treatment of polycythemia vera:
- Repeated phlebotomy (venesection) to lower the Hb%, hematocrits, and RBC cell mass.
- 500 mL of blood is removed every 2–3 days till the hematocrit reaches a desired level.
- Chemotherapy with chlorambucil, melphalan or cytosine arabinoside to reduce the number of RBCs.

Complications of polycythemia vera:
- Thrombophlebitis, myocardial, and cerebral infarctions.
- Thrombotic occlusion of the splenic, hepatic, portal, and mesenteric veins.
- Hemorrhage—nasal, intestinal, and cerebral, etc.
- Digital gangrene and necrosis.
- Gout—due to over production of uric acid.
- Congestive cardiac failure due to increased blood volume and hypertension.
- Acute leukemia may be a terminal complication of polycythemia vera.

LEUKEMIAS

Leukemia is a malignant disease of the blood-forming organs, characterized by increased proliferation of WBCs in the bone marrow at the cost of other hematopoietic cells. Although, leukemia is a disease of the WBCs, it often severely depletes the other major blood cell types; e.g. RBCs (causing anemia) and platelets (causing thrombocytopenia and hemorrhage), etc.

Despite overproduction of WBCs (which are the main defense cells of the body) there is often increased susceptibility to infection as these cells are immature and functionally inefficient.

Aleukemic leukemia

This is a rare type of leukemia characterized by a normal or below normal (less than 100/mm^3) of white blood cells in the blood despite leukemic changes in tissues.

In case of conventional leukemia the bone marrow produces abnormal, malignant WBC cells in high numbers, which are present in the peripheral blood too. However, in aleukemic leukemia the abnormal WBC cells mostly accumulate within the spleen, liver, lymph nodes, testes, brain, etc. and thus are not detectable in peripheral blood (which shows normal or abnormally low WBC cells).

Incidence

Leukemia accounts for 8% of all human cancers and is the common malignancy in children and young adults. One-half of all leukemiasis are classified as acute, with rapid onset and progression of the disease resulting in 100% mortality within days to months without appropriate therapy. The remaining leukemias are classified as chronic, which have a more indolent course.

Etiology

Although the exact cause of leukemia is unknown, several predisposing factors have been associated with this disease which include:

1. Chromosomal abnormality—presence of an abnormal chromosome, e.g. Philadelphia chromosome.
2. Exposure to high doses of radiation therapy
3. Exposure to certain chemicals, e.g. benzene, phenyl butazone and chloramphenicol, etc.
4. Chemotherapy
5. Pre-existing polycythemia vera
6. Genetic disorder (Down's syndrome)
7. Primary immune deficiency

8. Infection with human leukocyte virus (HTLV-1—human T-cell Leukemia virus-1).
9. Hereditary or familial susceptibility.

Classification of Leukemias (Box 17.1)

Leukemias are broadly classified into acute and chronic types.

Acute Leukemia

It is characterized by neoplastic proliferation of large number of abnormal and immature leukocytes in the marrow that spreads into tissues and infiltrate the lymph nodes, liver, spleen, and eventually all body systems.

In addition to this, production of other blood cells (i.e. red blood cells and platelets) is inhibited, which results in inadequate oxygen transport, thrombocytopenia, and immune system malfunction, etc.

According to the French–American–British (FAB) cooperative group, the acute leukemias are classified in the following.

Chronic Leukemia

These diseases have a gradual onset and a more protracted course than the acute forms. The white blood cells produced relatively are more mature and thus can better defend the body against infections.

Chronic leukemias are again classified into two types:
1. Chronic myelogenous leukemia
2. Chronic lymphocytic leukemia (CLL).

Clinical Features of Leukemias

- Acute leukemias occur commonly either in children aged between 2 years and 4 years and in adult patients aged 65 years or above. Chronic leukemias, on the other hand, occur in patients between the ages of 25 years and 60 years.
- Both types of leukemia occur predominantly among males.
- Patients often complain of fatigue, weakness, shortness of breath and severe pallor due to anemia.
- Easy bruising, epistaxis, petechiae, ecchymosis, and cerebral hemorrhage due to thrombocytopenia.
- Headache, vomiting, heat intolerance, and generalized pain in bone and joints, etc.
- Most of the patients may have the feeling of abdominal fullness due to hepatosplenomegaly.

Box 17.1	Classification of leukemias.
Acute leukemia	**Chronic leukemia**
Acute lymphocytic leukemia (ALL) L1—common childhood leukemia L2—adult ALL L3—rare subtype, blast cells Resemble Burkitt's lymphoma	Chronic myelogenous leukemia (CML)
Acute myeloblastic leukemia (AML) **Granulocytic** M1—myeloblastic leukemia without maturation M2—myeloblastic leukemia with maturation M3—hypergranular promyelocytic leukemia **Monocytic** M4—myelomonocytic leukemia M5—Monocytic leukemia **Erythroid** M6—erythroleukemia	Chronic lymphocytic leukemia (CLL)

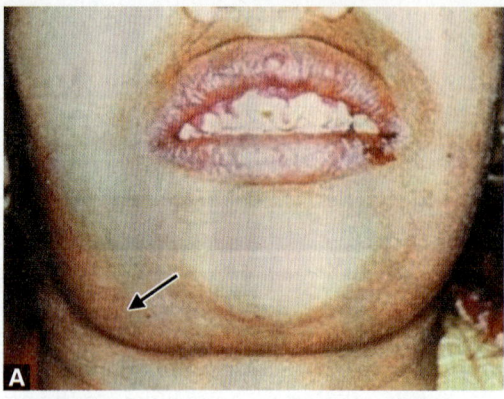 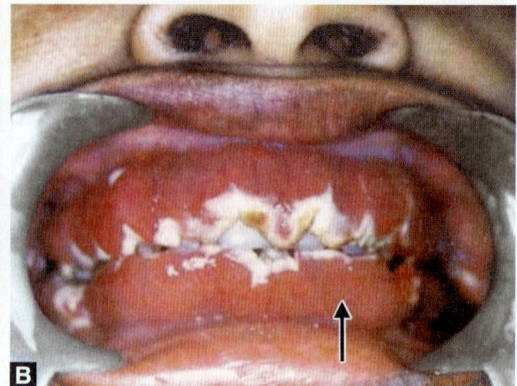

Figs. 17.2A and B: Submandibular lymph node swelling and severe gingival enlargement in a patient with acute myeloid leukemia.

- Persistent fever of unknown etiology, severe infections, e.g. pneumonia and septicemia, etc. due to depressed immunity Figures 17.2A and B.
- Weight loss and heat intolerance due to increased rate of body metabolism.
- Pain from infarction of the spleen.
- Leukemic cell infiltrations into the skin, Figure 17.3 mucosa, and other body organs.

Oral Manifestations of Leukemia

Oral manifestations in leukemia may be caused by the basic disease process itself or the secondary infections or due to local irritations aggregated by plaque, food debris, and ill-fitting dentures, etc.

- Gingival hyperplasia (due to leukemic cell infiltration) with ulceration and severe bleeding tendency.
- Diffuse hyperplastic gingivitis with cyanotic bluish discoloration of the gingiva.
- Tumor-like swellings in the gingiva, palate, and salivary glands due to deposition of leukemic cells.
- Oral mucosal pallor with petechiae, ecchymosis, hemorrhage, and hematoma formation in mouth Figure 17.4.
- Mucositis with frequent mucosal ulcerations, ulcers have pale margin.
- Recurrent secondary infections, e.g. candidiasis, histoplasmosis, aspergillosis and HSV infections, etc.

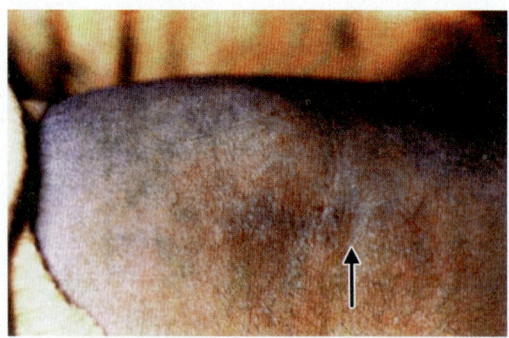 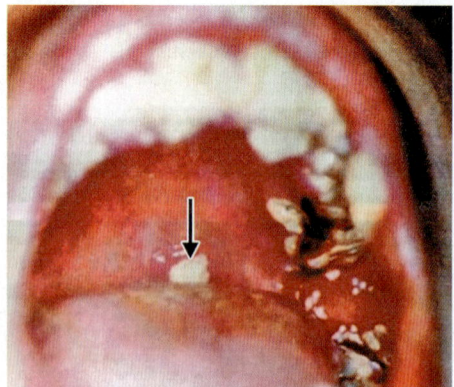

Fig. 17.3: Areas of ecchymosis of skin (extensor surface of hand) in the same patient.

Fig. 17.4: Necrotic ulcerations of oral mucosa in the patient with acute myeloid leukemia.

- Rapid loosening and spontaneous exfoliations of teeth due to destruction of periodontal ligament and alveolar bone.
- Post-extraction hemorrhage, delayed healing of socket after extraction and risk of development of osteomyelitis of the jaw.
- Involvement of dental pulp by leukemic cells produce atypical dental pain.
- Mental nerve neuropathy or the "numb chin syndrome".

Diagnostic Assessment

A comprehensive evaluation of all body systems is necessary for establishing the diagnosis and treatment plan for leukemia.

Complete Blood Count Values

- Complete peripheral blood count—WBC count may be greater than 20,00,000/mm^3.
- Bone marrow aspiration—abnormal increase in bone marrow cells with high proportion of leukocyte series.
- Lumbar puncture—to see the presence of leukemic cells in central nervous system
- Lymphangiogram—to determine the leukemic cells within lymph nodes.
- X-Rays:
  - Chest X-ray—to detect the mediastinal involvement.
  - Skeletal X-ray—to detect skeletal lesions.
  - MRI and CT scans—to detect lesions and sites of infection, especially in the head and neck areas.

Treatment

Antileukemic chemotherapy and radiotherapy. Repeated blood transfusions and administration of antibiotics.

AGRANULOCYTOSIS (GRANULOCYTOPENIA)

Agranulocytosis is a serious acute leukopenia characterized by a significant decrease in the number of granular leukocytes (chiefly the neutrophils).

Etiology

The disease commonly occurs among adult females and interestingly, it frequently affects the health professionals.

- Toxic effects of some drugs, e.g. sulfonamides, chloramphenicol, antihistaminics and chlorambucil, etc.
- Due to the hypersensitivity to drugs like aminopyrine.
- Long-term administration of analgesics (phenyl butazone), antithyroids, diuretics, cytotoxic drugs and anticoagulants, etc.
- Ionizing radiation, tuberculosis, typhoid fever, and malaria.

Clinical Features

- Fever, sore throat, weakness, bone pain, jaundice, and skin pallor.
- Persistent bacterial infections with regional lymphadenitis.
- Severe dysphagia, weak and rapid pulse, etc. are the other important features of the disease.
- Urinary tract infections with vaginal and rectal ulcerations are common.
- Early onset of pneumonia, sepsis and shock, etc. often with fatal outcome.

Oral Manifestations of Agranulocytosis

- Development of narcotizing ulcerations (agranulocytic angina) in the gingiva, soft palate, tonsils, lips, pharynx and cheek, etc.
- Oral ulcers are often deep, hemorrhagic and are often covered with a yellow or gray membrane; and characteristically there is absence of any red halo due to the lack of inflammation.
- Gingival bleeding, halitosis, excessive salivations and dysphagia often cause difficulty in taking food.
- Excessive tendency for developing secondary infections, which develop rapidly and soon become overwhelming. These lesions often resemble acute necrotizing ulcerative gingivitis (ANUG).

- Opportunistic fungal infections are also common in the mouth.

Histopathology

Biopsy taken from the oral ulcer reveals numerous bacterial organisms both on the surface and deep inside the tissue. Inflammatory response in the tissue is very little.

Diagnostic Assessment

Diagnosis of agranulocytosis is made on the basis of the following:
- WBC count reveals severe leukopenia (500–3,000/mm^3) with extreme reduction in neutrophil count (0–2%).
- Bone marrow examination reveals an absence of granulocytes, a maturational arrest of young developing cells or an increased number of myeloid precursors (signifying peripheral granulocyte destruction).
- Cultures of urine, blood, and materials taken from lesions in the throat and mouth, etc. are positive for bacteria (usually gram-positive cocci).
- A history of exposure to an offending agent, plus all the above findings (especially in case of a person, who medicates himself or herself) are generally diagnostic for agranulocytosis.

Treatment

Elimination of causative factors, antibiotics, vitamins, antipyretics, and high caloric soft diet.

■ CYCLIC NEUTROPENIA

Definition

Cyclic neutropenia is an idiopathic disease characterized by episodic defects in neutrophil maturation in the bone marrow, resulting in periodic fall in circulating neutrophils at regular intervals of 3–4 weeks. The condition is episodic in nature and is characterized by severe infections as the neutrophil count falls below the critical level, moreover the symptoms subside as the neutrophil count rises toward normal.

Clinical Features

- Cyclic neutropenia generally affects children and the patients often suffer from recurrent upper respiratory tract infections in uniformly spaced episodes.
- Patients develop short-term fever on regular basis along with anorexia, malaise, and lymphadenopathy, etc. which spontaneously resolve once the neutrophil count returns to normal.
- Aphthous-like ulceration in the mouth of short duration develop upon minor trauma, the areas commonly affected are lips, tongue, buccal mucosa, and oropharynx, etc.
- Oral ulcers often have an erythematous "halo" at the periphery.
- Cyclic neutropenia also characteristically produces rapidly progressive periodontal disease at an early age, which presents severe gingival recessions, rapid alveolar bone loss, and tooth mobility, etc.

Diagnostic Assessment

- Total WBC count decreases to 3,000 cells/mm^3 of blood in every month.
- The neutrophil count falls below a critical level of 500/mm^3 for 3–5 days and then it rises; the same cycle repeats in about every 3 weeks.
- Blood monocyte and eosinophil count increases as the neutrophil count falls.
- In cyclic neutropenia, the neutrophil count is always far below normal even during the remission period also.
- Oral ulcer histologically shows absence of infiltrating neutrophils.

Treatment

No specific treatment.

■ PURPURA

Purpura is defined as the extravasation of small amount of blood into the skin or mucous membrane, causing petechiae, ecchymosis or spontaneous bruising, etc. The disease purpura results from platelet disorder or occasionally due to vascular defects and is characterized by prolonged bleeding time (BT) but normal clotting functions.

Normal platelet count in our blood is 2.5–4 lac/cu mm; when the platelet count goes down below 100,000/mm³ of blood the condition is called purpura. At this level of platelet count spontaneous bleeding does not occur, rather it can occur only if the platelet count goes down below 20,000 per cu mm of blood.

Drugs, which may cause purpura
- Chloramphenicol
- Phenylbutazone
- Indomethacin
- Thiazide
- Diuretics
- Quinine
- Quinidine.

Types

The disease is of two types:
1. Idiopathic thrombocytopenic purpura (ITP).
2. Nonthrombocytopenic purpura.

Idiopathic thrombocytopenic purpura refers to thrombocytopenia caused by an unknown, possibly autoimmune disease. This disorder is characterized by premature destruction of platelets due to the formation of antibodies against them. The platelets are then destroyed by phagocytosis in the spleen or in the liver.

Normally, platelet cells survive 8–10 days within the circulation but in ITP, the platelet survival time is as brief as 1–3 days or less.

Nonthrombocytopenic purpura occurs due to the rupture of smaller blood vessels with resultant bleeding into the tissue.

Major forms of this disease are:
- Familial hemorrhagic telangiectasia
- Anaphylactoid purpura
- Toxic purpura.

Clinical Features of Purpura

- Purpura commonly occurs among adults below 40 years of age and females are more frequently affected than males.
- The disease is characterized by sudden and spontaneous occurrence of petechiae (Fig. 17.5) (*small pinpoint hemorrhage under the skin or mucosa*), ecchymosis (*escape of blood into tissues producing a large bruise*) or hematomas (blood-filled tumors) in the skin and mucous membrane (Fig. 17.6).
- Excessive bruising tendency, epistaxis, hematuria, melena, and hematemesis.
- Prolonged bleeding after surgery or injury.
- Purpuric spots on the skin, which do not blanch upon pressure.
- Bleeding into the diaphragm may result in pulmonary complications.

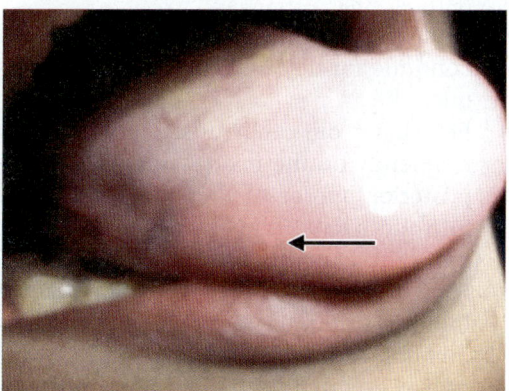

Fig. 17.5: Multiple petechial spots on the skin of a patient with thrombocytopenic purpura.

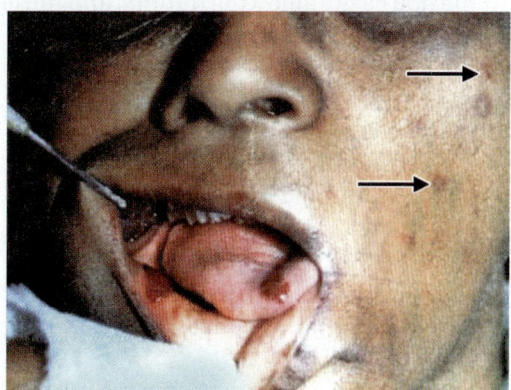

Fig. 17.6: Multiple petechial spots on the skin and gingival bleeding in a patient with purpura.

- Intracranial hemorrhage may produce paresthesia of the cranial nerves and hemiplegia.
- Bleeding into the muscles and joints with difficulty in movements.
- Interestingly, the spleen is not palpable and if it is palpable, leukemia should be suspected rather than purpura.

Oral Manifestations of Purpura

- Profuse gingival bleeding and development of blood blisters, which occur either spontaneously or upon slight provocation.
- Bleeding starts typically after a short delay following injury as platelets and vascular response provide initial phase of hemostasis.
- Persistent uncontrolled hemorrhage may continue for days and untreated patients often die.
- Petechiae or ecchymosis occurs very frequently on the palatal mucosa (where posterior border of the denture presses into the palatal mucosa), however other intraoral structures may also be involved.
- Excessive uncontrolled bleeding occurs following minor surgical procedures including dental extractions (however unlike hemophilia, bleeding in purpura ultimately stops spontaneously as a result of normal coagulation of blood).
- Submucosal hematomas often develop in the oral cavity following trauma, and these lesions appear as large and dark tumors.
- Bleeding into the facial muscles may cause difficulty in opening and closing the mouth.
- Bleeding into the temporomandibular joint results in pain and trismus.

Diagnostic Assessment

- Platelet count below 100,000/mm^3 of blood (normal platelet count is 2.5–400,000/mm^3 of blood).
- Spontaneous bleeding occurs if the platelet count goes below 20,000/mm^3.
- Prolonged bleeding time with normal coagulation time.
- Increased capillary fragility as demonstrated by "tourniquet test".
- Positive platelet antibody screening.
- Bone marrow aspirates contain normal or increased number of megakaryocytes.
- Examination of urine reveals proteinuria or hematuria.
- Gingival tissue biopsy with Periodic acid–Schiff stain reveals fibrin deposits within the small capillaries.

Treatment

By steroid therapy and repeated blood transfusions. Splenectomy and immunosuppressive drug therapy may be required.

HEMOPHILIA OR ROYAL DISEASE

Hemophilia is a potentially fatal inherited bleeding disorder characterized by profound hemorrhage due to the genetic deficiency of clotting factors. The disease occurs in males but is transmitted by females and the incidence rate is 1 in 8,000 to 10,000 populations.

The pathways of blood coagulation with the clotting factors of blood have been described in Flowchart 17.2.

Etiology and Pathogenesis (Flowchart 17.3)

- Heredity plays the most important role in the development of hemophilia and the disease has sex-linked recessive inheritance; most cases are caused by a mutation in the gene that encodes for one of the clotting factors.
- Since hemophilia gene is located on the X chromosome, hemophilia usually occurs in males, and females are the carriers of the disease.

Types

There are three major types of hemophilia.
- Hemophilia A (classic hemophilia): It is the most common type of hemophilia;

Flowchart 17.2: Pathways of blood coagulation and the clotting factors.

Clotting factors of blood

Factor I: Fibrinogen
Factor II: Prothrombin
Factor III: Tissue thromboplastin
Factor IV: Calcium ions
Factor V: Labile factor
Factor VII: Stable factor
Factor VIII: Antihemophilic factor
Factor IX: Christmas factor/plasma thromboplastin component (PTA)
Factor X: Stuart–Prower factor
Factor XI: Plasma thromboplastin antecedent (PTA)
Factor XII: Hageman factor
Factor XIII: Fibrin stabilizing factor
PL: Platelet membrane phospholipid
TF: Tissue factor

Pathways of blood coagulation

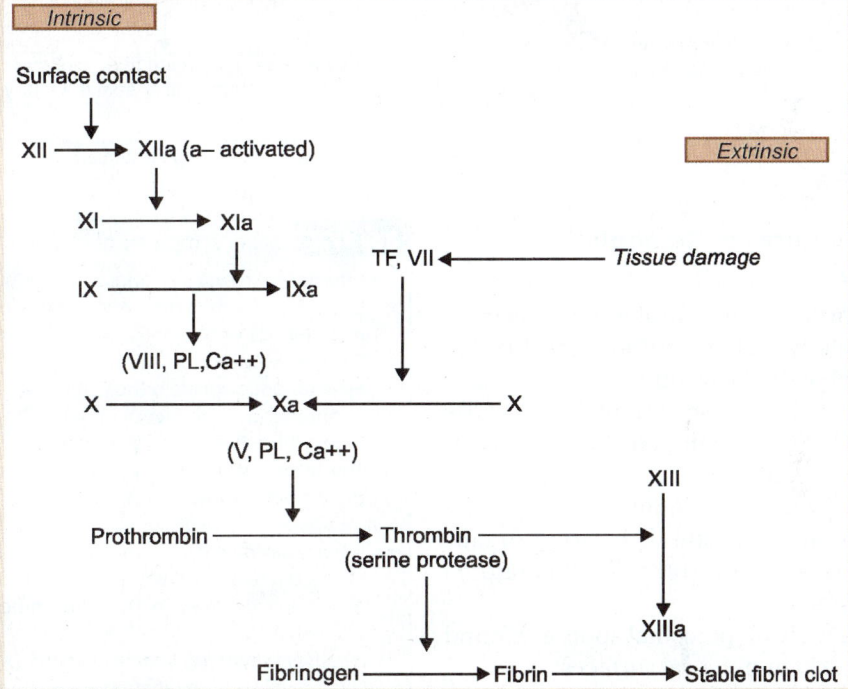

8 out of 10 hemophilic patients have hemophilia A and it occurs due to deficiency of clotting factor VIII.
- Hemophilia B (Christmas disease): It is a less common type of hemophilia, which occurs due to the deficiency of clotting factor IX.
- Hemophilia C: It is a mild form of hemophilia which occurs due to the deficiency of clotting factor XI (plasma thromboplastin antecedent that activates factor IX).
- Von Willebrand disease: It occurs due to the deficiency of von Willebrand factor (it binds to factor VIII and mediates platelet adhesion.

Since, the classic hemophilia constitutes about 80% of all hemophilias, the discussion on clinical features and treatments, etc. will be made mostly in reference to this entity.

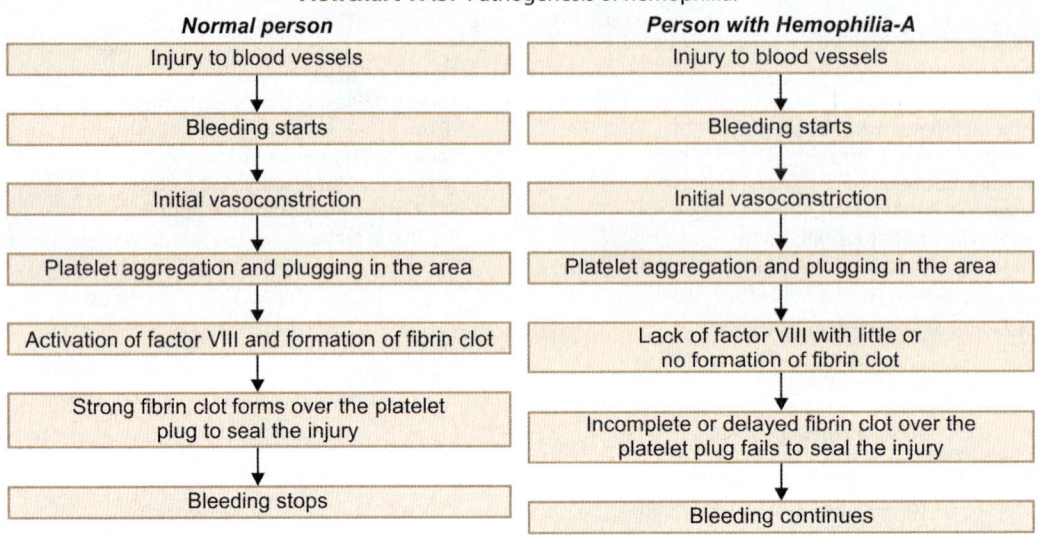

Flowchart 17.3: Pathogenesis of hemophilia.

Clinical Features of Hemophilia (Box 17.2)

- Easy bruising and prolonged bleeding, particularly after minor accidental, surgical or dental trauma.
- Bleeding into muscles and joints cause pain, swelling and difficulty in movement of the affected organ.
- Spontaneous bleeding into the subcutaneous tissue or internal organs leads to recurrent soft tissue hematoma formation.
- Interestingly no petechial spots are found on the skin or mucosal surfaces.
- Severe, sometimes fatal epistaxis after injury to the nose.
- Gastric hemorrhage may occur in case a gastric ulcer is present.
- Recurrent hemarthrosis (bleeding into the joints) occurs commonly in elbow, knee and ankle joints, etc. and untreated or recurrent cases may result serious joint deformity and permanent crippling.
- Patients often have spontaneous hematuria and intracranial hemorrhage.
- The disease is seldom diagnosed in infancy unless serious bleeding occurs from the umbilical cord or following circumcision.
- It is usually diagnosed after the child becomes active.

Box 17.2 Major symptoms of hemophilia.

Symptoms of external bleeding:
- Excessive bleeding from minor injury or injection needle prick or bite or from a mobile tooth.
- Easy bruising
- Spontaneous epistaxis (nose bleeds)
- Spontaneous gum bleeding
- Heavy bleeding from a minor cut
- The bleeding from the cut may stop for a short period but resumes soon.

Symptoms of internal bleeding:
- *Intracranial bleeding* (hemorrhage inside brain)—characterized by vomiting, blurred vision, extreme weakness in the extremities, fatigue, and convulsions.
- *Bleeding within large joints*—warm, painful, and swollen joints with difficulty in movements.
- *Blood in the urine* (from hemorrhage in the kidneys or bladder) and the urine typically looks "cola colored".
- *Coffee ground vomitus*—due to acute bleeding in the upper gastrointestinal tract (esophagus).
- *Tarry-black stools*—due to excessive bleeding in the stomach.
- *Large lumpy bruises* on the body due to bleeding into the large muscles of the body.

Oral Manifestation of Hemophilia

- Severe hemorrhage from the gingival tissue after surgical incision, curettage or dental extraction.
- Bleeding may even start after brushing the teeth with a hard toothbrush.
- Severe bleeding if not controlled may continue for weeks or until the patient dies.
- Slight trauma (e.g. common bumps or fall in case of small babies) may lead to ecchymosis or hematoma formations in the tongue, lips or palate, etc.
- Severe bleeding unexpectedly occurs from the tiny injection sites in the mouth.
- Internal bleeding into the glottis with subsequent airway obstruction; may occur following pterygomandibular-block-anesthesia, which may cause death of the patient.
- Recurrent subperiosteal hematoma with reactive new bone formation may cause tumor-like malformations of the jaw (such lesions are called pseudo-tumor of hemophilia).
- Hemophilic patients often carry a high caries index and severe periodontal disease.

Laboratory Investigations

- Clotting time is prolonged or sometimes it may test normal
- Platelet count and bleeding time is normal
- Prothrombin time is normal
- Prothrombin consumption—decreased
- Activated partial thromboplastin time is prolonged
- Thromboplastin generation—increased
- Genetic counseling and carrier detection by biologic and immunologic assays
- Blood grouping and cross matching
- Specific quantitative assays for factor VIII will determine the severity of the disease.

Common Complications in Hemophilia

- Airway obstruction due to hemorrhage into the neck and pharynx, down to glottis, occurs following inferior alveolar nerve block anesthesia.
- Even simple submucosal infiltration anesthesia may lead to serious consequences.
- Intestinal obstruction due to bleeding from the intestinal walls or into peritoneum.
- Compression of nerves with paralysis due to hemorrhage into deep tissues.
- Intracranial hemorrhage.
- Death may occur due to intracranial bleeding or from exsanguinations following any serious hemorrhage.

Treatment

- Immediate transfusion of factor VIII or IX concentrate is the primary treatment.
- Although plasma and cryoprecipitate contain factor VIII, the concentrates have known antihemophilic globulin (AHG) content and carry less risk of blood volume overload.
- As the procoagulant activity of AHG disappears rapidly, patients need transfusions every 12 hours until bleeding stops.
- Transfusion of packed RBCs or WBCs is used only to replace blood volume when there has been severe loss.
- Prophylactic transfusion of factor VIII to a level of 50% above normal is recommended in cases of minor injury or dental extractions.
- Topical bleeding can be temporarily controlled by applying pressure to the injured site or packing the area with fibrin foam, and by applying topical hemostatic agents such as thrombin.
- Analgesics and corticosteroids reduce joint pain and swelling.
- Joint immobilization and local chilling (packing ice around the joint) may give relief in case of hemarthrosis. If the pain is severe, it may be necessary to aspirate blood from the joint.
- In mild hemophilia, the use of intravenous desmopressin (acts by increasing factor

VIII activity) may eliminate the need of AHG.

BIBLIOGRAPHY

1. Aalto SM, Linnavuori K, Peltola H, et al. Immunoreactivation of Epstein-Barr virus due to cytomegalovirus primary infection. J Med Virol. 1998;56(3):186-91.
2. Anwar R, Miloszewski KJ. Factor XIII deficiency. Br J Hematol. 1999;107(3):468-84.
3. Ariens RA, Lai TS, Weisel JW, et al. Role of factor XIII in fibrin clot formation and effects of genetic polymorphisms. Blood. 2002;100(3):743-54.
4. Bradstock KF. The diagnostic and prognostic value of immunophenotyping in acute leukemia. Pathology. 1993;25:367-74.
5. Brink S, Hesseling PB, Amadhila S, et al. Platelet antibodies in immunothrombocytopenic purpura and Onyalai. S Afr Med J. 1983;60:855-8.
6. Brook AH, Bedi R, Chan Lui WY. Hemophilic pseudotumors of the mandible: report of a case in a one-year-old child. Br J Oral Maxillofac Surg. 1985;23:47-52.
7. Brown LD, Sebes JI. Sickle cell gnathopathy: radiologic assessment. Oral Surg Oral Med Oral Pathol. 1986;61:653-6.
8. Cannell H. The development of oral and facial signs in beta-thalassemia major. Br Dent J. 1988;164:50.
9. Carulli G, Sbrana S, Azzara A. Reversal of autoimmune phenomena in autoimmune neutropenia after treatment with rhG-CSF: two additional cases [letter; comment]. Br J Haematol. 1997;96(4):877-8.
10. Chisholm M. Tissue changes associated with iron deficiency. Clin Haematol. 1973;2(2):304.
11. Court-Brown WM, Doll R. Leukemia and aplastic anemia in patients irradiated for ankylosing spondylitis. Medical Research Council Special Report Series, No. 295. London. 1957.
12. Dallman PR. Manifestations in iron deficiency. Semin Hematol. 1982;19:19-30.
13. Delcourt-Debruyne EM, Boutigny HR, Hildebrand HF. Features of severe periodontal disease in a teenager with Chediak-Higashi syndrome. J Periodontol. 2000;71(5):816-24.
14. Dimopoulos MA, Panayiotidis P, Moulopoulos LA, et al. Waldenstrom's macroglobulinemia: clinical features, complications and management. J Clin Oncol. 2000;18(1):214-26.
15. Eddy TP. Non-infected diseases of malnutrition. In: Cruickshank R, Standard K, Russell HBL (Eds). Epidemiology and Community Health in Warm Countries. Edinburgh: Churchill Livingstone; 1976. pp. 331-55.
16. Edington GM, Gilles HM. Hemopoietic systems. In: Edington GM, Gilles HM (Eds). Pathology in the Tropics. London: Edward Arnold; 1969. pp. 404-512.
17. Edington GM, Gilles HM. The hemopoietic system. Pathology in the Tropics, 2nd edition. London: Edward Arnold; 1976;404-512.
18. Essien EM. Hemorrhagic disorders. Tropical Africa, Clin Haematol. 1981;3:917-32.
19. Filipovich AH, Stone JV, Tomany SC, et al. Impact of donor type on outcome of bone marrow transplantation for Wiskott-Aldrich syndrome: collaborative study of the International Bone Marrow Transplant Registry and the National Marrow Donor Program. Blood. 2001;97(6):1598-603.
20. Foerster J. Waldenstrom's macroglobulinemia. In: Lee GR, Foerster J, Lukens J, Paraskevas F, Greer JP, Rodgers GM (Eds). Wintrobe's Clinical Hematology, 10th edition. Baltimore, Md: Williams and Wilkins; 1999. p. 2681.
21. Fotos PG, Graham WL, Bowers DC, et al. Chronic autoimmune thrombocytopenic purpura. Oral Surg Oral Med Oral Pathol. 1983;55:564-7.
22. Girdhood RH. Diseases of the blood and blood forming organs. In: Macleod J (Ed). Davidson's Principles and Practice of Medicine. Edinburgh: Churchill Livingstone; 1978. pp. 607-11.
23. Greenberg MS. Clinical and histologic changes of the oral mucosa in pernicious anemia. Oral Surg Oral Med Oral Pathol. 1981;52:38-42.
24. Gunz FW. The epidemiology and genetics of the chronic leukemias. Clin Haematol. 1979;6:3-20.
25. Hagler L, Pastore RA, Bergin JJ. Aplastic anemia following viral hepatitis: report of two fatal cases and literature review. Medicine. 1975;54:139-64.
26. Hedley AG, Kumpel BM. The role of Rh antibodies in hemolytic disease of the newborn. Baillieres Clin Hematol. 1993;6:423-44.
27. Ichinose A. Physiopathology and regulation of factor XIII. Thromb Haemost. 2001;86(1):57-65.

28. Jacobs A. Epithelial changes in anemia East Africans. Br Med J. 1963;1:1711-2.
29. Jimenez E. Lymphomas and leukemias. Part 2.Topical America. Clin Haematol. 1981;10:894-915.
30. Kaito K, Kobayashi M, Katayama T, et al. Long-term administration of G-CSF for aplastic anemia is closely related to the early evolution of monosomy 7 MDS in adults. Br J Haematol. 1998;103(2):297-30.
31. Kaplan HS. On the etiology and pathogenesis of the leukemias: a review. Cancer Res. 1954;14:535-50.
32. Keusch GT, Acheson DW. Thrombotic thrombocytopenic purpura associated with Shigatoxins. Semin Hematol. 1997;34(2):106-16.
33. Layrisse M, Roche M, Baker SJ. Nutritional anemias. In: Beaton GH, Bengoa JM (Eds). Nutrition Prevention Medicine, WHO Monograph Series, No. 62. Geneva: World Health Organization; 1976. pp. 55-82.
34. Leavell BS, Thorup OA Jr. Fundamentals of Clinical Hematology. Philadelphia: WB Saunders; 1971. pp. 302-76.
35. Lewis EB. Leukemia, multiple myeloma and aplastic anemia in American radiobiologists. Science. 1963;142:1492-4.
36. Lynch MA. Hematologic diseases and related problems. Burkitt's Oral Medicine, 7th edition. Philadelphia: Lippincott; 1977. p. 431.
37. Mason RP, Fischer V. Possible role of free radical formation in drug-induced agranulocytosis. Drug Saf. 1992;7:45-50.
38. McGraw WT, Belch A. Oral complication of acute leukemia: prophylactic impact of a chlorhexidine mouth rinse regimen. Oral Surg Oral Med Oral Pathol. 1985;60:275-80.
39. Nathan DG, Oski FA. Hemophilia. Hematology of Infancy and Childhood. 1998;5:1631-45.
40. Okano M, Gross TG. Epstein-Barr virus-associated hemophagocytic syndrome and fatal infectious mononucleosis. Am J Hematol. 1996;53(2):111-5.
41. Pollack CV Jr. Emergencies in sickle cell disease. Emerg Med Clin North Am. 1993;11(2):365-78.
42. Poyton HG, Davey KW. Thalassemia: changes visible in radiographs used in dentistry. Oral Surg Oral Med Oral Pathol. 1968;25:564.
43. Ranasinghe AW. Effects of experimental iron deficiency anemia on epithelium of the hamster cheek punch. Unpublished D. Phil. Thesis, University of London; 1982.
44. Samual I, Rapaport L (Eds). Introducing to Hematology. Hagerstown, Maryland: Harper & Row; 1971.
45. Scully C, Cawson RA. Normal hematological values. Appendix to Chapter 1. In: Scully C, Cawson RA (Eds). Medical Problems in Dentistry. Bristol: Wright; 1982. pp. 15-20.
46. Soucie JM, Nuss R, Evatt B, et al. Mortality among males with hemophilia: relations with source of medical care. The Hemophila Surveillance System Project Ivestigators. Blood. 2000;96(2):437-42.
47. Srtoncek DF. Drug-induced immune neutropenia. Transfus Med Rev. 1993;7:268-74.
48. Streiff MB, Smith B, Spivak JL. The diagnosis and management of polycythemia vera in the era since the Polycythemia Vera Study Group: a survey of American Society of Hematology members' practice patterns. Blood. 2002;99(4):1144-9.
49. Werner EJ. Von Willebrand disease in children and adolescents. Pediatr Clin North Am. 1996;43(3):683-707.

CHAPTER 18

Periodontal Diseases

INTRODUCTION

The periodontium consists of several tissues namely the gingiva, the periodontal ligaments, the cementum, and the alveolar bone, etc. The periodontal diseases are a group of heterogeneous, chronic destructive inflammatory diseases of the periodontium.

Gingivitis: The term gingivitis is used to designate inflammatory lesions that are confined to the marginal gingiva.

Periodontitis: Once the inflammatory process from gingiva extends into the deeper tissues and causes destruction of the periodontal ligaments along with loss of alveolar bone; the disease is designated periodontitis.

EPIDEMIOLOGY

Although there is evidence that, at least, clinically several distinct types of chronic destructive periodontal diseases may exist. The term gingivitis is used to designate inflammatory lesions that are confined to the marginal gingiva. Once the lesions extend to include destruction of the connective tissue attachments of the tooth and loss of alveolar bone, the disease is designated periodontitis.

Chronic inflammatory periodontal diseases of varying severity affect practically all dentate individuals. Gingivitis is common in children, even by the age of 3 years, and early periodontitis may be detected in teenagers; in general, the extent and severity of disease increase with age. This does not imply that all gingivitis will eventually progress to periodontitis. Since the adoption of the Community Periodontal Index of Treatment Needs (CPITN), epidemiological data from various parts of the world can be compared. This has confirmed that virtually all adult individuals show some evidence of early periodontitis but the advance disease affects only about 10–15% of the population. Tooth loss as a result of periodontal destruction is uncommon before the age of 50 years unless the patient has some other systemic diseases (Table 18.1).

Etiology of periodontal diseases:
- Local factors
- Systemic factors

Table 18.1: Etiological factors of periodontal diseases.

Local factors	• Microorganisms • Calculus • Food impaction • Faulty restorations • Tooth malposition • Mouth breathing habit • Use of different drugs or chemicals.
Systemic factors	• Nutritional deficiency • Pregnancy • Diabetes • Allergy • Heredity • Immunological disorders • Psychogenic factors

Local factors in the etiology of periodontal diseases:
- Microorganisms
- Calculus
- Food impaction
- Faulty restorations
- Tooth malposition
- Mouth breathing habit
- Use of different drugs or chemicals.

Systemic factors causing periodontal diseases:
- Nutritional deficiency
- Pregnancy
- Diabetes
- Allergy
- Heredity
- Immunological disorders
- Psychogenic factors.

[Two important diseases caused by the same type of microorganisms—dental caries and periodontal diseases.]

The Role of Bacteria and Dental Plaque in Periodontal Disease (Box 18.1)

- Accumulation of plaque bacteria in mouth initiates periodontal disease while plaque control reestablishes periodontal health.
- Administration of antimicrobial agents can prevent gingivitis and periodontitis.
- Bacteria isolated from human dental plaque are capable of inducing periodontal disease when introduced into the mouths of gnotobiotic animals.

Box 18.1	Important microorganisms in periodontal disease.

- *Actinobacillus actinomycetemcomitans*
- *Actinomyces viscosus*
- *Capnocytophaga* group
- *Eikenella corrodens*
- *Fusobacterium nucleatum*
- *Porphyromonas gingivalis*
- *Prevotella intermedia*
- *Treponema*
- *Wolinella*

- Several species of pathogenic bacteria have been isolated from periodontal pockets.

Dental Plaque

Plaque is a thin, transparent film produced on the tooth surfaces and it consists predominantly of microorganisms suspended in salivary mucins and extracellular bacterial polysaccharides (glucans).

Acquired Pellicle

It is initial component of the dental plaque, which is made by the salivary glycoprotein and is formed just prior to the bacterial colonization.

Composition of acquired pellicle:
- Salivary glycoprotein
- Albumin
- Immunoglobulin G
- Immunoglobulin A.

The "Pioneering Organisms" in Dental Plaque

About 1 hour after the formation of acquired pellicle on the tooth surface, for the first time some organisms such as *S. sanguis, A. viscous, A. naeslundii* and *Peptostreptococcus*, etc. become attached to it. These organisms are called "pioneering organisms".

The Bacteria, which are Generally Present in Healthy Periodontal Tissues

Healthy periodontal tissues of humans are associated with a scanty flora located almost entirely supragingivally on the tooth surface. The microbial accumulations are 1–20 cells in thickness and comprise mainly gram-positive bacteria *Streptococcus* and *Actinomyces* species predominate, for example *S. sanguis, A. naeslundii*, A. viscosus, etc.

The Bacteria, which might be Present in Gingivitis

Members of the genus *Actinomyces* predominate, but there is a substantial increase in strict anaerobes and gram-negative organisms.

The Bacteria, which Predominate in Subgingival Tissue in Periodontitis

Microbial population in subgingival plaque in periodontitis comprises of gram-negative rods, motile forms, and spirochetes. Black–pigmented bacteroid group are the predominant cultivable organisms in most subjects and they have been reclassified as *Porphyromonas* or *Prevotella* species, for example, *Porphyromonas gingivalis*, *Prevotella melaninogenica*, and *Prevotella intermedia*, etc.

Common Bacteria causing Periodontal Disease

- *Actinomycetemcomitans*
- *Actinomyces viscosus*
- *Capnocytophaga group*
- *Eikenella corrodens*
- *Fusobacterium nucleatum*
- *Porphyromonas gingivalis*
- *Prevotella intermedia*
- *Treponema*
- *Wolinella.*

Calculus

It is the mineralized plaque, which is often seen on the tooth surface as hard deposits.

Calculus forms as the soft dental plaque gets mineralized due to the deposition of calcium and other minerals. These minerals often come from either the saliva or the blood serum. The calculus contributes to the development of periodontal diseases, either by harboring the plaque bacteria or by causing irritation to the gingival tissues (Fig. 18.1 and Box 18.2).

Other Local Factors

Local factors include the anatomy of teeth, gingiva, and alveolar bone, alignment and occlusal relationship of teeth, and proximal restorations, etc. and these factors may affect the accumulation and growth of plaque or interfere with its removal.

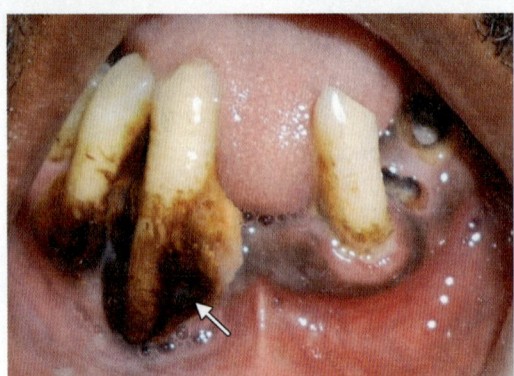

Fig. 18.1: Dental calculus causing gingival recession.

Box 18.2	Factors causing accumulation and stagnation of plaque.

- Calculus
- Food impaction
- Overhanging restoration
- Malocclusion
- Deep pockets
- Mouth breathing.

The Role of Systemic Factors

Although dental plaque is the essential factor in periodontal disease, there are many systemic factors, which may alter the host's response to local irritants and, therefore, could influence the development and progression of the lesion.

Several systemic factors have been associated with an increased incidence and severity of periodontal disease or with modifying the course of that disease.

Diabetes mellitus

Diabetes induced vascular changes (tiny vessels supplying the periodontium get obliterated due to atherosclerosis causing diminished blood supply) and defects in cellular defense mechanisms have been suggested as possible mechanisms, which increase the susceptibility of periodontal tissue to irritants from dental plaque.

Pregnancy and sex hormones
- Severity of a preexisting gingivitis increases in pregnancy from the second to the eight month of gestation and then decreases.
- There is overactivity of certain sex hormones during pregnancy, which results in altered tissue response to dental plaque and thus increase the susceptibility of the gingival tissue to get damaged by local irritants.
- The aggravation of gingivitis during pregnancy is related mainly to progesterone, which affects the function and permeability of the gingival microvasculature.
- Localized gingival hyperplasia also occurs during pregnancy (pregnancy tumor) (Fig. 18.2). Moreover, increased levels of gingivitis occurring around puberty and in some women taking oral contraceptives may also be related to the concentration of circulating sex hormones.

Nutrition
Nutritional deficiency particularly deficiency of protein and vitamin C in the diet can cause hemorrhagic gingivitis and generalized edematous enlargement of the gingiva.

Blood diseases
Acute leukemia is the most common blood disorder to seriously affect the periodontium, it often causes generalized gingival enlargement and gingival bleeding. Such changes in the gingiva occur mainly due to infiltration and packing of the tissues by leukemic cells, which eventually cause destruction of the periodontal ligaments and the alveolar bone.

Drugs
Therapeutic administration of certain drugs *(for the treatment of other diseases)* may cause abnormal changes *in the periodontium*, mostly in the form of tissue hyperplasia. *It is believed that these drugs often modify the response of the host (periodontal tissue) to local irritants and product from microbial plaque.*

The drugs which are commonly associated gingival hyperplasia include the following:
- Phenytoin sodium
- Cyclosporine
- Nifedipine
- Azathioprine
- Naproxen sodium
- Verapamil
- Estrogen and progesterone.

Immunodeficiency and periodontal diseases
Diminished cell mediated as well as humoral immunity can predispose to many periodontal diseases; it is particularly more commonly seen in HIV infected individuals. Such patients frequently develop:
- HIV-gingivitis—a linear gingival erythema, which is a fiery red band along the gingival margin and attached gingival with profuse bleeding tendency.
- Necrotizing ulcerative gingivitis—with typical destruction of interdental papilla.
- Rapidly progressing HIV periodontitis—advanced necrotic destruction of the periodontium, rapid bone loss, loss of periodontal ligament and sequestration, etc.

Smoking:
There is ample evidence that tobacco smoking is an important risk factor for the development and progression of periodontal diseases. Smoking probably impairs the

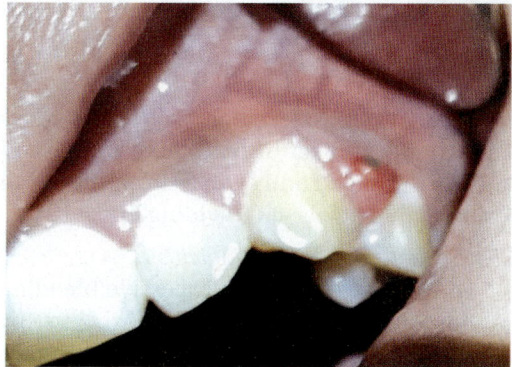

Fig. 18.2: Pregnancy tumor.

phagocytic function of polymorphonuclear neutrophils (PMN).

Factors which prevent the initiation and progression of periodontal diseases:
- Salivary factors
- Gingival crevicular fluid
- Epithelial barrier
- Transmigration of neutrophils
- Immune response.

PATHOGENESIS OF PERIODONTAL DISEASE

Host–parasite relationship—in healthy condition a balance exits between the challenge to the tissue from microorganisms in dental plaque and the host defense mechanisms. Disturbances in this host–parasite relationship lead to the development of periodontal disease, but the transition from healthy condition to gingivitis is not precisely identifiable (Table 18.2).

Potential for Tissue Regeneration and Repair

The host may be able to adapt to the imbalance in the relationship so that a new equilibrium is established and the disease may become arrested and remain stable over long periods of time. Transient imbalances in the host–parasite relationship are likely to occur frequently and yet the natural history of periodontal disease in humans usually spans decades, suggesting that equilibrium is rapidly restored and that for most of the time destruction is not continuous but is episodic in nature.

Table 18.2: Host–parasite relationship in periodontal disease.

Microbial plaque	Host defenses
Direct injury	Salivary factors
Toxic products	Crevicular fluid
Enzymes	Epithelial barrier
Antigenic challenge	Transmigrating of neutrophils immune response

Table 18.3: Stages of periodontal disease.

• The initial lesion	
• The early lesion	Gingivitis
• The established lesion	
• The advanced lesion	Periodontitis

The etiopathogenesis of periodontal disease following withdrawal of oral hygiene procedures and the accumulation of dental plaque has been described as occurring in four stages (Table 18.3).

The stages of periodontal diseases are broadly divided into two groups: (1) gingivitis and (2) periodontitis.
1. Gingivitis designates three stages:
   a. Initial lesion
   b. Early lesion
   c. Established lesion
2. Periodontitis designates only the advanced lesion.

Initial Lesion

The initial lesion of gingivitis develops within 2–4 days following the onset of plaque accumulation. The changes are histological and cannot be detected clinically.

Histologically it shows acute inflammatory response in the gingiva, characterized by vasodilatation with formation of both a fluid and cellular exudates and infiltration of polymorphonuclear neutrophilic (PMN) leucocytes in the subgingival connective tissue and intercellular spaces of the junctional epithelium.

Early Lesion

The early lesion develops within 4–7 days following the onset of plaque accumulation and overlaps with and evolves from the initial lesion with no clear-cut dividing line.

Clinical features of early gingivitis
- Gingival swelling with excessive bleeding tendency either spontaneously or by slight provocation (e.g. tooth brushing).

Periodontal Diseases

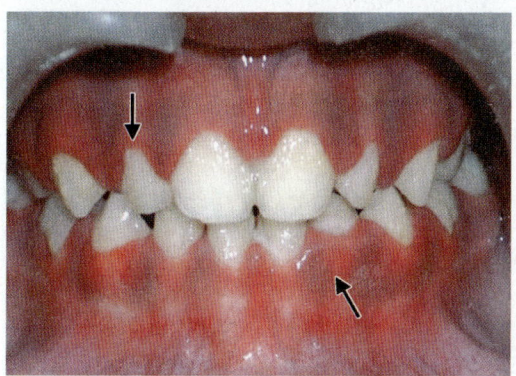

Fig. 18.3: Generalized gingivitis.

- The gingiva appears red or bluish red in color with a boggy or spongy consistency (Fig. 18.3).
- The gingival attachment level on the tooth surface remains does not change.
- There is no radiographic change in the underlying alveolar bone since it is a superficial lesion.

Established Lesion

- The established lesion of gingivitis develops within 2-3 weeks of the onset of plaque accumulation and evolves from the early lesion.
- Histologically, there is accentuation of the features of the initial lesion, but these changes are confined to a narrow band beneath the junctional and pathologically altered epithelium.
- There is further deepening of the gingival sulcus and further growth of subgingival plaque.
- The characteristic feature of the established lesion, which distinguishes it from the early lesion, is the shift in the inflammatory cell population within the connective tissue from predominantly lymphocytic (T cell) to predominantly plasma cell (B cell) type.
- There is continuing loss of collagen as the area of inflammation slowly expands.

Degradation of extracellular matrix
- Degradation of the extracellular matrix, especially collagen, in periodontal disease is a major event, since it ultimately results in loss of tooth.
- Destruction of collagen (extracellular matrix) in periodontal disease occurs as a consequence of its decreased rate of synthesis, increased rate of degradation, or a combination of both.
- Since collagen is synthesized by fibroblast cells, damage to these cells in the inflamed area would result in decreased synthesis.
- Increased degradation of collagen often results from enhanced collagenolytic enzyme activity, such as collagenase, stromelysin, and metalloproteinase, etc.

Common consequences of gingivitis
Gingivitis may have various consequences in different patients:
- It may remain stable for years in few patients
- It can progress slowly to periodontitis in some patients
- Occasionally it can have rapid progression with advanced bone loss at an early age.

Advanced Lesion—Chronic Periodontitis

- The advanced lesion corresponds to chronic periodontitis, a disease characterized by destruction of the connective tissue attachment of the root of the tooth, loss of alveolar bone, and pocket formation
- Plasma cells dominate the infiltrate at all stages of the advance lesions, although lymphocytes and macrophages are also present.

Early true pocket formation occurs in the following steps:
- Extension of gingival inflammation beneath the base of the junctional epithelium into the supra–alveolar connective tissue.

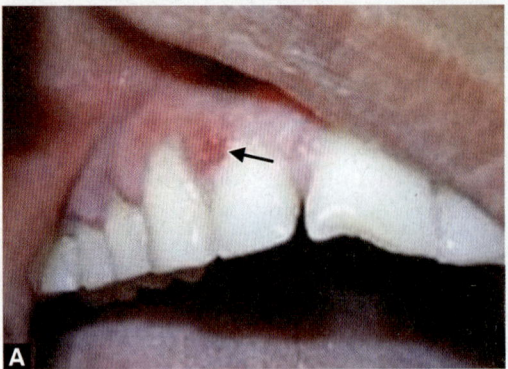 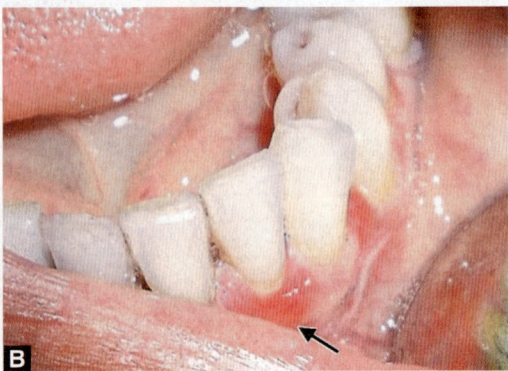

Figs. 18.4A and B: (A) Localized gingivitis. (B) Gingivitis with recession.

- Increase in the area and density of inflammatory infiltrate causes destruction of collagen in the supra-alveolar connective tissue.
- Loss of attachment of the collagen fibers from cementum on the root of the tooth.
- Loss of collagen attachment causes apical migration of the junctional epithelium on the root surface leading to early true pocket formation (Figs. 18.4A and B).

CLINICAL FEATURES OF PERIODONTITIS (TABLE 18.4)

Different types of periodontitis:
- Prepubertal periodontitis
- Juvenile periodontitis
- Rapidly progressive periodontitis
- Adult type periodontitis.

Table 18.4: Clinical classification of periodontitis.

Prepubertal periodontitis	A rare form affecting the deciduous dentition that may be localized or generalized. Genetic factors and a variety of medical conditions may be associated
Juvenile periodontitis	An uncommon form with onset in puberty and adolescence and relativity well-defined clinical features
Rapidly progressive periodontitis	An uncommon form with onset in late adolescence and early adulthood, characterized by episodes of localized or generalized periodontal destruction. Many cases have associated with defects in leukocyte function
Adult type periodontitis	The most common form of periodontitis typically seen in adults over the age of 30 years

Prepubertal Periodontitis

- It is a rare form of periodontitis affecting the deciduous dentition that may be localized or generalized. It is mostly genetic and there may be a variety of medical conditions associated with it.
- The Papillon–Lefèvre syndrome is characterized by skin lesions of palmar-plantar hyperkeratosis and severe periodontal destruction involving both the deciduous and permanent dentitions.
- It is probably transmitted as an autosomal recessive trait, but the mechanisms underlying the oral changes are uncertain, although a neutrophil abnormality has been reported.

Juvenile Periodontitis (Fig. 18.5)

Juvenile periodontitis is an uncommon form of periodontitis, which has onset in puberty or in adolescence; and which is not plaque dependent and exhibits relativity well-defined clinical features.
- The disease is characterized by rapid destruction of alveolar bone with vertical bone loss resulting in deep infrabony pockets.

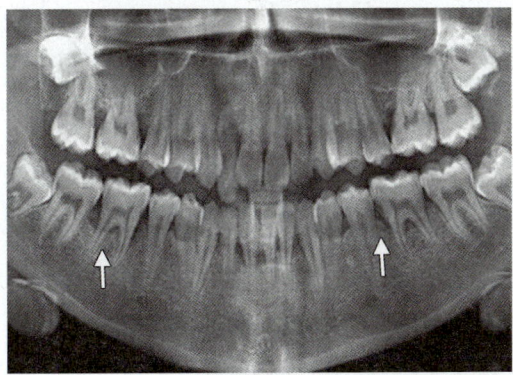

Fig. 18.5: Localized aggressive periodontitis with "arc-shaped" defect in both lower molar regions.

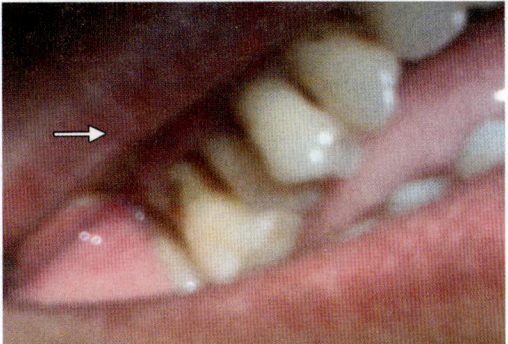

Fig. 18.6: Periodontitis causing recession.

- Initially, the permanent first molar and/or maxillary incisor teeth are affected, usually symmetrically, but the number of teeth involved increases with age.
- The pattern of involvement of teeth tends to follow their sequence of eruption.
- However, the subgingival flora in juvenile periodontitis is dominated by gram-negative anaerobic rods, particularly *Actinobacillus actinomycetemcomitans*. *Capnocytophaga* species and *Eikenella corrodens* may also be of etiological significance.
- In addition to a unique flora, host factors have also been implicated. In particular, a familial pattern has been found in several cases and there is increasing support for the suggestion that genetic factors are involved.
- Abnormalities in cell-mediated immunity and in PMN function have also been demonstrated.

Tetracycline is the drug of choice in the treatment of juvenile periodontitis.

Rapidly Progressive Periodontitis

- Less common than juvenile periodontitis, rapidly progressive periodontitis has an onset between puberty and 30 years of age but lacks well-defined characteristic.
- As the name suggests, the disease is very fast developing (occurs within a few weeks or months) and cause severe inflammation of the periodontium; affecting nearly the entire dentition with evidence of rapid bone destruction (Fig. 18.6).

Adult Type Periodontitis

- Adult type periodontitis is by far the most common form of chronic periodontal disease and is characterized by its chronicity (Fig. 18.7).
- Predominantly shows horizontal bone loss.
- Usually does not progress to tooth loss until after 50 years of age.
- The most common radiographic finding in chronic periodontitis is the destruction of alveolar bone with widening of the periodontal ligament space.

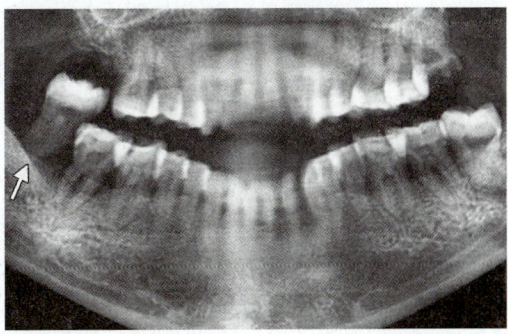

Fig. 18.7: Chronic periodontitis with bone loss.

Other conditions causing widening of periodontal ligament space
- Periapical abscess
- Current orthodontic therapy
- Trauma from occlusion
- Scleroderma
- Osteosarcoma of the jaw.

Factors affecting the prognosis of periodontal diseases
- Oral hygiene status
- Patient motivation
- Age of the patient
- Tooth factor
- Host resistance.

GINGIVAL HYPERPLASIA

An increase in the number of cells causing tissue growth is called hyperplasia while an increase in the size of cells causing tissue growth is called hypertrophy.

Gingival hyperplasia refers to the excessive, exuberant proliferation of gingival tissue causing swelling or overgrowth of the gingiva.

Gingival hyperplasia may be of two types:
1. Inflammatory hyperplasia (Fig. 18.8)
2. Fibrous hyperplasia.

Causes of Gingival Hyperplasia

Causes of inflammatory hyperplasia are as follows:
- Vitamin C deficiency (scurvy)
- Leukemia
- Chronic hyperplastic gingivitis
- Endocrine imbalance (puberty/pregnancy)
- Sarcoidosis
- Crohn's disease.

Causes of fibrous hyperplasia are as follows:
- Heredity (genetic)
- Drug intake (Figs. 18.9 and 18.10; Box 18.3)
- Orofacial angiomatosis
- Wegener's granulomatosis
- Idiopathic.

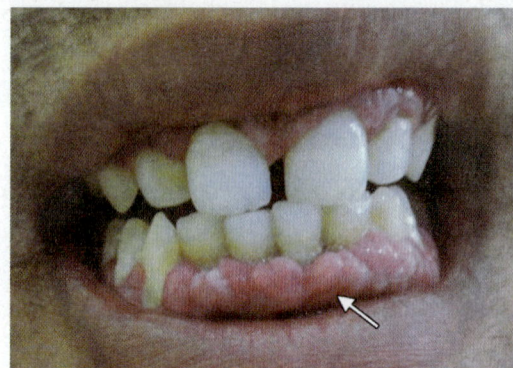

Fig. 18.8: Inflammatory gingival hyperplasia.

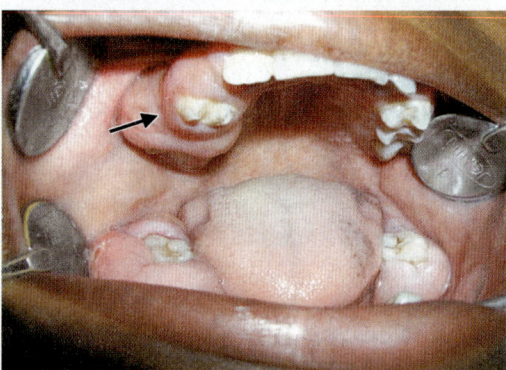

Fig. 18.9: Drug-induced gingival hyperplasia.

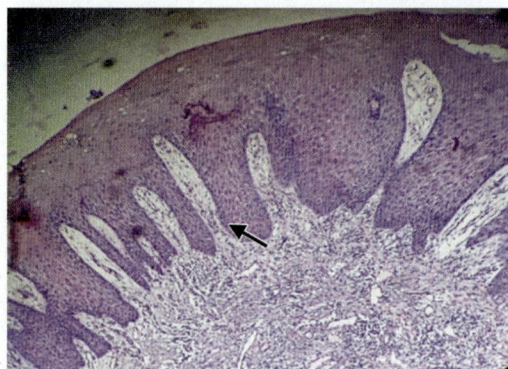

Fig. 18.10: Histopathology of drug-induced gingival hyperplasia.

Gingival Hyperplasia Associated with Vitamin C Deficiency

Vitamin C helps in the synthesis of collagen by helping in the hydroxylation of proline

> **Box 18.3** Common drugs associated with gingival hyperplasia.
>
> **Anticonvulsants**
> - Phenytoin
> - Carbamazepine
> - Ethotoin
> - Felbamate
> - Mephenytoin
> - Phenobarbital
> - Sodium valproate
>
> **Calcium channel blockers**
> - Amlodipine
> - Bepridil
> - Diltiazem
> - Nifedipine
> - Verapamil
>
> Cyclosporine
> Erythromycin
> Oral contraceptives

and glycine. Defective collagen synthesis in vitamin C deficiency produces scurvy and the disease will have the following manifestations:

- Swelling, ulceration, pain, and hemorrhage in the gingival.
- The crest of the interdental papillae appears "red or purple".
- The gingiva is often appears red and spongy and it is often necrosed.
- Gingival sulcus is often filled with blood clot and foul smell is often present in the mouth.
- Administration of vitamin C and improvement of the oral hygiene cures the disease.

Gingival Hyperplasia Associated with Leukemia (Fig. 18.11)

Acute leukemia commonly causes gingival hyperplasia, predominantly due to infiltration of malignant WBC cells into the gingival tissue.

Types of leukemias, which often cause gingival hyperplasia include:
- Acute monocytic leukemia
- Acute lymphocytic leukemia
- Acute myelocytic leukemia

Clinically the following manifestations develop:
- The gingiva becomes ulcerated, edematous, and swollen.
- It is usually painful, has a purplish color with extreme bleeding tendency.
- Pallor in the surrounding mucosa with petechiae or ecchymoses is often observed.
- The diagnosis is confirmed through hematological investigations.

Gingival Hyperplasia Associated with Endocrine Imbalance

Abrupt hormonal changes often take place in the body during puberty or pregnancy, etc. and these conditions are often associated with gingival hyperplasia.

Hormonal imbalance mostly increases the proliferative potential of the gingival tissue in response to the irritations caused by plaque bacteria and local irritants.

Clinically the following manifestations will develop:
- The gingiva becomes red, edematous, and swollen.
- It may or may not be painful but bleeds frequently.
- Sometimes, a localized "tumor-like" growth may develop on the gingiva during pregnancy and it is often known as "pregnancy tumor" (Fig. 18.12).

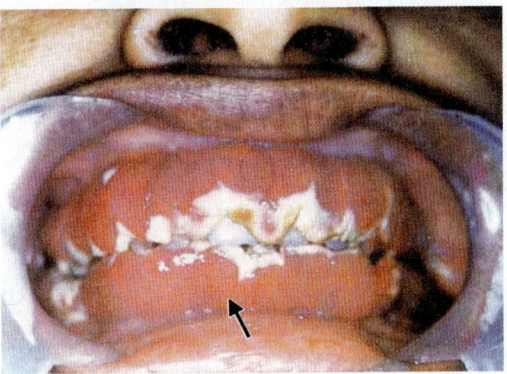

Fig. 18.11: Gingival hyperplasia in leukemia.

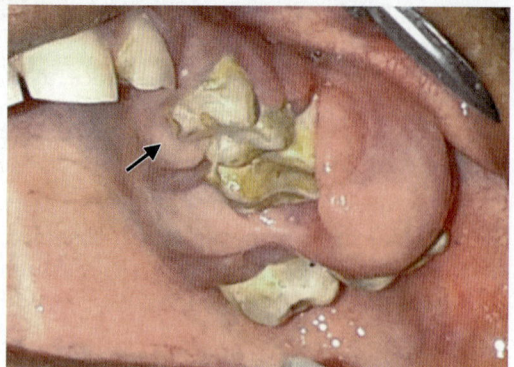 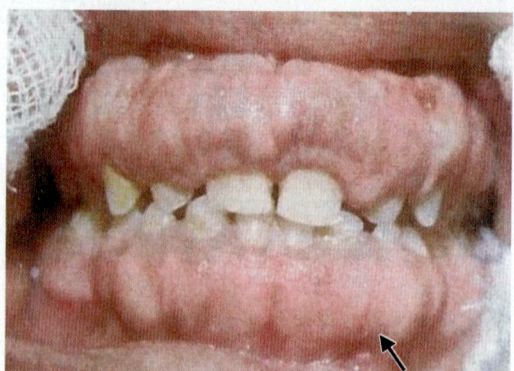

Fig. 18.12: Localized gingival hyperplasia.   **Fig. 18.13:** Dilantin hyperplasia of gingiva.

- The condition regresses spontaneously after the pregnancy period is over.

No treatment is required except oral prophylaxis and maintenance of oral hygiene.

Gingival Hyperplasia Associated with Crohn's Disease

The Crohn's disease is characterized by granulomatous superficial ulceration of the intestinal epithelium, with frequent development of multiple fistulas. The disease produces the following oral manifestations:
- Granular, erythematous swelling of the gingiva with ulceration and occasional bleeding tendency.
- "Cobble-stone" appearance of the buccal mucosa with many linear hyperpastic folds.
- Diffuse indurated swelling on the lips and multiple ulcerations on the palate.

Drug induced Gingival Hyperplasia

A large number of drugs can cause gingival hyperplasia and these are divided into the following groups:
- Anticonvulsants
- Calcium channel blockers
- Cyclosporine
- Erythromycin
- Oral contraceptives.

Dilantin sodium is an antiepileptic drug and it is the most common medicine to cause gingival hyperplasia (as its side effect) (Fig. 18.13).

Clinically the following manifestations develop in dilantin hyperplasia:
- The disease begins with painless enlargement of the interdental papilla.
- The swelling is rough, lobulated, and has a pebbly surface.
- The gingival tissue is of normal color and often there is an increase in stippling.
- It is firm and dense, with no tendency to bleed.
- The gingival growth ceases after the drug therapy is stopped.

Hereditary Gingival Hyperplasia

Hereditary or familial gingival hyperplasia occurs among several members of the same family (Fig. 18.14).

The gingiva is usually firm and resilient and is of normal color. Pain and hemorrhage, etc. are usually absent. In some patients, the gingival growth is so severe that it may cover up the entire crowns of the teeth and may even prevent the eruption of teeth in younger individuals.

Gingival Hyperplasia in Orofacial Angiomatosis

Angiomatous proliferation of the gingival blood vessels may sometimes cause gingival hyperplasia and in such cases, the gingiva

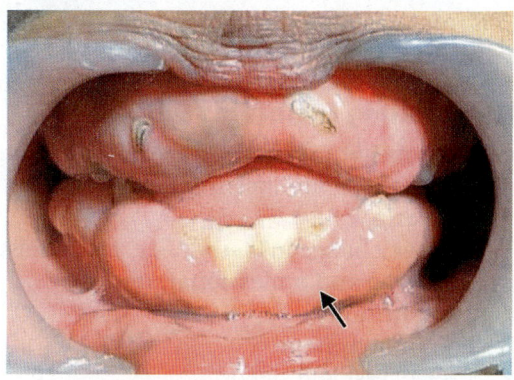

Fig. 18.14: Familial gingival fibromatosis.

clinically appears swollen and red. The enlargements may cause false gingival pocket formation on few occasions.

Gingival Hyperplasia in Wegener's Granulomatosis

Focal or diffuse gingival swelling can occur in Wegener's granulomatosis and the lesion is characterized by epithelial proliferation and dense inflammatory cell infiltration.

■ DESQUAMATIVE GINGIVITIS

Definition

Desquamative gingivitis refers to the condition in which the gingival epithelium sloughs spontaneously or can be scraped off with gentle rubbing (Fig. 18.15).

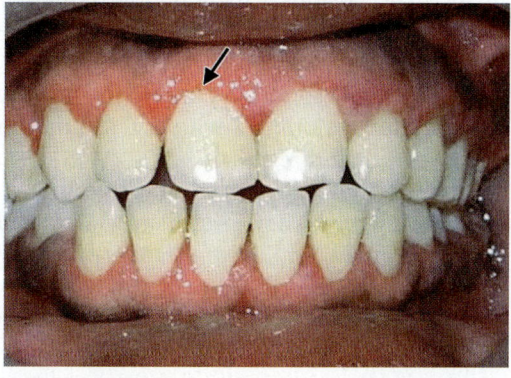

Fig. 18.15: Desquamative gingivitis.

Desquamative gingivitis is not a disease entity but a clinical term applied to the gingival manifestation of several different diseases.

Diseases, which might cause desquamative gingivitis.
- Benign mucous membrane pemphigoid
- Lichen planus
- Local hypersensitivity reactions to tooth pastes, cosmetics. chewing-gums and cinnamon, etc.
- Hormonal disturbances in menopausal females.

Clinical Features of Desquamative Gingivitis

- Clinically gingival tissue appears smooth, red, and edematous with loss of stippling; and there are areas of superficial ulceration, erosion or spontaneous desquamation of varying severity.
- Vesicles or bullae (filled with clear fluid or blood), white flecks or striae may also be seen depending on the underlying etiology.
- Severe pain, burning sensation, and difficulty in food intake are the common complaints.
- The involvement is patchy but the buccal and labial gingivae are more commonly affected than lingual or palatal tissues.
- The condition is more common in females (80%) than males and most cases occur after 30 years of age.
- The gingival reaction associated with chewinggum hypersensitivity (has also been referred to as "plasma-cell gingivitis"). The disease is characterized by widespread distribution of large numbers of plasma cells throughout the gingiva.

■ ACUTE NECROTIZING ULCERATIVE GINGIVITIS/VINCENT'S DISEASE/ TRENCH MOUTH

It is a rare microbial disease of gingiva characterized clinically by severe necrosis of

Flowchart 18.1: Stages of development of acute necrotizing ulcerative gingivitis.

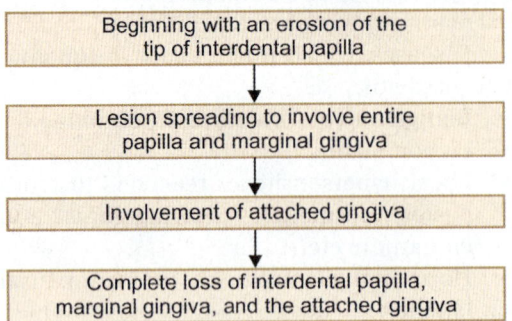

the gingival free gingival margin, the crest of gingiva, and the interdental papillae, etc. The condition is often associated with impaired host immune response.

Acute necrotizing ulcerative periodontitis (ANUP) is the advanced lesion of the same ulcerative process (ANUG) and occurs when the necrotizing process causes loss of epithelial attachment and spreads into the deeper tissues of periodontium, leading to periodontitis.

The stages of development of ANUG have been described in Flowchart 18.1.

Etiology

Acute necrotizing ulcerative gingivitis (ANUG) is a fusospirochetal disease and is caused predominantly by the fusiform bacilli and a spirochete called *Borrelia vincentii* (Box 18.4).

Interestingly, it has been observed that the disease affects multiple numbers of people staying under the same living conditions. This often gives a false impression of the contagious nature of this disease.

Precipitating Factors in ANUG

- Immunosuppression (AIDS and infectious mononucleosis)
- Smoking
- Sudden change in lifestyle, e.g. lack of rest and sleep and professional stress
- Malnutrition
- Poor oral hygiene
- Lack of rest and sleep
- Local tissue damage, local trauma
- Recent debilitating diseases (e.g. bacterial infections, diabetes, blood dyscrasia, etc.)
- Emotional and professional stress
- Down syndrome.

Clinical Features

- Acute necrotizing ulcerative gingivitis is most common in young adult males between the ages of 15 years and 35 years
- Stressed professionals like army recruits tend to suffer more (7%) from the disease than the normal population (1%).
- Moreover, young children suffering from malnutrition are also more vulnerable to the disease.
- Initially the gingiva becomes red, edematous, hemorrhagic, and painful.
- Later on, a sharply demarcated "punched-out" crater-like erosion of the interdental papillae occurs, which permanently destroys the tips of the interdental papillae of the gingiva.
- The gingiva is often covered by a gray "pseudomembrane" with accumulation of necrotic tissue debris.
- Patients have pronounced spontaneous bleeding tendency, exquisite pain, and an extremely unpleasant fetid odor in the mouth.
- Rarely, the gingival lesion may extend to the mucosal surfaces of soft plate and tonsils; and thereby resulting in the condition called necrotizing ulcerative stomatitis.

Box 18.4 Microorganisms often implicated in acute necrotizing ulcerative gingivitis.

- Borrelia vincentii
- Fusobacterium nucleatum
- Treponema denticola
- Prevotella intermedia
- Porphyromonas gingivalis

- Patients often develop headache, fever, malaise, and lymphadenopathy, etc.
- Often there is difficulty in taking food due to increased salivation and a metallic taste in the mouth.
- The necrotizing process may progress to involve and destroy the underlying periodontal ligaments and alveolar bone, and then the condition is called "necrotizing ulcerative periodontitis".
- Most of the patients develop systemic manifestations in the form of leukocytosis, tachycardia, and gastrointestinal disturbances, etc.
- When the necrotizing process of ANUG extends further through the oral mucosa and reaches to the extraoral skin surface, the condition is called "noma" or cancrum oris.

Histopathology
- The affected gingival tissue shows inflammation, ulceration, and extensive necrosis.
- The gingival stratified squamous epithelium is often replaced by a thick, fibrinopurulent "pseudomembrane" consisting of fusiform and spiral type microorganisms, PMN, and necrotic tissue debris, etc.
- The unaffected areas of the gingival tissue show a general lack of keratinization.
- The underlying connective tissue shows intense hyperemia and inflammatory cell infiltration by PMN.

Differential Diagnosis
- Primary acute herpetic gingivostomatitis
- Erosive lichen planus
- Cicatricial pemphigoid
- Drug allergy.

Treatment
- Local debridement of necrotic tissue with H_2O_2.
- Administration of metronidazole or tinidazole, tetracycline, and penicillin, etc.
- Oral hygiene motivation.

■ LATERAL PERIODONTAL ABSCESS

Definition
The lateral periodontal abscess is a localized area of suppurative inflammation arising within the periodontal tissue alongside a tooth and is distinct from the more common periapical abscess (Fig. 18.16).

Etiology
It develops under the following conditions:
- Occlusion in the opening of infra-bony periodontal pockets.
- Impaction of foreign material, such as food debris into a preexisting pocket.
- Following traumatic injury to a tooth.
- Lateral perforation of the root during endodontic therapy.

Clinical Features
- The affected tooth is extremely sensitive to palpation and tendered to percussion.
- Throbbing pain, redness, swelling, and tenderness of the overlying mucosa.
- Foul taste in the mouth with discharge of pus
- The tooth associated with lateral periodontal abscess is mostly vital.

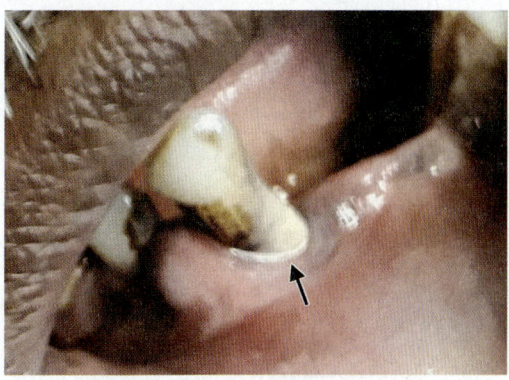

Fig. 18.16: Periodontal abscess.

Radiographic Features

There is often presence of a discrete radiolucent area along the lateral aspect of the root.

Treatment

- Drainage
- Antibiotics
- Elimination of the etiologic factors
- Surgical intervention

■ PERICORONITIS

Definition

Pericoronitis is inflammation of the soft tissue overlying the crown of an impacted or partially erupted tooth; and is seen commonly in association with mandibular third molars.

Pathogenesis

Pericoronitis mostly develops due to accumulation of bacterial plaque and food debris in the space between the crown of an impacted or partially impacted tooth and the overlying gum flap.

Clinical Features

- Edema, swelling, and pain in the gum flap around the tooth (Fig. 18.17).
- The pain is usually very severe and often radiates to the ear and floor of the mouth.
- Difficulty in closing the jaws due to swelling in the pericoronal tissue.

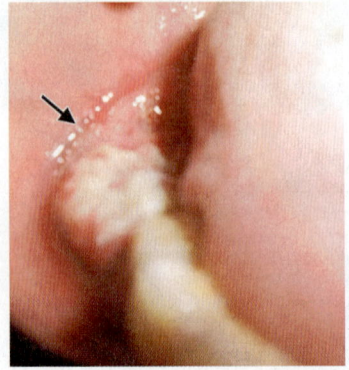

Fig. 18.17: Pericoronitis in relation to lower third molar.

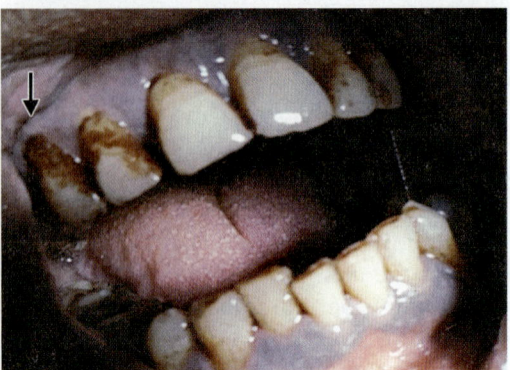

Fig. 18.18: Extrinsic stains of the teeth.

- Difficulty in opening the mouth due to trismus and dysphagia

Treatment

Treatment is done by antibiotic therapy, elimination of obstruction in the path of eruption of the involved tooth or extraction of the tooth whenever necessary.

■ STAINING OF TEETH

Extrinsic Stains of Tooth (Fig. 18.18)

Causes

- Tobacco
- Coffee, tea, and cold drinks, etc.
- Chromogenic microorganisms
- Mouth washes, e.g. chlorhexidine gluconate
- Mostly the brown, black, green or orange stains are produced by the chromogenic bacteria and these occur commonly on the labial surfaces of maxillary anteriors in children.

Common Stains in Teeth

Yellow-brown stains

Chlorhexidine produces yellow–brown discoloration, especially on the proximal surfaces of teeth near the cervical region.

Black-gray stains

These staining mostly occur due to amalgam restorations and are more intense in young individuals as they have more open dentinal tubules.

Brown or black stains
These stains are produced by sulfides or silver nitrates. Brown and black stains appear either as a thin line along the gingival margin or as wide band on the tooth surface. These stains are commonly seen on the teeth located adjacent to the salivary gland duct orifices.

Brown stains
Tobacco, tea and coffee, etc. often cause brown discoloration of teeth; smokers do have discoloration of lingual surfaces of mandibular incisors.

Green stains
Green stains are generally produced by metals, e.g. copper and nickel, etc. and these stains are usually seen on the labial surface of upper anterior teeth as a band and are probably caused by the blood pigments secondary to gingival hemorrhage. Green stains are produced due to excessive consumption of chlorophyll-containing foods.

Orange or yellow stains
Orange or yellow stains are formed on the gingival third of the teeth and are easily removed.

Intrinsic Stains of Tooth (Fig. 18.19)

The causes of intrinsic staining of teeth have been summarized in Table 18.5.

Table 18.5: Causes of intrinsic stains of the tooth.

Causes of intrinsic stain	Color change in tooth
Aging	Yellow-brown
Death of pulp (nonvital tooth)	Gray-black
Fluorosis	White-yellow or yellow-brown
Tetracycline	Yellow-brown
Minocycline	Blue-gray
Internal resorption	Pink
Dentinogenesis imperfecta	Blue-gray
Amelogenesis imperfecta	Yellow-brown
Congenital porphyria	Yellow or brown-red
Erythroblastosis fetalis	Yellow-green
Jaundice	Yellow-green
Lepromatous leprosy	Pink or red

BIBLIOGRAPHY

1. Axelsson P, Lindhe J. The significance of maintenance care in the treatment of periodontal disease. J Clin Periodontol. 1981b;8:281-4.
2. Baelum V, Fejerskov O, Karring T. Oral hygiene, gingivitis and periodontal breakdown in adult Tanzanians. J Periodontal Res. 1986;21:221-32.
3. Baelum V, Fejerskov O. Tooth loss as related to dental caries and periodontal breakdown in adult Tanzanians. Community Dent Oral Epidemiol. 1986;14:353-7.
4. Bailit HL, Braum R, Marynuil GA, et al. Is periodontal disease the primary cause of tooth loss in adults? J Am Dent Assoc. 1987;114:40-5.
5. Beck JD, Slade GD. Epidemiology of periodontal diseases. Curr Opin Periodontol. 1996;3:3-9.
6. Birkedal-hansen H. Role of cytokines and inflammatory mediators in tissue destruction. J Periodontal Res. 1993;28:500-10.
7. Birkedal-Hansen H. Role of metalloproteinases in human periodontal diseases. J Periodontol. 1993;64:474-84.
8. Brown RS, Beaver WT, Bottomley WK. On the mechanism drug-induced gingival hyperplasia. J Oral Pathol Med. 1991;20:201-9.
9. Buckley LA, Crowley MJ. A longitudinal study of untreated periodontal disease. J Clin Periodontol. 1984;1:523-50.

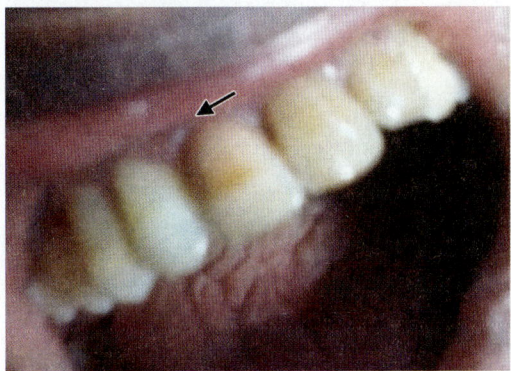

Fig. 18.19: Intrinsic stain on teeth.

10. Cawson RA, Odell EW. Essentials of Oral Pathology and Oral Medicine, 6th edition. Edinburgh: Churchill Livingstone; 1998.
11. Dickson GC. Long-term effects of malocclusion. Br J Orthodontics. 1974;1:63-8.
12. Enner J, Vogel JJ, Boyan-Salyers B, et al. Characterization of calculus matrix calcification nucleator. J Dent Res. 1979;58:619.
13. Ennever J, Vogel JJ, Riggan LJ, et al. Proteolipid and calculus matrix calcification in vitro. J Dent Res. 1977;56:140.
14. Frisken KW, Tagg JR, Laws AJ. Suspected periodontopathic microorganisms and their oral habitats in young children. Oral Microbiol Immunol. 1987;2:60-4.
15. Genco RJ, Christersoon LA, Zambon JJ. Juvenile periodontitis. Int Dent J. 1986;36:168-76.
16. Genco RJ, Slots J. Host responses in periodontal diseases. J Dent Res.1984;63:441-51.
17. Hallmon WW, Rossmon JA. The role of drugs in the pathogenesis of gingival overgrowth. A collective review of current concepts. Periodontol 2000. 1999;21:176-96.
18. Hardie JM. Oral microbiology: current concepts in the microbiology of dental caries and periodontal disease. Br Dent J. 1992;172:271-8.
19. Holdeman LV, Moore WEC, Cato EP, et al. Distribution of Capnocytophaga in periodontal microfloras. J Periodontal Res. 1985;20:475-83.
20. Ivanyi L, Lehner T. Lymphocyte transformation by sonicates of dental plaque in human periodontal disease. Arch Oral Biol. 1971;16:1117.
21. Kardachi BJ, Newcomb GM. A clinical study of gingival inflammation and renal transplant recipients taking immunosuppressive drugs. J Periodontol. 1978;49:307.
22. Loe H. The specific etiology of periodontal disease and its application to prevention. In: FA Carranza, EB Kenney (Eds). Prevention of Periodontal Disease. Chicago: Quintessence Publishing Co; 1981.
23. Mackler BF, Farner RM, Schur P, et al. IgG subclasses in human periodontal disease I Distribution and incidence of IgG subclass bearing lymphocytes and plasma cells. J Periodontal Res. 1978;13:109.
24. Manson JD. Juvenile periodontitis (periodontosis). Int Dent J. 1977;27:114.
25. McCarthy PL, Shklar G. Diseases of the Oral Mucosa, 2nd edition. Philadelphia: Lea and Febiger; 1980.
26. Neville BW, Damm DD, Allen CA, et al. Oral and Maxillofacial Pathology. Philadelphia: Saunders; 2002.
27. Newman MG. Carranza's Clinical Periodontology, 9th edition. Philadelphia: Saunders; 2002.
28. Orstavik D, Brandtzaeg P. Secretion of parotid IgA in relation to gingival inflammation and dental caries experience in man. Arch Oral Biol. 1975;20:701.
29. Robertson PB, Mackler BF, Wright TE, et al. Periodontal status of patients with abnormalities of the immune system II. Observations over a 2-year period. J Periodontol. 1980;51:70.
30. Saxen L. Juvenile periodontitis. J Clin Periodontol. 1980;7:1-19.
31. Soames JV, Southam JC. Oral Pathology, 3rd edition. London: Oxford University Press; 1999.
32. Tanner ACR, Haffergee C, Brathall GT, et al. A study of the bacteria associated with advancing periodontal disease in man. J Clin Periodontol. 1979;6:278.
33. van Palenstein Helderman WH. Microbial etiology of periodontal disease. J Clin Periodontol. 1981;8:261.

CHAPTER 19

Oral Aspects of Dermatological Disorders

■ INTRODUCTION

A large number of dermatological disorders may present with some oral lesions, either as a part of their manifestations or as the sole feature of disease. Most of these disorders have a diverse etiopathogenicity and, more importantly, few of them are potentially malignant in nature.

Diagnosis of dermal lesions usually depends on their oral and cutaneous manifestations, histopathology and immunohistochemistry, etc.

The features of some of the important dermatological diseases will be briefly discussed in this chapter.

■ HEREDITARY ECTODERMAL DYSPLASIA

Ectodermal dysplasias (EDs) are an inherited group of disorders that share in general developmental defects concerning more than one ectodermal derivatives. These tissues primarily are skin, hair, nail, eccrine glands, and teeth.

According to Freire-Maia (1971, 1977), ED is a congenital disorder characterized by alteration in two or more ectodermal structures, at least involving one in hair, teeth, skin, and sweat gland.

Hereditary ED is an inherited X-linked recessive disorder (with gene mapping on Xq12-q13.1; therefore, a male predominance is seen). The incidence rate in males is about 1 in every 100,000 births and nearly 17 females out of 100,000 are carriers of the disease. ED is characterized by defective formation of ectodermal structures of the body (e.g. skin, teeth, nails, sweat glands, sebaceous glands, and hair follicles).

Types
Types of ED are described as:
- ED1: Trichodysplasia (hair dysplasia)
- ED2: Dental dysplasia
- ED3: Onychodysplasia (nail dysplasia)
- ED4: Dyshidrosis (sweat gland dysplasia)

(The most common is the hypohydrotic or anhydrotic type of ED).

Clinical Features
- The disease occurs more frequently among males than females; patients have thin scalp hair, abnormal teeth, defective skin (peels off easily), inability to sweat, disturbed vision, and defective nails.
- The three most outstanding features of ED are:
  1. Hypohydrosis (lack of sweating)
  2. Hypotrichosis (absence of hair)
  3. Hypodontia (absence of teeth).
- The patients often have soft, dry, and smooth skin with little or no tendency for sweating (due to absence or scarcity of sweat glands). Lack of sweating causes difficulty in regulating body temperature because release of excess body heat (cooling down) through sweating is not possible and as a result patients often have

unexplained, recurrent high fever and they cannot endure warm temperature.
- Lack of hairs (hypotrichosis) is an important finding; the hair over the body skin, scalp, eyelashes and eyebrows are often fine, scanty and blond (Fig. 19.1). Patients frequently exhibit "pili torti" (kinky/twisted and brittle hair) on the scalp.
- The sebaceous glands are either sparse or absent (asteatosis).
- The skin all over the body is thin and dry, which may peel off easily; patients also exhibit fine wrinkling and hyperpigmentation over the periocular skin.
- Patients have malformed finger and toe nails, which are often abnormally thick, deformed, discolored and brittle. Sometimes nails may be completely absent or slow growing.
- Patients with ED always have a typical facial appearance characterized by depressed nasal bridge, frontal bossing and protuberant lips, etc. Since most of the patients have almost similar facial appearances, a large number of them can be mistaken as siblings.
- Dental defects are extremely important, which include complete or partial anodontia and enamel hypoplasia (involving both deciduous as well as the permanent dentitions). Canines are the only teeth which may be present in few patients, even then they look small and conical; on rare occasions, few other deformed teeth may erupt, e.g. small, tapered and conical incisors and little molars with smaller diameter (Figs. 19.2 and 19.3). Many patients need dentures from about the age of 2 years.
- Cleft lip and palate are common and popliteal pterygium (defect in face, skin, and genitalia) in few patients.
- Hypoplasia of salivary glands often causes xerostomia and it is often a constant feature of the disease. Moreover, absence of lacrimal glands may cause decreased secretion of tears and poor vision.

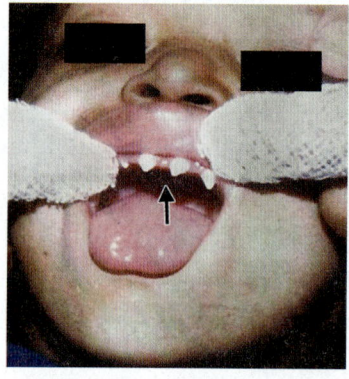

Fig. 19.2: Hereditary ectodermal dysplasia—patient showing formation of only few conical shaped teeth.

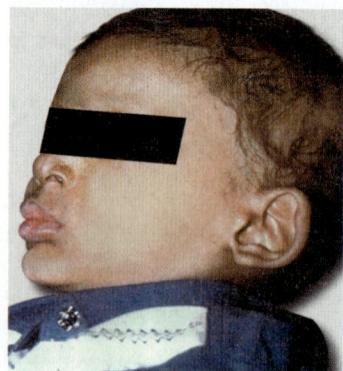

Fig. 19.1: Hereditary ectodermal dysplasia (typical facial profile).

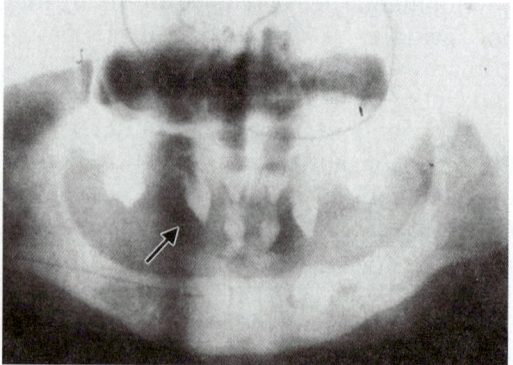

Fig. 19.3: X-ray showing partial anodontia in hereditary ectodermal dysplasia.

- The absence of mucosal glands in the upper respiratory tract, bronchi and esophagus often cause rhinitis, sinusitis, pharyngitis, etc. which may result in dysphagia and hoarseness of voice.
- Lack of development of breast and poor hearing are the rare features of ED.

Treatment

The typical clinical manifestations always confirm the diagnosis of this disease and there is no specific treatment for it. Artificial dentures (with soft liners) are constructed and are changed from time to time to cope up with the growth of the jaws and artificial saliva is given to keep the mouth moist.

> **Key Points of Hereditary Ectodermal Dysplasia**
> - Ectodermal dysplasia is a hereditary disorder characterized by defective formation of ectodermal structures of the body, e.g. skin, teeth, nails, sweat glands, sebaceous glands, and hair follicles.
> - Hypohydrosis, hypotrichosis, and hypodontia are the three most outstanding features of ED.
> - Hypohydrosis or lack of sweating causes difficulty in releasing the body heat through sweats and the patients thus always have high body temperature.
> - There is complete or partial lack of development of tooth and patients require artificial prosthesis from young age.
> - Xerostomia (dry mouth) is a constant feature due to decreased salivary secretion.
> - Patient have a typical facial appearance with depressed nasal bridge, frontal bossing, protuberant lips, etc.

PSORIASIS

Psoriasis is a common self-limiting, chronic inflammatory dermatological disease of unknown etiology. Some investigators believe that its occurrence is genetically determined. Psoriasis exhibits an increased proliferative activity of skin and mucous membrane.

Etiology

- The exact cause of psoriasis is unknown but patients do have genetic factor that seems to play a role, because as many as one-third of these patients have affected relatives.
- Abnormal immune reactions often trigger the disease because in psoriasis activated T lymphocytes abnormally produce cytokines, adhesion molecules, chemotactic polypeptides, and growth factors.
- Stress can also cause exacerbation of psoriasis.
- Psoriasis may also occur due to an increase in the turnover rate of dermal cells (from the normal turnover duration of 23 days to 3–5 days in affected areas).

Clinical Features

The disease occurs predominantly in the second and third decade of life. There is no sex predilection. Mental anxiety or stress often increases the severity of the disease.

Dermal Lesions of Psoriasis

- Skin lesions of psoriasis clinically appear as well-demarcated, painless, dry, erythematous patches with silvery scale on the surface.
- These lesions often develop on the skin over the elbows, knees, scalp, chest, face, etc.
- The lesions enlarge at the periphery and there may be periods of remissions and exacerbations.
- These skin lesions are often symmetrically distributed; these are more severe during the winter and the condition is much better during the summer.
- *Auspitz's sign*: In psoriasis, dry erythematous patches develop on the skin surface with silvery scales; upon removal of the scales, one or two tiny bleeding points often appear; this phenomenon is known as "Auspitz's sign" (*Auspitz sign occurs because the capillaries run very close to the surface skin in the affected areas and removal of the scale essentially pulls the tops of capillaries. This sign is also seen in Darier's disease and actinic keratosis*).

- *Nail lesions*: Nails exhibit yellow-brown discoloration with pitting, dimpling, crumbling and separation of nail plate from the nail bed.
- *Oral lesions*: In psoriasis, oral lesions may appear as erythematous patches with white scaly surfaces over the lips, palate, gingiva and cheek, etc. Some oral lesions may resemble the "geographic tongue".

Microscopic Findings

- The oral epithelium shows atrophy with hyperparakeratosis, absence of granular cell layer and elongation or clubbing of the rete pegs.
- Intraepithelial microabscess formation (abscess of Munro) is an important histological finding of psoriasis.
- There is always an increased mitotic activity seen in the psoriatic skin or mucous membrane.
- The subepithelial connective tissue shows many dilated capillaries and perivascular infiltrations of lymphocytes or histiocytes.

Treatment

No treatment is required as the disease undergoes spontaneous regression.

PITYRIASIS ROSEA

Pityriasis rosea is a rare mucocutaneous disease, which probably develops as a result of some viral infections.

Clinical Features

- The disease commonly occurs in children or young adults and it affects several people at a time.
- This disease often shows seasonal outbreaks and it is mostly noticed during spring or autumn.
- Pityriasis rosea clinically presents superficial, light red, macules or papules over the skin, which are preceded by a typical bright-red skin rash in the same area. Oral lesions present erythematous macules over the cheek, tongue and palate, etc.

HISTOPATHOLOGY

- The oral epithelium in pityriasis rosea exhibits hyperorthokeratosis or parakeratosis along with mild degree of acanthosis.
- Ulceration, hemorrhage and chronic inflammatory cell infiltration are found in the basal epithelium as well as in the juxta-epithelial connective tissue.

Treatment

Since, it is a self-limiting condition, no treatment is usually necessary.

INCONTINENTIA PIGMENTI

It is a relatively rare, serious type of inherited genodermatosis, which is transmitted as a sex-linked dominant trait.

Clinical Features

- The disease occurs mostly during infancy. Although it is more common among females, it is often lethal among males.
- Clinically the disease produces a typical slate-gray pigmentation of the skin after birth with formation of vesicles or bullae over the trunk and limbs. Teeth are often small and conical, while the oral mucosa exhibits patchy, plaque-like white lesions on the buccal mucosa.
- Patients may also have epilepsy, strabismus (misaligned eyes) with nystagmus (dancing eyes) and partial anodontia, etc.

Histopathology

- During the verrucous stage of the disease, intraepithelial vesicle formation is often seen with accumulation of large number of eosinophils.
- Dermal or submucosal accumulations of macrophages and melanin granules are also seen.

- White areas display hyperorthokeratosis or parakeratosis with acanthosis.
- Individual cell keratinization is also sometimes seen.

Treatment
No specific treatment is available.

ERYTHEMA MULTIFORME

Erythema multiforme is an acute self-limiting dermatitis characterized by a distinctive clinical eruption manifested by "iris" or "target" lesions over the skin surfaces *(multiforme means many forms)*. The disease occurs due to hypersensitivity reaction to certain infections and drugs; and in many cases, oral cavity is the only site of involvement.

Types of Erythema Multiforme
- *Erythema multiforme minor*: Characterized by localized eruption of the skin with mild or no mucosal involvement.
- *Erythema multiforme major*: Skin or mucosal erosions of severe and widespread skin and mucosal involvement with development of raised atypical "target" lesions (Fig. 19.4). Usually located on the extremities and/or over the face.
- *Stevens-Johnson syndrome*: Severe and widespread skin and mucosal involvement with development of flat atypical "target" lesions or purpuric macules. May be present on the trunk, face, and extremities.

Etiology
Although the exact etiology of erythema multiforme is obscure, some precipitating factors have been identified, which are shown in Table 19.1.

Pathogenesis
Erythema multiforme is characterized by keratinocyte injury mediated by skin-homing CD8+ cytotoxic T lymphocytes.

Clinical Features
- Erythema multiforme frequently occurs in young adults (15–40 years) and is

Table 19.1: Common causes of erythema multiforme.

Infections	- Herpes simplex (Type I and type II) infections - Tuberculosis - Infectious mononucleosis - Histoplasmosis
Drug hypersensitivity	- Barbiturates - Sulfonamides - Phenylbutazone - Salicylates - Oral pills
Hyperimmune reactions	Results formation of antigen-antibody complex against the sub-mucosal and dermal blood vessels.
Miscellaneous factors	- Radiation therapy - Crohn's disease - Vaccinations

Note: Following are the recent concepts in the etiology of the different forma of erythema multiforme:
- Erythema multiforme minor: Almost exclusively triggered by the herpes simplex virus infection.
- Erythema multiforme major: Mostly triggered by herpetic and Mycoplasma infections.
- Steven–Johnson syndrome: Drugs are the major cause.

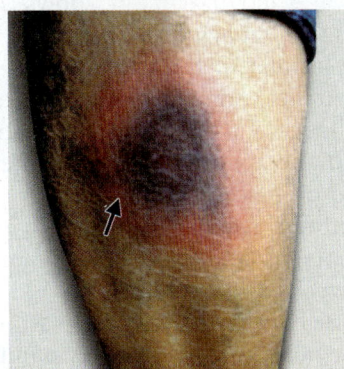

Fig. 19.4: Atypical "target lesion" in erythema multiforme.

more common in males; it is uncommon among children and older individuals; however, if it occurs in the older people, the possibility of an internal carcinoma should not be ruled out.
- The prodromal symptoms include mild fever, malaise, headache, cough, sore throat, etc. and they occur about 1week before the onset of the disease.
- Soon after rapidly developing round, erythematous macules, papules or vesicles appear over the skin in a bilaterally symmetrical pattern over the hands and arms, legs and feet, face and neck, etc.
- In severe cases, large bullae may also develop over the skin.
- The classic dermal manifestation of erythema multiforme is seen with the development of "target", "iris" or "bull's eye" lesions.
- The target lesions often appear on the skin of the extremities and they begin as dark red macules, usually 1–3 cm in diameter. They become slightly elevated and develop a characteristic bluish cyanotic center.
- There may be several concentric erythematous rings around the lesion separated by rings of near normal color on the skin, resulting from varying shades of erythema.
- Severe form of erythema multiforme may cause widespread sloughing and ulceration of the skin, and the mucous membrane of the entire body (Figs. 19.5 and 19.6). Severe form may also cause widespread necrosis.

(Milder cases, known as *erythema multiforme minor*, usually begin with the development of slightly elevated, round, dusky red patches on the skin of the extremities, mucosal involvement often absent).

Oral Manifestations

- Mucosal lesions occur most often in the lips, besides that tongue, buccal mucosa,

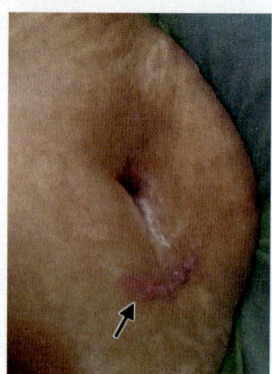

Fig. 19.5: Erythema multiforme showing erythematous skin lesions.

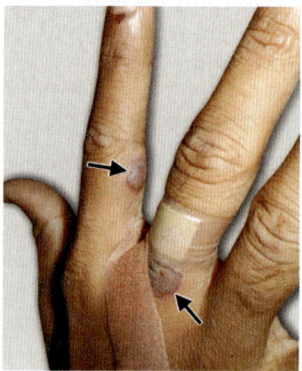

Fig. 19.6: "Target lesions" on the skin in erythema multiforme.

floor of the mouth and soft palate, etc. are also affected. Lip often shows swelling with hemorrhagic crusting.
- Oral lesions of the disease also consist of macules, papules or vesicles, etc.; the vesicles are often short-lived and they readily become eroded or ulcerated and bleed profusely. The new vesicles appear again and again in about every 10 days and the process may continue for nearly 3–4 weeks.
- The ulcers which form after the rupture of the vesicles are extremely painful with irregular borders and they are normally covered by a slough.

- The entire disease process may recur in a cyclic order at an interval of few months and the cycle may characteristically continue for 1–2 years, with increasing in severity after every recurrence.
- Patients often complain of foul smell in the mouth and difficulty in eating or swallowing, these often lead to severe weakness and dehydration.
- The cutaneous and mucosal lesions may occur either separately or simultaneously; in many cases, oral lesions are the only manifestation of the disease. Sometimes each attack on the skin is followed by several attacks on the oral mucosa.
- Gingival lesions are rare in this disease and this may help to distinguish between erythema multiforme and herpetic gingivostomatitis (the later disease shows severe gingival involvement).
- Patients with erythema multiforme may also develop secondary infection with tracheobronchial ulcerations and pneumonia, etc.
- Erythema multiforme is a self-limiting disease and it regresses spontaneously.

Precipitating Factors in Erythema Multiforme

- Stevens–Johnson syndrome
- Toxic epidermal necrolysis.

Stevens–Johnson syndrome is a severe, febrile form of erythema multiforme (also known as *erythema multiforme major*) with extensive involvement of skin; besides skin, there is also simultaneous involvement of conjunctiva, labial and oral mucosa, perianal area, and genitalia. This condition is often triggered by drugs; moreover, secondary infection in the affected areas may cause life-threatening sepsis.

Features of Stevens–Johnson syndrome:
- Skin lesions: Severe lesions are macules, papules, vesicles and bullae, etc.
- Mucosal lesions: Large vesicles or bullae with subsequent painful ulcerations and hemorrhage.
- Eye lesions: Photophobia, conjunctivitis, corneal ulceration and uveitis, etc.
- Genital lesions: Urethritis, balanitis and vaginal ulceration, etc.

Toxic epidermal necrolysis is another severe and potentially lethal variant of erythema multiforme, which causes extensive blistering, necrosis and sloughing of skin and mucosal surfaces. This often leads to fluid and electrolyte loss and secondary infections.

(The difference between Stevens–Johnson syndrome and toxic epidermal necrolysis is in the degree of skin involvement, with Stevens–Johnson syndrome having less than 10% of the body surface affected by the lesions whereas the toxic epidermal necrolysis shows more than 30% involvement of the body surface).

Histopathology

- The microscopic findings of erythema multiforme are often nonspecific.
- Histologically erythema multiforme presents severe nonspecific inflammation in the epithelium; with acanthosis, intra- or intercellular edema, widespread necrosis of the basal keratinocytes, vesicles or bullae formation within the epithelium and chronic inflammatory cell infiltration in the underlying connective tissue.
- An important finding in erythema multiforme is the intense inflammation and inflammatory cell infiltration along the dermal-epidermal junction together with necrosis and degeneration of basal keratinocytes; this phenomenon is often referred to as an *"interface dermatitis"*.
- With time, the lymphocytes from the connective tissue migrate upward into the epithelium (Fig. 19.7).

Differential Diagnosis

- Acute primary herpetic stomatitis
- Herpes zoster

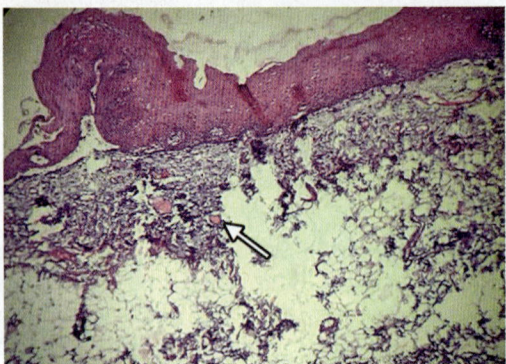

Fig. 19.7: Photomicrograph of erythema multiforme showing nonspecific ulceration.

- Aphthous ulcer
- Pemphigus
- Pemphigoid
- Erosive and bullous lichen planus.

Key Points of Erythema Multiforme

- Erythema multiforme is serious type of dermatological disorder characterized by extensive blistering and ulcerations of the skin and mucous membrane.
- Initially, the disease produces rapidly developing round, erythematous macules, papules or vesicles over the skin.
- These classic dermal lesions of erythema multiforme often characteristically appear as "target", "iris" or "bull's eye", etc.
- Vesicles also appear over the oral mucosa, which rupture and produce diffuse, extremely painful irregular ulcers with bleeding tendency.
- Stevens–Johnson syndrome is the most severe form of erythema multiforme, which simultaneously affect skin, mucosa, eyes, and genitalia.
- The disease can cause trachea-bronchial ulceration and pneumonia.
- Sometimes, erythema multiforme indicates the possibility of internal carcinoma.

Treatment

Topical and systemic steroid therapy, coupled with antibiotics, antihistaminics and analgesics, etc.

DERMATITIS HERPETIFORMIS

Dermatitis herpetiformis is a rare, intensely pruritic mucocutaneous disorder characterized by urticaria and grouped vesicles. Dietary gluten (sticky part of wheat flower) is believed to be responsible for the development of this disease.

Clinical Features

- The disease commonly occurs among teenagers and young adults, mostly in males.
- Initially there is pruritus with severe burning sensation of the skin, which involves extremities, buttock, face, periorbital regions and scalp, etc.
- Gradually, there is development of symmetrically distributed erythematous, papules or vesicles on the skin or mucous membrane, which often resemble *Herpes simplex* (hence the name dermatitis herpetiformis has been given).

Histopathology

- Disruption of the superficial epithelium with subsequent ulcerations are the common features.
- It characteristically exhibits aggregation of neutrophils and eosinophils at the apex of the connective tissue papilla with formation of microabscesses.
- As the microabscesses fuse together, subepithelial vesicles form, these vesicles may rupture to cause superficial ulcers and destruction of basement membrane.

Treatment

Gluten-free diet and administration of sulfapyridine.

KERATOSIS FOLLICULARIS (DARIER DISEASE)

Keratosis follicularis is a hereditary disorder of the skin and is characterized by the formation of multiple crusted, greasy lesions that often produce foul odor.

Clinical Features

- The lesions commonly develop over the face and neck of the young individuals.

- There is development of erythematous hyperkeratotic papules on the skin, which gradually turns grayish brown with age. Accumulation of keratin often gives a rough texture to these lesions; moreover bacterial desquamation of these keratins often produces foul smell from the lesion.
- In the oral cavity, multiple, small, normal colored or white flat-topped papules may appear on the gingiva, tongue, hard palate, cheek, etc.
- Numerous papules tend to be confluent, result in a cobblestone mucosal appearance.

Histopathology

Histologically the disease shows multiple clefts and lacunae within the epithelium; with narrow, elongated, "test-tube" like rete-ridges. Each epithelial cleft or lacunae contains two types of cells, namely the "corps grains" (grain-like keratinized epithelial cells) and "corps ronds" (eosinophilic cells).

Treatment

By high doses of vitamin A therapy or steroids.

ACANTHOSIS NIGRICANS

Acanthosis nigricans is a rare cutaneous disease, which usually affects the flexural surfaces of skin and it has an occasional oral mucosal component.

Types

The disease usually has three types:
1. *Benign type*: Present at birth or during puberty. It is inherited as autosomal dominant trait and is never associated with internal malignancy. The benign type of acanthosis nigricans often occurs in association with various disease conditions, e.g. diabetes mellitus, hypothyroidism, acromegaly, Crouzon syndrome, chronic steroid therapy, etc.
2. *Malignant type*: Usually develops after the age of 40 years and is invariably associated with internal malignancies like adenocarcinoma or lymphoma of the gastrointestinal tract.
3. *Pseudoacanthosis type*: It is the most common form of acanthosis nigricans and in this type, lesions develop around body creases as a result of obesity.

Clinical Features

- *Skin lesions*: They clinically present numerous, fine, velvety, confluent plaques with brownish pigmentation. These lesions predominantly occur on the flexural surfaces of skin over axilla, palms, soles, face, etc.
- *Oral lesions*: Oral lesions can be seen in the tongue, gingiva, lips and cheek, etc. and these oral lesions often occur in association with the malignant form of the disease.
- Tongue lesions are characterized by either hypertrophy of the filiform papilla or formation of a papillomatous growth.
- Lip is grossly enlarged (mainly the upper lip) and its surface is dotted with small papillomatous nodules especially at the commissure.
- Gingiva also exhibits hyperplastic changes and the lesions are clinically similar to that of the fibromatosis gingivae.

Histopathology

- Thickening of the epithelium with marked acanthosis.
- Hyper-orthokeratinization of the surface epithelium.
- Malignant form of the disease shows marked epithelial hyperplasia and acanthosis.

Treatment

There is no definitive treatment for this condition.

DYSKERATOSIS CONGENITA

It is a rare hereditary disorder of skin, which is inherited as a recessive trait.

Clinical Features

- Grayish-brown pigmentations of skin over the trunk, neck, and thighs.
- Facial skin appears red due to atrophic or telangiectatic changes.
- Formations of vesicles and bullae in the oral mucosa especially with occasional presence of leukoplakic or erythroplakic patches.
- Presence of systemic conditions like—mental retardation, dysphagia, deafness, thrombocytopenic purpura, aplastic anemia and hyperhydrosis of the palms and soles, etc.

Oral Manifestations

- Redness and atrophy of the facial skin with telangiectatic changes.
- Formations of vesicles and bullae in the oral mucosa with erosive changes in mucosa.
- Development of leukoplakic or erythroplakic patches in oral mucosa.
- Dysphagia
- Severe periodontal tissue destruction and loss of alveolar bone is often seen.
- Increased risk of development of squamous cell carcinoma from the leukoplakia lesions in the oral mucosa.

Histopathology

- Oral mucosa exhibits hyperortho or hyperparakeratosis and acanthosis.
- In many cases, there is presence of epithelial dysplasia.
- Skin lesions show increased vasculitis and increased number of melanin containing chromatophores.

Diagnosis

Presence of anemia, leukopenia, thrombocytopenia, Fanconi's syndrome, etc.

Treatment

No treatment is needed. Periodic evaluations of the oral lesions are required to look for any suspected malignant transformation.

■ WHITE SPONGE NEVUS

White sponge nevus is a hereditary disease of defective keratin formation and is characterized by formation of white, thickened, corrugated mucosal lesions in the oral cavity that often affects several members of the same family.

Etiology

In the 30-member family of keratin filaments, the pair of keratins known as keratin 4 and keratin 13 is specifically expressed in the spinous cell layer of mucosal epithelium. Novel mutation in the "keratin 4 gene" is believed to be the underlying cause of white sponge nevus.

Clinical Features

- The disease generally occurs at birth or during childhood and there is no sex predilection.
- Clinically, oral lesions exhibit symmetrically thickened, white, folded or corrugated diffuse plaques; which occur bilaterally over the cheek. The oral lesions are asymptomatic, soft and spongy with a peculiar opalescent hue.
- The lesion may also develop in other intraoral sites like palate, labial mucosa, tongue, gingiva, floor of the mouth, etc.
- Besides oral lesions, the disease may involve nasal, rectal or genital mucosae (Cannon's syndrome).

Differential Diagnosis

- Hereditary benign intraepithelial dyskeratosis
- Lichen planus
- Hyperplastic candidiasis
- Leukoplakia
- Verrucous carcinoma.

Histopathology

- Hyperparakeratosis of the epithelium with acanthosis and intercellular edema.

- Presence of some large "vacuolated" cells in the spinous cell layer with pyknotic nuclei.
- Presence of abnormally prominent epithelial cell membranes with a typical "basket-weave" appearance.
- There is no epithelial atypia or dysplasia seen in the epithelium.

Treatment

No treatment is required for this self-regressing disease.

POLYMYOSITIS

Polymyositis is an inflammatory myopathy of unknown etiology, which commonly affects the skin.

Clinical Features

- The acute form of the disease affects the people between the ages of 50 years and 60 years while the chronic form of the disease occurs in children between the ages of 5 years and 15 years.
- In both forms, there is a definite female predilection observed.
- The disease clinically presents muscle pain, fever, malaise, arthralgic pain and weight loss, etc.
- A violaceous skin rash commonly develops over the cheek, eyelids and hands, etc.
- Oral mucosa reveals erythematous patches having lichen planus like appearance with swelling and a high risk for malignancy.

Diagnosis

- Hypergammaglobulinemia
- Positive rheumatoid factor
- Positive antinuclear factor.

Treatment

There is no specific treatment for this condition.

AUTOIMMUNITY

Definition of autoimmunity: Autoimmunity is a condition in which structural and functional damage is produced by the action of immunologically competent cell or antibodies against the normal components of the body.

The immune system is supposed to protect the body from diseases, but autoimmunity does the opposite; therefore an autoimmune disease precisely means a pathological condition causing "injury to self" by the action of body's own cell-mediated or humoral immune systems. The specific area or the tissue in the body which is targeted in this disease is called the "site of election".

Criteria for Autoimmune Diseases

- Elevated levels of immunoglobulins
- Demonstrable autoantibodies
- Deposition of immunoglobulins or accumulation of lymphocytes/plasma cells in the site of election.
- Occurrence of more than one type of autoimmune lesion in an individual
- More susceptibility to females
- A genetic predisposition towards autoimmunity
- Chronic and often nonreversible nature of the disease
- Positive response from corticosteroid/other immunosuppressive therapies.

Mechanisms of Autoimmunity

1. *Antigenic alterations (neoantigens)*: Cells or tissues may undergo antigenic alteration due to physical, chemical or biological influences (e.g. radiation, drugs and infections, etc.). The altered antigens are called "neoantigens" which elicit immune response.
2. *Sequestrated (hidden) antigens*: Certain self-antigens may be present in the body in a hidden state and they remain unknown to the body's immune system since they are never exposed to the immune network; such antigens are called "sequestrated antigens". If sequestrated antigens get exposed due to injury and mix with the blood, then autoimmune reaction begins.

3. *Forbidden clones*: During the embryonic life, innumerable numbers of immunologically competent cells are produced in the body, which are capable of producing specific antibody patterns against all possible antigens. Any clone of cells formed during this process, carrying an abnormal pattern that may be reactive against self-antigens, is called a "forbidden clone" and it must be destroyed before birth; however, if a forbidden clone survives in intrauterine life or it evolves due to mutation in the later part of life then, it may be a potential threat for autoimmune disease.
4. *Cross-reacting foreign antigens*: Similar antigenic patterns may be shared by different organisms, for example, the antigen "M-protein" of *Streptococcus* and the human heart muscles share the similar antigenic characteristics. Because of this, repeated streptococcal infections may induce autoimmune reaction against heart muscles. That is why, caries vaccine produced from *Streptococcus mutans* surface antigen could not be successfully implemented.
5. *Polyclonal B cell activation*: An antigen usually activates only its corresponding B-cell but sometimes an antigen may stimulate multiple B cell clones, which results in formation of several additional immunoglobulins. These excess immunoglobulins often initiate autoimmune reaction in the body.
6. *Total disruption of immune system*: When body's control over the immune system is lost, the B cells might unnecessarily produce huge number of immunoglobulins; which can cause autoimmune reaction in the body.
7. *Altered T or B cell function*: When there is enhanced activity of T-helper cells and decreased function of T-suppressor cells, then the risk of autoimmune reaction becomes more.
8. *Malignancy*: When a cell undergoes malignant transformation, it acquires new surface antigens and often loses some normal antigens; this makes a malignant cell antigenically different from the normal cell of the host. Thus, in case of any cancer, the malignant tumor cells may induce autoimmune reaction in the body.

Common Autoimmune Diseases

- Hashimoto's disease (lymphadenoid goiter)—replacement of thyroid gland tissue by lymphoid tissue.
- Grave's disease (thyrotoxicosis)—formation of autoantibodies to thyroglobulin or thyroid membrane antigen.
- Addison's disease—autoimmune destruction of adrenal gland.
- Myasthenia gravis—formation of autoantibodies against acetylcholine receptor on the myoneural junctions of striated muscles. Failure of acetylcholine to combine with its receptor cause impairment of muscle contraction and excessive fatigability.
- Guillain-Barrè syndrome—formation of autoantibodies against the peripheral nerves.
- Pernicious anemia—two types of autoantibodies are formed in this disease: (1) one directed against the parietal cells of the gastric mucosa, and (2) other one directed against the "intrinsic factor" (thus preventing the absorption of vitamin B12 by the gastric mucosa, leading to anemia).
- Pemphigus—formation of autoantibodies to desmoglein (the intercellular adhesion protein) of the skin and oral epithelium.
- Pemphigoid—autoimmune destruction of the basement membrane zone of skin and oral epithelium.
- Systemic lupus erythematosus—multisystem disease with formation of various autoantibodies; e.g. against the cell nuclei (ANA), anti-DNA antibody, against

intracytoplasmic constituents, against thyroid glands and salivary glands, etc.
- Rheumatoid arthritis—formation of autoantibodies against the synovial membrane of the joints, which are called rheumatoid factor (RF).
- Sjogren's syndrome—autoimmune destruction of salivary and lacrimal glands (primary Sjogren's syndrome) and along with that rheumatoid arthritis (secondary Sjogren's syndrome).

■ PEMPHIGUS

Pemphigus is a group of uncommon, but potentially lethal vesiculobullous lesions of the skin and mucosa, which is characterized by the formation of vesicle (small fluid-filled blister 5 mm or less across) and bulla (large fluid-filled blister more than 5 mm across) that develop in cycles. In pemphigus, the vesicle or bulla form within the epithelium, which results in separation between cell layers above the level of basal cells. The term "pemphigus" is derived from the Greek word "*pemphix*" meaning bubble or blister. Few lesions may involve the eyes as well.

Types of Pemphigus
- Pemphigus vulgaris
- Pemphigus vegetans
- Pemphigus foliaceus (Brazilian pemphigus)
- Pemphigus erythematosus
- Paraneoplastic pemphigus.

Etiopathogenesis
An "autoimmune mechanism" plays the major role in the development of pemphigus. Actually, the patient develops immunoglobulin G (IgG) and complements in his or her body, which are specifically targeted against the intercellular cement substances (desmosomes) of the skin and mucous membrane.

Deposition of such autoantibodies in the skin or mucous membrane initiates an immune reaction, that eventually causes destruction and dissolution of the desmosomal attachments between the cells leading to the loss of adhesion between one cell to the other (acantholysis). Further accumulation of fluid in the region eventually leads to the development of intraepithelial vesicle or bullae that causes split within the epithelium above the basal layer (suprabasilar split).

According to another theory, which is known as the "protease theory", deposition of autoantibodies within the epithelium induces a proteolytic activity by activating the tissue plasminogens. This in turn generates proteolytic enzyme called "plasmin" that destroys the desmosomes.

Note:
- *Autoantibodies*: When specific antibodies are produced against some of the body's own tissues or cells or cellular components.
- In case of pemphigus, the antibodies are produced against the antigenic components of the desmosomes or the intercellular cement substances (desmoglein-3 and desmoglein-1).
- These autoantibodies attach to the desmosomal components and inhibit the molecular reaction that is responsible for cell to cell binding in the epithelium.

(Associations have been found between pemphigus vulgaris, myasthenia gravis and thymoma; and several drugs including penicillamine, rifampicin and captopril. Moreover, few cases of pemphigus are associated with internal malignancies, particularly of the hematolymphoid system, and the condition is often termed as *paraneoplastic pemphigus*) (Box 19.1).

Clinical Features of Pemphigus
Pemphigus Vulgaris (Figs. 19.8 and 19.9)
(In Latin, "vulgaris" means common).
- It is the most common type of pemphigus (above 80% of cases), which occurs

Essentials of Oral Pathology

Box 19.1 The site of vesicle/bulla formation in different vesiculobullous lesions.

Bulla at granular cell layer of the epithelium:
- Pemphigus foliaceous
- Pemphigus erythematous

Bulla at spinous cell layer (upper and mid-epidermis):
- Eczematous blisters
- Frictional blisters
- Viral blisters

Bulla at spinous layer (suprabasal area):
Pemphigus vulgaris

Bulla at basal cell area:
- Epidermolysis bullosa simplex
- Lichen planus
- Toxic epidermolysis necrosis

Bulla at lamina lucida of the stroma:
- Bullous pemphigoid
- Cicatricial pemphigoid
- Epidermolysis bullosa acquisita
- Dermatitis herpetiformis

Bulla at sub-laminar connective tissue:
- Epidermolysis bullosa dystrophica
- Erythema multiforme (dermal type)

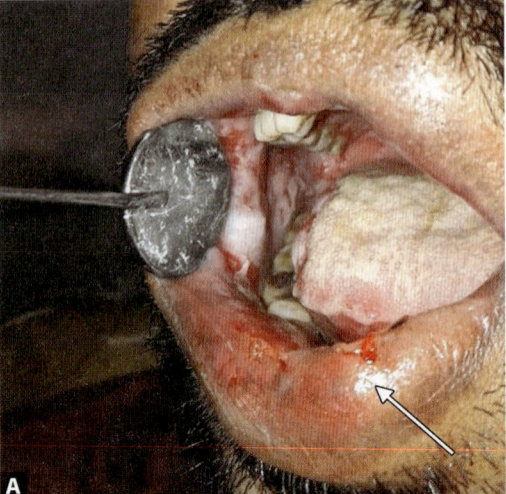
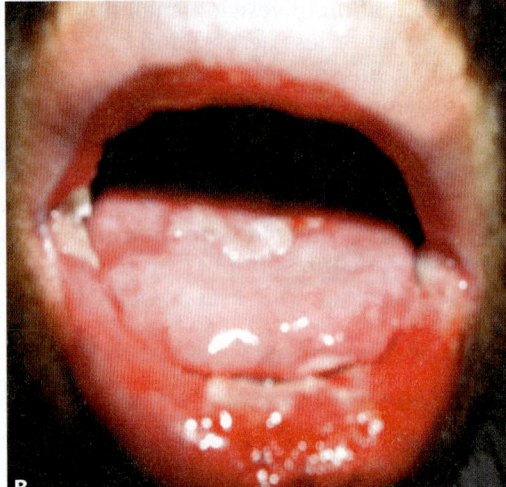

Figs. 19.9A and B: Pemphigus vulgaris–oral lesions.

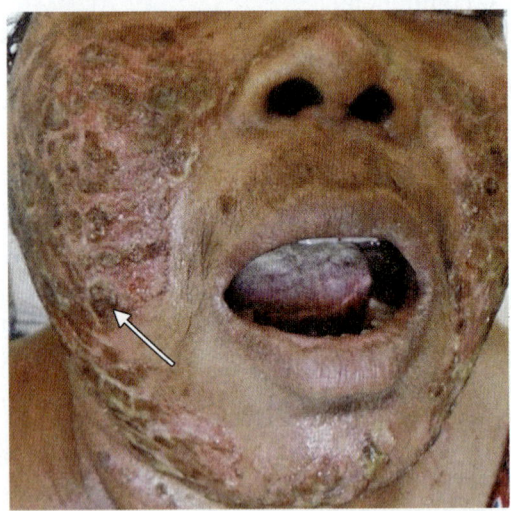

Fig. 19.8: Pemphigus vulgaris—skin lesions.

between the ages of 40 years and 70 years and it is more prevalent among females.
- Pemphigus involves mucosa and skin over the scalp, face, axilla, groin, trunk and points of pressure.
- The primary lesions are superficial vesicles or bullae that rupture easily and leave shallow erosions or ulcerations covered with serum and crust. Skin lesions of pemphigus usually heal by scar formation.
- Oral cavity is the most common site of initial involvement in pemphigus vulgaris and it may be the only site affected in about 25% cases. In over 60% cases of pemphigus vulgaris, oral lesions precede the skin lesions.
- Oral lesions in pemphigus vulgaris may involve any part of the oral cavity but

are more frequently found in those areas which are often subjected to trauma, e.g. buccal mucosa, gingiva and soft palate. Tongue lesions often appear as deep nonhealing fissures.

- The oral lesions often begin as *"bleb-like" blisters* filled with clear fluid or oral lesions may also occur in the form of diffuse gelatinous plaques. The oral lesions are often the first sign of the disease, and they are the most difficult to resolve with therapy. This has prompted the description of the oral lesions as *"the first to show, and the last to go".*
- The clear fluid of the vesicle later on changes into pus; oral vesicles rupture soon and give rise to extremely painful, superficial ulcers with ragged borders. The ulcerated area also exhibits boggy and shredded mucosa, which often bleeds profusely.
- Gentle traction or oblique pressure on the unaffected areas around the lesion causes denudation or stripping of the normal skin or mucous membrane, this phenomenon is known as *"Nikolsky sign".*
- Fluid from intact or recently ruptured vesicles may contain acantholytic cells (Tzanck cells).
- Pemphigus vulgaris sometimes shows a mild course, but in other cases, the disease may be fulminating in nature with widespread involvement of the oral mucosa, skin and eyes. Ocular lesions may develop in the form of bilateral conjunctivitis.
- Patients with oral pemphigus vulgaris often have sore mouth with severe pain, excessive salivation, bleeding, difficulty in taking food and an extremely foul smell in the mouth.
- When the cutaneous lesions are extensive, the disease may involve the entire body and in such cases, the patient's condition becomes as serious as a severely burnt case, especially in terms of fluid loss and risk for secondary infections. Such patient may die of dehydration and septicemia, etc.

Pemphigus Vegetans

This is an uncommon form of pemphigus, in which ordinary pemphigus vulgaris turns into a vegetative lesion especially in skin folds, where moist, papillomatous, proliferative verrucous type (wart-like) growths develop. These lesions are often studded with pustules and they do not form vesicles as seen in conventional pemphigus.

Oral lesions are present in about 50% of cases and mostly affect the tongue, lips and angle of the mouth.

This disease also produces serpiginous ulcers on the dorsum of tongue that often gives a typical appearance called "cerebriform tongue" (often resembles benign migratory glossitis). Rarely wart-like growth on the oral mucosa can be seen at the angle of the mouth. Pemphigus vegetans are highly persisting lesions and are often resistant to treatment.

Pemphigus Foliaceus (Brazilian pemphigus)

Pemphigus foliaceus is a rare, mild form of pemphigus, which occurs as endemic lesion in Brazil (hence called Brazilian pemphigus or "fogo selvagem"). It commonly affects older adults, in the scalp, face, chest and back regions; mucosal involvement is rare. In this form of pemphigus, the bulla forms in the very superficial layer of the skin (subcorneal blisters) and it is often associated with marked erythema of the involved skin. The bulla ruptures and the area dries up to leave masses of flakes or scales resembling an exfoliative dermatitis.

Pemphigus Erythematosus

It is considered to be a localized form of pemphigus foliaceus that selectively involve the facial skin of the malar region. The disease begins with vesicles or bullae concomitant with crusted patches.

Paraneoplastic Pemphigus

Paraneoplastic pemphigus is named so because this type of pemphigus occurs in association with many neoplastic conditions and it was recognized as a distinct entity in the year 1990. This disease is predominantly seen in association with Non-Hodgkin's lymphoma (NHL), chronic lymphocytic leukemia (CLL), and thymoma. Less frequently, it can occur along with bronchogenic and breast carcinomas.

It is believed that the tumor cells produce some proteins (plakin protein), which induce an autoimmune reaction in the body and resulting in the formation of autoantibodies. These autoantibodies target desmoglein-3 and desmoglein-1 and cause acantholysis.

Paraneoplastic pemphigus occurs more in males, often between the ages of 45 years and 70 years. Palmar and plantar bullae appear, which does not occur in other types of pemphigus; besides this, oral cavity is almost always involved, most commonly in the buccal mucosa, lips, oropharynx and nasopharynx, etc.

The disease produces vesicles and bullae in the mouth, which rupture and create painful, irregular, ragged ulcerations.

Histopathology of Pemphigus (Figs. 19.10 to 19.12)

Pemphigus is, histopathologically, characterized by the following features:
- Formation of intraepithelial vesicle or bullae that often results in a suprabasilar split or separation.
- Following this suprabasilar split in the epithelium, only a single layer of basal cells remain attached to the basement membrane at the bottom of the bulla; moreover, these cells are separated from each other laterally to form the characteristic "*row of tombstone*" appearance.
- Loss of intercellular bridges and collection of edema fluid result in acantholysis within the spinous cell layer, which causes disruption of the spinous cell layer.
- As a result of acantholysis, clumps of large hyperchromatic epithelial cells desquamate that are often seen lying free within the vesicular fluid, these desquamated cells are often rounded and smooth in appearance and are known as "Tzanck cells".
- Small number of polymorphonuclear neutrophil and lymphocytes may be found within the vesicular fluid, but there

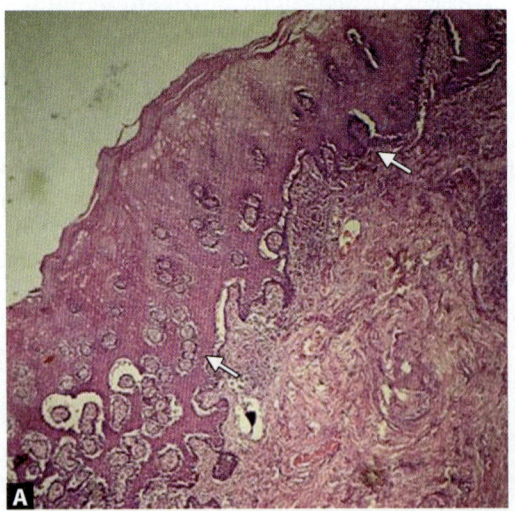 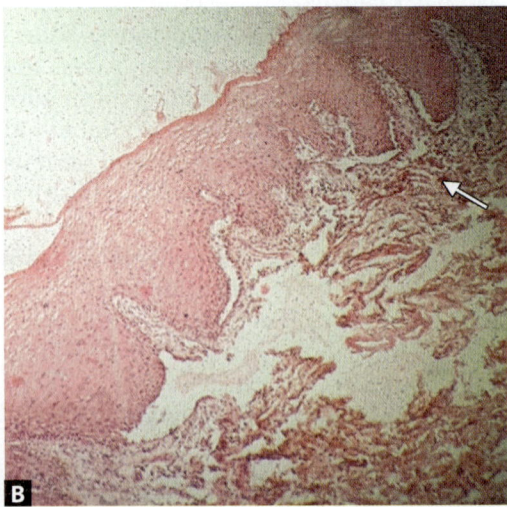

Figs. 19.10A and B: Photomicrographs of pemphigus vulgaris showing (A) intraepithelial vesicle; and (B) suprabasilar split in the epithelium.

Oral Aspects of Dermatological Disorders

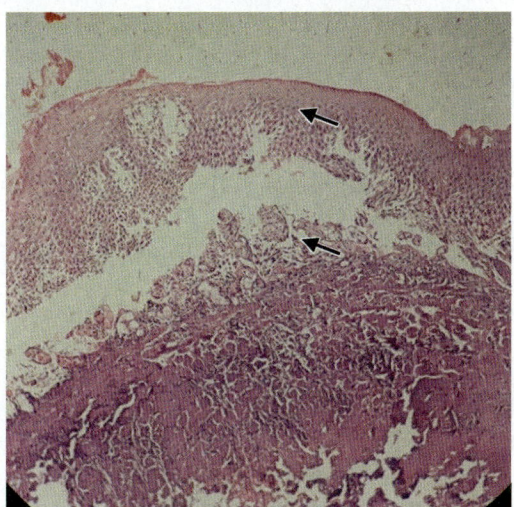

Fig. 19.11: Photomicrograph of pemphigus vulgaris showing acantholysis with intraepithelial vesicle formation.

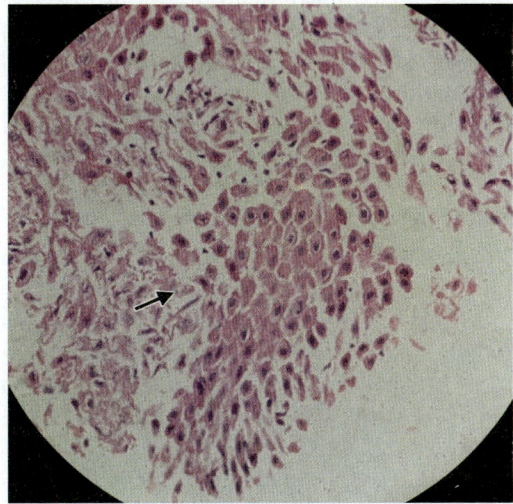

Fig. 19.12: Photomicrograph of pemphigus vulgaris showing acantholysis due to loss of desmosomal attachment between cells.

is minimum inflammatory cell infiltration in the underlying connective tissue (unlike any other vesiculobullous lesion).
- *Pemphigus vegetans* microscopically shows proliferative verruciform lesion in the epithelium with formation of characteristic "eosinophil microabscesses". Areas of acantholysis are also sometimes seen. (*Histologically, pemphigus vegetans looks very close to "pyostomatitis vegetans"*).
- *Paraneoplastic pemphigus* histologically exhibits intraepithelial acantholysis with suprabasal clefting, along with dyskeratosis of keratinocytes, liquefaction of basal cells and inflammatory cell infiltration.

The histological appearances indicate that there is an overlapping between paraneoplastic pemphigus and erythema multiforme.

Immunohistochemistry

- In pemphigus, direct immunofluorescence on frozen section of the perilesional tissue often demonstrate the deposition of specific immunoglobulins (IgG), within the intercellular junctions; less frequently, immunoglobulin M (IgM) and immunoglobulin A (IgA) are also seen.
- The intensity of the fluorescence is the greatest in the suprabasilar region (spinous cell layers), and gradually it becomes decreased towards the surface of the epithelium and it produces a characteristic "*chicken wire or fish-net*" *appearance*.

Key Points of Pemphigus

- ❖ Pemphigus is a vesiculobullous lesion of the skin and mucosa membrane, which occurs due to autoimmune destruction of the intercellular cement substance between cells.
- ❖ The disease produces rapidly developing vesicles or bullae on several areas of the skin and mucous membrane.
- ❖ Ruptured vesicles in the oral cavity often leave extremely painful, superficial erythematous ulcers with ragged borders.
- ❖ Gentle traction or oblique pressure on the unaffected areas around the lesion causes stripping of the normal skin or mucous membrane, this phenomenon is known as "Nikolsky's sign".
- ❖ Histologically, the disease is characterized by formation of intraepithelial vesicles or bullae, which causes separation of the epithelium above the basal cell layer.
- ❖ Loss of intercellular bridges and collection of edema fluid result in acantholysis within the spinous cell layer.

- Disruption of the spinous cells causes clumps of large hyperchromatic epithelial cells accumulating within the vesicular fluid; these desquamated cells are known as "Tzanck cells".
- The disease is treated by high dose of steroid therapy.

Levels of Autoantibody Deposition

Levels of autoantibody deposition in different vesiculobullous lesions (findings by direct immunofluorescence technique) are described in Box 19.2.

Differential Diagnosis
- Pemphigoid
- Erythema multiforme
- Bullous lichen planus
- Dermatitis herpetiformis
- Desquamative gingivitis
- Toxic epidermal necrolysis

Box 19.2 Levels of autoantibody deposition in the epithelium in various immune-mediated disorders.

- *Pemphigus vulgaris*: Intercellular deposition of IgG (IgG1 and 4) throughout the epidermis—chicken wire/fishnet appearance.
- *Cicatricial pemphigoid*: Linear deposits of complement (C3) and IgG, IgA at dermal-epidermal junction—"shore line appearance".
- *Bullous pemphigoid*: IgG (70–90%) and C3 (90–100%) deposition in a linear band at dermal-epidermal junction.
- *Epidermolysis bullosa acquisita*: Thick band of IgG and to a lesser extent C3, deposited linearly at the basement membrane zone.
- *Dermatitis herpetiformis*: Deposition of IgA at dermal-epidermal junction.
- *Erythema multiforme*: Granular deposits of IgG, C3, IgM, and fibrinogen present around dermal vessels or at dermoepidermal junction.
- *Systemic lupus erythematosus*: Deposition of IgG, IgM, or C3 in a shaggy or granular band at the basement membrane zone—"positive lupus band test."
- *Lichen planus*: Shaggy deposits at dermoepidermal junction of IgM (within scattered cytoid bodies), C3 and IgG along with fibrinogen deposition at the basement membrane zone.

- Aphthous ulcers
- Epidermolysis bullosa.

Treatment
- High dose of steroids
- Immunosuppressive drugs, e.g. azathioprine or methotrexate
- Antibiotics to prevent secondary infections
- Fluid and electrolyte balance must be strictly maintained.

PEMPHIGOID

Pemphigoid is a group of relatively uncommon, autoimmune vesiculobullous lesion, characterized histologically by the subepithelial bullae formation in the basement membrane zone (BMZ) of the skin and epithelium. Pemphigus and pemphigoid are the two most important autoimmune diseases of the skin and epithelium; the most significant difference between them is that in pemphigoid (a) "acantholysis" does not take place and (b) blistering occurs in the subepithelial tissue at the basement membrane zone.

Pathogenesis

Progression of the pemphigoid occurs in the following mechanisms (Flowchart 19.1).

Unlike pemphigus, pemphigoid lesions usually heal up by scar formation (cicatrization); however, the scarring mostly occurs in eye lesions and sometimes it can cause even blindness.

Although a large number of clinical variants of pemphigoid exist, the most common and the best understood among them are: (A) Benign mucous membrane pemphigoid (Cicatricial pemphigoid), and (B) Bullous pemphigoid.

The former lesion occurs commonly in relation to the mucous membrane, while the later one occurs frequently in relation to the skin. Pemphigoid is seen twice as common in females as in males and the mean age of occurrence is above 60 years. The disease is

Oral Aspects of Dermatological Disorders

Flowchart 19.1: Pathogenesis of pemphigoid.

Formation of autoantibodies in the body against hemidesmosomes, which binds basal keratinocytes to the basement membrane

↓

Bullous pemphigoid antigens (BPAGs) are components of hemidesmosomes; antibodies are commonly produced against one such component called BPAG2

↓

Once autoantibodies against BPAG2 are formed, they bind with the hemidesmosome in a continuous linear pattern along the dermal-epidermal junction

↓

After binding, autoantibodies cause activation of complements, which attract inflammatory cells (neutrophils and eosinophils) and initiate local inflammation

↓

Release of proteolytic enzymes (especially protease) by inflammatory cells

↓

Protease causes destruction of hemidesmosomal junctions of the basement membrane zone

↓

Formation of subepithelial vesicles or bullae with disruption of dermal-epidermal attachment

---

not life threatening and though, it often runs a chronic course for many years.

Benign Mucous Membrane Pemphigoid or Cicatricial Pemphigoid

Benign mucous membrane pemphigoid or cicatricial pemphigoid is an uncommon vesiculobullous condition that frequently affects the middle-aged or elderly females (40–60 years) (Fig. 19.13).

The most common site of occurrence is the oral mucous membrane, followed by the conjunctiva. Sometimes the disease also involves the nose, pharynx, larynx, esophagus, genitalia, etc. The name cicatricial pemphigoid has been given since scar formation is an important characteristic of this disease (although scarring occurs rarely); however, scars never form in eye lesions or lesions of the esophagus/larynx.

Clinical Features (Figs. 19.14A and B)
Oral lesions
- Oral cavity is often the first and, in most cases, the only site involved in cicatricial pemphigoid.
- In the mouth, it usually produces slowly progressive, mild erosion or desquamation of the gingival and palatal tissues.
- Erythematous changes occur in oral mucosa where vesicles or bullae arise subsequently.

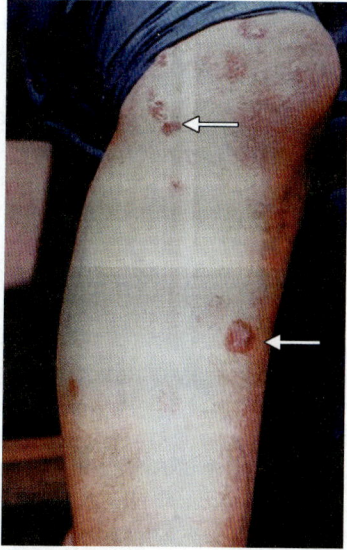

Fig. 19.13: Vesiculobullous lesion of skin in pemphigoid.

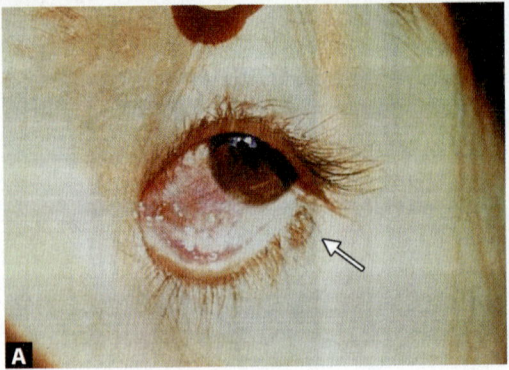 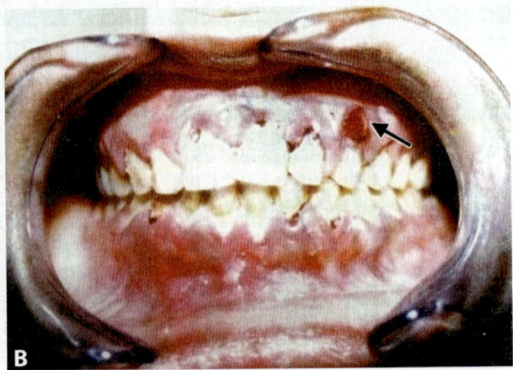

Figs. 19.14A and B: Vesicle formation in (A) eye; and (B) oral mucosa in pemphigoid.

- In severe cases, large vesicles or bullae may develop on the palate, cheek, alveolar mucosa or tongue, etc.
- Bullae are sometimes quite large in size (containing clear fluid) and they may remain intact for several days (In contrast to the vesicles or bullae of pemphigus, which do not persist and they rupture almost as soon as they form).
- Skin lesions occur in about 5% cases and mucosal lesions always precede the skin lesions.
- The mucosal bullae are often tense and are relatively tough because these are usually covered by a full thickness epithelium.
- Bleeding into the bullae can make them look like blood blisters.
- Once the bullae rupture, they leave large painful, eroded or ulcerated areas, which heal up slowly.
- Further erosions may occur in the adjoining areas and the process continues for long.
- The gingival lesions are very common (seen in about 90% cases) and they characteristically present either patchy erythema with mild discomfort or severe erythema, widespread desquamation, ulceration, etc.
- Sometimes, these gingival lesions are the only manifestations of pemphigoid and the so-called desquamative gingivitis can be the only manifestation of the disease.
- Pain and bleeding are the common complaints and Nikolsky's sign is strongly positive.
- Irritation from denture, calculus and plaque can exacerbate the condition.
- Secondary infection often occurs in preexisting pemphigoid lesions and oral lesions usually heal up by scar formation.
- Involvement of the pharynx, esophagus and larynx may produce discomforts like sore throat, dysphagia, strictures, etc.; some patients may develop septicemia.

Eye lesions
- Conjunctivitis
- Blister formation in the eye
- Corneal ulceration
- Swelling of the fornix and corneal opacity
- Fibrosis and scarring of the lacrimal ducts, which often leads to "dry eye".
- Scarring may cause adhesions between the bulbar and the palpebral conjunctiva (this is called as *symblepharon*).
- Scarring of the conjunctival mucosa may ultimately lead to eyelids turn inwards, termed as *entropion*.
- This causes eyelashes to rub against the cornea and is termed as *trichiasis*.

- Cornea then produces keratin (opaque material) as a protective mechanism that results in blindness.

Skin lesions

The skin lesions are rare in cicatricial pemphigoid and occasionally few large, tense and fluid-filled vesicles or bullae may appear over the face, scalp or neck.

Bullous Pemphigoid

Bullous pemphigoid occurs more commonly on the skin and it seldom affects the oral mucosa (only 10% cases). It is one of the most common autoimmune blistering conditions, occurring at an esteemed rate of 10 cases per million populations per year. The disease is characterized by the production of autoantibodies directed against components of the basement membrane.

Clinical Features

- Elderly people in the age group of 70 years and 80 years are usually affected, and there is no gender predilection.
- The skin lesions mostly occur on the inner aspects of the thighs, flexor surface of forearms, axillae, groin and lower abdomen.
- These lesions bullous pemphigoid also follow the usual clinical patterns of vesiculation, followed by ulceration and finally healing (without scarring).
- Skin lesions begin as red, eczematous plaques which eventually progress to the formation of bullae. The bullae are tense, containing clear fluid and are usually less than 2 cm in diameter (few can be as large as 4–8 cm in diameter). The bullae do not rupture easily (unlike the bullae in pemphigus) and heal without scarring.
- Skin lesions always precede the mucosal lesions and these mucosal lesions are always smaller than that of the cicatricial pemphigoid.

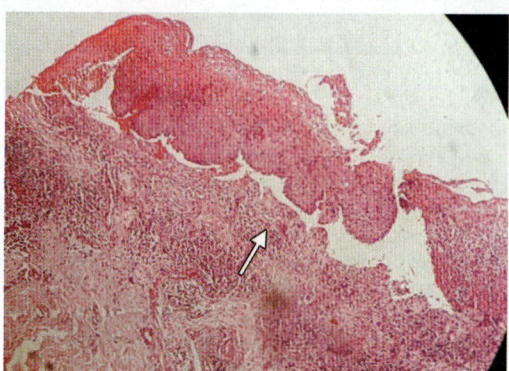

Fig. 19.15: Photomicrograph of pemphigoid showing subepithelial bullae formation.

- Bullous pemphigoid having oral lesions may be associated with internal malignancy.

Histopathology of Pemphigoid

- Extracellular edema and vacuolation in the basement membrane zone are the earliest histological changes in cicatricial pemphigoid.
- Gradually, there is formation of subepithelial vesicles or bullae (Fig. 19.15).
- The subepithelial bullae cause separation of the full thickness epithelium from the underlying lamina propria and thus the epithelium forms the roof of an intact bullae till it is ruptured.
- Acantholysis and epithelial degenerative changes are absent.
- In many cases, the entire surface epithelium may be lost due to positive Nikolsky's sign and the biopsy specimen may have only connective tissue.
- Polymorphonuclear neutrophils may be found within the vesicular fluid.
- Subepithelial connective tissue shows inflammatory cell infiltration by lymphocytes, macrophages and eosinophils in the perivascular areas.
- Blood vessels are often dilated and prominent in the superficial part of the lamina propria.

> **Key Points of Pemphigoid**
> - Pemphigoid is a relatively uncommon, autoimmune vesiculobullous lesion. It is characterized by subepithelial bullae formation in the basement membrane zone.
> - The disease produces large vesicles or bullae in the skin and mucous membrane, which rupture after a certain period and leave painful ulcers.
> - Pain, bleeding and secondary infection are the common problems caused by these ulcers.
> - Nikolsky's sign is typically positive in this disease.
> - Besides the dermal lesions, eye lesions also commonly develop in pemphigoid.
> - The eye lesions include conjunctivitis, blister formation in the eye, corneal ulceration, fibrosis of the lacrimal duct leading to dry eyes, etc.
> - Histologically, pemphigoid presents formation of subepithelial vesicles or bullae at the basement membrane zone which causes separation of full thickness epithelium from the underlying connective tissue.
> - Systemic steroid therapy is the treatment of choice.

Treatment

Systemic steroid therapy is the treatment of choice in both forms of the disease.

Differences between pemphigus vulgaris and bullous pemphigoid are described in Table 19.2.

■ EPIDERMOLYSIS BULLOSA

Epidermolysis bullosa is a generalized desquamating condition of the skin and mucosa, which characteristically exhibits formation of large blisters at sites of pressure, trauma or rubbing. It also causes extensive scarring and contractures in the skin along with some dental defects.

Pathogenesis

The disease occurs due to inherited defects in the structural proteins that give mechanical stability to the skin and mucous membrane; blisters form in the disease due to separation of the epithelium from the underlying connective tissue. Although hereditary form of the disease is more predominant, sometimes acquired form of the disease can also occur.

Types

Several forms of epidermolysis bullosa have been recognized, and these lesions are divided into two broad categories:
1. Hereditary epidermolysis bullosa
2. Acquired epidermolysis bullosa.

The hereditary forms of epidermolysis bullosa are again subdivided into four types:
1. Simplex type
2. Junctional type
3. Dystrophic (scarring) type
4. Mixed type.

There is only a single form of acquired epidermolysis bullosa, and it is named

Table 19.2: Difference between pemphigus vulgaris and bullous pemphigoid.

Pemphigus vulgaris	*Bullous pemphigoid*
• Autoantibodies are produced against the desmoglein-3 (desmosomes)	• Autoantibodies are produced against the hemodesmosomes at the basement membrane zone
• Occurs in younger people.	• Elderly people are more often affected
• Oral mucosa is a predominant site	• Oral mucosa is rarely affected
• Intraepithelial vesicle formation	• Subepithelial vesicle formation
• Vesicles are flaccid and rupture easily	• Vesicles are firm and stable
• Nikolsky's sign is positive	• Nikolsky's sign is negative
• Acantholysis occurs with appearance of "Tzanck cells"	• No acantholysis
• Immunofluorescence shows "net-like" IgG deposition pattern	• Immunofluorescence shows "linear" IgG deposition.
• Poor prognosis	• Good prognosis
• Tombstone appearance of the basal cells	• Eosinophilic infiltration seen in histology

as epidermolysis bullosa acquisita. This acquired form of the disease may be associated with multiple myeloma, diabetes mellitus, tuberculosis, amyloidosis, Crohn's disease, etc.

Clinical Features

- All forms of the disease are characterized by the formation of multiple vesicles or bullae on the pressure areas of the skin (i.e. elbows and knees).
- Dystrophic type is the most severe form of the disease and it may cause death secondary to septicemia.
- The bullae rupture and leave raw, painful ulcers, which heal up with scarring.
- The healing of skin lesions cause extensive scarring with pigmentation or depigmentation of the area.
- Nails often shed or exfoliate due to formation of blisters in the nail beds.
- The hereditary forms of the disease are usually very severe in nature and occur during infancy or early childhood, whereas the acquired form of the disease is common during adulthood only.
- Patients with hereditary epidermolysis bullosa may also exhibit stunted growth, mental retardation and ectodermal dysplasia, etc.
- The patients may have alopecia and claw-like hands due to repeated scarring and contractures.
- Many such patients die during childhood.

Oral Manifestations

- Rapidly developing, multiple, fragile and hemorrhagic blisters in the areas of trauma (particularly in the palate).
- The blisters rupture soon and leave painful ulcers, which heal with scarring.
- Repeated blistering and scarring around the oral cavity may result in decreased mouth opening (microstomia), ankyloglossia and loss of vestibular sulci.
- Some patients may develop perioral and perinasal crusted and hemorrhagic granular lesions.
- The dental changes include hypoplastic pitted enamel of the molar teeth, delayed eruption of teeth, increased caries susceptibility and increased periodontal diseases, etc.
- Sometimes oral lesions may transform into squamous cell carcinoma.

Histopathology

- Extensive destruction of the basal or the suprabasal layers of the oral epithelium results in the formation of vesicles or bullae.
- Bullae formation may also be seen within enamel organ of the developing tooth germ.
- Mucosal bullae formation occurs at different planes in various forms of epidermolysis bullosa and these are explained in the following sections (Table 19.3).

Treatment

- Systemic steroid therapy
- Immunosuppressive drug therapy
- Avoidance of trauma.

LUPUS ERYTHEMATOSUS

Lupus erythematosus is an autoimmune disorder, characterized by the destruction of tissue due to the deposition of autoantibody and immune complexes within it. Production of autoantibody, particularly the antinuclear antibody, is the hallmark of lupus erythematosus. The word "lupus" means "wolf" in Latin and the disease named so since the skin rash looked like a "wolf's bite".

Table 19.3: Mucosal bullae formation.

Disease types	Level at which bulla forms
Simplex type	Intraepithelial bullae
Junctional type	At the level of lamina lucida
Dystrophic type	At the level of sub-lamina densa
Acquired type	At the level of sub-lamina densa

Literally the term "lupus" also denotes "diseases affecting the skin", and "erythematosus" means reddening, therefore lupus erythematosus means a disease with reddening of skin.

Pathogenesis

Pathogenesis of lupus erythematosus is not clearly known. It is believed that autoimmune reactions cause changes within the basal cells of the skin or mucous membrane along with the collagen and vascular tissues. Autoantibodies to DNA and other nuclear and ribonuclear protein antigens are present in blood. The circulating autoantibodies cause cross reactivity with antigenic determinants on multiple tissues.

The disease occurs in two basic forms.
1. Systemic lupus erythematosus (SLE)
2. Discoid lupus erythematosus (DLE).

Systemic Lupus Erythematosus

Systemic lupus erythematosus frequently produces lesions in the skin and oral mucous membrane, and besides this, it also involves certain other body systems, e.g. kidney, joints and heart, etc.

Pathogenesis of Systemic Lupus Erythematosus

Genetics along with environmental factors play a role.

Persons will have susceptible gene exposed to UV rays (Sunrays) (Flowchart 19.2)

Clinical features of systemic lupus erythematosus

Skin lesions
- Systemic lupus erythematosus occurs in about 0.1–0.4% individuals.
- Skin lesions of SLE are characterized by the development of fixed, erythematous rashes that often have a "butterfly configuration" (Fig. 19.16) over the malar region and across the bridge of the nose.
- In some cases, the rashes may spread diffusely and have a wide area of skin involvement.

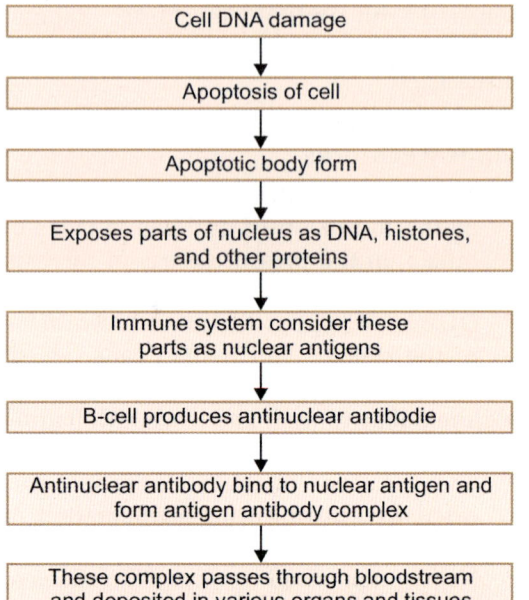

Flowchart 19.2: Pathogenesis of systemic lupus erythematosus.

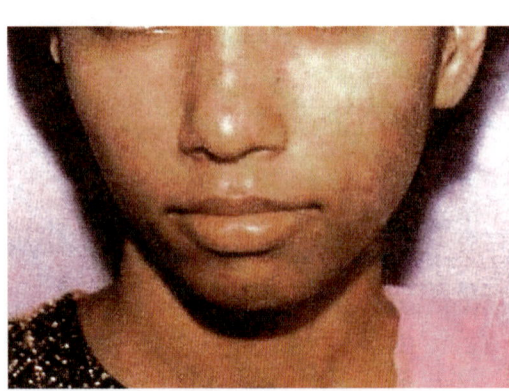

Fig. 19.16: Systemic lupus erythematosus patient showing erythematous rash on the facial skin.

- These skin rashes produce itching or burning sensation, which is often aggravated by the exposure to sunlight. The disease often causes hyperpigmentation of the skin.
- The diseases affect females five times more often than males and it is mostly detected in the fourth decade of life.
- Patchy or extensive loss of hair from the scalp is a very common (Fig. 19.17) clinical finding in lupus erythematosus (hair may grow once again after successful treatment in case of SLE, but not in case of DLE).

Oral lesions
- The bilateral malar rash often gives a "wolf-like" appearance of the face to the patient of SLE.
- Oral lesions occur in about 20% cases of SLE and these lesions usually appear as white, hyperkeratotic plaque-like areas and resemble lichen planus. Oral lesions mostly occur over the buccal mucosa, palate, gingiva, etc.
- Oral and nasopharyngeal ulcerations are recognized as the major diagnostic manifestations of SLE.
- There is often severe mucositis with burning sensations in the mouth; the affected mucosa is extremely tendered to palpation.

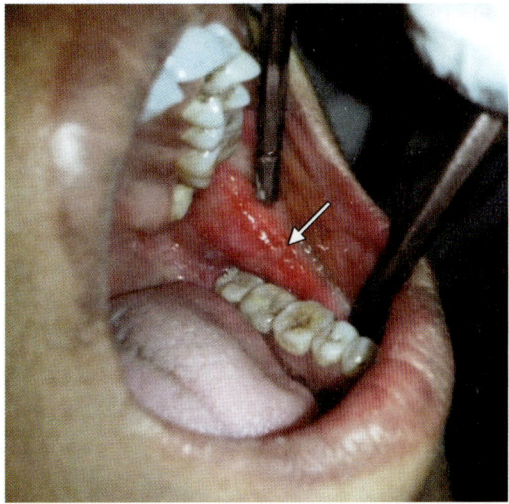

Fig. 19.18: Intense erythema in the oral mucosa with areas of ulcerations in systemic lupus erythematosus patient.

- An important feature is of SLE is the presence of shallow linear ulcers running parallel to the palatal gingiva. Oral ulcers are often painful and are surrounded by a red halo.
- Besides ulcerations, oral mucosa also has erythematous areas, hemorrhagic macules, petechiae and ecchymosis, etc. (Fig. 19.18).
- The vermillion border of the lower lip is sometimes affected and the condition is known as "lupus cheilitis".
- Secondary infections frequently occur to these mucosal lesions (mostly candidiasis).
- There may be involvement of salivary glands in SLE, which causes secondary Sjögren's syndrome and severe xerostomia.
- Besides xerostomia, patients may also suffer from altered taste sensations, sore mouth, chronic periodontal disease. In some cases, oral lesions may undergo malignant transformations.

Systemic manifestations of systemic lupus erythematosus

These are listed in Table 19.4.

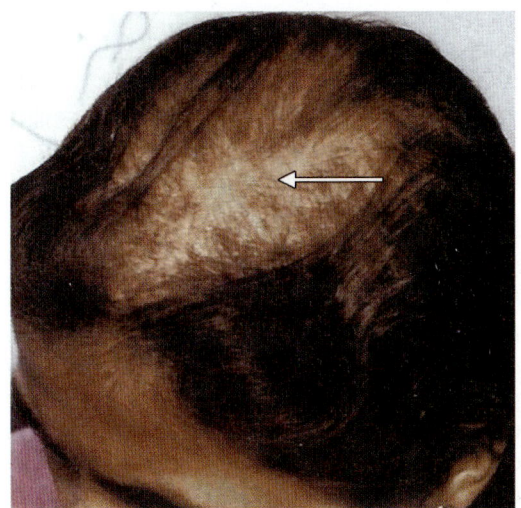

Fig. 19.17: Systemic lupus erythematosus patient showing loss of hair over the scalp.

Table 19.4: Systemic manifestations of systemic lupus erythematosus.

General symptoms	Fever, weight loss, fatigue, malaise, vomiting, diarrhea, anorexia, lymphadenopathy, etc.
Skin	Rashes with itching sensation and the malar rash often have butterfly configuration, photosensitivity
Serous membrane	Pleurisy and endocarditis
Lung problem	Pneumonitis
Gastrointestinal tract involvement	Pancreatitis, hepatomegaly and splenomegaly
Ocular disturbances	Conjunctivitis and retinal damage
Central nervous system disturbances	Neurosis, psychosis, seizures, depression, strokes and cranial nerve palsies
Hematologic disorders	Anemia, purpura and leukopenia
Cardiorespiratory problems	Vegetations in the heart valves (Libman–Sacks endocarditis) and myocarditis, pericarditis, pleurisy
Renal problems	Profuse proteinurea, nephritic syndrome and fibrinoid degeneration of the glomerular capillaries, which may lead to renal failure
Joint problems	Nondeforming arthritis and arthralgia
Mouth	Stomatitis and Sjögren's syndrome, oral ulcers
Disease often coexisting with systemic lupus erythematosus	Sjögren's syndrome, Raynaud's phenomenon, scleroderma, pemphigoid, erythema multiforme and pemphigus

Key Points of Lupus Erythematosus

- Lupus erythematosus is an autoimmune disorder, characterized by destruction of tissue due to the deposition of autoantibody and immune complexes within it.
- The disease occurs in two forms—SLE and DLE.
- SLE presents characteristic fixed, erythematous rashes with a "butterfly configuration" over the malar region and across the bridge of the nose.
- In the oral cavity, SLE produces white, hyperkeratotic plaque-like areas and resembles lichen planus. Involvement of salivary glands in SLE often results secondary Sjogren's syndrome and severe xerostomia.
- Systemic manifestations of SLE include hepatosplenomegaly, pneumonia, cardiac problem, renal problem, gastrointestinal disturbances, neural problem, etc.
- DLE clinically presents multiple white plaques with central atrophy, shallow ulcers, reddish purple erosions, etc.
- Histologically, SLE produces atrophy with hyperkeratinization and liquefactive degeneration of the basal cell layer of epithelium.
- Systemic steroid therapy is the treatment of choice in both forms of the disease.

Histopathology

The oral lesions present the following histopathological findings:

- Atrophy with hyperkeratinization of the oral epithelium
- Liquefactive degeneration of the basal cell layer
- Edema of the subepithelial connective tissue with vascular dilatations
- Lymphocytic infiltration is less severe than DLE and fibrinoid degeneration of the collagen fibers is more prominent.

Discoid Lupus Erythematosus

The term "discoid" means *"disk-shaped"* (resembling an ancient stone tool) and in DLE, there is often formation of disk-shaped macules on the skin. DLE also commonly produces oral lesions, but systemic manifestations are absent. DLE also occurs commonly among females and the usual age is the third and fourth decades of life. The disease commonly involves the skin over the back, chest and extremities, and the oral mucous membrane.

Clinical features of discoid lupus erythematosus

Skin lesions:
- These are slightly elevated, red or purple macules, which are often covered by a yellow or gray scale.
- Skin lesions of DLE also present a butterfly distribution over the malar region and across the nose.
- Upon forceful removal of the covering scale, numerous "carpet track" extensions of the pilosebaceous channels appear.
- Skin lesions in DLE usually enlarge at the periphery and in some cases, epidermoid or basal cell carcinoma may develop from these lesions.
- Involvement of scalp with loss of hair is also common.

Oral lesions (Figs. 19.19 and 19.20)
- The oral lesions of DLE closely resemble the oral lichen planus (Table 19.5) and they include multiple white plaques with central atrophy, shallow ulcers, reddish purple erosions, etc. The lesions initiate at a particular point and then gradually extend peripherally to cover a wider area.

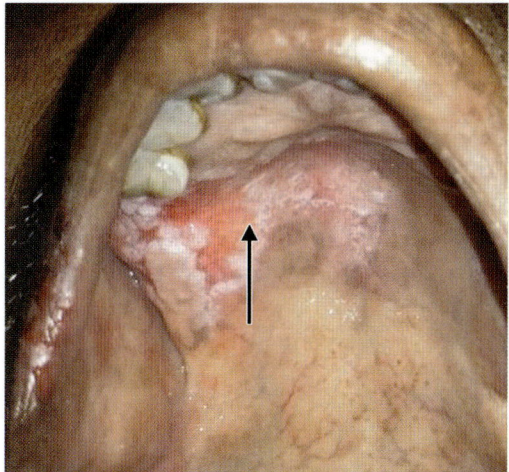

Fig. 19.20: Discoid lupus erythematosus showing white plaque with central atrophy and ulceration.

- Erythema or ulcerations in DLE may be surrounded by a white keratotic border, which can also have radiating striae.
- As the white plaque of the oral cavity extends peripherally, its central area becomes red and ulcerated while the border remains white and keratotic.
- These mucosal lesions frequently involve center of palate, cheek, upper lip and gingiva, etc.

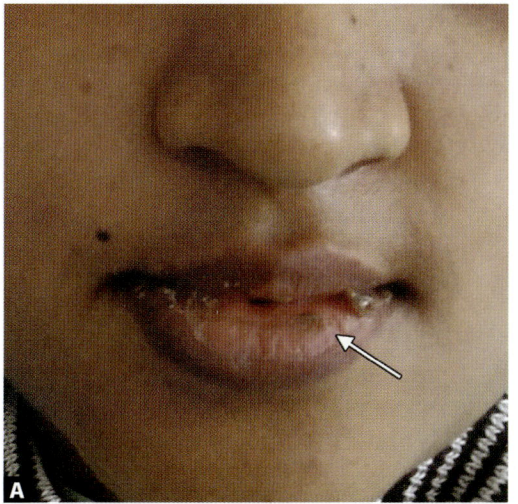
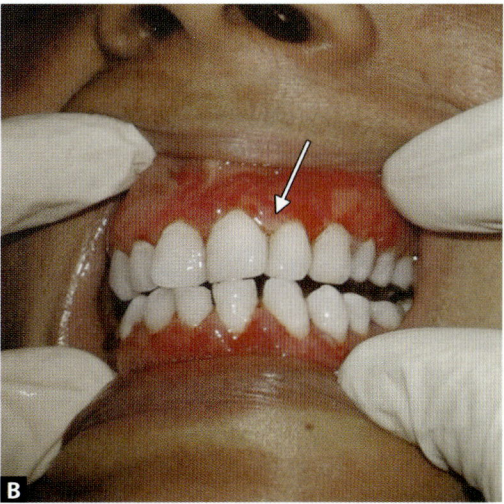

Figs. 19.19A and B: Discoid lupus erythematosus showing mucosal lesion in the (A) Lip; and (B) Gingiva.

Table 19.5: Differences between oral lesions of lichen planus and discoid lupus erythematosus (DLE).

Oral lichen planus	Oral lesion of DLE
Oral lesions often exhibit bilateral symmetrical distribution	Oral lesions does not have bilateral symmetrical distribution
External surface of the lip is not involved	External surface of the lip is frequently involved
Palatal lesions are rarely seen	Palatal lesions are very common
Pain and burning sensations are more common	Pain and burning sensations are not present
Epithelial rete pegs are thin and often have a "saw-tooth" like appearance	Rete pegs are hyperplastic and often form flame-like down growths into the underlying connective tissue. Rete pegs may even fuse together and create an appearance of pseudoepitheliomatous hyperplasia
Band-like infiltrations of inflammatory cells near the basement membrane zone	Band-like infiltrations of inflammatory cells present but its lower border tends to be less well defined and infiltrates often extend to the deeper tissues
BMZ shows duplication and fragmentation.	BMZ shows hyalinization

- Lip lesion often spread to the adjacent gingiva, which are often called kissing lesions. Small slit-like ulcers are often seen near the gingival margin.
- Pain and burning sensations are common in the mouth in DLE.

Histopathology

Oral lesions of DLE present the following histologic findings:
- Hyperortho or parakeratinization of the surface epithelium.
- The epithelium may be atrophic in some cases.
- Few lesions exhibit keratin plugging, acanthosis and pseudo-epitheliomatous hyperplasia.
- Liquefactive degeneration of the basal cell layer.
- Basophilic degeneration of the collagen with sign of hyalinization and perivascular lymphocytic infiltration in the lamina propria.
- Inflammatory cell infiltration typically extends deep into the connective tissue.
- PAS-positive thickening of the basement membrane zone and narrow blood vessels are seen, which occur due to deposition of antigen-antibody complex.
- Vasculitis occurs commonly in SLE but it is not seen in DLE.

Laboratory Investigations of Lupus Erythematosus

Lupus erythematosus cell inclusion phenomenon: It is a specific laboratory test for SLE. If the serum from a patient suffering from SLE is added to the buffy coat of normal blood, a typical lupus erythematosus cell will develop. These are neutrophil leukocytes, which have phagocytosed other leukocytes. Lupus erythematosus cell is characterized by a large, circular, basophilic inclusion within a neutrophil. Positive lupus erythematosus cell test is rare in DLE.

Other laboratory tests include the following:
- Antinuclear antibody test to determine if autoantibodies to cell nuclei are present in the serum.
- Anti-DNA antibody test determine if there are antibodies to genetic material in the cell.
- Complement proteins C3 and C4 test to examine specific levels.
- Polyclonal hyperactivity of the B-lymphocytes.
- Decrease in the number of suppressor cells.

- Blood examination reveals leukopenia, thrombocytopenia and hemolytic anemia.
- Hypergammaglobulinemia and profuse proteinuria.

Positive Antinuclear Antibody

Detection of antinuclear antibody by immunofluorescent technique is the most sensitive test for SLE. Although there may be other diseases, where antinuclear antibody may be positive and these include the following:
- Scleroderma
- Sjogren's syndrome
- Infectious mononucleosis
- Rheumatoid arthritis
- Patients receiving drug therapy, e.g. chlorpromazine, isoniazid and procainamide, etc.

Direct immunofluorescence test: This test will reveal the deposition of immunoglobulins (e.g. IgG, IgA, IgM and complement 3) in the basement membrane zone of the epithelium and skin, in case of both SLE and DLE.

Indirect immunofluorescence test: Reveals prominent circulating autoantibodies.

Other lab tests include: Erythrocyte sedimentation rate (ESR), C-reactive protein, liver and kidney function tests, creatine phosphokinase (CPK; muscle enzyme), urine protein or cellular cast, serum albumin.

Disease activity correlates with a rise in:
1. C-reactive protein binding
2. ESR
3. Anti-DNA
4. Liver and kidney function tests [aspartate amino transferase (AST), alanine amino transferase (ALT), blood urea nitrogen (BUN), creatinine]
5. CPK (muscle enzyme)
6. Urine protein or cellular casts.

Disease activity correlates with a fall in:
1. Complete blood count (white blood cells, hemoglobin, platelets)
2. Complement components
3. Serum albumin.

Treatment

Systemic steroid therapy is the treatment of choice in lupus erythematosus.

SCLERODERMA

Scleroderma or progressive systemic sclerosis is a complex multisystem autoimmune disease characterized by progressive diffuse subcutaneous fibrosis (sclerosis) of the skin, widespread submucous fibrosis in oral cavity and disorders in multiple internal organs including the gastrointestinal tract, lungs, heart, kidney, etc.

Pathogenesis

- Genetic, environmental and vascular factors are involved in scleroderma pathogenesis.
- Blood circulation insufficiency in the tissue because of the abnormalities in the arterioles and blood capillaries cause replacement of the normal connective tissue by the dense collagen bundles and this results in the fibrosis or sclerosis of the tissue.
- Antigens from the human leukocyte antigen histocompatibility complex, including HLA-B8, HLA-DR3, HLA-DR5, HLA-DR3, HLA-DR52, and HLA-DQB2, are involved in scleroderma.
- Apoptosis and the generation of free radicals may be involved in the pathogenesis.

Types

Scleroderma usually occurs in two basic forms:
1. Localized or morphea form
2. Generalized or diffuse form (it is the more common type).

The localized or "morphea" form of scleroderma is characterized by fibrosis with development of single or multiple, red or ivory colored, smooth, hard patches on the skin. Although, facial skin is frequently affected, it does not have any oral manifestations. Childhood "morphea" form of scleroderma may be responsible for the development of facial hemihypertrophy.

The generalized or diffuse form of scleroderma usually occurs among children or young adults, and it frequently affects females. Scleroderma is more prevalent in areas where silicosis is a common environmental hazard.

Clinical Features of Diffuse Scleroderma (Figs. 19.21 and 19.22)

- Females between the ages of 30 years and 50 years are very frequently affected by scleroderma.
- The disease begins with edema of the skin over the face, hands or trunk.
- The affected skin becomes thinned and stiff and it is fixed firmly to the underlying tissues, e.g. muscles, bones, etc.
- The affected skin is also marked by multiple telangiectasias and contractures.
- The skin often appears reddish and scaly, and it also frequently exhibits scarring.
- Fixation and stiffness of the skin causes progressive loss of mobility of hands and joints as well as restricted movements of many internal and external organs.

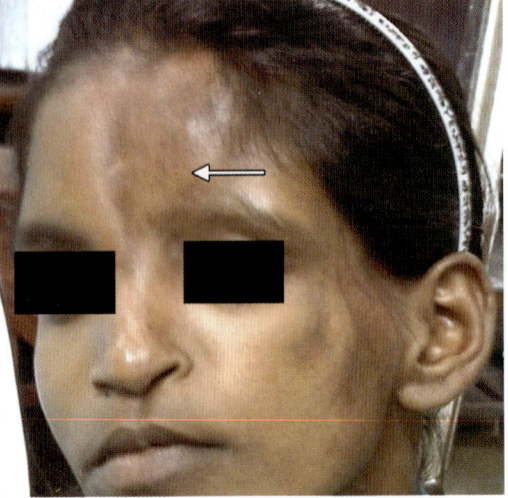

Fig. 19.21: Localized or morphea form of scleroderma involving facial skin.

- Resorption of terminal phalanges and flexion contractures often produce a typical "claw-like" appearance of the fingers. In this situation, the patient is unable to straighten the fingers.
- Ulcerations may occur on the fingertips due to fibrosis (abnormal collagen deposition) and reduced vascularity.

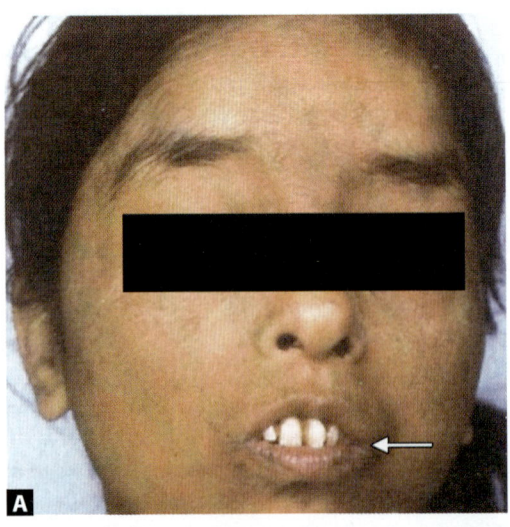
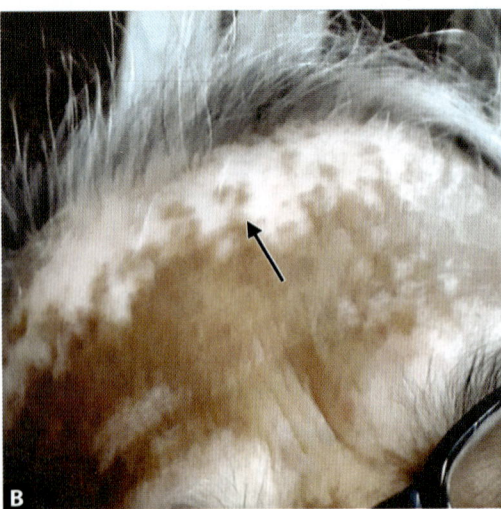

Figs. 19.22A and B: Diffuse scleroderma with (A) Rigidity of facial skin and microstomia; and (B) Loss of skin pigmentation.

- Widespread involvement of the disease causes wasting of muscles and body fat, with weakening of the limbs.
- Patients develop arthritis and arthralgia, along with neuralgia and paresthesia of the skin.
- As the disease progresses, the skin becomes yellow, gray or ivory white in color and it shows a waxy appearance.
- The skin gradually becomes thin or atrophic with areas of pigmentation and subcutaneous calcium deposition (calcinosis cutis).
- Due to fixation or toughness of the facial skin, "wrinkles" (lines of facial expression) do not form and eyes also become narrow. These cause a "mask-like" appearance of the face. This type of typical facial appearance or expression in scleroderma is also named as "Mona Lisa face".
- Atrophy of the ala of the nose often gives rise to a "pinched" appearance of the nose, which often produces a "mouse facies".
- Restriction of movements occurs in all the voluntary and involuntary muscles as a result of fibrosis, and later on, the patient becomes completely bedridden.
- Fibrosis of the viscera causes dyspnea, dysphagia, pulmonary hypertension, loss of vision, etc.
- Finally, all the internal organs, e.g. gastrointestinal tract, heart, lungs, kidneys, etc. become affected by the fibrosis and these organs gradually lose their respective functions. Among which, cardiac failure is the most threatening.
- CREST syndrome is often associated with scleroderma and it includes the following component features (Table 19.6).
- Besides this, scleroderma may also co-exist with some other systemic diseases like Sjögren's syndrome, rheumatoid arthritis, polymyositis, and lupus erythematosus.

Oral Manifestation of Diffuse Scleroderma

Facial Changes

- Mask-like expressionless face (Mona Lisa face) as wrinkles or lines of facial expression do not develop due to the stiffening of facial skin; complete loss of facial esthetics.
- Multiple telangiectatic spots may be seen on the facial skin.
- Patient may also have a "pinched" appearance of the nose, as the ala of the nose becomes atrophic due to fibrosis, this often gives the patient a typical "mouse facies".
- Constricted lip of the patient often produces another facial appearance, which is called "fish mouth" (Table 19.7).

Radiological Features

- There is generalized widening or thickening of the periodontal ligament space.

Table 19.6: Features of CREST syndrome.

C—Calcinosis cutis	Cutaneous deposition of calcium salts
R—Raynaud's phenomenon	When patient's hands and feet are exposed to cold temperature, the digits become dead white in appearance initially due to vasospasm and later on they become bluish due to venous stasis
E—Esophageal dysfunction	Fibrosis of the esophageal submucosa with stricture formation
S—Sclerodactyly	Abnormal collagen deposition causes stiffness and flexure of fingers with a claw-like deformity
T—Telangiectasia	Bleeding from superficial dilated capillaries produces multiple red macules on the skin, especially on the face

Table 19.7: Key points in oral manifestations of scleroderma.

Affected orofacial area	Signs and symptoms
Lips	"Pursed" lips with constriction of mouth opening
Mouth	Microstomia
Face	Mask-like expressionless face, no wrinkles on skin
Facial muscles	Weakness and muscle wasting
Oral mucosa	Edematous and atrophic, candidiasis often present
Salivary glands	Decreased salivary secretion (xerostomia), Sjögren's syndrome
Temporomandibular joint	Restricted movements with trismus, pain and clicking sound
Tongue	Stiffness with difficulty in speech and swallowing
Esophagus	Fibrosis and stricture causing increased gastroesophageal reflex
Gingiva	Becomes pale and firm
Palate	Loss or flattening of palatal rogue
Teeth	Premature loss of teeth due to advanced periodontitis and alveolar bone loss
Nerves	Trigeminal neuralgia (occasionally)

- Resorption of bone occurs in some areas of the condyle or ramus of mandible (often bilaterally) due to persistent pressure from the contracting facial skin, muscles and joints.
- In untreated cases, severe mandibular bone resorption occurs, which can lead to pathological fracture and even development of osteomyelitis.

Histopathology

- Atrophy of oral epithelium with flattening of the rete-pegs and areas of pigmentations.
- Thickening and hyalinization of the collagen fibers in lamina propria.
- Atrophy of the minor salivary glands and perivascular infiltration of inflammatory cells.
- Decreased vascularity in connective tissue with narrowing of vessels due to perivascular fibrosis.
- Thickening of the periodontal ligament due to increased synthesis of collagen and oxytalan fibers.
- Absence of sweat glands, sebaceous glands, and hair follicles facial in the skin.

Treatment

No specific treatment is available for scleroderma. Systemic steroid therapy may produce partial remission.

EHLERS–DANLOS SYNDROME

Ehlers–Danlos syndrome is a group of hereditary disorders characterized by defective or abnormal collagen synthesis in various body organs.

Clinical Features

- The patient often exhibits hypermobility of joints and increased laxity or hyperelasticity of the skin, and because of this, the patient is often referred to as the "rubber man".
- Excessive bruising tendency and defective wound healing occurs due to increased fragility of the skin and blood vessels.
- The skin is velvety, thin, and hyperextensible. Moreover, it shows an abnormal scarring response when subjected to minor injuries (Papyraceous scarring); and the scarred area of skin appears as "crumpled cigarette papers".

- Development of aortic aneurysm and its rupture is the common life-threatening factor for the patient.

Types of Ehlers-Danlos Syndrome
- *Type 1*: This is the classic and most severe form of the disease. It presents both hyperextensibility of joints and hyperelasticity of the skin; with easy bruisability. The skin often shows "cigarette-paper" scars.
- *Type 2*: Same as type I, but mild in nature.
- *Type 3*: Joint hypermobility is more prominent than skin change.
- *Type 4*: Excessive scars and hyperpigmentation of skin over the areas of bony prominence. The skin is so thin that the subcutaneous vessels are visible.
- *Type 5*: Patients may face sudden death due to rupture of large vessels and hollow organs.

Oral Manifestation
- Increased fragility of the oral mucosa
- Positive Gorlin's sign: Most patients can touch the tip of their nose with the tongue
- Bleeding from the gingiva and oral mocosa
- Mobility of teeth and marked periodontal weakness
- Retarded wound healing
- Enamel hypoplasia
- Loss of normal scalloping of the dentinoenamel junctions of the tooth
- Large pulp stones in the teeth and formation of irregular type of dentine
- Hypermobility and subluxation of the temporomandibular joint
- Difficulty in suturing the oral wounds due to extreme tissue fragility
- Easy bruising and bleeding following minor oral surgical procedures.

Laboratory Investigation
Clotting time is normal but the capillary fragility test is positive.

Treatment
No specific treatment is available.

BIBLIOGRAPHY
1. Accili D, Barbetti F, Cama A, et al. Mutations in the insulin receptor gene in patients with genetic syndromes of insulin resistance and acanthosis nigricans. J Invest Dermatol. 1992;98(6 Suppl):778-818.
2. Ahmed AR, Wagner R, Khatri K, et al. Major histocompatibility complex haplotypes and class II genes in non-Jewish patients with pemphigus vulgaris. Proc Natl Acad Sci USA. 1991;88(11):5056-60.
3. Anhalt GJ, Morrison LH. Bullous and cicatricial pemphigoid. J Autoimmun. 1991;4:17-35.
4. Arslanian SA. Type 2 diabetes mellitus in children: pathophysiology and risk factors. J Pediatr Endocrinol Metab. 2000;6:1385-94.
5. Basarab T, Dunnill MG, Munn SE, et al. Incontinentia pigmenti: variable disease expression within an affected family. J Eur Acad Dermatol Venereol. 1998;11(2):173-6.
6. Blaszczyk M, Jablonska S, Chorzelski TP, et al. Clinical relevance of immunologic findings in cutaneous lupus erythematosus. Clin Dermatol. 1992;10:399-496.
7. Brice SL, Huff JC, Weston WL. Erythema multiforme minor in children. Pediatrician. 1991;18:188-94.
8. Burgeson RE. Type VII collagen, anchoring fibrils, and epidermolysis bullosa. J Invest Dermatol. 1993;101:252-5.
9. Callen JP, Spencer LV, Burruss JB, et al. Azathioprine: An effective, corticosteroid-sparing therapy for patients with recalcitrant cutaneous lupus erythematosus or with recalcitrant cutaneous leukocytoclastic vasculitis. Arch Dermatol. 1991;127(4):515-22.
10. Cameli N, Picardo M, Pisani A, et al. Characterization of the nail matrix basement membrane zone: an immunohistochemical study of normal nails and of the nails in Herlitz junctional epidermolysis bullosa. Br J Dermatol. 1996;134(1):182-4.
11. Chan IS, Yancy KB, Hammerberg C, et al. Immune-mediated subepithelial blistering disease of mucous membrane. Arch Dermol. 1993;129:448-55.

12. Crawford EG, Burkes EJ, Briggaman RA. Hereditary epidermolysis bullosa: oral manifestations and dental therapy. Oral Surg Oral Med Oral Pathol. 1976;42:490-500.
13. D'Alise MD, Timmons CF, Swift DM. Focal dermal hypoplasia (Goltz syndrome) with vertebral solid aneurysmal bone cyst variant. A case report. Pediatr Neurosurg. 1996;24(3):151-4.
14. David-Bajar KM. Subacute cutaneous lupus erythematosus. J Invest Dermatol. 1993;100:2S-8S.
15. De Luca A, Terrone C, Tirri E. Vesical telangiectasias as a cause of macroscopic hematuria in systemic sclerosis. Clin Exp Rheumatol. 2001;19(1):93-4.
16. Eisen D. The clinical features, malignant potential, and systemic associations of oral lichen planus: a study of 723 patients. J Am Acad Dermatol. 2002;46(2):207-14.
17. Elder D, Elenitsas R, Jaworsky C, Johnson B (Eds). Lever's Histopathology of the Skin, 8th Edition. Philadelphia: Lippincott-Raven; 1998. p. 356.
18. Eversole IR Jacobsen PL, Stone CE. Oral and gingival changes in systemic sclerosis (scleroderma). J Periodontol. 1984;55:175-8.
19. Fagot-Campagna A, Pettitt DJ, Engelgau MM, et al. Type 2 diabetes among North American children and adolescents: an epidemiologic review and a public health perspective. J Pediatr. 2000;136(5):664-72.
20. Fine JD. Epidermolysis bullosa: Clinical aspects, pathology, and recent advances in research. Int J Dermatol. 1986;25:143-57.
21. George PM, Tunnessen WW. Childhood discoid lupus erythematosus. Arch Dermatol. 1993;129:613-7.
22. Gorsky M, Raviv E. Pemphigus vulgaris in adolescence. Oral Surg Oral Med Oral Pathol. 1994;77:620-2.
23. Haustein UF, Herrmann K, Bohme HJ. Pathogenesis of progressive systemic sclerosis. Int J Dermatol. 1986;25:286-93.
24. Hay KD, Reade PC. Spectrum of oral diseases induced by drugs and other bioactive agents. Current Therapeutics. 1983;24:81-103.
25. Jablonska S, Blaszczyk M. Sclerodema overlap syndromes. Adv Exp Med Biol. 1999;455:85-92.
26. Jablonska S, Blaszczyk-Kostanecka M, Chorzelski T, et al. The red face: lupus erythematosus. Clin Dermatol. 1993;11:253-60.
27. Koch P, Bahmer FA. Oral lesions and symptoms related to metals used in dental restorations: a clinical, allergological and histologic study. J Am Acad Dermatol. 1999;41(3 Pt 1):422-30.
28. Laman SD, Provost TT. Cutaneous manifestations of lupus erythematosus. Rheum Dis Clin North Am. 1994;20:195-212.
29. Lebbe C, Agbalika F. Pityriasisrosea and human herpesvirus 7, a true association? Dermatology. 1998;196(2):275.
30. Mutasim DF, Pelc NJ, Anhalt GJ. Cicatricial pemphigoid. Dermatol Clin. 1993;11:499-510.
31. Nicholls Ac, Valler D, Wallis S, et al. Homozygosity for a splice site mutation of the COLIA2 gene yields a non-functional pro(alpha)2(1) chain and an EDS/OI clinical phenotype. J Med Genet. 2001;38(2):132-6.
32. Norris DA, Pathomechanisms of photosensitive lupus erythematosus. J Invest Dermatol. 1993;100:58S-68S.
33. Porter SR, Kirby A, Olsen I, et al. Immunologic aspects of dermal and oral lichen planus: a review. Oral Surg Oral Med Oral Pathol Oral Radiol Endod. 1997;83(3):358-66.
34. Reichlin M. Progressive systemic sclerosis. Immunol Ser. 1991;54:275-87.
35. Rogers M. The "bar code phenomenon": a microscopic artefact seen in patients with hypohidrotic ectodermal dysplasia [letter]. Pediatr Dermatol. 2000;17(4):329-30.
36. Rook AH. Photopheresis in the treatment of autoimmune disease: experience with pemphigus vulgaris and systemic sclerosis. Ann N Y Acad Sci. 1991;636:209-16.
37. Roujeau JC. The spectrum of Stevens-Johnson syndrome and toxic epidermal necrolysis: a clinical classification. J Invest Dermatol. 1994;102:285-305.
38. Rowley AH, Shulman ST. Kawaski syndrome. Pediatr Clin North Am. 1999;46(2):313-29.
39. Schiodt M. Oral manifestations of lupus erythematosus. Int J Oral Surg. 1984;13:101-47.
40. Scully C, Beyli M, Ferreiro MC, et al. Update on oral lichen planus: etiopathogenesis and management. Crit Rev Oral Biol Med. 1998;9(1):86-122.

41. Sedano HO, Gorlin RJ. Epidermolysis bullosa. Oral Surg Oral Med Oral Pathol. 1989;67:555-65.
42. Shimizu H, Masunaga T, Ishiko A, et al. Autoantibodies from patients with cicatricialpemphigoid target different sites in epidermal basement membrane. J Invest Dermatol. 1995;104(3):370-3.
43. Stampien TM, Schwartz RA. Erythema multiforme. Am Fam Physician. 1992;46:1171-6.
44. Swaak AJ, Nossent JC, Smeenk RJ. Systemic lupus erythematosus. Int J Clin Lab Res. 1992;22:190-5.
45. Tsubota K, Satake Y, Kaido M, et al. Treatment of severe ocular-surface disorders with corneal epithelial stem-cell transplantation. N Engl J Med. 1999;340(22):1697-703.
46. Valdimarson H, Sigmundsdottir H, Jonsdottir I. Is psoriasis induced by streptococcal superantigens and maintained by M-protein-specific T cells that cross-react with keratin? Clin Exp Immunol. 1997;107 Suppl 1:21-4.
47. Weiss E, Schmidberger H, Jany R, et al. Palliative radiotherapy of mucocutaneous lesions in malignant acanthosis nigricans. Acta Oncol. 1995;34(2):265-7.
48. Williams, DM. Vesiculobullous mucocutaneous disease: Pemphigus vulgaris. J Oral Pathol Med.1989;18:544-53.
49. Wright JT, Fine JD, Johnson LB. Oral soft tissue in hereditary epidermolysis bullosa. Oral Surg Oral Med Oral Pathol.1991;71:440-6.
50. Yaghmai R, Kimyai-Asadi A, Rostamiani K, et al. Overlap of dyskeratosis congenital with the Hoyeraal-Hreidarsson syndrome. J Pediatr. 2000;136(3):390-3.
51. Yeh JS, Munn SE, Plunkett TA, et al. Coexistence of acanthosis nigricans and the sign of Leser-Trelat in a patient with gastric adenocarcinoma: a case report and literature review. J Am Acad Dermatol. 2000;42(2 Pt 2): 357-62.

CHAPTER 20

Diseases of the Nerves and Muscles

The different types of pain in the orofacial region are described in Box 20.1.

DISEASES OF THE NERVES

■ TRIGEMINAL NEURALGIA

Neuralgia can be defined as the pain along the distribution of nerves; and trigeminal neuralgia refers to an excruciating and often frightening painful disease, characterized by sudden, unilateral, brief, stabbing or lancinating type of recurring pain along the distribution of one or more branches of the trigeminal nerve.

Box 20.1	Different types of pain in the orofacial region.

A. *Pain in the teeth and supporting structures*
   - Pulpitis
   - Fracture of tooth
   - Cracked tooth syndrome
   - Apical periodontitis
   - Acute periapical abscess
   - Pericoronitis
   - Lateral periodontal abscess
   - HIV-associated periodontitis
   - Acute necrotizing ulcerative gingivitis

B. *Pain in the jaws*
   - Fractures
   - Osteomyelitis
   - Infected cyst
   - Osteoradionecrosis, malignant neoplasms
   - Sickle cell infarcts

C. *Pain in edentulous patients*
   - Trauma from denture

Contd...

Contd...
   - Mucosal disease below the denture
   - Jaw pathology
   - Glossodynia
   - Impacted tooth
   - Broken root of tooth erupting under the denture
   - Excessive vertical height of denture

D. *Postoperative pain*
   - Dry socket
   - Aerodontalgia
   - Fracture of jaw
   - Damage of temporomandibular joint
   - Postoperative osteomyelitis
   - Damage to the nerve during treatment

E. *Neurological pain*
   - Trigeminal neuralgia
   - Herpes zoster
   - Multiple sclerosis
   - Postherpetic neuralgia
   - Migrainous neuralgia
   - Causalgia
   - Intracranial tumors
   - Bell's palsy
   - Glossopharyngeal neuralgia

F. *Pain from extraoral sources*
   - Maxillary sinusitis
   - Meningitis
   - Carcinoma in maxillary antrum
   - Acute parotitis
   - Salivary calculi
   - Sjogren's syndrome
   - Malignant neoplasm of salivary gland
   - Otitis media
   - Cavernous sinus thrombosis
   - Myocardial infarction
   - Myofascial pain dysfunction syndrome (MPD)

G. *Psychological pain*
   - Atypical (psychogenic) facial pain
   - Burning mouth syndrome (BMS)

This is the most common neuralgia or nerve pain disorder and of the three branches of trigeminal nerve (ophthalmic, maxillary, and mandibular), the maxillary and mandibular branches are almost exclusively affected in trigeminal neuralgia.

Etiology or Risk Factors

- Mostly idiopathic
- Family history
- Traumatic compression of the nerve resulting in demyelination
- Biochemical change in the nerve cells
- Abnormal blood vessel causing compression of the nerve at the point exit from the cranial foramen
- Multiple sclerosis
- Hypertension
- Female gender.

Clinical Features

- This condition often causes severe, unilateral, and "lancinating" type of pain in the orofacial region that is usually radiating in nature.
- The disease usually occurs among middle-aged people (40–60 years of age) and it occurs more in females than males.
- Most of the patients give the history of excruciating pain attacks, which feels like sharp stabbing or like an electric shock.
- The most interesting characteristic of pain in trigeminal neuralgia is that it lasts for only a few seconds or minutes and then disappears promptly. Between the attacks, the people are relatively pain free.
- Presence of the "trigger zone" is a definitive indicator of trigeminal neuralgia; these are specific zones or areas on the facial surface, which triggers severe pain as the patient touches or gives pressure on them.
- Trigger zones may also get stimulated and the pain might start while washing the face, toothbrushing, talking, eating, chewing, smiling, shaving, or even if a strong wind or breeze touches the face (Box 20.2).

Box 20.2 Major triggers of trigeminal neuralgia.
- Eating, talking, chewing, and swallowing
- Stress and tiredness
- Touching, shaving, and laughing
- Brushing and cleaning teeth
- Strong breeze, hot and cold weather and rain
- Tilting or bending head

- Often the people with trigeminal neuralgia remain panicked as the sharp intermittent pain interferes with common daily activities, e.g. eating, talking, shaving, etc.
- Patients are often scared of taking foods or drinks because of the fear of unpredictable horrific pain. Many of them suffer from insomnia, irritability, anticipatory anxiety, depression, etc. and even suicidal tendency is also not uncommon.
- The pain in trigeminal neuralgia may also produce spasmodic contractions of the facial muscles and because of this characteristic muscle spasms, the condition is also called "tic douloureux".
- The pain may involve any part of the face on either side, depending upon which branch of the trigeminal nerve is affected. Generally, maxillary branch is more often affected than the mandibular branch (ophthalmic branch is least affected).
- If maxillary branch is involved, the pain occurs in the cheekbone, entire nose, upper lips and teeth of upper jaw. Whereas, if mandibular nerve is involved, the pain occurs in lower cheek, lower lip, lower teeth, and jaw.
- However, right side of the face is affected more frequently than the left side and it rarely crosses the midline.
- Surprisingly, there is no detectable disease or pathology present in the jaw in patients with trigeminal neuralgia (Box 20.3).

Histopathological Findings

In trigeminal neuralgia, focal areas of myelin degeneration can be seen within the Gasserian ganglion or along the course of the nerve.

| Box 20.3 | Clinical features of trigeminal neuralgia can be described in the name of Greek philosopher Socrates. |

- *S-site*—Unilateral facial pain
- *O-onset*—Sudden onset
- *C-characteristic*—Electric shock like lancinating and superficial pain
- *R-Radiating pain*—Radiate from the angle of mouth to:
  - *Ear*—Involving mandibular division
  - *Eye*—Involving maxillary division
  - *Nostril*—Involving ophthalmic division
- *A*—Associated with spasticity, wincing, tic douloureux
- *T-Time*—Lasts for few seconds to 1–2 minutes
- *E-Exacerbating factor*—Spontaneous, smiling, eating, chewing, swallowing, touch, face washing, face makeup, toothbrushing, kissing
- *S-Severity*—Severe pain

Laboratory Diagnosis

- History of the patient and absence of neurological findings usually establish the diagnosis beyond doubt.
- Magnetic resonance imaging (MRI) may be suggested for detection of any space occupying lesion or any large vessel compressing the nerve root.
- Computed tomography (CT) scan and MRI of the head and neck region are also advised to rule out suspected brain tumor, meningitis, or any other neurological abnormality.

Key Points of Trigeminal Neuralgia

- Trigeminal neuralgia refers to severe, excruciating pain along the distribution of any branch of trigeminal nerve on one side of the face.
- The "lancinating" or excruciating pain in trigeminal neuralgia lasts for only a few seconds or minutes and then promptly disappears.
- Often the burst of pain attacks are precipitated by touching some "trigger zone" on the face. Presence of this trigger zone is a definitive indicator of trigeminal neuralgia.
- The trigger zones on the face may get stimulated by any of the common actions, e.g. washing the face, toothbrushing, talking, eating, chewing, smiling, shaving, etc.
- The disease occurs more frequently among middle-aged females and maxillary or mandibular branch of the trigeminal nerve is often involved.
- Pain in trigeminal neuralgia often characteristically produces spasmodic contractions of the facial muscles.

Differential Diagnosis

- Multiple sclerosis
- Migraine
- Glossopharyngeal neuralgia
- Myofascial pain
- Cluster headache
- Temporomandibular joint disorder
- Intracranial hemorrhage
- Acute pulpitis.

Treatment

Trigeminal neuralgia can be treated by the following methods:

- Peripheral neurectomy
- Injection of alcohol or boiling water into the Gasserian ganglion
- Injection of steroid or anesthetic in the ganglion
- Electrocoagulation of the same ganglion
- Administration of carbamazepines, methylcobalamin (vitamin B12) and benzodiazepines. etc.
- A recent treatment called microsurgical decompression of trigeminal root being tried with good results.

■ SPHENOPALATINE NEURALGIA

Sphenopalatine neuralgia is a distinctive syndrome of headache, characterized by a unilateral radiating pain in the region of the eye, maxilla, ears, teeth, cheek, nose, etc.

Types

There are two types of sphenopalatine neuralgia:
1. Episodic
2. Chronic.

Clinical Presentation

- The pain begins very rapidly; it persists for few minutes to few hours and then disappears.
- Generally, 1–3 short attacks of pain occur in a day.
- The condition often simulates toothache, however, unlike the trigeminal neuralgia, no "trigger zone" is present in this case.
- Sphenopalatine neuralgia occurs more frequently among females and sometimes it may be associated with other symptoms like sneezing, nasal discharges and watering of the eyes, etc.
- Interestingly, in some patients, the onset of pain is exactly at the same time every day and hence, it is referred to as the "alarm clock" headache.

GLOSSODYNIA AND GLOSSOPYROSIS

Glossodynia refers to the painful tongue, while glossopyrosis means burning sensation of the tongue.

Etiology of Glossodynia and Glossopyrosis

- Vitamin deficiency
- Anemia (especially pernicious anemia)
- Hormonal disorder, e.g. diabetes and hypothyroidism
- Xerostomia
- Gastrointestinal disturbances (hyper- or hypoacidity)
- Psychogenic factor, e.g. cancer phobia, chronic anxiety, and depression
- Trigeminal neuralgia
- Referred pain from tooth
- Angioneurotic edema
- Heavy metal poisoning, e.g. mercurialism
- Moeller's glossitis
- Postmenopausal syndrome
- Oral thrush
- Cervical nerve injury.

Clinical Features

- Glossodynia usually occurs among the middle-aged or elderly people, mostly among females.
- The sensations which are commonly encountered in this disease are pain and burning, itching or stinging sensations of the mucous membrane covering the tongue.
- However, in glossodynia, the tongue appears normal and, clinically, there are no apparent lesions, e.g. discoloration or ulcerations, which can precipitate the symptoms.
- The pain is low or absent during morning, however, it gradually builds up as the day progresses.

Treatment

Topical anesthetics, analgesics, muscle relaxants and sedatives, etc. are given in case of glossodynia, although permanent remission is difficult to achieve. Low doses of benzodiazepines, tricyclic antidepressants, or anticonvulsants may also be effective.

AURICULOTEMPORAL SYNDROME (FREY'S SYNDROME)

Frey's syndrome occurs due to anomalous repair of the damaged auriculotemporal nerve following injury, which results in the innervations of sweat glands by the parasympathetic salivary fibers.

The patients with this syndrome typically exhibit flushing and sweating in the temporal area during meals. Moreover, this can happen even when the patient sees or thinks or talks about certain foods that cause increased salivation. The condition usually occurs following the surgical procedures like removal of the parotid gland or resection of the ramus of mandible, etc.

GLOSSOPHARYNGEAL NEURALGIA

Glossopharyngeal is the 9th (ninth) cranial nerve, which supplies the pharynx, throat muscles, tonsils, and tongue. Glossopharyngeal neuralgia manifests itself by repeated episodes of sharp, shooting pain in the throat, ear, tonsillar area and the posterior part of the tongue, etc.

Triggering Factors
- Chewing
- Coughing
- Talking
- Swallowing
- Laughing.

Etiology
The exact etiology of this syndrome is not clearly known and the probable initiating factors could be the following—abnormal blood vessels pressing down on glossopharyngeal nerve, growth at the base of the skull, and tumor or infection in the mouth, etc.

Clinical Features
The intensity of pain is nearly similar to that of trigeminal neuralgia and often there is a "trigger zone" present in the tonsillar fossa region. Glossopharyngeal neuralgia mostly affects the older individuals; the pain occurs unilaterally, lasts for few seconds to few minutes. Frequency of the pain often varies; it can repeat 5–10 times every hour and may continue for weeks or months. Patients pulse is often slow, and fainting may occur if the pain is severe.

There are two types of glossopharyngeal neuralgia:
1. Pharyngeal type
2. Tympanic type.

Pharyngeal type of glossopharyngeal neuralgia: Causes pain in the pharynx and posterior tongue, which radiates to the ear, eyes and maxilla, etc.

Tympanic type of glossopharyngeal neuralgia: Pain occurs along the distribution of the tympanic branch of glossopharyngeal nerve and causes pain in the ear (tympanic membrane).

BELL'S PALSY (FACIAL NERVE PARALYSIS)

Bell's palsy refers to the paralysis of facial nerve resulting in inability to control the facial muscles on the affected side of the face. The condition is named after Scottish anatomist Charles Bell who first described it.

Functions of Facial Nerve
- Blinking, closing eyes, smiling, frowning, lacrimation, salivation, and perception of taste.

Etiology of Bell's Palsy
The disease may be precipitated by the following conditions:
- Change in the atmospheric pressure, e.g. while flying or diving, etc.
- Malignant tumors of the parotid gland and brain
- Stroke, meningitis, head injury, multiple sclerosis, and lyme disease
- Surgical procedures in the parotid region
- Infections, e.g. acute otitis media and herpes simplex virus infection
- Melkersson–Rosenthal syndrome
- Exposure to cold (often cold breeze hitting one side of face through open car window)
- Following incorrect pterygomandibular block anesthesia
- Ischemic damage of the facial nerve.

Clinical Features (Figs. 20.1A and B)
- Bell's palsy commonly affects the middle-aged females and mostly the condition occurs unilaterally.
- The paralysis is often rapidly progressing and it can be either complete or partial.
- The patient cannot close the eye on the affected side due to loss of muscle control,

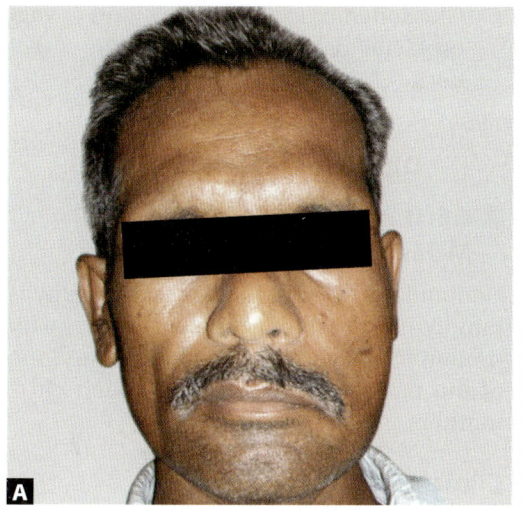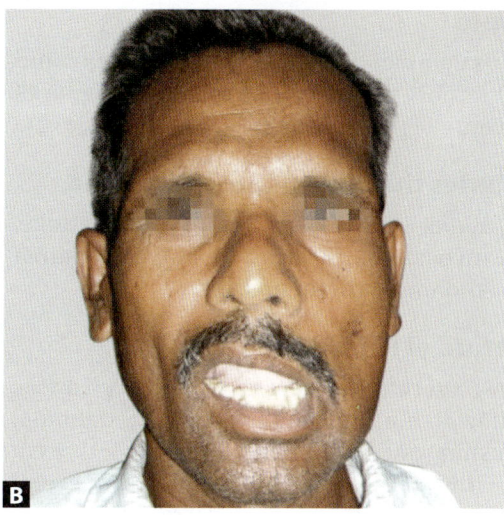

Figs. 20.1A and B: Bell's palsy.

which results in irritation in the eye with constant watering. If the eye remains open for long, conjunctival dryness and ulceration may occur.
- Change in facial appearance due to drooping of corner of the mouth on the affected side due to loss of control over the facial muscles.
- The corner of the mouth on the affected side does not raise during smile and this gives the patient a typical "mask-like" expressionless appearance.
- Loss of facial muscle function also cause constant drooling (uncontrolled drop of saliva) from the corner of the mouth.
- Most of the patients complain of difficulty in speech (they have a slurred speech), difficulty in taking foods and there may be even loss of taste sensations.
- The patients cannot raise their eyebrows and there is no wrinkle formation in their forehead.
- Bell's palsy patients fail to blow whistles by their mouth when they try (Box 20.4).
- Recurrent attacks of Bell's palsy can be associated with "Melkersson–Rosenthal syndrome", which also have other features like cheilitis granulomatosa, fissured tongue and edema of the face, etc.

Treatment

There is no specific treatment for Bell's palsy. Administration of histamine or nicotinic acid has been beneficial in some cases. Physiotherapy is also helpful in some patients. The eye on the involved side has to be protected from infections by using protective glasses, eye drops, ointments, etc.

CAUSALGIA

Causalgia refers to the burning pain in the area of previous injury or surgical procedures, which results from damage to the peripheral nerve. In the oral cavity, it can occur following tooth extraction.

Criteria of Causalgia

- Pain is spontaneous, severe, and persistent.
- It should be present for at least 5 weeks.
- Pain should be felt distal to the proximal nerve injury.

Types

Causalgia can be of two types—(1) major and (2) minor; the difference is in the degree of severity of pain.

Injuries that Might Cause Causalgia

- Bullet injury, head injury, polio, stroke, myocardial infarction, surgical trauma and tooth extractions, etc.

Nature of Pain in Causalgia

The pain can be of several types, which are as follows--burning, tingling, searing, stabbing, crushing and lightening, etc.

The pain arises within a few days to several weeks after the tooth extraction, although the oral wound has already been completely healed up by that time. Pain in causalgia is most commonly felt in the limbs.

Factors Precipitating the Pain in Causalgia

- Emotional stress, visual stimulation, auditory stimulation, and physical stimulation.

■ EAGLE'S SYNDROME

The "Eagle's syndrome complex" was first described by Eagle and hence it is called Eagle's syndrome. It is characterized by the following features:

- Elongation of the styloid process or ossification of the styloid ligament causing dysphagia and pain in the throat, pharynx and ear, etc.

Box 20.4	Common Causes of Paresthesia or Anesthesia of the Lip
- Inferior alveolar nerve block - Injury or fracture of the jaw - Acute osteomyelitis - Malignant or metastatic tumor of mandible - Exposed mental foramen - Herpes zoster - Multiple sclerosis - Tetany	

- Glossodynia, headache and vague orofacial pain and pain on the side of neck.

DISEASE OF THE MUSCLES

■ GENERALIZED FAMILIAL MUSCULAR DYSTROPHY

Generalized familial muscular dystrophy is a rapidly progressing muscular disease, which predominantly affects the children and most of the patients are the sons of their carrier mothers.

Clinical Features

- The earliest manifestation of the disease is inability of the child to stand, run or walk even after attaining a standard age.
- Most of the kids fall rapidly while making an attempt to stand or walk by themselves and this happens due to the weakness of the muscles of extremities.
- In severe cases, all the muscles of the body including those of the facial, masticatory or ocular groups become involved.
- In generalized familial muscular dystrophy, most of the patients die by the age of 20 years due to pulmonary infections related to the respiratory muscle weaknesses.

Oral Manifestations

- Malocclusion
- Open-bite or cross-bite
- Macroglossia
- Expanded dental arch.

Histopathology

Histologically, the involved muscles reveal gradual loss of muscle fibers, which are replaced by connective tissue or fat.

Laboratory Diagnosis

Elevation of serum creatine kinase is a significant laboratory finding.

Treatment
There is no satisfactory treatment for this disease.

MYASTHENIA GRAVIS
Myasthenia gravis is one of the best known autoimmune diseases, in which antibodies are produced against acetylcholine receptors of the muscle end plate of the neuromuscular junctions. This results in an impairment of acetylcholine signal transmissions across the neuromuscular junction, thereby causing muscle weaknesses and pronounced fatigability. In some cases, antibodies are formed against muscle specific tyrosine-kinase protein (MuSK protein), which regulates the concentration of cholinergic receptor or neuromuscular junction.

Clinical Features
- *Age group*: Bimodal age distribution. In younger patients, females are more than males, and in older patients, males are more than females.
- This disease commonly affects middle-aged females.
- The patients often experience difficulty in mastication and deglutition.
- Dropping of the jaw, slurring of speech, loss of taste sensation, and dysphagia.
- Limited facial expression (lost smile).
- Dry mouth along with ulceration of the tongue, buccal mucosa, and palate.
- Dropping of head, diplopia, ptosis, weight loss, and exhaustion.
- Atypical facial pain and candidiasis.
- Hyperplasia of thyroid gland and waddling gait.
- Many patients die of respiratory failure but few patients survive and lead a relatively normal life.
- Younger female patients of myasthenia gravis usually have thymic hyperplasia whereas thymoma is more common in older patients.

Abnormal conditions with which myasthenia gravis is often associated are
- Systemic lupus erythematosus
- Sjogren's syndrome
- Progressive systemic sclerosis.

Treatment
Intramuscular administrations of physostigmine improve the strength of the affected muscles readily, but the remission is temporary.

MYOSITIS OSSIFICANS
Myositis means inflammation and degradation of the muscles. Myositis ossificans is a skeletal muscle disease of unknown etiology, which is characterized by the formation of bone (calcification) and connective tissues within the muscles.

Types
- *Nonhereditary type*: This is the common type, in which ossification occurs following injury.
- *Hereditary type*: It is known as myositis ossificans progressive and in this type, the ossification occurs without injury.

Ossifications of the muscle may occur following an inflammatory process and the disease can involve either a single muscle (focal) or the entire group of muscles (generalized).

Clinical Features
- Myositis ossificans occurs frequently among children and young adults.
- Most patients develop a single or multiple, soft, fluctuant or firm, nodular, painless swellings on the body, which often arise following trauma to the affected area.
- In the later stages, some of the nodules disappear while the remaining nodules become bony hard and they often exhibit an overlying red skin.
- The condition can be painful especially when the affected muscle is used for any work.

- In the orofacial region, the masseter muscle is often affected by this disease, which results in trismus and difficulty in food intake.
- Eventually, the entire group of muscles in the body becomes ossified and this transforms the patient into a rigid organism.
- In many cases, the abnormal bone within the muscle becomes resorbed spontaneously.

Treatment

There is no treatment possible for this disease; surgical treatment has limited success.

BIBLIOGRAPHY

1. Anniversary special issue, on 102nd birth anniversary celebration of R. Ahmed; West Bengal state Dental journal; 2013.
2. Argoff CE. A focused review on the use of botulinum toxin for neuropathic pain. Clin J Pain. 2002;18(6 Suppl):S177-81.
3. Ash Jr M. Oral Pathology, 6th edition. Philadelphia: Lea and Febiger; 1992.
4. Banovac K. The effect of etidronate on late development of heterotopic ossification after spinal cord injury. J Spinal Cord Med. 2000;23(1):40-4.
5. Buchanan J, Zakrzewska J. Burning mouth syndrome. Clin Evid. 2002;(7):1239-43.
6. Callen JP. Relation between dermatomyositis and polymyositis and cancer. Lancet. 2001;357(9250):85-6.
7. Cawson RA. Oral Pathology and Diagnosis—Color Atlas with Integrated Text, 1st edition. Philadelphia: Saunders; 1987.
8. Cepeda MS. Defining the therapeutic role of local anesthetic blockade in complex regional pain syndrome. A narrative and systematic review. Clin J Pain. 2002;18(4):216-33.
9. Edlich RF, Hammarskjold M. Multiple Sclerosis. In: Tintinalli JE (Ed). Emergency Medicine. New York: McGraw-Hill; 1997.
10. Ellerin BE, Helfet D, Parikh S, et al. Current therapy in the management of heterotopic ossification of the elbow: a review with case studies. Am J Phys Med Rehabil. 1999;78(3):259-71.
11. Eversole LR. Clinical Outline of Oral Pathology: Diagnosis and Treatment. Shelton, CT: People's Medical Publishing House-USA; 2011.
12. Goaz PW. Oral Radiology: Principles and Interpretations. St. Louis: Mosby; 1987.
13. Hill CL, Zhang Y, Sigurgeirsson B. Frequency of specific cancer types in dermatomyositis and polymyositis: A population-based study. Lancet. 2001;357(9250):96-100.
14. Jackson EM, Bussard GM, Hoard MA, et al. Trigeminal neuralgia: A diagnostic challenge. Am J Emerge Med. 1999;17(6):597-600.
15. John Macleod. Davidson's Principles and Practice of Medicine, 14th edition. Edinburgh: Churchill Livingstone; 1984.
16. Kemler MA, Rijks CP, De Vet HC. Which patients with chronic reflex sympathetic dystrophy are most likely to benefit from physical therapy? J Manipulative Physiol Ther. 2001;24(4):272-8.
17. Lynch MA, Brightman VJ, Greenberg MS. Burket's Oral Medicine-Diagnosis and Treatment, 9th edition. Philadelphia: Lippincott Williams & Wilkins; 1994.
18. Mendizabal JE, Umana E, Zweifler RM. Cluster Headache: Horton's Cephalalgia Revisited. South Med J. 1998;91:606-17.
19. Ogutcen-Toller M, Uzun E, Incesu L. Clinical and magnetic resonance imaging evaluation of facial pain. Oral Surg Oral Med Oral Pathol Oral Radiol Endod. 2004;97(5):652-8.
20. Prabhu SR, Daftary DK, Johnson NW. Oral Diseases in the Tropic. New York: Oxford University Press; 1992.
21. PRISMS Study Group. Randomised, double-blind, placebo-controlled study of interferon [beta] -1a in relapsing/remitting multiple sclerosis (Abstract). Lancet. 1998;352:1498-504.
22. Regezi JA, Sciubba JJ, Jordan R. Oral Pathology: Clinical Pathologic Correlations. St. Louis: Saunders; 2016.
23. Sapp PJ, Eversole LR, Wysocki JP. Contemporary Oral and Maxillofacial Pathology. St. Louis: Mosby; 2004.
24. Scala A, Checchi L, Montevecchi M, et al. Update on burning mouth syndrome: overview and patient management. Crit Rev Oral Biol Med. 2003;14(4):275-91.
25. Shafer WG, Hine MK, Levy BM. A Textbook of Oral Pathology, 4th edition. St. Louis: WB Saunders Co.; 1983.

26. Shear M. Cysts of the Oral Region, 3rd edition. Oxford: Wright; 1992.
27. Soames JV, Southam JC. Oral Pathology, 3rd Edition. New York: Oxford University Press; 1998.
28. Tencate AR. Oral Histology: Development, Structure, and Function, 3rd edition. Ontario, Canada: Mosby; 1989.
29. The Lippincott Manual of Nursing Practice, 2nd edition. Philadelphia: JB Lippincott Company; 1978.
30. Wood NK, Goaz PW. Differential Diagnosis of Oral Lesions, 4th edition. St. Louis: C.V. Mosby; 1991.
31. Zvartau-Hind M, Din MU, Gilani A, et al. Topiramate relieves refractory trigeminal neuralgia in MS patients. Neurology. 2000;55(10):1587-8.

CHAPTER 21

Oral Manifestations of Generalized Diseases

VITAMIN DEFICIENCIES (TABLE 21.1)

Table 21.1: Signs and symptoms of vitamin deficiencies.

Name of the disease	Important oral manifestations
Vitamin A deficiency	Hyperkeratosis of oral epithelium, decreased salivary flow and dryness of mouth
Hypervitaminosis A	Cortical thickening of bone, mucosal pigmentations, hemorrhages, retardation of growth
Vitamin B$_1$ (Thiamine) deficiency	Edema of the tongue, loss of papillae, pain and paresthesia
Niacin deficiency	Stomatitis and bleeding in the oral mucosa, glossitis and Sandwith's bald tongue (red, smooth and raw tongue)
Riboflavin deficiency	Reddening and inflammation of tongue with cyanosis and ulceration (magenta glossitis), angular cheilitis, sore throat, swelling and erythema of oral mucosa
Nicotinamide deficiency	Glossitis, stomatitis and gingivitis
Vitamin B$_{12}$ deficiency	Glossitis, aphthous ulcer
Pyridoxine deficiency	Cheilitis and glossitis
Folic acid deficiency	Glossitis, aphthous ulcer
Vitamin C deficiency	Widespread petechiae and ecchymosis of the oral mucosa along with hyperemia, edema and ulceration. Generalized enlargement of gingiva with spontaneous bleeding. Severe periodontal inflammation, alveolar bone loss, tooth mobility and premature loss of teeth. Failure of wound healing
Vitamin D deficiency	Delayed tooth eruption, malpositioning of teeth, retardation of mandibular growth, development of class II malocclusion. Increased susceptibility to jaw fracture due to minimum injury
Vitamin K deficiency	Increased gingival bleeding, lack of blood coagulation after surgery

Contd...

IMPORTANT CAUSES OF LYMPHADENOPATHY (TABLE 21.2)

Table 21.2: Causes of lymphadenopathy.

Infections	Neoplasms
Bacterial infections: • Oral, tonsil, face and scalp • Tuberculosis • Syphilis • Cat-scratch disease • Lyme disease	*Primary:* • Hodgkin's disease • Non-Hodgkin's lymphoma • Leukemia
Viral infection: • Herpetic stomatitis • Infectious mononucleosis • HIV infections	*Secondary:* • Carcinoma of oral, salivary gland and nasopharyngeal • Malignant melanoma

Contd...

Infections	Neoplasms
	• Mesenchymal tissue neoplasms
Parasitic infections: • Toxoplasmosis	*Miscellaneous conditions:* • Sarcoidosis • Drug reactions • Connective tissue diseases

BLOOD DYSCRASIAS (TABLE 21.3)

Table 21.3: Oral manifestations due to blood dyscrasias.

Name of the disease	Important oral manifestations
Leukemias	Enlargement, bleeding and necrosis of gingiva, ecchymosis, necrosis and ulceration of oral mucosa, profuse bleeding upon trauma or following extraction of tooth.
Agranulocytosis	Gangrenous ulceration of the gingiva, buccal mucosa, soft palate and lip. Delayed wound healing. Severe secondary infections.
Polycythemia	Petechiae, ecchymosis, hematoma formation and ulceration of the mucosa, gingiva and tongue. Spontaneous gingival bleeding. Purplish red discoloration of tongue, cheek and lips.
Multiple myeloma	Pain and swelling of the jaw, numbness of the lips, multiple punched-out radiolucencies in the jaw bone, formation of epulis and unexplained mobility of teeth.
Iron deficiency anemia	Mucosal atrophy and pallor, bald tongue with atrophic glossitis. Angular cheilitis, glossodynia and increased risk of candidiasis.
Plummer–Vinson's syndrome	It is a rare condition characterized by iron deficiency anemia, dysphagia and glossitis. Other features of the disease include atrophy of the tongue papilla with smooth red surface, glossodynia, increased risk of oral precancer and cancer, angular cheilitis and difficulty in wearing prosthesis.
Pernicious anemia	Erythematous oral mucosa with burning sensation, beefy red tongue with depapillation (Hunter's glossitis), focal areas of atypical mucosal erythema.
Folic acid deficiency anemia	Depapillation of tongue with glossitis and glossodynia, aphthous-like ulceration.
Aplastic anemia	Purpura, spontaneous gingival bleeding, ulceration and bad breath, etc. Severe mucosal pallor.
Erythroblastosis fetalis	Black, brown or bluish pigmentations of teeth, protrusion of upper teeth, osteoporosis of bone, thinning of lamina dura.
Thalassemia	Protrusion of upper teeth, osteoporosis of bone, thinning of lamina dura, prominent premaxilla and cheek bone, Mongoloid facies.
Sickle cell anemia	Mucosal pallor, "stepladder-like" arrangement of bony trabeculae between the roots of the teeth, pain in the mandible with lip paresthesia. Osteoporosis of the jaw bone including the alveolar bone.
Purpura	Gingival bleeding, petechiae and ecchymosis.
Hemophilia	Petechiae, hemarthrosis, excessive bleeding upon trauma or extraction of tooth.
Hereditary hemorrhagic telangiectasia	Cherry red, pin-point or large lesions resembling a crushed spider in the mucosa. The lesion blanches on pressure.

METABOLIC DISORDERS (TABLE 21.4)

Table 21.4: Oral manifestations due to metabolic disorders.

Name of the disease	Important oral manifestations
Diabetes mellitus	Severe periodontitis with loosening of teeth, gingivitis and painful gingiva, burning mouth syndrome, delayed wound healing, mucosal ulceration, acetone breath, increased risk of infection, bilateral non-tendered enlargement of parotids (diabetic sialadenitis), xerostomia, gingival hyperplasia, candidiasis and atrophy of tongue papillae.
Amyloidosis	Macroglossia with smooth, brawny and indurated tongue, localized, yellow, nonulcerated nodules on the oral mucosa. Hoarseness of voice, dry mouth, claudication of the jaw, petechiae and ecchymosis of the oral mucosa.
Hurler's syndrome	Short and broad mandible, coarse lips, delayed eruption of teeth, multiple radiolucencies in the jaw bone, diastema, hyperplastic dental follicles.
Jaundice	Icterus (diffuse yellow pigmentation) of the palatal and sublingual area.
Hypophosphatesia	Premature loss of primary teeth, especially deciduous incisors. Delayed eruption of permanent teeth, premature loss of permanent teeth, thin cortex and lamina-dura of bone, decreased enamel thickness and large pulp size of tooth.
Hypophosphatemia	Bone pain, muscle weakness, poorly formed teeth, large pulp chambers of teeth with pulp horns extending up to the dentino-enamel junction, increased incidences of periodontal and periapical abscess formation with sinus tract. Deformity of tooth enamel with microclefts helps in early pulp exposure.
Protein-energy malnutrition	Oral mucosal pallor, atrophy of the tongue papilla, enamel hypoplasia, glossitis, angular cheilitis, generalized stomatitis, fissuring of lips, delayed wound healing.
Chronic alcoholism	Inflammatory gingival lesion with bleeding tendency.
Chronic steroid therapy	Obesity of the upper part of the body, "buffalo-hump" or round shouldered person, mooning of the face, secondary oral infections due to depressed immunity, osteoporosis.
Uremic stomatitis	It occurs due to renal failure and is characterized by development of multiple ragged white plaques on the buccal mucosa, tongue and floor of the mouth. Unpleasant taste in the mouth, oral burning sensation and odor of ammonia or urine in the mouth.

HEAVY METAL POISONING (TABLE 21.5)

Table 21.5: Oral manifestations due to heavy metal poisoning.

Name of the metal	Oral manifestations
Arsenic	Vomiting, diarrhea, hyperpigmentation, hyperkeratosis of oral mucosa
Lead	Excessive salivation, metallic taste and a dark lead line along the gingival margin

Contd...

Contd...

Name of the metal	Oral manifestations
Bismuth	Burning sensations of the oral mucosa, metallic taste and a bismuth line (similar to lead line) along the gingival margin
Mercury	Stomatitis, increased salivation, glossitis and enlargement of salivary glands
Phosphorus	Progressive osteomyelitis of the jaws
Silver-amalgam	Gray-black discoloration of the oral mucosa
Graphite	Gray-black mucosal color change
Lead-mercury	Gray oral mucosa

■ ENDOCRINE DISTURBANCES (TABLE 21.6)

Table 21.6: Important oral manifestations of endocrine disturbances.

Name of the disease	Important oral manifestations
Pituitary gigantism	Enlargement of jaw bone, enlargement of oral soft tissues, increased vertical height of jaw bone, macroglossia, true macrodontia, early eruption of teeth and hypercementosis, etc.
Pituitary dwarfism	Underdeveloped face and jaws, delayed shedding of primary teeth and delayed eruption of permanent teeth, delayed root completion of teeth, microdontia and absence of third molars
Acromegaly	Increased mandibular growth with development of class-III malocclusion, diastemas, anterior open bite, increased soft tissue growth with macroglossia, periodontitis, gingivitis and hypercementosis, etc.
Cushing's syndrome	Mooning of the face (face becomes round due to excessive deposition of fat within the facial tissues),

Contd...

Contd...

Name of the disease	Important oral manifestations
	osteoporosis of bone, loss of lamina dura, increased risk of infection due to lowered immunity, increased incidences of pathological fractures of bone
Hypoparathyroidism	Hypocalcemia, tetany, delayed eruption of teeth, pitting enamel hypoplasia, extensive bone resorptions. Positive Chvostek's sign and persistent oral candidiasis
Hyperparathyroidism	Loosening of teeth, *brown tumors in the jaws*, loss of lamina dura, radiograph shows ground glass appearance of the bone (due to severely decreased bone density) and multicystic jaw lesions, bone and joint pain, peptic ulcer, hypercalcemia, renal calculi. Massive enlargement of jaw
Imbalance of sex hormones	*Puberty*—puberty gingivitis
	Menstruation—gingivitis, cyclical ulceration of the oral mucosa, gingival bleeding
	Menopause—dry mouth, burning tongue
Pregnancy	Gingival bleeding, pregnancy tumor (epulis)
	Aggravated gingivitis, recurrent aphthous ulcer
	Vomiting, hypo- or hypertension
Addison's disease	Yellow to brown pigmentations of oral mucous membrane due to increased melanin production
Hyperthyroidism	Premature eruption of teeth and loss of deciduous dentition, osteoporosis of the jaw bones

Contd...

Contd...

Name of the disease	Important oral manifestations
Cretinism	Retarded tooth eruption or complete failure of tooth eruption, delayed exfoliation of deciduous teeth, malocclusion, macroglossia, macrocheilia, drooling of saliva, delayed closure of bony sutures, etc.
Myxedema	Thick lips, macroglossia and swollen face

■ GRANULOMATOUS DISEASES (TABLE 21.7)

Table 21.7: Important oral manifestations due to granulomatous diseases.

Name of the disease	Important oral manifestations
Syphilis	Oral chancres in primary syphilis, *mucous patches* in secondary syphilis, *gumma* in tertiary syphilis and *Hutchinson's triad* in congenital syphilis
Tuberculosis	Oral tuberculous ulcer, tuberculous gingivitis, and osteomyelitis, scrofula
Sarcoidosis	Enlargement of salivary glands, circumscribed nodules in the soft palate, gingiva and cheek, etc.
Histoplasmosis	Ulceration and nodular growth on the gingiva, tongue or palate that often simulates a carcinoma
Candidiasis	White or grayish white "curdled milk"-like patches on the oral mucosa, which leave raw painful, bleeding surfaces upon their removal
Actinomycosis	Enlargement of mandible with many pus discharging sinuses, the pus contains small yellowish sulfur granules

Contd...

Contd...

Name of the disease	Important oral manifestations
Crohn's disease	Recurrent aphthous stomatitis, diffuse nodular swelling of the lips and cheeks, cobble-stone appearance of the oral mucosa. Linear granulomatous ulcer on buccal vestibule
Ulcerative colitis	Recurrent aphthous ulcer, pyostomatitis vegetans, hemorrhagic ulcers
Pyostomatitis vegetans	Multiple linear yellow pustules over the buccal and labial mucosa, soft palate and undersurface of the tongue
Celiac disease	Recurrent aphthous stomatitis

■ DERMATOLOGICAL DISEASES (TABLE 21.8)

Table 21.8: Oral manifestations due to dermatological diseases.

Name of the disease	Important oral manifestations
Ectodermal dysplasia	Anodontia, salivary gland aplasia with xerostomia, depressed nasal bridge, frontal bossing, dry skin, unexplained pyrexia, hoarseness of voice
Pemphigus	Vesicle or bullae formation in oral mucosa, vesicles rupture with subsequent ulcer formation, Nikolsky's sign is positive, pain with bleeding and secondary infection
Pemphigoid	Vesicle or bullae formation, desquamation of the gingiva
Epidermolysis bullosa	Multiple bullae in the area of trauma, hypoplasia of teeth
Ehlers–Danlos syndrome	Increased fragility of skin, gum bleeding, tooth mobility, delayed wound healing, enamel hypoplasia

Contd...

Contd...

Name of the disease	Important oral manifestations
Lichen planus	Patchy white lesions on the oral mucosa that present lace-like radiating striae at the periphery, burning sensations and mucosal pigmentations often develop
Scleroderma	Atrophy of the oral mucous membrane with stiffening and fixation, depapillation of tongue, difficulty in deglutition, and widening of the periodontal ligament space
Psoriasis	Erythematous patches with white scaly surface on the oral mucosa
Lupus erythematous	Multiple white plaques in oral mucosa with dark-reddish purple margins. Erythematous skin rash on the face with a butterfly configuration across the bridge of the nose
Keratosis follicularis	Multiple small papules on the oral mucosa

■ BONE DISEASES (TABLE 21.9)

Table 21.9: Important oral manifestations due to bone diseases.

Name of the disease	Important oral manifestations
Paget's disease of bone	Enlargement of the jaws, loosening of teeth and diastema formation, "cotton-wool" type radiographic features of the bone, hypercementosis of teeth and pulp calcification, etc.
Osteopetrosis	Delayed tooth eruption, retarded healing of the extraction wound, spontaneous jaw fractures, etc.
Osteogenesis imperfecta	Frequent bone fractures, blue sclera, in case of associated dentinogenesis imperfecta feature like obliteration of pulp chambers, excessive tooth wear and short roots, etc.

Contd...

Contd...

Name of the disease	Important oral manifestations
Caffey's disease	Sudden jaw swelling that disappears in 3–12 months, cortical thickening, and bulging of the lower border of mandible
Fibrous dysplasia	Enlargement of the jaws, hypergonadism in females and café-au-lait spots on the skin, etc., ground-glass radiographic appearance of bone
Fluorosis	Lustless opaque white teeth with mottling or pitting, opaque hypomineralized areas of tooth which may stain yellow to dark brown, decreased caries incidence

■ ACUTE LETHAL TYPE INFECTIOUS DISEASES (TABLE 21.10)

Table 21.10: Important oral manifestations due to acute lethal type infectious diseases.

Name of the disease	Important oral manifestations
Rabies	Excessive salivation, facial palsy, hydrophobia, difficulty in deglutition.
Tetanus	Lockjaw, risus sardonicus
Anthrax	Malignant edema of the lip, oral mucosa, larynx and pharynx
	Malignant pustule formations in the labial and palatal mucosa
Meningitis	Bleeding from the mouth, stomatitis, mouth ulcers, foul breath, loss of taste sensation, coating on the tongue

■ HELMINTHIC DISEASES (TABLE 21.11)

Table 21.11: Important oral manifestations due to helminthic diseases.

Name of the disease	Important oral manifestations
Tapeworm infections	*Teniasis:* Edematous mucosal ulcerations, gingival bleeding
	Cysticercosis: Well-defined, painless, fluctuant swelling over the lips, tongue and cheek, which often resembles mucoceles

Contd...

Contd...

Name of the disease	Important oral manifestations
	Hydatid cyst: Small, progressively increasing, painless, well-defined, soft fluctuant swelling on the tongue
Roundworm infections	*Trichinosis:* Bilateral gingival swelling, swelling of the tongue and myelohyoid muscle
	Ascariasis: Submental swelling, mucosal pigmentations, toxic manifestations from worm by-products, e.g. facial edema and urticaria, etc.
	Filariasis: Edematous swelling of the lips and tongue
Protozoal infections	*Tripanosomiasis:* Unilateral facial edema with crepitations, widening of the transverse diameter of face, salivary gland swelling, cervical and preauricular lymphadenopathy
Leishmaniasis	Ulcerations of the oral mucosa, progressive destructions of soft palate, uvula and gingiva
Toxoplasmosis	Aphthous stomatitis, pharyngitis, lymphadenopathy, facial palsy

■ RENAL DISEASES (TABLE 21.12)

Table 21.12: Important oral manifestations due to renal diseases.

Name of the disease	Important oral manifestations
Renal failure	Bad odor or smell of ammonia in the mouth, gingivitis, stomatitis, xerostomia, parotitis, mucosal erythema, oral thrush, bacterial plaques, mucosal ulcerations, purpura, giant-cell lesions (secondary to hyperparathyroidism) mucosal pallor due to anemia
Renal osteodystrophy	Demineralization of maxillary and mandibular bone, loss of trabeculations, total or partial loss of lamina dura, ground-glass radiolucency of bone

Contd...

Contd...

Name of the disease	Important oral manifestations
Kidney transplantation	Xerostomia, metallic taste, mucosal pallor, low grade gingival inflammation, increased bleeding tendency from gingiva and oral mucosa, petechiae or ecchymosis, erosive glossitis, staining of teeth, bone demineralization, gingival hyperplasia

■ NEURAL DISEASES (TABLE 21.13)

Table 21.13: Problems due to neural diseases.

Name of the disease	Problems
Multiple sclerosis	Anesthesia or paresthesia of all branches of trigeminal nerve, nonspecific neuralgia, glossopharyngeal neuralgia
Epilepsy	Gingival hyperplasia due to intake of phenytoin sodium, hirsutism, lymphadenopathy
Cerebral palsy	Class II malocclusion with open bite is often seen, severe caries and periodontal diseases, severe tooth erosion, enamel hypoplasia, bruxism, mouth breathing, drooling, delayed tooth eruption, traumatic damage of teeth, disturbance in swallowing

■ SEXUALLY TRANSMITTED DISEASES (TABLE 21.14)

Table 21.14: Oral manifestations due to sexually transmitted diseases.

Name of the disease	Important oral manifestations
Syphilis	*Oral chancres*—in primary syphilis
	Mucous patches—in secondary syphilis
	Gumma—in tertiary syphilis
	Hutchinson's triad—in congenital syphilis
Gonorrhea	Gonococcal stomatitis with ulcerations of the oral mucosa, gingivostomatitis with red, yellow or greenish discoloration of the tissue
Granuloma inguinale	Extensive superficial ulcerations in the oral mucosa with ill-defined margins

CARDIOVASCULAR DISEASES (TABLE 21.15)

Table 21.15: Oral manifestations due to cardiovascular diseases.

Name of the disease	Important oral manifestations
Congestive cardiac failure	Cyanosis of the lips, tongue, and other parts of oral mucosa
Coarctation of aorta	Enlargement of the mandibular artery and its branches supplying the teeth, enlargement of the dental pulp, excessive hemorrhage after tooth extractions
Congenital heart disease	Generalized bluish discoloration of the gingiva, severe marginal gingivitis, bleeding gums, delayed eruption of teeth
Hypertension	Uncontrolled hemorrhage following oral surgical procedures, gingival hyperplasia due to intake of nifedipine, oral mucosal ulcers due to intake of methyldopa, dryness of mouth due to use of diuretics
Stroke	Impaired speech, facial paralysis, poor oral hygiene, inability to wear artificial prosthesis

GENETIC DISORDERS (TABLE 21.16)

Table 21.16: Important oral manifestations due to genetic disorders.

Name of the disease	Important oral manifestations
Down's syndrome	Small mouth, large tongue, conical teeth, high arched palate, microdontia, delayed eruption of teeth
Apert's syndrome	Cleft palate, cleft uvula, malocclusion, high palatal vault
Achondroplasia	Hypoplastic maxilla, mandibular prognathism, malocclusion
Cleidocranial dysplasia	Midfacial hypoplasia, high-arched palate with or without cleft, delayed eruption of teeth, multiple impacted or unerupted supernumerary teeth

Contd...

Contd...

Name of the disease	Important oral manifestations
Cruzon's syndrome	Anodontia, peg-shaped teeth, palatal cyst
Marfan syndrome	TMJ-dysarthrosis, high arched palate, cleft palate
Pierre–Robin syndrome	Cleft palate, micrognathia, glossoptosis
Trisomy-13 syndrome	Cleft lip, cleft palate

ALLERGIC CONDITIONS (TABLE 21.17)

Table 21.17: Important oral manifestations due to allergic reactions.

Name of the disease	Important oral manifestations
Contact allergy	Multiple vesicles followed by ulcerations, in the oral mucosa, swelling and fissuring of the lips
Systemic allergy	*Type-I*—anaphylactic shock
	Type-II, III, IV—lichenoid reaction, pemphigus, pemphigoid and erythema multiforme, etc.

GENERAL MANIFESTATIONS OF ORAL DISEASES (TABLE 21.18)

Table 21.18: General manifestations due to oral diseases.

Diseases produced	Oral diseases responsible for such conditions
Cavernous sinus thrombosis and meningitis	Cavernous sinus thrombosis and meningitis occurs in rare cases, when the infections from the "danger zone" of the face reach the cavernous sinus and the meninges
	Clinical features: Exophthalmos, loss of vision, photophobia, lacrimation, fever, chills and vomiting
Septicemia	Extraction of infected teeth without antibiotic coverage may lead to septicemia or even death

Contd...

Contd...

Diseases produced	Oral diseases responsible for such conditions
Oral infections	Fever, malaise, leukocytosis, headache and lymphadenopathy, etc. may develop when there is presence of a dentoalveolar abscess or osteomyelitis of the jaw
Subacute bacterial endocarditis	In case of careless tooth extraction in a cardiac patient without proper antibiotic therapy, the *Streptococcus beta–haemolyticus* group of organisms may spread from the oral cavity to the heart and produce SABE
Hypovolemic shock	Excessive hemorrhage from the oral cavity following tooth extraction may produce hypovolemic shock
Malignant oral tumors	Malignant oral tumors, e.g. squamous cell carcinoma, malignant melanoma, osteosarcoma and lymphoma, etc. can metastasize to the distant areas of the body and kill the patient
Loss of teeth	If the lost teeth in the oral cavity are not replaced by artificial dentures, the patients' ability to masticate adequate nutritious food is decreased and nutritional deficiency symptoms develop
Oral foci of infection	The infected dental pulp, dental abscess, periodontal abscess, inflamed gingiva, etc. harbor microorganisms and hence are called oral foci of infections. The microorganisms from these oral foci may produce secondary infections in the distant parts of the body
Transitory bacteremia	Extraction, scaling or any other minor oral surgical procedure may cause spread of bacteria from the oral cavity into the circulation. This type of bacteremia lasts for about 30 minutes

BIBLIOGRAPHY

1. Anniversary special issue, on 102nd birth anniversary celebration of R. Ahmed; West Bengal state Dental journal; 2013.
2. Cawson JW, Eveson RA. Oral pathology and diagnosis-color atlas with integrated text, 1st edition. Portsmouth, New Hampshire: William Heinemann Medical Books Limited; 1987.
3. Eversole LR. Clinical outline of oral pathology: diagnosis and treatment. New York: People's Medical Publishing House; 2001.
4. Eveson JW, Shear M. Cysts of the Oral Region, 3rd edition. Oxford: Butterworth-Heinemann Ltd.; 1992.
5. Lynch MA, Brightman VJ, Greenberg MS. Burket's oral medicine–diagnosis and treatment, 9th edition. Philadelphia: Lippincott Williams and Wilkins; 1994.
6. Macleod J. Davidson's Principles and Practice of medicine, 14th edition. Philadelphia: Churchill Livingstone; 1977.
7. Neville B, Damm DD, Allen C, et al. A Text Book of Oral Pathology, 4th edition. New York: Elsevier; 2015.
8. Philip SJ, Eversole LR, Wysocki JP. Contemporary oral and Maxillofacial pathology. St. Louis: Mosby; 2003.
9. Prabhu SR, Daftury DK, Johnson NW. Oral diseases in the tropic. Oxford: Oxford University Press; 1992.
10. Regezi J, Sciubba J, Jordan R. Oral Pathology, 6th edition. New York: Elsevier; 2011.
11. Soames JV, Southam JC. Oral Pathology, 3rd edition. New York: Oxford University Press; 1998.
12. Tencate AR. Oral Histology: development, structure, and function, 3rd edition. St. Louis: Mosby; 1989.
13. The Lippincott Manual of Nursing Practice, 2nd edition. Philadelphia: JB Lippincott Company; 1978.
14. White SC, Goaz PW. Oral radiology: principles and interpretations. Philadelphia: Elsevier Health; 2014.
15. Wood NK, Goaz PW. Differential Diagnosis of Oral Lesions, 4th edition. St. Louis: Mosby; 1997.

CHAPTER 22

Syndromes Related to Oral Diseases

DEFINITION OF SYNDROME

It is a combination of signs and symptoms occurring commonly enough to constitute a distinct clinical entity. A syndrome also means a set of symptoms, which collectively indicate or characterize a disease, a psychological disorder or other abnormal condition. Some investigators state that "a disease which has more than one identifying features or symptoms is a syndrome".

A large number of syndromes occur as symptom complexes in association with many oral diseases; some of them are very common while few others are extremely uncommon entities.

It is important to remember that once a single component feature of a syndrome is found in a patient, care should always be taken to look for other possible symptoms, which might be present elsewhere in the body so that an early and accurate diagnosis of a syndrome could be made, whenever it is present. Early diagnosis of a syndrome is always important since severity of a disease can be much more when it is occurring in association with a syndrome rather than when it is occurring as a single entity.

In the following section, salient features of some important "oral disease-related syndromes" will be discussed (Table 22.1).

Table 22.1: Salient features of some important oral disease-related syndromes.

Name of the syndrome	Important features
Acquired immunodeficiency syndrome	Severe reduction in T-lymphocytes due to human immunodeficiency virus, breakdown of cell mediated immunity as well as humoral immunity, overwhelming opportunistic infections and neoplasms, etc.
Acute radiation syndrome	A syndrome caused by exposure to a whole body dose of over 1 gray radiation, features include erythema, nausea, vomiting, fatigue, diarrhea, petechiae, bleeding from oral mucosa, hypotension and tachycardia
Adrenogenital syndrome	Pseudohermaphroditism, sexual precocity, virilism in women or feminization in men, premature eruption of teeth, if the disease begins in early life
Albright syndrome	Polyostotic fibrous dysplasia of bone, café-au-lait spots on the skin, endocrine disturbances, e.g. precocious puberty
Aldrich syndrome	Thrombocytopenic purpura eczema, increased susceptibility to infection, otitis media, petechiae, ecchymosis
Amelo-onycho-hypohydrotic syndrome	Severe hypoplastic-hypocalcified enamel, subungual hyperkeratosis, defective nails, hypofunction of the sweat glands, seborrheic dermatitis
Andersen syndrome	Craniofacial and skeletal anomalies, hyperuricemia, diastolic hypertension, maxillary hypoplasia, mandibular prognathism, malocclusion

Contd...

Contd...

Name of the syndrome	Important features
Angio-osteohypertrophy syndrome	Port-wine stains on the face, varices, hypertrophy of bone including jaw bones, facial asymmetry, malocclusion, altered eruption pattern of teeth
Anorexia-cachexia syndrome	Systemic response to cancer occurring as a result of a poorly understood relationship between anorexia and cachexia, manifested by malnutrition, weight loss, muscular weakness and toxemia
Apert syndrome	Early synostosis of cranial sutures, triangular facial defects, high arched palate, syndactyly and mandibular prognathism. Shovel-shaped incisors, malocclusion, parrot-beak type nose
Ascher's syndrome	Acquired double lip, blepharochalasis and nontoxic thyroid enlargement. Recurrent edema of both eyelids
Baby bottle syndrome	The condition occurs in children those who drink excessive sugar containing milk or other drinks by feeding bottle for a longer period of time (especially if the milk is kept in mouth overnight). There will be multiple numbers of caries in several teeth
Beckwith's hypoglycemic syndrome	Macroglossia, neonatal hypoglycemia, umbilical hernia, postnatal gigantism
Behcet's syndrome	Oral ulceration, genital ulceration, photophobia, conjunctivitis, uveitis, pyoderma and arthralgia
Bernard–Soulier syndrome	It is a bleeding disorder due to some platelet defects and is characterized by normal platelet aggregation to adenosine diphosphate (ADP) and collagen but an abnormal response to fibrinogen. Increased bleeding time and decreased platelet count
Bing–Neel syndrome	Hyperglobulinemia with central nervous system (CNS) involvement on a toxic infectious basis. Encephalopathy, hemorrhage, stroke and convulsions
Baelz syndrome	A rare disease of children or adolescents, characterized by enlargement, hardening and finally eversion of the lip leading to exposure of the opening of accessory salivary glands
Berry's syndrome	Mandibulofacialdysostosis evident at birth
Book's syndrome	Premature whitening of hair, hyperhydrosis of palms and soles, aplasia of premolars and third molars
B-K mole syndrome	A hereditary condition characterized by the presence of large pigmented nevi. It often carries a very high risk for development of melanoma
Bloch-Sulzberger syndrome	Erythematous, vesiculobullous lesion on the trunk and extremities. The initial lesion disappears, following which a lichenoid, papillary or verrucous lesion develops. Finally, a brownish-gray macule develops over the skin. Delayed tooth eruptions, conical tooth crowns, extra cusp, and anodontia
Blepharonasofacial syndrome	Mental retardation, microcephaly, joint disorders, hypoplastic maxilla and protruding lips
Bowen syndrome	Craniofacial anomalies, hypotonia, hepatomegaly, micrognathia, protruding tongue, high arched palate, increased serum iron level
Brittle bone syndrome	Fragile bones, clear blue sclera, deafness, loose ligaments, open fontanelles, repeated fractures of bone, opalescent teeth with short roots and obliterated pulp chambers
Burning mouth syndrome	Acute intense pain and burning sensation in the mouth, altered taste sensation and xerostomia, no clinically detectable lesion in the mouth, middle-aged women are commonly affected

Contd...

Contd...

Name of the syndrome	Important features
Caffey–Silverman syndrome	Development of a tender, deeply placed soft tissue swelling in bone especially mandible, increased cortical thickening of bone, severe malocclusion, fever, pseudoparalysis, dysphagia, anemia, leukocytosis
Candidiasis endocrinopathy syndrome	Chronic oral candidiasis, hypoparathyroidism, hypothyroidism, hypoadrenocorticism, diabetes mellitus, enamel hypoplasia
Carotid artery syndrome	Pressure or impingement on the external or internal carotid artery by elongated or deviated styloid process or calcified stylohyoid ligament. It often causes pain in the pharyngeal region
Cerebrocostomandibularsyndrome	Thoracic deformity with barking cough, mandibular micrognathia, palatal defects, absence of uvula or even soft palate, mental retardation
Chinese restaurant syndrome	Throbbing headache, lightness of the jaw, neck and shoulders, light-headedness, etc. after taking Chinese foods. These symptoms occur as a result of transient arterial dilatation due to ingestion of "monosodium glutamate" which is sometimes used liberally for seasoning the Chinese foods
Coffin–Lowry syndrome	Incapability of speech, severe mental deficiency, muscle, ligament and skeletal abnormality
Cri-dui-chat syndrome	Hypertelorism, microcephaly, mental retardation and a plaintive cat-like cry
Chediak–Higashi syndrome	It is a progressive systemic disorder with oculocutaneous albinism, photophobia, nystagmus, severe gingivitis, oral ulcer, glossitis, pancytopenia and histiocytic inclusions in different organs
Costen's syndrome	Intermittent or continuous impairment of hearing, stuffy sensation in the ear, tinnitus, otalgia, dizziness, headache, glissodynia
Cowden's syndrome	Multiple papules on the lips and gingiva, papillomatosis of the oral mucosa resulting in a "cobble-stone" appearance, follicular keratosis of the perioral, perinasal and periorbital skin, variety of neoplastic changes in many organs
CREST syndrome	This phenomenon is a variant of progressive systemic sclerosis characterized by calcinosis cutis, Raynaud's phenomenon, esophageal dysfunction, sclerodactyly, and telangiectasia
Cushing syndrome	It occurs due to hyperadrenocortism with development of adiposity, mooning of the face, buffalo hump, abnormal hair distribution in the body, vascular hypertension, glycosuria, osteoporosis, hypertrichosis
Cross syndrome	Microphthalmia, gingival enlargement, corneal clouding, hypopigmentations, white hair and blond skin
Cracked tooth syndrome	This syndrome is characterized by development of a crack in a restored or an unrestored tooth due to excessive occlusal forces. There will be sharp pain on biting, the pain can mimic trigeminal neuralgia and the crack cannot be detected by the radiograph
Crouzon syndrome	Craniosynostosis without syndactyly, early synostosis of bone, triangular frontal defect, mandibular prognathism and high-arched palate, nasomaxillary retrusion with mouth breathing
Down syndrome	Small slanting eyes with epicanthal folds, mongoloid facies, flat face, large anterior fontanelle, open sutures, sexual underdevelopment, open mouth with macroglossia, mental retardation and cardiac abnormalities

Contd...

Contd...

Name of the syndrome	Important features
Eagle's syndrome	Elongation of the styloid process of temporal bone or ossification of styloid ligament causing dysphagia, glossodynia, sore throat and pain along the distribution of the external carotid artery. The pain starts at the tonsillar area during mandibular movements, radiates to the temporomandibular joint (TMJ) or base of the tongue and interestingly it subsides as the jaws are closed
Edwards syndrome	Mental retardation, small eyes, prominent occiput, micrognathia, cleft palate and uvula, the index finger overlaps the third finger and fifth finger overlaps the fourth
Ehlers–Danlos syndrome	Hyperelasticity of skin, hyperextensibility of joints, increased capillary fragility, easy bruising of the skin and mucosa, delayed wound healing, increased bleeding tendency
Ellis-Van Creveld syndrome	Dwarfism, polydactyly, cardiac malfunction, dysplasia of hair and nails, hypodontia, fusion of the mid-portion of the upper lip to the anterior maxillary alveolar ridge and hypoplasia of teeth
Epidermal nevus syndrome	Cutaneous nevi extending upto oral mucosa and gingiva, mental deficiency, skeletal abnormality, hypoplastic teeth
EEC (ectrodactyly-ectodermal dysplasia-clefting) syndrome	Ectodermal dysplasia, hypopigmentation of skin and hair, cleft palate, cleft lip and tooth abnormality
Fanconi's syndrome	Aplastic anemia, bone abnormality, microcephaly, hypogenitalism, generalized olive-brown pigmentation of skin
Fetal-alcohol syndrome	This abnormal condition occurs in children born of women, who were chronically alcoholic during pregnancy. The features include maxillary hypoplasia, prominent forehead and mandible, short palpebral fissures, microcephaly and mental retardation
Fragile X syndrome	X-linked mental retardation, macroorchidism, large ears, long narrow face, cleft palate, mitral valve prolapse
Floppy infant syndrome	Hypotonia, generalized muscle weakness, reduced tendon reflexes, inability to sit, stand or walk due to generalized weakness
Focal dermal hypoplasia syndrome	Focal absence of dermis with herniation of the subcutaneous fat into the defect, atrophy and pigmentation of skin, telangiectasias, papillomatosis, syndactyly. Microdontia, enamel hypoplasia, cleft lip and palate
Frey's syndrome	It occurs as a result of damage to the auriculotemporal nerve with subsequent reinnervations of sweat glands by parasympathetic salivary fibers. The features include flushing and sweating of the temporal area during taking foods
Gardner's syndrome	Multiple polyposis of large intestine (colon), osteomas of bone, multiple epidermoid or sebaceous cysts of the skin, desmoid tumor, multiple impacted supernumerary and permanent teeth
Gorlin–Goltz syndrome	Basal cell carcinoma of the skin, multiple odontogenic keratocysts, bifid ribs, hypertelorism, mental retardation, hypogonadism, multiple basal cell nevi
Goldenhar syndrome	Unilateral microstomia, mental retardation, hypoplastic zygomatic arch, downward slanting of palpebral fissures, malformed pinna, high arched palate, cleft palate and uvula
Grinspan syndrome	It occurs in association with lichen planus and consists of lichen planus of skin and mucosa, vascular hypertension, and diabetes mellitus

Contd...

Contd...

Name of the syndrome	Important features
Gorlin-Chaudhry-Moss syndrome	Craniofacial dysostosis, patent ductus arteriosus, hypertrichosis, hypotonia, hypoplasia of labia majora
Gilles de la Tourette syndrome	Spontaneous erratic behavior of the patient, incoherent facial expression and verbalizations, tendency for self-mutilation (often the oral tissues) by the use of teeth and finger nails along with movement of the jaw
Heerfordt's syndrome	Painless, firm enlargement of the parotid and other glands due to sarcoidosis, uveitis of the eye, fever, vomiting, facial palsy, xerostomia, malaise, gastrointestinal disturbances
Horner's syndrome	It occurs due to ipsilateral brainstem lesion causing miosis or contraction of pupil, ptosis of the upper eyelid, anhydrosis and vasodilatation over the facial or periorbital skin causing flushing
Horton's syndrome	Unilateral paroxysm of intense pain in the eye, maxilla, ear, mastoid region, base of the nose and beneath the zygoma. Absence of trigger zone, occurrence of pain everyday exactly at the same time
Hurler's syndrome	Inherited mucopolysaccharide metabolism effect characterized by prominent forehead, saddle nose, hypertelorism, macroglossia, puffy eyelids, corneal clouding, short broad mandible, gingival hyperplasias, multiple cyst-like osteolytic lesions of the jaws, dwarfism, deafness
Hunter syndrome	Mild but similar features like Hurler's syndrome but without corneal clouding, death usually occurs before age of 15 years
Hutchinson–Gilford syndrome	Alopecia, atrophic skin with areas of pigmentation, prominent veins with loss of subcutaneous fat, high pitched squeaky voice, young boys with wizened old man-like look. Small mandible, delayed eruption of teeth, excessive secondary dentin formation
Hand–Schuller–Christian syndrome	Punched-out bone destruction in the skull, exophthalmos, diabetes insipidus, premature exfoliation of teeth
Hajdu-Cheney syndrome	Short stature, long nose, low frontal hairline, disintegration of the terminal phalanges of fingers and toes. Premature loss of teeth, susceptibility to multiple fractures of bone
Hallermann–Streiff syndrome	Small face, microphthalmia, beak-like nose, strabismus, double cutaneous chin with central furrow, hypodontia, microstomia, retained deciduous teeth
Hyoid syndrome	Elongation of the greater cornu of hyoid bone with impingement on adjacent laryngeal tissue, pain in the lateral neck and carotid area when the neck is turned to one side, pain during swallowing. Ipsilateral referred pain in the ear, syncope, patient always feels as if a foreign body is lodged in the throat
Happy Puppet syndrome	Jerky puppet-like movements of the body, peculiar open mouthed appearance, frequent laughter, mental and motor retardation and seizures
Jaffe-Lichtenstein syndrome	Multiple bone lesions of fibrous dysplasia, skin pigmentations
Jugular foramen syndrome	Dysphagia, hoarseness of voice, glossopharyngeal neuralgia like pain, palatal weakness, vocal cord paralysis
Jadassohn-Lewandowsky syndrome	Bilateral oral white lesions involving the tongue and buccal mucosa, laminated thickening of the finger and toenail

Contd...

Contd...

Name of the syndrome	Important features
Jaw-winking syndrome	Exaggerated opening of the eye on moving of the mandible in a contralateral direction, ptosis of the affected eye at rest, normal pupillary reflexes
Klinefelter's syndrome	This syndrome occurs in males, whose sex chromosome constitution includes one or more extra chromosomes. The patient may develop taurodontism. Small testes, azoospermia and infertility
KBG syndrome	Macrodontia, mental retardation, unusual facies, short stature
Lacrimal-auricular-dental and digital syndrome	Lacrimal duct obstruction with overflow of tears, cup-shaped deformed ear with loss of hearing, peg-shaped teeth, enamel hypoplasia and medial/lateral deviation of fingers
Larsen syndrome	Prominent forehead with frontal bossing, flat midface, depressed nasal bridge, hypertelorism, congenital (bilateral) dislocation of tibia or femur with displaced patella, cleft palate
Laugier–Hunziker syndrome	Acquired pigmented macules in the lips, oral cavity and fingers
Marfan's syndrome	Disproportionately long thin extremities, spidery fingers, long and narrow face, hyperextensibility of joints, kyphosis or scoliosis, recurrent joint dislocations (Figs. 22.1A to C) **Figs. 22.1A to C:** Marfan's syndrome—(A) Long narrow face; (B) Spidery fingers; (C) High arched palate.
Morquio's syndrome	Severe enamel hypoplasia with gray and pitted enamel, severe bone changes, mild corneal clouding, aortic regurgitation, pigeon breast
Marin-Amat syndrome	This condition occurs usually after peripheral facial paralysis and is characterized by automatic closing of the eye during forceful wide mouth opening like—chewing, etc. Tears may also flow
Myofascial pain dysfunction syndrome	This condition occurs in relation to the TMJ and is characterized by the following features—pain, muscle tenderness, clicking sound in TMJ, limitation of jaw movements, but no pain in the joint when palpated through the external auditory meatus
Median cleft face syndrome	Hereditary defect of abnormal midline development of face and head characterized by hypertelorism, median cleft of the lip, premaxilla and palate, cranium bifidum occultum, malocclusion
Melkersson–Rosenthal syndrome	Cheilitis granulomatosa, facial paralysis and scrotal tongue, persistent unilateral edema of the orbit and eyelid
Multiple endocrine neoplasia syndrome (MEN-I)	Tumors or hyperplasia of the pituitary, parathyroids, adrenal cortex and pancreatic islets. Peptic ulcer or gastric oversecretion

Contd...

Contd...

Name of the syndrome	Important features
Miescher's syndrome	Diffuse swelling of the lip. Scaling, fissuring, vesicle or pustule formation on the vermillion border. It is a monosymptomatic form of Melkersson–Rosenthal syndrome
Mikulicz's syndrome	Painless, chronic bilateral hypertrophy of the parotid or lacrimal glands accompanied by enlargement of the lymph nodes, xerostomia. The syndrome represents some generalized septic disease, e.g. lymphomas and tuberculosis
Mobius syndrome	Congenital facial diplegia, expressionless face due to facial paralysis, inability to close the eyes due to paralysis of the abducens, swollen lips, deafness, epilepsy, etc
Mucocutaneous lymph node syndrome	Fever, bilateral congestion of ocular conjunctiva, edema of the extremities, dryness and fissuring of the lips, strawberry-like redness and swelling of the tongue, acute nonpurulent swelling of the lymph node
Myxoma syndrome	Perioral pigmented macules, soft tissue myxomas and endocrinopathies
Murray-Puretic-Drescher syndrome	Gingival fibromatosis, tumors of the head, trunk and extremities, mental retardation, suppurative skin lesions, flexion contractures
Mohr syndrome	Short stature, digital deformities, midline cleft lip, bifid tip of nose, high arched palate, and hypodontia. Lingual, facial and mandibular deformity
Middle fossa syndrome	The condition occurs due to a tumor in the region of the Gasserian ganglion and causes hyperesthesia, paresthesia, paralysis of the ocular muscles, deviated mandibular opening, unilateral soft palate paralysis
Muir–Torre syndrome	Multiple sebaceous neoplasms, keratoacanthoma
Magic syndrome	Mouth and genital ulcers with inflamed cartilage
Munchausen syndrome	A factitious disorder with habitual seeking of hospital admission for apparent acute illness, patient often gives a plausible and dramatic history of the disease which is entirely false
Myelodysplastic syndrome	A group of bone marrow disorder preceding to development of acute myelogenous leukemia, characterized by abnormal hematopoietic stem cells, anemia, neutropenia and thrombocytopenia
MEN-III syndrome	Medullary carcinoma of thyroid, pheochromocytoma, café-au-lait pigmentation of skin, neurofibromatosis
Maffucci's syndrome	Multiple hemangiomas of the skin and oral mucosa, multiple chondromas of the jaw bone
Nagar syndrome	Hypoplasia of malar bones, antimongoloid obliquity, palpebral fissures, defective hearing, cleft palate, micrognathia
Neck-tongue syndrome	Unilateral upper nuchal or occipital pain with or without numbness in the area, simultaneous numbness of the tongue on the same side, malocclusion
Noonan syndrome	Congenital heart disease, chest deformity, mental retardation, short stature, facial bone anomalies, cryptorchidism
Occipital condyle syndrome	Occipital pain, which is exacerbated by neck fixation, weakness of the hypoglossal nerve
Oculoglandular syndrome of Parinaud	Localized granuloma of the eye, preauricular lymphadenopathy. It occurs in association with cat-scratch disease

Contd...

Contd...

Name of the syndrome	Important features
Oral-facial-digital syndrome	Cleft of the tongue, upper lip, palate and mandibular alveolar process, micrognathia, depressed nasal bridge, frontal bossing, digital malformation, thick fibrous bands in the lower mucobuccal fold eliminating the sulcus, supernumerary canines and premolars, small hands and feet
Oromandibular limb hypogenesis syndrome	Ocular hypotelorism, cranial nerve palsy, hypodactyly of hands and feet, hypoglossia, cleft palate, conical shaped mandibular incisors
Otopalatodigital syndrome	Deafness, cleft palate, generalized bone dysplasia, prominent supraorbital ridge, frontal bossing
Orbital syndrome	It occurs due to malignant disease of the orbit, supraorbital pain and hyperesthesia, blurred vision or diplopia, ptosis, ophthalmoplegia
Paraneoplastic syndrome	A symptom complex arising in a cancer-bearing patient that cannot be explained by local or distant spread of the tumor
Patau syndrome	Microcephaly, microphthalmia, ocular hypertelorism, deafness, polydactyly, heart anomalies, cleft lip and cleft palate
Pfeiffer syndrome	Craniosynostosis, turribrachycephaly, broad thumbs, halluces, midface hypoplasia, mandibular prognathism, high arched palate
Papillon–Lefevre syndrome	Hyperkeratosis palmoplantaris, generalized hyperhydrosis, fine body hair, peculiar dirty-colored skin, aggressive periodontitis with severe destruction of alveolar bone, gingival hyperplasia
Paratrigeminal syndrome	Severe pain or headache in the area of trigeminal distribution with sign of ocular sympathetic paralysis. Onset of pain is sudden, middle-aged males are frequently affected
Parry–Romberg syndrome	Atrophy of the skin, subcutaneous tissue, bone and cartilage causing hemifacial deformity, trigeminal neuralgia, loss of hair and vitiligo on the affected side. Contralateral Jacksonian epilepsy
Plummer–Vinson syndrome (Paterson–Kelly syndrome)	Dysphagia, smooth, red, depapillated painful tongue. Lemon tinted pallor of skin, cracks and fissures on the corner of the mouth, atrophy of the filiform and fungiform papillae of tongue
Portsmouth syndrome	Bleeding disorder due to defective platelet aggregation. The condition shows normal ADP-induced platelet aggregation but an abnormal or absent collagen-induced aggregation. Severe bleeding tendency, easy bruisability, epistaxis
PFAPA syndrome	Periodic fever, aphthous stomatitis, pharyngitis and adenitis
Pierre Robin syndrome	Cleft palate, micrognathia, glossoptosis and congenital heart disease. Absent gag reflex, airway obstruction due to falling back of tongue on the posterior pharyngeal wall due to micrognathia
Peutz-Jeghers syndrome	Recurrent abdominal pain due to familial intestinal polyposis, cutaneous pigmentation in perioral region, precocious puberty, gastrointestinal bleeding and pigmentation of the buccal mucosa
Riley–Day syndrome	Congenital absence of tongue papilla, vasomotor dysfunctions, loss of reflexes, feeding problems, lack of pain and taste sensations
Reiter's syndrome	Urethritis, arthritis, conjunctivitis, keratotic macules and papules on the skin
Ramsay Hunt syndrome	Facial paralysis, pain in the external auditory meatus and pinna of the ear, vesicular eruptions in the oral cavity and oropharynx, hoarseness of voice, tinnitus, vertigo

Contd...

Syndromes Related to Oral Diseases

Contd...

Name of the syndrome	Important features
Rubinstein–Taybi syndrome	Developmental retardation, broad thumbs and great toes, delayed or incomplete descent of testes in males
Rieger's syndrome	Hypodontia, enamel hypoplasia, protruding lower lip, maxillary hypoplasia, blue sclera, coloboma, malformed anterior teeth, microdontia
Rutherford syndrome	Congenitally enlarged gingiva, delayed tooth eruption, curtain-like superior corneal opacities and mental retardation
Sipple's syndrome (MEN-II)	Parathyroid hyperplasia or adenoma, pheochromocytomas of the adrenal medulla, medullay carcinoma of thyroid, no peptic ulcer, no pancreatic tumor
Sjogren's syndrome	Dry eyes, keratoconjunctivitis sicca, xerostomia, parotid swelling, burning pain in the oral, nasal and pharyngeal mucosa, rheumatoid arthritis
Scheuthauer-Marie-Sainton syndrome	Open fontanelle of the skull, partial or complete absence of clavicles, underdeveloped maxilla, multiple impacted or unerupted permanent or supernumerary teeth
Stevens-Johnson's syndrome	It is a severe expression of erythema multiforme characterized by widespread vesiculation, denudation, sloughing and necrosis involving the skin, oral mucous membrane, eyes and genitalia (Figs. 22.2A to C)
	Figs. 22.2A to C: Stevens–Johnson's syndrome "target lesion" on the skin and mucosal lesions.
Sturge–Weber syndrome	Orofacial and meningeal angiomatosis with secondary mental deficiency, intracranial calcifications, seizures, hemiplegia, nevus, gingival enlargement (Figs. 22.3A to C)
	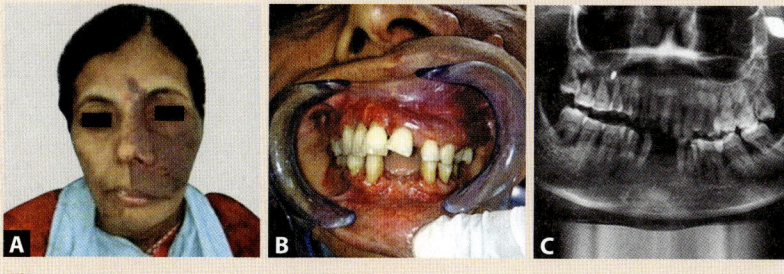 **Figs. 22.3A to C:** Sturge–Weber syndrome showing (A) Port-wine stain; (B) Gingival swelling and angiomatous lesions in gingiva or mucosa; (C) X-ray with destruction of alveolar bone.
Sanfilippo's syndrome	Severe CNS defects, mild somatic disturbances, enamel hypoplasia, excessive dentinogenesis with obliteration of pulp chambers
Sweet's syndrome	Acute onset of fever, leukocytosis, erythematous papules and plaques in the skin, predominantly neutrophilic infiltrates in the dermis without leukocytoclastic vasculitis, internal malignancy

Contd...

Contd...

Name of the syndrome	Important features
Sweat retention syndrome	Extravasation of sweat or saliva in the tissue with subsequent inflammation, keratin plug formation in sweat glands and accessory salivary glands
Syndrome of crocodile tears	This abnormal condition occurs following facial nerve paralysis, herpes zoster and operative trauma in the cranium. It seems to occur due to straying of the regenerating autonomic nerve fibers, some of those destined for salivary glands go to the lacrimal gland instead, resulting in a salivary-lacrimal reflex. It is characterized by spontaneous lacrimation occurring parallel with normal salivation during meals
Treacher Collins syndrome	Treacher Collins syndrome presents brachycephaly, hypoplasia of malar bone and mandible. Small external ear. Antimongoloid palpebral fissures and drooping of eyelids, typical narrow face and microstomia (Figs. 22.4A to C)

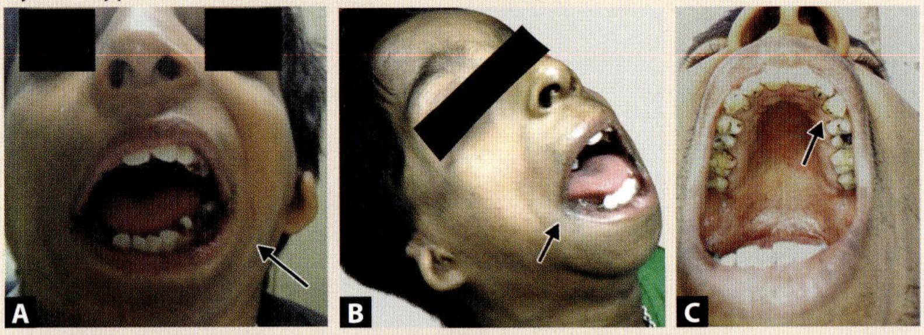

Figs. 22.4A to C: Antimongoloid palpebral fissures, small external ear, hypoplasia of the facial, especially malar and mandibular bones. Microstomia and typical narrow face.

Turner syndrome	Short stature, cubitus valgus, webbed neck, sexual infantilism, renal disorders, micrognathia, premature eruption of teeth
Trotter's syndrome	Nasopharyngeal tumor often producing trigeminal neuralgia-like pain in the mandible, tongue and side of the head in association with middle ear deafness
Tricho-dento-osseous syndrome	Tightly curled and kinky hair, osteosclerosis, hypoplastic hypocalcified enamel, many unerupted teeth and taurodontism, diastema, microdontia
Urbach–Wiethe syndrome	Pathologic accumulation of glycoprotein in most bodily tissues, hoarseness of voice, multiple papules and nodules in the body, intracranial calcifications, hypodontia
Van Buchem syndrome	Excessive deposition of endosteal bone throughout the skeleton, facial swelling, visual acuity, occasional facial paralysis and deafness
Vander Woude syndrome	The simultaneous occurrence of pits of the lower lip, cleft lip or cleft palate
Von-Recklinghausen's syndrome	Multiple neurofibromatosis in the body including oral cavity, pigmentation and hirsutism, risk of malignant transformation of one or more lesions
Waterhouse–Friderichsen syndrome	This syndrome occurs due to acute adrenal cortical insufficiency and is characterized by acute meningitis, septicemia, pronounced purpura, bilateral adrenal hemorrhage fever, coma, etc. Death usually occurs within 48–72 hours
Weber-Cockayne syndrome	It is a localized form of epidermolysis bullosa characterized by recurrent bullous eruptions of hands and feet
Whistling face syndrome	Sunken eyes, true ocular hypertelorism, antimongoloid obliquity of palpebral fissures, small nose, micrognathia, protruding lips as seen during whistling, high arched palate

Contd...

Contd...

Name of the syndrome	Important features
Wolf–Hirschhorn syndrome	Microcephaly, ocular hypertelorism, cleft palate, micrognathia and low-set ear
XXXXY syndrome	Hypoplastic midface, short stature, mental retardation, taurodontism, cleft uvula, hypertelorism
Zimmerman–Laband syndrome	Gingival fibromatosis with defects in ear, nose, bone and nails, frog-like fingers and nails, hyperextensible joints and hepatosplenomegaly
Zinsser syndrome	Oral leukoplakia, dystrophic nails, hyperpigmentation of skin, pancytopenia, aplastic anemia
Zinc deficiency syndrome	Defective taste bud function secondary to zinc deficiency

BIBLIOGRAPHY

1. Anniversary special issue, on 102nd birth anniversary celebration of R. Ahmed, West Bengal State Dental Journal, 2013.
2. Ash Jr M. Oral Pathology, 6th Edition. Philadelphia: Lea and Febiger; 1992.
3. Cawson RA. Oral Pathology and Diagnosis—Color Atlas with Integrated Text, 1st edition. Philadelphia: Saunders; 1987.
4. Eversole LR. Clinical Outline of Oral Pathology: Diagnosis and Treatment. Shelton, CT, USA: People's Medical Publishing House; 2011.
5. Goaz PW. Oral Radiology: Principles and Interpretations. St. Louis: Mosby; 1987.
6. Lynch MA, Brightman VJ, Greenberg MS. Burket's Oral Medicine-Diagnosis and Treatment, 9th edition. Philadelphia: Lippincott Williams & Wilkins; 1994.
7. Macleod J. Davidson's Principles and Practice of Medicine, 14th edition. Edinburgh: Churchill Livingstone; 1984.
8. Prabhu SR, Daftary DK, Johnson NW. Oral Diseases in the Tropic. New York: Oxford University Press; 1992.
9. Regezi JA, Sciubba JJ, Jordan R. Oral Pathology: Clinical Pathologic Correlations. St Louis: Saunders; 2016.
10. Sapp PJ, Eversole LR, Wysocki JP. Contemporary Oral and Maxillofacial Pathology. St. Louis: Mosby; 2004.
11. Shafer WG, Hine MK, Levy BM. A Textbook of Oral Pathology, 4th Edition. St. Louis: WB Saunders Co.; 1983.
12. Shear M. Cysts of the Oral Region, 3rd edition. Oxford: Wright; 1992.
13. Soames JV, Southam JC. Oral Pathology, 3rd edition. New York: Oxford University Press; 1998.
14. Tencate AR. Oral Histology: Development, Structure, and Function, 3rd edition. Ontario, Canada: Mosby; 1989.
15. The Lippincott Manual of Nursing Practice, 2nd edition. Philadelphia: JB Lippincott Company; 1978.
16. Wood NK, Goaz PW. Differential Diagnosis of Oral Lesions, 4th edition. St. Louis: CV Mosby; 1991.

CHAPTER 23

Important Classifications of Oral Diseases

INTRODUCTION

Classifications of diseases are important, since they not only help in understanding the disease in a better way, but also provide guidelines regarding the diagnosis and prognosis of a particular disease belonging to a specific group or category. In a sense, classifications of diseases are as useful as the classifications of the animals and plants made in the field of biology. While making the classification, some diseases are categorized from others and put into certain specific groups on the basis of their clinical features or radiological features or biological behavior, etc. However, the most important criteria in this regard will be the histopathological nature of diseased tissue that can determine, finally, regarding which category a particular disease will belong to while making their classification. In the following section, some important classifications of oral diseases are discussed.

WHITE LESIONS OF THE ORAL CAVITY

Hereditary Conditions

- Leukoedema, white sponge nevus, keratosis follicularis, and pachyonychia congenita
- Hereditary benign intraepithelial dyskeratosis, dyskeratosis congenita
- Incontinentia pigmenti and tylosis syndrome.

Leukoplakia and Malignancies

- Chronic cheek biting
- Frictional keratosis
- Leukoplakia-homogenous, ulcerative, and nodular types
- Hairy leukoplakia, actinic cheilitis, carcinoma in situ, and squamous cell carcinoma
- Verrucous carcinoma, smoker's palate, and verruciform xanthoma.

Dermatosis

Lichen planus and lupus erythematosus.

Inflammation

Koplik spots of measles, mucous patches of syphilis, chemical burns, candidiasis, and dentifrice associated slough.

Miscellaneous Conditions

- Fordyce's granules, dental lamina cyst, Bohn's nodules, and Epstein's pearls
- Oral submucous fibrosis, ectopic lymphoid nodules, geographic tongue, and papilloma
- Parulis, lipoma, systemic sclerosis, hairy tongue, and Heck's disease
- Oral lesions of chronic renal failure and Paterson–Kelly syndrome.

RED-BLUE LESIONS OF THE ORAL CAVITY

Developmental Lesions

Hemangioma and median rhomboid glossitis.

Reactive Lesions

Pyogenic granuloma and peripheral giant cell granuloma.

Pre-neoplastic and Neoplastic Lesions

Erythroplakia, nodular leukoplakia, Kaposi's sarcoma, squamous cell carcinoma, field cancerization and angiosarcoma.

Metabolic Conditions

- Vitamin C and vitamin B complex deficiency
- Pernicious anemia, iron-deficiency anemia, and burning mouth syndrome.

Infective Conditions

- Scarlet fever, atrophic candidiasis, and lymphonodular pharyngitis
- Infectious mononucleosis, herpetic ulcers, and aphthous ulcer.

Immunological Abnormalities

Plasma cell gingivitis, drug reactions, and allergic mucositis.

Petechiae or Ecchymosis

Suction petechiae, thrombocyte disorders, hereditary hemorrhagic telangiectasia and ecchymosis.

Miscellaneous Conditions

- Bullous and erosive mucosal disorders, radiation mucositis, and xerostomic mucositis
- Traumatic wound, dermatitis herpetiformis, mucosal burns, and nonspecific mucositis
- Hematoma and mucocele.

PIGMENTED LESIONS OF THE ORAL CAVITY

Benign Melanocytic Lesions

- Racial pigmentations, physiologic pigmentations, and smoking associated pigmentations
- Ephelis, Lentigo, oral melanotic macules, nevi, and hematoma.

Neoplastic Conditions

- Melanoma, multiple neurofibromatosis, and neuroectodermal tumor of infancy
- Hemangioma and Kaposi's sarcoma.

Pigmentations due to Exogenous Deposits

Amalgam tattoo, graphite tattoo, heavy metal pigmentations, and drug-induced pigmentations.

Miscellaneous Conditions

- Peutz–Jeghers syndrome, Addison's disease, and pigmented lichen planus
- Hairy tongue, HIV-associated oral pigmentations, and mucocele
- Endocrinopathic pigmentations and Café-au-lait pigmentations.

CLASSIFICATION OF VESICULOBULLOUS DISEASES

Viral Disease

- Herpetic gingivostomatitis, herpes labialis, and recurrent herpetic stomatitis
- Herpangina, hand-foot-mouth disease, *Varicella zoster*, and measles.

Immunologic Conditions

- Pemphigus, pemphigoid, erythema multiforme, and dermatitis herpetiformis
- Linear immunoglobulin A (IgA) disease, epidermolysis bullosa acquisita, contact vascular stomatitis, and bullous lichen planus.

Hereditary Conditions

Epidermolysis bullosa (inherited form), Hailey–Hailey disease, and Darier's disease.

Miscellaneous Conditions

Impetigo and oral blood blisters.

CLASSIFICATION OF ULCERATIVE CONDITIONS

Infective Lesions (Table 23.1)

Table 23.1: Infective lesions.

Bacterial diseases	Viral diseases	Fungal diseases
Syphilis	Acute herpetic Gingivostomatitis	Sporotrichosis Histoplasmosis
Gonorrhea	Herpes labialis	Cryptococcosis
Tuberculosis	Herpangina	Mucormycosis
Leprosy	HIV infections	
Actinomycosis	Infectious mononucleosis	
Noma	Herpes zoster	
ANUG	Measles	
Nonspecific mixed bacterial infections		

Traumatic Conditions

Mechanical, thermal, chemical, radiation injuries, and factitious injury.

Immunologic Disorders

- Aphthous ulcer, Behcet's syndrome, Reiter's syndrome, and erythema multiforme
- Pemphigus, pemphigoid, contact allergy, and ulcerative lichen planus
- Discoid lupus erythematosus.

Systemic Diseases

- Leukemia, agranulocytosis, cyclic neutropenia, and pernicious anemia
- Gluten enteropathy, Crohn's disease, and uremic stomatitis.

Necrotic Conditions

Midline lethal granuloma, Wegner's granulomatosis, malignant reticulosis, and osteoradionecrosis.

Malignant Conditions

Squamous cell carcinoma, antral carcinoma, and verrucous carcinoma.

Miscellaneous Lesions

Angular cheilitis, congenital lip pits, commissural pits, necrotizing sialometaplasia, and oroantral fistula.

CLASSIFICATION OF DISCOLORATION OF TOOTH

Extrinsic Stains

- Substances in the diet, smoking, habitual chewing of tobacco, betel nut, etc.
- Medicaments, e.g. chlorhexidines or dentifrices and chromogenic microorganisms.

Intrinsic Stains

- Changes in structure or thickness of dental tissues
    - Enamel hypoplasias, fluorosis, amelogenesis imperfecta, and enamel opacities
    - Enamel caries, dentinogenesis imperfecta, and dentin dysplasia (Type II)
    - Age changes in dental tissues.
- Diffusion of pigments into dental tissues after their formation
    - Extrinsic stains, endodontic materials, and products of pulp necrosis.
- Pigments incorporated during formation of dental tissues
    - Bile pigments in biliary atresia and hemosiderin pigments in erythroblastosis fetalis
    - Porphyrins in porphyria, tetracycline stains, and postmortem pink tooth.

CLASSIFICATION OF GIANT CELL LESIONS

Neoplasms

- Giant cell tumor of the bone, central giant cell granuloma, and peripheral giant cell granuloma
- Giant cell epulis, brown tumor of hyperparathyroidism, and giant cell fibroma
- Malignant fibrous histiocytoma, osteoblastoma, and chondroblastoma
- Hodgkin's lymphoma.

Other Lesions where Giant Cells may be Present

- Osteoblastoma, chondroblastoma, and aneurysmal bone cyst
- Fibrous dysplasia of bone, cherubism, tuberculosis, and fibrous histiocytoma
- Sarcoidosis, Hodgkin's disease, and calcifying epithelial odontogenic cyst
- Eosinophilic granuloma, Letterer–Siwe disease, and giant cell arteritis
- Pulse granuloma, histoplasmosis, and brown tumor of hyperparathyroidism.

■ CLASSIFICATION OF VERRUCAL-PAPILLARY LESIONS OF ORAL CAVITY

Reactive Lesions

- Papillary hyperplasia of palate, condyloma latum, squamous papilloma, and oral warts
- Oral papillomatosis, condyloma acuminatum, and Heck's disease.

Neoplasms

Keratoacanthoma, verrucous carcinoma, pyostomatitis vegetans, and verruciform xanthoma.

■ CLASSIFICATION OF FIBRO-OSSEOUS LESIONS

- Fibrous dysplasia of bone, ossifying fibroma, and cementing fibroma
- Central giant cell granuloma and brown tumor of hyperparathyroidism
- Paget's disease of bone, cherubism, and aneurysmal bone cyst
- Hemorrhagic bone cyst, focal condensing osteitis, and bony exostoses
- Focal osteoporotic bone marrow defect (FOBMD)
- Fibrous defect (nonossifying fibroma) of the mandible and osteogenesis imperfecta
- Osteoporosis, vanishing bone disease (massive osteolysis), and infantile cortical hyperostosis
- Histiocytosis X, condylar hypertrophy, acromegaly, and Fragile X syndrome
- Cleidocranial dysplasia, achondroplasia, rickets, scurvy, and Hurler's syndrome
- Garre's osteomyelitis.

■ CLASSIFICATION OF VASCULAR TISSUE DISEASES

- The arteritides
  - Polyarteritis nodosa
- Midfacial granuloma syndrome
  - Wegener's granulomatosis, Stewart-type midfacial granuloma, giant cell arteritis, and radiation arteritis
- Vascular hamartomas
  - Hemangiomas and lymphangiomas
- Telangiectases
  - Hereditary hemorrhagic telangiectasia and radiation telangiectasia
- Vascular tumors
  - Leiomyoma, leiomyosarcoma, hemangiopericytoma, hemangioendothelioma, Kaposi's sarcoma, angiolymphoid hyperplasia with eosinophils, and Kimura's disease.

■ CLASSIFICATION OF DISEASES OF THE HEMOPOIETIC TISSUES AND LYMPHORETICULAR SYSTEM

- Anemia, sickle cell disease, thalassemia, leukopenia, purpura, leukemia, lymphoma, mycosis fungoides, multiple myeloma, solitary plasmacytoma, and pseudolymphoma
- Amyloidosis, infectious mononucleosis, and angiofollicular lymphoid hyperplasia.

■ CLASSIFICATION OF STOMATITIS

- Infective stomatitis
  - Primary herpetic stomatitis, herpes labialis, chicken pox, and infectious mononucleosis
  - Hand-foot-and-mouth disease, herpangina, candidiasis tuberculosis, and syphilis

- Stomatitis immunologically mediated or of dubious origin
  - Aphthous stomatitis, Behcet's syndrome, lichen planus, lupus erythematosus, pemphigus vulgaris, pemphigus vegetans, pyostomatitis vegetans, cicatricial pemphigoid, desquamative gingivitis, bullous erythema multiform epidermolysis bullosa, dermatitis herpetiformis, Reiter's syndrome, Cowden's syndrome, and acanthosis nigricans.

CLASSIFICATION OF SEVERE INFECTIONS OF THE OROFACIAL TISSUES

- Acute cellulitis and space infections. Ludwig's angina, cavernous sinus thrombosis, herpes zoster, actinomycosis, histoplasmosis, phycomycosis cryptococcosis, aspergillosis, and blastomycosis
- Cat scratch disease, cancrum oris, midline lethal granuloma, osteoradionecrosis, acute osteomyelitis of the jaws, acute infections in AIDS patients, and other immunocompromised conditions.

CLASSIFICATION OF CHRONIC OROFACIAL PAIN

Neuralgias

Primary trigeminal neuralgia (tic douloureux), herpes zoster, postherpetic neuralgia, geniculate neuralgia, glossopharyngeal neuralgia, superior laryngeal neuralgia, and occipital neuralgia.

Pain of Muscular Origin

- Cervical osteoarthritis and temporomandibular joint (TMJ) disorders
  - TMJ rheumatoid arthritis
  - TMJ osteoarthritis
  - Myofacial pain dysfunction syndrome
- **Eagle's syndrome, fibromyalgia, cervical sprain or hyperextension, and** primary vascular disorders
- Migraine, cluster headache, and hypertensive vascular changes.

Psychogenic Pains

Generalized Pain Syndrome

Post-traumatic pain and causalgia

Lesion of the Ear, Nose, and Oral Cavity

Maxillary sinusitis, otitis media, Odontalgia: Pulpitis, periapical pathology, periapical abscess, periodontal pathology, cracked tooth syndrome, and occlusal trauma.

Other Conditions

Cyst and tumors, osteitis, mucocutaneous diseases, salivary gland diseases, atypical facial pain, and glossodynia.

CLASSIFICATION OF DISEASES OF TONGUE

Developmental Disorders

Aglossia, hypoglossia, cleft tongue, ankyloglossia, fissured tongue, scrotal tongue, median rhomboid glossitis, benign migratory glossitis, hairy tongue, lingual thyroid, thyroglossal duct cyst, microglossia, macroglossia, and bald tongue.

Disorders in Lingual Papillae

Hairy tongue, oral thrush, chemical burns, white sponge nevus, vesiculobullous lesions, lichen planus, leukoplakia, hairy leukoplakia, vitamin deficiency, Hunter's glossitis, atrophic glossitis in Plummer–Vinson's syndrome or Paterson–Kelly syndrome, glossitis due to syphilis, pigmentations, traumatic ulcers, infectious diseases, lingual varicosities, and lingual hematoma.

Diseases Affecting Body of the Tongue

- Amyloidosis, lingual abscess, muscular dystrophy, hypoglossal nerve palsy, and actinomycosis
- Cysticercosis, trichinosis, neck-tongue syndrome, glossoptosis, glossopyrosis,

glossodynia, infarcts in the tongue, and angioneurotic edema.

Benign Tumors
Traumatic fibroma, pyogenic granuloma, granular cell tumor, hemangioma, lymphangioma, neurofibroma, and salivary gland tumor.

Malignant Tumors
Squamous cell carcinoma, verrucous carcinoma, and malignant fibrous histiocytoma.

CLASSIFICATION OF GINGIVAL ENLARGEMENTS

Focal Gingival Enlargements
Pyogenic granuloma, fibroepithelial polyp, parulis, denture irritation peripheral giant cell granuloma, peripheral fibroma, giant cell fibroma fibrous histiocytoma, malignant fibrous histiocytoma, fibrosarcoma, squamous cell carcinoma, exostosis, gingival cyst, eruption cyst, and congenital epulis of newborn.

Generalized Gingival Enlargements
- Inflammatory enlargements
  - Scurvy, puberty, pregnancy, oral contraception, acute leukemias, hormonal imbalance, Crohn's disease, and Wegener's granulomatosis
- Fibrous overgrowths of the gingiva
  - Hereditary gingival fibromatosis, drug-induced gingival fibromatosis (due to phenytoin sodium, cyclosporine nifedipine and verapamil), chronic hyperplastic gingivitis, orofacial angiomatosis and idiopathic
- Syndrome associated gingival enlargements
  - Rutherford syndrome, Zimmerman-Laband syndrome, Cowden syndrome, tuberous sclerosis syndrome, Gorlin-Goltz syndrome, Murray–Puretic–Drescher syndrome, Cross syndrome, Ramon syndrome, lysosomal storage disease, acanthosis nigricans, and epidermal nevus syndrome.

CLASSIFICATION OF TASTE DISORDERS
Gustatory-olfactory confusion in patients with hyposmia, post-upper respiratory tract infection, damage to olfactory nerve, poor oral hygiene, heavy dental plaque, poorly maintained prosthesis, gingivitis, periodontitis, radiotherapy, sialadenitis, sialolithiasia, xerostomia, Sjogren's syndrome, metabolic byproducts of ingested foods and medications, mucositis, pericoronitis, dry socket, bacterial, viral and fungal infections of mouth, septic tonsil, diabetic ketoacidosis, metal poisoning, corrosion of metallic restotarions or prosthesis, old age, loss of taste buds, glossitis, lichen planus, leprosy, surgical damage to glossopharyngeal and facial nerves, chemotherapy, head injury and brain lesions affecting central taste pathways, epilepsy multiple sclerosis, hypothyroidism and hyperthyroidism adrenal insufficiency, hepatic disease, pregnancy, demyelinating diseases, metabolic disorders, and diabetes mellitus.

CLASSIFICATION OF NECK SWELLINGS
- Lateral neck swelling
  - Lymphadenitis—nonspecific, bacterial, viral, fungal
  - Metastatic carcinoma to lymph nodes
  - Lymphoma
  - Parotid lesion (neoplasms, mumps, Sjögren's syndrome)
  - Metabolic diseases
  - Carotid body tumor
  - Epidermoid cyst
  - Cystic hygroma
- Midline neck swelling
  - Thyroglossal duct cyst

- Thyroid tumor
- Dermoid cyst.

CLASSIFICATION OF YELLOW CONDITIONS OF ORAL MUCOSA

Fordyce granules, superficial abscess, superficial nodules of tonsillar tissue acute lymphonodular pharyngitis, lipoma, lymphoepithelial cyst, epidermoid and dermoid cysts, pyostomatitisvegetans, jaundice or icterus, lipoid proteinosis, carotenemia, and pseudoxanthoma clasticum.

ANATOMIC RADIOLUCENCIES OF JAW BONES

- Structures related to mandible
  - Mandibular foramen
  - Mandibular canal
  - Mental foramen
  - Lingual foramen
  - Airway shadow
  - Mental fossa
  - Midline symphysis
  - Medial sigmoid depression
- Structures related to maxilla
  - Intermaxillary suture
  - Incisive canal
  - Incisive foramen
  - Nasal cavity
  - Naris
  - Nasolacrimal duct or canal
  - Maxillary sinus
  - Greater palatine foramen.
- Structures common to the jaw
  - Pulp chamber
  - Root canals
  - Periodontal ligament space
  - Marrow space
  - Nutrient canals
  - Developing root crypt.

RADIOLUCENT LESIONS OF THE PERIAPICAL REGION

Periapical granuloma, periapical cyst, periapical abscess, periapical scar, surgical defect, dentigerous cyst, cementoma stage I, periodontal pathology, traumatic bone cyst, benign nonodontogenic tumor, malignant nonodontogenic tumor, ameloblastoma, aneurysmal bone cyst, ameloblastic fibroma, hemorrhagic bone cyst, buccal cyst, cementifying fibroma (early stage), ossifying fibroma (early stage), osteoblastoma, cementoblastoma, Gaucher's disease, central giant cell granuloma, hemangioma, brown tumor of hyperparathyroidism, histiocytosis X, leukemic cell invasion, lingual mandibular salivary gland depression, mandibular infected buccal cyst, odontoma (early stage), periodontal cyst, solitary/multiple myeloma, and metastatic tumor.

CLASSIFICATION OF PERICORONAL RADIOLUCENT LESIONS

Dentigerous cyst, follicular space around the crown of an impacted tooth, ameloblastoma, calcifying epithelial odontogenic cyst, adenomatoid odontogenic tumor, ameloblastic fibroma, calcifying epithelial odontogenic tumor, envelopmental odontogenic keratocyst, Ewing's sarcoma, histiocytosis X, teratoma, odontogenic carcinoma, odontogenic fibroma squamous odontogenic tumor, squamous odontogenic tumor, squamous odontogenic tumor, squamous odontogenic tumor, odontogenic myxoma, odontoma in pericoronal area, ossifying fibroma, paradental cyst, pseudotumor of hemophilia, nonodontogenic malignant tumors, and salivary gland tumors.

CLASSIFICATION OF INTERRADICULAR RADIOLUCENT LESIONS

- Periodontal pocket, lateral radicular cyst, lateral periodontal cyst, furcation involvement, odontogenic keratocyst (collateral type), traumatic bone cyst, globulomaxillary cyst, odontogenic tumors, nasopalatine duct cyst, benign nonodontogenic tumors, median mandibular cyst, and paradental cyst.

CLASSIFICATION OF MULTILOCULAR RADIOLUCENT LESIONS OF THE JAWS

Odontogenic keratocyst, ameloblastoma, central giant cell granuloma, central hemangioma, neurilemmoma, giant cell tumor of hyperparathyroidism, cherubism, odontogenic myxoma, aneurysmal bone cyst, calcifying epithelial odontogenic tumor, calcifying epithelial odontogenic cyst, ameloblastic fibroma, lymphoma, central ossifying fibroma, central mucoepidermoid tumor, central odontogenic and nonodontogenic fibroma, chondroma, chondrosarcoma, eosinophilic granuloma, immature odontoma, neuroectodermal tumor of infancy, and osteomyelitis.

MIXED RADIOLUCENT-RADIOPAQUE LESIONS ASSOCIATED WITH TEETH

- Rarefying and condensing osteitis
- Periapical cementoma—intermediate stage
- Cementifying and ossifying fibroma
- Calcifying and keratinizing odontogenic cyst
- Cementoblastoma—intermediate stage
- Foreign bodies
- Generalized (nodular cemental masses) Paget's disease
- Odontoma—intermediate stage
- Osteomyelitis—chronic
- Adenomatoid odontogenic tumor
- Keratinizing and calcifying odontogenic cyst
- Ameloblastic fibro-odontoma
- Calcifying epithelial odontogenic tumor
- Odontogenic fibroma
- Eruption sequestrum.

MIXED RADIOLUCENT-RADIOPAQUE LESIONS NOT NECESSARILY ASSOCIATED WITH TEETH

Chronic osteomyelitis osteoradionecrosis, fibrous dysplasia, Paget's disease– intermediate stage, cementifying and ossifying fibromas, osteogenic sarcoma, osteoblastic metastatic carcinoma, chondroma and chondrosarcoma, ossifying subperiosteal hematoma, adenomatoid odontogenic tumor, ameloblastic fibrodentinoma, ameloblastic fibro-odontoma, calcifying epithelial odontogenic tumor, central hemangioma, Ewing's sarcoma, intrabony hamartoma, keratinizing and calcifying odontogenic cyst, lymphoma of bone, malignant tumors with superimposed osteomyelitis, sclerosing cemental masses, osteoblastoma (intermediate), and osteoid osteoma.

MULTIPLE SEPARATE RADIOPAQUE LESIONS OF THE JAWS

- Tori and exostosis
- Multiple retained roots
- Multiple socket sclerosis
- Multiple mature cementomas
- Multiple periapical condensing osteitis
- Multiple embedded or impacted teeth
- Cleidocranial dysplasia
- Multiple hypercementosis
- Calcinosis cutis
- Cretinism (unerupted teeth)
- Cysticercosis
- Gardner's syndrome (osteomas)
- Idiopathic hypoparathyroidism
- Maffucci's syndrome
- Multiple calcified nodes
- Multiple chondromas (Ollier's disease)
- Multiple odontomas
- Multiple osteomas of skin
- Multiple phleboliths
- Multiple sialoliths
- Myositis ossificans
- Paget's disease—intermediate stage
- Sickle cell sclerosis.

GENERALIZED RADIOPACITIES OF THE JAWS

- Sclerotic cemental masses
- Paget's disease—mature stage
- Osteopetrosis

- Albright's syndrome
- Caffey's disease (infantile cortical hyperostosis)
- Fluorosis
- Gardner's syndrome
- Metastatic carcinoma of prostate
- Multiple large exostoses and tori
- Osteogenesis imperfecta.

CLASSIFICATION OF CAUSES OF TRISMUS

Intra-articular
- Traumatic arthritis, infective arthritis, rheumatoid arthritis, and dislocation
- Intracapsular fracture
- Fibrous or bony ankylosis following trauma or infection.

Extra-articular
- Adjacent infection, inflammation of TMJ (e.g. mumps, pericoronitis, submasseteric abscess, impacted 3rd molar, tonsil or peritonsillar infection)
- Extracapsular fractures (mandible, zygoma, middle third)
- Overgrowth (neoplasia) of the coronoid process
- Fibrosis from burns or irradiation
- Hematoma/fibrosis of medial pterygoid (e.g. following inferior dental block)
- Myofascial pain-dysfunction syndrome
- Drug-associated dyskinesia and psychotic disturbances
- Tetanus, tetany, rabies, jaw fracture, hysteria, parotitis, osteomyelitis, poliomyelitis, and strychnine poisoning.

CLASSIFICATION OF HAMARTOMATOUS LESIONS OF ORAL AND MAXILLOFACIAL REGION

Odontogenic Origin
Adenomatoid odontogenic tumor, squamous odontogenic tumor, ameloblastic fibro-odontoma, odontoma, peripheral odontogenic fibroma.

Nonodontogenic Origin

Vascular Origin

Hemangioma and lymphangioma.

Osseous Origin

Cemento-osseous dysplasia and fibrous dysplasia.

Skin or Mucosal Malformation

Melanocytic nevi.

Neural Origin

Neurofibromatosis.

Syndrome Associated

Peutz-Jeghers syndrome, Cowden disease (multiple hamartoma syndrome) and Maffucci syndrome.

Salivary Gland Origin

Adenomatoid hyperplasia of mucous glands.

Hard Tissue Origin

Osteochondroma and osteochondromatosis and nasal chondromesenchymal hamartoma.

CLASSIFICATION OF ORAL GRANULAR CELL LESIONS INCLUDING ODONTOGENIC AND NONODONTOGENIC TUMORS

Odontogenic Neoplasms
- Granular cell ameloblastoma
- Central and peripheral granular cell odontogenic tumor/granular cell ameloblastic fibroma/central granular cell odontogenic fibroma
- Calcifying epithelial odontogenic tumor
- Granular cell odontogenic cyst (variant of lateral periodontal cyst).

Nonodontogenic Neoplasms

Granular cell tumor, congenital epulis of newborn, leiomyoma, rhabdomyoma, neurilemmoma, granular cell traumatic neuroma, paraganglioma, dermatofibroma alveolar soft part sarcoma, malignant granular cell tumor, rhabdomyosarcoma, Hodgkin's lymphoma, basal cell carcinoma, angiosarcoma, dermato-fibrosarcoma

- Salivary gland diseases (oncocytic lesions): Sialadenosis, oncocytosis, warthin's tumor, oncocytoma, canalicular adenoma, acinic cell carcinoma, mucoepidermoid carcinoma, epithelial-myoepithelial carcinoma, oncocytic carcinoma, salivary duct carcinoma
- Melanocytic lesions: Pigmented basal cell carcinoma, malignant melanoma, nevus, melanocytic macule
- Histiocytic lesions: Langerhans cell histiocytosis, verruciform xanthoma, xanthogranuloma, atypical fibroxanthoma
- Reactive lesions: Gingival hyperplasia
- Metastatic lesions: Granular cell variant of renal cell carcinoma, metastasis from carcinoma of breast, metastatic malignant melanoma, and metastatic oncocytic carcinoma of thyroid.
- Miscellaneous: Granular cell lichen planus.

CLASSIFICATION OF GRANULOMATOUS DISEASES

- Infection:
    - Bacterial
        - Tuberculosis, leprosy, actinomycosis
    - Fungal
        - Histoplasmosis, blastomycosis, phycomycosis, aspergillosis candidiasis, and cryptocoecosis
    - Spirochetal
        - Syphilis
    - Parasitic
        - Leishmaniasis, myiasis, and toxoplasmosis
- Traumatic etiology
    - Pyogenic granuloma and reparative granuloma
- Foreign body etiology
    - Oral foreign body reactions (suture, hair, amalgam, endodontic sealer, hyaluronic acid, etc. Cholesterol granuloma, cocaine-induced midline granuloma and gout
- Neoplastic
    - Histiocytosis X, eosinophilic granuloma, Hand-Schuller-Christian disease, Letterer–Siwe disease, benign fibrous histiocytoma, necrotizing sialometaplasia, and polymorphic reticulosis
- Unknown etiology
    - Sarcoidosis and Crohn's disease
- Autoimmune and vascular disease
    - Wegener's granulomatosis, systemic lupus erythematosus, and Sjögren's syndrome
- Developmental
    - Milkersson–Rosenthal syndrome
- Congenital chronic granulomatous disease of childhood.

BIBLIOGRAPHY

1. Anniversary special issue, on 102nd birth anniversary celebration of R. Ahmed; West Bengal State Dental Journal, 2013.
2. Ash Jr M. Oral Pathology, 6th edition. Philadelphia: Lea and Febiger; 1992.
3. Cawson RA. Oral Pathology and Diagnosis—Color Atlas with Integrated Text, 1st edition. Philadelphia: Saunders; 1987.
4. Eversole LR. Clinical Outline of Oral Pathology: Diagnosis and Treatment. Shelton, CT, USA: People's Medical Publishing House; 2011.
5. Goaz PW. Oral Radiology: Principles and Interpretations. St. Louis: Mosby; 1987.
6. Lynch MA, Brightman VJ, Greenberg MS. Burket's Oral Medicine-Diagnosis and Treatment, 9th edition. Philadelphia: Lippincott Williams & Wilkins; 1994.
7. Macleod J. Davidson's Principles and Practice of Medicine, 14th edition. Edinburgh: Churchill Livingstone; 1984.

8. Prabhu SR, Daftary DK, Johnson NW. Oral Diseases in the Tropic. New York: Oxford University Press; 1992.
9. Regezi JA, Sciubba JJ, Jordan R. Oral Pathology: Clinical Pathologic Correlations. St. Louis: Saunders; 2016.
10. Sapp PJ, Eversole LR, Wysocki JP. Contemporary Oral and Maxillofacial Pathology. St. Louis: Mosby;2004.
11. Shafer WG, Hine MK, Levy BM. A Textbook of Oral Pathology, 4th edition. St Louis: WB Saunders Co.; 1983.
12. Shear M. Cysts of the Oral Region, 3rd edition. Oxford: Wright; 1992.
13. Soames JV, Southam JC. Oral Pathology, 3rd edition. New York: Oxford University Press; 1998.
14. Tencate AR. Oral Histology: Development, Structure, and Function, 3rd edition. Ontario, Canada: Mosby; 1989.
15. The Lippincott Manual of Nursing Practice, 2nd edition. Philadelphia: JB Lippincott Company; 1978.
16. Wood NK, Goaz PW. Differential Diagnosis of Oral Lesions, 4th edition. St. Louis: CV Mosby; 1991.

INDEX

Page numbers followed by *b* refer to box, *f* refer to figure, *fc* refer to flowchart, and *t* refer to table.

A

Abacavir 397
Abfraction 355
Abrasion 355
  causes of 357, 357*b*
  habitual 357, 358
  occupational 357, 358
  of teeth 357*f*
    treatment 359
  prosthetic appliances 357, 358
  ritual 357, 358
  toothbrush 357
Abscess 460
  of munro 626
  subperiosteal 477
Acantholysis 635, 639*f*, 640
  with intraepithelial vesicle formation 639*f*
Acanthomatous ameloblastoma 275, 288
Acanthosis nigricans 72, 631
  benign type 631
  malignant type 631
  treatment 631
  types 631
Achondroplasia 574, 675, 691
Acid 428
  acetic 431
  acetylsalicylic 506
  aspartic 431, 532
  butyric 431
  demineralization, rate of 432*b*
  fastness 370
  glutamic 431
  lactic 431
  mycolic 370
  produced in caries 431*b*
  propionic 431
  role of 431
  trichloroacetic 506
Acidic foods and beverages 359
Acidogenic theory 427
  limitations of 433
Acini, replacement of 236
Acinic cell carcinoma 261, 262
  treatment 263
Acinic cell tumor 259, 263*f*
  of palate 262*f*
Ackerman's tumor 106
Acquired anomalies 1
Acquired causes 590

Acquired immunodeficiency syndrome 209, 390, 464, 677
  related complex 394*b*
  treatment of 397
Acquired macroglossia, causes of 22
Acquired micrognathia 13
Acquired pellicle 607
Acquired syphilis 374
Acquired syphilitic lesions, histopathology of 377
Acridine-binding method 103
Acromegaly 13, 539, 671
  treatment 539
Actinic keratosis 106, 625
Actinic radiation 104, 198, 200
Actinobacillus actinomycetemcomitans 607, 613
Actinomyces israelii 379, 430, 431, 460 466
Actinomyces naeslundii 430, 431, 460
Actinomyces viscosus 430, 431, 607
Actinomycosis 379, 380*f*, 419, 672, 690
  abdominal 379
  predominantly 379
  treatment 381
  types 379
Acute radiation syndrome 677
Addison's disease 4, 395, 545, 634, 671, 689
Adenocarcinoma 91, 91*f*, 237, 245, 249, 259, 261-263, 264*f*
  of maxilla 263*f*
  polymorphous low grade 249, 264*f*
  treatment 264
Adenoid cystic carcinoma 98, 249, 256, 257, 257*f*, 258*f*, 261
  of palate 257*f*
  treatment 259
  typical 257*f*
Adenolymphoma 252, 253
Adenoma 67
Adenomatoid odontogenic tumor 269, 279, 280*f*, 281*f*, 282*f*, 284, 321, 338
  enucleated specimen of 281*f*
  of mandible 280*f*
  origin 279
  radiologically 281*f*
  treatment 282
Adenosine triphosphate 528
Adenosquamous carcinoma 91

Adenosquamous cell carcinoma 97, 97*f*
Adipose tissue
  neoplasms of 69
  origin, benign 129
Adrenal androgens 544
Adrenal cortex liberates 544
Adrenocortical hormone, hyperfunction of 546
Adrenocortical insufficiency, chronic 545
Adrenogenital syndrome 677
Aerodontalgia 456
Aglossia 21
Agnathia 12
Agranulocytic angina 597
Agranulocytosis 464, 597, 669
  treatment 598
Airborne infections 370
Airway shadow 694
Albers-Schönberg disease 570
Albright syndrome 4, 561, 677
Albumin 323, 329
Alcohol 80, 198, 199
  amount of 80
  consumption of 78
  inferior quality of 80
  mechanism of action of 80
  quality of 80
  quantity of 80
Alcoholism, chronic 360, 464, 670
Aldosterone 544, 545
Aldosteronism 545
Aldrich syndrome 677
Allergic conditions 544, 675
Allergic dermatitis 400
Allergic reactions 675*t*
Allergy, systemic 675
Alpha-fetoprotein 103
Alveolar bone 367
  grafting 363
Alveolar nerve, inferior 153*f*
Alveolar osteitis 520
Alveolar rhabdomyosarcoma 162, 188
Alveolar ridge 90
  malignant melanoma of upper and lower 110*f*
Amalgam 227*f*
  tattoo 112
Amelanotic melanomas 110
Ameloblastic carcinoma 93, 300, 301*f*
  radiograph of 301*f*
Ameloblastic fibrodentinoma 269

Ameloblastic fibroma 269, 288, 289f, 321, 339, 345
  of mandible 288f
  radiograph of 288f
  treatment 289
Ameloblastic fibro-odontoma 269, 289, 289f, 321, 339
  radiograph of 290f
  treatment 290
Ameloblast-like cells 273
Ameloblastoma 106, 126, 269, 271-274, 276, 276f, 285, 296, 313, 322, 336, 339, 345, 364f
  basal cell type of 276, 276f
  bone destruction in 272f
  desmoplastic type of 276
  early 332
  etiology 270
  histogenesis of 270
  malignant 300
  of mandible 271f
    intraoral swelling 271f
  peripheral 275f
  radiograph of 271f, 272f
  root resorption in 272f
  simple 271
  treatment 277
  types of 270
  unilocular 321
  Vicker and Gorlin criteria for 322b
Amelogenesis imperfecta 40, 49, 53, 55, 64, 355
  hypocalcification type 54
  hypomaturation type 54, 54f
  hypoplastic type 54, 54f
  treatment 55
  types of 53, 54, 54f
Amelogenesis, defective 50t
Amelo-onycho-hypohydrotic syndrome 677
American Joint Committee on Cancer 164
Amlodipine 615
Amphotericin-B, administration of 420
Amyloidosis 23, 533, 670
  systemic 534
  treatment 534
  types 533
Andersen syndrome 677
Anemia 464
  causing 594
Aneurysmal bone cyst 120, 126, 271, 272, 296, 306, 313, 336, 345-347, 566
  aspiration 347
  macroscopy 347
  pathogenesis 347
  treatment 347
Angiolipoma 130, 130f
Angiolymphoid hyperplasia with eosinophilia 32
Angioneurotic edema 506, 506f

Angio-osteohypertrophy syndrome 678
Angiosarcoma 162
Angiotensin-converting enzyme 384
Angular cheilitis 531, 690
  in riboflavin deficiency 532f
Angular stomatitis 496
Anisonucleosis 204
Ankyloglossia 24
  causes of development 24
  complete 24
  partial 24
  treatment 24
  types 24
Ankylosing spondylitis 581
  treatment 581
Ankylosis
  bilateral 580
  true 579
  types of 579
Anodontia 35, 497, 505
  complete 35, 35f
  etiology 35
  partial 35, 36
  total 36
  true 35
  types 35
Anomalies
  developmental 230
  hereditary developmental 1
  types of developmental 1t
Anorexia 382, 541
  cachexia syndrome 678
Anthrax 673
Antibacterial action, direct 436
Antibody-mediated hemolytic disorders 590
Anticipatory anxiety 659
Antigens, hidden 633
Antihemophilic globulin 603
Antinuclear antibody 583
Antioxidants 208
Anti-Rh agglutinins 593
Anti-Sjögren's syndrome 239
Antitubercular drugs 373
Antoni A tissue 148
Antoni B tissue 148
Antrolith 140
Aorta, coarctation of 675
Apert's syndrome 19, 675, 678
Aphthous ulcer 373, 408, 409b, 410b, 517, 630
  etiological factors in 408b
  etiology 408
  herpetiform type of 410f
  histopathology of 410
  minor 409, 409f
  of lip, major 410f
  treatment of 411
  types 409
Apical periodontitis
  chronic 458
  primary acute 458

Apicectomy 523
Aplasia 230
Aplastic anemia 485, 587, 589, 669
  common symptoms 589
  etiology 589
  oral manifestations 589
  treatment 589
Apparent macroglossia 23
Aptyalism 243
Aquamous cell carcinoma
  adenoid 97
  adenomatoid 97f
Arachnia propionica 460
Arched palate, high 572f, 573f
Areca nut 215f
Arecoline to produce arecoidene 79
Arising de novo 346
Arrested caries 439f
  of dentin 439
  of enamel 439
Arsenic 504
Arthritis, systemic juvenile 579
Arthroplasty 581
Ascher's syndrome 678
Aspergillosis 596
Aspergillus flavus 397
Aspirin 506
  burn 506f
Asymptomatic infections, chronic 393
Atazanavir 398
A-thalassemia 590
Atmospheric pollution 81
Atresia 232
  biliary 503
Atrophic candidiasis 212
  acute 414, 416
  chronic 414
  of palate 414f
Atrophic glossitis 225
Atrophic mucositis 588
Attrition 355
  causes of pathological 356
  pathological 355
  physiological 355
  treatment of 357
  types of 355
Auriculotemporal syndrome 661
Auspitz's sign 625
Autogenous transplantation 523
Autoimmune disease 396, 634, 640
  criteria for 633
Autoimmune theory 427, 434
Autoimmunity 633
  mechanism of 633
Autosomal dominant disorder 563
Azathioprine 609

B

B cell
  function, altered 634
  neoplasms, mature 174
Baby bottle syndrome 678

Index

Bacteremia 483, 489
Bacteria 607, 608
Bacterial agents 489
Bacterial infections 370, 396, 668
  nonspecific mixed 690
  specific 370
Bacterial plaque, role of 432
Bacterial sialadenitis 230, 237
  acute 237
  chronic 238
Bacteroides 466
Baelz syndrome 678
Balanitis 629
Bald tongue 588f
Ballooning degeneration 404
Basal cell adenoma 250, 251, 251f
  membranous type 251
  solid type 251
  trabecular type 251
  tubular type 251
Basal cell carcinoma 104, 105, 105f, 259, 276, 697
  of skin 105f, 312f
    multiple 311
  origin 104
  pigmented 112
  syndrome 309
    nevoid 309, 310, 310b, 311
  treatment 106
  types of 104b
Basal cells of lining epithelium, arrangement of 315f
Basaloid cell 97
Basement membrane
  reduction in thickness of 206
  zone 640
Basilar hyperplasia 204f
  of epithelium 205f
Basket cells 230
Basket weave 11
Bay cyst 324, 324f
Beckwith's hypoglycemic syndrome 678
Behcet's syndrome 409, 411, 678
  eye lesions 411
  genital lesions 411
  oral lesions 411
  skin lesions 411
  treatment 411
Bell stage
  early 268
  late 268
Bell's palsy 662, 663, 663f
  etiology of 662
  treatment 663
Benzene 594
Benzodiazepines 660
  doses of 661
Bepridil 615
Bernard-Soulier syndrome 678
Berry's syndrome 678
Bifid tongue 24

Biliary cirrhosis, primary 240
Bilirubin 504
Biliverdin 504
Bing-Neel syndrome 678
Biopsy 509
  causes of failure of 516b
  contraindications of 510
  excisional 510, 510f, 511f
  incisional 511, 512f
  indications of 509
  multiple 511
  performing 514b
  report 515
  specimen, fixation of 515b
  types of 510, 510b
  wound 518f
    fresh 518f
    healing of 518, 519f
Biphasic tumor 96
Bird facies 553
Birth injuries 52
Bismuth 504, 671
B-K mole syndrome 678
Black-gray stains 620
Bleeding
  symptoms of external 602
  symptoms of internal 602
  within large joints 602
Blepharonasofacial syndrome 678
Bloch-Sulzberger syndrome 678
Blood 391, 394
  cell types 594
  coagulation, pathways of 601
  diseases 609
  disorders 544
    common 587t
  dyscrasias 669, 669t
  hemoglobin 587
  in urine 602
  picture 178
  pigments 504
  products 391
  vessels 68
Blood-borne infections 484
Blue nevus 76
B-lymphocytes 173
B-lymphocytic origin 178
Body of mandible, fracture wound in 521f
Bohn's nodules 333
Bone 98, 394
  abscess, chronic 141
  appearance 570
  basic
    function of 552
    structure of 552
  benign neoplasm of 138
  callus, formation
    of primary 521
    of secondary 521
  cancer 164
    staging system of 164

  causing swelling of maxilla 554f
  composition of 552fc
  cortical plates of 271b
  dead 467f
  destruction, severe 168f
  disease 552, 673, 673t
    vanishing 575
  formation within lesion 168f
  infarct 169
  loss
    in jaw, severe 542f
    irregular 462f
  marrow biopsy 178
  peripheral cuffing of 122f
  pieces of 520
  radiolucency, simple 372
  resorbing activity 317, 323, 330
  resorption 553
  scan 178
Bony ankylosis, true 579
Bony artifact 297, 331
Bony myxomas 128
Book's syndrome 678
Borrelia vincentii 388, 618
Botryoid odontogenic cyst 336, 336f
  treatment 337
Bovine facies 553
Bowen syndrome 678
Brain 98
  infection 419
Branchial cleft cyst 138
Brazilian pemphigus 637
Brittle bone
  disease 566
  syndrome 678
Brodie's abscess 465
Bronzing hyperpigmentations 546
Brush biopsy 103, 514
Bruxism 355, 356, 491, 583
  causing severe attrition of teeth 492f
  treatment 493
  types of 492
Buccal mucosa 3, 83, 89, 217f, 227f, 406f, 647
  carcinoma of 89
  malignant melanoma of 110f
  preleukoplakia of 198f
  with exophytic growth, carcinoma of 90f
Buffering action 428
Buffering capacity 435
Bulimia 360
Bull neck 486f
Bull's eye 628
  lesions 628
Bull-dog nose 377
Bullous lichen planus 630, 640
  of lip 225f
Bullous pemphigoid 640, 643, 644, 644t
  treatment 644

Burkitt's lymphoma 93, 162, 178, 178f, 179, 180, 180f, 271, 395, 398
  sporadic 179
  treatment 181
  types of 179
Burning mouth syndrome 678
Burning tongue 587

C

Cachectic facies 553
Café-au-lait
  pigmentation 149
  skin pigmentations 559, 561
Caffey's disease 566, 573, 673
Caffey-Silverman syndrome 679
Calcifying epithelial odontogenic
    cyst 120, 126, 271, 284, 285, 321, 337, 337f-339f, 339, 345, 691
    classification of 338b
    pathogenesis 338
    treatment 340
  tumor 282, 283f, 284f, 285, 285f, 296, 339
Calcifying odontogenic cyst 269, 306, 309
Calcinosis cutis 653
Calcitonin 526
Calcium 526
  abnormal deposition of 527
  dietary source 526
  dystrophic calcification 527
  homeostasis 552
  pathologic calcifications 527
  types 527
Calcospherites 56
Canalicular adenoma 250, 251
Cancer
  cells, survival of 102
  multiple 85
  self-healing 73
Cancrum oris 388, 619
Candida 199
Candida albicans 26, 413
Candida associated angular cheilitis 415, 415f
Candidal endocarditis 416
Candidal hyphae 206, 417f
Candidal infections, chronic 199
Candidal meningitis 416
Candidal septicemia 416
Candidiasis 81, 198, 199, 207, 225, 413, 517, 596, 672
  acute 414
  chronic 197, 209, 414
  development of 413b
  endocrinopathy syndrome 416, 679
  histopathology of 416
  pathogenesis 413
  syndrome associated 415
  systemic 414, 416
Canine fossa infection 478
  treatment 478

Canine regions, swelling on upper 280f
Cannon's disease 10
Cannon's syndrome 632
Capillary hemangioma 134f
Capnocytophaga
  group 607
  species 613
Carbamazepine 615, 660
Carbohydrate
  metabolism, disturbances in 535
  role of 428
  types of 428, 429t
Carcinoembryonic antigen 103
Carcinogenesis 80
Carcinogenic agents 80
Carcinoma 67
  causing destructive 85f
  ex pleomorphic adenoma 91, 255, 261
  in floor of mouth 84f
  in situ 206, 210, 211, 211f
    treatment 211
Carcinosarcoma 67, 96, 255
Cardiac disease 593
Cardiac failure, congestive 675
Cardiorespiratory problems 648
Cardiovascular diseases 675, 675t
Caries
  activity tests 445
  factors with
    high 436
    low 436
  in animals, experimental 447
  pit and fissure 64, 437, 437f, 441
  proximal 441f
  radiation of 441f, 501
  smooth surface 64
  vaccine 447
Cariogenic bacteria, essential qualities of 430b
Cariogenic carbohydrate 429b
Cariogenic microorganisms, common 430b
Carious tooth with pulp exposure, X-ray of large 451f
Carotid artery
  internal 102
  syndrome 679
Cartilage tissue, benign neoplasm of 141
Cartilaginous tissue, neoplasms of 70
Cartilaginous tumor, benign 67
Causalgia 663
  criteria of 663
  factors precipitating pain in 664
  injuries that might cause 664
  nature of pain in 664
  types 664
Causative microorganisms 485
Cavernous hemangioma 134f
Cavernous sinus
  thrombosis 462, 483, 486, 675
    treatment 487

Cavity, pathological 306
Celiac disease 409, 672
Cell
  cycle, stage of 499
  dead 520
  keratinization, individual 204
  of origin 94
  peripheral 325
  proliferation, excessive 317, 323, 329
  rest 308
    of Malassez 269, 325, 332, 340
    of Serres 269, 270, 309, 332, 334
Cellular atypia 203, 203f
Cellular cementum, especially 367
Cellular layer, changes in 203
Cellular pleomorphism 204
Cellulitis 483, 484f
  acute 483
  development of 462
  treatment 485
Cemental tear 491
Cementicles 368
Cementifying fibroma 120, 281, 288, 298f, 558
Cementoblastoma 269, 299, 300f, 470
  macroscopy 300
  of right side of mandible, benign 299f
  origin 299
  radiograph of benign 299f
  treatment 300
Cementoma 296, 297f, 331
  mature 470
  treatment 297
Cementum
  changes in 368
  disturbance in structure of 63
  primary 63
Central atrophy and ulceration 649f
Central caseous necrosis 373, 373f
Central cementifying fibroma 141, 297 of mandible 298f
Central giant cell granuloma 120, 123, 125, 125t, 271, 272, 296, 331, 336, 345, 566
  causing 124f
  pathogenesis 126
  treatment 126
Central hemangioma 171, 272
Central jaw lesions 176
Central nervous system disturbances 648
Central neurilemmoma 296
Central odontogenic fibroma 126, 294
  of left mandible 294f
  treatment 295
Central ossifying fibroma 117, 118f, 141, 345
  of mandible 118f
  treatment 120
Centroblasts 177
Cerebral palsy 674

Index

Cerebriform tongue 637
Cerebrocostomandibular syndrome 679
Cervical
  lymph nodes 265
  sprain 692
Cervicofacial actinomycosis 379
Chalk stick-type fracture 555
Chancre 374
Chediak-Higashi syndrome 679
Cheek
  biting, chronic 688
  hemangioma of 132*f*
Cheilitis glandularis 5, 6, 6*f*
  etiology 5
  treatment 7
  types 6
Cheilitis granulomatosa 7, 663
  pathogenesis 7
  treatment 8
Chelation 434
Chelitis granulomatosa 7*f*
Chemical burn 207, 237, 417, 506
  types of 506
Chemical injuries 503
Chemotherapy 402
Cherubism 120, 126, 272, 562, 563, 564*f*, 565*f*, 574, 575
Chewing habits, abnormal 356
Chickenpox 400-402
  diagnosis 402
  treatment 402
Chinese restaurant syndrome 679
Chipmunk facies 553
Chloramphenicol 597, 599
Cholesterol clefts 329, 329*f*
Chondroblastoma, benign 142
Chondroblasts, malignant 166*f*
Chondroid change 248
Chondroma 67, 141, 249
  treatment 142
Chondromyxoid 248
  fibroma 296
Chondrosarcoma 165, 165*f*, 166*f*, 171, 172
  histological grading of 167*t*
  mesenchymal 167
  of left maxilla 166*f*
  periosteal 165
  primary 165
  secondary 165
  treatment 167
  variants of 166
Chromosome, abnormal 594
Chubby face 553
  in cherubism 564*f*
Church spires 107
Chvostek's sign 544
Cicatricial pemphigoid 411, 640, 641
Ciliary nerve 403
Circulating tumor cells 514

Circulatory factors 517
Clear cell
  chondrosarcoma 166
  odontogenic carcinoma 302
Cleft face syndrome, median 19, 682
Cleft in lower lip 21
Cleft in upper lip, isolated 19*f*
Cleft lip 16, 17, 311
  and palate, bilateral 19*f*
  bilateral complete 21*f*
  classification of 17*t*
  development of 19*t*
  etiology of 17
  isolated 19, 19*f*
  monogenic inheritance of 18
  pathogenesis 18
  unilateral 19*f*, 20*f*
Cleft palate 16, 17, 20, 40, 311
  bilateral complete 21*f*
  classification of 17*t*
  common syndromes with 19
  development of 19*t*
  etiology of 17
  isolated 19
  monogenic inheritance of 18
  pathogenesis 18
  unilateral 19*f*, 20*f*
Cleft tongue 24
Clefts in orofacial region, congenital malformations causing 18*b*
Cleidocranial dysplasia 19, 40, 568, 569, 675, 691
  origin 569
  treatment 570
Cloaca 465
Clostridia 590
Clostridium tetani 386, 386*f*
Clotting factors 601
Cluster headache 660
Clutton's joints 377
Coarse facies 553
Cobblestone 10, 241*f*
Coccidioides immitis 417, 417*f*
Coccidioidomycosis 417
  oral manifestation 417
  treatment 418
Codman's triangle 171, 172
Coffee ground vomitus 602
Coffin-Lowry syndrome 679
Coin-like circular skin rashes of secondary syphilis 375*f*
Cold sores 400
Collagen diseases 544
Columnar oncocytes 254
Common autoimmune diseases 634
Common wart 405
Complete blood count 583
Complex odontoma 171, 269, 470
Complex odontome 291*f*
  excised specimen of 292*f*
Compound nevus 76
Compound odontoma 269

Concrescence 43, 44, 64
Condensing osteitis 297, 469
Condylar hyperplasia 578
Condyloma acuminatum 405
Condyloma lata 375
Cone biopsy 513
Congenital anomalies 1
Congenital macroglossia, causes of 22
Congenital syphilis, clinical features of 376
Conjunctivitis 642
Connective tissue 509
  changes 218
  neoplasms 230
  stroma 218, 284
  supra-alveolar 611
Constitutional diseases 394
Contact allergy 213, 675
Containing clear fluid 642
Cooley's anemia 591
Core biopsy 513
  vacuum-assisted 513
Core needle biopsy 513
Corneal cells 241
Cortex, duplication of 473, 473*f*
Cortisol 544
Corynebacterium diphtheriae 382
Costen's syndrome 679
Costochondral grafting 581
Cotton-wool appearance 555, 555*f*
Cow's milk 370
Cowden's syndrome 72, 679, 693
Coxsackie virus 408
  infections 407
Cracked tooth syndrome 679
Cramp-like pain, severe 534
Craniofacial dysostosis 569
Craniopharyngioma 339
Crest syndrome 653, 679
  features of 653*t*
Cretinism 539, 672
Crevicular fluid 610
Cribriform pattern 258
Cri-dui-chat syndrome 679
Crocodile tears, syndrome of 686
Crohn's disease 7, 411, 614, 616, 672, 690, 693, 697
Cross syndrome 679, 693
Crouzon syndrome 19, 631, 679
Crumpled cigarette papers 654
Cruzon's syndrome 675
Cryptococcal meningitis 397
Cryptococcosis 419, 419*f*
  oral manifestation 419
  treatment 420
Cryptococcus neoformans 397
Cushing's syndrome 546, 671, 679
  clinical features of 546*b*
  oral manifestations of 546*b*
Cutaneous anomalies 311
Cutaneous lesions 221

Cyclic neutropenia 409, 598
  treatment 598
Cyclosporine 609, 615
Cylindroma 258
Cyst 310, 317, 348, 362, 472
  abscess 326
  aggressive nature of 318
  branchial 31
  classification of 306
  contents of 306
  developmental 306
  enlargement of 317, 329
    mechanism of 317b
  epithelium, keratinization pattern of 318
  fluid, osmolarity of 317, 323, 329
  in jaw 363
  inflammatory 306
  lining
    corrugated nature of 318
    nature of 318
  nonepithelial 307
  nonodontogenic 307, 340
  normal 279t
  odontogenic 306
  of dental lamina 333
  of incisive papillae 343
  of maxillary antrum, surgical ciliated 352f
  of oral region 232, 306
  of salivary gland 347
    etiology 347
    pathogenesis 347
    treatment 349
  of tissue
    of face 307
    of mouth 307
    of neck 307
  primordial 308
  types of 333
Cystic epithelial cells 322
Cystic epithelium 328f
  metaplasia of 336
Cystic fluid 314, 327
  in dentigerous cyst 321
  in odontogenic keratocysts 314f
  in radicular cyst 328f
Cystic hygroma 136, 137, 137f, 351
  treatment 138
Cystic lesion 347
  in tongue 23
Cystic lining epithelium 330
Cysticercosis 349
Cystine trypticase agar 379
Cytologic smear 400
Cytology, exfoliative 103, 515, 516, 516f
Cytomegalovirus infection 161, 404
  treatment 404
Cytoplasms 10
Cytotoxic drug therapy 505f
  oral manifestations of 504

D

Dancing eyes 626
Darier's disease 625, 630, 689
Daughter cyst 315f, 319f
Davis and Ritchie classification 17
De novo lesions 79
Deciduous incisor teeth, upper 438f
Deciduous teeth 57f
  premature exfoliation of 40
  retained 40
Defense cells 102
Dens evaginatus 48, 49
  of maxillary lateral incisors 48f
  pathogenesis 48
  treatment 48
Dens in dente 46, 47f, 64
  radicular 47f
  treatment 48
  types 46
Dens invaginatus 46, 49
  causing pulp exposure 454f
Dental anomalies 311
Dental calculus 608f
Dental caries 355, 426, 426f, 428, 430-432, 436t, 450
  acidogenic theory 427
  arrested caries 439
  backward caries 440
  chronic caries 439
  clinical aspects of 437
  clinical types 437
  contributing factors in 434
  epidemiology of 426
  forward caries 440
  incipient caries 437
  initiation of 433b
  major theories of 427b
  nursing bottle caries 438, 439
  pathophysiology of 427
  prevention of 435, 436
  proteolytic theory of 433
  radiation caries 440
  rampant caries 438, 439
  recurrent caries 440
  root caries 440
  sequelae of 444fc
  smooth surface caries 437
Dental erosion, prevention of 361
Dental factors 78, 80
Dental floss 358
Dental follicle 269
  enlarged 321
Dental lamina 268, 307, 309, 334
  cyst 333
    treatment 334
    remnants of 286
Dental pain 450
Dental papilla 268
  formation of 268
Dental plaque 428, 607, 608
Dental procedures 579

Dental pulp 366
Denticles 366
Dentigerous cyst 272, 281, 308, 313, 318, 321, 322, 322b, 322f, 339
  in early stage 320f
  lateral 332, 340
  long-standing 322
  of mandible 320f
  pathogenesis of 319, 319fc
  radiograph of 320, 320f
  treatment of 324
  X-ray of 321f
Dentin 63
  biochemical property of 59
  changes in 368
  disturbances in structure of 56
  dysplasia 60, 61f, 64
    defective dentin in 62f
    types 60
  irregular reactionary 444
  of two separate teeth, merger of 42f
  protective responses of 444
  pulp complex 450
  regular reactionary 444
  subtransparent 443
  tissues 268
  transparent 443
Dentinal abnormality 60
Dentinal caries 431
Dentinal changes 60
Dentinal tubules 443f
Dentinoenamel junction, loss of scalloping at 59f
Dentinogenesis imperfecta 49, 56, 57f, 58, 59, 59f, 64, 355
  classification 56
  in permanent teeth 57f
  treatment 59
Dentinogenic ghost-cell tumor 285, 339
  of maxilla 286f
Dentin-pulp complex, disease of 450
Dentoalveolar abscess 460
Dentobuff 445
Denture
  hyperplasia 496
  related injuries 496
  sore mouth 496
  stomatitis 496
Depressed nasal bridge 572f
Depression 659
Dermal calcinosis 311
Dermal lesions, diagnosis of 623
Dermatitis herpetiformis 225, 630, 640
  treatment 630
Dermatofibroma 112
Dermatologic conditions 544
Dermatological diseases 672, 672t
Dermatological disorders 623
  oral aspects of 623
Dermatomyositis 240

Dermoid cyst 351, 352*f*
  in midline of floor of mouth 351*f*
  treatment 352
Desmoplastic ameloblastoma 276*f*
Desmoplastic fibroma 114, 120, 271
  treatment 115
Desquamative gingivitis, clinical
    features of 617
Destructive inflammatory disease,
    chronic 606
Destructive periodontal diseases,
    chronic 606
Dextran 429
Diabetes 464, 547
  insipidus 538
    causes 538
    treatment 538
  juvenile 547
  mellitus 485, 547, 608, 631, 670
    complications of 548*b*
    insulin-dependent 547
    noninsulin-dependent 547
    oral manifestations of 548*b*
    treatment of 549
    types of 547
Diabetic ketoacidosis 548
  features of 549
Diabetic nephropathy 548
Diabetic neuropathy 548
Diabetic retinopathy 548
Diarrhea 395
  chronic persistent 397
Diastolic pressure, decreased 541
Didanosine 397
Diet factor 436
Diet, composition of 436
Dietary carbohydrates 428, 430
Dietary deficiency 198, 199
DiGeorge syndrome 543
Dilaceration 44, 64
Diltiazem 615
Dimorphism 413
Diphtheria 382
  treatment 383
Discoid lupus erythematosus 207,
    225, 417, 646, 648, 649*f*, 650*t*
  clinical features of 649
Discrete cemental masses in periapical
    area 297*f*
Disseminated infections 395
Distomolars 37
Diuretics 599
Dog-like facies 553
Down's syndrome 19, 23, 137,
    572, 572*f*, 594, 618, 675,
    675, 679
  oral manifestations of 572
  treatment 573
  with macroglossia 573*f*
Drug addiction 464
Dry eye 642
Dry mouth 243

Dry socket 520
  possible causes of 520*b*
  treatment 521
Ductal epithelium, metaplasia of 241*f*
Ductal proliferation and stroma 247*f*
Dull facies 553
Dysgeusia 244
Dyskeratosis 204
  congenita 631
    treatment 632
Dysphagia 632
Dysplasia 203
  cytological changes of 204
  histological classification of 204
  in epithelium, architectural changes
    of 204
  severe 204*f*, 211*f*, 213*f*
Dystrophic calcification 527
  pathogenesis of 527

E

Eagle's syndrome 664, 680, 692
Eburnated dentin 439
Ecchymosis 689
  of skin 596*f*
Ectoderm 351
Ectodermal dysplasia 623, 672
  hereditary 623, 624*f*, 625
  treatment 625
  types of 623
Ectopic salivary glands, common
    locations of 232
Edematous, acute 483
Edwards syndrome 19, 680
Egg shell crackling 271
Ehlers-Danlos syndrome 311, 654,
    672, 680
  treatment 655
  types of 655
Eikenella corrodens 607, 613
Elbows 645
Electrical burns of mouth,
    complications of 497*t*
Electrical pulp test 457
Elephant foot 107
Elephantiasis nostras verrucosa 6
Ellis-Van creveld syndrome 680
Elsahy-Waters syndrome 19
Embedded tooth 41
Embryonal rhabdomyosarcoma 164,
    188, 189*f*
Emtricitabine 397
Enamel 63
  acquired disturbances of 50
  after tooth formation, causes of loss
    of 355*b*
  caries 441
  changes in 368
  disturbance in structure of 50
  epithelium, reduced 323, 340
  formation 50
    hereditary disturbance of 53

hypocalcification 50
hypoplasia 51, 51*f*, 52, 385
  generalized 51, 52*f*
  pitted 406
opacity, idiopathic 50, 51*f*
organ 307
pearl 49
solubility test 446
Encephalitis 395
Enchondroma 566
Enchondromatosis, multiple 165
Endocarditis, subacute bacterial 676
Endochondromas 142
Endocrine
  disorders 22
  disturbances 671, 671*t*
  imbalance 614, 615
  neoplasia syndrome, multiple 682
Endoderm 351
Endodontic-periodontic lesions 474
Endosteal hyperostosis 571
Endothelial myeloma 162
Environmental enamel
    hypoplasia 49
Enzymatic mechanisms 317
Enzyme-linked immunosorbent
    assay 397
Eosinophil microabscesses 639
Eosinophilic cells 631
Eosinophilic cytoplasms 252
Eosinophilic enameloid
    material 282*f*
Eosinophilic granular cells 252
Eosinophilic granuloma 93, 120, 172,
    536, 536*f*, 562, 566
  radiograph of 536*f*
  treatment 536
Eosinophilic perivascular cuffing 566
Epidermal nevus syndrome 680
Epidermoid carcinoma 146
Epidermoid cell 261*f*
Epidermolysis bullosa 49, 55, 644,
    672, 689
  pathogenesis 644
  treatment 645
  types 644
Epilepsy 626, 674
Epistaxis 85
Epithelial barrier 610
Epithelial cell 249, 338
  neoplastic proliferation of 289*f*
  rests of Malassez 324
Epithelial dysplasia 197, 203, 204
  degree of 208
  features of 204*b*
  grades of 204
  in leukoplakia 206*b*
  mild 205, 205*f*
  moderate 205, 205*f*
  severe 205, 206*f*
Epithelial hyperplasia 203*f*
Epithelial mucin 248

Epithelial odontogenic tumor,
 benign 286
Epithelial overgrowths 91
Epithelial progenitor cells 230
Epithelial root sheath of hertwig 269
Epithelial tissue 71
 neoplasms 230, 245
 origin 71
  malignant neoplasms of 77
  neoplasms of 69t
Epithelial tumor
 benign 67, 231
 malignant 231
Epithelioid cells 373f, 377
Epithelioid fibrosarcoma,
 sclerosing 155
Epithelium
 changes in thickness of 203
 tangential section of 96f
Epstein's pearls 333
Epstein-Barr virus 78, 239, 405
 diseases 398
 infection 179, 405
Epulis fissuratum 496, 497f
Erosion 355
 clinical features of 360
Erosive lichen planus 212, 630
 turning into carcinoma 226f
Eruption abnormalities, types of 39
Eruption cyst 309, 331, 339
 origin 331
 treatment 331
Eruption hematoma 331
Eruption of teeth
 disturbances in 38
 factors causing delayed 39
Erythema multiforme 400, 627, 627f,
 629, 630, 640
 causes of 627t
 major 627, 629
 minor 627, 628
 oral manifestations 628
 treatment 630
 types of 627
Erythematous maculopapular skin
 rash 406f
Erythematous patch 25
Erythroblastosis fetalis 504, 587,
 593, 669
 oral manifestation 593
 pathogenesis 593
Erythromycin 615
Erythroplakia 82, 197, 211, 212, 213f
 etiology 212
 of cheek 212f
 speckled 212
 treatment 213
Esophageal dysfunction 653
Esophagitis 360, 654
Estrogen 609
Ethambutol 373
Ethotoin 615

Ewing's sarcoma 93, 162, 163, 163f,
 164, 167, 168, 173t, 190, 473
 jaws lesions of 163
 of maxilla 163f
 origin of 162
Ewing's tumor 162
Exanthematous disease 52
Excisional biopsy
 advantage of 511
 limitations of 511
 procedure of 511f
Exfoliative cytology
 indications of 517b
 technique of 516
Exostoses 140
Extracellular matrix, degradation
 of 611
Extracellular polysaccharide 429
Extracted mesiodens 38f
Extraction wound, healing of 519
Extralateral incisors 37
Extramedullary plasmacytoma 187
Extrapulmonary tuberculosis 370, 371
Eye 393, 394
 blister formation in 642
 lesions 642
 misaligned 626
 toward heaven 564
 vesicle formation in 642f

F

Face 654
 development of 1
Facial changes 653
Facial deformity 497
Facial hemiatrophy 15, 15f
 radiograph of 15f
 treatment 16
Facial hemihypertrophy 14, 14f
 etiology 14
 of left side 14f
 oral manifestations 15
 radiograph of 14f
 treatment 15
Facial muscles 654, 659
Facial nerve
 functions of 662
 paralysis 662
Facial skin
 erythematous rash on 646f
 impetigo on 381f
 rigidity of 652f
 scleroderma involving 652f
Factitious injuries 495
False ankylosis 579
Familial fibrous dysplasia 563
Familial gigantiform cementoma 297
 origin 298
 treatment 299
Familial gingival fibromatosis 617f
Familial mucocutaneous
 candidiasis 415

Familial muscular dystrophy,
 generalized 664
Familial rickets 530f
Fanconi's syndrome 589, 632, 680
Fat-soluble vitamin 531
Felbamate 615
Fessas bodies 592
Fetal-alcohol syndrome 680
Fever, low-grade 382
Fibrinogen 323, 329
Fibroblast cells, malignant 155
Fibroepithelial polyp 148, 349, 389, 389f
Fibrolipoma 130
Fibroma 67, 112, 113f, 144, 146,
 148, 249
 irritation 113f, 114f
 ossifying and cementifying 120f
 treatment 114
Fibromatosis 129
 gingivae 11, 11f
 treatment 12
Fibromyalgia 692
Fibromyxoid appearance 249
Fibro-osseous lesions, classification
 of 691
Fibrosarcoma 129, 154, 155, 155f,
 172, 273
 anaplastic form of 155
 developing in mandible 154f
 high-grade 155
 intermediate grade 155
 of maxilla 154f
 primary 154
 secondary 154
 treatment 156
 types of 154
Fibrosis, peripheral 373
Fibrous ankylosis
 intra-articular 580
 true 580
Fibrous callus, formation of 521
Fibrous connective tissue
 benign neoplasm of 112
 neoplasms of 69
Fibrous dysplasia 119, 126, 169, 347,
 464, 560f, 563, 673
 disseminated juvenile 563
 immature 473
 of bone 120, 558, 562, 563f, 566
 of mandibular lesions 560f
 of maxillary lesions 560f
Fibrous histiocytoma 120, 129
 benign 126, 127f, 697
 malignant 93, 97, 156, 156f, 157f, 690
 of mandible, benign 127f
Fibrous hyperplasia, causes of 614
Fibrous tissue 236, 575
Filiform papilla 28
Fine needle aspiration cytology
 249, 513
 aspirated sample after 513f
 procedure of 513f

Fish mouth 653
Fish-like face 553
Fissured tongue 25, 25f
　etiology 25
　treatment 25
Fistulas 2
Floor of mouth 83
　carcinoma of 88
Floppy infant syndrome 680
Florid osseous dysplasia 298, 558
Fluid deprivation test 538
Fluoride
　action 435
　and mottling 52
　role of 436
Fluorosis 504, 673
Focal dermal hypoplasia
　　syndrome 72, 680
Focal enamel hypoplasia 50
Focal epithelial hyperplasia 9
Focal gingival enlargements 693
Focal infection 488
　mechanism of 488
Focal microdontia 32, 34
Focal reversible pulpitis 451
　etiology of 451b
Focal sclerosing osteomyelitis 140, 300
　chronic 469, 470f
Fogo selvagem 637
Folic acid 532, 586
　deficiency 532, 668
　　anemia 669
　　causes of 532
Follicular ameloblastoma 273, 274f, 275f
Forbidden clone 634
Fordyce's granules 8, 8f, 9
　cheek 8f
　lip 8f
　treatment 9
Foreign body
　etiology 697
　reaction 373
Formalin fixative, biopsy sample in 515f
Fracture
　bone, abnormally healed 574
　callus 172
　jawbone, healing of 521
　pathological 85, 271
Fragile X syndrome 680
Frenal tag 3
　treatment 3
Frey's syndrome 661, 680
Frog-like face 553
Frontal bossing 377
Frozen section biopsy 513
Fungal agents 489
Fungal infection 370, 393, 413
　deep 396, 417
Furrowed tongue 25
Fusion 41
　causes 41
　complete 42
　incomplete 42
　treatment 43
　types of 43
Fusobacterium necrophorum 388
Fusobacterium nucleatum 607, 618

G

Galactose 429
Galvanic reactions 200
Galvanism 198, 200
Gap arthroplasty 581
Gardner's syndrome 40, 139, 680
Gargoyle facies 553
Garre's osteomyelitis 163, 164, 172, 298, 472, 473, 562, 691
　of mandible 472f, 473f
Gasserian ganglion 659
Gastritis 360
Gastroesophageal reflux disease 360
Gastrointestinal infections 395
Gastrointestinal problems 544
Gastrointestinal system 394
Gastrointestinal tract involvement 648
Gaucher's disease 537
Gemination 41, 64
　problems in 41
　treatment 41
Genetic disorders 675, 675t
Geniculate neuralgia 692
Genital herpes 401
Genital lesions 629
Genital ulcers 409
Genitalia 394
Geographic tongue 27, 28, 28f, 209, 626
　etiology of 27
　treatment of 28
Gestational diabetes 549
　cause of 549
Ghost cells 337, 338, 339f
Ghost tooth 49, 62, 64
Giant cell 120, 691
　epulis 690
　fibroma 113, 115, 145
　　treatment 115
　granuloma 126, 543
　　peripheral 113, 120, 121f, 122f, 123, 148
　　radiograph of central 124f
　Langhans type of 374f
　lesions
　　classification of 690
　　of oral cavity, common 120b
　multinucleated 345
　periostitis 473
　tumor 690
　　of bone 120, 123, 125, 125t, 126, 169, 347, 555, 562
　type 169
Gigantism 538
　oral manifestations of 539b
Gilles De La Tourette syndrome 681
Gingiva 286, 647, 654
　atrophic lichen planus of 224f
　attached 90
　carcinoma of 90, 90f
　developmental defects of 11
　dilantin hyperplasia of 616f
　mucosal lesion in 649f
　swellings of 283
Gingival acrylic splints, placement of 12
Gingival bleeding 599f
Gingival cyst 309, 333, 333t, 334, 334f
　treatment 335
Gingival enlargement 11
　classification of 693
　generalized 693
　severe 596f
Gingival fibromatosis 11
Gingival hyperplasia 596, 609, 614-617
　causes of 614
　common drugs with 615b
　drug induced 614f, 616
　hereditary 616
　in leukemia 615f
　localized 616f
Gingival inflammation 611
Gingival involvement, severe 629
Gingival lesion 161f
Gingival recession 608f
Gingival tissue 11
Gingivectomy wound, healing of 518
Gingivitis 396, 606, 607, 610
　aggravation of 609
　clinical features of early 610
　common consequences of 611
　desquamative 617, 617f, 640, 642
　generalized 611f
　in diabetic patient, severe 548f
　localized 612f
　with recession 612f
Gland
　acini, replacement of 238
　minor 245
　neoplasms 246
　suprarenal 544
　type 245
Glandular fever 405
Glandular odontogenic cyst 335, 335f, 336f
Glenoid fossa 578
Globulin 323, 329
Globulomaxillary cyst 281, 332, 340, 341, 341f
　treatment 341
Glossal central papillary atrophy 25
Glossitis 587
Glossodynia 587, 550, 661, 664
　etiology of 661
Glossopharyngeal neuralgia 660, 662
　etiology 662
　pharyngeal type of 662
　triggering factors 662
　tympanic type of 662

Glossoptosis 692
Glossopyrosis 588, 661
   etiology of 661
Glucocorticoid 544
   function of 544
   indications of 545
   therapy 549
Glycosaminoglycans 56, 321, 552
Goblet cells 323
   mucous secreting 328, 335
Gohn complex 373
Goldenhar syndrome 19, 680
Gonorrhea 378, 674, 690
   clinical presentation of 378
   diagnosis of 379
   oral manifestations of 378
   symptoms of 378b
   treatment 379
Gorlin cyst 337
Gorlin's sign, positive 655
Gorlin-Chaudhry-Moss syndrome 681
Gorlin-Goltz syndrome 311, 311b, 312b, 680, 693
   association with 318
Graft reaction 225
Gram-negative rods 457
Gram-positive rods 457
Granular cell
   ameloblastoma 275
   myoblastoma 144, 145
   tumor 91, 145, 146f, 697
      origin 145
      treatment 146
Granulation tissue 458
Granulocytopenia 597
Granuloma 332, 458
   inguinale 674
Granulomatous diseases 672, 672t
   classification of 697
Graphite 671
Grave's disease 634
Grenz zone 127
Grinspan syndrome 680
Guillain-Barrè syndrome 634
Gumma 376
Gunshot injuries 484

H

Hailey-Hailey disease 689
Hair
   absence of 623
   dysplasia 623
   follicle 9, 352f
   grips 358
   lack of 624
   over scalp, loss of 647f
Hair-bearing areas 104
Hairy leukoplakia 396, 398, 692
Hairy tongue 29, 29f
   treatment 29
Hajdu-Cheney syndrome 681
Hallermann-Streiff syndrome 681

Halo mole 76
Halo nevus 76
   on facial skin 76f
Hamartoma 153
Hamartomatous anomalies 1
Hamartomatous lesions, classification of 696
Hand-foot-and-mouth disease 408, 691
Hand-Schuller-Christian
   disease 535, 697
   syndrome 681
Hank's balanced salt solution 522
Hansen disease 384
Happy puppet syndrome 681
Hard palate, hemangioma of 132f
Hard tissue 274
   origin 696
Hashimoto's disease 634
Headache 382
Healing phase
   early 518
   late 519
Heart 393
   disease, congenital 675
Heck's disease 9, 688
Heerfordt's syndrome 242, 681
Helicobacter pylori infections 173
Helminthic diseases 673, 673t
Helminthic infections 393
Hemangioendothelioma 158, 158f, 159, 159f
   treatment 159
Hemangioma 112, 131, 131t, 135, 136t, 138, 160, 162, 165
   capillary 134
   cavernous 134
   central 133, 135
   growth pattern 131
   intramuscular 132
   macroscopic findings 134
   radiographic appearance of central 134
   strawberry 132
   treatment 135
Hemangiomatous
   ameloblastoma 276, 277f
Hemangiopericytoma 158, 159, 160f, 168
   treatment 160
Hemarthrosis 580, 583
Hematologic disorders 648
   oral aspects of 586
Hematolymphoid tumors 231
Hematoma 112, 172
   on face due to injury 492f
Hemifacial hyperplasia 23
Hemochromatosis 529
Hemolysis 590, 592
Hemolytic anemia 587, 589
   causes 590
   oral manifestations 590
   treatment 590

Hemolytic jaundice 592
Hemophilia 600, 669
   A 600
   classic 600
   common complications in 603
   etiology 600
   major symptoms of 602b
   oral manifestation of 603
   pathogenesis of 602
   treatment 603
   types 600
Hemopoietic tissues, classification of diseases of 691
Hemorrhage 594
   intracranial 660
Hemorrhagic bone cyst 344, 346
Hemorrhagic telangiectasia, hereditary 112, 669
Herpangina 407
   treatment 408
Herpein 398
Herpes labialis 399f, 400
Herpes simplex 517, 630
   infection of facial skin 398f
   virus 78, 199
      diseases 398
      infections 398, 401
Herpes virus 398
   infections 398
Herpes zoster 363, 401, 402, 402f, 403, 517, 629
   diagnosis of 404
   infection 362
Herpetic eczema 400
Herpetic gingivostomatitis
   acute 399
   primary 399, 399f
Herpetic infections 400
Herpetic stomatitis
   acute primary 629
   primary 691
Herpetic ulcers 411
Herpetiform ulcer 410
Hertwig epithelial root sheath 325
Hippocratic facies 553
Histoplasma capsulatum 397, 418, 418f
Histoplasmosis 418, 419f, 596, 672
   oral manifestations 418
   treatment 419
Hodgkin's disease 691
   types of 183
Hodgkin's lymphoma 120, 173, 174, 181, 181b, 181f, 182, 182f, 182t, 184, 184t, 402, 690, 697
   feature of 181
   histological types of 183
   staging system of 183t
Homogenous
   erythroplakia 212
   leukoplakia 201f, 207

Index

transplantation 523
ulcerative leukoplakia 201f
Honey-comb appearance 272, 272f
Hormonal imbalance 198, 199, 363
Hormone
  adrenal 544
  adrenocorticotropic 545
  disorder 544
  female sex 199
  metabolism, disturbances in 537
  pancreatic 547
Horner's syndrome 681
Host reaction 225
Human androgen receptor gene 245
Human blood cells, types of 586, 586fc
Human cytomegalovirus diseases 398
Human immunodeficiency virus 78, 208, 370
  infection 396, 402, 409, 464, 485
    pathogenesis of 391
  stages of 392t
  structure of 391f
  verruca of mouth in 396f
Human papillomavirus 78, 106, 199
  infection 405
Human T-cell lymphotropic virus 239
Hunter's glossitis 587, 692
Hunter's syndrome 681
Hurler's syndrome 535, 670, 681
  treatment 535
Hutchinson's freckle type 111
Hutchinson's incisors 52
Hutchinson's teeth 377
Hutchinson's triad 377
Hutchinson-Gilford syndrome 681
Hyaline ring 282
Hyalinized stroma 248
Hydrocephalus 377
Hydrochloric acid preparations 360
Hydrophobia 412
Hydrostatic pressure 317, 323, 330
Hyoid syndrome 681
Hypercementosis 63, 64, 64f, 65f, 367
  etiology of 367t
  microscopy 367
Hyperextension 692
Hyperglycemia 547
Hyperkeratinization 203
Hypermineralized bone 557f
Hyperorthokeratinization 203
Hyperorthokeratinized epithelium 202f
Hyperparakeratinization 203
Hyperparakeratinized epithelium 202f
Hyperparathyroidism 296, 313, 360, 362, 541, 542f, 543b, 558, 562, 566, 575, 671
  after treatment 543f
  brown tumor of 120, 126, 562
  multiple giant 543f
  treatment 543
Hyperphosphatemia 528

Hyperpigmented black papules 222f
Hyperpituitarism 362, 538, 541
Hyperplasia 203, 372f
  pseudoepitheliomatous 146
Hyperplastic
  candidiasis, chronic 415, 415f, 416
  epithelium 416
  gingivitis, chronic 614
  pulpitis, chronic 455
Hypertension 675
Hyperthyroidism 671
  causes 541
  oral manifestations of 541b
  treatment 541
Hypertrichosis 15
Hypervitaminosis A 668
Hypocalcemia 52
Hypocementosis 64
  causes 64
Hypodontia 36
Hypoglycemia 537, 549
Hypoglycemic coma and death 548
Hypomaturation 54
Hypoparathyroidism 49, 543, 671
  causes 543
  juvenile 60
  oral manifestations of 544b
  treatment 544
Hypophosphatasia 60, 362, 528, 670
  cytotoxic agents 60
  dentinal changes 60
Hypophosphatemia 60, 362, 528, 670
  causes 528
Hypopituitarism 537
  causes 537
  dwarfism 537
  oral manifestations of 537b
Hypothyroidism 23, 362, 539, 631
  causes 539
  general features of 540
Hypotrichosis 624
Hypovolemic shock 676

I

Immune-mediated chronic inflammatory disease, multisystem 239
Immune-mediated diseases 230, 238
Immunity 437
  suppression of 102
Immunofluorescence test
  direct 651
  indirect 651
Immunosuppression 81, 161
Impaction of tooth, factors causing 40
Incisional biopsy
  advantage of 511
  limitation of 512
  performing 512
Incisive canal cyst 342

Incisors
  palatal aspect of upper central 37f
  teeth, fusion of 42f
Incontinentia pigmenti 626
  treatment 627
Indinavir 398
Indomethacin 599
Infantile cortical hyperostosis 573
  oral manifestations 573
  treatment 574
  types 573
Infantile osteopetrosis 570
Infected dentin 443, 443f, 444f
Infected postextraction wound 484
Infections 517
  acute 392
  chronic 78
  focus of 488
  primary sources of 484t
  route of spread of 238, 486
  space 462, 477-479, 483
  spreading into neck, space 478f
Infectious diseases, acute lethal type 673, 673t
Infectious mononucleosis 398, 405, 651
  treatment 405
Infective lesions 230, 237, 690, 690t
Inflammatory cell 518
  infiltration, chronic 206
Inflammatory dermatological disease, chronic 625
Inflammatory disease 464
Inflammatory disorders 581
Inflammatory enlargements 693
Inflammatory gingival hyperplasia 614f
Inflammatory hyperplasia of tissue 135
Inflammatory periodontal diseases, chronic 606
Inflammatory resorption, internal 365
Infraorbital area, large swelling in 90f
Infratemporal space infection 478
Insomnia 659
Insulin
  importance of 547
  resistance 547
Interradicular radiolucent lesions, classification of 694
Intestinal polyposis, hereditary 3
Intra-alveolar carcinoma, primary 93, 112, 271, 302
Intracellular polysaccharides 429
Intracranial bleeding 602
Intracytoplasmic myofibrils 143
Intradermal nevus 75
Intraluminal unicystic ameloblastoma 278, 279
Intramucosal nevus 75
Intramuscular lipomas 131
Intraoral lesion 278f
Intraoral nevus, benign 112

Intraosseous hemangioma 347
Intraosseous mucoepidermoid
    tumor 336
Intraosseous odontogenic cysts 335
Intraspinal seeding 98
Intrinsic stain, causes of 621
Invasion, local 67
Involucrum 465
Ionizing radiation 81, 501*t*
Iris 628
Iron 528
    absorption 528
    deficiency anemia 80, 587, 588,
        588*f*, 669
        causes 588
        oral manifestation 588
        treatment 589
Irritation, chronic 198, 200, 200*f*
Ischemic heart disease 548

J

Jacob ulcer 104
Jadassohn-Lewandowsky
    syndrome 681
Jaffe-Lichtenstein syndrome 559, 681
Jaffey's type 559
Jaundice 376, 670
Jaw
    and teeth, smaller size of 15*f*
    bone
        anatomic radiolucencies of 694
        development of 1
        malignancies, detection of 92*b*
        metastatic tumor of 473
        pathological fracture of 92*f*
        tuberculous lesions of 372
    carcinoma of 92*f*
    cysts, clinical significance of 307
    fracture, healing of wound after 522*f*
    generalized radiopacities of 695
    malignancy 92
    metastatic tumors of 190
        treatment 191
    multiple separate radiopaque
        lesions of 695
    torus in 16
Jaw-winking syndrome 682
Joint problems 648
Joint space, obliteration of 581*f*
Jugular foramen syndrome 681
Junctional nevus, treatment 76
Juxtacortical lesions 165
Juxtacortical osteosarcoma 172

K

Kaposi's sarcoma 112, 135, 158, 160,
    161, 161*f*, 162*f*, 213, 395, 397,
    398, 404, 691
    endemic 161
    etiology 161
    nodular stage 162

of gingiva 161*f*, 397*f*
patch stage 161
plaque stage 162
treatment 162
Keratin 203
    flakes 316
    horn 106, 107*f*
    pearls 275
    plugging 74
Keratinization pattern 318
Keratinized epithelial cells, grain-
    like 631
Keratinocytes 203
Keratoacanthoma 73, 74*b*, 74*f*
    causes 73
    development of 73
    of lower lip 72*f*
    origin 73
    treatment 74
Keratoconjunctivitis 400
    sicca 241
Keratocyst 40, 312, 313, 313*t*
    collateral type of 288, 313
    envelopmental type of 313
    extraneous type of 313
Keratosis
    follicularis 630, 673
        treatment 631
    frictional 207, 496
Kernahan and Stark symbolic
    classification 17
Kidney
    diseases 485
    transplantation 674
Kissing disease 405
Kissing lesions 650
Klestadt's cyst 341
Klinefelter's syndrome 682
Knob-like enlargement 64
Koilocytes 10, 72
Koplik's spots 406, 406*f*

L

Labial fibrous bands 217*f*
Lacrimal auricular-dental and digital
    syndrome 682
Lacrimal glands 238
Lactobacillus 431
    acidophilus 430, 431
Lamina propria 226
    fibrosis of 218*f*
Lamivudine 397
Langerhans cell
    disease 120
    histiocytosis 162
Langhans type giant 385
Laparotomy 178
Larsen syndrome 19, 682
Laser Doppler flowmetry 457
Laser radiation 503
Laugier-Hunziker syndrome 682

Lead 504
Leiomyoma 143, 145, 148
    intraosseous 143
    treatment 144
    types 144
Leiomyosarcoma 187
    treatment 188
Leishmaniasis 419, 674
Leonine face 385, 553
Leontiasis ossea 554
Lepra cells 385
Lepromas 385
Leprosy 384, 690
    diagnosis 385
    facial skin in 384*f*
    oral manifestations of 385*b*
    treatment 385
Lesion 496
    location of 169
    of ear 692
    of nose 692
    of oral cavity 692
    slow-growing 313
    superficial 348
Lethal granuloma, midline 387
    treatment 387
Letterer-Siwe disease 536, 697
    treatment 537
Leukemia 164, 395, 594, 614, 615, 669
    acute 464, 595
        lymphocytic 595
        myeloblastic 595
    chronic 595
        lymphocytic 595
        myelogenous 595
    classification of 595*b*
    complete blood count values 597
    diagnostic assessment 597
    etiology 594
    incidence 594
    oral manifestations of 596
    treatment 597
    types of 594
Leukoderma aquisitum
    centrifugum 76
Leukoedema 10, 207, 209
    treatment 210
Leukopenia 632
Leukoplakia 197, 199, 203, 207, 224,
    417, 688
    classification of 201*b*
    clinical classification of 201
    clinical features of 200
    clinical type of 207
    development of 200
    erythroplakia 197, 510
    etiological factors of 198*b*
    etiology of 198
    histopathology 202
    homogenous ulcerative 201
    in khaini chewing 199*f*

nodulospeckled 202
nonhomogenous 201
of cheek 213*f*
of tongue 200*f*
patches of 212
proliferative verrucous 202
speckled 207
staging system of 207*b*
treatment of 208
verrucous 202
Lichen planus 207, 209, 220, 220*f*, 222*f*, 225, 225*f*, 226*f*, 417, 510, 640, 673
atrophic type 224
bullous type 224
clinical types of 223
cutaneous lesions of 221
dysplastic changes in 226*f*
erosive type 223
leukoplakia 692
of cheek 222*f*
pigmented 689
plaque type of 224, 224*f*
process of 221*fc*
reticular type 223
treatment 227
ulcerative type 223
Lichenoid reaction 224, 227, 227*f*
Liesegang rings 285
Linea alba 494
Lingual mandibular salivary gland 232
Lingual papillae, disorders in 692
Lingual thyroid nodule 29
treatment 30
Lingual varices 27, 27*f*
treatment 27
Lion-face 553, 554
Lip 101, 654
and palate, anomalies of 2
anesthesia of 664*b*
carcinoma of 86, 86*f*
deformities 497
double 2, 3*f*
clinical features 2
treatment 3
mucosal lesion in 649
nevus on 72*f*
pits 2
clinical features 2
treatment 2
upper 3*f*
Lipid metabolism, disturbances in 535
Lipoblast 129
cells, malignant 158
Lipoma 129, 130*f*, 138, 249, 254, 349
on buccal mucosa 130*f*
treatment 131
Liposarcoma 156, 157, 158*f*
in floor of mouth 157*f*
treatment 158
types of 158

Lipschutz bodies 400
Lipstick sign 244
Liquid biopsy 514
Liquid biopsy, principle of 514
Liver 98, 394, 485
biopsy 178
scan 178
Lopinavir 398
Low calcium levels in plasma, effects of 526*b*
Lower incisors, concrescence in 43*f*
Ludwig's angina 462, 483, 485, 485*b*, 692
causing 486*f*
pathogenesis of 485
treatment 486
Lues maligna 375
Luminal unicystic ameloblastoma 278, 278*f*
Lumpy bruises, large 602
Lung 98, 393
problem 648
Lupus erythematosus 240, 645, 648, 650
cell inclusion phenomenon 650
pathogenesis of 646
systemic 640, 646, 646*f*, 647*f*, 648*t*, 665
treatment of 651
Lymph node
enlargement of 239
metastasis 88*t*
metastatic 101*f*
regional 102
swelling in sarcoidosis 383*f*
syndrome, mucocutaneous 683
tuberculosis of 372
Lymphadenoid goiter 634
Lymphadenopathy 382
causes of 668, 668*t*
generalized 376
persistent generalized 394, 396
Lymphangioma 23, 136, 138*f*
capillary 136
cavernous 136
cystic 136
of commissure 137*f*
of tongue 137*f*
types of 136*t*
Lymphatic vessels, benign neoplasm of 136
Lymphocytes 183, 373, 380
Lymphocytic leukemia, chronic 638
Lymphoepithelial carcinoma 97
Lymphoepithelial cyst 31
benign 351
treatment 32
Lymphoid aggregates, reactive 31
Lymphoid elements 254*f*
Lymphoid tissue
neoplasms of 70
of stroma 253

Lymphoma 91, 162, 164, 168, 173, 174, 395
classification of 173
development of 173
groups of 173
malignant 254
of bone, primary 93, 176
Lymphoreticular system 691

M

Macrodontia 34
causes 34
focal 35
localized 35
relative generalized 35
true generalized 35
types 35
Macroglobulinemia 240
Macroglossia 22, 23, 23*f*, 23*t*
causes 22, 22*b*
treatment 24
types 22
Macrognathia 13
treatment 14
true 13
types 13
Maffucci's syndrome 142, 165, 683
Maggot infection 420
Magic syndrome 409, 683
Magnesium 80
Malaise 382
Malformed crown of tooth, causes of 49
Malignant transformation, symptoms of 77*b*
Malocclusion 497
Mandible 21
expansion of lower border of 272*f*
infection of space of body of 482
metastatic tumor of 190*f*
multicystic lesions in 565*f*
odontome of 291*f*
on left side, overgrowth of 14*f*
pathological fracture of 92*f*
unicystic ameloblastoma of 278*f*
Mandibular bony expansion in cherubism, severe 565*f*
Mandibular canal 694
Mandibular condyle
hyperplasia of 578
hypoplasia of 578
Mandibular cysts, large 313
Mandibular foramen 694
Mandibular gingiva 90
Mandibular macrognathia 13*f*
Mandibular swelling
bilateral 564*f*
causing large 283*f*
Mandibular third molar 319
macrodontia of 34*f*
Mandibulofacial dysostosis 574
treatment 574

Manganese 80
Marble bone disease 570
Marfan's syndrome 19, 571, 571f, 572f, 675, 682
  oral manifestations 572
Marginal gingiva 12
Marin-Amat syndrome 682
Mask-like face 553
Massive extraoral growth 86f
Massive facial swelling 320
  spreading 484f
Massive osteolysis 575
  treatment 575
Massive swelling 163f
  of maxilla 156f
Matrix metalloprotease 553
Maxilla
  surgical ciliated cyst of 352
  swelling
    in anterior 280f
    of left 124f
Maxillary antrum 307
  carcinoma of 90, 90f
  invasion into left 160f
Maxillary bone
  destruction of 264f
  expansion of 554f
Maxillary branch 659
Maxillary canine 280
Maxillary gingiva 389f
Maxillary lesions 346
Maxillary processes 17
Maxillary sinusitis 487
  treatment 488
Maxillary teeth 358
Maxillary tumors 271
Mazabraud syndrome 559
McCune-Albright syndrome 559, 561
Measles 406, 464
  treatment 406
Meckel's cartilage 165
Melanocytic lesions, benign 689
Melanoma 109b
  acral lentiginous 109
  amelanotic 110
  clinical diagnosis of 111b
  grades of malignant 112, 112t
  lentigo maligna 109
  malignant 109, 111f
    treatment 112
  mucosal lentiginous 109
  superficial spreading 109
  types of 112
Melanophages 76
Melanotic freckle of Hutchinson 109
Melanotic neuroectodermal
  tumor 151
Melkersson-Rosenthal syndrome 7, 232, 662, 663, 682
Meningitis 395, 673, 675
Meningoencephalitis 401

Menopause 550
Menstruation 550
Mental foramen 694
Mental retardation 377, 572
Mental space infections 479
  treatment 479
Mephenytoin 615
Mercury 504, 671
Mesenchymal chondrosarcoma 164, 167, 167f
  treatment 168
Mesenchymal tissue
  malignant neoplasms of 154
  origin, neoplasms of 69t, 112
Mesiodens 37f
Mesoderm 351
Metabolic disorders 670, 670t
  oral aspects of 526
Metal poisoning 504t
  heavy 670, 670t
  oral manifestations of 504
Metastasis 68, 97, 98
  mechanism of 98
  routes of 98
  step-by-step mechanism of 100t
Metastatic calcification 527
Metastatic carcinoma 93, 164, 262, 313, 558
Methylcobalamin 660
Microbiological test 446
Microdontia 32, 33
  causes 33
  generalized 32
  of lateral incisor 33f
  of upper third molar 33f
  true generalized 33
  types 33
Microglossia 22
  with bifid tongue 22f
Micrognathia 12, 40
  causes 12
  congenital 13
  of mandible 12f
  of maxilla with high-arched palate 12f
  true 13
  types 12
Micrometastasis 99
Microorganisms 428, 607b
  role of 430
Microstomia 497, 645, 652f
Middle fossa syndrome 683
Miescher's syndrome 683
Migraine 660
Migratory glossitis 28
  benign 27, 637
Mikulicz's disease 230, 238, 239
  treatment 239
Mikulicz's syndrome 239, 683
Miliary tuberculosis 371
Milk sugar 429
Miller's chemicoparasitic theory 427

Mineral metabolism, disturbances in 526
Mineralocorticoids 544, 545
  function of 544
Minerals 552
Mitosis
  excessive 93
  higher rate of 102
Mitotic index 499
Mobius syndrome 683
Mohr syndrome 683
Molar
  infection causing cellulitis, third 484f
  lower third 314f
  regions, lower 613f
  teeth, concrescence of 43f
Molybdenum 80
Mona Lisa facies 553
Mongoloid facies 553, 572f
Monila 413
Moniliasis 413
Monkey-like face 553
Monogenic defect 18
Monomorphic adenoma 249, 251f, 259
  lip 250f
  treatment 251
  types of 250
Mononuclear cells 380
Monostotic fibrous dysplasia 559
Moon's molars 377
Moon-like face 553
Morquio's syndrome 55, 682
Moth-Eaten radiolucency 92f
Mottling of enamel, clinical features of 53
Mouse facies 653
Mouth 654
  dryness of 231
  electrical burns in 497
  opening
    complete lack of 580f
    restricted 214f
  thermal burns in 497
  ulcers 409
Mucin pools 335
Mucocele 113, 135, 138, 347, 348
  on lower lip 348f
  types of 350
Mucocutaneous candidiasis 414
  localized 415
Mucocutaneous disease 626
Mucocutaneous infections 395
Mucoepidermoid carcinoma 91, 237, 249, 259
Mucoepidermoid tumor 245, 254, 259, 259f-262f, 263
  high-grade 261
  low-grade 261
  treatment 262
Mucogingival junctions 12

Index

Mucopolysaccharidoses 55
Mucormycosis 397, 420
    oral manifestations 420
    treatment 420
Mucosa
    atrophy of 218*f*
    violent rubbing of 495
Mucosal atrophy 197
Mucosal bullae formation 645*t*
Mucosal malformation 696
Mucous cells 261*f*
Mucous extravasation cyst 230, 347-349, 349*f*, 349*t*
Mucous membrane
    hemangioma of 131
    pemphigoid 225
        benign 641
Mucous retention cyst 230, 254, 347-349, 349*f*
Mucous-filled area, large 350
Muir-Torre syndrome 73, 683
Mulberry molars 52, 377
Multicentric cancer 85
Multilocular radiolucency 147*f*, 271*f*
Multilocular radiolucent lesions of jaws, classification of 695
Multiple myeloma 93, 162, 183, 184*b*, 185, 185*f*, 186, 186*b*, 186*f*, 313, 669
    pathogenesis of 184*fc*
    treatment 187
Multisystem disease 634
Mumps 406
    complications 407
    treatment 407
Munchausen syndrome 683
Mural unicystic ameloblastoma 278, 279
Murray-Puretic-Drescher syndrome 683, 693
Muscle
    attachments, areas of 477
    benign neoplasm of smooth 143
    disease of 658, 664
    tissue, neoplasms
        of smooth 70
        of striated 70
Muscular origin, pain of 692
Myasthenia gravis 634, 635, 665
    treatment 665
Mycobacteria 370
    atypical 393
    drug-resistant 370
Mycobacterium avium intracellulare 393
Mycobacterium bovis 370
Mycobacterium tuberculosis 370
Mycotic infections, deep 373
Myelodysplastic syndrome 683
Myeloid leukemia, acute 596*f*
Myeloma 164

Myoepithelial carcinoma 252
Myoepithelial cells 230
Myoepithelioma 251
    malignant 252
Myofascial pain 660
    dysfunction 584*t*
    syndrome 583, 682
Myofibroma 115
    treatment 116
Myositis ossificans 665
    hereditary type 665
    nonhereditary type 665
    treatment 666
    types 665
Myxedema 539, 540, 672
    diagnosis 540
    general symptoms 540
    oral manifestations of 540*b*
    treatment 541
Myxochondroid stroma of tumor 247*f*
Myxoid chondrosarcoma 166, 167*f*
Myxoid lipoma 131
Myxoma 120, 126, 127, 128*f*, 144, 249, 269
    of anterior mandible 128*f*
    of maxilla 128*f*
    syndrome 683
    treatment 128

N

Nager syndrome 19, 683
Nail
    dysplasia 623
    lesions 626
Naproxen sodium 609
Nasal bleeding 85
Nasal process, lateral 17
Nasoalveolar cyst 341
Nasociliary nerve 403
Nasolabial cyst 341, 342*f*
    origin 341
    treatment 342
Nasopalatine duct 343
    cyst 342, 343, 343*f*, 344*f*
    treatment 344
Nasopharyngeal carcinoma 398
Nasopharyngeal type carcinoma 97
Natural killer cell neoplasms 174
Neck swelling
    classification of 693
    midline 693
Neck-tongue syndrome 683, 692
Necrotic tissue 520
Necrotizing sialometaplasia 236, 237
    pathogenesis 236
    treatment 237
Necrotizing ulcerative
    gingivitis, acute 405, 597, 617, 618*b*
    periodontitis 619
        acute 618
    stomatitis 618

Negri body 413
Neisseria gonorrhoeae 379
    bacteria 378
Nelfinavir 398
Neoantigens 633
Neonatal herpes 401
Neonatal teeth 39*f*
Neoplasm 67, 393, 579, 690
    benign 67, 68*t*, 69, 71, 144
    characteristics of 67
    malignant 67, 68*t*, 69, 109, 188
Neoplastic cells 285
    of chondrosarcoma 166
Neoplastic disorders 230
Neoplastic lesions 689
Neoplastic tissues 248
Nerve 654
    deafness, eighth 377
    diseases of 658
Nervous system disorder 360
Neural diseases 674, 674*t*
Neural origin 696
Neural tissue
    benign neoplasm of 146
    neoplasms of 70
Neuralgias 692
Neurilemmoma 146-148, 148*f*, 151*t*, 271
    of mandible 147*f*
    treatment 148
Neuroblastoma 162, 164, 190
Neuroectodermal tumor 151, 164
    of infancy 151*f*, 152*f*
Neuroendocrine carcinoma 91
Neurofibroma 113, 129, 144-146, 148, 149, 150*f*, 151*t*
    multiple 149
    of tongue 149*f*
    origin 149
    treatment 150
Neurofibromatosis 23
    of skin 149*f*
Neurogenic sarcoma 156, 189, 190*f*
    cells 190
    of jaw 189*f*
    of maxilla 189*f*
    origin 189
    treatment 190
Neurolemmoma 147*f*
Neurologic diseases 394
Neurological anomalies 311
Neurological disorders 396
Neurological pain 658
Neurosyphilis 376
Neutropenia 411
Nevus 74
    cells 72*f*, 75
    function of 75
    preexisting 77*b*
    types of 75*b*
    unius lateris 72

Niacin 532
    deficiency 668
        clinical features of 532
Nicotinamide deficiency 668
Niemann-Pick disease 537
Nifedipine 609, 615
Nikolsky's sign 637, 639
Nitrosonornicotine 80
N-nitrosodimethylamine 79
N-nitrosonornicotine 79
N-nitrosopyrrolidine 79
Nodular fasciitis 128, 156
    treatment 129
Nodular sclerosis 183
Nodulospeckled leukoplakia of
        cheek 202f
Noma 388, 619, 690
Non-Hodgkin's lymphoma 173-175,
        176f, 177, 177f, 178, 184, 184t,
        271, 638
    of mandible 175f, 176f
    of maxilla 175f
    staging system of 176t
Nonkeratinized epithelium 203
Nonlethal type, severe 567
Non-neoplastic disorders 230
Nonodontogenic lesions 339
Nonodontogenic neoplasms 68, 697
Nonodontogenic origin 696
Nonodontogenic tumors 696
Nonossifying fibroma 691
Noonan syndrome 683
North American blastomycosis 420
Nuclear hyperchromatism 111, 204
Nuclear pleomorphism 204
Nuclear remnant in keratin 202f
Nuclear-free zones 148
Numb chin syndrome 191, 597
Nursing bottle caries 439t
Nutritional deficiency 51, 214,
        409, 609
Nystagmus 626

O

Occipital condyle syndrome 683
Occupational erosions 360
Occupational hazards 78, 81
Ocular diseases 544
Ocular disturbances 648
Oculodento-osseous dysplasia 55
Oculoglandular syndrome of
        Parinaud 683
Odontoameloblastoma 269
Odontoblast 56
    cells 445
    defective function of 533
Odontogenic carcinoma 269, 301
Odontogenic cells 32
Odontogenic cysts 40, 307t, 308, 308t
Odontogenic ectomesenchyme 269
Odontogenic epithelial cells 273, 308
Odontogenic epithelium 269

Odontogenic fibroma 269, 293, 294f
    mandible 294f
    origin 293
    peripheral 293
    treatment 293
Odontogenic ghost cell carcinoma 339
Odontogenic infections 477
    sequelae of 483b
Odontogenic keratocyst 126, 271, 272,
        308, 310, 310f, 312f-314f, 315,
        316, 318b, 321, 336, 695
    in mandible, multiple 312f
    intraoral lesion in 311f
    lining of 315f
Odontogenic lesions 339
Odontogenic myxoma 295, 295f,
        296f, 313
    origin 295
    treatment 296
Odontogenic neoplasm 68, 268, 696
    malignant 300
    peripheral 113
Odontogenic origin 696
Odontogenic sarcomas 269, 302
Odontogenic tumor 40
    classification of 269
Odontomas 140, 285, 339
Odontomes 38, 40, 281, 290, 292, 319
    complex 290
    compound 290, 291
    treatment 292
    types 290
Oligodontia 36
Ollier's disease 165, 695
Ollier's syndrome 142
Oncocytes 252
Oncocytoma 249, 252, 254
    malignant 252
    treatment 253
Oncogenes 82
Onion-skin 264
Opalescent dentin, hereditary 56
Opalescent teeth 568
Oral and maxillofacial region 696
Oral cancer 78, 91, 103, 197, 220, 512
    etiology of 78
    prevention of 104
    primary prevention 104
    secondary prevention 104
    special aspects of 85
    treatment of 91b, 103
Oral candidiasis 395
    classification of 414t
Oral carcinoma 93b
Oral cavity 101, 229, 393, 477, 636, 691
    benign neoplasm of 67
    chemical injuries of 491
    malignant neoplasms of 67
    pigmented lesions of 689
    red-blue lesions of 688
    teratoma of 153f
Oral complications of scarlet fever 382

Oral disease 675t, 677
    classifications of 688
    general manifestations of 675
    pre-existing 78
    related syndromes 677t
Oral epithelial lesions 509t
Oral epithelium, basal layer of 318
Oral facial digital syndrome 19, 684
Oral foci of infection 488b, 676
Oral granular cell lesions, classification
        of 696
Oral hairy leukoplakia 208, 397f
    treatment 209
Oral infection 484, 676
    chronic 81
    extensive 546f
    spread of 477
    to distant sites, spread of 477b
Oral lesions 221, 626, 641
    of gonorrhea 379f
    of Hodgkin's lymphoma 182
    of leiomyomas 188
    of lichen planus 222, 650t
    of scurvy 533f
    of tuberculosis 371
    pre-existing 82
Oral leukoplakia 82, 198, 207b
    staging system of 206
Oral lichen planus 197, 199, 650
Oral lymphoid tissue, anomalies of 31
Oral maggot infection 421f
Oral melanomas 110
Oral melanotic macule 4, 4f, 112
    treatment 5
Oral microflora, modify 446
Oral mucosa 244, 654
    anomalies of 8
    blanching of 217f
    classification of yellow conditions
        of 694
    inflammation of 588
    intense erythema in 647f
    necrotic ulcerations of 596f
    papillomatosis of 72
    vesicle formation in 642f
Oral mucosal
    lesions, classification of 199b
    ulcer 505f
Oral myasis 420
Oral neoplasms, classification of 67,
        68
Oral nevus 74
Oral precancerous lesions 197
Oral soft tissue infections 484
Oral squamous carcinomas 199
Oral squamous cell carcinoma 82, 98b
    clinical presentation of 82
Oral structures, formation of 17t
Oral submucous fibrosis 197, 214,
        214f, 217f-219f
    etiology of 214b
    features of advanced 217

pathogenesis of 216*fc*
staging of 219
Oral transplants 485
Oral tuberculous lesions 373
Oral tumors, malignant 676
Oral wounds
 healing of 509, 516
 self-inflicted 495
Orbital syndrome 684
Organ transplant 402
 recipients 544
Organisms, factors relating to 477
Orofacial
 angiomatosis 616
 cellulitis 484, 484*t*
 clefts 16
 pain, classification of chronic 692
 region 1, 488, 658
  types of pain in 658*b*
 tissues
  classification of 692
  severe infections of 692
Oromandibular limb hypogenesis syndrome 684
Oropharyngeal carcinoma 86*f*
Orthodontic force 367
Orthokeratin 203
Orthopantomogram 441, 441*f*
Osseous anomalies 311
Osseous tissue, neoplasms of 70
Ossifying fibroma 119*f*, 120, 281, 473, 558
 enchondroma 562
 of maxilla, aggressive 118*f*
 types 119
Osteitis
 deformans 553
 fibrosa cystica, generalized 543
Osteoarthritis 581
 erosion of head of condyles in 582*f*
 treatment 582
Osteoblast 552
 cells 533, 552
 malignant 170*f*
Osteoblastic osteosarcoma 170*f*, 473
Osteoblastoma 126, 140, 141*f*, 172, 300, 347, 470
Osteochondroma 169
Osteoclast 553
 activating factor 330, 459
 cells 520
Osteoclastoma 120, 123, 126
Osteocytes 552
Osteogenesis imperfecta 169, 566, 567, 567*f*, 673
 oral manifestations of 568
 treatment 568
Osteoid 552
 osteoma 140, 300
  treatment 141
Osteo-integrated implan*t*, healing around 523, 524*f*

Osteolipoma 130
Osteolytic phase of osteosarcoma 575
Osteoma 138, 139*f*, 140*f*, 470, 574
 central 138
 endosteal 138
 exophytic 138
 of mandible 139*f*
 of maxilla 139*f*
 periosteal 138
 presentation 139
 radiographic features 139
 treatment 140
 types 138
Osteomyelitis 93, 462-464, 464*b*, 465, 472, 477, 484, 488, 574
 acute 463
  suppurative 271, 313, 465
 chronic 169, 463, 472
  nonsuppurative 141
  suppurative 468, 468*f*
 classification of 463*b*
 development of 597
 etiology of 464
 idiopathic 463
 of jaw, acute 466*f*
 of right mandible 467*f*
 pathogenesis of 464, 465*fc*
 radiation induced 463
Osteopetrosis 464, 558, 570, 574, 673
 treatment 571
 types 570
Osteophytic lipping 581
Osteoplasia 276
Osteoporosis 529
Osteoradionecrosis 501, 502
 grades of 502*b*
 treatment 503
Osteosarcoma 168*f*, 169, 171, 173*t*, 190, 271, 300, 558
 classic 170
 clinical features of 169
 fibroblastic type of 169
 low-grade 562
 of jaw 168*f*
 of lower jaw 168*f*
 of mandible 168*f*
 small cell 162, 164
 telangiectatic type of 169
 treatment 172
 types of 169, 170, 171*f*
Osteosclerosis 469
Otitis media, acute 662
Otopalatodigital syndrome 19, 684
Owl-eyecells 404
Oxyphilic adenoma 252

P

Paan chewing, mucosal changes due to 79*f*
Paget's disease 154, 553, 554*f*, 555, 555*f*, 556, 557*f*

of bone 13, 64, 165, 169, 298, 300, 313, 363, 367, 464, 553, 562, 673, 691
 oral manifestations of 556
Pain
 in acute pulpitis, characteristics of 453*b*
 syndrome, generalized 692
 types of 453
Palatal erythema 213
Palatal space infection 478
 source of 478
 treatment 478
Palate 647, 654
 carcinoma of 89, 89*f*
 destruction of 257*f*
 hemangiopericytoma of 160*f*
Palmar keratosis 311
Pancytopenia 589
Paper electrophoresis 314
Papillary cystadenoma lymphomatosum 253
Papillary hyperplasia of palate 496
Papillary palatal hyperplasia 496
Papillary squamous cell carcinoma 97
Papilloma 71
 histopathology of 71*f*
 multiple 72
 on palate 71*f*
 treatment 73
Papillomatosis 72
Papillon-Lefèvre syndrome 612, 684
Papules, flat-topped 631
Papyraceous scarring 654
Paradental cyst 340
 origin 340
 treatment 340
Parakeratin 203
 plugging 74
Paramolars 37
Paramyxovirus infection 406
Paraneoplastic pemphigus 635, 638, 639
Paraneoplastic syndrome 684
Parasympathetic salivary fibers 661
Parathormone 541
Parathyroid
 gland 543
 hormone 526
Paratrigeminal syndrome 684
Paresthesia 169, 346
 causes of 664*b*
Parosteal osteosarcoma 172
Parotid gland 233, 245
Parotid lesion 249, 693
Parotid lymph node, enlarged 252, 254
Parotid space infection 479
 treatment 479
Parotid stone 234
Parotid tumors 246
Parry-Romberg syndrome 684
Patau syndrome 684

Paterson-Brown-Kelly syndrome 220
Paterson-Kelly syndrome 684, 692
Paul-Bunnell test 405
Peg-shaped laterals 49
Pemphigoid 400, 511, 517, 630, 634, 640, 642f, 643f, 644, 672
   histopathology of 643
   pathogenesis of 641fc
Pemphigus 400, 511, 630, 635, 672
   clinical features of 635
   erythematosus 637
   foliaceus 637
   histopathology of 638
   types of 635
   vegetans 637, 639
   vulgaris 411, 517, 635, 636f, 638f, 639f, 640, 644, 644t
   oral lesions 636f
Peptic ulcer 360
Peptostreptococcus 430
   intermedium 471
Periapical abscess 331, 460, 463, 477, 484, 488
   acute 461f
   chronic 461f
   complications of acute 462
   etiological factors of 460b
   treatment 463
Periapical cemental dysplasia 296
Periapical cyst 297, 324, 463, 694
Periapical granuloma 297, 331, 458, 459f, 463, 694
   treatment 460
Periapical infection, extraoral spread of 462f
Periapical inflammation 63, 362, 367
Periapical lesions 463f
Periapical region, radiolucent lesions of 694
Periapical tissues 450
   diseases of 458
Periarteritis nodosa 240
Pericoronal abscess 484
Pericoronal radiolucent lesions, classification of 694
Pericoronitis 40f, 477, 479f, 484, 488, 620
   simple 340
   treatment 620
Peridens 37
Perineural invasion 259
Perineural sheath 98
Periodontal abscess 332, 477, 484, 488, 619, 619f
Periodontal cyst, lateral 281, 288, 309, 313, 332, 332f, 333f, 340
   pathogenesis of lateral 332f
Periodontal disease 606, 606t, 607, 609, 610t
   common bacteria causing 608
   dental plaque in 607
   prognosis of 614
   progression of 610
   role of bacteria in 607
   stages of 610
   systemic factors causing 607
Periodontal ligament tissue 332
Periodontal surgery 363
Periodontal tissues, healthy 607
Periodontitis 396, 606, 610
   adult type 612, 613
   causing recession 613f
   chronic 611
   clinical classification of 612t
   juvenile 612
   primary acute apical 458
   rapidly progressive 612, 613
   types of 612
   with bone loss, chronic 613f
Periosteal chondromas 142
Periosteal osteosarcoma 172
   of maxilla 173f
Peripheral ossifying fibroma 113, 116, 116f, 117f
   origin 116
   treatment 117
Peripheral tall columnar cells 282f
Permanent tooth 362f
Pernicious anemia 586, 587, 634, 669
   oral manifestation 587
   treatment 588
Petechiae 689
Petechial spots on skin, multiple 599f
Peutz-Jeghers syndrome 3, 4, 684, 689
   treatment 4
PFAPA syndrome 684
Pfeiffer syndrome 684
Pharyngeal space infection
   complications lateral 481
   lateral 481
   source of lateral 481
   treatment lateral 481
Phenol 506
Phenylbutazone 597, 599
Phenytoin 615
   sodium 609
Philadelphia chromosome 594
Phoenix abscess 460
Phosphorus 528, 528b, 671
Phycomycosis 420
Pierre-Robin syndrome 19, 675, 684
Pigmented cellular nevus 74
   treatment 75
Pilomatricomas 339
Pindborg's tumor 271, 273, 282, 534
Pituitary dwarfism 671
Pituitary gigantism 13, 538, 671
Pituitary gland 539
Pituitary insufficiency 537
   treatment 538
Pityriasis rosea 626
Plantar hyperkeratosis 312f
Plantar keratosis 311
Plaque
   disruption 446
   stagnation of 608b
Plasma cell 329, 373, 380
   in multiple myeloma, typical 186f
   myeloma 169
   proliferation of numerous 186f
Plasmacytoid pattern 252
Plasmin 635
Plasmodium falciparum 590
Platelets 594
Platybasia 555
Pleomorphic adenoma 245, 246, 247f, 248f, 249, 252, 254, 259, 262, 263
   clinical features 246
   histological types of 249b
   malignant 254
   of minor salivary glands of palate 246f
   of parotid gland 246f
   origin 245
   preexisting 255
   treatment 249
Pleomorphic lipomas 131
Pleomorphic rhabdomyosarcoma 188
Plethoric facies 553
Plexiform ameloblastoma 273, 273f, 274f
Plicated tongue 25
Plummer-Vinson's syndrome 78, 82, 220, 588, 669, 684, 692
Pneumocystis carinii pneumonia 394
Pneumonia 394, 596
Pocket cyst 324
Polyclonal B cell activation 634
Polycythemia 587, 669
   vera 593, 594
      complications of 594
      treatment of 594
Polydipsia 538
Polyhedral tumor cells 284f
Polymorphonuclear neutrophils 518
Polymyositis 240, 633
   treatment 633
Polyostotic fibrous dysplasia 559
Polyuria 538
Porphyria 534
   congenital 503
   erythropoietic 534
   hepatic 534
   types 534
Porphyromonas 460, 466, 608
   gingivalis 607, 608, 618
Portsmouth syndrome 684
Port-wine stain 133, 133f, 135
Postherpetic neuralgia 692
Postradiation sialadenitis 230, 236
Potter facies 553

Pregnancy 360, 609, 671
  tumor 609f, 615
Preleukoplakia 198, 199
Premature eruption 39
  types 39
Premaxilla 340
Pre-neoplastic lesions 689
Prepubertal periodontitis 612
Presecretory ameloblasts 268
Prevotella 460, 466
  intermedia 388, 607, 608, 618
  melaninogenica 608
Primordial cyst, collateral type
  of 332
Progeria 549
Progesterone 609
Proliferative periostitis 472
Proliferative verrucous
  leukoplakia 206f
Propionibacterium acnes 471
Protease 392
  inhibitor 398
Protein
  abnormal 185
  energy malnutrition 670
  metabolism, disturbances in 533
Proteolytic chelation theory 427, 434
Proteolytic enzymes 433
Proteolytic theory 427, 433
  limitations of 434
Protozoal infections 393, 674
Provirus 391
Psammoma bodies 119f
Psammomatoid 119
Pseudoanodontia 35
Pseudocyst 306, 345
Pseudomacrognathia 13
Pseudomembranous candidiasis,
  acute 414, 414f, 416
Pseudomicrognathia 12
Pseudomonas aeruginosa 394
Pseudo-tumor of hemophilia 603
Psoriasis 625, 673
  cause of 625
  dermal lesions of 625
  treatment 626
Psychogenic pains 692
Psychological pain 658
Pterygomandibular space
  infection 478
  sources of 479
  treatment 479
Ptyalism 243
  etiology of 243
Pulmonary actinomycosis 379
Pulmonary tuberculosis 370, 371
Pulp 63, 452f
  calcification 365
    causes of 366b
    pathogenesis of 366fc
    types of 366t

chambers of teeth, obliteration
  of 59f
cold test 457
degeneration 451
diffuse linear calcifications of 366
dry gangrene of 454
heat test 457
miscellaneous diseases of 451
necrosis 451, 456
palpation 457
percussion 457
polyp 455, 455f
  contributing factors for 455b
  treatment 456
protective responses of 444
response, clinical test for evaluation
  of 457
stones 366, 527f
  attached 366
  free 366
  interstitial 366
  types of 366
therapy, direct 451
tissues 268
vitality tests 457, 457b
Pulpal diseases 450
Pulpal infections, bacteriology of 457
Pulp-dentin complex, effective 435
Pulpitis
  acute 452, 660
  chronic 454, 469
  classification of 451t
  etiology of acute 453b
  irreversible 451
  reversible 451
Pulpless teeth, intracoronal bleaching
  of 363
Pulse granuloma 473
Punch biopsy 512
  advantages of 512
  limitations of 512
  procedure of 512
Punched-out ulcer 376
Purpura 598, 599, 599f, 669
  causes of 599
  oral manifestations of 600
  treatment 600
  types 599
Pus discharging sinus 461f
Pyemia 483, 489
Pyknotic nuclei with keratin 202f
Pyogenic granuloma 135, 162, 388,
  389, 389f, 390f
  treatment 389
Pyostomatitis vegetans 639, 672
Pyridoxine deficiency 668

Q

Quasi-malignant 158
Quinidine 599
Quinine 599

R

Rabies 412, 673
  treatment 413
Radiation
  in blood, effects of 501
  in embryo, effects of 502
  in fetus, effects of 502
  injury 498
    factors determining degrees
      of 499b
  on blood vessels, effects of 500
  on bone, effects of 501
  on cells, effects of 499
  on muscles, effects of 500
  on oral mucosa, effects of 500
  on organs, effects of 499
  on salivary glands, effects
    of 500
  on skin, effects of 500
  on teeth, effects of 501
  on temporomandibular joint,
    effects of 500
  on tissues, effects of 499
  therapy 355
Radicular cyst 308, 324, 327f-329f,
  330, 332, 340
  arcading 330
  of mandible 326f
  of maxilla 326f
  pathogenesis of 325fc
  treatment 331
  true 324, 324f
  types 324
Radiolucent-radiopaque lesions,
  mixed 695
Radiotherapy 402
  treatment, dose selection 498
Rampant caries 438f, 439t
Ramsay Hunt syndrome 684
Ranula 350, 350f
  plunging type of 350
  treatment 351
  types of 350
Raspberry tongue 382
Raynaud's phenomenon 653
Recurring pain, types of 658
Red blood cell 331, 595
Reed-Sternberg giant cells
  173, 182
Regional odontodysplasia 62
  treatment 63
Reiter's disease 409
Reiter's syndrome 411, 684
  treatment 412
Renal diseases 674, 674t
Renal failure 674
Renal osteodystrophy 49, 674
Replantation, causes of failure
  of 523
Reproductive system 394

Residual carbohydrates 435
Residual cyst 309, 327, 327f, 331
Resorption
  idiopathic external 363
  internal 64
    replacement 365
  types of internal 365
Respiratory tract infection,
    upper 399
Resting cells 308
Restore tooth surface 447
Rete pegs, flattening of 218f
Reticulosis, malignant 690
Retrocuspid papilla 12
Retropharyngeal space
    infection 482
Rhabdomyoma 144, 145
  treatment 145
Rhabdomyosarcoma 156, 188, 190
  of palate 188f
  treatment 189
  types 188
Rheumatic condition 544
Rheumatoid arthritis 582, 651
  treatment 583
Rheumatoid factor 635
Rhomboid glossitis, median 25, 26,
    26f, 688
Riboflavin 531
  deficiency 668
    clinical features of 531
Ricketic facies 553
Rickets 530
  oral manifestations of 530b
Rieger's syndrome 685
Rifampicin 373
Right maxillary antrum, carcinoma
    of 93f
Riley-Day syndrome 684
Risus sardonicus 386
Ritonavir 398
Rodent ulcer 104, 105
Root
  ankylosis 64
  external resorption of 362f
  formation of 269
  fracture 491
  of teeth, malformation of 63
  resorption in dentigerous cyst,
    causes of 324
Rootless teeth 61f
Round cell
  sarcoma 162
  tumors, common 162
Roundworm infections 674
Royal disease 600
Rubeola 406
Rubinstein-Taybi syndrome 685
Rushton bodies 329
Russell bodies 329
Rutherford's syndrome 11, 685

S

Saddle nose 377
Saliva
  hypersecretion of 243
  retention of 233
  viscosity of 435
Salivary buffering capacity test 445
Salivary duct system 229
Salivary enzymes 435
Salivary epithelium 245
Salivary function, role of 361
Salivary gland 229, 232, 245t,
    538, 654
  acini 262
  agenesis of 230
  aplasia 230
  carcinomas of 264
  change in 244
  congenital absence of 230
  cysts 232
  disease 229, 396, 398, 697
    classification of 230
  excised 235f
  functional unit of 229
  hypoplasia of 232
  major 229
  minor 229
  miscellaneous disorders of 242
  neoplasms 106, 113, 135, 146, 244,
    245t
    malignant 254, 259
  origin 696
  reactive lesions of 232
  tissue 236, 241f
    neoplasms of 70
  treatment 232
  tuberculosis of 372
  tuberculous lesions of 372
  tumor 231f, 349, 351
    different malignant 261t
Salivary immunoglobulins 435
Salivary neoplasms, benign 249
Salivary reductase test 445
Salivary tumors, common 246
Salivation, excessive 243
Salt-and-pepper effect 591
Sand dunes, series of 62
Sanfilippo's syndrome 55, 685
Sapho syndrome 471
Saquinavir, consists of 398
Sarcoidosis 120, 373, 383, 614,
    672, 691
  oral manifestations 383
  treatment 384
  with nodular growths on
    palate 384f
Sarcoma 67, 98
Sarcomatoid carcinoma 96
Satellite cyst 318
Scanning electron microscopy 331
Scar 580

Scarlet fever 381
  oral manifestations 382
  systemic complications of 382
  treatment 382
Scheuthauer-Marie-Sainton
    syndrome 19, 685
Schirmer test 242
Schwann cell 145, 148, 148f
Schwannoma 120, 146
Sclerodactyly 653
Scleroderma 651, 673
  diffuse 652f
  oral manifestations of 654t
  pathogenesis 651
  treatment 654
  types 651
Sclerosing osteomyelitis 558
  chronic 141
  diffuse 470, 471f
    involving left mandible, diffuse 471f
Sclerosing sialadenitis, chronic 236
Sclerosing sialometaplasia,
    chronic 230
Sclerosis
  multiple 660, 674
  progressive systemic 665
  systemic 240
Sclerosteosis 571
Sclerotic cemental masses 140
Screwdriver-shaped incisors 377
Scrofula 371, 371f
Scrotal tongue 25, 573f
Scurvy 614
Sebaceous adenoma on cheek 9f
Sebaceous glands 8, 352f
  and hair follicles 153f
  lobules of 8f
Seborrheic dermatitis 395
Seborrheic keratitis 112
Seborrheic keratosis 106
Self-regressing disease 633
Sentinel lymph node 84
Septicemia 462, 483, 489, 596, 675
  clinical features of 489
  complications in 489
Sequestrated antigens 633
Sequestrum 467f
Sex hormones 544, 609
  imbalance of 549, 671
Sexually transmitted disease 373,
    674, 674t
Shell teeth 58
Shingles 402, 403
Shrunken uvula 217f
Sialadenitis 237, 238f, 263, 693
Sialolipoma 131
Sialolithiasis 230, 233, 235, 693
  diagnosis of 234
  treatment 235
Sialoliths 233, 234
  composition of 234

Index

Sialo-odontogenic cysts 335
   origin 335
   treatment 336
Sialosis 242, 538
   treatment 243
Sicca syndrome 240, 242
Sickle cell anemia 587, 592, 669
   treatment 593
Sickle cell crisis 592
Sideropenic dysphagia 197, 220
Silver 504
   amalgam 671
   nitrate 506
Sinus histiocytosis 138
Sinusitis 394
Sipple's syndrome 685
Sjögren's syndrome 173, 230, 238-240,
      240*t*, 241, 241*f*, 582, 635, 647,
      651, 653, 665, 685, 693, 697
   primary 239, 240, 242, 635
   secondary 240, 535
   symptoms of 240
Skin 98, 394, 696
   epidermal cyst of 311, 311*f*
   eruption 505*f*
   hemangioma of 131
   in erythema multiforme 628*f*
   in leprosy, burn-out shiny patches
      on 385*f*
   lesions 636*f*, 643
   overlying tumor, erythema of 175*f*
   pigmentation, loss of 652*f*
   vesiculobullous lesion of 641*f*
Sleep apnea, obstruction 23
Small cell carcinoma, metastatic 168
Smokeless tobacco 78
Smoking, frequency of 78
Snarling facies 553
Snuff Dipper's cancer 106
Snyder test 445
Soap-bubble appearance 272, 272*b*
Sodium
   salt 241
   valproate 615
Soft palate 83
Soft tissue 331, 337
   of mouth, overlying 466*f*
   tumors 231
Solitary bone cyst 120, 344, 345
   treatment 345
Solitary plasmacytoma 187, 187*f*
   of palate 187*f*
   treatment 187
Sore mouth 496
Sphenopalatine neuralgia 660
   types 661
Spherule enclosing endospores 417*f*
Spidery fingers 571*f*
Spiking resorption 170
Spindle cell
   carcinoma 96, 96*f*
   component 97

lipoma 130
pattern 252
Spinous cell layer 339
Spongiotic abscess 28
Squamous cell 94
   carcinoma 77, 84, 74*b*, 82, 83*t*, 85,
      86*f*, 91, 92, 92*f*, 93, 94, 94*f*, 95,
      95*f*, 95*t*, 96, 96*f*, 97, 102, 103,
      106, 108, 108*t*, 208*f*, 237, 249,
      261, 262, 271, 288, 313, 373, 395,
      419, 517
   basaloid 97
   differentiation of 94
   early 212
   histologic grading of 94
   metastasis of 99*fc*
   of cheek 512*f*
   of floor of mouth 88*f*
   poor prognosis in 96*b*
   malignant 97
Squamous intraepithelial
   neoplasia 203
Squamous metaplasia 275, 275*f*
   of tumor cells 248*f*
Squamous odontogenic tumor 286,
      287, 287*f*
   of right maxilla 287*f*
   origin 286
   treatment 288
Stafne's bone cyst 313, 345,
      346, 346*f*
   treatment 346
Stains
   black 621
   brown 621
   yellow-brown 620
Staphylococcus 379
   aureus 237, 381, 395, 464
Starches produce 430
Stavudine 397
Stellate reticulum cells 268
Stephan's curve 428, 432
Steroid 544
   crisis 545
   diabetes 549
      cause of 549
   therapy 546*f*
      chronic 631, 670
      indications of 544*t*
      long-term 485, 545*b*
Stevens-Johnson's syndrome
      627, 629, 685
Still's disease 582
Stimulate salivary flow 446
Stomach 394
Stomatitis 396
   classification of 691
   nicotina 197, 213, 213*f*
   treatment 214
Strabismus 626
Strawberry tongue 382
Streaming fashion 155

Streptococcal infections 381
   treatment 381
Streptococcus 379, 447, 634
   milleri 430, 431
   mitior 430, 431
   mutans 430, 431, 446, 634
      colonization mechanism of 431*b*
   pyogenes 237, 381, 483, 590
   salivarius 430, 431
   sanguis 430, 431
Streptomycin 373
Striated muscle, benign neoplasm
      of 144
Stroke 675
Stromal tumor 263
Sturge-Weber syndrome 133, 685
Subepithelial bullae formation 643*f*
Sublingual glands 245
Sublingual space infection 480, 481*f*
   treatment 481
Submandibular duct, sialolith in
      left 233*f*
Submandibular gland 245
   tumors 257
Submandibular lymph node 98, 181*f*
   carcinoma spreading into 84*f*
   swelling 596*f*
Submandibular nodes 86
Submandibular salivary gland 233,
      237
Submandibular sialolithiasis 234
Submandibular space infection 480
   acute 480*f*
   contents 480
   source of 480
   treatment 480
   with extraoral sinus 480*f*
Submasseteric space infection 482, 483*f*
   source of 483
   treatment 483
Submental space infection 479
   source of 480
   treatment 480
Submerged teeth 41, 493
   treatment 494
Sucrose 429, 429*b*
   chelation theory 427, 434
Sulfonamides 597
Sulfur granules 380
Sun-burst appearance 166*f*
Sun-ray appearance 171*b*
Supernumerary teeth 36, 37*f*, 40, 49, 64
   common locations 37
   lingual to lower premolars 37*f*
   multiple 37*f*
   treatment 38
   types 37
Sutton nevus 76
Swallow saliva 386
Sweat
   gland dysplasia 623
   retention syndrome 686

Sweating, lack of 623
Sweet's syndrome 685
Swiss-cheese 257f
Symblepharon 642
Syphilis 81, 197-199, 225, 373, 464, 672, 674, 690
  clinical features of 374
  congenital 49, 51, 374, 376
  early congenital 376
  late 375
  mucous patch of 417
  oral manifestations of
    primary 374b
    secondary 375b
    tertiary 376b
  primary 374, 377
  secondary 374, 375, 377
  tertiary 374, 375, 377
Syphilitic
  chancre 488
  glossitis 376
  leukoplakia 376
  patches 207
  ulcer 237
Systemic diseases 360b
Systemic lupus erythematosus
  clinical features of 646
  pathogenesis of 646, 646fc

T

T cell
  function, altered 634
  neoplasms, mature 174
Tachycardia 541
Tall columnar cells 275f
Talon cusp 48, 49
  treatment 49
  X-ray 49f
Tapeworm infections 673
Target cells 590, 592
Target lesion 627f, 628f
Tarry-Black stools 602
Taste disorders, classification of 693
Taurodontism 45, 45f, 64
  treatment 46
Teeth 654
  abfraction of 359, 359f
  abnormalities of 32
  abrasion of 357
  absence of 623
  age changes in 368
  and gum problems 244
  ankylosis of 493
    symptoms with 493
    treatment 493
  attrition of 355, 356f
  bearing, dentigerous means 318
  brushing 610
  care, postextraction 522
  causes of
    intrinsic stains of 621, 621t
    premature loss of 492t

chalky-white appearance of 437
classification of discoloration of 690
common stains in 620
composition of 435
decay, cause 431b
development 1
  in rickets, lack of 530f
dilaceration of 45f
displacement of 122f
disturbance in
  number of 35
  shape of 41
  size of 32
  structure of 50
erosion of 359, 360b, 361f
  extrinsic factors 359
  intrinsic factors 360
  medications 360
  preventive treatment 361
  restorative treatment 361
  treatment 361
external resorption of 64, 362, 365, 365t
extrinsic stains of 620, 620f
factor 434
follicle, enlarged 340
formation of 269
formative cells 308
forming cells 32
fractures of 491
functionless 367
fusion of 41f, 49
gemination of 49
habitual grinding of 356
impacted 40, 363
in caries 432b
in internal resorption, pink 364f
injury with loss of vitality of 491f
internal resorption of 364, 365, 365t
intrinsic stain on 621, 621f
loss of 676
morphology of 435
mottling of 53f
position of 435
premature
  extraction of 356
  loss of 61f
prick 358
proximal walls of 358
radiograph of fusion of 42f
regressive alterations of 355
reimplantation of 362, 363
remineralization of 436
repair 367
replantation of 522
resorption of 361, 361t
root resorption, types of 361
  local causes 362
  systemic causes 362
rotation of 40
small conical-shaped 38f
staining of 620

structural defects in 356
transplantation of 523
unerupted 367
Telangiectasia 653
Temporal pouch infection 479
  source of 479
  treatment 479
Temporomandibular joint 654
  ankylosis of 579, 579t, 580f, 581, 581f
  causing microstomia, ankylosis of 580f
  diseases of 578
  disorder 660
  neoplasia of 584
Tenofovir 397
Teratoma 153
Tetanolysin 386
Tetanospasmin 386
Tetanus 385, 386, 673
  antitoxin, injection of 387
  treatment 387
Tetracycline 505
  staining 505f
  oral manifestations of 505
Thalassemia 587, 590, 591, 669
  classic 591
  intermedia 591
  major 591
  minor 590
  oral manifestations of 592
  trait 591
  treatment 592
Therapeutic radiations, types of 498
Thiamine 531
  deficiency 668
Thiazide 599
Third molars, impacted 40f
Throat
  diphtheric patch in 383f
  muscles 662
Thrombocytopenia 395, 594, 632
Thrombocytopenic purpura 599f
Thrombophlebitis 486, 594
Thymoma 635
Thyroglossal tract cyst 30
  origin 30
  treatment 31
Thyroid
  hormone, secretion of 539
  stimulating hormone 539
Tic douloureux 659
Tissue
  biopsy, procedure of 514
  nature of 499
  neoplasms of mixed 70, 153
  processing 515
  sample after biopsy 512f
  spaces 98
  types of 517
Tobacco 198
  carcinogenic effect of 78
  chewing form of 198

Index

habits, types of 199*b*
 in carcinogenesis, action of 79
 pouch keratosis 208
  of buccal vestibule 208*f*
 role of 78
 smoking 78
Toluidine blue test 103
 methods 103
Tongue 414*f*, 654
 anterior part of 87
 atrophic lichen planus of 224*f*
 biting habits, chronic 209
 carcinoma of 87
  posterolateral border of 87*f*
 classification of diseases of 692
 diseases affecting body of 692
 healing of wound in 519*f*
 lesions 587, 631
 painful 587, 588
 papillomatosis of 71*f*
 problems 244
 tie 24, 24*f*
Tonsillar pillars, near 83
Toothbrush abrasion 357*f*
Toothbrush injury 494
 causing traumatic ulcer 494*f*
Toothpick injury 494
Torpid facies 553
Torus mandibularis 16*f*
Toxemia 483, 489
Toxic epidermal necrolysis 629, 640
Toxoplasmosis 674
Transitory bacteremia 676
Transplantation
 causes of failure of 523
 criteria of successful 523
 types of 523
Transverse clefts 444
Trauma 355, 362, 472, 517
Traumatic arthritis, acute 583
Traumatic atrophic glossitis 494
Traumatic bone cyst 306, 331, 344, 347
Traumatic disorders 578
 treatment 579
Traumatic malocclusion 469
Traumatic neuroma 152, 153*f*
 treatment 153
Traumatic ulcer 237, 373, 411, 417, 495, 496
 causes of 495
 on tongue 495*f*
 treatment 495
Treacher-Collins syndrome 19, 574, 578, 686
Trench mouth 617
Treponema 607
 denticola 618
 pallidum 51, 374, 376
Trichiasis 642
Tricho-dento-osseous syndrome 686
Trigeminal nerve, branches of 659

Trigeminal neuralgia 658-660, 660*b*, 662
 major triggers of 659*b*
 treatment 660
Trigeminal root, microsurgical decompression of 660
Trismus, classification of causes of 696
Trotter's syndrome 686
Tubercular gingivitis 372*f*
Tuberculosis 120, 138, 370, 374*b*, 394*b*, 419, 672, 690
 oral manifestations of 372*b*
 types of 371
Tuberculous bacilli 373
Tuberculous gingivitis 372
Tuberculous lesions 371
 histopathology of 373
Tuberculous lymph node 372*f*, 373*f*
Tuberculous lymphadenopathy 371, 371*f*
Tuberculous nodules 372
Tuberculous osteomyelitis 372, 372*f*
Tuberculous patches 372
Tuberculous tonsillitis 372
Tuberculous ulcer 237, 372
Tuberous sclerosis syndrome 693
Tubular sclerosis 444
Tularemia 373
Tumor 67, 260, 310, 363, 396
 benign 245*t*
 calcification within 284*f*
 cells 87, 103, 248, 282
  duct-like proliferation of 281*f*
  malignant 98
 high-grade 261
 histology 169
 incidence of 245
 jaw 363
 low-grade 260
 malignant 245*t*
  mixed 256*f*
 markers 103
 metastatic 68, 93, 191*f*, 470
 mixed 254
 of palate, malignant mixed 255*f*
 primary 101
 secondary 68, 231
 suppressor genes 82
 tongue 22
Turbid dentin 443
Turner's hypoplasia 50
Turner's syndrome 137, 686
Turner's tooth 49, 50*f*
Typhoid fever 464
Tzanck cells 637

U

Ulcer 396, 408, 411
 slit like 650
Ulcerative colitis 672
Ulcerative gingivitis 618*fc*
Ulcerative leukoplakia 207

Ulcerative lichen planus
 of tongue 223*f*
 on buccal mucosa 224*f*
Ultraviolet radiation 80
Unicystic ameloblastoma 277, 278*f*, 279, 279*t*, 281, 315, 315*f*
 of mandible 278*f*
 origin 277
 treatment 279
 types of 277
Upper central incisor, macrodontia of 34*f*
Upper lip, development of 2, 16
Urbach-Wiethe syndrome 686
Uremic stomatitis 670
Urethritis 629
Urinary tract infection 464
Uvula elongata 5, 5*f*
 treatment 5

V

Vaginal ulceration 629
Valley fever 417
van Buchem disease 571
van Buchem syndrome 686
van der Woude syndrome 686
Varicella zoster 401, 689
 virus 398
  diseases 398
  factors causing reactivation of 402*b*
  infections 401
Vascular disorders 548
Vascular endothelium, neoplasms of 158
Vascular hamartomas 691
Vascular malformation 131, 131*t*
 of palate 132*f*
Vascular origin 696
Vascular tissue
 diseases, classification of 691
 neoplasms of 69
 origin, benign neoplasm of 131
Vascular tumors 691
Ventral tongue 83
Verapamil 609, 615
Verocay bodies 148, 148*f*
Verruca vulgaris 405
 on genitalia 395*f*
 on lower lip 403*f*
 on skin 395*f*
Verrucal-papillary lesions, classification of 691
Verrucous carcinoma 91, 106, 107, 107*f*, 108*f*, 108*t*, 207
 of gingiva 107*f*, 108*f*
 treatment 109
Verrucous leukoplakia 209
Vesiculobullous diseases, classification of 689
Vesiculobullous lesions 636*b*
Vincent's disease 617
Violaceous plaque 161

Viral disease 689
Viral infections 198, 199, 370, 390, 393, 668
 of oral mucosa 395
Viral load 392
Viral sialadenitis 230
Viruses 81
Vitamin 436
 A 80, 436, 531, 531b, 668
  deficiency of 51, 214
  doses of 208
  functions 531
  in body, excess 531
 B complex 436, 531
  deficiency of 214
 B1 deficiency 668
 B12 586, 634, 660
  absorption of 586
  deficiency 668
  injections of 588
 B3 532
 B9 532
 C 80, 360, 532, 614
  deficiency of 51, 214, 533, 614, 668
  functions of 532b
 D 80, 436, 527, 529
  deficiency of 51, 668
  dependent rickets 60
  functions of 529b
  metabolic pathway of 529fc
  resistant rickets 49, 60
 deficiencies 668
  signs of 668t
  symptoms of 668t

E 80, 531
 deficiency, features of 531
K 436, 533
 deficiency 668
 metabolism, disturbance in 529
Vomiting 382
von Ebner's glands 229
von Recklinghausen disease 149, 543, 561
von Recklinghausen syndrome 686
von Willebrand disease 601

W

Waldeyer ring 31
Warthin's tumor 246, 249, 253, 254f
 of parotid gland 253f
 treatment 254
Waterhouse-Friderichsen syndrome 545, 686
Waxy papules 105
Weber-Cockayne syndrome 686
Wegener's granulomatosis 373, 387, 614, 617, 690, 691, 693
 treatment 388
Whistling face syndrome 686
White blood cell 331
White lesions of
 leukoedema on cheek 210f
 oral cavity 688
White patch 222f
White plaque 649f
White sponge nevus 10, 207, 209, 632
 electron microscopic study 11
 treatment 11, 633

Whole body radiation, effects of 501
Wickham striae 221
Wilms' tumor 15
Wolf-Hirschhorn syndrome 687
Wolf-like face 553
World Health Organization
 classification of
  lymphomas 174t
Wound
 in factitious injuries, characteristics of 496b
 location of 517
 mobility of 517
 of extraction socket before healing 519f

X

Xerostomia 240, 243, 243t, 383, 435, 538, 693
 causes of 243t
 clinical features of 244
 common effects of 243
 diagnosis of 244
XXXXY syndrome 687

Z

Zalcitabine 397
Zidovudine, consisting of 397
Zimmerman-Laband syndrome 687, 693
Zinc 80, 529
 deficiency
  effects of 529
  syndrome 687
Zinsser syndrome 687